MODERN MEDICINE

Modern Medicine

SECOND EDITION

A Textbook for Students

EDITED BY

Alan E. Read, MD(Lond), FRCP
*Professor of Medicine, University of Bristol, and sometime
Examiner in Medicine to the Universities of Bristol,
Cambridge, Dundee, London, Newcastle, Manchester, Lagos,
Khartoum, and to the Welsh National School of Medicine and
the Royal College of Physicians of London*

D. W. Barritt, MD(Lond), FRCP
*Physician and Cardiologist, Bristol Health District
(Teaching), and Examiner in Medicine to the Universities of
Bristol, Lagos and to the Royal College of Physicians of
London*

R. Langton Hewer, FRCP
*Neurologist, Frenchay Hospital and Bristol Health District
(Teaching)*

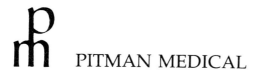 PITMAN MEDICAL

First published 1975
Second edition 1979

Catalogue Number 21 3208 81

Pitman Medical Publishing Co Ltd
P O Box 7, Tunbridge Wells,
Kent, TN1 1XH, England

Associated Companies

UNITED KINGDOM
Pitman Publishing Ltd, London
Focal Press Ltd, London

CANADA
Copp Clark Pitman, Toronto

USA
Fearon Pitman Publishers Inc, San Francisco
Focal Press Inc, New York

AUSTRALIA
Pitman Publishing Pty Ltd, Melbourne

NEW ZEALAND
Pitman Publishing NZ Ltd, Wellington

British Library Cataloguing in Publication Data

Modern Medicine. – 2nd ed.
  1. Pathology 2. Medicine
  I. Read, Alan Ernest
  II. Barritt, Donald Walker
  III. Hewer, Richard Langton
  616   RB111   79–40625

ISBN: 0–272–79530–5

Text set in 10/11½ pt VIP Palatino, printed
and bound in Great Britain at
The Pitman Press, Bath

Contents

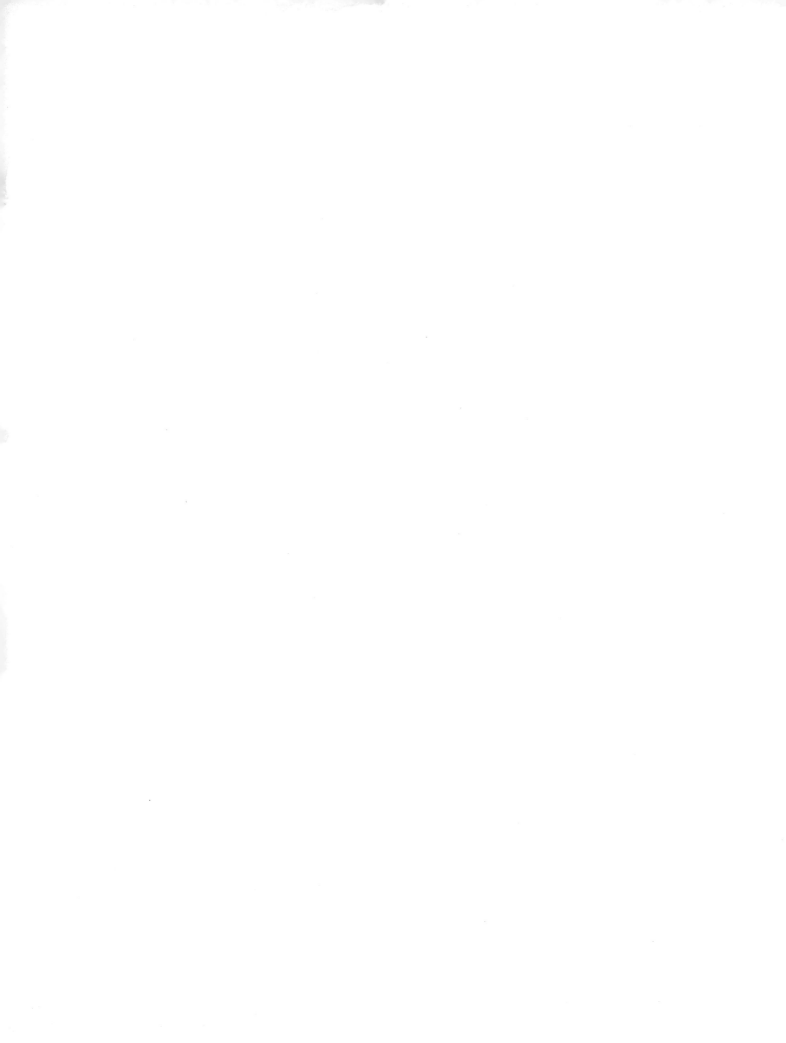

Preface

No book was so bad but some good might be got out of it – PLINY THE YOUNGER, *AD 61–105*

It is customary to offer some excuse for writing a new textbook of medicine. No other than Sir William Osler, that most distinguished of clinicians, recognised that they had some worth. He likened the study of medicine without the use of a textbook to that of venturing to sea without navigational charts. He was also wise enough to point out, however, that a study of medicine limited to textbooks alone was, in sea-faring terms, like never going to sea at all. There seems, therefore, to be some reason why a medical student should have some short, but selective, account of medicine to act as a 'navigational aid' during the initial and often difficult clinical appointments. One recognises, too, that the textbook becomes of declining value as experience and clinical expertise allow the student to acquire something that no textbook can provide, namely the ability to think and fathom clinical situations for themselves.

Textbooks of medicine abound. Many, however, are massive, expensive and their length too great for the average undergraduate to absorb. Others attract by their conciseness and cheapness. These tend, however, to be scrappy, incomplete and may give an unjustifiably dogmatic view of medicine. Both types are in our experience generally poorly illustrated and uninteresting to read. Both suffer from 'ageing' so that they are often seriously out-of-date the day they appear on the booksellers' shelves.

Our textbook hopefully avoids some of these problems. It is not unduly long when one considers the ever-increasing amount of information the present-day medical student must absorb. We hope, too, that the illustrations are meaningful, for we are certain that one good diagram is worth many pages of text. Neither have we been too 'wordy' when describing signs and symptoms, which we have usually tabulated. There would seem little point, to our minds, for using lengthy accounts of these phenomena when the first clinical appointment in medicine and any one of a number of excellent practical manuals will provide all that is necessary as regards instruction in eliciting signs and knowing about patterns of symptoms. We have included a fairly comprehensive account of molecular and inherited disease as, though rare, these disorders illustrate the enormous progress being made by biochemists and geneticists in this most exciting fringe of medicine. We hope, therefore, that students will forgive us this one 'luxury'. We have also included a section on dietetics and tables of normal values in clinical measurements so that students will be able to appreciate biochemical and other abnormalities readily without referring to other texts. Neither, at least at the time of writing this foreword, are we unduly out-of-date.

Above all, we have tried to give adequate space for the presentation of the problems of the cause, prevention and treatment of disease. Prevention is becoming of paramount importance because many of the major diseases we deal with can be prevented, and important clues as to the aetiology of others is now available from epidemiological and ecological surveys. A 'wind of change' is also blowing through the world of therapeutics resulting from a realisation of the important contributions the clinical pharmacologist can make. Adequate description of the drug treatment of disease is therefore essential.

The modern medical student finds every specialist branch of medicine and surgery making claims on him and competing for his time. There is a great danger that the student will be completely submerged in a wealth of seemingly disconnected facts. No specialist subject must take a greater part of the valuable curriculum time than it deserves. General medicine must remain the sheet anchor of the medical teacher's approach so that the subject shall remain as fresh and as exciting as it has been to the teachers who have experienced it.

We sincerely hope that this book by members of the teaching staff of the University of Bristol and our clinical colleagues in the United Bristol Hospitals will help students to enjoy the exciting journey that clinical medicine will present for them and that *this* navigational aid will allow them a fair and tranquil passage.

Many colleagues have helped us and in particular we would like to thank
Professor Russell Fraser,
Dr D. C. E. Speller,
Miss Phillipa Champion, Chief Dietician, United Bristol Hospitals,
Mr Leonard Clarke, Senior Technician, Department of Cardiology, United Bristol Hospitals,
Mr John Eatough, Superintendent Photographer, University of Bristol,
Miss Angela Manzi,
Mrs Christine Davis.

A.E.R.
D.W.B.
R.L.H.

PREFACE TO THE SECOND EDITION

We have been encouraged by the success of this book and have launched our second edition but with some changes. We were mindful of the need to include more material on drug reactions and the important topic of the care of the chronic sick, whilst there has been a major revision or a complete rewrite of all the surviving chapters. Some colleagues have left Bristol for further fields and new contributors have taken their place. Our aim is still to provide a concise and readable textbook principally for the student studying for the final MB. Again good illustrations are, we feel, a major requirement for this purpose.

Our thanks are due to many kind friends, both past and present contributors, the staff of Pitman Medical and the long-suffering medical students who have been persuaded to read this book.

A.E.R.
D.W.B.
R.L.H.

List of Contributors

D. W. Barritt
MD (London), FRCP, Consultant Cardiologist, Bristol and Weston Health District (T).

R. E. Barry
BSc, MD (Bristol), MRCP, Consultant Senior Lecturer in Medicine, University of Bristol.

P. Brown
BSc, MB (Bristol), MRCP, Lecturer in Medicine, University of Bristol.

J. R. T. Colley
BSc, MD (London), FFCM, Professor of Community Medicine, University of Bristol.

T. J. David
MB, PhD (Bristol), MRCP, Tutor in Paediatrics, University of Bristol.

F. Fakunle
MB (Ibadan), MRCP, Consultant Senior Lecturer in Medicine, Ahmadu Bello University Hospital, Zaria, Northern Nigeria.

W. A. Gillespie
MA, MD (Dublin), FRCPI, FRCP, DPH, FCPath, Emeritus Professor of Clinical Bacteriology, University of Bristol.

R. R. M. Harman
MB (London), FRCP, Consultant Dermatologist, Bristol and Weston Health District (T).

M. Hartog
DM (Oxon), FRCP, Reader in Medicine, University of Bristol.

R. F. Harvey
MD (London), MRCP, Consultant Physician, Frenchay Hospital, Bristol.

D. A. Heath
MB (Birmingham), FRCP, Reader in Medicine, University of Birmingham.

K. W. Heaton
MA, MD (Cantab), FRCP, Reader in Medicine, Consultant Senior Lecturer in Medicine, University of Bristol.

M. I. V. Jayson
MD (London), FRCP, Professor of Rheumatology, University of Manchester.

R. Langton Hewer
MB (London), FRCP, Consultant Neurologist, Bristol and Weston Health District (T) and Frenchay Hospital, Bristol.

G. Laszlo
MA, MD (Cantab), FRCP, Consultant Physician, Bristol and Weston Health District (T).

J. C. Mackenzie
BA, MB (Cantab), MRCPE, DRCOG, DIH Consultant Nephrologist, Bristol and Weston Health District (T) and Southmead Hospital, Bristol.

A. J. Marshall
MD (Bristol), MRCP, Tutor in Medicine, University of Bristol.

R. E. Midwinter
BSc, MD (Bristol), FFCM, Consultant Senior Lecturer in Community Medicine, University of Bristol.

H. G. Morgan
MA, MD (Cantab), FRCP, FRCPsych. Professor Elect, Department of Mental Health, University of Bristol.

A. E. Read
MD (London), FRCP, Professor of Medicine, University of Bristol.

C. J. C. Roberts
MB (London), MRCP, Lecturer in Clinical Pharmacology, University of Bristol.

G. L. Scott
BA, MD (Cantab), FRCP, Consultant Haematologist, Bristol and Weston Health District (T).

A. E. Tinkler
MA, MD (Dublin), DPH, Emeritus Consultant in Genitourinary Medicine, Bristol and Weston Health District (T).

J. Verrier Jones
BA, BCh (Oxon), FRCP, Professor of Rheumatology, Rush Presbyterian—St. Lukes Medical Centre, Chicago, USA.

R. V. Walley
BA, MD (Cantab), Consultant Physician, Southmead Health District, Bristol.

G. Walters
MD, FRCP, FRCPath, Consultant Chemical Pathologist, Bristol and Weston Health District (T).

R. P. Warin
MD (Leeds), FRCP, Consultant Dermatologist, Bristol and Weston Health District (T).

Gary M. James
MMAA, prepared special illustrations.

Health and Disease

1

R. E. MIDWINTER and J. R. T. COLLEY

The doctor who wishes to practise good clinical medicine must be able to make decisions. When a patient consults him, it is necessary to decide whether or not the patient is ill. If he is ill, a decision has to be made about what sort of illness is involved. Then the most suitable treatment must be selected. Often in hospital practice the first decision has already been made by someone else, usually the referring doctor. Much of the undergraduate clinical curriculum is devoted to helping future doctors to choose between various diagnoses, and selecting the most appropriate treatments. Comparatively little time is spent on helping them to make decisions about whether or not people are ill, or on how to distinguish between what is normal or abnormal.

THE CLINICAL SPECTRUM

In the field of health care, normality and health are synonymous. Both states are difficult to define and are, therefore, not easy to measure. The World Health Organisation has defined health as 'a state of complete physical, mental and social well-being and not merely the absence of disease or infirmity'. This is an idealistic definition and, if it were possible to quantify any of these terms, perhaps few people could be regarded as truly healthy. However, in the population at any one time the majority of people will probably have no detectable abnormality and would, therefore, be regarded as normal. Some of the remainder will be apparently normal and yet would possess some characteristic like, for example, overweight which would put them in a high risk category in relation to the future chances of developing disease. Others will possess some precursor morbid state like atheroma, which has not yet given rise to any clinical circulatory impairment. A further group will show, on examination, signs of disease not previously recognised and not yet giving rise to symptoms. Some will have overt, recognisable signs and symptoms of disease and a few will have such advanced disease that they are in the process of dying. There is thus a 'clinical spectrum' of disease in populations, ranging from health to terminal illness. In general

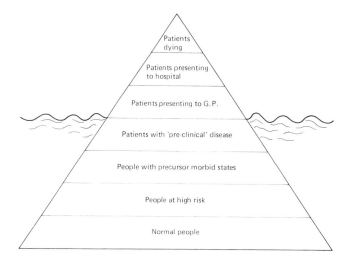

Fig. 1.1 The clinical iceberg.

it is only those with recognised disease that tend to be seen as patients in hospital. They represent the tip of what has become known as the 'clinical iceberg'. Much disease, and most people who are at high risk of developing disease, remain undetected in the community (Fig. 1.1).

Table 1.1 Symptoms self-treated and doctor-treated (Wadsworth, Butterfield and Blaney, 1971)

Groups of symptoms	Per cent of all symptoms	Per cent self-treated	Per cent doctor-treated
Respiratory	26	63	37
Mental	21	80	20
Locomotor	15	61	39
Gastrointestinal	11	78	22
Central nervous system	8	59	41
Skin	5	73	27
Cardiovascular system	4	58	42
Accidents	3	78	22
Others	7	47	53
	100	72	28

Source: Journal of the Royal College of General Practitioners, Report from General Practice 16: 1973. Present state and future needs of general practice.

Table 1.2 Persons consulting for minor illnesses in a year in a hypothetical average practice of 2,500

Conditions	Consultations per 2,500 patients
Minor illness	
General	
Upper respiratory infections	500
Emotional disorders	300
Gastrointestinal disorders	250
Skin disorders	225
Specific	
Acute tonsillitis	100
Acute otitis media	75
Cerumen	50
Acute urinary infections	50
'Acute back' syndrome	50
Migraine	30
Hay fever	25

Source: Journal of the Royal College of General Practitioners, Report from General Practice 16: 1973. Present state and future needs of general practice.

Table 1.3 Persons consulting for acute major illnesses in a year in a hypothetical average practice of 2,500

Conditions		Consultations per 2,500 patients
Acute major (life-threatening) illness		
Acute bronchitis and pneumonia		50
Severe depression		12
Acute myocardial infarction		7
Acute appendicitis		5
Acute strokes		5
All new cancers		5
Cancer of lung	1–2 per year	
Cancer of breast	1 per year	
Cancer of large bowel	2 every 3 years	
Cancer of stomach	1 every 2 years	
Cancer of bladder	1 every 3 years	
Cancer of cervix	1 every 4 years	
Cancer of ovary	1 every 5 years	
Cancer of oesophagus	1 every 7 years	
Cancer of brain	1 every 10 years	
Cancer of uterine body	1 every 12 years	
Lymphadenoma	1 every 15 years	
Cancer of thyroid	1 every 20 years	
Suicidal attempts		3
Deaths in road traffic accidents		1 every 3 years
Suicide		1 every 4 years

Source: Journal of the Royal College of General Practitioners, Report from General Practice 16: 1973. Present state and future needs of general practice.

Table 1.4 Some leading causes of death: England and Wales 1975

Category	Number of deaths	Percentage of all deaths
Ischaemic heart disease	154,412	26
Neoplasms	123,728	21
Cerebrovascular disease	77,060	13
Chronic bronchitis, emphysema and pneumonia	74,103	13
Accidents, poisoning, violence	20,859	4
All causes	582,841	100

Source: OPCS Mortality Statistics for 1975, England and Wales. London: HMSO, 1977.

Many people with health problems do not consult a doctor. They either treat themselves or seek help from a neighbour or perhaps the local chemist (Table 1.1).

Of the people who do seek medical advice and help, most will first of all consult a general medical practitioner. Most illness that is dealt with at this primary health care level is of a minor nature and does not require referral to hospital (Table 1.2).

Serious acute illness, on the other hand, is seen much less often in general practice (Table 1.3).

Patients with these sorts of problems or whose illness is difficult to diagnose will tend to be sent to hospital for either out-patient or in-patient treatment. Thus the hospital clinician is confronted with a highly selected sample of patients and disease states. A house surgeon working in a general hospital may see and deal with two or three cases of acute appendicitis each day, whereas a general practitioner will only come across four or five cases in the course of a year.

The tip of the 'iceberg' are those who are in a terminal state. The conditions which account for most of the deaths taking place in England and Wales are shown in Table 1.4.

The importance of a disease in medical practice, in terms of how common and how severe it is, thus varies markedly from one level of presentation to another. A full table of death rates by cause per million persons for England and Wales is to be found at the end of this chapter (Table 1.10).

WHAT IS NORMAL?

Distribution of Clinical Measurements

Clinicians need yardsticks by which to assess normality and abnormality. A paediatrician confronted by a child who is small for his age will have to decide whether the smallness is of such a degree that it indicates or represents a disease state, or whether the child is simply below average height and is otherwise well. Height, like weight, is one measurement made in the clinical examination of a child as an index of disease or non-disease.

Children grow throughout childhood, so height in general increases with age. Yet if the heights of a group of boys of the same age are measured, it will be obvious that some will be very small, and some very tall, but the majority will fall towards the middle of the height range. If a frequency distribution of the heights of a sample of boys of the same age were plotted, the curve would look something like that shown in Fig. 1.2.

The curve would tend to have a symmetrical inverted bell shape. The average height for any age is easy to determine and is of some use as a clinical yardstick. Comparatively few boys are, however, of exactly average height. The majority are either just below or just above average, while successively decreasing numbers

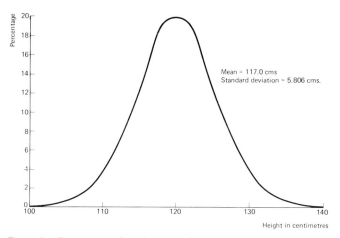

Fig. 1.2 Frequency distribution of heights of a sample of boys and girls aged six years.

are taller or shorter and a very few are very small or very tall. This kind of frequency distribution is very like a mathematical curve called the curve of normal distribution.

Measure of Scatter

A further yardstick – a measure of scatter – is also needed as a clinical aid. It is possible to measure the average amount of scatter that exists about this mean. The measure of scatter or dispersion is called the standard deviation and has a rather complex mathematical formula. In practice it is an easy measure to calculate and it can be a very valuable yardstick. Within the area of the curve that lies between the arithmetic mean plus or minus one standard deviation (SD) lie about 68 per cent of the individual measurements that go to make up the curve (Fig. 1.3). Within the area encompassed by the mean plus or minus two standard deviations lie 95 per cent of the values, and within plus or minus three standard deviations, 99.7 per cent.

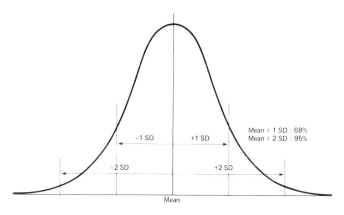

Fig. 1.3 The normal distribution curve.

Is the Measurement Abnormal?

The chance of an individual measurement lying outside the range of the mean ±1 SD is about one in three, outside ±2 SD one in twenty, and outside ±3 SD, about three in a thousand. If a child is examined and his height is found to be outside the range of the mean height for his age ±2 SD, the odds are one in twenty that he could still be part of the normal population and simply very small or tall. It is more likely, however, that he is not part of the normal population but is part of a different population of very small or very tall children who are thus 'abnormal'. In clinical medicine the mean ±2 SD is often used somewhat arbitrarily to indicate what has become known as the normal range of attributes possessing this type of frequency distribution.

If all pathologically small children were so small that their heights did not overlap the normal range, it would be very easy to devise a simple cut-off point to separate the normal from the abnormal. In practice, however, this seldom happens and the small 'abnormal' distribution is 'lost' in the tail of the normal distribution. In this circumstance, if the yardstick mean ±2 SD is used as a clinical guide to distinguish normality from abnormality, what happens is shown diagrammatically in Fig. 1.4. Here, while the cut-off point distinguishes most 'abnormals', it does so at the cost of incorrectly labelling some 'normals' as 'abnormal'.

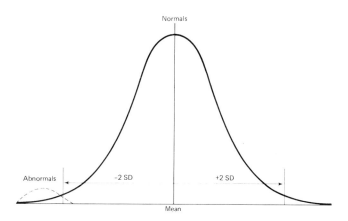

Fig. 1.4 'Normal' and 'abnormal' distributions.

MEASUREMENT IN CLINICAL PRACTICE

MAKING A DIAGNOSIS

The clinician's main task when presented with an ill patient is to formulate diagnoses and, where indicated, institute treatment. The process by which a diagnosis is made can be relatively simple, as in a child with suspected chickenpox. Here, knowledge that the child has never had the disease, has been in contact with a case, that the incubation period is appropriate, with physical signs of fever and a typical rash, will lead to a rapid and firm diagnosis. In contrast, many of the chronic diseases of middle and old age often present complex diagnostic problems. In part this is due to their wide range of possible clinical manifestations and degrees of severity. An example is cerebrovascular disease. This can present as a massive and life-threatening hemiplegia with prolonged loss of consciousness; at the other extreme it may present as episodes of transient and minor disturbance of vision. Both these manifestations can also be produced by pathology other than cerebrovascular disease. The process of arriving at a diagnosis under these circumstances can be highly complicated, relying upon several different sources of evidence. Past history, present symptoms, results of physical examination, biochemical, haematological and other tests would all contribute to a final diagnosis. The clinician assesses individual findings for their deviation from what is thought normal, and in so doing constructs particular patterns of findings that suggest a diagnosis, or several possible diagnoses. In clinical practice it is unusual for a diagnosis to be made on a single finding.

As so much weight is placed upon clinical findings in arriving at diagnoses, and thus deciding on the appropriate treatment, some indication is needed of the precision with which clinicians make these assessments. This becomes of particular importance when an individual physical sign or biochemical test does not depart greatly from what is considered normal.

Suppose that the precision with which the physical sign was measured, or the biochemical estimation was made, is poor. This may lead to a patient receiving a treatment that was not needed, or not receiving a treatment that could have given benefit; both outcomes being unsatisfactory for the patient. A further aspect involves the follow-up of patients. Here the clinician may be attempting to gauge whether, for example, a treatment is improving, worsening or making no difference to the patient's condition. If the clinician relies on a measurement with a poor precision to indicate progress, he may be led astray in concluding from an apparent change in the measurement that the patient's condition has changed, when in truth this may not have happened. It is necessary to know how inherently variable the clinical measurements are that are used to make diagnoses and to assess the results of treatment.

SOURCES OF VARIATION IN CLINICAL MEASUREMENTS

There are two main sources of variation in clinical measurements (Fig. 1.5). The first arises from the underlying true or biological variation. For example, systolic blood pressure in an individual varies from occasion to occasion, often quite widely and in a fairly unpredictable way.

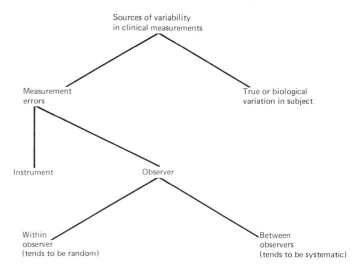

Fig. 1.5 Variation and clinical measurement.

The second source of variation is that associated with the measurement of the attribute itself. This variation can be partly due to the imprecision of the instrument being used, to inconsistencies in the clinician making the measurement, and when several clinicians assess the same patient, to differences in their techniques of measurement.

The underlying biological variation, imprecision of the measurement technique and inconsistencies in the individual clinician tend to be random. This is of importance in clinical medicine as the greater the random variation of a measurement the less confidence can be placed upon it.

Variation between clinicians has been extensively studied and is usually systematic. This means that an individual clinician may tend consistently either to over-report, or under-report, findings compared with another clinician. This can be seen in Fig. 1.6 where four doctors independently assessed men for the presence of cough, sputum and history of bronchitis. The four doctors agreed well on the proportion of men who had a history of bronchitis but agreed very poorly on the proportion with cough and sputum. Dr. A. assessed 12 per cent of the men as having sputum while Dr. D. found 40 per cent.

Systematic differences such as these have been found, for example, in the assessment of chest signs, heart size, heart sounds, retinal pathology, liver size, peripheral arterial pulses, and reading of chest X-rays. Attention is drawn to this aspect of clinical measurement simply to alert the reader to the potential size and sources of differences that may be found in certain clinical measurements.

MINIMISING MEASUREMENT VARIATION

The true, or biological variation may be reduced if the factors that influence what is being measured are

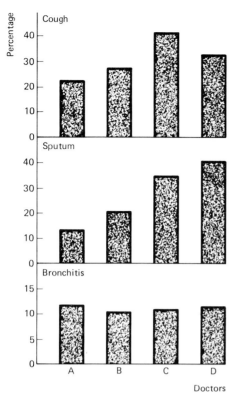

Fig. 1.6 Observer variation in assessing the presence of chest symptoms and past history of bronchitis.

From: Cochrane A. L., Chapman P. J. and Oldham P. D. (1951) Observer errors in taking medical histories, *The Lancet* i: 1007–1009.

known. Blood pressure can change for a number of reasons, for example, whether the subject is lying, sitting or standing. By strictly defining the circumstances under which blood pressure is measured, variation due to posture can be minimised. A further aid is to make repeat measurements on the subject and take the mean.

Between observer differences may also be reduced by defining precisely the criteria required before reporting that a clinical sign is present. In the examples above, where the doctors disagreed on the presence of cough and sputum, an agreed definition of what constituted a cough, or production of sputum would have produced better agreement on the proportions of men with these symptoms. The Medical Research Council produced a set of standard questions to aid the investigation of chronic bronchitis. Those on cough are as follows:

The investigation of chronic bronchitis

1. Do you usually cough first thing in the morning in the winter?
2. Do you usually cough during the day or during the night in the winter?
If 'Yes' to 1 or 2
3. Do you cough like this on most days for as much as three months each year?

THE EPIDEMIOLOGICAL APPROACH TO MEDICINE

POPULATIONS AND DISEASES

The medical student starting clinical practice will be confronted with a succession of patients with often unrelated problems. After a while, patterns will begin to take shape as experience is gained. It will become apparent that people with similar problems have several characteristics in common. Thus will begin an awareness of the epidemiological approach to medicine. The recognition that some types of people are more at risk of developing a particular disease than others leads one to question why this should be so.

Epidemiology may be defined as the study of the distribution and determinants of disease in populations. The study of disease patterns in human populations is an early step in a chain of processes that ends in identifying the cause of disease. If cause can be identified, then it may be a relatively easy matter to prevent a disease from occurring. It makes sense to prevent, rather than to try to treat, often inadequately, the late effects of disease processes. Yet at present, and in most countries, far more money is spent on 'curative medicine' than on 'preventive medicine'.

Sources of Data

To study the distribution of disease in populations, mortality and morbidity information must be available or obtainable. In developed countries, information about numbers and causes of death is collected and published routinely. Numbers of deaths are usually measured accurately; the accuracy of cause of death is less certain. Information about illness, or morbidity statistics, is also collected and published. However, for many reasons, including the difficulty of defining illness, the quality of morbidity information is more variable. Mortality and morbidity statistics provide numerators for measuring disease frequencies in populations. It is necessary to relate them to denominators which are population measurements. These demographic statistics are also collected and published routinely in developed countries. Censuses are held primarily for legal and administrative purposes and the information collected is also of use in health care, not only as denominators for rates but also for health care planning purposes. Some developing countries have vital statistical information relating to the populations of city areas but not for the whole country, while others have little or no routine information available at all.

Time, Place, Persons

It has been known since the time of Hippocrates that personal, place and time factors influence whether or not people become ill.

5

Age and Sex. Of the personal factors, age is one of the most important. In developed countries death rates, except in the first year of life, are very low until middle age or late middle age, when they begin to rise steeply (Fig. 1.7).

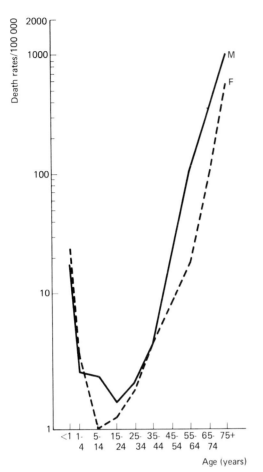

Fig. 1.7 Death rates from pneumonia and bronchitis in the Netherlands, 1969.

From: Respiratory disease in Europe. Report on a study (1974). Regional Office for Europe. WHO: Copenhagen.

Because of this marked association, the age structure of populations must be taken into account when attempts are made to compare death rates. Various standardisation techniques are available to make this possible. In developing countries, death rates in the first few years of life are usually very high: in some areas more than 50 per cent of children die before the age of five. Infant mortality rates – deaths in the first year of life – are a useful index of the 'healthiness' or otherwise of a country.

The sex of an individual is also an important determinant of health or disease. The male appears to be the biologically weaker sex, and death rates are higher for males than for females at almost every age.

Ethnic and Cultural Factors. These factors have important influences, though it is often difficult to separate their individual effects. Death rates among the non-white population of the United States are higher, age for age, than among the white. The differences are mostly explainable in terms of a poorer total environment rather than in 'racial' terms. Few Seventh Day Adventists die of lung cancer; cigarette smoking is not encouraged in that sect.

Social Class. Some striking patterns emerge when social class and morbidity or mortality are examined. Table 1.5 shows standardised mortality ratios (SMRs) for various causes of death by social class for men aged 15 to 64 in England and Wales. These figures are standardised for age, and 100 is the average experience for the whole population of employed men between those ages.

Table 1.5 SMR and social class: men aged 15 to 64, England and Wales 1959 to 1963

| Cause of death | Social class | | | | |
	I	II	III	IV	V
Malignant neoplasm, all sites	73	80	104	102	139
Stomach cancer	49	63	101	114	163
Lung cancer	53	72	107	104	148
Coronary disease	98	95	106	96	112
Non-syphilitic aortic aneurysm and dissecting aneurysm	132	110	105	91	89
Bronchitis	28	50	97	116	194
Stomach	46	58	94	106	199
Appendicitis	104	79	104	105	108
Motor vehicle accidents	72	78	103	107	157
Suicide	91	94	87	103	184
All causes	76	81	100	103	143

Source: The Registrar General's Decennial Supplement, England and Wales 1961. Occupational Mortality Tables. London: HMSO, 1971.

Occupation. Occupation affects health in a variety of ways. First, there are jobs which are dangerous in that physical, chemical or biological hazards are directly involved. Second, there are jobs that are relatively poorly paid, so that in societies where health care or education have to be purchased directly, individuals and their families are at a disadvantage. There are also occupations that are mentally stressful but which demand little physical activity, a combination which may lead to an increased likelihood of the development of coronary artery disease. The Office of Population Censuses and Surveys in England and Wales publishes after each census an Occupational Mortality Supplement which is an excellent source of information, although occupational mortality figures must be interpreted with caution. Table 1.6 shows the risk by occupation of death from coronary artery disease.

Marital Status. Marital status, and morbidity and mortality experiences are related. Death rates in England and Wales in divorced people are about twice those of

Table 1.6 SMRs by occupation: coronary disease, men aged 15 to 64, England and Wales 1959 to 1963

	SMR
Farmers	63
University teachers	65
Dentists	75
Lorry drivers	96
Electricians	101
Medical practitioners	118
Clerks	121
Service, sport and recreation workers	122
Nurses	131
Coal-mine face-workers	144
Telephone operators	164
Police officers	165
Armed forces	346
Company directors	758

Source: The Registrar General's Decennial Supplement, England and Wales 1961. Occupational Mortality Tables. London: HMSO, 1971.

married people of the same sex and age. For specific causes of death, such as road traffic accidents, there may be a threefold difference in risk. Death rates for single persons are higher than for the married. While these differences are statistically significant ones, this does not necessarily mean that the relationships are causal. For instance, the higher death rates among single people may be partly due to the fact that individuals with physical or mental handicap are less likely to marry than are those without.

Geography. Patterns of disease and death tend to vary throughout the world. The patterns are largely determined by the state of economic and other development of the country concerned. In developing countries the major problems are those of infections, parasitism and undernutrition, though little reliable data are available for what amounts to about 70 per cent of the world's population. Health services in developed countries, on the other hand, will deal mainly with diseases of ageing populations, of wear and tear, of stress and over-indulgence. Tables 1.7 and 1.8, taken from the World Health Organisation's Annual Report for 1972, compare and contrast the leading causes of death in England and Wales and in the Philippines.

Less obviously explained geographical variations in disease patterns occur within countries. There are often

Table 1.7 Death rates per 100,000 population, England and Wales 1972

Ischaemic heart disease	309.3	(22.7)
Cerebrovascular disease	167.1	(12.1)
Lung cancer	64.6	(2.0)
Bronchitis, emphysema, asthma	61.0	(14.5)
Stomach cancer	25.4	(2.5)
Breast cancer	22.9	(1.6)
Motor vehicle accidents	14.1	(2.9)
Diabetes mellitus	10.8	(2.6)
All causes	1207.0	(732.0)

( ) = Corresponding rates for Philippines 1972.
Source: World Health Statistics Annual 1972, Vol. I Vital Statistics and Causes of Death. WHO Geneva, 1975.

Table 1.8 Death rates per 100,000 population, Philippines 1972

Ill-defined and unknown causes	96.3	(2.6)
Bronchopneumonia	88.1	
Respiratory tuberculosis	73.3	(2.0)
Gastroenteritis (not neonatal)	42.1	
Ill-defined neonatal conditions and immaturity	39.9	(4.1)
Avitaminosis etc.	31.4	(0.5)
Infections of the newborn	17.0	
Tetanus	9.3	(0.0)
Lobar pneumonia	7.2	
All causes	732.0	(1207.0)

( ) = Corresponding rates for England and Wales 1972.
Source: World Health Statistics Annual 1972, Vol. I Vital Statistics and Causes of Death. WHO Geneva, 1975.

quite striking local variations even from one small neighbourhood to another. Some of these reflect differences in general between the urban and rural environment. In England and Wales, death rates from chronic bronchitis and emphysema are considerably higher in towns than in rural areas (Fig. 1.8).

The excess urban deaths are partly 'explained' by the greater degree of air pollution experienced by town dwellers. Other local differences are less easy to 'explain'. Table 1.9 shows that the risk of dying from stomach cancer is almost three times greater in North and West Wales than in many rural areas of Central and Eastern England.

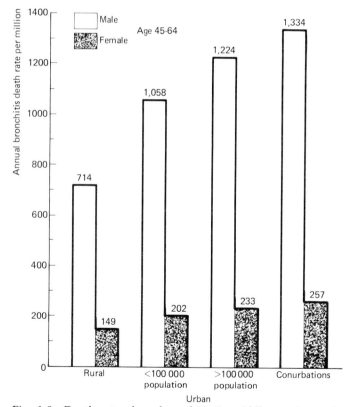

Fig. 1.8 Death rates from bronchitis in middle age in rural and urban areas, England and Wales 1959 to 1963.

From: Air Pollution and Health. A report for the Royal College of Physicians (1970). Pitman: London.

Table 1.9 Stomach cancer: SMR by administrative county, England and Wales 1961

	SMR
West Sussex	66
Dorset	71
Buckinghamshire	77
Gloucestershire	89
Cornwall	92
London	100
Staffordshire	109
Cumberland	115
Glamorganshire	127
Durham	133
Cardiganshire	142
Caernarvonshire	150
Denbighshire	161

Source: The Registrar General's Decennial Supplement, England and Wales 1961. Area Mortality Tables. London: HMSO, 1965.

Time Trends. Variations in disease patterns also occur with time. Fig. 1.9 shows how lung cancer deaths in males have increased dramatically in Britain during this century and how some of the factors that have been suspected as being causal have varied over the same period. The only factor that precedes the rise in lung cancer mortality by the right time interval and increases in parallel is cigarette consumption.

This variation is a long term one. Others occur over short periods of time. Epidemics of infectious diseases have been of importance since early in man's history and are still familiar events in most countries of the world. Epidemics of non-infectious disease may also occur. Fig. 1.10 illustrates the sudden increase in deaths that occurred during the week or so of the great London Smog in December 1952.

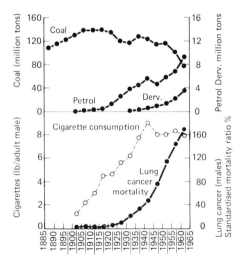

Fig. 1.9 Trends in fuel used, cigarette smoking and lung cancer mortality in men.

From: Air Pollution and Health. A report for the Royal College of Physicians (1970). Pitman: London.

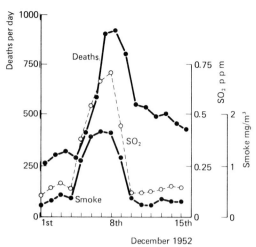

Fig. 1.10 Death and pollution levels in the fog of December 1952.

From: Air Pollution and Health. A report for the Royal College of Physicians (1970). Pitman: London.

Many of the excess deaths were of elderly people already chronically ill. However, the death rate from bronchitis in persons under 45 was also higher than expected.

THE SEARCH FOR CAUSATION

Making and Testing Hypotheses

Once disease patterns in populations are identified, the clinician will try to explain their existence by making up a suitable hypothesis. This must then be tested rigorously and scientifically. There are several approaches to such hypothesis-testing. Retrospective or case studies are usually attempted in the first instance. If, for example, it is suspected that cigarette smoking causes lung cancer, then the smoking histories of patients with lung cancer will be investigated. If all, or the great majority, smoke cigarettes, then this is the first step towards establishing a causal link. However, it may simply be that the majority of the population smokes cigarettes anyway.

The next logical step is to look at the smoking histories of patients with problems other than lung cancer who are matched as closely as possible in terms of their personal and other characteristics. If as a group they smoke less heavily, then this is useful additional information linking cigarette smoking and lung cancer. This is the case control study. Studies such as these are usually fairly easy to undertake and may not involve a great deal of time and effort. They are, however, dependent on the accuracy of history-taking and recording and they do not enable their investigator to measure the magnitude of the risk involved. This is only assessable by means of a prospective or cohort study. A prospective study, designed to test a possible relationship between cigarette smoking and lung cancer, would identify a group of smokers and ideally would match them by as many other characteristics as possible with a group of non-smokers. These two groups could then be followed up carefully so that year by year the risks of developing lung cancer in each group can be assessed. The prospective approach often involves the expenditure of much time and effort and may be impracticable where rare conditions are involved. Such studies may establish the existence of strong statistically significant links between what is thought to be cause and what is thought to be effect.

The final stage in the unravelling of aetiology is aimed at establishing that the links are causal and not merely some secondary association through another as yet undiscovered factor. For example, a prospective study may show a high risk of cigarette smokers developing lung cancer over a period of years compared with a low risk for non-smokers. This phenomenon may still be explained by a hypothesis which states that people who are genetically more likely to develop lung cancer are also more likely to smoke cigarettes. In this example, a great deal of further work has been done to show that this is unlikely to be the case and that cigarette smoking and lung cancer are indeed causally linked.

If the cause of a disease is established, then at least in theory it becomes possible to prevent its occurrence. Prevention often involves the clinician in trying to alter people's behaviour patterns towards risk factors. The role of such health education in clinical medicine is an important one, but it is also a difficult area in which to work. Even when the cigarette smoker is confronted with the mass of evidence linking smoking and disease, there is usually strong resistance towards changing the habit.

EVALUATING TREATMENT

Preventing disease from happening in the first place, or primary prevention, is not always possible even when the cause is known. Much of clinical medicine is involved with trying to treat already established disease processes. Sometimes the treatment is curative (secondary prevention). Often, in the absence of a known cure, treatment is aimed at trying to prevent signs and symptoms from getting worse (tertiary prevention). Measuring the effectiveness of treatment is one of the greatest challenges in modern medicine. Recent advances in therapeutics have been so rapid that there has been a tendency to introduce new therapies either before their effectiveness has been tested properly or before the natural history of the disease process is fully understood. If a new treatment is introduced prematurely, it is often then either difficult or impossible to test adequately its validity. Properly constructed clinical trials, carried out before the widespread introduction of new forms of treatment, should be a routine part of the practice of clinical medicine.

CONTROLLED CLINICAL TRIALS

There have been few therapies that have stood out, from the start, as major advances. Examples are penicillin, quinine in the treatment of malaria, and lime juice in scurvy. Unfortunately most new therapies at best confer some small, but often worthwhile, advantage over existing treatments. Because such benefits may be small it is of importance to identify them correctly; in the same way unwelcome effects need to be detected. The basis upon which new treatments are evaluated involves comparison of their effects with the effects of either an existing treatment, or where appropriate an inert substance or placebo. The sequence in making such an evaluation, by conducting a controlled clinical trial, is set out in Fig. 1.11.

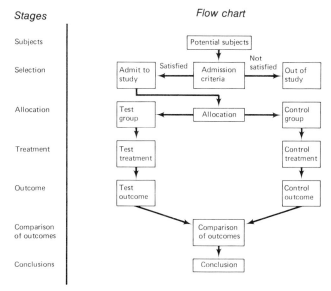

Fig. 1.11 Controlled clinical trials.

Criteria for Entry and Treatment Allocation

Potential subjects are first assessed to see whether they satisfy various criteria for entry to the study. Those that pass this are admitted to the study for allocation either to the test group, i.e. to have the new treatment, or to a control group who have the existing treatment or placebo. One of the primary requirements in any controlled clinical trial is to construct comparable groups to receive the new and the existing treatment. Here the allocation procedure is crucial and the preferred method would be random allocation of subjects to test or control group. Random allocation refers to the procedure whereby subjects are allocated to the test or control group by chance; thus removing biases that might arise should the investigator exercise judgement in deciding to which group a subject should be allocated. Trials that employ random allocation are referred to as randomised controlled clinical trials.

Very occasionally a systematic allocation of treatment, such as allocating subjects alternately to test or control group, may be preferred, usually on grounds of simplicity. In some circumstances serious bias may be introduced by this technique. Whichever method is used, the comparability of the group should always be checked after allocation.

Assessment of Outcome

Results of treatment, or outcomes, are the means by which the value of the test treatment is assessed. Outcomes in the test and control groups are compared and conclusions drawn on the advantages or otherwise of the test treatment. Problems may arise in making this assessment. Occasionally a subject, knowing which treatment he had received, may exaggerate or minimise its effects. For example, the subject may be firmly of the view that aspirin is useless, and in a trial of a new analgesic with aspirin as a control tend to exaggerate the beneficial effects of the new analgesic. In these circumstances it would have been an advantage if the subject had not known which treatment he had received, an arrangement sometimes referred to as a 'single-blind trial'. A somewhat similar problem can arise with the investigator. Here, with knowledge of what treatment the subject has received, he may find difficulty in being wholly objective when measuring outcome and unwittingly introduce bias into his assessment. To overcome potential bias a 'double-blind' assessment can be made when neither subject nor investigator is aware of which treatment the subject has received.

Applications of the Technique

Controlled clinical trials are usually thought of as pharmacological experiments designed to measure the effect of a drug, vaccine, or therapeutic agent. This definition is too narrow. As well as including drug trials, they now embrace studies designed to evaluate the health effects of changes in human behaviour (e.g. the health effects of losing weight, taking more exercise) and the health effects of changes in delivery of medical care (e.g. the early detection of cervical cancer on length of survival, early postoperative discharge on subsequent morbidity).

Ethics

Controlled clinical trials are experiments on human beings. This raises certain ethical issues. When is such a trial justified? A general answer would be when there is genuine doubt of the value of a treatment. In fact it may be unethical in these circumstances not to perform a controlled clinical trial. Is a subject's informed consent necessary before participating in a trial? There is no agreed answer, but the legal view may be that it is necessary.

CHECK LIST FOR DESCRIBING A DISEASE

It is often useful when describing a disease to ask a series of questions. A check list of such questions is given below.

Check list for describing a disease

How common?
Who affected?
Where?
Is incidence changing?
What is its spectrum of severity?
Are its causes known?
Are there effective treatments?
Can the disease be prevented?

---

1. **How Common Is It?** Diseases which appear to be common in hospital practice may be uncommon in the population as a whole. Diseases common in the population may be diagnosed and treated in general practice and thus seldom can be seen in hospital.

2. **Who Are Affected?** What are the personal characteristics of people with the disease? Do they form a common pattern?

3. **Where?** Is there any geographic variation in the incidence or prevalence of the disease?

4. **Is the Incidence Changing?** The disease may be increasing in importance and effect, or it may be declining naturally. Such background trends may complicate the interpretation of the effectiveness of treatment.

5. **What Is Its Spectrum of Severity?** This involves the concept of the 'clinical iceberg'. For example, few people die from brucellosis in the United Kingdom. Estimates of the number of clinical cases of brucellosis vary from about one hundred to about one thousand each year. However, the greater proportion of veterinary practitioners and farm-workers and many people living in rural areas have antibodies to *Brucella abortus* antigen.

6. **Are its causes known?** If they are, then prevention or effective treatment may be possible.

7. **Are there effective treatments?** What is the evidence that new or even current usual treatments are really effective? Does the published work on evaluation stand up to a rigorous scientific scrutiny?

Table 1.10 Death rates per million persons, England and Wales 1975: all causes and selected causes

All causes	11,825
Infections and parasitic diseases	61
Tuberculosis	26
Neoplasms	2,510
Oesophagus	68
Stomach	243
Large intestine	213
Rectum	115
Trachea bronchitis, lung	667
Breast (female)*	461
Cervix uteri*	85
Bladder	83
Hodgkins disease	15
Myeloid leukaemia	35
Endocrine etc. disease	143
Diabetes mellitus	103
Diseases of blood-forming organs, etc.	37
Mental disorders	41
Diseases of nervous system, etc.	126
Multiple sclerosis	16
Motor neurone disease	14
Diseases of circulatory system	6,080
Chronic rheumatic heart disease	122
Hypertensive disease	164
(Hypertensive renal disease)	10
Ischaemic heart disease	3,133
(Acute myocardial infarction)	2,153
Cerebrovascular disease	1,564
Diseases of respiratory system	1,650
Influenza	29
Pneumonia	974
Bronchitis, emphysema, asthma	529
Diseases of digestive system	301
Stomach ulcer	37
Duodenal ulcer	41
Appendicitis	6
Cirrhosis of liver	37
Cholecystitis	8
Acute pancreatitis	13
Diseases of genito-urinary system	160
Nephritis and nephrosis	61
(Chronic nephritis)	50
Calculus	4
Hyperplasia of prostate†	40
Diseases of skin, etc.	8
Diseases of musculoskeletal system, etc.	56
Accidents, poisoning, violence	423
Motor vehicle traffic accidents	117
Suicide, etc.	75
Homicide	10

* Per million females.
† Per million males.
Source: OPCS Mortality Statistics, Cause, England and Wales 1975. London, HMSO, 1977.

SUGGESTED FURTHER READING

Barker, D. J. P. and Rose, G. (1976) *Epidemiology in Medical Practice.* Edinburgh: Churchill Livingstone.

Morris, J. N. (1975) *Uses of Epidemiology.* Edinburgh: Churchill Livingstone.

Bradford Hill, A. (1977) *A Short Textbook of Medical Statistics.* London: Hodder and Stoughton.

Bourke, G. J. and McGilivray, J. (1975) *Interpretation and Uses of Medical Statistics.* Oxford: Blackwell Scientific Publications.

8. **Can the disease be prevented?** Often, if the cause of a disease is known, then prevention may be possible. This may involve inoculation or vaccination in the case of an infectious disease; it may involve controlling insects in the case of a parasitic disease like malaria; with lung cancer, changing people's attitudes and altering cigarette smoking behaviour may be the effective approach.

Infectious Diseases 2

R. V. WALLEY

FACTORS LEADING TO INFECTION

An infection requires the invasion of a susceptible patient by a pathogenic micro-organism. The organism, which may come from another patient or from a carrier, must be present in sufficient numbers to overcome the patient's resistance. A person may carry micro-organisms, commonly in the throat or bowel, without showing any sign of the disease. The carrier state may follow a clinical illness or a subclinical infection without signs or symptoms. The patient's resistance, and so his susceptibility to infection, will depend on inherent factors and immunological state. Of the first we know little. Of the second we know that immunity is increased by natural infection, transfer of maternal antibodies and artificial immunisation. It is little developed in the premature and newborn infant and is depressed by certain drugs such as corticosteroids and azathioprine, and by certain diseases such as Hodgkin's disease, affecting the reticuloendothelial system and antibody production (*see* page 407) (Fig. 2.1).

The invasion of the body is by two main routes: the respiratory tract by droplet infection; the alimentary

ALIMENTARY TRACT

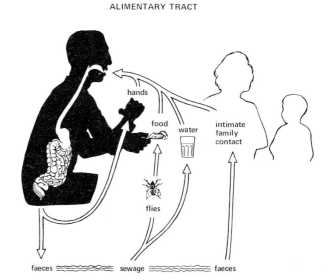

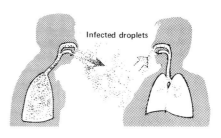

RESPIRATORY TRACT

Fig. 2.2   Principal routes of spread of infection.

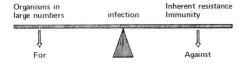

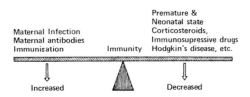

Fig. 2.1   Infection and immunity – the balance of power.

tract by faecal contamination, usually of food or water (Fig. 2.2). Having invaded the patient, a period of time elapses before the symptoms and signs of the disease develop, the incubation period. During this period the micro-organism is multiplying, probably in the reticuloendothelial system. The length of the incubation periods of common diseases which vary by a few days, may be grouped as follows:

THE CLINICAL ILLNESS

In a few diseases, such as rubella, anterior poliomyelitis and other enterovirus infections, the infection may be subclinical in most cases and detectable only by isolation of the organism or the appearance of specific antibodies. In the majority of infections the micro-organism, or its toxins, are widely distributed throughout the body at the end of the incubation period, giving rise to a viraemia, a septicaemia, or a toxaemia. To these are ascribed certain features common to most infections. Fever is almost invariable. It is due to the reaction of the temperature regulating centre in the hypothalamus to the micro-organism. The centre also reacts to any foreign protein. The fever is accompanied by complaints of headache, shivering, aching pain in the back and legs, and tiredness. Children commonly vomit and go to sleep. Adults lose their appetite. The loss of appetite is accompanied by a catabolic state which leads to weight loss. The features of the disease then appear in an orderly way with a pattern peculiar to the particular disease. Recognition of that pattern aids diagnosis. For example, the rash of measles appears on the third or fourth day after the onset with fever, cough etc., while the rash of rubella may be the first sign of the disease.

Rashes in infectious diseases

Diagnosis depends on:
  day of onset
  distribution
  character of lesion

As the illness develops, so do the patient's defence mechanisms. These include phagocytosis of organisms by the reticuloendothelial system and the development of cellular and humoral immunity. With many infections, particularly with the common virus infections, this leads to a recovery in the uncomplicated case, coinciding with a rise in the level of the specific antibody. With the subsidence of the illness the patient enters the convalescent period of tissue recovery and weight gain, when the antibody level is at its highest. It lasts for a period ranging from a few days after a mild attack of measles, to some weeks after a severe attack of typhoid.

LABORATORY AIDS TO DIAGNOSIS

Confirmation of the diagnosis of infectious disease is best made by isolation of the causative organism. In bacterial infections this can be done in twenty-four to forty-eight hours, and enables treatment to be given with the antibiotic to which the organism is sensitive. The isolation of viruses by growth on tissue culture takes one to three weeks and positive results can only be expected in one-third to two-thirds of cases. The tissue culture has to be selected on which the suspected virus will grow. To do this the virologist must have clinical information on the type of infection. More rapid methods have been developed in recent years enabling identification of the virus in a few hours. Some viruses, such as that of smallpox, vaccinia and chickenpox can be identified under the electron microscope. Some viruses have first to be tagged with specific antiserum labelled with fluorescence or radioactivity. Then the fluorescence may be seen under the light microcope (herpes simplex, influenza and parainfluenza viruses, respiratory syncytial virus) or by detecting the radioactivity.

Confirmation of the diagnosis can also be made by demonstrating a rising level of specific antibodies in the blood taken at ten-day intervals. The finding of a raised level of antibody titre in a single specimen only may be due to previous infection or immunisation.

Examination of the white blood cells may aid the diagnosis in some diseases. Thus, a leucopenia is common in typhoid, brucellosis and influenza, and a leucocytosis in generalised pneumococcal, staphylococcal and streptococcal infections. Atypical mononuclear cells are the rule in glandular fever, but occasionally occur in brucellosis, toxoplasmosis, infectious hepatitis and cytomegalic infection.

TREATMENT

Virus Infections

Certain antiviral drugs are at present being introduced and they seem promising in their limited field, such as methisazone for the prevention of smallpox and iododeoxyuridine for the treatment of herpetic infection of the eye, but, in general, there are no effective antibiotics for virus infections. Some benefits can be obtained from intravenous injection of specific human immunoglobulins, obtained from convalescent donors. This has been used in the treatment of chickenpox in immunosuppressed patients. Otherwise treatment has, therefore, to be on symptomatic and general lines providing the best conditions for natural recovery. Bed rest is advisable during the febrile period.

The fluid intake should be sufficient to achieve a good urinary output, about 2.5 litres in adults. A high calorific intake is desirable, in view of the increased metabolic rate due to the fever, but it is difficult to achieve because the patient's appetite is poor. Carbohydrate foods are most acceptable and protein intake has to be mainly in the form of milk and milk foods. During the convalescent period the appetite recovers and the weight loss can be made good with a fuller diet.

Bacterial Infections

Although the general lines are the same in bacterial infections, specific treatment with the correct antibiotic in full doses takes first place. To select the correct antibiotic the sensitivity of the causative organism must be known, preferably from results of bacteriological culture. It is undesirable to prescribe antibiotics when fever and general features are the only signs of infection, for frequently such an infection is due to a virus and subsides in a few days, while antibiotics have harmful side effects. Furthermore, if the infection is bacterial in origin premature use of antibiotics may delay diagnosis. Only if the patient appears to be very ill as shown by such features as high and prolonged fever, rigors, delirium or coma, or circulatory collapse, should antibiotics be given after taking specimens for bacteriological examination such as blood and cerebrospinal fluid. In very severe infections of this nature, intravenous fluids and corticosteroids may be necessary as supportive therapy.

For further information *see* Chapter 25 – Principles of Antimicrobial Chemotherapy.

PREVENTION OF INFECTIOUS DISEASES

For the community as a whole, the control of the spread of infectious diseases is achieved by such public health measures as the provision of clean food and water, the hygienic disposal of sewage, and avoidance of overcrowding. To facilitate this control, the notification of the most important infectious diseases has been made compulsory under the Public Health Act. These diseases include:

Common – measles, scarlet fever, whooping-cough, infective hepatitis, tuberculosis, dysentery, food poisoning.

Rare – anthrax, smallpox, leptospirosis, tetanus, diphtheria, typhoid fever, acute poliomyelitis, acute meningitis.

Immunisation

For the protection of the individual, particularly against those diseases spread by droplet infection of the respiratory tract, specific active immunisation is necessary. Table 2.1 gives an example of the programme that is widely used in Great Britain at the present time.

Table 2.1   Immunisation schedule

Age	Disease	Type of vaccine	Mode of administration
6 m	Diphtheria	Diphtheria toxoid	Intramuscular injection
	Tetanus	Tetanus toxoid	
	Whooping-cough	H. pertussis, killed organism	
	Poliomyelitis	Live attenuated virus	Oral
8 m	Repeat above	As above	As above
12 m	Repeat above	As above	As above
13 m	Measles	Live attenuated virus	Subcutaneously or intramuscular injection
4 y	Diphtheria		
	Tetanus	As above	As above
	Poliomyelitis		
13 y	Rubella (girls only)	Live attenuated virus	Subcutaneously or intramuscular injection
14 y	Tuberculosis	BCG Live attenuated organism	Skin inoculation with Heaf gun

When considering the advisability of active immunisation in any particular instance it is axiomatic that all methods have harmful side effects. These side effects have to be weighed against the likelihood of catching the infection and the severity of the resulting illness. For example, smallpox vaccination in Great Britain is only advisable for those at special risk, e.g. health workers and travellers, for reactions to it are sometimes unpleasant and on rare occasions fatal and the risk of catching smallpox in Great Britain is negligible. The desirability of whooping-cough vaccination has been questioned recently since on very rare occasions brain damage occurs, while the disease itself at the present time has a low incidence and mortality due in part to immunisation. However, if the community were not protected, whooping-cough would become more common and itself cause more brain damage and death on a much wider scale than immunisation. Passive immunisation by the use of specific human immunoglobulin may be used to prevent disease when there is no time to immunise actively, as with tetanus or rabies, or when there is no antigen available, as with hepatitis, types A and B. Although the protection is immediate, it only lasts for three to six months.

Isolation

Isolation of the infected patient can only be effective in preventing the spread of the disease in the community when the disease is not endemic. Then, combined with active immunisation, it may help control an outbreak introduced from abroad as it has in the past with smallpox. Isolation is generally used to prevent the spread of the disease in hospital to other patients and, if possible, to the attendants. In hospital, isolation is combined with barrier nursing. The aim of this technique is to provide a sterile barrier around the isolation room. Inside the room it is assumed that everything is contaminated with the infectious agent to a greater or lesser degree. Everything removed from the room has to be rendered free from contamination by washing, or, if possible by autoclaving or incineration. The technique is imperfect but is successful with diseases spread by the faecal-oral route, such as typhoid fever.

When the disease is highly infectious and is spread by air-borne droplet infection, as is the case with chickenpox or smallpox, success is more difficult to achieve. It is necessary to control airflow patterns, sterilising the outflow. When, in addition, there is no immunisation available to the attendants and the disease has a high mortality, as with Lassa and Marburg virus disease, isolation and barrier nursing are carried to their logical extreme. The patient is isolated in an airtight plastic tent ventilated with fresh air, the outflow being extracted through a filter capable of extracting virus particles. Everything is taken from the tent in sealed plastic bags which are either incinerated or autoclaved.

MEASLES

Definition

A virus infection involving the skin and the mucous membranes of the respiratory tract, the eyes and the mouth.

Background

The disease is spread by droplet infection from the respiratory tract. It is highly infectious for four days before and five days after the appearance of the rash. Most infections occur in childhood, but not in the first six months of life for, during this period, the child is usually protected by antibodies that have crossed the placenta from the mother.

Pathology

A mononuclear reaction with accompanying giant cells is widespread throughout the respiratory tract and affected skin.

Symptoms and Signs

Prodromal stage
Fever, cough.
Red, running eyes, lids swollen.
Koplik spots: pinhead, grey on the buccal mucosa.

Eruptive stage
Rash.
Signs of bronchitis.
Misery.

Rash of measles	
Onset:	fourth day of disease.
Distribution:	on the face, spreading to the trunk and limbs.
Lesions:	blotchy, irregular, maculopapular, deep red, occasionally some petechiae.
Duration:	four days.

Complications

Obstructive laryngitis – rare, a tracheotomy may be needed.
Bronchopneumonia – usually due to secondary bacterial infection, rarely to the virus itself
Otitis media – due to secondary bacterial infection.
Encephalitis – rare (*see* page 548).
Pansclerosing encephalitis – a very rare progressive fatal condition, occurring some years after the acute illness, brought on by a defect of cellular immunity (*see* page 547).

Differential Diagnosis

Scarlet Fever. Sore throat present. Rash erythematous.

Rubella. Rash of similar character but less marked. No prodromal stage.
Both the above illnesses are milder than measles.

Drug Rashes. Generalised maculopapular rash. (History of taking drugs such as ampicillin.)

Basis of Treatment

All that is required are general measures, unless bronchopneumonia or otitis media occur, when intramuscular penicillin should be given.

Prevention

This can be achieved by immunisation with a live attenuated virus (*see* Table 2.1). Febrile reactions occur occasionally. Passive immunity can be conferred by injecting human gammaglobulin within five days of exposure, and this may be required if the child has severe intercurrent disease, e.g. fibrocystic disease of the pancreas, renal failure, etc.

RUBELLA (GERMAN MEASLES)

Definition

A mild virus infection of childhood and adult life but the cause of widespread damage to the fetal tissues when transmitted congenitally.

Background

Spread by droplet infection from the respiratory tract, rubella is infectious for about ten days before and four days after the appearance of the rash. About half the infections are subclinical. If a woman becomes infected in the first three months of her pregnancy there is a one in five chance of congenital infection of the fetus, with severe results. After four months the danger is negligible. Subclinical and overt infection of the mother are equally dangerous. In cases of diagnostic difficulty, great help may be obtained from studies of rubella antibodies in the serum.

Symptoms

Often the patient does not feel ill.

Signs

Rash.
Conjunctival injection.
Enlarged suboccipital glands.

Rash of rubella	
Onset:	first day of disease.
Distribution:	on the face, spreading to the trunk, rarely the limbs.
Lesions:	small, maculopapular, light pink in colour.
Duration:	One to two days.

Complications

Mild arthritis.
Meningoencephalitis – rare.
Congenital defects such as deformity of the eye (cataract), the heart (patent ductus, pulmonary stenosis, coarctation of the aorta) or the ear (deafness). In addition, the newborn child may have a prolonged illness during which the rubella virus is widespread throughout the body with extensive clinical manifestations. These include low birth weight, purpura, anaemia, myocarditis, chronic hepatitis, bone changes and mental defect (Fig. 2.3).

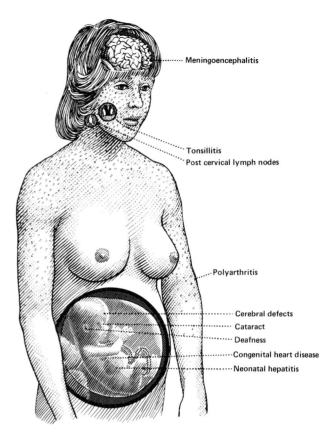

Fig. 2.3 The clinical features and complications of rubella.

Investigations

Culture of the virus from the throat. Detection of an antibody rise after a ten-day interval.

Basis of Treatment

The illness in adults and children requires little treatment and there is nothing that can be done to halt the congenital disease. Prevention is, therefore, crucial.

Prevention

A live attenuated virus vaccine has recently been introduced and found effective (see Table 2.1).

Prevention of congenital deformity caused by rubella
1. Immunisation of young girls.
2. When a pregnant woman is exposed to rubella:
Confirm the diagnosis in the contact case.
Check the duration of the pregnancy.
Check the immune state of the mother by antibody levels.
If the mother has been infected therapeutic abortion should be considered.

MUMPS

Definition

A virus infection involving the salivary glands principally, but frequently affecting the meninges and the testes.

Background

Spread by droplet infection, mumps appears to be less infectious than chickenpox or measles but, since many infections are subclinical, this is hard to judge. The patient is infectious a few days before and a few days after the parotid swelling.

Pathology

Oedema of the cells lining the ducts and lymphocytic infiltration occur in the parotid gland. Similar changes occur in the testes and partial atrophy may follow.

Symptoms

Fever.
Pain in neck.
Dry mouth.
Pain on eating.

Signs

Swollen, tender parotid enlargement (usually, but not always bilateral).
Inflamed parotid duct orifices.
Other salivary glands may be involved.

The symptoms and signs are often worse in adults.

Complications (Fig. 2.4)

Meningoencephalitis (see page 548). This occurs after the parotitis or may be the only manifestation of the disease.
Arthritis – rare.
Orchitis – occurs after puberty; even when bilateral it rarely causes sterility.
Oophoritis.
Pancreatitis – causes abdominal pain, vomiting and resolves without treatment.

Investigations

The virus can be cultured from the throat. A rising titre to the S and V antibodies of mumps can be detected during the illness.

Basis of Treatment

This is on general and symptomatic lines. Some relief of the considerable pain of orchitis may result from the administration of prednisolone 15 mg three times a day.

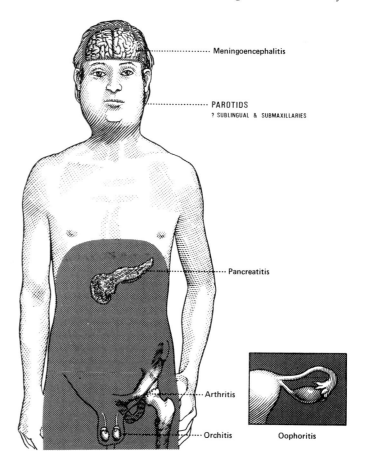

Fig. 2.4   The clinical features and complications of mumps.

Prevention

An effective vaccine is available, but is rarely used since the disease is mild in childhood and uncommon in adults.

CHICKENPOX (VARICELLA)

Definition

A virus infection involving primarily the skin and mucous membranes of the mouth and, on rare occasions, other organs.

Background

Chickenpox is spread by droplet infection and is highly infectious one day before and seven days after the appearance of the rash. Most cases occur in childhood and are mild. After an attack of chickenpox the virus may persist in the body, lying dormant, only to reappear when immunity falls later in life, in certain diseases such as Hodgkin's disease, or in patients receiving immunosuppressive drugs. It then causes herpes zoster (*see* page 550).

Pathology

Degeneration occurs in the prickle cells of the epidermis with the out-pouring of oedema fluid forming the vesicles. The vesicle fluid rapidly becomes turbid with polymorphonuclear leucoctyes. Giant cells and inclusion bodies are present.

Symptoms and Signs

Irritating rash (see Fig. 2.5 and Table 2.2).
Fever.
Constitutional upset.

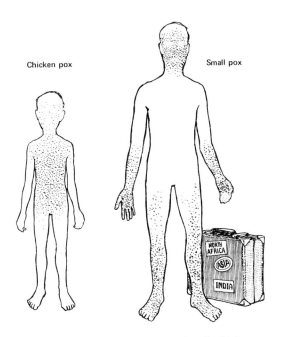

Chicken pox   Small pox

NORTH AFRICA
ASIA
INDIA

Fig. 2.5 The distribution of the rash of chickenpox and smallpox.

Complications

Pyogenic lesion of the skin due to secondary infection with staphylococci.
Encephalitis (*see* page 548) – rare.
Pneumonia, caused directly by the virus – rare. (Pneumonia may result in scattered pulmonary calcification and resultant diagnostic confusion when chest X-ray is performed later in life.)
Fatal generalisation of the disease in patients receiving steroid or other immunosuppressive drugs – rare.

Differential Diagnosis

Impetigo. Vesicles larger than chickenpox occur in clusters, irregular distribution.

Papular urticaria. The papule has a small horny vesicle. No constitutional upset.

Smallpox.

Basis of Treatment

Bed rest during the febrile period is all that is usually required. When the rash is severe, calamine lotion with 1 per cent phenol may relieve irritation.

HERPES ZOSTER (*see* page 550).

SMALLPOX (VARIOLA)

Definition

An infection involving the skin and mucous membranes of the mouth accompanied by a toxic and often fatal viraemia.

Background

Smallpox is close to being eliminated from the world. At the present time it only occurs in Somalia and Ethiopia. Elimination has been possible since clinical diagnosis is straightforward in the non-immune, and vaccination provides excellent immunity. The disease is highly infectious from the onset of the fever when the virus is transmitted by droplet infection, until the last crust has separated, since the crust contains virus particles. The mortality is high, around twenty to thirty per cent in outbreaks in Great Britain.

Symptoms and Signs

Intense toxaemia at the onset.
Rash.

Investigations

Provisional identification of the virus from the lesions in a few hours with the electron microscope. Culture of the virus from the lesion in three days.

Differential Diagnosis (*see* Table 2.2 and Fig. 2.5)

Chickenpox presents the most frequent problem.

Basis of Treatment

General measures only are available. Care of the skin is especially important.

Table 2.2 Rashes of chickenpox and smallpox

	Chicken pox	Smallpox
Onset:	on first or second day, toxaemia slight or absent	on third or fourth day, severe toxaemia present before rash.
Distribution:	centripetal: on face and trunk first	centrifugal: on hands and feet and face first.
Lesions:	small, superficial vesicles, papules and pustules also are present	deep, larger lesions progressing regularly from macule to papule vesicle, pustule and crust. (Morbilliform – prodromal rash occurs.)
Duration:	four to seven days	progresses over 9 days, lasts two weeks or until death.

Prevention

Early diagnosis and isolation in special hospitals play an important role in Great Britain. This is the responsibility of the community physician who must be informed immediately if smallpox is suspected. Mass vaccination, which has enabled the disease to be abolished from this country, is no longer recommended since the risks of its complications (see Table 2.3) outweigh the risks of the disease. Vaccination is limited to those at special risk, such as health workers and foreign travellers. The protection given by a successful vaccination is acquired after six days and continues reliable for one year and remains good for three years and then wanes. Immediate protection against smallpox is given by the drug methisazone.

Table 2.3 Complications of vaccination

Complications	Contraindications
Eczema-vaccinatum – sometimes fatal	Infantile eczema
Generalised vaccinia	Corticosteroid and immuno-suppressive therapy Hypogammaglobulinaemia Hodgkin's disease Leukaemia
Fetal infection	Pregnancy
Encephalitis – sometimes fatal	

HERPES SIMPLEX

Definition

A virus infection of the mouth and lips occurring first in childhood, and in some subjects recurring throughout life. The infection is sometimes widespread in the body.

Background

Two-thirds of the population are infected with the virus in childhood by way of the respiratory tract, but few show signs of this, apart from the presence of specific antibodies in the blood. A small proportion of those with antibodies harbour the virus throughout life, in the posterior root ganglia. These people suffer from recurrent lesions of the lips. The virus can be cultured without difficulty and the diagnosis of uncommon manifestations confirmed in this way.

Pathology

The deeper layer of the mucous membranes and the skin show a ballooning degeneration of the cells with the formation of oedema fluid. Giant cells and inclusion bodies occur.

Symptoms and Signs

Acute stomatitis in infants aged one to three.
Fever.
Painful vesicles in the mouth.

Acute generalised infections of the newborn. Rare, usually fatal.
Encephalitis. Rare (see page 548).

Recurrent Herpes. Vesicles appear on the lips and neighbouring skin at the start of many infections such as colds, pneumonia, meningitis or even on exposure to sunlight.

Herpetic Whitlow. Often on nurses fingers: painful.

Genital Herpes. Painful vesicles appear on the vulva in women and on the penis in men.

Eczema Herpeticum. Vesicles appear on the skin of infant and child. Sometimes fatal.

Differential Diagnosis

Oral Thrush. In infants this has the appearance of curds on the oral mucous membrane.

Basis of Treatment

An antiviral agent iododeoxyuridine may be useful for local infection in the eye, but is toxic and not satisfactory for generalised infection. Treatment has, therefore, to be on general lines.

INFECTIOUS MONONUCLEOSIS (GLANDULAR FEVER)

Definition

A virus infection involving the lymphatic tissues and tonsils, causing a mononucleosis in the blood.

Background

The disease is caused by the Epstein Barr virus which infects eighty per cent of the population, mostly in childhood. The great majority of the infections are subclinical. The clinical illness is common in adolescents and young adults when the infecting dose of the virus – spread by kissing – is high. The illness lasts three weeks and sometimes is followed by a period of malaise lasting two to four months.

Pathology

There is a proliferation of mononuclear cells in the lymph nodes, spleen, and sometimes in other organs.

Symptoms

Sore throat.
Fever.

Signs

Generalised lymphadenopathy (small, mobile, painless).
Enlarged tonsils with exudate.
Splenomegaly.
Sometimes rash, and jaundice due to hepatitis.
Lasts 2 to 3 weeks, but may need prolonged convalescence.

Investigations

The white blood count shows an increase in lymphocytes and abnormal mononuclear cells. Diagnostic of infectious mononucleosis is a rise in heterophil antibodies to sheep red cells, the Paul-Bunnel test.

Complications

Hepatitis appears in the second week – not uncommon.
Drug rash – almost invariable if the patient is treated with ampicillin.
Encephalitis – rare.
Peripheral neuritis – this is acute and widespread in some cases producing a Guillan-Barré syndrome – rare.
Haemolytic anaemia – rare.
Rupture of the spleen – rare.

Differential Diagnosis

Tonsillitis due to other causes (see Diphtheria, page 24).

Basis of Treatment

Antibiotics have no effect on the throat and treatment is on general and symptomatic lines. Should tonsillar swelling threaten to obstruct the breathing, corticosteroids given by injection will give relief in a few hours.

ENTEROVIRUS INFECTIONS

Definition

Infections caused by the Coxsackie and Echo groups of viruses of which there are many antigenic types. These viruses can be isolated best from the faeces, hence their name. (The poliovirus is an enterovirus; the illness it causes is described on page 548.)

Background

These viruses are present in the stool during the acute illness and for some time afterwards. They can also be isolated from the throat during the acute attack. The spread of infection is from person to person, probably both by droplet infection and by the faeces. Subclinical infections are much more common than clinical disease.

Clinical Features

Infections with these viruses may cause a number of febrile illnesses. Both the Coxsackie and Echo groups cause aseptic meningitis (see page 547), and nonspecific febrile illnesses, sometimes accompanied by a transient macular rash. In addition the Coxsackie group cause a number of well defined disease patterns (see Table 2.4).

Table 2.4 Coxsackie virus infections

Group A	
Herpangina:	sore throat, grey papules on the pharynx becoming ulcerated.
Hand, foot and mouth disease:	vesicles 3 to 8 mm in diameter in the mouth and on the hands and feet.
Group B	
Bornholm disease:	acutely painful myositis of the thoracic, less commonly of the abdominal muscles. Onset sudden, lasting a few days.
Pericarditis	
Myocarditis	
Neonatal infection:	myocarditis, sometimes meningoencephalitis with a high mortality.

Investigations

The viruses can be isolated from the throat and faeces. A rise in specific antibody can be detected during the acute illness.

Basis of Treatment

This must be on symptomatic lines, as there is no satisfactory antiviral agent.

RABIES

Definition

A viral encephalitis, primarily of wild animals. The disease may spread to cats and dogs and, rarely, hence to man.

Pathology

Neuronal necrosis of the central nervous system, particularly in the thalamus and substantia nigra. Typical inclusion bodies (Negri bodies) are present.

Background

The disease is endemic in Africa and in the east. Recently it has spread in foxes from eastern Europe, reaching France and Belgium but not, as yet, the British Isles. The disease is spread by biting, the virus being in the saliva. Dogs and cats are infectious ten days before and during the illness. The dog changes its behaviour, becoming restless and wild, biting without provocation. Later it becomes paralysed, froths at the mouth and dies within ten days of the onset. The incubation period in man is usually one to three months, making post infection immunisation possible, but the period ranges from ten days to two years.

Symptoms

Headache, vomiting and fever for two to three days, then tingling in the affected limb.
Fearful excitement.

Signs

Increased muscular tone.
Jerky movements.
Increased salivation, then choking fits at the sight of water (hydrophobia).
Convulsions.

Investigations

Diagnosis in life depends on the clinical picture. After death the virus can be grown from the brain which shows typical changes (*see above*).

Basis of Treatment

Sedation.
Measures to maintain a clear airway.

Prognosis

Always fatal when the illness is fully developed.

Prevention of rabies

Quarantine of animals entering Great Britain.
In endemic areas:
  Control of foxes.
  Immunisation of people at risk, e.g. nurses, doctors, dog handlers.
  Immunisation of dogs and cats.
Post exposure:
  Cleaning the wound with soap and water or alcohol or quaternary ammonium compounds (e.g. Cetrimide).
  Confirm the diagnosis in the animal.
  Immunisation of patient.
  Administration of antiserum in cases of greatest risk.

LASSA AND EBOLA (MARBURG) VIRUS FEVER

Definition

Two recently identified virus infections with a high mortality, endemic in Africa. There is a danger that they may be imported to Great Britain and Europe.

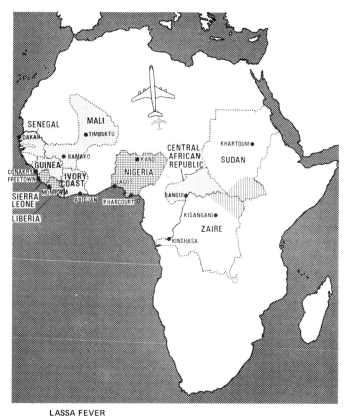

LASSA FEVER

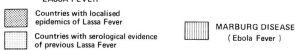
Countries with localised epidemics of Lassa Fever

Countries with serological evidence of previous Lassa Fever

MARBURG DISEASE
(Ebola Fever)

Fig. 2.6   Lassa and Ebola (Marburg) fever. Endemic regions of Africa.

Background (Fig. 2.6)

Lassa fever is endemic in West Africa where the disease is spread primarily by a particular species of rat, not present in Great Britain. However, close human contact can spread the disease. Also, the blood, containing large amounts of virus is particularly infectious. In Africa many infections are subclinical. Ebola virus disease occurs in the southern Sudan and Zaire. It is spread in a similar fashion. The possibility of the diagnosis of these two diseases must be considered in any patient developing a fever within twenty-one days after leaving the above areas. Owing to the serious nature of the disease and infectivity, such patients have to be admitted to special isolation units and investigated by designated high security laboratories.

Symptoms and Signs

Similar in both diseases.
Insidious onset malaise, fever, anorexia.
Tonsillitis, pharyngitis with small ulcers.
Diarrhoea, vomiting, abdominal pain.
Cough, chest pain, pleural effusion.
Fatal cases develop haemorrhagic features.
A maculopapular rash occurs in Ebola virus infections on the fourth day of the disease.

Investigations

The virus can be isolated from the blood.
(*Caution:* This should only be in a specially designated laboratory.)

WHOOPING-COUGH (SYN. PERTUSSIS)

Definition

An illness of infants and children, characterised by a spasmodic cough and caused by *Bordetella pertussis.*

Background

Whooping-cough is a prolonged illness developing over the course of two weeks and lasting on average six weeks. It is most serious in the first year of life when the spasms are exhausting and interfere with feeding. They may result in apnoea and convulsions, causing brain damage and death.

Pathology

The mucous membrane of the respiratory tract shows inflammatory and necrotic changes with the production of much mucus. The mucus tends to block the smaller bronchioles causing areas of collapse. The brain may show anoxaemic changes.

Symptoms and Signs (Fig. 2.7)

Upper respiratory catarrh.
Coughing spasms ending in a whoop caused by deep inhalation. These may cause vomiting, apnoea, cyanosis, convulsions.
Fever is present only in the first few days.

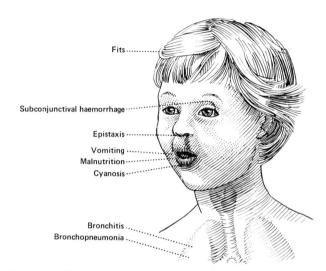

Fig. 2.7 Clinical features and complications of whooping-cough.

Investigations

Bordetella pertussis can be cultured from a pernasal swab in the early stage. A lymphocytosis of 80 per cent with a total count of 20,000 or more is present.

Complications (Fig. 2.7)

Conjunctival haemorrhage.
Segmental collapse of the lung due to secondary infection.
Brain damage due to anoxia.
Bronchopneumonia.

Basis of Treatment

The aim of treatment is to keep the child nourished during a long disease with vomiting. When the spasms cause cyanosis the child should be nursed in an oxygen tent. Antibiotics do little to relieve the disease, but the secondary pneumonia is treated with penicillin intramuscularly.

Prevention

A moderately effective vaccine is available which can be given with diphtheria and tetanus immunisation. It rarely causes convulsion and brain damage. The matter is discussed on page 14.

STREPTOCOCCAL INFECTIONS

Background

The beta haemolytic streptococcus is the cause of a number of different types of infection in man, including scarlet fever, erysipelas, tonsillitis, peritonsillar infection, local infections and septicaemia. The infecting streptococcus commonly belongs to Lancefield group A. All Griffiths types of this group are capable of producing an erythrogenic toxin and, so, of causing scarlet fever. Immunity to the toxin will follow scarlet fever, but bacterial immunity will be limited to one type of streptococcus. The patient, therefore, will be susceptible to infection with other types, though immune to scarlet fever.

Rheumatic fever and nephritis commonly occur two to three weeks after tonsillitis, but can occur after any streptococcal infection. They are the result of an immune reaction to the streptococcus.

The spread of streptococcal infection is commonly by droplet infection, in which throat carriers, numbering five to eight per cent of the population, play an important part.

SCARLET FEVER

Definition

A childhood infection caused by the erythrogenic toxin of the beta haemolytic streptococcus.

Symptoms and Signs

Fever.
Sore throat with enlarged tonsils sometimes covered with exudate.
Enlarged tender cervical lymph glands.
Rash (see below).
Furred tongue with red papillae, peeling to become bright red.

Rash of scarlet fever	
Onset:	second day of disease.
Distribution:	on the face, trunk and upper-thighs.
Lesion:	erythema with raised red spots, pallor around the mouth.
Duration	1 to 3 days.

Investigations

Culture of the streptococcus from the throat.

Complications

Purulent rhinitis and otitis media.
Acute glomerular nephritis and rheumatic fever occur after ten days.

Differential Diagnosis

Measles. Prodromal stage with cough. Rash appears on the third day, maculopapular.

Rubella. Rash maculopapular. Clinical differentiation may be difficult.

Drug Rash. Irregular maculopapular rash on the trunk, often irritating.

Basis of Treatment

Penicillin is the drug of choice for all streptococcal infections.

ERYSIPELAS

Definition

An infection of the skin accompanied by a marked toxaemia occurring in middle age and tending to recur.

Symptoms and Signs

Fever.
Toxaemia.
Rash (see below).

Rash of erysipelas	
Onset:	second day of disease.
Distribution:	on the bridge of the nose, spreading to the forehead and eyelids, or on the shin.
Lesion:	red raised skin; large vesicles may follow.
Duration:	the rash continues to spread until treated.

Differential Diagnosis

Ophthalmic Herpes Zoster: The vesicular lesions are painful and limited to one side of the face.

Basis of Treatment

Intramuscular penicillin.

PERITONSILLAR INFECTION (SYN. QUINSEY)

Symptoms

Severe sore throat.
Difficulty in swallowing.

Signs

Trismus.
Swelling of the pillar of the fauces on one side, extending towards and often across the midline.

Basis of Treatment

Intramuscular penicillin.
An abscess may form and require incision.

DIPHTHERIA

Definition

A severe toxic illness caused by the infection of the throat, nose or skin by *Corynebacterium diphtheriae*. The disease has been almost completely eradicated in Great Britain by immunisation.

Background

The illness is spread by droplet infection from other patients or throat carriers. The organism grows on the tonsils, producing a toxin which is spread throughout the body, giving rise to other features of the disease. The patient remains infectious as long as the organism is present in the throat.

Pathology

The membrane in the throat consists of leucocytes, cellular debris and organisms enmeshed in coagulated serum. The other organs show the nonspecific changes of toxaemia. The cardiac muscle shows microscopic damage and the heart is dilated.

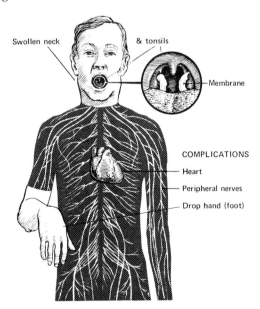

Swollen neck   & tonsils

Membrane

COMPLICATIONS
- Heart
- Peripheral nerves
- Drop hand (foot)

Fig. 2.8   Diphtheria.

Symptoms and Signs (Fig. 2.8)

Sore throat with enlarged tonsils covered with yellow green exudate which may spread to the palate, pillars of the fauces and pharynx.
Marked enlargement of the cervical lymph glands with oedema of the neck.
Slight fever.
Marked toxaemia.

Nasal Diphtheria. Bloody nasal discharge with little toxaemia.

Laryngeal Diphtheria. Laryngeal obstruction with little toxaemia.

Investigations

The diagnosis is confirmed by isolation of the organism from the throat. Some strains are avirulent and, when the clinical condition gives rise to doubts, virulence tests should be performed.

Complications (Fig. 2.8)

Cardiac failure. This is due to myocarditis – in fatal cases it is associated with heart block. It occurs in the second or third week.
Peripheral neuritis. Palatal paralysis is common in the third week. Generalised paralysis may later cause death from respiratory failure.
Laryngeal obstruction. This may necessitate a tracheotomy.

Differential Diagnosis

Streptococcal Tonsillitis. Fever greater, toxaemia less.

Glandular Fever. Prolonged fever but little toxaemia. Lymphatic glands and spleen enlarged.
(If diphtheria is prevalent it must be excluded in these cases by culture of a throat swab.)

Basis of Treatment

Intramuscular penicillin 0.25 mega units six-hourly will eliminate the organism but has no effect on the established disease caused by the toxin. Since this is fixed to the tissue, antitoxin also has limited effect but should be given in doses of 20,000 to 100,000 units intramuscularly depending on the extent of the membrane. Since the antitoxin is prepared from horse serum it may give rise to an allergic reaction, serum sickness occurring after ten days with rash and joint pains or, more rarely, immediate anaphylactic shock. This may be fatal and requires immediate treatment with 1/1,000 adrenaline, 1 ml injected intramuscularly (*see* page 126). A test dose of 0.1 ml of the antitoxin given subcutaneously may enable sensitive subjects to be detected without causing serious reaction. They can then be desensitised. Heart failure and respiratory failure may require treatment.

Prevention

Immunisation should be carried out in childhood (*see* Table 2.1) with toxoid given in conjunction with the tetanus and pertussis vaccine. If immunisation is considered later in life, it is advisable to Schick test the individual first. This measures susceptibility to infection. Diluted diphtheria toxin solution, 0.1 ml is injected subcutaneously into one arm and 0.1 ml of heated toxin solution into the other as a control. If there is no skin reaction to the toxin, the subject has a protective level of antibody. If there is a reaction, either he is susceptible or he is sensitive to the protein material in the toxin solution. In that case there will also be a reaction to the control solution.

If an outbreak of the disease occurs the contacts should be protected by active and passive immunisation.

INFECTIVE DIARRHOEA IN GREAT BRITAIN

Definition

A number of bacteria, the salmonellae, shigellae, certain staphylococci, *Clostridium perfringens* (*welchii*) and *Bacillus cereus* give rise to an illness in which diarrhoea, sometimes accompanied by vomiting, is the principal feature. These illnesses have much in common and will be described together.

Background

Infective diarrhoea is spread by faecal contamination, usually of food or water. Faecal contamination results from a patient or carrier handling certain foods, such as prepared meat, fish or milk products, which are capable of supporting rapid bacterial growth if their temperature is around 37°C. Water may be contaminated by infected sewage. When it is, the resultant outbreak is explosive and widespread. The case is infectious from the start of the diarrhoea until the stool is clear of organisms, usually some time after the clinical illness.

Prevention of these diseases is achieved by breaking the chain of the spread of infection, by public health measures. Cases and carriers must be detected. They can then avoid infection by personal hygiene (washing hands, etc.) and by not preparing food for others. The other important measures are proper sewage disposal, the provision of clean water and hygienic conditions for handling food.

Symptoms

Fever.
Diarrhoea.

Abdominal pain of a colicky nature.
Sometimes vomiting.

Signs

Abdominal tenderness.
Signs of fluid and electrolyte loss.

Investigations

The stools should be cultured on two occasions to identify the causative organism. To establish freedom from infection, when this is necessary, six consecutive negative results must be obtained, for excretion is sometimes intermittent.

Differential Diagnosis

Acute Appendicitis. Pain is constant and the predominant feature. An acutely tender spot is felt abdominally or rectally.

Ulcerative Colitis. The diarrhoea is prolonged, well over one week and the faeces contain blood.

Basis of Treatment

An adequate fluid intake should be assured. With severe diarrhoea and vomiting this may have to be by intravenous infusion with electrolyte control. The diet, if taken, should be light with a low residue. Symptomatic treatment of the diarrhoea is rarely effective but, if the condition is distressing, codeine phosphate 30 mg three times daily or Lomotil (diphenoxylate with atropine) tablets, two four times a day may be tried.

The particular features of the different conditions will now be considered.

SALMONELLA FOOD POISONING

There are many salmonella species and all cause the same type of illness. The diarrhoea starts with fever twelve to forty-eight hours after eating the infected food and lasts from a few days to a week. Occasionally, the organism enters the bloodstream causing a septicaemia. Most cases have clear stools in a few weeks, but some carry the organism for six to nine months.

Specific Treatment

Unless there is a septicaemia, antibiotics have little effect on the clinical condition or carrier state and, in fact, may prolong the carrier state. For a septicaemia, ampicillin is a suitable antibiotic.

SHIGELLA INFECTION: BACILLARY DYSENTERY

Shigella sonnei causes most of the infection in this country. Infecting toddlers and children, it is more commonly spread from case to case in the family or at school than by food. The disease is usually mild and self-limiting. Bloody diarrhoea, fever and toxaemia are rare with *Shigella sonnei*, but occur more commonly with *Sh. flexneri* and *Sh. shiga* infections. *Sh. shiga* is not to be found in this country and bacillary dysentery in this sense is now more a tropical disease spread by water.

Specific Treatment

Neomycin 1 g three times daily by mouth and streptomycin 1 g twice daily by mouth for six days are satisfactory in the clinical illness and for clearing the stool. The carrier state is not so persistent as with salmonella infections.

STAPHYLOCOCCAL TOXIN FOOD POISONING

Certain phage types of staphylococci are capable of producing an enterotoxin which will withstand boiling. As is common with all staphylococci, these may be carried in the nose, and from this site contaminate food in preparation. Here they grow and produce their toxin which, when the food is eaten, gives rise to profuse vomiting and sometimes diarrhoea in two to four hours. The illness is often prostrating, but lasts only twelve hours.

Specific Treatment

None.

CLOSTRIDIUM PERFRINGENS (WELCHII), AND BACILLUS CEREUS FOOD POISONING

These organisms also cause a toxin food poisoning similar but less severe than that caused by staphylococci. *B. cereus* may contaminate cooked rice when it is kept warm for long periods in Chinese restaurants.

Specific Treatment

None.

TYPHOID AND PARATYPHOID FEVER

Definition

A septicaemia originating from invasion of the small bowel by *Salmonella typhi* or *S. paratyphi* B.

Background

These diseases are spread by the same routes as other salmonella infections, though spread by contaminated water supply is more common. In addition to stool carriers, urinary carriers occur occasionally and both

may continue to excrete for life. Typhoid fever is not epidemic in this country and paratyphoid fever is rare. Patients are more usually infected after a stay in Southern Europe or North Africa and the popularity of overseas holidays means that there is an increasing risk from this source (Fig. 2.9). Illness caused by *Salmonella paratyphi* A and C have the characteristics of food poisoning. They are rarely imported from the East.

Pathology

The organism first invades the lymphatic tissue of the small intestine (Peyer's patches) and then the bloodstream. Proliferation of the endothelial cells, derived from the reticuloendothelial systems, is present, particularly in the lymphoid tissue of the small bowel wall, in the mesenteric lymph glands and in the spleen. This eventually causes inflammatory foci with necrosis and, in the case of the bowel wall, ulceration and perforation.

Symptoms

Insidious onset of headache, malaise, cough, fever.

In second week. Abdominal pain, distension, diarrhoea.

Signs (Fig. 2.9)

Few.
Mounting pyrexia, relatively slow pulse.

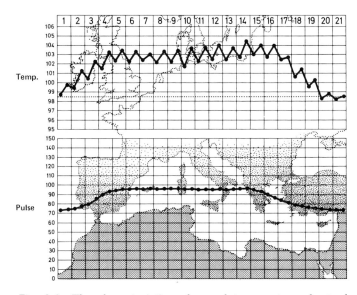

Fig. 2.9 The characteristic pulse and temperature chart of typhoid fever. (The background stippling shows the potentially dangerous 'package holiday' zone.)

After 7 days. Frequent rash, splenomegaly, deterioration with delirium, profound weakness.

Investigations

The organism can be cultured from the blood at the start of the illness and from the stools and urine towards the end of the first week.

The agglutination titre of specific H and O antibodies, the Widal reaction, begins to rise in the second week and continues for the next two weeks. The finding of a single raised titre may be due to immunisation or to a previous attack. A Vi antibody level of more than 1/5 usually indicates that the organism is present, either in the acute or carrier state.

In about half the cases the white blood count shows a leucopenia of 4,000 or below, in which lymphocytes predominate.

Complications

These appear in the second or third week. They are many, the common ones being bronchopneumonia and perforation, or haemorrhage from the small bowel.

Differential Diagnosis

Diseases causing persistent high fever without physical signs.

Basis of Treatment

Chloramphenicol is the most effective antibiotic. It is given in divided doses of 4 g a day until the temperature falls, when the dose is reduced to 2 g a day, the whole course lasting a fortnight. The dosage and length of treatment are important in reducing the number of relapses. These used to recur frequently before chloramphenicol was introduced, the illness, having made what appeared to be a natural recovery, started all over again, the blood becoming positive once more. The general measures of treatment are those of infective diarrhoea. The urine as well as the stool must be negative on culture for the patient to be proved free of the infection. A few urinary and stool carriers clear with a course of ampicillin, but those that are still positive after six to twelve months remain so for life.

Prevention

The public health measures are those already described for infective diarrhoea. The individual who is likely to be exposed to infection, e.g. doctors, nurses, travellers, can be protected by TABT vaccine. Two intradermal injections are given at intervals of four weeks, with reinforcing injections at intervals of one to two years. Intradermal is much to be preferred to intramuscular injection for it causes minimal febrile reaction and yet stimulates a satisfactory antibody response. The protection achieved is about 75 per cent effective.

CHOLERA

Definition

An enteritis caused by infection with the *Vibrio cholerae* causing violent diarrhoea with dehydration and collapse.

Background

Cholera is spread largely by faecal contamination of water. It is endemic in the Far East, particularly in India and Pakistan. The last outbreak in Great Britain occurred in the late nineteenth century. However, in the last few years the disease has spread to the Middle East, Turkey, North Africa and Spain. The cases have been of the mild form of the disease caused by the El Tor biotype. An occasional mild case has occurred in Great Britain and the diagnosis should be considered in patients returning from the above areas with diarrhoea.

Pathology

The small intestine is primarily involved and the disease process does not extend outside it. The exotoxin of the *V. cholerae* causes the mucosa to lose large quantities of sodium, potassium and bicarbonate, although there is no loss of proteins.

Symptoms

Acute diarrhoea.
(Stool volume 20 to 30 litres/day – clear 'rice water' stools).
Muscle cramps.

Signs

Dehydration, stupor, cyanosis.
Hypotension.
Note: El Tor biotype gives milder picture.

Investigations

Diagnosis is confirmed by isolation of the *V. cholerae* from the faeces. The culture media in use for isolating the common faecal pathogenic bacteriae occurring in Great Britain will not grow *V. cholerae* and a special medium has to be used. For this reason the laboratory must be informed of the suspected diagnosis.

Basis of Treatment

Intravenous infusion of water and electrolytes in amounts that replace their loss is the essential method of treatment. The initial dehydration may be corrected in a few hours. Ringer lactate solution (Hartman's Solution, BPC) is satisfactory as a general rule, but in the individual case, intravenous therapy should be controlled by estimation of the blood electrolytes. It may be found necessary to give additional potassium either by mouth or by intravenous infusion. When the vomiting has ceased, in addition to the above treatment, tetracycline 250 mg six-hourly should be given by mouth. This reduces the volume of diarrhoea and clears the stool of organisms.

Prevention

Proper sewage disposal and purification and a clean water supply has abolished endemic cholera in Western Europe and North America. A vaccine-killed *V. cholerae* given in two doses at seven to twenty-eight days interval, will protect the individual in 75 per cent of the cases for the period of six months. The booster dose is then required.

BRUCELLOSIS

Definition

Primarily a disease of cattle, brucellosis in man is a low-grade septicaemic illness.

Background

In Great Britain, *Brucella abortus* commonly causes abortion in cows. (*Brucella melitensis* causes a similar disease in goats and man.) The majority of infections in man arise from drinking infected, unpasteurised milk. Subclinical infections are common in farm workers and veterinary surgeons, but clinical infections are rare.

Symptoms

Fever (intermittent) with headaches.
Slight weight loss.
Lassitude.

Signs

Splenomegaly frequent.

Investigations

Blood culture in an atmosphere of 10 per cent carbon dioxide. Rise in specific antibody level in the blood.

Complications

These are rare but, since brucellosis is a septicaemia, many organs, particularly the joints, heart and liver, may be specifically affected, producing osteitis of the spine, arthritis, endocarditis and hepatitis (Fig. 2.10).

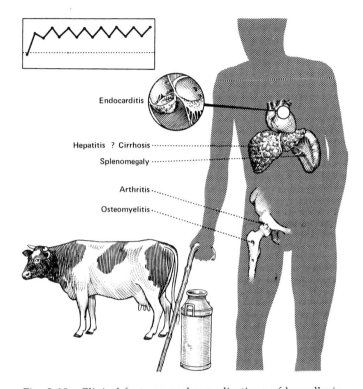

Fig. 2.10   Clinical features and complications of brucellosis.

Basis of Treatment

Streptomycin 0.5 g intramuscularly twice a day for fourteen days, combined with tetracycline 1 g twice a day are effective. The disease can be prevented in man by the pasteurisation of all milk and the eradication of the disease in cattle.

LEPTOSPIROSIS (WEIL'S DISEASE)

Definition

An uncommon septicaemic infection due to the spirochaete, *Leptospira icterohaemorrhagica*, involving the liver and kidney.

Background

Leptospira icterohaemorrhagica is a natural pathogen of rats and man is infected from their urine. Thus, sewer and farm workers are particularly at risk, while potholing and swimming in infected water represent other hazards. *Leptospira canicola*, which mainly infects dogs, causes an aseptic meningitis similar to that caused by viruses.

Pathology

The bile-staining of the tissues and haemorrhages are evident, the microscopic haemorrhages of the muscles being diagnostic of Weil's disease. The liver shows little change and the kidney only nonspecific tubular damage.

Symptoms and Signs (Fig. 2.11)

Jaundice.
Conjunctivitis.
Bleeding into the skin, lungs and gut.
Tender muscles (myositis).
Oliguria.
Bronchopneumonia.

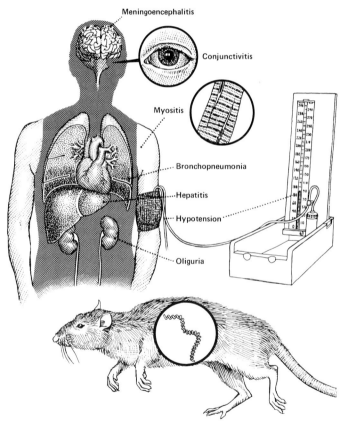

Fig. 2.11 Clinical features and complications of Weil's disease.

Investigations

Isolation of the organism from guinea pig inoculation.
Specific antibodies in the blood, the level rising over ten days.

Leucocytosis – in contrast to leucopenia of Type A hepatitis.
Raised blood urea.
Red blood cells and casts in the urine.

Differential Diagnosis

Viral hepatitis.

Basis of Treatment

It remains unproven whether antibiotics alter the course of the disease. However, present opinion favours giving penicillin. Death from renal failure can be prevented by haemodialysis.

UNCOMMON INFECTIOUS DISEASES

A number of infectious diseases, uncommon in Great Britain, may have to be considered in diagnosis when the more common infections have been excluded. Four are described here, paired together on the grounds of their clinical presentation.

PSITTACOSIS AND Q-FEVER

Background

Psittacosis, caused by chlamydia, a small organism more akin to the bacteria than the viruses, is primarily a disease of birds such as parrots, budgerigars, and pigeons. The organism is present in the discharges and faeces of the infected bird, which spread the disease to man. Case to case infection is uncommon. Q-fever is primarily a disease of cattle, sheep and goats, caused by *Coxiella burneti*. Spread to man may be by inhalation or by milk.

Symptoms

High fever.
Chills and sweats.
Headache and muscular pains.
Cough.

Signs

Signs of patchy lung consolidation.

Complications (Fig. 2.12)

Q-fever. Endocarditis – rare. Hepatitis.

Investigations

Diagnosis depends on the direction of a rising agglutination titre for the appropriate organism.

Basis of Treatment

Tetracycline 0.5 g four times a day is effective in both diseases.

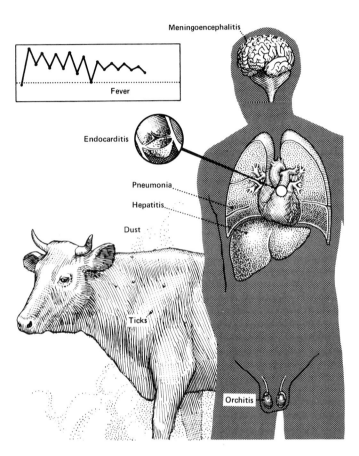

Fig. 2.12 Clinical manifestations and complications of Q-fever.

CYTOMEGALIC VIRUS INFECTION AND TOXOPLASMOSIS

Background

Toxoplasma gondii, a protozoan 3 to 6 μ in size, causes widespread infection in animals, while the cytomegalic virus infection is limited to man. Antibody studies of these agents give evidence of subclinical infection in about a quarter of the population, but clinical disease is rare.

These parasites seem to be well adapted to man as a host, who usually suffers only if there are other predisposing factors such as treatment with immunosuppressive drugs, lack of immunological response in the fetus, or massive infection with the cytomegalic virus in a blood transfusion.

Symptoms and Signs

Adult Infection
Fever.
Enlarged glands.

Congenital Infection (often fatal).
Jaundice, enlarged liver.
Respiratory distress.
Convulsions.
Choroidoretinitis.
Brain damage if the child survives.
Brain calcification (toxoplasmosis only).

Investigations

Rising titre of specific antibody. Detection of atypical mononuclear cells in the blood in both conditions. Cytomegalic virus culture from urine.

Basis of Treatment

When the disease is severe, as in infants, pyrimethamine with sulphonamides may be effective in toxoplasmosis but there is no drug that influences the course of cytomegalic virus infection.

INVESTIGATIONS OF PYREXIA OF UNDETERMINED ORIGIN

Definition

These are certain febrile patients in whom initial examination does not provide sufficient evidence for a diagnosis to be made. This article outlines the investigations of these patients.

Background

The range of infections likely to be the cause of the fever varies in different parts of the world. This article deals with those most likely to occur in Great Britain. Since rapid travel by air is common they will include the serious infections which might be imported from abroad.

History

Additional information should be sought concerning:
1. Contact with febrile illness.
2. Occupation which might lead to infection.
   farm worker – brucellosis, leptospirosis
   bird fancier – psittacosis
3. Foreign travel.
   malaria
   typhoid fever
   Lassa fever

30

Ebola virus fever
amoebiasis
4. Drug therapy which might itself cause fever.
5. Immune state, including past infections, immunisation and immunosuppressive drugs.

Physical Examination

Although initial examination has revealed nothing significant, physical signs may well appear as the disease progresses and must be looked for daily, e.g. enlarged spleen and glands, rashes, heart murmurs. Rectal examination should not be forgotten.

Laboratory Investigations

These have been grouped in three stages together with the relevant infection (*see* Table 2.5, 2.6 and 2.7). Stage I will be appropriate for all patients. History and examination may point to investigation in Stage II or III.

It may well become apparent before the above investigations have been completed that the cause of the fever is not an infection. The non-infectious causes may be grouped as follows:

Table 2.5   Stage I investigation – general

Chest X-ray	Segmental pneumonia
White blood count	
Leucocytosis	Pyogenic infections with
	Staph. aureus
	Strep. pyogenes
	Strep. pneumoniae
	E. coli, etc.
Leucopenia	Typhoid fever
	Brucellosis
	Influenza and some other
	virus infections
'Atypical'	Glandular fever
mononuclear cells	Toxoplasmosis
	Cytomegalovirus infection
	Brucellosis
Blood culture	Septicaemia including
(repeated on three	typhoid fever
occasions)	brucellosis
	endocarditis

Neoplasms. e.g. widespread secondary deposits with small primary tumour in the lung, bowel or pelvis; hypernephroma; multiple myeloma; leukaemia; reticuloses.

Collagen Disease. e.g. rheumatoid arthritis; disseminated lupus erythematosus; polyarteritis nodosa. These conditions are described elsewhere.

Finally, it should be realised that a significant proportion of patients recover without the cause of their fever being found.

Table 2.6   Stage II investigation – specific tests for infection

Isolation of the organism

Bacterial infections	Typhoid fever – from blood, stool, urine
	Brucellosis – from blood
	Tuberculosis – from sputum, urine
Viral infections	Respiratory infection –
	from milk saline throat swabs
	Cytomegalovirus infections – from urine
	Enterovirus infection – from stool
Protozoa	Malaria – from blood film
	Amoebiasis – from stool

Specific blood antibody estimation, repeated if necessary at ten-day interval

Bacterial infection	Typhoid fever
	Brucellosis
	Leptospirosis
	Syphilis
Viral infection	Influenza and other respiratory infections
	Enterovirus infections
	Psittacosis
	Q-fever
	Mycoplasma infections
	Toxoplasmosis
	Glandular fever (Paul-Bunnel test)
Specific tissue	Tuberculosis – Mantoux test
immune response	

Table 2.7   Stage III investigation – local infections

Localisation of abscess in:

Brain	EMI scan
Tooth	X-ray
Subphrenic region	X-ray screen
Liver	Ultrasonic scan
Subphrenic region	Intravenous pyelogram
Pelvic region	Rectal examination
	Pelvic examination
Spine and bones	X-ray

SUGGESTED FURTHER READING

General

Christie, A. B. (1974) *Infectious Diseases*. Edinburgh: Livingstone. (A critical review with a full bibliography.)
Mims, C. A. (1977) *The Pathogenesis of Infectious Disease*. London: Academic Press.

Lassa Fever

Fuller, J. G. (1974) *Fever!* London: Harte Davis, McGibbon. (A vivid account of the outbreaks of Lassa fever in which the virus was first isolated, written primarily for the layman.)
Memorandum on Lassa fever (1976) London: H.M.S.O.

Rabies

Memorandum on Rabies (1977) London: H.M.S.O.

Rheumatic Diseases

M. I. V. JAYSON

3

Rheumatic complaints in Britain lead to a loss of some 35 million working days a year; this is several times that due to industrial disputes and, therefore, represents not only a major health burden, but also an important economic loss to the community. 'Rheumatism' is a loose term that cannot be defined, but, in general, it includes painful disorders of the locomotor system and especially of the joints. Rheumatology includes inflammatory and degenerative disorders of the joints and connective tissues. Degenerative changes in the joints (osteoarthrosis) are dealt with only briefly, as full descriptions may be found in orthopaedic textbooks. The systemic disorders of connective tissue are dealt with in Chapter 7.

Assessment of any rheumatic patient includes a full history not only about the arthritis and the patient's general health, but also about the patient's home and work circumstances to elucidate practical problems that may be remediable. A full general examination should be performed. There are many systemic manifestations of connective tissue diseases that must be identified. The pattern of distribution of arthritis is important and may help to distinguish between different types of disease. Careful examination of involved joints will indicate which particular joint structures are involved. Joint swelling can be due to an effusion, synovial hypertrophy or bony swelling. The skin over the joint may be warm and erythematous due to underlying inflammation. In advanced arthritis there may be ligamentous instability, and various deformities may occur. There is often severe wasting of the muscles controlling damaged joints. Details of the methods of examination of individual joints are well explained in *Outline of Orthopaedics* by J. Crawford Adams (Churchill Livingstone, 1976).

The principal symptoms in arthritis are joint pain and stiffness. Pain receptors are not present in articular cartilage so that, despite the gross damage that occurs, the symptoms must arise elsewhere. It is likely that changes in the joint capsule, such as altered physical properties, and the irritant effect of the inflammatory enzymes and kinins are responsible. Pain may also be produced in the periosteum and from within the bone epiphysis.

RHEUMATOID ARTHRITIS

Definition

Rheumatoid arthritis is a chronic generalised inflammatory disorder which principally involves the synovial joints and tendon sheaths producing a symmetrical poly-arthritis. Recurrent inflammation may eventually lead to permanent joint damage and typical deformities.

Background

The cause of rheumatoid arthritis is unknown. It is classed among the group of 'auto-immune' diseases in which the patient has become sensitive to and developed immune reactions against his or her own tissues. There is an association with other auto-immune conditions such as pernicious anaemia and thyroid disease, and abnormal antibodies are often found in the patient's serum. These antibodies react with the patient's own immunoglobulins producing immune complexes which are deposited in the joints and elsewhere leading to inflammation. The precipitating events leading to the development of autoantibodies have not been elucidated. The hypothesis is that certain micro-organisms could be responsible. They act as the initiating factor but then a self-perpetuating inflammatory cycle develops. For this reason, culture of synovium in late disease is unlikely to reveal the responsible organism. Various micro-organisms such as mycoplasmas and diphtheroids have been found in rheumatoid tissues and an intensive study is now being made of viruses as possible aetiological factors. In most studies, organisms have been found in a higher percentage of rheumatoid than normal tissues, but they are not uniformly present and are occasionally found in other types of joint disease. It seems likely that the organisms identified so far are merely commensals flourishing in an appropriate environment rather than themselves being responsible for development of the disease.

Rheumatoid arthritis effects about two per cent of males and five per cent of females, the prevalence increasing with advancing age. Although the mean onset is at about 40 years, it may begin at any age. Five to ten per cent of patients have a family history of rheumatoid arthritis and there is an association with the tissue type HLA-DRW 4. Until recently the disease was thought to be restricted to temperate zones, but it has now been identified in all parts of the world. However, it does seem rare in primitive populations.

Pathology

The principal pathological events are inflammation most marked in the synovium, nodules, and vasculitis. The earliest changes appear in the synovium with inflammatory swelling and proliferation. The synovium spreads as a sheet of pannus across the cartilage eroding the articular surface so that eventually the cartilage is destroyed. In advanced disease, erosions and cysts appear in the underlying bone and in weight-bearing joints the articular surface may collapse. Microscopy of the synovium shows diffuse infiltration and focal aggregation of lymphocytes and plasma cells and synovial lining cell hyperplasia. Nodules may appear almost

anywhere, but are most common subcutaneously in sites exposed to trauma and most often appear on the extensor surfaces of the forearms (Fig. 3.1). They show central areas of necrosis surrounded by palisades of histiocytes and chronic inflammatory cells. Inflammatory changes appear in the walls of blood vessels leading to obstruction and peripheral ischaemia. This vasculitis is most common on the fingers but may occur elsewhere.

Symptoms and Signs (Fig. 3.1)

The disease may begin with joint symptoms and systemic manifestations such as malaise, weight loss and pyrexia. Arthritis predominantly effects the limb joints (Table 3.1) and only infrequently the spine. The initial symptoms and signs (Table 3.2) are due to inflammatory effusions and synovial hypertrophy. In more advanced disease, when there is loss of joint cartilage, destruction of the articular surfaces and malfunction of both tendons and muscles, characteristic deformities occur (Table 3.3).

Table 3.1 Order of frequency of joint involvement in rheumatoid arthritis

1. Metacarpo-phalangeal, proximal-interphalangeal of fingers, metatarso-phalangeal.
2. Wrist, knee.
3. Elbow, ankle.
4. Hip, shoulder, neck.

Table 3.2 Early rheumatoid arthritis

Symptoms	Signs
Morning stiffness	Joint hot, swollen, tender
Joint pain	Synovial thickening
swelling	Joint effusions
tenderness	Tendon sheath effusions
loss of function	Loss of movement

Table 3.3 Advanced rheumatoid arthritis

Joints	Loss of range of movement
	Fibrous or bony ankylosis
	Instability
	Deformities, e.g. Fixed flexion – knees, elbows
	Ulnar deviation of fingers
	Swan-neck deformity of fingers
	Valgus deformity – ankles, knees
Tendons	Nodular tenosynovitis, 'Trigger finger'
	Tendon displacement, e.g. In ulnar deviation of fingers
	Tendon rupture, e.g. 'Dropped finger'
Other	Muscle wasting
	Subcutaneous nodules at pressure points, e.g. Elbows

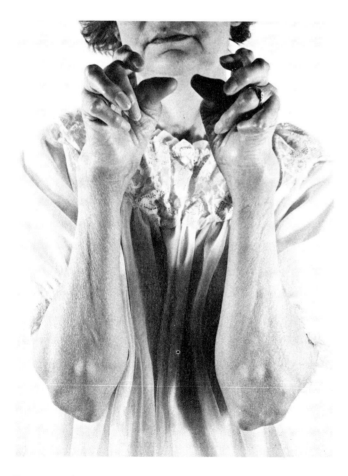

Fig. 3.1 Rheumatoid arthritis, showing ulnar deviation of the fingers with flexion deformity of the proximal interphalangeal joints and hyperextension of the interphalangeal joints of the thumbs. Rheumatoid nodules and swelling of the wrists (synovial hypertrophy) are also shown.

Virtually every body system may be involved in rheumatoid arthritis. The more important complications are listed in Table 3.4. They are not common and usually only appear in severe disease.

Table 3.4 Systemic manifestations of rheumatoid arthritis

General	Malaise and pyrexia
	Anaemia
	Anorexia and weight loss
	Amyloidosis and renal failure
Vascular	Raynaud's syndrome
	Digital arteritis – small ischaemic lesions on finger tips
	Subacute arteritis, e.g. peripheral neuropathy
	Necrotising arteritis – widespread involvement of large vessels
Cardiac	Pericarditis
	Myocarditis
	Coronary arteritis
Respiratory	Pleurisy and pleural effusions
	Fibrosing alveolitis (diffuse interstitial pulmonary fibrosis)
	Rheumatoid nodules in the lungs
	Caplan's syndrome (massive pulmonary fibrosis in pneumoconiosis with rheumatoid arthritis)
Neurological	Carpal tunnel syndrome (due to median nerve compression at the wrist)
	Peripheral neuropathy – arteritis
	Mononeuritis multiplex – arteritis
	Spinal cord damage – cervical spine involvement
Skin	Rheumatoid nodules
	Ulcers – arteritis
Eyes	Kerato-conjunctivitis sicca (Sjogren's syndrome)
	Scleritis and scleromalacia perforans
Spleen	Splenomegaly and leucopenia (Felty's syndrome)

Investigations

1. The blood sedimentation rate and plasma viscosity are increased and there is often an anaemia.
2. Serological studies reveal the presence of an abnormal protein (rheumatoid factor) which is an antibody directed at IgG and is capable of agglutinating sheep erythrocytes previously sensitised with a sub-agglutinating dose of anti-sheep cell serum (Rose-Waaler test) or sensitised latex particles (Latex test). Rheumatoid factor is found in approximately 80 per cent of rheumatoid patients, but is sometimes present in other chronic inflammatory diseases.
3. X-rays of the joints show soft tissue swelling and peri-articular osteoporosis in early disease, and later, loss of joint space with erosions and cysts in the bone ends.

Differential Diagnosis

1. **Osteoarthrosis.** A degenerative joint disease without inflammatory changes which often affects the terminal inter-phalangeal joints of the fingers. X-rays show loss of joint space, sclerosis of the bone ends and osteophytes.

2. **Gout.** Recurrent attacks of very acute arthritis, eventually leading to chronic joint damage and associated with a raised serum uric acid.

3. **Pyrophosphate Arthropathy.** A form of poly-arthritis with features ranging from degenerative changes to recurrent very acute attacks resembling gout, and associated with the deposition of calcium pyrophosphate in the joints which may be recognised on radiographs.

4. **Ankylosing Spondylitis.** Usually starts in young males, and principally involves the spine rather than the peripheral joints.

5. **Reiter's Disease.** Urethritis, conjunctivitis and arthritis, usually following sexual contact but sometimes dysentery.

6. **Psoriatic Arthritis.** An asymmetrical chronic inflammation of the joints associated with psoriasis of the skin.

Basis of Treatment

General. In acute arthritis, considerable improvement can be obtained by complete bed rest. Immobilisation of an acutely inflamed joint in a splint will also lead to rapid subsidence of local inflammation and, provided the period of immobilisation is not over-prolonged, the range of joint movement will not be impaired. Attention must be paid to the patient's posture to prevent and correct flexion deformities in those in whom such changes are developing. Flexion of the knee, hips and other joints are often the result of improper positioning of the joints in bed and failure to adopt preventive measures.

Anaemia should be investigated and if any specific cause is found, appropriate therapy administered. Many rheumatoid patients however, suffer from chronic anaemia with a low serum iron, which is resistant to iron therapy and is due to iron being deposited in the inflamed synovium. This anaemia will improve when the arthritis is controlled.

Obesity should be corrected, but otherwise, diet does not influence the course of rheumatoid arthritis.

Physiotherapy. When acute inflammation has subsided, physiotherapy may be helpful. Measures are directed at restoring muscle power, maintaining and improving the range of joint movement, and restoring function.

Drug Therapy. The principal aims of treatment are to relieve pain (analgesia), suppress inflammation (anti-inflammatory), and provoke a remission of the disease (anti-rheumatic).

Anti-inflammatory analgesic drugs. Aspirin in low doses is an analgesic, but when taken in larger amounts also has anti-inflammatory properties and will objectively diminish signs of acute arthritis. Soluble calcium aspirin (up to 5 g a day) is usually given, but if there is gastrointestinal intolerance, enteric-coated preparations are available. Side effects include dyspepsia, gastrointestinal bleeding (which may be occult and produce an insidious anaemia), allergic reactions and tinnitus. Tablets containing phenacetin alone or mixed with aspirin or other analgesics must be avoided as long continued administration of phenacetin may lead to renal papillary necrosis (*see* page 243). Phenylbutazone (100 mg three times a day) and indomethacin (25 mg four times a day) are very effective analgesic anti-inflammatory drugs. Both of these can produce gastrointestinal irritation with perhaps ulceration, haemorrhage or perforation. Phenylbutazone may cause blood dyscrasias, skin rashes and fluid retention. Morning headaches frequently complicate indomethacin administration and necessitate reduction in dosage. The propionic acid derivatives such as, ibuprofen, naproxen and many others have fewer side effects and are nearly as effective.

Anti-rheumatic drugs. Gold prepared as a soluble salt, sodium aurothiomalate, is effective in producing remissions of rheumatoid arthritis. It is given by intramuscular injection. Test doses of 10, 25 and then 50 mg are given at weekly intervals and if all is well 50 mg is continued weekly until there is remission, or to a total of 1,000 mg. Benefit does not usually appear until about half way through the course. Once the patient is in remission the dose can be reduced, or the interval between injections extended, so that the remission can be prolonged indefinitely. If there is no remission by 1,000 mg then the gold should be stopped. Toxic reactions are common, and if they occur the drug should be withdrawn. The principal side effects are pruritis, skin rashes, which are macular when mild, but which can proceed to an exfoliative dermatitis, stomatitis, blood dyscrasias and renal damage with proteinuria. It is essential that the patient is questioned regarding pruritis and any infections, examined for a skin rash, and the urine and blood tested on the occasion of each gold injection. In particular, the blood checks must include haemoglobin, white cell and platelet counts. Toxic reactions are treated by immediate drug withdrawal and, if necessary, a gold-chelating agent, such as dimercaprol (British anti-Lewisite).

Penicillamine is capable of dissociating rheumatoid factor and was therefore tried for rheumatoid disease. It is effective, but probably not by this means. The drug must be introduced in low dosage, 125 or 250 mg/day, and then the dose slowly increased at monthly intervals to a maximum of 750 mg/day or until there is a response. Side effects – rashes, thrombocytopenia, proteinuria, gastrointestinal upsets and loss of taste – are common, but usually disappear on drug withdrawal. Blood and urine checks must be weekly at first but later can be monthly.

A similar remission after two or three months treatment may be obtained with the anti-malarial drugs, chloroquine (250 mg daily) and hydroxychloroquine (200 mg twice a day). The important complications are in the eye with retinal deposits and macular degeneration which may be irreversible, and corneal deposits which clear when the drug is withdrawn. The eyes should be examined at six-monthly intervals, and particularly if any visual symptoms develop. Other side effects include a neuromyopathy and bleaching of the hair.

Corticosteroids and adrenocorticotrophic hormone (ACTH). These drugs dramatically relieve all signs of inflammatory activity in rheumatoid arthritis. However, it is difficult, if not impossible, to withdraw steroids from most patients established on this treatment without provoking acute exacerbations of arthritis. When steroids are administered for many years side effects become very common and rheumatoid patients appear particularly prone to develop osteoporosis, gastric intolerance and dermal atrophy. ACTH is more likely to produce hypertension and fluid retention, and has to be given by injection, but it does not lead to adrenal suppression. Other side effects, too, appear to be less frequent than with oral steroids.

This group of drugs should be avoided if at all possible and should only be administered for severe disease when more conservative therapy has failed. Systemic complications of rheumatoid arthritis may also suggest their use. The normal maximum dose is 7.5 mg of prednisolone or its equivalent daily.

When a single joint is acutely inflamed a long-acting corticosteroid can be injected directly into the synovial cavity with considerable relief. Strict asepsis is essential as rheumatoid joints are very susceptible to secondary infection.

Immunosuppressive drugs. Recent studies suggest that in very severe disease, and with systemic complications, immunosuppressive drugs, such as azathioprine (2.5 mg/kg/day) may be useful. Careful and frequent monitoring of the blood count and of liver and kidney function is essential.

Immunorestoration. In rheumatoid arthritis there is some evidence of loss of activity of suppressor T lymphocytes leading to overactivity of B lymphocytes. Immunorestoration with drugs such as levamisole may restore T cell activity and lead to control of the disease. Haematological side effects may occur and the use of this drug must be monitored closely.

Surgery. The place of early synovectomy in acute disease is not fully established. It is helpful for relieving inflammation in perhaps one or two joints and it seems likely that it will prevent development of permanent damage. Reconstructive surgery is often performed for badly damaged joints. Joint replacement (arthroplasty) can be very successful for severe hip, knee, and metacarpophalangeal joint disease. An unstable painful joint may be fused (arthrodesis) or a malalignment corrected (osteotomy). Other procedures include replacement and repair of displaced and ruptured tendons.

Rehabilitation

Once deformities are established and accepted, considerable improvement in the patient's ability to cope can be obtained by retraining and the use of various aids and appliances. Occupational therapists are specifically trained for this type of assessment which is aimed at restoring function to the patient not just in hospital, but also at home and at work.

Prognosis

The long term course of rheumatoid arthritis is very variable. Many patients never develop sufficient symptoms to attend hospital and, of those that are seen, the disease will remit in at least half leaving little or no residual deformities. Probably no more than ten per cent of hospital patients may ultimately become severely crippled. The prognosis is worst in those who develop early radiological erosions, rheumatoid nodules, and high titres of rheumatoid factor.

JUVENILE CHRONIC POLY-ARTHRITIS (STILL'S DISEASE)

Definition

Juvenile chronic poly-arthritis refers to a group of different forms of poly-arthritis developing in children below the age of sixteen years. The different types are described but in some patients there is overlap between the groups.

Disease Types

Oligo-arthritic. This usually occurs in children under the age of five years, more commonly in girls than boys. It affects a small number of joints, most often the knee, and the arthritis will resolve completely leaving little or no residual damage. However, it is this group that are at particular risk of developing eye involvement with chronic uveitis and permanent visual damage.

Juvenile Ankylosing Spondylitis. A form of lower limb arthritis, predominately occurring in boys of twelve years or older and often associated with acute uveitis. Many possess the tissue type HLA 27 (*see below*) and develop the changes of ankylosing spondylitis in later life.

Systemic Type. An acute illness with poly-arthritis, pyrexia, a maculopapular rash, lymphadenopathy and severe malaise.

Poly-articular. Acute arthritis affecting multiple joints.

Juvenile Rheumatoid Arthritis. Typical rheumatoid arthritis with positive tests for rheumatoid factor occurring in children.

Others. Rarely, other forms of connective tissue disease may occur in children.

Differential Diagnosis

Rheumatic Fever. This does not usually occur under the age of five. The arthritis tends to flit from joint to joint. It is now very rare in Britain.

Acute Leukaemia. This can present with bone and joint pain, high pyrexia and gross lymphadenopathy. The white cell count and lymph node biopsy provide the diagnosis.

Scurvy. This is associated with swellings around the joints, but is distinguished by the radiographic changes and other clinical findings.

Basis of Treatment

Rest.
Prevention of deformities with splints.
High doses of salicylates (30 to 40 mg/kg/day), or other non-steroidal anti-inflammatory drugs.
Corticosteroids – no long term advantages over salicylates. (They produce premature fusion of epiphyses and cessation of growth, and should be avoided whenever possible. If essential they should be given on alternate days.)

Prognosis

In most cases the disease remits completely leaving little if any residual signs of joint damage. Some patients, however, suffer from permanent deformities and also from growth defects due to premature fusion of epiphyses. Others develop chronic arthritides of rheumatoid or ankylosing spondylitis types. In late cases amyloidosis may occur and lead to renal failure. Close watch must be kept for ocular complications and iridocyclitis is the principal indication for local or systemic steroids.

HLA 27 AND ARTHRITIS

The understanding of a group of forms of inflammatory arthritis was dramatically enhanced by the recognition of certain surface antigens on leucocytes. One of these, HLA (human leucocyte antigen) 27, is specifically associated with ankylosing spondylitis and somewhat less frequently with other related conditions (Table 3.5).

Table 3.5 HLA 27 and arthritis

Groups	Prevalence of HLA 27 (%)
Normal population	5–8
Ankylosing spondylitis	95
Reiter's syndrome	90
Psoriatic spondylitis	50
Spondylitis of ulcerative colitis	66
Spondylitis of Crohn's disease	53

There is considerable overlap between many of these conditions (Fig. 3.2) such that sometimes it is not possible to make a specific diagnosis. There is also an increased incidence of these conditions in the families of patients with one of them.

Possible reasons why people possessing the tissue type HLA 27 are at increased risk of developing these disorders are:

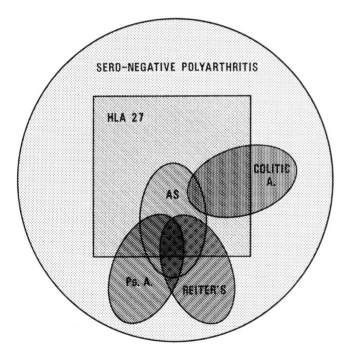

Fig. 3.2 Venn diagram to show the relationships between tissue type HLA 27, ankylosing spondylitis and the other conditions.
PsA = psoriatic arthropathy; As = ankylosing spondylitis.

1. **Genetic Marker.** The gene on the sixth chromosome responsible for this tissue type is physically located adjacent to the gene responsible for susceptibility to these diseases.

2. **Receptor Site.** Certain micro-organisms could attach directly to the cell surface antigen responsible for this tissue type and so lead to disease.

3. **Molecular Mimicry Theory.** The molecular configuration responsible for tissue type HLA 27 is similar to that of certain bacteria so that the subject, being tolerant to his own tissues is unable to mount an adequate antibody response allowing infection to multiply.

ANKYLOSING SPONDYLITIS (MARIE STUMPEL'S DISEASE)

Definition

An inflammatory disease of the joints in the spine starting with sacro-iliitis and spreading upwards with ossification of the paraspinal ligaments leading to loss of spinal movement.

Background

Ankylosing spondylitis most often occurs alone, but may occur in association with Reiter's syndrome, psoriasis, ulcerative colitis and Crohn's disease. On occasions, these latter diseases predominate and the spinal involvement appears as a complication.

Ankylosing spondylitis is about eight times as frequent in males as in females and usually starts at between 15 and 30 years of age, so that it is a common cause of backache in young men.

Pathology

Inflammation occurs in the entheses, the sites of insertion of ligaments into bone, and also in the synovium of joints. Inflammation of the enthesis heals by calcification and ossification producing a bony spur, the tip of which is now the enthesis. In this way progressive ossification of ligaments occurs. The pathological changes start in the sacro-iliac joints and spread to involve the apophyseal joints and the ligaments of the spine. These changes lead to increased spinal stiffness and, in gross cases, complete rigidity. Similar changes less commonly affect the other joints, but may occur in the hip and knee.

Symptoms and Signs

The initial symptoms are:
Low back pain and stiffness aggravated by rest and relieved by exercise.

Malaise and weight loss in the acute stage.

Limitation of spinal movements in all directions and of chest expansion.

Acute peripheral arthritis may occur in the hips and knees or elsewhere.

Pain under or behind the heels due to plantar fasciitis or Achilles tendinitis.

In advanced cases characteristic deformities appear (Fig. 3.3).

Investigations

1. The blood sedimentation rate or plasma viscosity is raised but rheumatoid factor tests are negative.

2. Radiographs of the sacro-iliac joints show bilateral changes with patchy erosions and sclerosis and loss of definition of the joint margins. Eventually, the joint surfaces may fuse. The 'bamboo' and 'tramline' spines are due to ossification of the longitudinal spinal ligaments. Ligamentous ossification can also be seen as plantar spurs in the Achilles tendon and around the ischial tuberosities.

3. The tissue type HLA 27 is found in about 95 per cent of cases and may be helpful if the diagnosis is uncertain (*see* Table 3.5).

Complications

These can be mechanical or inflammatory and are listed in Table 3.6.

Table 3.6   Complications of ankylosing spondylitis

Mechanical	
Rigid spine	→ Liability to fracture
Costovertebral joint	→ Respiratory insufficiency
involvement	and chest infections
	Upper lobe fibrosis
Inflammatory	
Iritis	→ Blindness
Aortitis	→ Aortic incompetence
Inflammation of the	→ Ulcerative colitis and
bowel	Crohn's disease
Amyloid disease	

Differential Diagnosis

1. **Degenerative Disease of the Spine, Prolapsed Intervertebral Discs and Spondylolisthesis.** These conditions produce back pain, but usually only flexion of the spine is limited. Gross degenerative disease may prevent all spinal movements but can be distinguished by the radiographs. The blood sedimentation rate is normal.

2. **Tuberculosis and Brucellosis.** These can produce unilateral sacro-iliitis, but ankylosing spondylitis is always bilateral.

Basis of Treatment

The aim of therapy is to preserve spinal mobility and to prevent limitation of movement and deformity by vigorous and regular physiotherapy. Breathing exercises should be included. It is most important that the patient appreciates that these exercises must be performed every day and indefinitely. They should become part of his way of life.

Nocturnal symptoms often can be relieved by sleeping on a firm mattress. This will also help to prevent

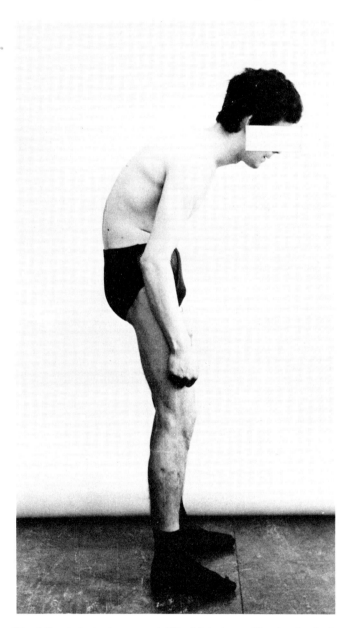

Fig. 3.3   Ankylosing spondylitis. Note loss of lumbar lordosis and severe dorsal kyphosis with extension of the neck.

deformity. Analgesics should be administered so as to allow the patient to perform a full painless range of movements. Aspirin, phenylbutazone, indomethacin and the propionic acid derivaties are particularly useful. Radiotherapy to an inflamed joint can produce a local remission but makes no difference to the long term prognosis and is associated with an increased incidence of leukaemia, so it is avoided whenever possible. Corticosteroids are occasionally used, particularly if there is sight-threatening iritis.

Prognosis

In most cases the disease eventually becomes inactive. It is essential to ensure that there is little residual disability and no serious deformity when this stage is reached.

PSORIASIS AND ARTHRITIS

Four types of joint inflammation occur with psoriasis.

PSORIASIS AND RHEUMATOID ARTHRITIS

These are both common conditions and it is, therefore, hardly surprising that they sometimes coincide. The arthritis is exactly the same as rheumatoid arthritis elsewhere.

PSORIATIC ARTHROPATHY

An acute inflammatory, often asymmetrical, arthropathy. In contrast with rheumatoid arthritis, the terminal interphalangeal joints of the fingers and toes are frequently involved, and are usually associated with corresponding psoriatic nail involvement. Occasionally, joints may be severely destroyed with gross reabsorption of the bone ends (arthritis mutilans).

PSORIASIS AND THE SPINE

Both psoriasis and psoriatic arthropathy are associated with sacro-iliitis and low back pain. In advanced cases this may develop into ankylosing spondylitis.

PSORIASIS AND HYPERURICAEMIA

Extensive psoriasis may be associated with a high rate of purine metabolism in the skin which may be sufficient to produce hyperuricaemia and, occasionally, acute gout.

REITER'S SYNDROME

Definition

A triad of non-specific urethritis, arthritis and conjunctivitis.

Background

Most cases in this country occur in the promiscuous and follow sexual contact, but others follow dysentery. It is believed that the syndrome is precipitated by some infection, but bacteriological and virological studies have not consistently demonstrated any organisms. The condition must not be confused with gonococcal arthritis, a suppurative arthritis following gonorrhoea and from which the gonococcus can be cultured. Subjects possessing the tissue type HLA 27 are at greater risk of developing Reiter's syndrome.

Reiter's syndrome is most frequent in young males (aged 15 to 30) and is uncommon in females.

Symptoms and Signs

Following urethritis, conjunctivitis and then arthritis develop. The joint involvement can be very acute and is most frequent in the knees, ankles and feet. Spontaneous remissions are common, but relapses are frequent and may eventually lead to permanent joint damage and deformity.

Complications

Sacro-iliitis and spinal changes identical with ankylosing spondylitis may develop.
Plantar fasciitis and Achilles tendinitis.
Keratodermia blenorrhagica – a rash virtually identical with pustular psoriasis and showing a propensity for the palms and soles.
Ulceration of the buccal mucosa and the glans penis (circinate balanitis).
Heart block, aortitis, and aortic incompetence.

Basis of Treatment

In the acute stage, bed rest, physiotherapy and anti-inflammatory drugs are used. A course of antibiotics such as tetracycline is usually given, but although this controls the urethritis it is doubtful whether it influences the arthritis.

ARTHRITIS OF ULCERATIVE COLITIS AND CROHN'S DISEASE

Both ulcerative colitis and Crohn's disease are associated with:
1. An acute inflammatory poly-arthritis, most commonly affecting the joints of the lower limbs, whose activity is directly related to the activity of bowel inflammation.
2. Sacro-iliitis and ankylosing spondylitis. Spinal involvement does not correlate with activity of the

bowel disease and may precede it. There is an increased incidence of the tissue type HLA 27.

POLYMYALGIA RHEUMATICA

Definition

A systemic disorder of the elderly, with limb girdle pain and stiffness often associated with giant-cell arteritis.

Background

The aetiology of this syndrome is unknown but altered immunological reactions to the arterial wall may play some part. There is a significant association with giant-cell arteritis.

Symptoms and Signs

The condition usually affects the elderly but may occur in the middle-aged. The predominant symptoms are of increasing limb girdle stiffness, pain and limitation of movements. Symptoms are worst on awaking and ease up during the morning. In severe cases, the patient may have great difficulty in raising the arms or in rising from a chair. There may also be malaise, weight loss, pyrexia and night sweats.

Complications

Histological evidence of giant-cell arteritis has been found in up to 50 per cent of cases of polymyalgia rheumatica. This disease may manifest clinically as temporal arteritis with tenderness and loss of pulsation of the temporal arteries and with risk of visual and neurological damage (*see* page 522).

Investigations

1. The blood sedimentation rate and plasma viscosity are considerably increased.
2. X-rays of the spine, shoulders and hip joints are of little help as they commonly show degenerative changes in this age group that are of no relevance. There are no specific features on radiographs of the joints in this condition.

Basis of Treatment

Prednisolone (15 mg/day) rapidly controls the symptoms and the blood sedimentation rate. Much higher doses (60 mg/day) are necessary if there is clinical evidence of temporal arteritis. Treatment must be started immediately as permanent visual loss can develop whilst awaiting the results of investigations. Throughout therapy, the sedimentation rate should be monitored closely as an index of disease activity. When under control the steroid dose should be slowly reduced with the aim of ultimate withdrawal.

Prognosis

The disease will usually remit after one to three years. Steroids must be continued throughout the period of disease activity to prevent the development of arteritis.

CRYSTAL DEPOSITION DISEASE

In certain types of joint disease, crystals are deposited and phagocytosed by polymorphonuclear leucocytes. Lysosomal enzymes, kinins and other inflammatory substances are released and produce a very acute inflammatory reaction. Gout, pyrophosphate arthropathy and calcific periarthritis are all examples of crystal deposition diseases. Different crystals can be identified by polarised light microscopy and by X-ray diffraction.

GOUT

Definition

A systemic disorder with an increase in the serum uric acid levels and deposition of monosodium urate crystals in the joints and elsewhere and characterised by very acute recurrent arthritis, eventually leading to chronic joint damage.

Background

Purines and pyrimidines are metabolised in the body and converted by a complicated metabolic pathway into uric acid (Fig. 3.4). Monosodium urate is freely filtered

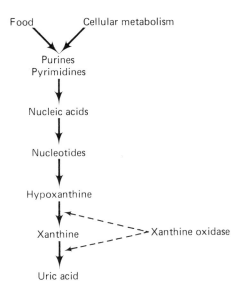

Fig. 3.4   The production of uric acid.

by the renal glomeruli, but completely reabsorbed in the proximal renal tubules. Urate is re-secreted by the distal tubules and lost from the body in the urine. Increase in the serum level of uric acid can be due to either increased production or to diminished excretion.

Either or both of these mechanisms may be involved in primary (idiopathic) or secondary gout and the renal excretion of uric acid can vary accordingly. Secondary gout is rare and the various causes are shown in Table 3.7. Of particular importance is iatrogenic gout due to over-production of uric acid by aggressive chemotherapy for acute leukaemia destroying vast masses of white cells. Certain drugs, particularly oral diuretics, act on the renal tubules and cause uric acid retention.

Table 3.7 Causes of secondary gout

Increased uric acid production	Polycythaemia rubra vera Chemotherapy for acute leukaemia Rare enzyme defects
Diminished uric acid excretion	Renal failure Renal tubular defects (lead poisoning) Drugs – thiazides, pyrazinamide

Primary gout is often familial and is much more common in males, usually beginning between 30 and 60 years of age. It is relatively rare in females and then almost always starts after the menopause. Increased serum uric acid levels and gout are associated with higher social class, higher intelligence, obesity and alcohol intake.

Pathology

In acute gout, strongly negative birefringent needle-shaped crystals of monosodium urate are found in the synovial fluid and identified by polarised light microscopy. Later, solid chalky deposits, known as tophi and consisting of monosodium urate, may be found in the joints disrupting the bone ends, in the subcutaneous tissues, and in the kidneys.

Symptoms and Signs

Recurrent attacks of very acute arthritis usually begin in the great toe (podagra), but may occur in any synovial joint. The joint becomes extremely swollen, red and exquisitely tender. Later, chronic changes occur with permanent swellings and deformities (Fig. 3.5).

Tophaceous deposits may occur in the subcutaneous and periarticular tissues, particularly in the hands, the olecranon bursa, and the helix of the ear, and may ulcerate to discharge chalky white material.

Investigations

1. The serum uric acid is elevated.
2. In acute gout, radiographs show no bony changes,

but in advanced disease there are 'punched out' cystic areas near the joint surfaces due to urate deposits.
3. Polarised light microscopy of synovial fluid or of tophaceous material will show the typical crystals.
4. The haemoglobin, white blood cell count and blood urea should always be measured to exclude secondary causes of gout.

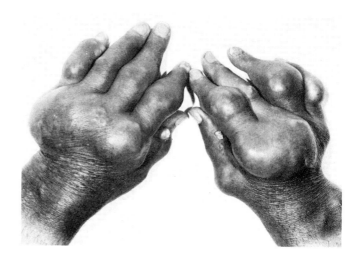

Fig. 3.5 Chronic tophaceous gout. Gross swelling with ulceration over tophi on thumbs.

Complications

Urate may be deposited in the renal parenchyma or as urinary tract calculi with renal colic. Calculi may be produced by uricosuric therapy. Fortunately, renal failure and hypertension are rare complications.

There is an association of hyperuricaemia and gout with coronary artery disease. Whether this is due to some effect of elevated urate levels on platelet adhesiveness and turnover, due to an association of hyperuricaemia with abnormal lipids in the blood, or simply due to gout being more frequent in the obese is uncertain.

Differential Diagnosis

Rheumatoid Arthritis. The arthritis is not so acute in onset, is usually polyarticular and symmetrical and often begins in the hands. The Rose-Waaler test is positive and the serum uric acid is normal.

Pyrophosphate Arthropathy (Chondrocalcinosis). Similar very acute arthritis may occur, but the serum uric acid is normal and calcification of the articular cartilage is seen on radiographs (*see below*). The great toe is not usually involved.

41

Suppurative Arthritis. Extreme pain and swelling in the affected joints can stimulate gouty arthritis, but there is no previous history of similar attacks and pus from which organisms can be cultured can be aspirated from the joint.

Basis of Treatment

Acute Attack. Colchicine (0.5 mg every hour up to 5 mg, or until the pain is relieved) is specific for gout and provides relief within a few hours, but this may not be obtained until sufficient has been taken to produce gastrointestinal side effects. It acts by inhibiting polymorph phagocytosis of uric acid crystals. Phenylbutazone (100 mg three times a day initially), indomethacin (100 mg three times a day initially), or propionic acid derivatives are also very effective in relieving acute arthritis. Aspirin should be avoided as it has a dual effect on the kidney, both increasing and reducing renal excretion of uric acid.

Interval Treatment. This is aimed at lowering the serum uric acid, either by reducing its formation or by increasing its renal excretion. Uric acid is formed from xanthine and hypoxanthine by a reaction catalysed by the enzyme xanthine oxidase (*see* Fig. 3.4). Allopurinol (200 to 400 mg/day) lowers the serum uric acid by inhibiting this enzyme and is both effective and safe. Probenecid (1 to 2 g/day) or sulphinpyrazone (400 mg/day) reduces proximal tubular reabsorption of urate and therefore increases the urinary uric acid loss. They are contraindicated when the gout is secondary to renal disease or if urate calculi are already present. During the first two months of treatment with either type of drug, prophylactic colchicine, phenylbutazone or indomethacin should be given as, otherwise, mobilisation of urate from the tissue may provoke very acute attacks of gout.

A strict diet, low in nucleoproteins can lower the uric acid by up to 1 mg per cent, but, as the drugs now available are very effective, dietary restrictions are rarely indicated. Excessive obesity or alcohol intake may be associated with gout and should be corrected if possible.

Prognosis

With proper treatment it is possible to control virtually every case of gout. Usually this must be continued for life.

PYROPHOSPHATE ARTHROPATHY (CHONDROCALCINOSIS, PSEUDO-GOUT)

Definition

A disorder of the joints associated with the deposition of calcium pyrophosphate dihydrate (CPPD) in articular cartilage.

Background

The fundamental biochemical defect is unknown, but CPPD is deposited in the joints partly because of overproduction but also because of a deficiency of the enzyme pyrophosphatase. The condition is usually idiopathic and may then be familial, but it is sometimes associated with haemochromatosis, hyperparathyroidism, gout, diabetes mellitus and acromegaly.

Symptoms and Signs

Pyrophosphate arthropathy affects adults of both sexes. It is most common in the knee but may effect any synovial joint.

Most typical is an extremely acute arthritis resembling acute gout (pseudo-gout). However, it may present as a progressive degenerative arthritis, with or without acute exacerbations.

The radiological changes may be chance findings in asymptomatic joints.

Investigations

1. Radiographs show calcification of the superficial layer of the articular cartilage.
2. On polarised light microscopy, weakly positive birefringent crystals of CPPD are found in the synovial fluid, and larger deposits may be identified by X-ray diffraction.
3. Screening tests should be performed to exclude possible associated conditions.

Basis of Treatment

Symptoms can be controlled with anti-inflammatory analgesic drugs such as phenylbutazone and indomethacin or by intra-articular injection of a long-acting corticosteroid. Unfortunately, specific treatment of the associated diseases does not influence the course of pyrophosphate arthropathy.

CALCIFIC PERIARTHRITIS

Definition

A recurrent periarthritis due to deposits of calcium hydroxyapatite around the joints.

Symptoms and Signs

Calcific periarthritis affects adults of any age and both sexes. It is a systemic disorder and is found in multiple sites, but most commonly in the supraspinatus tendon above the shoulder. There is recurrent extremely acute periarticular inflammation which can easily be confused with an acute arthritis.

X-rays reveal transient soft tissue calcification which may completely disappear when the condition is in remission.

Basis of Treatment

There is no specific therapy but anti-inflammatory drugs, local injection with steroid, and surgical aspiration of persistent deposits may all be useful.

DEGENERATIVE JOINT DISEASE (OSTEOARTHROSIS)

Definition

Degenerative changes occurring in joints, often following sustained stress, previous injury or disease.

Background

Degenerative changes in joints begin with fibrillation (surface roughening) of the joint cartilage. The cartilage becomes worn away and there is sclerosis of the underlying bone. Hypertrophy of the joint margins produces osteophytes which may be palpable. Although the pathological changes are primarily degenerative there may be superimposed inflammatory episodes due to abnormal stresses on the synovium or possibly the presence of crystals of calcium hydroxyapatite in the joint fluid. Secondary fibrosis and contracture of the capsule may occur.

Osteoarthrosis may be part of the ageing process. Predisposing factors include joint damage by previous trauma, disease such as rheumatoid or septic arthritis, and excessive stresses such as poor joint alignment and obesity. The simple concept of osteoarthrosis as a wear-and-tear phenomenon, however, is being increasingly questioned. Sometimes osteoarthrosis develops in multiple joints with no obvious cause and is then termed 'primary generalised osteoarthrosis'. The terminal interphalangeal joints of the fingers are often involved with osteophytes, known as Heberden's nodes. As these are non-weight bearing joints, wear-and-tear is unlikely. Such changes may well develop in relationship to biochemical defects and may be genetically determined. An example of this is ochronosis, in which generalised osteoarthrosis follows deposition in the joint of a pigment derived from polymerised homogentisic acid due to deficiency of homogentisic acid oxidase in the liver (*see* page 621).

Symptoms and Signs

Symptoms usually develop in the middle-aged or elderly, with gradually progressive pain, stiffness and loss of movement.

The hip and knee are the most common of the peripheral joints affected, but sometimes the terminal interphalangeal joints of the hands are involved producing Heberden's nodes. Similar changes are found in the spine with degenerative changes in the apophyseal joints and intervertebral discs.

Investigations

1. The erythrocyte sedimentation and plasma viscosity rates are normal unless the osteoarthrosis is secondary to some inflammatory condition.
2. Joint radiographs show loss of cartilage space, subchondral sclerosis, sometimes with bone cysts, and marginal osteophytosis.

Basis of Treatment

Initial therapy is palliative with analgesics, physiotherapy and weight reduction. The same analgesic drugs are used as in rheumatoid arthritis. For advanced cases surgery may be helpful. Useful procedures include joint replacement (arthroplasty), joint fusion (arthrodesis), and realignment of bones (osteotomy). Total replacement of the hip with both femoral head and acetabular prostheses is particularly successful.

LOW BACK PAIN

The Structure of the Spine

The spine bears the brunt of all the mechanical stresses and strains of the body. It acts as the supporting structure for the soft tissues and the limbs, so it is hardly surprising that it is liable to a wide variety of mechanical disturbances. The spine represents a superb example of engineering. It bears the weight of the body, protects the spinal cord and yet it is capable of bending and straightening for a life-time. No artifical structure has ever been constructed with similar specifications.

The lumbar spine consists of five vertebrae, mounted one on top of the other with a lumbar lordosis. The sacrum below is tilted backwards. The structure is intrinsically unstable but is strengthened by very powerful spinal muscles and ligaments. The vertebral bodies are separated from those above and below by the intervertebral discs. Each contains an outer ring of tough fibres, termed the annulus fibrosus, that spiral up and down and interlace with one another to form an extremely strong lattice. Within the annulus is the soft gelatinous nucleus pulposus which is semi-fluid and under relatively high pressure in younger subjects. It is the strength of the annulus which prevents prolapse or herniation of the nucleus pulposus. The vertebral arches behind are joined by the apophyseal joints. These are synovial joints with a very limited range of gliding movements. The spinal cord passes down through the spinal canal behind the vertebral bodies to the level of the second lumbar vertebra. A pair of nerve roots emerge from the canal at each level passing through the intervertebral foramina in close proximity to the intervertebral discs.

Causes of Lumbar Pain

A classification of the causes of lumbar pain is shown in Table 3.8.

Table 3.8 Causes of low back pain

1. Pain arising in the spine:	
Structural	Prolapsed intervertebral disc
	Lumbar spondylosis
	Hyperostotic spondylosis
	Congenital anomalies
	Developmental (Scheuermann's osteochondritis)
	Non-specific
Inflammatory	Ankylosing spondylitis and related spondylopathies
	Rheumatoid arthritis (rare in lumbar spine)
	Infections (TB, brucellosis, typhoid, staphylococcal etc.)
Neoplastic	Primary and secondary tumours
	Reticulosis and myelomatosis
Bone disease	Osteoporosis
	Osteomalacia
	Paget's disease
2. Pain referred to back:	
Lumbar	Posterior duodenal ulcer
	Pancreatic disease
	Kidney disease
	Aortic aneurysm
Sacrum	Gynaecological disease
	Rectal disease

Investigation of Back Pain

A full clinical examination should be performed including a pelvic examination where necessary. The patient's spine should be X-rayed. The erythrocyte sedimentation rate is used as a screening test for inflammatory or neoplastic disease of the spine. Other tests are the serum level of calcium (raised in hyperparathyroidism, myelomatosis and various neoplastic conditions), alkaline phosphatase (raised in any condition with bone damage), acid phosphatase (raised in prostatic carcinomatosis), and serum protein electrophoresis (abnormal in myelomatosis).

PROLAPSED INTERVERTEBRAL DISC

Definition

Posterolateral herniation of the nucleus pulposus often associated with stress, and impinging upon nerve roots producing local and referred symptoms and signs. The term 'slipped disc' is not only inaccurate but also conveys a false idea of the nature of the problem.

Background

Often after some trivial exercise the nucleus pulposus herniates through the annulus fibrosus usually at a weak point – its posterolateral aspect – impinging on ligaments or nerve roots. There is now evidence that such prolapse only occurs in discs that are previously abnormal and that the healthy annulus can withstand such loads. Due to the positions of the vertebrae, the stresses discs transmit, and the amount of movement occurring, the L4/5 and L5/S1 discs are at the greatest risk of prolapse and can damage the L5 and S1 roots respectively.

Prolapsed intervertebral disc occurs most frequently in subjects between 20 and 40 years. In older people with more advanced degeneration the fluid contents of the nucleus are reabsorbed leaving fibrous material which is less likely to extrude. Prolapse occurs more commonly in males, presumably because they undertake heavier manual work more likely to lead to disc damage.

Symptoms

Acute. Severe back pain. Pain and paraesthesiae in the appropriate root distribution, e.g. down back of leg to foot. Aggravation of pain by movement, coughing, straining etc.

Chronic. Recurrent attacks which may lead to persistent pain and weakness.

Signs

Patient adopts a 'sciatic scoliosis' in a reflex attempt to avoid pressure on nerve roots.
Movements of the spine are limited. Reduced straight leg raising (Leségue's test).
Sensory and motor loss and loss of ankle jerk in appropriate nerve root distribution (*see* page 502).

Investigations

1. There are no immediate radiological changes as the disc is radio-translucent, but later the disc space may narrow.
2. Myelography or radiculography is performed if an operation is contemplated and will demonstrate a filling defect.

Basis of Treatment

Drugs. Sufficient analgesics should be given to control the symptoms. For very severe pain pethidine may be required, but otherwise aspirin, phenylbutazone, indomethacin or one of the propionic acid derivatives should be used.

Rest. Complete bed rest on an orthopaedic bed or a firm mattress supported by fracture boards is essential until the severe pain is relieved. Continuous spinal traction immobilises the spine, but does not 'suck back' the prolapse into the disc space. If symptoms persist a surgical corset or plaster-of-Paris jacket protects the spine against movements.

Injections. Epidural injections of local anaesthetic, perhaps mixed with corticosteroids, may sometimes relieve the acute symptoms. Painful areas can be directly infiltrated with local anaesthetic and corticosteroid.

Manipulation. The value of this is still unproven. Some patients improve dramatically. The evidence to date suggests that manipulation can hasten improvement in some patients but makes no difference to the long term prognosis.

Surgery. The prolapse is exposed and removed together with the remains of the offending disc. This is only rarely necessary and is performed for severe pain that has failed to improve after three months of conservative treatment. It is important to perform surgery if there is cauda equina compression with sphincter involvement or muscle wasting due to persistent nerve root damage.

Remobilisation. Exercises should be practised to strengthen the spine and the patient should be instructed on the correct ways to bend and lift.

Employment. The type of work should be assessed to determine whether it can be modified to minimise further stresses to the spine.

LUMBAR SPONDYLOSIS

Definition

Structural changes involving intervertebral disc degeneration, apophyseal joint osteoarthrosis and osteophyte formation around the discs and joints.

Background

Degenerative changes are very common chance findings in symptomless patients. Their significance is often doubtful and alternative diagnoses must be considered before attributing back pain to these radiological changes.

Symptoms

Recurrent low back pain aggravated by exercise. Pain in legs due to compression of nerve roots by osteophytes.

Signs

Stiffness of the spine particularly on flexion.

Basis of Treatment

Analgesics. For example, aspirin, phenylbutazone, indomethacin and propionic acid derivatives.

Physiotherapy. With local heat and exercises. Traction and manipulation may relieve the symptoms but their long term value is not proven.

Spinal Supports. Surgical corsets are used to prevent excessive spinal movement in patients with recurrent symptoms or who undertake heavy work.

Attention must be paid to posture, seating, bed, work etc.

HYPEROSTOTIC SPONDYLOSIS

Definition

A primary overgrowth of osteophytes without narrowing of the associated intervertebral disc spaces.

Background

This condition is more common in elderly men and sometimes in association with diabetes. It is most frequent in the dorsal spine and may spread to the lumbar and cervical regions. The osteophytes fuse together and the spine becomes rigid, and clinically but not radiologically resembles advanced ankylosing spondylitis.

NON-SPECIFIC BACK PAIN

Background

Many patients suffer recurrent back pain with a full range of spinal movements. The symptoms may be aggravated by poor posture, as when standing or when seated in a poorly designed chair. It is difficult to attribute the symptoms to the radiological changes.

Many names are given for this condition including fibrositis, postural backache, ligamentous strain, and lumbo-sacral strain. They all suggest specific pathologies which are unproven. It would seem preferable to call them all 'non-specific back pain' until they are better understood.

Treatment

Analgesics, adjustment of posture and physiotherapy.

SUGGESTED FURTHER READING

Ehrlich, G. E. (1973) *Total Management of the Arthritic Patient.* Philadelphia and Toronto: Lippincott.

Jayson, M. (1976) *The Lumbar Spine and Back Pain.* London: Pitman Medical.

Scott, J. T. (1978) *Copeman's Textbook of Rheumatology.* Edinburgh: Churchill Livingstone.

Gastroenterology

4

A. E. READ

DISORDERS OF THE ALIMENTARY TRACT

MAJOR SYMPTOMS

Disorders of the alimentary tract are common. There can be few who have not suffered from occasional dyspepsia or diarrhoea. The patent medicine purveyors dispense a large number of mixtures both active and inactive which are offered for the relief of alimentary symptoms. Such a state of affairs exists because of the ignorance of the cause of the majority of symptoms, and though great strides are being made in the understanding of the complex factors, humoral, nervous and emotional, which control the function of the intestines and their associated glands, much still remains unanswered. Some of the symptoms of alimentary disease and some disease processes depend on an improper balance of intestinal neuromuscular co-ordination. These include achalasia of the cardia, Hirschsprung's disease, irritable bowel syndrome, etc.

Abdominal Pain

Abdominal pain is the most common symptom of alimentary disease. Suggestion of its alimentary origin is given by its relationship to alimentary functions such as swallowing, the digestion of food, and relief by vomiting, as well as its relationship to defaecation.

Confusion may result from the fact that somatic pain is often referred from both superficial and deep structures, not only in the abdominal wall but from the chest wall, spine, meninges, and pleural cavity.

Visceral pain mechanisms are several in origin – the more easily understood is that arising from obstruction to the intestinal tube, or the bile ducts. This gives rise to pain which waxes and wanes and which, in the case of the small bowel, is felt characteristically in the centre of the abdomen (intestinal colic), though rather vaguely localised. Other varieties of visceral pain result from localised inflammation ischaemia or necrosis, in which case the pain may be localised, too, with overlying muscle spasm. The liver capsule, when stretched by expansion of the hepatic parenchyma, such as may result from hepatic congestion and hepatic neoplasia, or the inflammatory reaction associated with acute hepatitis or acute hepatic abscess may give rise to local pain and tenderness.

Dysphagia

Difficulty with the swallowing process so that the transit of food and/or fluid from pharynx to stomach is delayed is caused by a wide variety of disorders. It is an

Table 4.1 Causes of dysphagia

Functional	Neurological	Extrinsic pressure on oesophagus	Mucosal and muscular disease of oesophagus	Strictures and foreign bodies
Globus hystericus (belief that there is an impacted object in the oesophagus).	(a) Damage to medulla, e.g. vascular disease of brain, progressive muscular atrophy, polymyelitis, etc.	Retropharyngeal abscess. Thyroid enlargement. Aortic aneurysm. Carcinoma of bronchus.	Post-cricoid web. Systemic sclerosis. Candidiasis. Pharyngeal pouch. Oesophageal diverticulum, etc.	Carcinoma (oesophagus or gastric fundus). Impacted foreign body, e.g. fish or meat bones.
	(b) Damage to or interruption of, oesophageal nerve plexuses – Achalasia, Chagas' disease, etc.	Enlarged hilar glands, e.g. reticulosis. 'Rolling' hiatus hernia, etc.	Oesophageal spasm. 'Corkscrew' oesophagus. Myasthenia gravis, etc.	Peptic oesophagitis with stricture or ulcer. Stricture following corrosives.

important symptom and certainly one that should never be dismissed without proper investigation. Of the most important lesions, carcinoma (page 85) and achalasia must be described separately (*see* Table 4.1).

ACHALASIA OF THE CARDIA

Definition

A disorder of oesophageal neuromuscular co-ordination which results in inco-ordinated oesophageal contractility and, in particular, in impaired relaxation of the oesophageal sphincter.

Background

There is a degeneration of the myenteric nerve plexus. This is present both in the body and sphincter region of the oesophagus. In the latter area loss of β adrenergic inhibiting activity means that the unopposed a adrenergic receptors sustain circular muscle contraction in this region, with resultant tonic oesophageal contraction. In the body of the oesophagus, degenerative changes in ganglion cells result in a loss of postganglionic parasympathetic fibres and disordered peristalsis.

The cause is not known, and it is equally distributed between the sexes. It is commonest in middle age. Among theories for its causation are degenerative changes in the vagal nucleus in the brain stem, and psychological factors. A similar type of picture is produced in the rare disease (Chagas' disease) caused by a trypanosome (*T. cruzi*) which also causes a degeneration of oesophageal nerve plexuses.

Pathology

There is dilatation of the oesophagus above the contracted segment and in long term cases the oesophagus is lengthened and tortuous. Stagnation of contents leads to ulceration and, in some, carcinoma. Aspiration of food and oesophageal contents into the lung may result in lung abscess – chronic inhalation pneumonia, etc. (Fig. 4.1).

Symptoms

Slowness in completing a meal.
Dysphagia (particularly for solids) and often intermittent *and*
Choking and regurgitation after meals.
Retrosternal pain, often severe, nocturnal and of uncertain cause.
Loss of weight.
Occasionally, arthralgia and pain due to pulmonary hypertrophic osteoarthropathy.

Signs

None, except wasting.
Mild anaemia.

Investigations

1. A barium meal shows a characteristic smooth, funnel-shaped deformity of the oesophagus with variable dilatation of the gullet above the contracted segment.
2. There may be a mediastinal shadow on plain X-ray with a visible fluid level within the dilated gullet. Evidence of pulmonary infection due to aspiration may be present. The gastric gas bubble characteristically is absent.
3. Endoscopy is valuable (after aspiration of oesophageal contents) in the diagnosis of the disorder, largely to exclude a carcinoma. It allows the recognition of secondary oesophagitis and complicating carcinoma.
4. Occasionally, hypertrophic pulmonary osteoarthropathy may be seen in X-rays of the forearm bones.
5. The denervated oesophagus shows enhanced (and painful) contraction following subcutaneous injection of mecholyl 15 mg (Cannon's law).

Complications

These include carcinoma, and aspiration pneumonia.

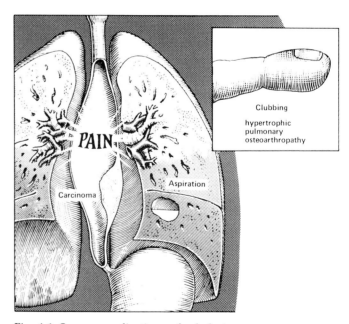

Fig. 4.1 Some complications of achalasia.

Differential Diagnosis

From carcinoma of the oesophagus and benign stricture.

48

Basis of Treatment

Opinion is divided, and treatment consists either of multiple dilatations with a hydrostatic or mechanical (Stark) dilator which is operated under radiological control, or by means of a surgical operation that incises the muscle in the lower contracted oesophageal segment down to the mucosa (Heller's operation). The operation is best performed by the trans-thoracic route and provides satisfactory relief of symptoms in the majority treated in this way. Oesophageal reflux is a possible complication and the risk of carcinoma does not disappear completely.

INDIGESTION (DYSPEPSIA) (Fig. 4.2)

This term is widely used and it is essential that both patient and student appreciate what they mean by its use. In general, indigestion refers to pain, abdominal discomfort, or oral passage of wind related to the taking of food. Surveys have shown that up to 30 per cent of apparently normal subjects may suffer from it in varying degrees. The pain may be felt in the chest or abdomen, the discomfort described as tightness or fullness. There are many causes of indigestion, some such as gastric cancer and ulcer are important, and others trivial, due to gastric atony or hyperactivity associated with acute and chronic neurosis.

The commonest causes of indigestion are gastritis, peptic ulceration, and hiatus hernia, but a wide variety of organic and functional causes may be operative. These are described separately.

VOMITING (Table 4.2)

Closure of the pylorus, relaxation of the cardia, and strong contractible movements of the abdominal muscles result in violent expulsion of the gastric contents. This may be a protective phenomenon for the expulsion of gastric irritants, but also may be a sign of local ulcer or cancer, particularly where there is pyloric stenosis. Vomiting is then likely to be massive in volume with stale food residue.

Various other acute abdominal disorders may be accompanied by vomiting. On the whole, the precise

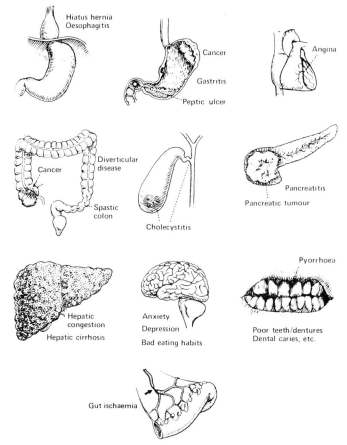

Fig. 4.2 Some causes of 'indigestion'.

cause for this is unknown but there is often severe abdominal pain (so there may be an element of reflex vomiting secondary to the pain) while a localised ileus – a common cause of small bowel distension – may be partially responsible.

Drugs such as digitalis, cytotoxic drugs, toxic disorders such as uraemia and hypercalcaemia, and a variety of neurological disorders may also be responsible. These neurological disorders include conditions of increased intracranial pressure, e.g. cerebral tumour and abscess – of meningitis, and of disorders of the vestibular apparatus and a variety of psychiatric and neurotic illnesses. Vomiting is a symptom that must always be

Table 4.2 Causes of vomiting

Functional	Obstructive-oesophageal gastric or small bowel	Metabolic	Drugs	Neurogenic	Reflex
Psychogenic vomiting. (A diagnosis by exclusion only.)	Either intra- or extraluminal e.g. in the small bowel due to ileus, in the stomach due to pyloric ulcer or cancer, etc.	Uraemia, pregnancy, hyponatraemia, hypercalcaemia, porphyria, etc.	Digitalis, cytotoxic drugs (and X-irradiation), etc.	Raised intracranial pressure. Meningitis. Ménière's syndrome. Migraine, etc.	Associated with severe pain, e.g. myocardial infarction, intestinal perforation, acute pancreatitis, etc.

taken seriously and investigated in a concise and intelligent way. Vomiting due to psychiatric disease is a diagnosis reached only by exclusion.

DIARRHOEA (Table 4.3)

Of all the alimentary disorders this is the commonest. It must be admitted that in many cases the reason for this symptom is difficult to determine, though with greater understanding of intestinal pathophysiology some causes are becoming more clearly demarcated. Suffice it to mention several examples where this is so.

1. In ileal disease and resection there is the possibility that irritative bile salts and metabolites may be formed by bacterial action in the colon following failure of bile salt absorption at specific ileal sites. A copious watery diarrhoea that responds to a bile salt chelating agent may result (cholerhoeic enteropathy).
2. The diarrhoea of the blind loop syndrome also seems to be due to bile salt depletion secondary to bacterial inactivation of bile salt conjugates in the stagnant blind loop.
3. Though the malabsorption of fat may partially explain the diarrhoea of malabsorption, a failure of glucose and disaccharide absorption and a consequent failure of sodium absorption (glucose is essential for function of the Na carrier pump) means that electrolyte and osmotic factors add to malabsorption diarrhoea.
4. The loss of function of microvilli (which contain sugar-splitting enzymes – disaccharidases) results from a variety of non-specific injurious agents, e.g. coeliac disease, skin disease, etc. Disaccharidase deficiency results from this 'brush border disease'. Sugars such as lactose are malabsorbed because they are incompletely split to their monosaccharide components, e.g. lactose fails to be split to glucose and galactose. An osmotic diarrhoea with acidic stools results from bacterial breakdown of lactose in the colon. A congenital form of this disease, alactasia – where lactase is absent from the 'brush border' – causes milk intolerance in those of African and Mediterranean origin. The congenital disorder is rare, however, in Caucasians, but an acquired deficiency may result from the secondary 'brush border' damage accompanying severe skin disease, coeliac disease, gastroenteritis, etc.

5. Pressure studies of luminal pressures in the gut have helped to explain the diarrhoea of diseases such as ulcerative colitis and Crohn's disease. In these situations, colonic muscular activity may be reduced so that intestinal resistance to faecal flow is lessened. Reference will be made to the possible relationship between increased intestinal activity and the irritable bowel syndrome.
6. In infective diarrhoeas, it may well be that bacterial toxins increase the outpouring of water and sodium from the bowel lumen. Such an abnormality has been noted in cholera and may play a similar part in the pathogenesis of the diarrhoea of infective gastroenteritis. The mechanism here seems to be a stimulation of cyclic AMP, which then causes fluid outpouring. Tumours of the pancreas, which have a similar effect, are thought to secrete hormones such as VIP (vasoactive intestinal polypeptide) – (pancreatic cholera). This is quite distinct from the Zollinger-Ellison syndrome (*see* page 88).

Basis of Treatment

Drugs useful in the treatment of diarrhoea – that is apart from that due to blind loop syndrome and cholerhoeic enteropathy where antibiotics and cholestyramine may be helpful – include:

Codeine phosphate, 30 mg to 60 mg three times daily.
Diphenoxylate (Lomotil), 5 mg three times a day (possibly dangerous in liver disease – a morphine derivative).

Table 4.3 Causes of diarrhoea

	Colonic		Small bowel		Central
Mucosal	Ulcerative colitis Crohn's disease dysentery, carcinoma, etc.	Mucosal	Coeliac disease/Sprue. Alactasia, etc.	Functional	Anxiety, etc.
		Gut or gastric resection			
Muscular	Diverticular disease, Purgative abuse (cathartic colon), etc.	Postvagotomy			
		Secretory			
Nervous	Spastic colon (abnormal motility), etc.		Excess acid or intestinal secretion e.g. Zollinger-Ellison syndrome, and 'pancreatic cholera' (pancreatic VIP-producing tumour).		
Secretory	Villous papilloma.				
Abnormal flora	Antibiotics, etc.	Reduced transit time Abnormal flora	Carcinoid syndrome. Thyrotoxicosis, etc. Blind loop syndrome. Gastroenteritis. Cholera, etc.		

Loperamide – a safer drug without sedative properties – 4 mg by mouth to start and 2 mg three times daily.
Kaolin and Morphine Mixture, BPC, 15 ml three times daily.

There is some suggestion that these drugs by increasing bowel wall contraction could aggravate diverticular disease.

In acute infective diarrhoea starvation, liberal fluids, if necessary intravenously, form the basis of treatment. There is no evidence to suggest that antibiotics (sulpha drugs, streptomycin, and neomycin) are required in any but moderate or severe gastroenteritis and even some to suggest that recovery may in some cases be delayed, and bacterial resistance encouraged. Further, antibiotics may cause pseudomembranous colitis and even possibly precipitate ulcerative colitis. Clindamycin and lincomycin are particularly dangerous in this respect.

IRRITABLE BOWEL SYNDROME

Definition

A condition due to abnormal neuromuscular function in the large bowel and usually associated with abdominal pain and altered bowel function.

Pathology

There are no pathological changes, but there is considerable evidence to suggest that this disorder may be a forerunner of diverticulosis coli.

Background

It is well recognised that a number of these patients have a chronic neurosis. Nevertheless, motility and pressure studies have demonstrated increased muscular activity and pressure changes in the sigmoid colon following such stimuli as food or prostigmine. Muscle hypertophy may be associated, and the high intracolonic pressure generated by segments of the colon could be responsible for herniation of the mucosa between the taenia coli – diverticular disease. Some patients with diarrhoea may have an abnormality of bile salt metabolism with an exaggerated ileal loss of fluid.

Symptoms

Cramping abdominal pain, often after food.
Bloating.
Altered bowel habit:
  Constipation.
  Small pellet-like faeces (rabbit stools).
  Passage of mucus per rectum.
  Diarrhoea.

Signs

Nil, or occasionally tenderness over the colon.
Sigmoidoscopy normal, but air insufflation may produce pain similar to that which patients complain of.

Investigations

It is essential to examine and investigate all patients with abdominal pain and alteration of bowel habit by:
1. Routine haemoglobin blood film and plasma viscosity.
2. A search for occult blood in the stools.
3. Sigmoidoscopy.
4. Barium studies of the colon, and where symptoms are related to meals, by barium studies of the stomach and small bowel too.

All these investigations are normal in patients with this disorder unless there are complicating diverticulae, and although helpful information may be obtained by manometric and motility studies these are not usually performed. The diagnosis is essentially by exclusion, but this does not mean that any short cuts should be taken.

Differential Diagnosis

Usually this is not difficult unless the history is short, when large bowel cancer is the most important. In cases where symptoms are of longer duration, peptic ulcer (relation of pain to food), Crohn's disease and diverticular disease must be considered.

Basis of Treatment

By far and away the most important part of treatment is thorough physical examination of the patient, exclusion of organic disease by meticulous investigation, and a careful explanation of the findings to the patient.

Those who suffer from this disorder are usually amenable to the suggestion that the disorder is due to an overactivity of the bowel muscle – that there is no serious organic disease, such as cancer, present and, further, that the disorder is not one where cancer develops later. Full radiological examination is essential to make certain of these facts, but once performed, a firm policy of avoiding further investigation must be adhered to, that is, unless there are obvious changes in symptoms suggesting some other disorder. Reassurance is particularly important because it has been shown that symptoms do persist and that routine medical treatment is relatively ineffective.

Nervous tension is treated, when possible, with chlordiazepoxide 5 mg three times daily, and advice is given about cutting down on stressful situations that can be important precipitates of symptoms. Antispasmodics, e.g. propantheline 15 mg three times daily, or better, mebeverine 100 mg three times daily, can be used. The latter drug is said to have a specific action on the colon and therefore to be free of troublesome side effects such as dry mouth, difficulty with vision, etc.

Probably the most important and effective therapy is with compounds that increase faecal bulk for example, Isogel 5 g three times daily and All Bran. A high fibre diet is a more physiological way of achieving this end and a beneficial response to its use is often seen. This may on occasions be quite dramatic. In those who suffer from diarrhoea, codeine phosphate 30 mg three times daily or diphenoxylate 5 mg three times daily are usually effective, but a watch must be kept for the aggravation of pain by these compounds which are potent muscle constrictors.

Prognosis

Though benign, the disease tends to cause persistent symptoms, and patients are likely to be constant attenders at surgeries and out-patient departments. Tactful, but firm, handling can be helpful to the patient and can avoid unnecessary and repeated investigation. Diverticular disease with all its surgical complications is a possible long term development.

CONSTIPATION (Table 4.4)

The passage of hard stools such that the patient has difficulty or discomfort in emptying the bowel constitutes constipation. At the same time, stool number is also reduced, but not invariably so.

A wide variety of lesions may be responsible, ranging from painful disorders of the anal canal to hypercalcaemia. A further division resulted from studies of Sir Arthur Hurst, who recognised that most causes of constipation were due to suppression of the normal rectal stimulus to defaecation which comes from filling the rectal ampulla with faeces. This form is likely to occur if a regular daily, unhurried attempt is not made to empty the rectum.

Basis of Treatment

The treatment is that of the cause, but so often no pathology is found and then only symptomatic treatment is required. The nature of the muscular dysfunction causing the disorder must be explored. Usually, this is a failure on the part of the patient to appreciate the normal sensation of rectal distension and the resulting normal call to stool. A bowel action is most likely after meals (usually breakfast) so that a skipped or hurried breakfast, and an insufficient allowance of time for bowel emptying soon suppresses the normal evacuation reflex, and with this stools become dry and hard and more difficult to expel. A vicious circle then begins.

Patients must be encouraged to take a diet with a high roughage content, and to make positive and unhurried attempts to empty the bowel after meals. Above all they must be told that constipation is not a disorder that will do them serious harm and it is one in which retraining can bring back a normal bowel rhythm. Students must remember that 'normality' as applied to bowel actions can be from three motions a week to three a day, and that constipation is present only where there is discomfort, difficulty or undue straining in emptying the bowels. The majority of patients are controlled by a regime such as this plus simple aperients. Remember that abuse of purgatives may result in an atonic and completely 'paralysed' bowel and that the resulting watery diarrhoea may be a potent cause of severe and dangerous potassium deficiency. Beware too of the patient who becomes constipated having had a normal bowel routine before. Though this may happen after a debilitating illness or pregnancy one must always think of causes such as colonic and rectal carcinoma and remember the 'medical' causes such as myxoedema and hypercalcaemia.

Useful drugs include:

Senna. An anthracene purgative which, like the others of this group, acts on the large bowel musculature, though absorption is from the small bowel.
Preparations: Senokot tablets one or two on alternate days.

Table 4.4 Causes of constipation

Physical inactivity	Endocrine	Psychosis	Drugs	Neurological	Colonic and rectal obstruction	Painful anal conditions
e.g. bed rest, pregnancy, etc.	Myxoedema. Hyperpara-thyroidism.	Depression. Dementia.	Aludrox. Codeine Opiates.	Lesions of sacral plexus, e.g. tumour, trauma.	Carcinoma. Diverticular disease, etc.	Fissure. Prolapsed piles, etc.
				Lesions of colonic nerve plexuses, e.g. Hirschsprung's disease.		

Bisacodyl (Dulcolax). Direct stimulant of colonic muscle effective by mouth or as a suppository. Dose 10 mg.

Glycerine suppositories, which can be administered by the patient, and a plain water or soapy water enema may be required in refractory cases will all help, together with a high fibre diet with added bran.

In extreme cases hard faecal masses may be removed manually, and in all constipated patients a rectal examination must be performed before purgatives are prescribed. In very exceptional cases removal of redundant atonic bowel or ileo-rectal anastomosis may be the only means of making the patient's existence tolerable.

One form of constipation due to neuromuscular inco-ordination needs special description.

HIRSCHSPRUNG'S DISEASE

Definition

A disorder of colonic neuromuscular function associated with a deficiency of colonic nerve ganglia.

Background

Deficiency of colonic nerve ganglia is a congenital lesion. The affected area may be a segment a few centimetres long or there may be a deficiency in the whole of the colon, rarely spreading to involve part or all of the small bowel. The disorder is presumably due to a deficient migration of cells from the neural crest. Histochemical studies reveal abnormal nerve fibres in the muscle layers of the gut. There is a family history in some cases, and in those with 'short segment' disease the sex ratio male:female is 5:1.

Pathology

The colon is grossly dilated usually above a constricted segment in the rectum or sigmoid colon. There is a secondary putrefactive enterocolitis with ulceration and bleeding of the distended bowel.

Symptoms

Gross constipation from birth – overflow diarrhoea.
Failure to thrive.
Vomiting.

Signs

Wasting.
Gross abdominal distension with visible peristalsis.

Investigations

1. Plain radiography demonstrates a distended colon ending in an unexpanded rectum. Demonstration of a narrowed segment may be possible with a barium enema.
2. A full thickness rectal biopsy taken 1 cm above the anal canal will not only confirm the diagnosis, but may also be used to confirm the upper limit of the diseased segment. Though a suction biopsy technique has been used, open operation, the taking of a specimen from the muscle layer 2 cm or more in length, multiple sections and histochemical stains are all required to make a firm diagnosis.
3. Manometric studies of the colon may in future be helpful in making a diagnosis and may eventually replace diagnostic biopsy.

Basis of Treatment

Following bowel washouts, improvement of nutrition and anaemia, the treatment is essentially surgical. Usually, initial colostomy or ileostomy is required, followed by definitive surgery. Definitive surgery is of several types, but basically the diseased segment is pulled down into the rectum and resected, while bowel continuity is then effected by reanastomosis.

ALIMENTARY BLEEDING

Definition

Loss of blood from the alimentary tract may take the form of rectal bleeding (fresh blood in the stools), melaena (the passage of altered blood in the stools) and haematemesis, when blood either fresh or altered is vomited. Combinations of these are possible, and in massive upper gastrointestinal bleeding all may be present together. Sometimes, blood loss may be minute and detectable only by biochemical tests – occult bleeding.

Pathology

A variety of pathological lesions may cause alimentary bleeding. By far the most important are disorders of the oesophagus, stomach, and duodenum, so that blood loss commonly occurs as haematemesis and melaena, or combined. The common gastric and duodenal pathologies are acute and chronic peptic ulceration, while in the oesophagus there may be a hiatus hernia, often with chronic ulceration in the hernial sac. Portal hypertension causing bleeding from varices forms a relatively small percentage of all bleeds. A list covering common and less common causes is contained in Table 4.5.

The pathology of these conditions is covered elsewhere, but an explanatory note is needed concerning Mallory/Weiss syndrome which is associated with bleeding from a longitudinal mucosal tear at the oesophagogastric junction. It often, but not always, complicates prolonged retching in, for example, the alcoholic. It is diagnosed with certainty by endoscopy.

Symptoms

These vary with the severity and speed of bleeding. In general, massive bleeding from the duodenum, stomach and oesophagus causes haematemesis and melaena. Melaena alone can result from bleeding anywhere from the oesophagus to the ascending colon. Bleeding from areas below this is usually associated with fresh blood in the stools.

Acute Haemorrhage. (a) Vomiting – haematemesis – dark red or coffee ground material. (b) Melaena – dark, loose, tarry stools.
Associated symptoms – faintness, thirst, sweating, palpitations, abdominal discomfort.

Chronic Haemorrhage. Symptoms of anaemia – dyspnoea, fatigue, etc.

Signs

Acute Haemorrhage. Shock – tachycardia, sweating, pallor, low blood pressure. Stools show frank blood and/or melaena.

Chronic Haemorrhage. Signs of chronic anaemia.
Note. In any patient with intestinal bleeding it is important to look for evidence of chronic liver disease (*see* Fig. 4.3) and for evidence of conditions such as pseudoxanthoma and hereditary telangiectasia.

Investigations

1. Estimation of the haemoglobin in acute intestinal haemorrhage may be erroneous and for 24 hours or more the haemoglobin will be well maintained because of the delay in haemodilution.
2. The blood urea is often elevated and this is due to pre-renal uraemia (low renal blood flow).
3. Radiology. Provided the patient's condition is reasonable, transportation to the X-ray department and examination of the upper alimentary tract, using a small amount of barium, is a valuable early procedure in the diagnosis of the cause of the upper intestinal bleeding. Double contrast techniques may further increase accuracy. This is generally more satisfactory than the use of ward techniques of radiology which usually produce indifferent results.
4. Endoscopy. Modern fibre-optic instruments are well tolerated by the patient and have facilities for biopsy, cytology, and photography. Provided there is initial gastric lavage with ice cold saline, visualisation is usually good and there is no doubt that a most valuable diagnostic tool is now available with the introduction of machines that can visualise oeophagus, stomach and duodenum. Further, they are able to detect lesions such as acute erosions which cannot be detected radiologically.

These last two techniques (radiology and endoscopy) should be used to complement each other.

In patients with chronic intestinal bleeding the above techniques may be supplemented by:
(a) Serial examination of the stools to detect occult bleeding, using guaiac, or, in certain cases, by estimating the loss of faecal radioactivity following ^{51}Cr labelling of the patient's red blood cells.

Table 4.5 Causes of acute gastrointestinal bleeding

Cause	Incidence%	Others	Incidence%	Rare but important
Chronic duodenal ulcer	35	Portal hypertension	4	Diverticular disease of the colon.
Chronic gastric ulcer	17	Carcinoma of stomach	3	Meckel's diverticulum.
Acute gastric and duodenal ulcers	25 (80)			Mallory-Weiss syndrome.
Hiatus hernia	3			Rendu Osler Weber disease (hereditary telangiectasia) (*see* page 412).
				Pseudoxanthoma elasticum (a hereditary condition associated with friable connective tissue. The skin is coarse and yellow – and in the optic disc angioid streaks occur).
				Angiodysplasia. Recently described, this condition can only be demonstrated by intestinal arteriography and careful histology of resected specimens of gut. The microabnormalities of the intestinal blood vessels are a cause of intestinal bleeding and where other causes cannot be found such a diagnosis should be considered.
				Blood dyscrasias, burns, acute pancreatitis, aneurysms of intestinal arteries, etc.

(b) By a 'string' test, which involves swallowing a marked tape weighted at one end and noting either the area of blood-staining on withdrawal of the tape or the area of fluorescein-staining following intravenous injection of this dye. In each case the area of staining is related to the position of the tape on plain radiography of the abdomen.

(c) Other radiological techniques to outline the small or large bowel may be required, for example, small bowel meal and enema, and in patients who are actively bleeding use has been made recently of coeliac axis angiography, which may detect the pooling of blood in the bowel lumen at the actual point of haemorrhage.

Basis of Treatment

The aim of treatment in examples of acute upper intestinal bleeding is to replace blood loss, in order to stave off circulatory failure and, in the event of being unable to keep up with blood loss by blood transfusion, to intervene surgically to prevent further bleeding. Treatment must take priority over investigation, but it is important to try to determine the cause by taking a careful history to include previous illness, ingestion of alcohol and drugs (aspirin in all its forms, butazolidine and cortisone) and of previous dyspepsia such as might suggest a chronic ulcer or hiatus hernia. A history of previous jaundice is also important. The points in the physical examination worth recording are illustrated in Fig. 4.3. These will include any evidence of bleeding tendency. The clinical assessment must include serial estimations of the blood pressure and pulse, but these can be misleading. A low diastolic pressure and evidence of poor peripheral skin blood flow as shown by pale, cold, waxy hands, are signs of importance in assessing the severity of haemorrhage.

Following this initial assessment and the estimation of the haemoglobin, grouping and matching blood, blood transfusion may clearly be indicated and at this stage a valuable method of monitoring its effectiveness is by measuring the central venous pressure (CVP) by means of a fine catheter introduced into the superior vena cava via a brachial vein. A fall in CVP may indicate that rebleeding has occurred, and, hence that there is possibly a need for transfusion before there are any changes in systolic blood pressure or pulse rate. Further, CVP estimations help prevent overloading the circulation by over-transfusion. This is particularly important in the elderly with latent heart disease.

Sedation with heroin 10 mg is preferable to morphine because of the lesser risk of vomiting and the less profound depressant effect on the circulation. These drugs must be avoided if there is any suggestion of bleeding associated with liver disease, even if the bleeding is thought to be due to an ulcer rather than varices. In patients who are bleeding from proven peptic ulcers or from a haemorrhagic gastritis, treatment with an H_2 blocker, cimetidine, is recommended, particularly if bleeding has not responded to other therapy or the patient is considered to be too ill or too frail for surgery.

The patient is allowed water and milk drinks by mouth from the start and, following initial replacement of blood, the risk of a recurrence and the possibility of this causing serious circulatory collapse or other complications are assessed as far as is possible.

On the whole, the following are associated with a high risk of serious complications and, therefore, tend to be indications for early surgery.

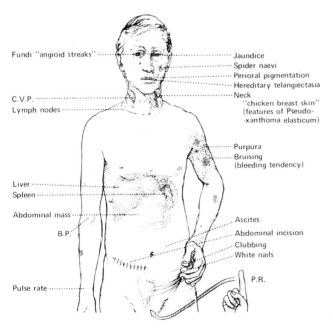

Fig. 4.3 In acute gastrointestinal bleeding look for these features.

Indications for early surgery

1. Age over 50.
2. Haematemesis (this suggests rapid bleeding).
3. Bleeding from a known chronic gastric ulcer.
4. Signs of shock and need for six or more units of blood to restore circulatory equilibrium.
5. A second haemorrhage in hospital.

In the event of these factors being present or of there being a history of previous intestinal bleeding, early emergency surgery is anticipated and it is essential for a surgeon to be alerted if such a sequence of events occurs. In many hospitals all cases of intestinal haemorrhage are seen conjointly by physician and surgeon, and co-operation of this sort from the early stages is most valuable.

Rebleeding under treatment or failure to control an initial bleed, particularly when the conditions previously listed are present, is an indication for surgical intervention. It is at this stage that the results of endoscopy and radiology are vital in planning the type and nature of the operation.

There has been a tendency of late to deal with bleeding chronic ulcers by local ligation of bleeding vessels with a vagotomy and pyloroplasty rather than a formal gastrectomy. On occasions, a bleeding site may not be found or multiple gastric erosions may necessitate a gastric resection.

Prognosis

The prognosis is variable and in patients under 40 the mortality is less than five per cent, so that it may be permissible to press on with blood transfusion in the hope that bleeding will eventually stop. The risk to life rises sharply over the age of 60 and the mortality in the elderly is twenty per cent. Further, despite apparent advances in treatment and the use of liberal blood transfusion, these figures are not decreasing. This is again a reason for electing for early surgery in this high-risk group.

THE COMMON UPPER GASTROINTESTINAL DISORDERS

GASTRITIS

Definition

An acute or chronic inflammatory disorder of the stomach mucosa of uncertain cause and with no specific clinical picture.

Background

There are two quite separate disorders to be considered here.

Acute Gastritis. A response of the gastric mucosa to a variety of injurious agents, some taken by the patient, e.g. alcohol, various drugs (particularly aspirin and cortisone, tobacco, etc.), which lead to superficial damage and even acute ulceration of the stomach. With removal of the stressful substance or situation, the gastric mucosa returns to normal, though with recurrent insults, permanent damage may occur.

Atrophic Gastritis (Chronic Gastritis). This is quite distinct and though it may follow repeated bouts of acute gastritis, it seems likely that the most important cause is an autoimmune destruction of the gastric mucosa. In certain patients this can be extreme enough to produce total gastric atrophy, when pernicious anaemia may also be found. In others the disease does not extend to this stage, and though investigation may show impaired vitamin B_{12} absorption, the clinical features of pernicious anaemia do not develop. Atrophic gastritis is not uncommon in the elderly, so that the

severity of the disorder is an expression of both auto-immune 'potency' and duration of the damaging process. Environmental factors such as smoking, the taking of unduly hot tea, and habitual analgesic intake may also play a part. Patients with atrophic gastritis show a high incidence of parietal cell antibodies in the serum, and in those with vitamin B_{12} malabsorption two types of intrinsic factor antibody are also commonly found. The name atrophic gastritis is erroneous, as studies have shown increased rather than decreased cellular losses from the gastric mucosa.

Pathology

In acute gastritis there is an acute inflammatory and haemorrhagic destruction of the superficial parts of the gastric mucosa with, in some examples, one or many small and acute ulcers (or erosions). In chronic atrophic gastritis there is atrophy of the glands, lymphocytic infiltration of the stroma between the glandular elements, and a change in the epithelium of these glands which become more like those of the intestine 'intestinal metaplasia'.

ACUTE GASTRITIS

Symptoms

None, or
Pain – epigastric.
Nausea and vomiting, and in patients who have developed gastric erosions – haematemesis and melaena.

These symptoms may follow hours after taking gastric irritants such as alcohol, analgesics, corticosteroids, or staphylococcal endotoxin (staphylococcal food poisoning).

Signs

Nil, or epigastric tenderness.

CHRONIC ATROPHIC GASTRITIS

Symptoms

None, or chronic epigastric pain, anorexia, nausea, vomiting, 'non-ulcer' dyspepsia.

Signs

Nil.
Occasionally, the features of pernicious anaemia.

Investigations

1. A barium meal is essential to exclude peptic ulcer, hiatus hernia, gastric carcinoma, etc. Occasionally,

chronic atrophic gastritis is severe enough to be associated with X-ray changes – 'the bald tubular stomach'.

2. Fibre-optic endoscopy with biopsy offers the most satisfactory way of diagnosing acute gastritis (particularly erosions) and determining the presence of histological changes. It is important, too, in determining the presence of chronic ulcer and cancer, when gastritis is particularly common.

3. Serum may be tested in chronic atrophic gastritis for parietal cell and intrinsic factor antibodies. There may also be evidence of other autoimmune disease and appropriate serum abnormalities, e.g. thyroid, adrenal.

4. A Schilling test may show impaired vitamin B$_{12}$ absorption, fully corrected by intrinsic factor administration.

Complications

There is an increased risk of gastric cancer in those with chronic atrophic gastritis.

Differential Diagnosis

This includes peptic ulcer, cancer, hiatus hernia, spastic colon, cholecystitis, etc.

Basis of Treatment

In patients with acute gastritis, care must be taken to avoid gastric irritants, either singly, or, in particular, the combination of alcohol and aspirin (a not uncommon treatment for acute coryza). This combination can lead to severe gastric bleeding in susceptible patients. In chronic atrophic gastritis a search for irritant factors is also important, and though treatment with alkalis may be started it may not necessarily help symptoms. Reassurance is important as is a careful search for other forms of upper gastrointestinal disease. It is wrong to attribute symptoms to gastritis unless all other disorders have been excluded.

Vitamin B$_{12}$ is obviously required if there is malabsorption of this substance.

HIATUS HERNIA (Fig. 4.4)

Definition

The presence of a pouch of gastric mucosa within the thoracic cage.

Background

This is of unknown cause, but presumably, as with other herniae, the factors to be considered are weakness of the hernial orifice – in the right crus of the diaphragm – and the effects of raised intra-abdominal pressure. With respect to the former, little is known apart from

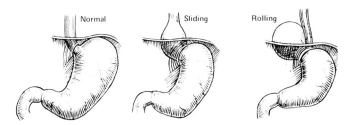

Fig. 4.4 Types of hiatus hernia.

the normal laxity that results from ageing, while in the latter, obesity, multiple pregnancies, and straining such as might result from constipation are important. A hiatus hernia is often associated with reflux of gastric contents into the oesophagus, and it has been shown that some are associated with pyloric incompetence so that bile salts may also be partially responsible for oesophagitis. A recent tendency has been to blame the presence of oesophageal reflux more to an abnormally low resting pressure in the lower oesophageal sphincter (LOS) than to the presence of the hernia *per se*.

Pathology

The hernial sac may be large or small, the former being found in the 'rolling' type of hernia. The oesophagus above the hernial sac often shows inflammatory change or frank mucosal haemorrhage. Chronic oesophagitis may lead to fibrosis and stricture formation. In some examples the lower oesophagus is lined by gastric rather than squamous epithelium. In these cases a peptic ulcer may be a complication and this may, of course, occur in the pouch of herniated gastric mucosa.

Symptoms

None, or

Heartburn – burning pain radiating from epigastrium to upper chest made worse by bending, lying flat and, occasionally, by food.

Waterbrash – regurgitation of fluid into the mouth.

Dysphagia – which may be progressive in patients with a stricture.

Haematemesis and/or melaena or occult bleeding.

Less commonly, and usually in rolling hernia, severe left chest pain and flatulence. These attacks may mimic myocardial disease.

Signs

None, but patients may be noted to be obese or to have increased their weight.

Investigations

1. A barium meal will demonstrate both a hernia and reflux of gastric contents into the oesophagus.

2. Endoscopy with biopsy will identify oesophagitis.
3. Studies of gastric secretory function may define those with hypersecretion or pyloric incompetence.

Differential Diagnosis

When there is stricture formation this will include carcinoma and achalasia.

Note: An accompanying duodenal ulcer may cause symptoms and aggravate those of peptic oesophagitis.

A further problem is the distinction of the chest pain of oesophagitis from angina. Indeed both may be present together.

Basis of Treatment

Symptoms are often dramatically improved by making the patient lose weight, even if they are not strikingly obese. A weight loss of a stone is often sufficient to bring about a dramatic improvement in heartburn and dysphagia. Alkalis and local anaesthetics are helpful, and commonsense advice about avoiding stooping (e.g. gardening, etc.) and sleeping with the head of the bed on blocks are followed by an equally convincing improvement. It is important that patients should stop smoking and avoid anticholinergic drugs. Both may reduce LOS tone and promote reflux, and may avoid what is otherwise technically very difficult surgery. Some cases of 'acid' regurgitation may result from the damaging effects of bile salts either alone or with acid. Pyloric regurgitation is a feature of these cases, and surgery aimed at diverting bile away from the duodenum via a long intestinal loop may be helpful.

In patients who have disabling symptoms not relieved by such a regime, surgery (vagotomy, pyloroplasty and hernia repair) should be considered. Difficulty may arise in complicated cases from oesophageal stricture, peptic ulcer with haemorrhage, and sometimes recurrent chest infection from aspiration. As long as there are no contraindications, this group of patients are best treated by elective surgery as emergency surgery for these complications may be very difficult. It seems likely, however, that the introduction of cimetidine will prove very useful in the treatment of peptic strictures secondary to a hiatus hernia.

CHRONIC PEPTIC ULCER

Definition

The presence of a chronic simple ulcer in the stomach, duodenum, or, in rare situations, in ectopic gastric epithelium found in a Meckel's diverticulum, or in the lower oesophagus, constitutes peptic ulceration. In reality, two distinct forms – gastric and duodenal ulcer of differing aetiology – constitute the vast majority of these lesions.

Background

Chronic Gastric Ulcer. This must be considered as a chronic ulcer, perhaps due to local loss of mucosal defence mechanisms. It is well recognised that there is hypo- rather than hypersecretion of gastric acid and that the disease shows a familial (genetic) predisposition with a slightly increased tendency to occur in those of blood Group O. It is certainly commoner in those of the lower social groups, often accompanied by chronic respiratory disease, though the reason for this is not understood. The stomach in which a chronic gastric ulcer develops often shows chronic gastritis (*see* page 56), perhaps further evidence of mucosal abnormality, while there is a very small but definite risk of malignancy. Recent studies have confirmed that reflux of duodenal contents into the stomach is present in some patients with chronic gastric ulcer, and in the duodenal contents, bile salts have been singled out as possible mucosal damaging agents. Whether or not there could be a defect in protective gastric mucus is unknown. There also seems to be an abnormality of gastric emptying which slows this, and the resultant stasis could, with the addition of biliary regurgitation, be an important aetiological factor in gastric ulcer production.

Chronic Duodenal Ulcer. In contrast, a duodenal ulcer is often associated with gastric hypersecretion (>30 mEq acid/hr following pentagastrin stimulation) and with a raised basal level. There is, however, an overlap between normal subjects with hypersecretion and those with chronic duodenal ulcer. There is also a genetic predisposition with a higher incidence among men as opposed to women (3:1) compared with gastric ulcer. Chronic duodenal ulcer is commonest in those with blood Group O who are non-secretors (no blood group activity in intestinal secretions) and is also seen more commonly in the middle and upper social classes. Though a high gastric acid and pepsin output may be important, nervous tension and anxiety may have some part to play in the aetiology and there is much experimental data to support nervous tension as a cause of experimental peptic ulcer. A recent trend has been to shift part of the blame to the possibility of defective neutralisation of acid by impaired pancreatic and intestinal bicarbonate production, with resultant deficient neutralisation. Unlike gastric ulcer, duodenal ulcer is not complicated by malignancy.

It is estimated that about one in ten people have a chronic peptic ulcer at some time in their lives, at least in the United Kingdom, but there are enormous regional differences.

Pathology

Ulcers are of variable size, from a few mm to 10 cm or more. Duodenal ulcers are usually in the cap, but can be in the second part of the duodenum or in the prepyloric area. Gastric ulcers are usually on the lesser curve, at the junction of the antrum and the acid-secreting body of the stomach. Antral and greater curvature ulcers are likely to prove malignant. Histologically there is loss of superficial epithelium, variable penetration with fibrosis, and in the vessels in the ulcer base there is endarteritis obliterans.

Symptoms

Pain.
  Site – epigastric, rarely chest (GU) or lower abdomen, localised unless ulcer penetration.
  Character – dull, burning.
  Precipitants – food, interval usually half to three hours *p.c.*, and in the latter case often referred to as occurring before meals.
  Relief – alkalis, food, vomiting.
  Periodicity – bouts commonly last two to three weeks with intervals of freedom of several weeks, occasionally months or years.
Note: The characteristics of the pain rarely allow differentiation into GU or DU.
Vomiting. Usually relieves pain; may therefore be self-induced; if massive think of pyloric stenosis.
Flatulence, loss of weight, anxiety, etc., and other symptoms are variable.
Heartburn. Due to associated hypersecretion (DU) or pyloric regurgitation (GU). Beware of the patient with a high penetrating GU who complains of vague chest pain with uncertain relation to food, often considered to be 'fibrositis' or even angina pectoris.

Signs

There is in a patient with an uncomplicated ulcer only one physical sign; namely, localised epigastric tenderness. Signs of associated diseases must be carefully looked for, e.g. chronic bronchitis, polycythaemia, hyperparathyroidism, etc.

Investigations

1. The most helpful is a barium meal, which is likely to pick up three-quarters of all chronic GUs, and may suggest the presence of a simple or malignant ulcer as well as detecting complications, such as an hour-glass stomach or pyloric stenosis. Satisfactory visualisation of duodenal ulcers is less frequent.
2. Endoscopy, using a fibre-optic gastroduodenoscope, allows visualisation, biopsy, cytology and photography of gastric and duodenal lesions. Further, healing can be checked by repeating endoscopy. Malignant change may be found in one to seven per cent of GUs. Multiple biopsies should be obtained at endoscopy so that this can be detected early and dealt with surgically.
3. Examination of the stools for occult blood, the blood

for anaemia and a raised plasma viscosity are non-specific and in the case of the plasma viscosity no certain indicator of possible neoplastic change in a GU.
4. Acid secretion studies (*see* page 94) are of little value in the average case as the overlap with normal subjects is considerable and, in the case of chronic refractory DU, do not really help in the selection of the type or extent of surgery required. In cases of bizarre duodenal and jejunal ulceration, basal and maximally stimulated acid studies may show high values with reduction of the ratio of basal/stimulated secretion in the Zollinger-Ellison syndrome.

Complications (*see* Fig. 4.5)

GASTRIC ULCER

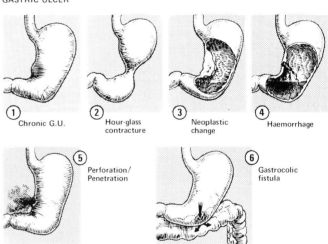

DUODENAL ULCER

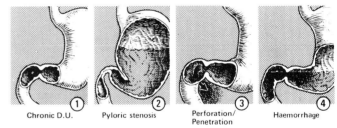

Fig. 4.5 The complications of gastric and duodenal ulcer.

Differential Diagnosis

1. From other causes of dyspepsia such as :
Hiatus hernia – history of reflux and heartburn, radiology helpful.
Cholecystitis – history of very acute pain with long episodes of freedom.
2. From gastric or colonic or pancreatic carcinoma – suspect in anyone in middle age with symptoms of pain and weight loss, related to meals.
Investigate fully if a barium meal is negative.
3. From nervous dyspepsia and spastic colon syndrome – make these diagnoses by exclusion only.

4. Rarely, from cardiac pain or disease of chest wall (fibrositis).

Basis of Treatment

Gastric Ulcer. Because of the difficulty of being quite certain that an ulcer in the stomach is not initially malignant, or the small possibility that malignant change will ensue, gastric ulcers are (rightly) treated with respect. Treatment should be intensive, with bed rest (preferably in hospital), administration of a nutritious diet, with antacids such as Aludrox, Magnesium Trisilicate Mixture, BPC, etc., for pain and the abolition of smoking. There is little to be gained, unless pain is severe, from a bland, uninteresting 'gastric' diet. Sedation may be important if the patient is anxious and extra vitamin C may help ulcer healing. The period of treatment should extend over six weeks, and healing, as judged by a repeat barium meal and/or endoscopy, with multiple biopsies, should be well advanced before ambulation is allowed. Persisting symptoms and poor or absent healing are evidence in favour of surgical intervention. The above regime can be reinforced by the administration of a steroid synthesised from glycyrrhizinic acid which is, in turn obtained from liquorice – carbenoxolone sodium. This latter compound is, however, not found in liquorice itself. The agent, which has anti-inflammatory properties, is marketed as Biogastrone and is administered in a dose of 100 mg three times daily. Investigations using a double-blind technique have confirmed its ability to produce a significant increase in healing of chronic GU compared with a control group. Possible complications are associated with its sodium-retaining and potassium-losing properties and these consist of fluid retention and hypertension (dangerous in those with latent heart disease) and fatigue and, occasionally, plain or voluntary muscle paralysis due to hypokalaemia. Because of these problems and the more recent introduction of cimetidine, which is probably more effective than Biogastrone, it is possibly safer to use the latter at least in elderly patients as a means of healing gastric ulcers. It is given in a dose of 200 mg three times daily with a bedtime dose of 400 mg.

On occasions, it may be justifiable to treat patients with gastric ulcers by an ambulant regime supplemented with Biogastrone, and in any case there is uncertainty whether Biogastrone is able to speed healing of the hospitalised ulcer patient.

Surgery. This is indicated for complications as well as for known malignant ulcers or failure of healing in an otherwise well patient. Prior to surgery it is important to make sure that the patient's general condition is improved. This may entail correction of anaemia, removal of septic teeth, treatment of chronic chest infection, etc. The surgical operation currently used is a limited partial gastrectomy. In this way the whole of the ulcer is available for detailed histology.

Duodenal Ulcer. Bed rest at home or in hospital, sedation, cessation of smoking and the administration of frequent meals with alkalis for pain form the basis of treatment. There is no risk of neoplasia, so that insistence on complete healing is less necessary. In any case, radiology may often not show an ulcer crater and it is difficult to detect changes in a duodenal cap that merely shows deformity. There is, therefore, little to be gained by re-X-raying duodenal ulcer patients unless, for example, symptoms change and complications such as pyloric obstruction ensue.

The above treatment can be reinforced by antispasmodic drugs such as probanthine, but there is no evidence that they help to increase the rate of healing. A dose of probanthine (15 mg) and a glass of milk last thing at night may ensure a pain-free night. It is usual for a patient with ulcer symptoms to show a marked decrease in symptoms within a few days of starting hospital rest. If symptoms do not improve it is worthwhile making certain that the patient really is having bed rest and not just sitting around at home or in the ward and that he is not smoking. It is occasionally worthwhile giving a milk/alkali drip intragastrically to relieve pain, though, again, there is no evidence to suggest that healing is accelerated. Cimetidine is able to heal duodenal ulcers and, except where symptoms are mild when used on a long term basis it probably offers a method as effective as surgery for keeping them healed. In the opinion of the author, surgery is to be preferred for ulcer therapy for those who are young and otherwise fit and for whom there is no contraindication to operation.

Surgery. This is indicated:
(a) If after a period of bed rest and medical treatment, including cimetidine, there are subsequently further severe symptoms.
(b) If complications such as recurrent bleeding or pyloric stenosis occur.
Obviously, patients must be reviewed individually, and factors such as recurrent absence from work, inability to take regular meals, or residence away from first-class surgical facilities may be those that influence the decision to embark on early surgery.

The surgical operation used is generally vagotomy (either total or selective) with pyloroplasty, or a highly selective vagotomy without drainage.

COMPLICATIONS OF PEPTIC ULCER AND GASTRIC SURGERY OF IMPORTANCE TO THE PHYSICIAN

PYLORIC STENOSIS

Vomiting, particularly if voluminous and containing stale food residue, wasting, and visible gastric peristalsis suggest this diagnosis, which can be confirmed radiologically. It is usually due to scarring from a duodenal ulcer or gastric carcinoma. Correction of potassium deficiency (due to K lost in vomit and secreted in excess by the kidneys because of the alkalosis) must be fully corrected and, after daily gastric lavage to empty the stomach and re-establish gastric tone, surgery (vagotomy, gastroenterostomy or gastrectomy) is required.

RECURRENT ANAEMIA DUE TO IRON OR VITAMIN B₁₂ DEFICIENCY (*see* Fig. 4.6)

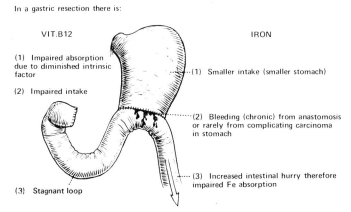

In a gastric resection there is:

VIT.B12

(1) Impaired absorption due to diminished intrinsic factor

(2) Impaired intake

(3) Stagnant loop

IRON

(1) Smaller intake (smaller stomach)

(2) Bleeding (chronic) from anastomosis or rarely from complicating carcinoma in stomach

(3) Increased intestinal hurry therefore impaired Fe absorption

Fig. 4.6 Anaemia and partial gastrectomy.

Patients after gastrectomy must be followed-up and the haemoglobin measured and deficiency corrected. In particular, vitamin B₁₂ deficiency may first be manifest with neurological and neuro-psychiatric symptoms. Vague symptoms such as paraesthesiac weakness and confusion must lead to investigation of vitamin B₁₂ status and its correction.

BONE DISEASE (*see also* page 197).

This is common in the elderly gastrectomised subject. Though this operation is now less frequently carried out and even when employed is less radical – virtually being confined to gastric ulcer patients – the legacy of gastrectomised patients is considerable. The major lesion is osteomalacia, which causes bone thinning, with pain and difficulty with walking (due to accompanying myopathy). Radiology is helpful in showing pseudo-fractures, as is bone biopsy. Biochemical changes include a low serum phosphate and calcium and raised alkaline phosphatase. The disease arises from vitamin D deficiency due largely to impaired intake and impaired absorption, while in elderly patients, lack of sunshine (enforced inactivity) is a further factor. Beware of any patient who has had gastric surgery and who appears with 'rheumatism'; the disorder may be easily corrected by vitamin D.

CANCER AND ANASTOMOTIC ULCER

There is a certain amount of evidence to show that the mucosal atrophy in the gastric remnant after gastric surgery may proceed to neoplastic involvement, so that gastric cancer must always be considered in any patient with persisting postoperative symptoms. Anastomotic ulcer is seen particularly in those who have had gastric resection for duodenal ulcer, while the possibility of a Zollinger-Ellison syndrome must also be borne in mind.

NUTRITION

Nutrition is impaired after gastric resection because of impaired intake and by malabsorption (Fig. 4.7). Patients may also have distressing symptoms such as palpitations, sweating and faintness (dumping syndrome) due to rapid entry of hyperosmotic fluid into the small bowel and possible release of hypotensive kinins from the gut into the blood. This may be so severe that it requires surgical correction. A late dumping syndrome is caused by excessive insulin secretion due to increased emptying of food into the small bowel, with resultant symptoms of hypoglycaemia.

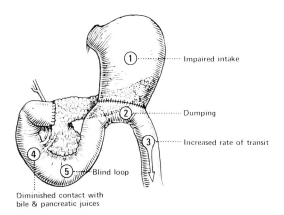

① Impaired intake

② Dumping

③ Increased rate of transit

④

⑤ Blind loop

Diminished contact with bile & pancreatic juices

Fig. 4.7 Malnutrition following gastric surgery.

OTHER COMMON GASTROINTESTINAL DISORDERS

JAUNDICE (ICTERUS)

Definition

The retention of bile pigments in the tissues as a result of liver disease, biliary obstruction, haemolysis, or combinations of these factors.

Background

Bile pigments are produced by the breakdown of haemoglobin from degenerate red blood cells. Most are produced in the reticuloendothelial system where iron and globin are removed prior to the remaining tetra-pyrolle ring being cleaved with the production of a chain structure–bilirubin. A small percentage (10 to 15 per cent) of bilirubin is derived from other sources and from structurally related haem compounds, e.g. iron-containing enzymes, cytochromes, etc.

Transport to the liver is by loose attachment to serum albumin, and entry into liver cells may involve the action of two (or perhaps more) specific receptor proteins called, at the moment Y and Z. The most fundamental process that occurs in liver cells is conjugation with glucuronic acid to form bilirubin diglucuronide. This is freely water-soluble, which allows its excretion in urine, while its insolubility in lipid prevents its absorption by the small intestinal mucosa. Conjugation is carried out in the microsomes of the smooth endoplasmic reticulum (SER) of the liver, and excretion of conjugated bilirubin is into biliary canaliculi, small tubules which link with the rest of the biliary apparatus but which are formed by specialised portions of adjacent liver cells.

Bacterial breakdown of bilirubin diglucuronide in the large gut produces stercobilinogen and stercobilin, the major pigment of the faeces. Reabsorption of a fraction of this results in a recirculation to the liver (entero-hepatic circulation) where the fraction excreted in the urine, known as urobilinogen, forms a valuable pointer to the presence of hepatobiliary disease as it can easily be estimated using Ehrlich's aldehyde reagent.

Jaundice can be classified as prehepatic (haemolytic), posthepatic (obstructive) and due to liver cell disease (hepatic). In view of the key role of the microsomes of the SER, it is also possible to divide jaundice into two varieties, premicrosomal (i.e. haemolytic and hepatic) and postmicrosomal (obstructive).

Pathology

The diseases responsible for jaundice can be either of the liver cell, the biliary apparatus, or those associated with increased red cell destruction. Liver cell diseases are often due to infection, e.g. viral hepatitis, or the action of certain drugs. A rare but important group of cases of liver cell jaundice are due to congenital disorders of bilirubin metabolism, e.g. Gilbert's disease, Dublin-Johnson syndrome (see Table 4.6).

Biliary obstruction may be intra- or extrahepatic. In the former, this results from a variety of causes including the action of a number of drugs (different from those causing liver cell disease) and involvement of the liver by multiple intrahepatic metastases. The major causes of extrahepatic obstruction are biliary stones, neoplasms of the ampulla of Vater or pancreas and biliary strictures. There is a fundamental distinction between intra- and extrahepatic biliary obstruction, the biliary apparatus being dilated in the latter case, and collapsed in the former. Treatment is also fundamentally different in that the former does *not* respond to surgery. Chronic biliary obstruction may, in time, lead to hepatic fibrosis and cirrhosis.

Table 4.6 The congenital hyperbilirubinaemias

Feature	Najjar and Crigler	Gilbert	Rotor	Dublin-Johnson
Pigment in blood	Unconjugated	Unconjugated	Conjugated	Conjugated
Pigment in urine	No	No	Yes	Yes
Severity	+++ (fatal)	+−++	+	+
			Benign	
Familial	Yes	Yes	Yes	Yes
Age group	Infancy	Any	Any	Any
		Usually first noted in childhood		
Liver histology	Normal	Normal	Normal	Pigment (melanin) in liver
Nature of defect	Lack of hepatic transferase (no conjugation)	Partial lack of conjugation + defective hepatic uptake	Defective bilirubin uptake and storage	Defective bilirubin excretion
Associated disorders	Kernicterus	–	Non-filling gall bladder (X-ray)	Non-filling gall bladder
Treatment	Nil	Nil usually required Severe cases respond to phenobarbitone	Nil	Nil

Symptoms

In Haemolytic (Prehepatic) Jaundice:
1. Jaundice (mild).
2. Symptoms of anaemia.
3. Of the cause of haemolysis, e.g. joint pains, skin rashes in SLE.

In Liver Cell (Hepatic) Jaundice:
1. Jaundice – mild, moderate or deep.
2. Skin irritation (rarely persistent).
Note: In chronic or fulminant cases further symptoms are – ankle swelling (oedema), abdominal swelling (ascites) – bleeding tendency – encephalopathy.

In Obstructive (Posthepatic) Jaundice:
1. Jaundice – mild, moderate or severe.
2. Persistent pruritus.
3. Symptoms of the cause, e.g. abdominal pain (gall stones, carcinoma) loss of weight (carcinoma), etc.
Note: In all three types of jaundice a history of the taking of drugs may be of diagnostic importance – check with the patient's relatives and general practitioner.

Signs

Haemolysis:
Pallor – mild jaundice; splenomegaly.
Faeces dark. Urine dark on standing due to increased urobilin.
(*Note:* No bilirubin in urine.)

Hepatic Jaundice:
Liver enlarged, sometimes small.
Bruising, oedema, ascites.
Hepatic foetor.
Flap.

Cutaneous stigmata of chronic liver cell disease (spiders, clubbing, etc., *see* page 69).
Faeces lighter than usual. Urine dark (conjugated bilirubin).

Obstructive Jaundice:
Jaundice – mild, moderate or severe.
Hepatomegaly.
? Gall bladder enlarged in neoplastic obstruction below cystic duct, i.e. +ve Courvoisier's sign (palpable gall bladder).
Faeces light. Urine dark (conjugated bilirubin).
Also in neoplasia:
Enlarged lymph nodes (supraclavicular).
Ascites.
Pelvic involvement (rectal examination).
In chronic cases:
Pigmentation.
Tender bones.
Xanthomata (subcutaneous cholesterol deposits).

Investigations

These are best considered by reference to Table 4.7. Further tests may be required in individual cases, for example in haemolytic disease, to discover the cause of haemolysis. In liver cell disease detection, of hepatitis B virus (HBV), a Paul Bunnel test and spirochaetal antibody tests (Weil's disease) may be important in acute cases, while in chronic liver cell disease, tests for LE cells and immunological reactions such as antinuclear factor and DNA binding antibodies may be found in chronic active hepatitis. In obstructive jaundice, tests for faecal occult blood, barium studies of the duodenal loop and a plain film to detect radio-opaque gall stones may be helpful.

Table 4.7 Investigations of jaundice

Test	Haemolytic	Hepatic	Obstructive
Blood count	Anaemia (evidence of haemolysis)	Normal (unless chronic)	Normal (unless blood loss)
Liver function tests			
Bilirubin	↑ (+)	↑ (+ − + + +)	↑(+ − + + +)
Alk. phosphatase	Normal	Normal or ↑	↑(usually >30 KA units)
Other enzymes			
SGPT	Normal	↑ + + +	↑+
LDH			
Flocculation tests, e.g. thymol turbidity	Normal	Increased	Normal or slightly increased +ve test for lipoprotein X (LPX)
Others	To detect haemolysis and its cause (*see* page 384)	HBV ⎱ Paul Bunnel ⎰ acute ANF ⎰ SM antibodies, etc. ?Biopsy	Occult blood in stools Plain film of abdomen Barium meal Ultrasound Transhepatic cholangiography ERCP

Liver biopsy is hazardous in the jaundiced patient and should be performed only if diagnostic information cannot be obtained in any other way. It is indicated where liver function tests fail to categorise jaundice as either due to obstruction or liver cell disease. A satisfactory biopsy will usually make this distinction and in obstructive cases it may be valuable in the differentiation of intrahepatic obstruction from the extrahepatic variety. The differentiation is of more than academic importance as the latter is an indication for surgical treatment. Scintiscanning, using a compound excreted in the bile, for example [131]I Rose Bengal, may be helpful in confirming the patency or otherwise of the biliary tract, while scintiscanning using a compound taken up by the reticuloendothelial system, may identify filling defects in the liver associated with intrahepatic tumours.

Three further investigations may be valuable in patients with biliary obstruction:

1. Transhepatic cholangiography. A very fine needle introduced through the liver punctures the dilated biliary system, which can be visualised and obstruction identified. Such a procedure is often performed prior to biliary tract surgery. In patients with intrahepatic biliary obstruction, where the biliary apparatus is collapsed, transhepatic cholangiography may be unsuccessful and this, too, may have some diagnostic importance in patients with biliary obstruction of unknown cause. Cholangiography in the jaundiced patient may also be performed by:
2. Cannulation of the ampulla of Vater by direct vision at fibre-optic duodenoscopy (ERCP).
3. Ultrasonic scanning of the liver may be used to detect enlarged intrahepatic bile ducts in patients with extrahepatic biliary obstruction, whilst they are normal in size where there is intrahepatic obstruction. This is a useful screening test which may be followed by transhepatic or endoscopic cholangiography, depending on the results of ultrasonic scanning.

Mention must be made of two procedures which may both be of therapeutic and diagnostic importance in the jaundiced patient. A trial of five days corticosteroid therapy (40 mg prednisolone daily) is indicated in patients with presumed intrahepatic obstructive jaundice. A fall in serum bilirubin of 8 per cent or more/day (40 per cent in five days) suggests obstruction due to viral hepatitis (so called 'cholangiolitic' hepatitis).

A laparotomy is dangerous in those with liver cell disease, but is indicated in those with persistent obstruction, particularly if evidence points to this being due to extrahepatic biliary obstruction. The dangers of laparotomy in jaundiced patients are haemorrhage and postoperative renal failure. The former is corrected by vitamin K, by intramuscular injection, and there is some evidence to suggest that intravenous mannitol may have some prophylactic value against renal failure, at least in elderly deeply jaundiced patients with biliary obstruction.

VIRAL HEPATITIS

Definition

A number of viruses cause acute hepatic damage, but usually this title refers to three major and separate clinical disorders, the result of infection by three or more different viruses – virus A, virus B and the recently introduced 'non-A, non-B' type.

Virus A. The virus of infective hepatitis is associated with a generally mild sporadic and sometimes epidemic disorder commonest in young children and with an excellent prognosis (Fig. 4.8).

The virus can now be detected in the stools and specific antibodies found in the serum.

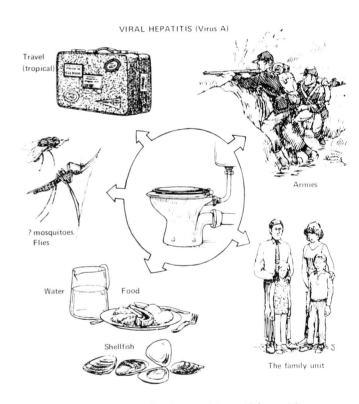

Fig. 4.8 The aetiology of infective (virus A) hepatitis.

Virus B. The virus of syringe or serum hepatitis is introduced by contaminated blood or blood products, by transfusion, injection or by contamination of hypodermic needles. The infection thought clinically indistinguishable from virus A infection carries a higher mortality and in over 80 per cent of patients hepatitis B surface antigen (HBsAg) is found in the blood in the acute phase.

Background (Fig. 4.8)

Infective hepatitis is commonest in the young and is a family disease, depending on close contact between its members, so that opportunities may then exist for faecal-oral transmission of the virus. Armies in the field, where personal hygiene may be poor, and travelling to the tropics, are particularly at risk. Contamination of food (shellfish) and water (contamination by sewage) may occasionally be responsible, while a possible reservoir exists in certain non-human primates.

Pathology

In classical cases the liver shows patchy necrosis, maximal in the centrilobular zones, with a mononuclear portal infiltrate. In patients with obstructive features (see below) there may be cholestasis and in those with massive necrosis, the liver is reduced in size with a wrinkled capsule and virtual disappearance of liver cells from the microscope field. In cases of this severity, where there is survival, a coarse multilobular cirrhosis may follow.

Symptoms

Incubation period 2 to 6 weeks, usually 14 days.
Preceding the jaundice (4 to 5 days):
  Anorexia, lassitude, nausea.
  Abdominal pain.
  Distaste for cigarettes.
With onset of jaundice which reaches a maximum intensity quickly:
  Icterus.
  Pale stools.
  Dark urine.
  Transient itching.

Signs

Pyrexia.
Icterus (but note patient can be anicteric).
Enlarged and tender liver.
Enlarged spleen (about 30 per cent).
Sometimes cervical (particularly right-sided) lymphadenopathy.

Investigations

1. A blood count shows a mild anaemia and leucopenia with a normal platelet count.
2. Liver function tests show abnormalities suggesting a liver cell cause for the jaundice.
(a) The serum bilirubin is raised and in severe cases may be over 300 μmol/l (18 mg/100 ml).
(b) The serum alkaline phosphatase is either normal or slightly raised but on some occasions may be greater than 30 KA units (when the temptation to assume that the jaundice is obstructive should be resisted).
(c) The serum shows a normal albumin level unless the disease runs a protracted course, while the β and γ globulins are raised. In laboratories where flocculation tests are still performed these are positive, due to the increased globulins.
(d) The liver enzymes are extremely helpful and values for LDH and transaminases are raised. In moderately severe cases this elevation of transaminases is greater than 300 units/l, while values of 1 to 2,000 units/l are not uncommon. Raised levels are found even when the patient is not jaundiced.
3. The prothrombin time may be increased (bleeding tendency) and this is often not corrected by vitamin K therapy.
4. Liver biopsy, which is indicated only if there is difficulty in differentiating jaundice from that due to obstruction, shows scattered foci of liver cell damage with a tendency to centrilobular localisation and a marked mononuclear cell infiltrate in the portal zones which are enlarged.

Complications

The complications of infective hepatitis are many, but the serious ones, aplastic anaemia, massive hepatic necrosis and chronic liver disease (cirrhosis), are all rare. The following are brief comments on them.

Common Complications:
Posthepatitis syndrome
Symptoms – Fatigue, anorexia depression, hepatic tenderness persisting often after clinical and biochemical evidence of acute liver disease have gone.
Aetiology – Probably psychosomatic.
Treatment – Reassurance.

Rare Complications:
Progression to chronic liver disease and hepatoma (see page 68).
Symptoms – Persisting jaundice with splenomegaly, ascites and cutaneous evidence of chronic liver disease. Patients may appear to recover completely from hepatitis only to present with cirrhosis or its complications many years later.
Aetiology – Probably persistence of the responsible virus and/or immunological change.

Acute hepatic necrosis
Symptoms – Deepening jaundice, confusion, noisy delirium and coma, bleeding tendency and oliguric renal failure. Death. Liver progressively smaller on clinical examination.
Aetiology – Massive necrosis of liver cells and collapse of reticulin.

Treatment – By full anticoma regime (*see* page 71), corticosteroids, ?exchange blood transfusion or hepatic assistance using pig or other liver for perfusion by patient's blood.

Aplastic anaemia

Symptoms – Anaemia, leucopenia and thrombocytopenia, leading to haemorrhages, infection, and death, follow viral hepatitis.

Aetiology – Presumably marrow damage secondary to viral infection.

Obstructive jaundice, 'cholangiolitic' hepatitis. Cause uncertain, but symptoms and liver function tests are those of obstruction rather than liver cell disease. Distinction from extrahepatic obstruction may be difficult, but liver biopsy and a dramatic fall in serum bilirubin after corticosteroids (five days of 40 mg prednisone) may be helpful. Laparotomy occasionally required when cholangiography and surgical biopsy are essential.

Persistent unconjugated hyperbilirubinaemia. Cause presumably related to impaired uptake of unconjugated bilirubin into the liver cell. It is of diagnostic importance only.

Differential Diagnosis

Infective hepatitis is no respector of age, though it is commonest in school children and teenagers. The importance of recent travel abroad (poor hygiene) and exposure to patients with jaundice or obscure febrile illness is obvious. The ingestion of shellfish is important in patients in the USA but not in Great Britain.

The important differential diagnoses are drug jaundice where the history may be the only helpful clue (all other clinical, biochemical and pathological tests being non-helpful), alcoholic hepatitis and Weil's disease. (In the latter, the polymorph nuclear leucocytosis, acute course and myositis and evidence of renal involvement, together with a history of exposure to rats, are important (*see* page 29). Other virus infections, notably infective mononucleosis (sore throat, generalised lymphadenopathy, skin rash, positive Paul Bunnel reaction) and cytomegalovirus infection are the most important. Obstructive jaundice should not be a diagnostic problem unless viral hepatitis is followed by a prolonged cholestatic phase.

Basis of Treatment

Prophylaxis. Obviously, the maintenance of high standards of personal hygiene are important, and in prevention of epidemics such standards among personnel such as food handlers are vital. It has been demonstrated that an intramuscular injection of human gammaglobulin 0.06 ml/kg will protect against the disease in those who are exposed to it, e.g. travellers, medical attendants, etc.

Careful disposal of faeces and urine are important in patients with the disease, but in fact the major infectivity of faeces occurs prior to the onset of jaundice, and provided care is taken there is no reason why jaundiced cases should not be treated in a general medical ward. Great care must be taken with blood samples as, in the acute stage, a viraemia is present, and if the possibility of hepatitis is present in a jaundiced patient, laboratory and medical staff must treat and transport samples with caution.

Management. The average case is treated with rest in bed, a high protein diet (provided there is no evidence of acute hepatic failure with hepatic encephalopathy). When the patient feels well (and usually this is so once jaundice has passed its peak) he is allowed up to toilet. A low fat diet is of no therapeutic value, but many patients are nauseated by fat, in which case restriction is common sense. Antibiotics are of no value.

Certain physical signs and symptoms should be carefully noted. Deepening jaundice, persistent anorexia and vomiting, and continuing pyrexia are signs of worsening hepatic disease. Daily estimates of liver size are important in the early diagnosis of acute hepatic necrosis as also is frequent estimation of the serum bilirubin and detection of a polymorph leucocytosis. Diminishing jaundice and a return of urobilinogen excretion in the urine (urobilinogen is absent from the patient's urine in the acute phase of the disease) are both favourable signs, as also is the patient's return of appetite and strength.

If jaundice does not fade, and if the patient remains unwell, there is good evidence that corticosteroids will produce not only a sense of well-being in the patient, but a decrease in jaundice and improvement of liver function tests. Relapse is, however, a danger of such treatment which should not be an excuse for abandoning bed rest. Dosage is 20 to 40 mg of prednisolone daily, reducing as the serum bilirubin falls, with continuation of treatment for at least a month.

Patients who have had hepatitis may complain of persisting weakness and ill health for weeks or months. Reassurance is important, and most can return to work following a month's convalescence. It is traditional to ban alcohol for three to six months. This is probably a reasonable way of conveying to the patient the impression that the illness is one that can produce severe debility and where some common sense is required in the convalescent period. Relapse is in any case seen in less than ten per cent of patients and does not usually signify a greater likelihood of progression to chronic liver disease.

VIRUS B (SERUM) HEPATITIS

The major distinctions between serum hepatitis and infective hepatitis concern their mode of transmission.

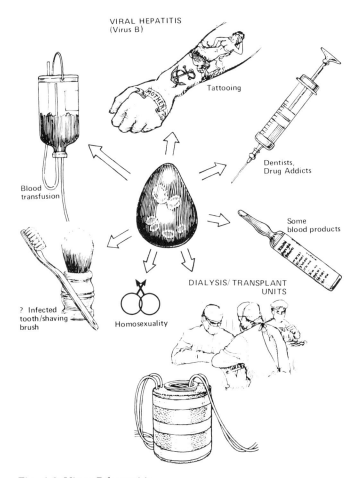

VIRAL HEPATITIS (Virus B)

Tattooing

Dentists, Drug Addicts

Some blood products

DIALYSIS/ TRANSPLANT UNITS

Homosexuality

? Infected tooth/shaving brush

Blood transfusion

Fig. 4.9 Virus B hepatitis.

Background (Fig. 4.9)

Transmission of this disease depends on the inoculation of serum, blood plasma or blood products (particularly fibrinogen) into susceptible subjects. In Great Britain 1 in 1,000 units of blood screened for transfusion is infected but in countries such as the USA a higher risk results because of payment to donors and the higher prevalence of drug addicts among them. The risk is high where multiple units of blood are required, e.g. for cardiac surgery. Tattooing, dental treatment, narcotic addiction, and renal dialysis units are further associations with the disease and it is more common in homosexuals.

In general, this disease affects an older group than infective hepatitis and one where there is often underlying disease. The prognosis is therefore worse, and a mortality of twenty per cent is recorded in some surveys. Protection from the disease with γ globulin is less effective. In the following respect the clinical and investigational features of the two diseases also differ:
1. In serum hepatitis the incubation period is up to six months, and the mean time to symptoms about seven weeks.

2. The blood gives a positive test for HBV or HBsAg, or both, in the acute phase. It is then highly infective. Hepatitis B antibody, HBsAb appears in the serum and normally with recovery HBsAg is cleared. It has been shown that at least four sub-types of HBsAg exist, and these being geographically determined may be useful in epidemiological studies. The centre of the virion or core, which is derived from the hepatocyte nucleus is designated HBc and the antibody to this agent is core antibody, HBcAb. 'e' antigen seems to determine the infectivity of the agent. HBsAg may be found in the serum by electron microscopy in spherical and tubular forms and as the complete virus particle (Dane particle) of core and outer coat. The former is derived from liver cell nuclei and the latter added from hepatocyte cytoplasm (Fig. 4.10).

The components of the hepatitis B virus (HBV)	
Antigens	**Antibodies**
(a) Core antigen (HBc) from liver cell nucleus indicates viral replication.	(a) Core antibody (HBcAb) indicates recent infection.
(b) Surface antigen (HBsAg) from liver cell cytoplasm indicates active infection or carrier state.	(b) Surface antibody (HBsAb) indicates past or present infection.
(c) 'e' antigen (HBe) determines infectivity.	(c) 'e' antibody (HBeAb) protective against infection.

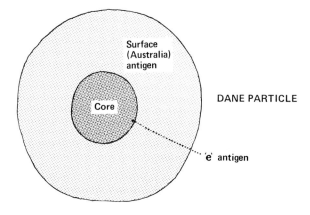

Fig. 4.10 Diagrammatic representation of components of hepatitis B virus (HBV).

Great importance is currently attached to the screening of all blood donors for HBV (by immunological and electron microscopy techniques), so that those carrying the antigen are vigorously eliminated from blood donor lists. Carriage of HBV may presumably last for many years without apparent long term effects on the carrier. On the other hand, various types of chronic liver disease, including hepatoma, are being recognised in conjunction with the persistence of HBV.

CIRRHOSIS OF THE LIVER

Definition

A chronic liver disease with many causes, both known and unknown, in which fibrosis of the liver is accompanied by formation of regeneration nodules and by variable liver cell damage.

Background

Cirrhosis is the end result of certain forms of chronic liver cell damage. Injury leads to cell necrosis which, in turn, is followed by regeneration of remaining 'healthy' liver cells. The end result of this regeneration is the formation of regeneration nodules, i.e. areas of liver tissue with an abnormal structure, blood supply, and function. Further, compression of hepatic venous radicles by expanding regeneration nodules is a major cause of the portal venous hypertension that complicates some cases of hepatic cirrhosis. The change resulting in the cirrhotic process may be clinically obvious and cirrhosis may follow an attack of viral hepatitis, but such progression is unusual and, in fact, many patients with cirrhosis have no clinical history of an acute bout of liver cell disorder. It is therefore obvious that the chronic liver injury is often of low-grade activity and that clinical manifestations of liver disease may occur only when the cirrhotic process is complete.

Cirrhosis may complicate liver disease due to or associated with:
1. Viral hepatitis, though this is rare. Persistence of the virus(es) or secondary immunological damage could be responsible factor(s).
2. Alcoholism – but cirrhosis is rare, while fatty infiltration is common. The factors necessary for progression from one to the other are unknown, but bouts of severe liver cell damage 'acute alcoholic hepatitis' are important.
3. Chronic active hepatitis which, on fairly strong evidence, is associated in many cases with an autoimmune disorder, progresses inexorably to cirrhosis. Other cases may be caused by drugs or persistent HBV infection.
4. Cirrhosis is part of the syndrome of haemochromatosis, though the cause of the liver disease in most is unknown.
5. It is also part of the clinical picture of Kinnier Wilson's disease, where copper deposition may be the cause, and of congenital fibrocystic disease, where biliary obstruction and infection are important aetiological factors.
6. A chronic obstruction of the biliary tract, either of the common bile duct or of the minor ductules in the liver,

is also a cause of cirrhosis (biliary cirrhosis). The former is usually due to a biliary stricture, the latter to auto-immune damage to biliary apparatus (primary biliary cirrhosis).

Other causes of cirrhosis include a_1 antitrypsin deficiency, and chronic congestive cardiac failure, 'cardiac' cirrhosis.

Cirrhosis is a balance between cell injury and replacement and, under certain circumstances, in patients with cirrhosis, liver tumours result from uncontrolled cellular regeneration. Thus, a hepatoma is an important complication of some varieties of cirrhosis.

Pathology

The liver may be larger or smaller than normal with an uneven nodular surface. The nodularity is due to areas of regeneration which may be large, 'macronodular cirrhosis', or small, 'micronodular cirrhosis'. In some, smaller (up to 5 mm) and larger (up to several cm) regeneration nodules may be present, giving a 'mixed' picture.

Symptoms

There may be no symptoms of cirrhosis, the disease being discovered by some abnormality of the blood count or plasma viscosity or liver function tests.

The following may be symptoms:
Jaundice – usually mild and of the liver cell type, except in biliary cirrhosis.
Fluid retention. Ascites or ankle swelling, due to hypoalbuminaemia, and retention of sodium and water related to secondary hyperaldosteronism.
Mental confusion or stupor, due to poisoning of deep centres in the brain by products of bacterial breakdown of protein that are not detoxified by the damaged liver. These escape into the peripheral (systemic circulation) via collateral vessels which link the portal and systemic circulations and which result from portal hypertension. An intestinal haemorrhage, haematemesis or melaena due to rupture of oesophageal varices, which, in turn, are due to obstruction of blood flow through the liver and opening up of portal systemic collaterals, including those at the lower end of the oesophagus.

Haemorrhage in the cirrhotic patient is extremely dangerous, and though it may occur from varices, an ulcer, or gastritis (the latter two are also common in the cirrhotic), whatever the site the risk is of the precipitation of liver failure and death.
Less common presentations include deep jaundice, infections, diabetes, etc.

Signs (Fig. 4.11)

The cutaneous stigmata of liver disease are of importance.

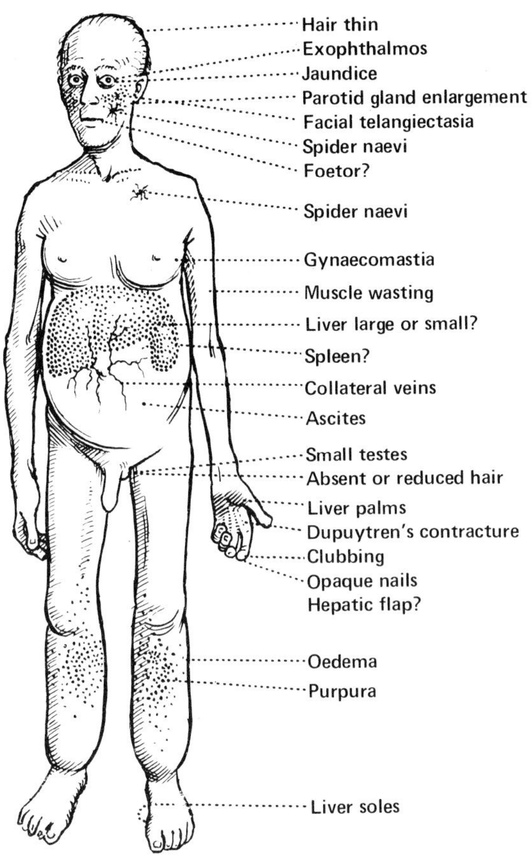
Hair thin
Exophthalmos
Jaundice
Parotid gland enlargement
Facial telangiectasia
Spider naevi
Foetor?
Spider naevi
Gynaecomastia
Muscle wasting
Liver large or small?
Spleen?
Collateral veins
Ascites
Small testes
Absent or reduced hair
Liver palms
Dupuytren's contracture
Clubbing
Opaque nails
Hepatic flap?
Oedema
Purpura
Liver soles

Fig. 4.11 The possible stigmata of hepatic cirrhosis.

Clubbing is of uncertain cause and seen most commonly in primary biliary cirrhosis.

Spider naevi consist of a dilated subcutaneous arteriole with a series of radiating vessels around it. They are found in normal people and are of diagnostic importance only when there are many (>5) and when they are large. They are particularly common on exposed surfaces – face, neck, hands, arms, etc. – and are usually found on the trunk only above the nipples. They, and the erythematous palms (liver palms) found in cirrhosis, presumably depend on the presence of a vasodilator material in the bloodstream.

White, or opaque nails, sparse body hair and gynaecomastia in males, and, in the case of alcoholic cirrhosis. Dupuytren's contractures and enlarged parotid glands may be further cutaneous signs.

Other physical signs may include –

An enlarged, firm nodular liver (*Note:* the liver may also be small and percussion is therefore important).

Splenomegaly and dilated abdominal wall veins (portal hypertension).

Ascites.

Ankle swelling.

Icterus.

Anaemia.

A flapping tremor of the extended hands, hepatic fetor in the breath, confusion and stupor signify the presence of neurological complications, i.e. hepatic encephalopathy.

Investigations

1. There is often anaemia (normochromic), leucopenia and thrombocytopenia. These three are often related to splenic enlargement (hypersplenism).
2. Liver function tests show the following:

S. bilirubin	– mildly raised (see other types of cirrhosis).
Alk. phosphatase	– raised.
S. albumin	– lowered.
S. globulins	– raised.
S. transaminases, LDH, etc.	– raised.

3. Radiographs of the barium-coated oesophagus show varices and they may appear as filling defects in the gastric fundus, too. They may be detected by endoscopy.
4. A liver biopsy (which may be difficult to perform) may result in a small fragmented biopsy, but often gives clear evidence of cirrhosis.
5. Removal of bromsulphthalein (BSP) from the bloodstream by the liver is impaired so that a standard BSP test (5 mg of dye/kg body weight IV) shows a 45-minute retention in blood of more than five per cent.
6. Certain immunological reactions may be positive, e.g. rheumatoid factor, ANF, false positive WR, etc. These are related to the abnormally high globulins.

Complications

Variceal Haemorrhage. Reducing liver blood flow may rapidly produce hepatic failure (ascites, encephalopathy, deepening jaundice). Haemorrhage must be treated by liberal transfusion, the administration of vitamin K to correct coagulation problems, and vasopressin which, when given in an intravenous drip, reduces splanchnic arteriolar inflow and results in cessation of variceal bleeding. Sedatives and hypnotics must be avoided.

If the patient is thought to be suitable for surgical therapy a Sengstaken tube (a pneumatic tube which compresses oesophageal and gastric varices) may be passed and positioned to control haemorrhage. Operation is usually directed at the varices (oesophageal ligation), and with cessation of haemorrhage the patient may then require an elective portocaval or spleno-renal anastomosis (Fig. 4.12).

All shunt operations suffer from the fact that they deprive the damaged liver of portal blood. In this way they potentiate liver damage despite their beneficial effect of stopping variceal haemorrhage. The Warren distal spleno-renal shunt has been designed to encourage maintenance of portal venous blood flow, though technically a difficult operation to perform (Fig. 4.13).

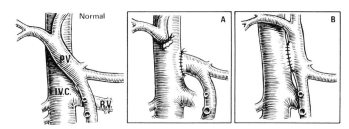

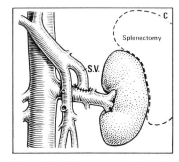

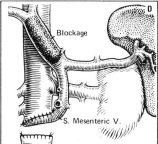

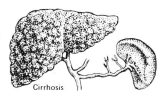

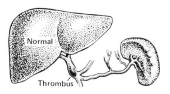

Fig. 4.14 Intra- and extrahepatic portal hypertension.

Cirrhosis	*Extrahepatic obstruction*
Abnormal liver	Normal liver
Abnormal liver function tests	Usually normal liver function tests
Prognosis for bleeding – poor	Prognosis for bleeding – good
Aetiology varied	Aetiology usually sepsis
Age group – adult	Age group – often children

Fig. 4.12 Shunt operations for portal hypertension.
A. End to side portocaval shunt
B. Side to side portocaval shunt
C. Spleno-renal shunt
D. Cavo-superior mesenteric shunt for extraheptic portal vein obstruction.
IVC = Inferior vena cava
PV = Portal vein
RV = Left renal vein
SV = Splenic vein.

Bleeding from oesophageal varices may occur because of portal venous occlusion often related to previous sepsis; the liver is then normal (Fig. 4.14). Though bleeding may be very troublesome and repeated, the prognosis for life is better because of the rarity of liver failure. Normal liver function tests, normal liver biopsy and the demonstration of a pressure difference between the portal venous pressure (intrasplenic pressure) and hepatic venous pressure (hepatic vein catheter) are

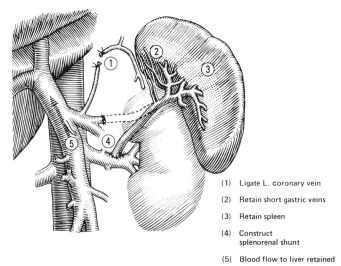

(1) Ligate L. coronary vein
(2) Retain short gastric veins
(3) Retain spleen
(4) Construct splenorenal shunt
(5) Blood flow to liver retained

Fig. 4.13 The Warren (distal spleno-renal) shunt.

helpful diagnostic aids, as may be a splenic venogram (injection of radiological contrast medium into the spleen with subsequent visualisation of the portal vein).

Ascites. This may appear slowly with gradually diminishing liver cell function or more rapidly after an acute liver insult such as an infection or an intestinal haemorrhage.

Symptoms. Abdominal swelling; abdominal pain; dyspnoea.

Physical signs. Distension of the abdomen; dullness to percussion in the flanks with central resonance; a fluid thrill (if ascites is tense); shifting dullness in both flanks.

There are also signs of chronic liver disease present with signs of effusion or collapse at the lung bases.

Differential diagnosis. Important differential diagnoses are ascites due to:
Carcinomatosis.
Meig's syndrome (in women).
Hypoproteinaemia (nephrotic syndrome, etc.).
Abdominal tuberculosis.
Heart failure (chronic severe right-sided failure, e.g. constrictive pericarditis).
Myxoedema (rarely).

Treatment. Treatment is with diuretics, that is unless the patient is acutely dyspnoeic or in great discomfort in which case a small paracentesis is indicated. A low sodium regime and a combination of diuretics which includes both frusemide, spironolactone or triamterene is often required. Too rapid a diuresis may be complicated by hepatic encephalopathy as may the biochemical disturbances (hyponatraemia and hypokalaemia) which accompany them.

Chronic ascites in liver disease is a sign of progressive liver cell damage. There is a 50 per cent two-year mortality, despite effective diuretic therapy.

Portosystemic Encephalopathy. Attacks of stupor, confusion and, eventually coma are a well-recognised complication of hepatic cirrhosis. The brain is poisoned by products of protein digestion and a variety of clinical signs may be recognised, including features of Parkinsonism, cerebellar ataxia, paraplegia, as well as bouts of coma. Thus, it may mimic a variety of neurological disorders. Hepatic fetor, a sweetish and not unpleasant though highly characteristic smell to the breath, and slow flapping tremor of the extended fingers are helpful signs, as is progressive slowing of the EEG rhythmic activity.

Important precipitants of hepatic encephalopathy are:

An intestinal haemorrhage.
Diuretic therapy.
Narcotic drugs.
Dietary (high protein) indiscretion.
In chronic cases a large portosystemic shunt, e.g. a portocaval anastomosis.

Treatment is by absolute protein restriction – intravenous carbohydrate (glucose 20 per cent) feeding and sterilisation of the large gut by neomycin, and the induction of diarrhoea with purgatives and colon washouts. In chronic cases protein restriction (50 g/day), neomycin 1 g six-hourly and lactulose (a non-absorbable disaccharide) may be helpful, and on occasions by-pass of the colon by ileo-rectal anastomosis may produce a dramatic improvement.

Hepatoma. Progressive deterioration of liver cell function, pain and an enlarging liver, perhaps with bouts of intestinal bleeding from varices, should suggest in a cirrhotic the possibility of a hepatoma. The presence of *a* feto protein in the patient's serum (detected immunologically) may be diagnostically helpful. These tumours metastasise locally, but unfortunately are often multicentric in origin. Treatment is unsatisfactory, but some relief of pain can be obtained with cytotoxic therapy.

In certain parts of the tropics and sub-tropics a high percentage of hepatoma patients may show positive HBsAg reactions for hepatitis B virus (HBV). The tumour can occur in an otherwise normal liver and it is far more common in male than female cirrhotics. In this respect it is of interest that the administration of androgenic hormones can, in susceptible males, produce this tumour.

Infection in the Cirrhotic – Diabetes. Infection of ascitic fluid must always be thought of in the ill cirrhotic with ascites, who presents with impending hepatic coma. Aspiration – culture and effective antibiotic therapy – may be life-saving. A tendency to diabetes is shown by abnormal glucose tolerance, and is seen in nearly one-third of cirrhotics. This may account for the not unusual finding of urinary infection. In the alcoholic, pneumococcal pneumonia and tuberculosis are common.

SPECIAL TYPES OF CIRRHOSIS (*see below*)

Cryptogenic	
Cause	Unknown – may follow drugs or hepatitis.
Age and sex	Female > male, middle age.
Presentation	Discovered accidentally or following onset of complications, e.g. bleeding, varices, jaundice, ascites, hepatic encephalopathy.
Diagnostic features	Non-specific.
Treatment	Of complications only.

Chronic active hepatitis	
Cause	Viral hepatitis (some are HBV +ve). A second type seems to be immunological and a third due to drugs, e.g. Aldomet.
Age and sex	The immunological variety is commonest in young adult females.
Presentation	With jaundice, hepatosplenomegaly and (in females) amenorrhoea. The immunological variety is a *multisystem disease* and there may be arthralgia, skin rashes, renal involvement, ulcerative colitis, etc.
Diagnostic features	(a) The liver biopsy is characteristic (plasma cell infiltrate, piecemeal necrosis, etc.). (b) There are immunological markers such as +ve LE cells, +ve DNA binding, +ve smooth muscle antibodies, etc. (c) The presence of multiorgan involvement may aid diagnosis.
Treatment	With corticosteroids clinical and biochemical evidence of liver cell damage reversible. Azathioprine may enable one to reduce the corticosteroid dosage which may produce some side effects.

Primary biliary cirrhosis

Cause	Probably an immunological destruction of small intrahepatic bile ducts.
Age and sex	Almost entirely a disease of middle-aged females.
Presentation	Usually with the features of mild obstructive jaundice and hepatosplenomegaly.
Diagnostic features	(a) Early on the liver biopsy may show granulomata related to damaged bile ducts. (b) The serum shows M (antimitochondrial antibodies in >90%per cent of cases and often to high titre. (c) Metabolic bone disease (vitamin D deficiency), peptic ulcer and Sjogen's syndrome and renal tubular acidosis are complications.
Treatment	To prevent complications (vitamin K injections and cholestyramine to treat pruritis.

Haemochromatosis

Cause	In the genetic form an inborn and excessive absorption of iron. A second form occurs in alcoholics who drink red wine (high iron content) and in patients with refractory anaemia.
Age and sex	Much more common in males – usually middle-aged or elderly. Primary forms show HLA A_3 in 70 per cent of cases.
Diagnostic features	Skin pigmentation, hepatomegaly, diabetes, hypogonadism. Elevated serum iron, transferrin and ferritin. Hepatoma more common than in most cirrhoses. Increased iron found in liver, bone marrow and urine.
Treatment	Venesection at weekly intervals until iron stores normal.

Alcoholic cirrhosis

Cause	Alcohol, but the precise cause of the cirrhosis, which is not found in all heavy alcoholics, is unknown.
Age and sex	More common in males, but incidence in women rising.
Presentation	If there is accompanying alcoholic hepatitis there is fever, leucocytosis, hepatomegaly and jaundice. Otherwise, it may present with intestinal bleeding or ascites. Other features include Dupuytren's contractures parotid enlargement, peripheral neuropathy and delirium tremens (DTs). Histologically fatty change, alcoholic hepatitis and cirrhosis may all be found, The perinuclear cytoplasm of some hepatocytes may show. Mallory's alcoholic hyaline – common in, but not specific for, alcoholic liver disease.
Treatment	Obvious, but very difficult.

Wilson's disease

Cause	An inherited disorder of copper metabolism with resultant copper deposition in the tissues.
Age and sex	In children and young adults.
Diagnostic features	Signs of cirrhosis in a young person, particularly if there is evidence of tremor, involuntary movements, Kayser-Fleischer rings. A high urinary and liver copper and a low copper-binding protein caeruloplasmin. Aminoaciduria, bone disease and haemolytic anaemia are further features.
Treatment	Chelation of copper with D penicillinamine produces marked CNS improvement.

MALABSORPTION SYNDROMES

Definition

A series of acquired and congenital disorders of the small bowel associated with impaired absorption of carbohydrate, protein, fats, vitamins, electrolytes and water, either singly or collectively, with resultant variable clinical presentation.

Background

The small bowel, by means of its length, mucosal folds, villi and microvilli is ideally adapted for the absorption of nutriments from the intestinal lumen. Three major processes are involved.

Simple Diffusion. A process of limited importance except for low molecular weight water-soluble substances. The process requires no chemical energy and is equally well achieved in any part of the small bowel, where it can occur only if there is a concentration gradient from intestinal lumen to bloodstream, i.e. it is 'downhill'.

Active Transport. This is the mechanism responsible for the bulk of absorption, i.e. fat, protein, carbohydrate, water, electrolytes. It may be concentrated or performed with greater facility in one region of the small bowel.

The process occurs against a concentration gradient – it requires chemical energy, and, in some instances, is thought to involve participation by a 'carrier protein' system (which is Na-dependent) to transport nutriments across the enterocyte from luminal to serosal surface.

Facilitated Diffusion. The importance of this process is unknown, but the name is given to the absorptive process which occurs at a rate faster than could be explained by diffusion alone, but which still cannot occur against a concentration gradient.

Absorption of Individual Nutriments

Fats (mainly dietary, long-chain triglycerides) undergo lipolysis (lipase) to long-chain fatty acids and monoglycerides. These cross the luminal border of the enterocyte as micelles – packages of fat held in solution by bile salts and lecithin. Inside the cell re-esterification to neutral fat takes place and absorption is as chylomicrons into the portal lymphatics.

Carbohydrates. Polysaccharides are split to disaccharides (amylase). Enzymes in the brush border (microvilli) split the dietary disaccharides (lactose, sucrose, maltose) to monosaccharides. These are absorbed by active transport and with the help of a sodium-dependent carrier.

Proteins. These are split to polypeptides, peptides and amino acids, of which the L forms are most avidly absorbed. There seems to be competition between individual amino acids for absorption, presumably because of carrier competition. Absorption of peptides is also possible, and in the neonate whole protein can be absorbed as such. The enzymes responsible for protein absorption are the peptidases and trypsin. The latter is secreted as an inactive precursor from the pancreas (trypsinogen) and an intestinal activatory, enterokinase, produces the active enzyme.

A special note must be made of the specific site of absorption of vitamin B_{12} in the ileum. At this site vitamin B_{12} is split from its binding with intrinsic factor and is absorbed in its free state, before being rebound to transcobalamin. Vitamin B_{12} deficiency may therefore result from ileal resection – such as may occur with Crohn's disease. Bile salts – di- and trihydroxy conjugates with glycine or taurine – also depend on the integrity of the ileum for their absorption. Ileal disease produces depletion of the bile acid pool, luminal bile salt deficiency, and steatorrhoea, while leakage into the colon because of lack of an ileal absorptive mechanism produces an irritative watery colonic diarrhoea, 'cholerhoeic enteropathy'.

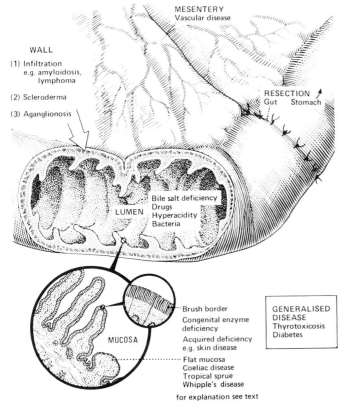

Fig. 4.15 The causes of malabsorption.

Pathological Anatomy

There are many causes of malabsorption (Fig. 4.15); they may be classified as follows:

In the Gut Lumen:

Deficiency of bile (bile salts) and pancreatic juice due to hepatic disease (usually cirrhosis) or pancreatic disease (usually chronic pancreatitis or, in childhood, fibrocystic disease of the pancreas). Certain drugs, e.g. neomycin, may produce malabsorption by interfering with bile salt function in the gut lumen, as does the hyperacidity of the Zollinger-Ellison syndrome.

Gut or stomach resection, which acts by reducing absorptive surface, increasing intestinal hurry and, in the case of gastric or ileal resection, interferes with vitamin B_{12} absorption.

A blind or stagnant loop syndrome. The area of stagnation in the small gut (which has a variety of causes, some of which are the aftermath of gastric or intestinal surgery) acts by encouraging bacterial growth which, in turn, deconjugate bile salts, rendering them less effective agents for fat absorption. The resultant luminal deficiency of conjugated bile salts and the inactivation of vitamin B_{12} results in both steatorrhoea and megaloblastic anaemia.

In the Gut Wall:

Abnormalities, either genetic or acquired, of the brush border result in malabsorption due to deficiency of carbohydrate splitting enzymes (disaccharidases). The increased luminal concentration of disaccharides then causes an osmotic diarrhoea, intestinal hurry, and steatorrhoea. Genetic and acquired deficiency of lactase (alactasia) is the most important member of this group of conditions.

Villous 'atrophy', badly named because there is probably, in many cases, increased cell loss rather than diminished production, is a feature of coeliac disease, tropical sprue and, possibly, an occasional complication of a number of other diseases, including neoplasia. Tropical sprue, which is endemic in parts of the Far East, is probably the result of bacterial damage to the small gut mucosa and it responds to folic acid and antibiotic treatment, though vitamin B_{12} deficiency is an important complication of tropical sprue. Whipple's disease is also infective in origin though the precise organism(s) has not been identified. Steatorrhoea is then accompanied by fever, joint pains, pigmentation of the skin, and lymphadenopathy. The villi may be swollen with material of bacterial origin which stains with the PAS (Periodic Acid Schiff) reagent.

Infiltration of the gut wall by amyloidosis – tumour, e.g. Hodgkin's disease, are also causes of malabsorption.

Extramural Disease. The lymphatics and blood vessels of the mesentery may become diseased either due to blockage or congenital absence of lymphatics (lymphangiectasia) or, in the case of the blood vessels, by disease of small blood vessels (polyarteritis nodosa) or atheronematous or thrombotic occlusion of the superior mesenteric arteries.

Certain Generalised Diseases. Severe skin disease, thyrotoxicosis, Addison's disease and hypogammaglobulinaemia (increased bacterial population of small gut) may also be associated with steatorrhoea.

Symptoms

Because of the wide variety of deficiencies that may result from malabsorption it is clear that symptomatology may be variable.

Diarrhoea, often with the characteristics of steatorrhoea (pale offensive sticky stools which may float and also require flushing several times to clear the toilet). (*Note:* steatorrhoea may be present when patients declare their stools to be normal.) Personal inspection is important. One unformed bowel motion a day may constitute the only abnormality of bowel function.

Ankle oedema, and on occasions ascites, signify malabsorption of protein or excessive faecal loss from mucosal exudation, or diminished production from accompanying liver disease (fatty infiltration).

Fatigue, lassitude and shortness of breath signify the presence of anaemia due to iron folate or B_{12} deficiency. A smooth tongue and, in the case of vitamin B_{12} deficiency, symptoms of paraesthesiae, ataxia and motor weakness suggest subacute combined degeneration of the cord. Deficiency of fat-soluble vitamins, particularly vitamins D and K, gives rise to bone pains (osteomalacia) and a haemorrhagic state with bruising, bleeding gums, etc.

Abnormalities of the absorption of water may be associated with nocturia.

Skin rashes of various types are often associated with malabsorption; one (dermatitis herpetiformis) is specifically associated with coeliac disease. Apart from this, pigmentation, eczema, and less specific abnormalities may occur.

Electrolyte abnormalities due to increased potassium, magnesium and calcium loss, and sodium and water retention, produce weakness, lethargy, muscular paralysis and tetany. Muscle weakness may affect intestinal smooth muscle with abdominal distension, vomiting, and a syndrome resembling intestinal obstruction.

Abdominal pain and gurgling are common in these patients, particularly if associated with malabsorption and intestinal strictures, e.g. Crohn's disease.

Signs

Clubbing.
Wasting.
Pallor.
Smooth tongue.
Neurological signs, e.g. peripheral neuritis.
Bone tenderness.
?Abdominal scars to suggest possible blind loop from previous surgery.
Oedema.
Distended 'boggy' abdomen on palpation.

Investigations (see page 95)

1. Anaemia is proven and characterised by blood film, marrow and serum iron, vitamin B_{12} and folate estimations.
2. Xylose absorption is low (and therefore renal excretion low) if 5 g of these substances are given by mouth. A two-hour and five-hour excretion figure may help distinguish upper from lower small bowel disease. Normal >23 and 35 per cent excretion, respectively.
3. A fat balance on a fixed dietary intake of fat shows increased daily excretion (>23 mmol (5 g)/24 hours) and in severe cases is usually greater than 200 mmol (44 g)/day. In cases of blind loop syndrome or pancreatic disease, repetition of the test showing diminished fat excretion after antibiotics or pancreatic extract therapy helps to support these diagnoses.
4. A Schilling or Dicopac test shows diminished vitamin B_{12} absorption in severe coeliac disease (ileal

involvement), gastric resection, tropical sprue and blind loop syndrome. The latter shows correction after antibiotic therapy.
5. Intestinal biopsy with a Crosby capsule or similar apparatus is of most value in the diagnosis of subtotal villous atrophy – usually, in Britain, due to coeliac disease. Histology may also be very helpful in other rare diseases, e.g small bowel amyloidosis, Whipple's disease and lymphangiectasia.
6. Serum electrolyte determinations are important in the detection of potassium and magnesium deficiency and in the diagnosis of metabolic bone disease (osteomalacia). This may be verified by bone biopsy.
7. Radiology is of value as a screening test when flocculation of the barium medium used may be suggestive of the presence of malabsorption, but on occasions these signs may be present without evidence of malabsorption. Radiology is, however, extremely effective in the detection of any area of localised abnormality associated with malabsorption, such as Crohn's disease or a stagnant loop syndrome. Radiology of bones (signs of osteomalacia), chest (e.g. fibrocystic disease), or abdomen (calcification of the pancreas) may all be helpful.

Individual types of malabsorption will require extra investigations to verify their presence, for example:

1. Blind Loop (Stagnant Loop) Syndrome:
Urine for increased bacterial breakdown products of dietary tryptophan, i.e. indoxyl sulphate (indican).
Culture (aerobic and anaerobic of intestinal juice).
Chromatography of intestinal juice for deconjugated bile salts.
A breath test following ^{14}C labelled bile salts (^{14}C glycocholate) may detect increased and early excretion of [14]CO_2 in the patient's breath.

2. Pancreatic Deficiency:
Tests of exocrine (Lundt test meal and pancreozymin/secretin test) and endocrine (glucose tolerance) function.
Sweat test (to exclude fibrocystic disease).
Scintiscanning.
ERCP.

3. Whipple's Disease:
Small bowel biopsy and culture.
Lymph node biopsy.

4. Alactasia:
Lactose and glucose/galactose tolerance tests. Small bowel biopsy for histology and enzyme studies.
The blood glucose should rise 20 mg or more after 50 g of lactose if lactase is present in normal amounts in the gut wall. A confirmatory rise of glucose/galactose should also be obtained after a load of each, confirming the absence of monosaccharide malabsorption. A barium X-ray showing malabsorption pattern can often

be shown in lactase-deficient subjects by adding lactose to the radio-opaque medium. A breath test using ^{14}C lactose may in alactasia show reduced and delayed $^{14}CO_2$ excretion.

5. Lymphangiectasia of the Gut:
Small bowel biopsy.

Basis of Treatment

Most patients with malabsorption need dietary treatment in order that diarrhoea may be controlled. Further, adequate supplement of fat-soluble vitamins and haematinics are required to prevent important deficiencies. A basic diet for patients with malabsorption would therefore be low in fat (40 g/day) and would allow a high intake of protein (>100 g/day). Carbohydrate may cause increased osmotic diarrhoea and colonic fermentation so that it needs to be supplied in normal or reduced amounts. In patients with lactase deficiency (brush border disease) a diet low in milk and dairy products reduces the intake of dietary milk sugar (lactose) and can help in the control of diarrhoea in this condition. A basic low fat, high protein diet is well tolerated but is expensive for the patient and must be reinforced with vitamin D 100,000 units intramuscularly each month, vitamin K 10 mg intramuscularly once a month and with ferrous sulphate and folic acid. Vitamin B_{12} supplements are required in patients with a blind loop syndrome and in those with ileal disease or resection. There are also a few patients with severe coeliac disease associated with ileal mucosal damage where it is also required. Failure of diarrhoea to respond to fat restriction is an indication for oral codeine phosphate (30 mg three times a day) or diphenoxylate (Lomotil) 5 mg three times daily or loperamide 2 mg three times a day. Failure of the patient's condition to respond to fat restriction, particularly if there is gross wasting, would be an indication for using oral medium chain triglycerides which can be absorbed, in the absence of bile salts and lipase, directly into the blood (portal) stream. A suitable preparation is obtained from coconut oil in a daily dosage of 90 ml.

Severe diarrhoea in patients with ileal disease or resection should suggest the possibility of bile salts entering the colon and producing watery explosive diarrhoea (cholerrhoeic enteropathy). This may respond dramatically to the oral bile salt chelating agent cholestyramine (4 g three times daily before meals). It is valueless for other types of diarrhoea.

Other varieties of malabsorption demand special treatment. A gluten-free diet is indicated only in coeliac disease, there being no other condition where a beneficial effect is obtained. Antibiotics are particularly valuable in tropical sprue, Whipple's disease, and in patients with a blind loop syndrome. Sulphonamides, tetracycline, ampicillin and lincomycin (the latter being particularly valuable in the treatment of anaerobic bacterial colonisation of a stagnant loop syndrome) may be given in one or more courses, while in other cases surgical correction may be possible. Lincomycin may cause severe diarrhoea in some patients where it produces a membranous enterocolitis. It must be used with great caution. Pancreatic steatorrhoea responds to oral replacement therapy and preparations such as Nutrizym, which can be taken as one to two tablets with each main meal, are very useful.

COELIAC DISEASE (NON-TROPICAL SPRUE; GLUTEN-SENSITIVE ENTEROPATHY)

Definition

A disorder of the small bowel associated with malabsorption and accompanied by small intestinal mucosal damage and sensitivity to dietary gluten.

Background

The precise cause of this disorder is unknown, but a certain number (about 30 per cent) of patients have suffered from childhood coeliac disease and in 5 to 10 per cent there is evidence of genetic predisposition. The distribution of the HLA antigens in coeliac disease differs from that in normals and an increased incidence of HLA B8 and HLA DW3 is found. The classical observation by Dicke in Holland during the Second World War indicated that the disease was aggravated by wheat germ protein, gluten. The cause of the abnormal reaction to this protein is unknown, but currently there would appear to be two possibilities. One has been that intestinal mucosal deficiency of a peptidase allows the absorption of harmful peptides which cause mucosal damage. Certainly, estimations of various mucosal enzymes are low, but correction of the disease by gluten restriction is associated with elevation of mucosal peptidase levels to normal, which makes primary enzyme deficiency unlikely. More likely is the second possibility, that gluten produces a cellular type of immune damage in the intestinal mucosa, and it is this reaction which alters the mucosa. There is evidence that lymphoreticular function is abnormal in a percentage of patients with coeliac disease, a factor that might explain a tendency to neoplastic disease in some patients. It has been estimated that 1:2,000 of the population in England have coeliac disease, but mild cases may be undiagnosed.

Pathology

The essential pathology is confined to the small intestine, which shows thinning of the wall and dilatation. Changes are maximal in the jejunum and decrease distally. In some cases the gut may be pigmented, 'brown bowel syndrome' (a possible manifestation of vitamin E deficiency). The mucosa of the small bowel

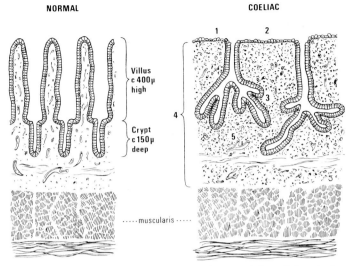

Fig. 4.16 The coeliac mucosa. 1. An abnormal 'brush border'; 2. Loss of villi; 3. Increased depth of crypts; 4. Increased mucosal thickness; 5. An inflammatory exudate.

shows loss, or gross stunting, of villi with deep hyperplastic crypts and increased cellular infiltrate in the lamina propria (Fig. 4.16) resulting in increased thickness of the submucosal layer. Under the microscope there is disorganisation of the columnar epithelial lining, and damage to the brush border (microvilli). In chronic cases the spleen and lymphoid tissue may be atrophic (spleen 5 to 10 g in weight).

Though in the past the villous deformity has been termed 'atrophy', there is good evidence to show a hyperdynamic state of cellular maturation and exfoliation.

Symptoms

There may be few symptoms in mild cases or when the onset has been insidious. A history of family involvement is important, as is the enquiry for childhood involvement. The age of onset is variable, usually from 30 onwards. Symptoms may be referable to:
Diarrhoea. Stools are loose, pale, bulky, offensive and possibly difficult to flush away. There may be only one stool daily and, as patients often declare that motions are 'normal', do not be put off.
Loss of weight and strength. These result from intestinal loss, together with anorexia, and may be profound. Hypokalaemia may be a further cause of weakness.
Tiredness, palpitations and dyspnoea may be symptoms of anaemia. This is due to failure to absorb haematinics and to their loss from cell exfoliation. Folate and iron deficiency are particularly common. Vitamin B$_{12}$ deficiency is less common, because often the ileum is normal.
Skin rashes of various types, including eczema and more specifically dermatitis herpetiformis may be seen, and vitamin B deficiency may cause skin lesions and glossitis.
Bone disease and tetany may be due to a combination of vitamin D deficiency due to malabsorption, increased calcium loss in intestinal secretions and impaired parathyroid function. In the bones, a combination of osteoporosis, osteomalacia, and secondary tertiary hyperparathyroidism may be seen.
Oedema. Ankle oedema and, more rarely, ascites may accompany the hypoproteinaemia of severe coeliac disease.
Chronic aphthous ulceration of the mouth may occur.

Some patients may only become symptomatic when they are stressed in various ways (Fig. 4.17).

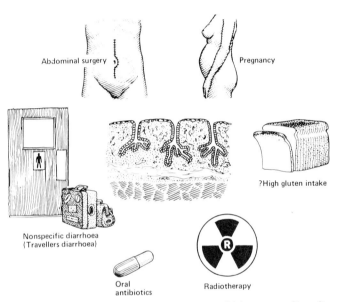

Fig. 4.17 Some events that may 'unmask' latent coeliac disease.

Signs

The following physical signs may be found:
General: Wasting, oedema, pigmentation, finger clubbing, anaemia.
Abdomen: Distension 'doughy'.
Tongue: Glossitis – looks red, smooth and raw.

Investigations

In mild cases physical signs may be non-existent and special procedures may be required.
1. A blood count, serum iron, folate, vitamin B$_{12}$, and bone marrow puncture help to identify the presence and characteristics of anaemia. Most untreated patients have a low serum and red cell folate which are worthwhile screening tests.
2. Xylose absorption, glucose tolerance test, fat balance and intestinal radiology to identify a malabsorption process.
3. Small intestinal biopsy (Crosby capsule) to identify

the disease as coeliac disease. (*Note:* In Great Britain severe mucosal 'atrophy' in a jejunal biopsy usually denotes coeliac disease, as tropical sprue is rare).

4. Serum electrolytes (particularly serum potassium), calcium, phosphorus, alkaline phosphatase and possibly bone needle biopsy to detect mineral deficiency and latent and manifest bone disease. This may also be detected by radiology.

5. Serum proteins and immunoglobulin determinations. Both a low serum albumin and IgM deficiency are commonly seen.

Complications (Fig. 4.18)

COMMON		UNCOMMON
Anaemia		Depression
Bone disease & electrolyte (K) deficiency		Neuromyopathy
		Neoplasia
Wasting		Intestinal pseudo-obstruction
Tetany		
Infection		Infertility

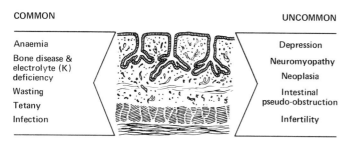

Fig. 4.18 The complications of coeliac disease.

The complications of this disease are many. Some have been mentioned and form part of the malabsorptive process. Others are of unknown cause and in particular, malignant lymphoma and neurological disorders fall into this category. Malignant disease usually involves the gut, is rapidly fatal, and may be related to incomplete treatment by gluten restriction. It causes abdominal pain, perforation (due to rupture of neoplastic ulcers), and a return of the symptoms of malabsorption. Various neurological sequelae are described, including proximal myopathy, cerebellar degeneration, peripheral neuritis, depression, epilepsy, etc. These complications, with the exception of depression, may not respond to gluten restriction. Of special importance is a small group of patients with coeliac disease who fail to respond to gluten restriction. In fact, some or all of these patients may not have coeliac disease, for some histological differences have been commented on by Creamer who claims that these patients may have a thinner mucosa with absent Paneth cells and shallow crypts. Paneth cells may in some way control cellular differentiation in the crypts of Lieberkühn, and in coeliac disease there is a greater exfoliation of cells into the gut lumen than normal. Certainly, the mucosa is hyperactive in most patients, cell loss returning to normal with gluten restriction, and this may be of some diagnostic importance in telling classical coeliac disease from other diseases where the mucosa is flat but not hyperactive.

Of recent interest has been the observation that two-thirds of patients with the skin disorder dermatitis herpetiformis (DH) have malabsorption which in some cases is associated with a flat intestinal mucosa and a complete response to gluten withdrawal. The probable explanation lies in a genetic predisposition to both disease, DH and coeliac disease being located in adjacent chromosomal loci.

Differential Diagnosis

This is best considered by studying the list of disorders associated with malabsorption. Intestinal biopsy and, in particular, a clinical and histological response to gluten restriction are the most important factors.

Abdominal distension and vomiting in the severely ill coeliac may make the diagnosis of intestinal obstruction likely. Surgical therapy must be avoided, if possible, in these circumstances.

Basis of Treatment

The basis of treatment is the removal of gluten from the diet. This means that all articles made from wheat flour, including bread, pastry, biscuits, are forbidden and replaced by similar products made from gluten-free flour. A host of tinned goods contain sauces, and thickenings made with flour and these are similarly excluded. Even one biscuit made with wheat flour may be enough to induce a relapse, but otherwise if the diagnosis is correct the patient responds by recovering lost weight, a disappearance of diarrhoea, and a loss of the deficiencies produced by malabsorption. Improvement is usually obvious within two to three weeks, but, especially in adults, this may be delayed for up to six months. In elderly patients with mild symptoms there may be a place for treatment without gluten restrictions. The regime then includes:

A low fat (<40 g/24 hour) and high protein (>100 g/24 hour) diet.
Extra iron, calcium and folic acid.
Extra vitamin D by IM injection.

Until the relationship of neoplasia to gluten restriction is decided, it is wise to insist that most coeliacs stay on full gluten restriction for life. In any case it is important to review patients regularly, to make sure with a dietician that gluten restriction is complete. In childhood, it is mandatory because of the danger of failure of growth, but there is a danger that the teenager enjoying the natural remission of the disease that is seen after puberty may decide to give up dietary treatment. In female patients a relapse in pregnancy is a common complication (*see* Fig. 4.17).

In those with severe symptoms and a failure of gluten restriction the diagnosis must be reviewed, the degree of gluten restriction checked, and complications such as neoplasia considered. Corticosteroids are then useful, and a full response to these agents can sometimes be obtained. Much helpful information on dietary and other matters for ambulant patients can be obtained by their joining the local Coeliac Society.

Prognosis

Patients responding to therapy should have a normal span of life, but the risk of oesophageal and abdominal neoplasia is always a possibility even twenty or more years after the diagnosis has been made. The tumour in the abdomen is usually a non-Hodgkin lymphoma arising in the small gut wall. It is rapidly fatal and produces symptoms due to intestinal obstruction and perforation.

CROHN'S DISEASE

Definition

A chronic granulomatous disease of the small and large bowel of uncertain cause which tends to affect multiple segments, to produce thickening of the bowel wall, and to be complicated by abscess and fistula formation.

Background

First identified by Crohn, Ginzburg and Oppenheimer in the USA in 1932, this disease is world-wide, commoner in whites than non-whites and certainly commoner in Jews. There has been much speculation about its aetiology, but at the time of writing great interest centres about the possibility that the disease is due to a transmissable agent, presumably a virus, for it can be produced in mice by inoculation of Crohn's tissue from sufferers with the disease.

Other factors may be important. Cases within a family group or in identical twins which are well recorded may suggest common genetic or environmental factors; the latter would include, for example, susceptibility to infection. There has been much work suggesting the importance of immunological factors, notably from a study of the pathology (lymphoid infiltration and granuloma formation) and from impaired delayed hypersensitivity (skin testing with tuberculin, sarcoid antigen and DNCB (dinitro-1-chlorbenzene), etc.).

The low incidence of serum antibodies to a variety of organs does not, however, suggest an autoimmune basis.

There may well be some aetiological significance in the production, in the experimental animal, of lesions similar to Crohn's disease by oral feeding of sand and talc. Lymphatic obstruction and oedema may result, and these are important histological features of Crohn's disease where submucosal oedema contributes to the thickening of the bowel. Infection of the bowel by *Yersinia enterocolitica* produces a similar type of lesion, and this disease must be excluded by serology. The disease seems uncommon in England, but commoner in Scandinavia and North Europe.

Pathology

Commonest in the ileum, and perhaps related to the abundant lymphoid tissue, the disease is submucosal and though deep ulceration may occur, the striking feature is thickening of the gut wall with reduction of the intestinal lumen. The histology shows prominent granulomata with giant cells in up to two-thirds of cases, oedema, and lymphocyte and plasma cell infiltration. Skip areas, i.e. areas of normal bowel separated by segments of thickened bowel, are characteristic of the disease. There may be extensive lymph node involvement.

Table 4.8 Crohn's disease

		Symptoms	Signs
Two-thirds	Ileal	Malaise pyrexia Colic diarrhoea Anorexia Weight loss	Nil or palpable RIF mass Anal disease
	Jejunal	Malaise pyrexia Colic diarrhoea Anorexia Malabsorption (steatorrhoea, sore tongue, oedema, etc.)	Abdominal mass Anal disease
One-sixth	Large bowel	Diarrhoea Urgency of defaecation Weight loss Bleeding	Anal disease Palpable colon Abnormal mucosa on sigmoidoscopy Hyperaemia Oedema Ulceration Cobblestone mucosa
One-sixth	Large and Small bowel	As in large bowel	

Symptoms and Signs

The disease can affect any part of the gut from oesophagus to anus, but in general the types set out in Table 4.8 are recognised.

The diagnosis may on occasions be very difficult and the clinical presentation can be as a pyrexia of unknown origin, as a problem of weight loss and hypoproteinaemia, as failure of growth in children, as oedema, or as a lesion mimicking acute appendicitis, ulcerative colitis (colonic Crohn's) or even duodenal ulcer. Involvement of perianal skin, and the mouth, where ulcers and hypertrophic gingivitis may occur, are now well recognised manifestations outside the gut.

Investigations

1. A blood count may show anaemia (due to iron, folic acid and, in ileal disease, vitamin B_{12} deficiency). Sometimes a non-specific normochromic anaemia is found.

The plasma viscosity is nearly always raised and there may be a polymorphonucleocytosis. The faecal occult blood may be positive.

2. In patients with jejuno/ileal disease the biochemical features of malabsorption (e.g. steatorrhoea, diminished D-xylose excretion, etc.) may be present.

3. The liver function tests may be abnormal, either because of fatty infiltration of the liver or hepatic cirrhosis.

4. Radiology of the intestinal tract may show abnormal mucosal patterns with gross narrowing in some areas (string sign). In other areas there may be an abnormal mucosa or a non-specific picture of malabsorption. Sharp fissures and fistula formation may produce further changes, and in the large bowel a coarse mucosal pattern, stricture formation, and ulceration are typical.

5. Biopsy. Helpful diagnostic information may be obtained from diseased bowel or from the rectum (mucosal biopsy) or anal ulcers and skin tags, even when the rectum and large bowel are apparently unaffected. A peroral small bowel mucosal biopsy is, on the other hand, rarely of value. In large bowel disease, anal lesions are present in 80 per cent of patients and some sort of histological help may often be obtained. Laparotomy may be required for diagnosis.

Complications and Associated Disorders (see Fig. 4.19)

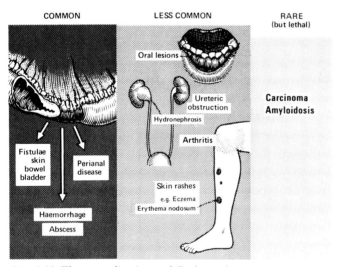

Fig. 4.19 The complications of Crohn's disease.

Differential Diagnosis

When radiological findings of small bowel Crohn's disease are clear-cut there is usually no diagnostic problem, but without this evidence, and particularly where there is malabsorption, a list of conditions may be simulated (see page 74). On the whole, the rule malabsorption + pain = Crohn's, is not a bad rule in the UK. In large bowel disease, the differentiation from ulcera-

tive colitis may on occasions be not only difficult but impossible. In more classical cases the features are easily distinguishable. In the large bowel in particular, neoplasms and diverticular disease must be excluded. Yersinia enterocolitica infection and intestinal tumours and tuberculosis also need careful consideration.

Basis of Treatment

Medical and surgical treatment both have a part to play in the treatment of this disease and patients are best treated by a team comprising an interested physician and surgeon.

In acute disease it is important to rest the patient in bed, and equally important to make sure that nutrition is adequate to prevent and combat hypoproteinaemia and wasting. A high protein diet with extra supplements of protein in the form of Casilan, added vitamins (particularly vitamin B_{12} for ileal disease or resection), haematinics and, in patients with steatorrhoea, the introduction of medium-chain triglycerides and reduction in normal dietary fat may all be required. If anorexia is severe, intravenous feeding and albumin infusions may bring about a dramatic improvement.

The decision whether or not to use corticosteroids depends on the severity of the patient's symptoms and the degree of relief of symptoms by simpler means. Diarrhoea often responds to codeine phosphate, and abdominal colic to antispasmodic drugs, but persistence of symptoms and systemic effects may be an indication for their use. They should certainly be considered:

(a) When general ill health is present despite control of other symptoms.

(b) In the presence of malabsorption or extensive bowel disease.

(c) Following previous surgery when symptoms have recurred.

In general, patients with large bowel disease often complicated by fistula formation and perianal infection do poorly on corticosteroids, while many patients with small bowel disease show a remarkable improvement. Treatment begins with oral prednisolone 30 to 40 mg daily, reducing to 5 to 15 mg daily. Complications include abscess formation, fistula formation and, in young patients, retardation of growth. Long term treatment is often required, though in some it may be possible to employ multiple short courses. There is no good evidence to suggest that salazopyrine has a part to play in the treatment of this disease. Recently, severe cases refractory to corticosteroids have been treated with some success with immunosuppressive drugs, for example, azathioprine.

Surgery is best avoided unless there is evidence of intestinal obstruction, fistula formation, or abscesses. Occasionally, surgery is required in order to verify the diagnosis and to treat obstruction or infection, but in general it is best reserved until after corticosteroid therapy has been tried. Resection is now preferred to short-circuiting, provided sufficient healthy bowel can be left behind and that division of a small or large bowel is through healthy tissue. On the whole, the chances of recurrence are less after resection than after a diversion operation. In the case of colonic disease, resection with anastomosis to healthy bowel is usually possible, but in total colonic disease or with disease restricted to the rectum, ileostomy may be the only feasible surgical therapy. Ileal disease may, on occasions, mean a resection of ileum as well, and ileostomy dysfunction and nutritional difficulties may then be encountered. In disease confined to the colon, recurrence in the small bowel is unusual, and ileostomy is more easily embarked on. In general, chronic perianal fistulae and sepsis will not heal unless diseased bowel is removed.

Prognosis

Crohn's disease tends, in a high percentage of cases, to be progressive. Thus, of those severe enough to come to laparotomy 50 per cent will have further trouble and of these about 25 per cent will require further surgery. This is then adequate reason for reserving surgery until the indications for it are clear-cut. Patients particularly at risk for recurrent disease are those where there is disease of a considerable length of small bowel, or extensive lymph node involvement, or, possibly, when the patient is young.

Though many patients will lead a stormy existence and require corticosteroids and/or surgery, in many cases the disease eventually remits.

ULCERATIVE COLITIS

Definition

An acute inflammatory disease of the colonic mucosa associated with diarrhoea and rectal bleeding and a tendency to progress to chronic disease.

Background

Early workers, impressed no doubt by the acute inflammatory reaction in the colon in bacillary dysentery, thought this disease was of bacterial origin, but no pathogen either bacterial or viral has been isolated. There followed a period in which the disease was attributed directly to psychological causes, which was backed up by the observed, and perhaps not surprising, degree of mental disturbance seen in the ill, colitic patient. It is now recognised that much of this change is the result rather than the cause of the disease, though chronic stimulation of the parasympathetic nerve supply to the colon in the experimental animal can produce hyperaemia and ulceration of the large gut.

Present thought concerning this disease centres about its being caused by immunological damage, though psychological factors are of importance in relapses and

there is an important increased familial incidence of the disease. Roughly, 1 in 1,000 of the population are affected, and evidence in support of autoimmunity comes from the identification of serum antibodies to extracts of germ-free colonic mucosa in patients with the disease and, also, evidence that the lymphocytes from the blood of colitics produces cytopathological changes in tissue culture of colonic cells. Further support comes from the increased evidence of other 'allergic' and autoimmune disorders in the patients and their relatives, and from the response to immunosuppressive therapy. The disease is commoner in women than men (ratio 3:2) and though no age group is exempt the majority of patients are between 20 and 50 years of age at the start of the disease. A second smaller peak of incidence is seen in the elderly. Jews seem to have an increased incidence of the disease which is, on the whole, one of the developed rather than the developing countries.

Pathology

The colonic mucosa is inflamed and haemorrhagic. There may be ragged mucosal ulceration. The extent of the disease is variable, ranging from rectal to total colonic involvement. Due to incompetence of the inflamed ileo-caecal valve, there may be inflammation and dilatation of the terminal ileum. Histology shows loss of superficial epithelium, crypt abscesses, i.e. polymorph infiltration around the gland crypts, with rupture and spreading inflammation either into the gland lumen or under the mucosa. There is congestion and polymorph infiltration of the mucosa, spreading through, in severe examples, to the peritoneal coat. Surviving islands of mucosa may undergo hyperplastic change in chronic cases (pseudopolypi), while with total colonic involvement of some duration, gland metaplasia and premalignant polypoid changes may be seen with frank carcinoma, often multicentric.

Symptoms

These are proportional to the severity and extent of the colonic disease. The disease can be of acute catastrophic onset or of a continuous or remittent type. Attacks may occur following psychological disturbances such as the stress of pregnancy (usually the postpartum period), examinations, broken love affairs, bereavements, etc. The symptoms are:

Diarrhoea, up to ten or more stools containing blood and mucus.

Pain, hypogastric, relieved by defaecation and associated with urgency.

Weakness and wasting due to hypokalaemia, dehydration, and anorexia.

Fatigue, dyspnoea, and lassitude due to anaemia.

In proctitis, constipation with rectal bleeding may be present.

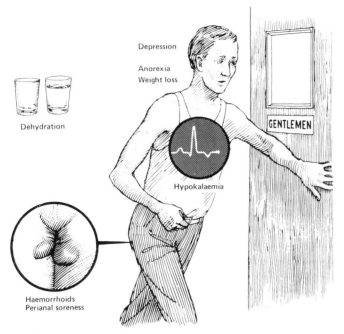

Fig. 4.20 The complications of diarrhoea.

Signs

These may be few and confined to pyrexia, pallor, wasting, clubbing of the fingers and abdominal tenderness over the colon. The colon is not usually palpable unless there is constipation or the diagnosis is Crohn's disease. There may be hepatomegaly and further signs produced by complications.

Investigations

1. Sigmoidoscopy. The diagnosis is suggested by the history and verified by the sigmoidoscopic findings. This is because the disease involves the rectum in nearly all cases. Involvement of the colon proximal to this site and without rectal involvement is usually a sign of Crohn's disease.

At sigmoidoscopy the rectal mucosa has lost its vascular pattern, is congested, friable, and shows a granular appearance. Frank ulcers are not usually conspicuous. Biopsy is helpful in mild cases and where there is confusion with Crohn's disease.

2. Barium enema. The extent of the disease is determined by barium enema examination or by colonoscopy. The colon becomes tubular, lacking haustral folds, and may show mucosal irregularity due to superficial ulcers on radiological examination. The abrupt demarcation between the diseased and normal bowel is often striking.

3. The degree of systemic illness is suggested by:

(a) Fever.

(b) A blood count – a low haemoglobin, increased white blood count and polymorph leucocytosis are signs of active disease.

(c) Serum proteins – low albumin, raised a_2-globulins indicate severe disease.

(d) Electrolytes. Low serum potassium is an indication of loss due to diarrhoea and poor intake from anorexia.

(e) Liver function tests other than the proteins, such as alkaline phosphatase, serum bilirubin and SGOT may all be abnormal if there is secondary hepatic disease.

Complications

Diarrhoea alone can cause complications but in ulcerative colitis these are numerous and can be local – in the gut, and systemic when their aetiology is uncertain (Figs. 4.20, 4.21).

Local. Perianal sepsis, haemorrhoids and fistulae are common, but the presence of the latter should alert one to the possibility of Crohn's disease. They may occur at any stage of the colitis.

Perforation. This is a serious complication usually seen in the patient with a first attack of severe total disease. Corticosteroid drugs are not causative, but may mask the symptoms. Treatment is surgical.

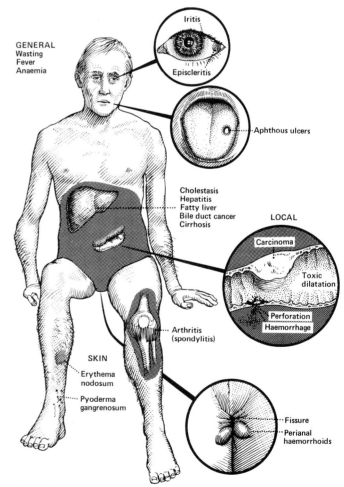

Fig. 4.21 Some complications of ulcerative colitis.

Haemorrhage. Massive haemorrhage is also a feature of severe disease. Treatment is by transfusion. Surgery may rarely be required.

Toxic dilatation. A most important complication for the physician to be aware of. The features are:
(a) Cause:
(i) Destruction of muscle and nerve plexuses by penetrating disease of the colonic wall.
(ii) Aggravating factors may be anticholinergic drugs, hypokalaemia, sigmoidoscopy and barium enema. Occasionally, incomplete faecal evacuation may be a cause.
(b) Symptoms:
'Toxaemia' – confusion.
Abdominal distension, abdominal pain, fever, vomiting, and sometimes diminution of diarrhoea. Serial plain radiographs are extremely helpful in making the diagnosis before distension is gross, and the increasing calibre of the gas-filled colon and, later, the ileum are well seen.
(c) Treatment:
Nasogastric decompression of the gut – complete cessation of oral feeding, IV therapy with fluids, electrolytes (especially potassium), antibiotics and corticosteroids is the initial treatment. If no clinical or radiological improvement is seen in 48 hours, surgery is indicated as an emergency. Perforation may complicate this situation; the mortality is about 25 per cent.

Carcinoma. This fatal complication occurs in patients with long-standing total colitis. It is seen in 20 per cent of patients after twenty years' total disease. There is grave diagnostic difficulty, and the tumour is often multicentric. Repeated barium enemas may not be helpful, though it has recently been claimed that premalignant change may be seen in rectal biopsy material. Undoubtedly, the prophylaxis of this fatal complication is colectomy for those with total disease of ten or more years' duration. The cancer risk in those with subtotal colitis is not much greater than in the general population and, thus, even with chronic disease there is no extra indication for surgery. An immunological test for serum colonic carcinoma antigens is available, but is not helpful in early diagnosis.

General:
(a) Anaemia is due to blood loss and marrow failure.
(b) Venous thrombosis, which is difficult to treat with anticoagulant drugs in the face of colonic bleeding, may cause fatal pulmonary embolism.
(c) Liver disease is of various forms, some of them 'autoimmune' in type, others related to wasting and portal bacteraemia. Fatty liver (the commonest), viral hepatitis, cirrhosis, chronic active hepatitis, cholestasis, bile duct cancer, and sclerosing cholangitis may all

occur. Colectomy may not prevent continuing liver damage.
(d) Skin involvement – erythema nodosum – pyoderma gangrenosum and leg ulcers usually occur when colitis is active.
(e) Arthritis, usually of the knees or ankles, coincides with attacks of colitis. Arthritis responds to colectomy. Ankylosing spondylitis, which also occurs, is not amenable to surgery, and ulcerative colitis is an important 'cause' of ankylosing spondylitis, particularly in females. HLA B27 is found in those who suffer from spondylitis.
(f) Eye lesions occur in about four per cent of sufferers, usually iritis or episcleritis.
(g) Mouth ulcers may also occur.

Differential Diagnosis

The important disorders to be considered are:
1. Dysentery and amoebiasis, usually in those who have returned from abroad.
2. Crohn's disease and colonic carcinoma and the rare case of radiation colitis.
3. In the elderly, ischaemic colitis may be a further possibility.

Radiology, sigmoidoscopy, colonoscopy and biopsy usually provide the answer, but there may be considerable confusion in distinguishing Crohn's disease of the colon from ulcerative colitis, and histological examination may not be helpful. Antibiotics are associated with diarrhoea and lincomycin and clindamycin in particular cause an acute membranous enterocolitis which can mimic ulcerative colitis.

Basis of Treatment

In acute cases, admission to hospital, correction of anaemia with iron therapy, and blood transfusion are required. A search for precipitating psychological factors is sometimes rewarding, and a sympathetic but firm liaison between patient and attending physician is important. Psychotherapy is occasionally required and sedation may be helpful. In severe examples of the disease, intravenous therapy with electrolyte solutions and added potassium are essential to combat intestinal losses. Antibiotics have little place in therapy except perhaps intravenously when acute dilatation of the colon has occurred.

Diarrhoea is treated with codeine phosphate, loperamide, or Kaolin and Morphine Mixture, BPC, and abdominal pains with antispasmodic drugs, for example Pro-Banthine 15 mg three times a day, remembering, however, the possible part that such therapy may play in the precipitation of toxic dilatation.

If bed rest, with a high protein diet supplemented with vitamins, intravenous therapy, correction of anaemia, and symptomatic treatment of diarrhoea fail to restore the patient quickly to good health, then there is no doubt that corticosteroid drugs (either ACTH or cortisone) are indicated. It was shown in the MRC trial of the early 1950s that corticosteroids produce a remission rate of 40 per cent in acute colitis, with a slightly higher figure for first attack remissions. Somewhat higher figures have been obtained with higher doses. Dosage should be prednisone 60 mg in divided doses daily, or 80 to 100 units of ACTH gel – or its equivalent as Synacthen. These drugs are diminished in dosage as a response is obtained. In acute disease, local corticosteroid therapy into the rectum, and salazopyrine are not so effective as in the chronic disease. The former is to be avoided because of the risk of toxic dilatation, and the latter because it may produce nausea, vomiting, and anorexia. In less severe cases, where out-patient treatment is possible, systemic corticosteroids may not be necessary. Then, rectal installation of corticosteroid enemas once, before retiring, may be enough, with anti-diarrhoeal measures to control the disease. This can be given most conveniently as Predsol enemas (i.e. prednisone 21-phosphate 25 mg in a disposable container) which, after simple instruction regarding positioning, can be used and retained by most patients.

The stand-by for chronic disease is oral salazopyrine, a combination of sulphapyridine and salicylic acid 2 or 3 g daily in divided doses. Though not infrequently producing anorexia and nausea, severe side effects, acute haemolytic anaemia and skin rashes, are uncommon. The best place for treatment with this drug seems to be as a way of preventing relapses in chronic disease and thus allowing patients to stop or reduce corticosteroid therapy.

Once the patient has been diagnosed as suffering from frank colitis a regular system of out-patient follow-up appointments is necessary to assess the severity and extent of the disease, regulate the dose of drugs, and to prevent complications of therapy. The establishment of a firm patient-doctor relationship, if possible with the same clinician at each appointment, is also important. Further barium and sigmoidoscopic studies are required to assess progress and detect possible carcinomatous change.

Patients with proctitis may need treatment for constipation rather than diarrhoea and are best treated with stool-softening agents such as a high fibre diet with added bran, with long term salazopyrine and rectal corticosteroid therapy in the form of enemata or suppositories. Even long term local therapy with prednisone runs some chance of suppressing adrenal corticosteroid rhythm and this type of therapy does not necessarily prevent relapses. Recently, in patients resistant to corticosteroids, there has been a tendency to use immunosuppressive therapy in the form of azathioprine, but this must be used only after careful consideration and when other treatments have failed to control or have produced dangerous side effects in the

patient with severe disease. Similarly, beneficial effects can be produced with oral sodium cromoglycate (Intal).

Surgery. This is indicated in the following situations:
1. In acute disease:
(i) For complications such as perforation and acute toxic dilatation of the colon.
(ii) For severe disease failing to respond to full medical treatment.
2. In chronic disease:
(i) If the patient's disease produces chronic ill health and loss of employment. Evidence of systemic complications is an important factor to be considered here.
(ii) In chronic total colitis, even if symptoms are not particularly severe, as a way of preventing or treating colonic carcinoma.

The operation is a removal of the colon with ileostomy (ileostomy and subtotal colectomy). In most cases the rectal stump is retained, to be removed at a second operation six months later. Impotence may follow this operation in young males and this may be an indication for retaining the rectal stump for a longer period of time, providing regular review is undertaken to detect rectal cancer.

Life with an ileostomy, provided it is fashioned correctly and sited properly (in the waistline to the left of the umbilicus) is perfectly compatible with a full and entirely normal life. In women, pregnancy is not contraindicated. Ileal effluent is collected in an adherent ileostomy bag changed every 48 hours and emptied through an opening at its lower end four-hourly.

The unfortunate patient may, particularly in the early months after surgery, have one or several bouts of ileostomy dysfunction with profuse loss of intestinal contents and resultant dehydration and mineral loss. This requires urgent correction.

Usually, the chronically ill colitic patient is vastly improved and entirely happy with the results of surgery, with gain in weight, and vigour and a vast improvement in mental adjustment to disease. The Ileostomy Association, a society composed of ex-patients who have had an ileostomy performed, is a helpful way of introducing patients in whom one is contemplating recommending surgery to well-adjusted members.

The alternative operation, ileo-rectal anastomosis and colectomy, should be mentioned. It is only occasionally possible, when the rectum is not severely diseased, but it obviously has the advantage that it is a way of preserving the normal excretory mechanism.

GASTROINTESTINAL CANCER

Though largely the province of the surgeon, at least as far as treatment is concerned, it is essential to include in a textbook of medicine for students an account of the symptomatology and pathology of the common gastro-intestinal tumours, as these are not uncommonly first seen by the physician where they may masquerade as cases of anaemia (due to intestinal blood loss), indigestion, and jaundice.

It is also important that the student tries to appreciate the magnitude of the problem of intestinal cancer, perhaps by remembering that over 40,000 new cases of primary cancer of the alimentary canal and accessory glands (pancreas, gall bladder, liver) occur in England and Wales each year (population, *c* 48 million) and, therefore, in this respect outnumber both bronchial and mammary tumours and, at the same time, account for about one-quarter of all malignant tumours. A brief review of the important lesions follows.

CARCINOMA OF THE OESOPHAGUS (*c* 2,500 new cases a year in England and Wales)

Usually, it is squamous cell, but occasionally an adenocarcinoma from gastric epithelium in the lower oesophagus, which causes stenosis of the oesophagus.

Background

The following are known to be important in the aetiology of oesophageal cancer:

(a) **Cancer of Upper Oesophagus:**
Chronic iron deficiency.

(b) **Cancer of Middle and Lower Oesophagus:**
Alcoholism.
Smoking.
Achalasia of the cardia.
Tylosis (a severe form of icthyosis – congenital thickening of the skin.
Coeliac disease.
The striking geographical variation and, in particular, the very high incidence in some African tribes, e.g. the South African Bantu, may be related to the ingestion in large amounts of home-produced alcoholic beverages. A similar finding around the Caspian Sea may be due to opium chewing.

Symptoms

Progressive, often painless dysphagia.
Loss of weight.
Sometimes 'vomiting' after meals (regurgitation of food).

Signs

None before spread to glands, liver, lungs, etc.

Investigations

1. Barium meal.
2. Endoscopy with biopsy.
3. Occasionally, lymph node biopsy.

Basis of Treatment

Carcinoma of the upper third is best treated by radiotherapy; the lower and middle third by surgical excision and re-anastomosis, or by replacement of the oesophagus by a colonic segment. Inoperable cases may be treated by intubation with a plastic tube to relieve dysphagia. This can now be inserted endoscopically without a formal operation.

Prognosis

Poor – if resection is possible, the five-year survival is 10 to 20 per cent.

CARCINOMA OF THE STOMACH (*c* 12,000 new cases/year)

An adenocarcinoma in most instances, with a variable stromal response so that polypoid, ulcerating, or diffusely infiltrating ('leather bottle stomach') forms are seen. Small early carcinomata found in the mucosa only, 'superficial cancer of the stomach', are also being found by endoscopy.

Background

The following are known to be of some aetiological importance:

(a) **Chronic Atrophic Gastritis and Gastric Atrophy.** The gastric cancer risk in pernicious anaemia is 10 to 20 times that in normal subjects. A significant increase is also present following gastrectomy when gastritis is found in the gastric stump.

(b) **Chronic Gastric Ulcer.** The risk is small, but unpredictable – even healing may occur in a malignant gastric ulcer. Most ulcerated cancers of the stomach are, however, neoplastic from the onset.

(c) **Gastric Polyps.** A small but definite risk of malignant change exists.

(d) **Blood Group A.** Confirmed by many observers – note increase of blood group A in pernicious anaemia. ?Related to change in gastric mucus structure or function.

Important epidemiological differences in incidence are found:
(a) Where the organic content of the soil is high (confirmed in certain parts of Wales and Netherlands).

(b) In the lower socio-economic groups where the incidence is high compared with executive and professional classes.

(c) In certain world populations. A very high incidence is found in Japan and Iceland, and a higher incidence in blacks in the USA compared with whites. Though dietary factors, e.g. high fish intake, could account for the finding in the first two groups, a better explanation is a genetic (hereditary) influence.

(d) Hereditary factors. In families of gastric cancer sufferers there is a four-fold increase of gastric cancer – genetic similarity is thus an important factor, perhaps tying in well with blood group studies.

Symptoms

Weight loss and weakness.
Epigastric pain or discomfort.
Vomiting.
Anorexia.
Dysphagia (fundal lesions).
Note: These may differ in no way in the early stages from simple 'indigestion'.

Signs

None, or
Loss of weight.
A palpable epigastric mass.
Enlarged left supraclavicular lymph nodes (Virchow's gland).
In advanced cases:
Malignant ascites.
Pelvic involvement (Krukenberg tumours).
Pyloric stenosis.
Jaundice (hepatic secondary deposits).

Investigations

1. Barium meal is likely to diagnose about 80 per cent of gastric cancers. Ulcers are often very difficult to diagnose as benign or malignant and another difficulty is the diffusely spreading variety ('leather bottle stomach') and those which are superficial only.
2. Fibre endoscopy with biopsy has a higher success rate.
3. Exfoliative cytology previously performed 'blind' on the aspirated gastric contents and now directly at endoscopy is worthwhile, provided a pathologist, skilled in cytology, is available.
4. Indirect evidence may be obtained from the occult blood reaction of the stools. The plasma viscosity is often, but not always, raised and achlorhydria may be present, but it is emphasised that achlorhydria is found in only 65 per cent of patients with gastric cancer and in any case is also a finding in 25 per cent of the general population over 50 years of age.

In patients in whom any doubt exists as to the presence or not of a gastric neoplasm, diagnostic laparotomy is indicated. In those with chronic peptic ulcer it is important to insist on complete healing before concluding that a gastric cancer is not present, and even then there may be doubt.

Basis of Treatment

Treatment is surgical, either partial or total gastrectomy, depending on the site and extent of the tumour. Unfortunately, total removal is often not possible, and for the 40 per cent in whom curative resection is possible five-year survival ranges from 14 to 60 per cent, depending on whether there are lymph node deposits. Superficial gastric cancer has a much more hopeful outlook, 90 per cent surviving five years after surgery.

CARCINOMA OF THE COLON AND RECTUM
(*c.* 17,000 new cases/year)

Background

An adenocarcinoma producing a local tumour, ulcer or stricture. Fifty per cent of large bowel cancer occurs in the rectum, while of the remainder there is a roughly equal distribution of growths between the ascending transverse and descending colons. There is little to be gained in a textbook of medicine from dividing these two major sites of growth, i.e. rectal and colonic.

The following are important aetiological factors:
(a) Total involvement of the colon by ulcerative colitis is associated with a rising incidence of colonic cancer. After 20 years of total colonic involvement the incidence is 20 per cent. The growths are often multiple.
(b) A rare familial disease, familial polyposis – inherited as a dominant autosomal lesion – is associated with an almost 100 per cent incidence of large bowel cancer in adult life. Prophylactic colectomy is therefore important.
(c) It becomes increasingly recognised that there is an important relationship between large bowel adenomatous polyps and carcinoma. They frequently occur together, and although there is no absolute proof that one is the precursor of the other, the polyp and the colonic carcinoma may well be grades of the same neoplastic change.
(d) The vast majority of colonic carcinomas are of no known cause. A recent theory to account for the higher incidence in Europe as opposed to Africa and India has been the greater anaerobic bacterial population in the gut in the former, perhaps related to dietary differences, particularly fat and fibre intake. This would give rise to altered bile salt deconjugation and degradation by anaerobic bacteria, with the possible production of potentially carcinogenic agents. Increased bowel transit time associated with a diet low in fibre would ensure prolonged mucosal contact with carcinogens.

Symptoms

None, or very few in the early stages.
Change in bowel habit – constipation and diarrhoea.
Pain – cramping and diffuse.
Fatigue, dyspnoea due to anaemia.
Loss of appetite and weight.
Particularly with rectal growths, blood and mucus in stools, sensation of incomplete evacuation.
Late symptoms include wasting, jaundice and ascites due to peritoneal and hepatic secondaries.

Signs

Pallor.
An abdominal mass.
In rectal carcinoma a mass in the rectum, blood and mucus on the finger cot.
(*Note:* 50 per cent of rectal cancers are palpable with the finger.)

Investigations

1. Sigmoidoscopy should demonstrate all rectal and many sigmoid growths. Its efficiency can be improved by examination under an anaesthetic and by fibre-optic colonoscopy. Biopsy of suspicious lesions is extremely helpful.
2. Barium enema is most helpful in the diagnosis of sigmoid and other colonic growths. Difficulties may arise because of incomplete preparation or inability of patients to retain barium. Difficulty is experienced, particularly with caecal tumours, where it is often impossible to tell the difference between faeces and a polypoid tumour.
3. The presence of positive OB tests in the faeces and of anaemia are non-specific, but the presence of intestinal bleeding without evidence of a lesion in the upper alimentary tract must alert one to the possibility of a tumour in the colon. Laparotomy may in such circumstances be the only feasible way to proceed.
4. A valuable test of the future may be the detection by simple immunological tests of colonic cancer antigens in the serum, but early promise has not been upheld and early disease is not so identifiable.

Basis of Treatment

In the case of colonic cancer this is essentially surgical, by resection of the right transverse descending or sigmoid colon with re-anastomosis. In those with colonic obstruction, proximal colostomy is followed by resection and re-anastomosis. In patients with rectal carcinoma, either abdominoperineal resection of the rectum with proximal colostomy or low anterior section (segmental resection) with primary anastomosis may be performed. This latter is indicated where there is 5 cm of uninvolved bowel and perirectal tissue below the lesion.

Prognosis

A 50 per cent five-year survival is usually quoted for colonic carcinoma, but early detection (so often difficult in view of the paucity of symptoms) is critical. Rectal cancer, depending on the spread of the tumour to neighbouring lymph nodes, has a five-year survival ranging from 30 to 70 per cent and is much influenced by the pathological grading of the tumour.

Villous Papilloma. These large tumours often become locally malignant. They are of concern to the physician because their mucus secretion contains abundant potassium, so that potassium depletion occurs, which causes apathy, muscular weakness, ileus, etc. It is a cause of potassium deficiency that must be thought of and felt for by rectal examination.

CANCER OF THE PANCREAS/AMPULLA OF VATER AND COMMON BILE DUCTS
(*c.* 4,000 new cases/year)

Adenocarcinoma in over 90 per cent of cases. There is no known aetiological factor either genetic or acquired, but a rising incidence in developed countries suggests the importance of diet, smoking and alcohol.

Pathology

Lesions in the pancreas are of the head, body or tail, while carcinomata of the bile duct are commonest below the cystic duct and in the common hepatic duct, particularly near the bifurcation.

Symptoms and Signs

Carcinoma of the head of the pancreas/ampulla of Vater and the common bile duct cause obstructive jaundice (*see* page 63). Differentiation between them is difficult, but ampullary lesions may particularly cause intestinal bleeding and radiological abnormalities of the duodenal loop. Carcinoma of the head of the pancreas, in addition to obstructive jaundice, may be associated with obstruction of the pancreatic duct system (raised serum amylase and onset of diabetes). Both these lesions may be associated with a positive Courvoisier's sign. Carcinoma of the hepatic duct above the cystic duct is not associated with gall bladder enlargement. Clear distinction between these lesions can usually be made via transhepatic cholangiography which is often performed prior to laparotomy, or, where facilities exist, by transduodenal catheterisation of the bile duct at fibre-optic duodenoscopy. Carcinoma of the body and tail of the pancreas are notoriously difficult to diagnose. Symptoms are vague: dyspepsia, flatulence, loss of weight, and backache. Sufferers are often labelled as neurotic, and with persistence of symptoms, a severe depressive illness may ensue. Physical signs are negligible and usually occur only when there is widespread dissemination. X-ray studies, for example coeliac axis angiography, may be helpful, but probably most help is from pancreatic, ultrasonic or computerised tomography (CT) scanning.

Basis of Treatment

All patients with obstructive jaundice must receive vitamin K 10 mg intramuscularly for several days to correct coagulation disorders. Postoperative renal failure is a further possible hazard and may possibly be prevented by the use of intravenous dextran.

Surgical resection is the only feasible treatment. Carcinoma of the head of the pancreas or ampulla, if resectable by a Whipple's operation (pancreatico-duodenectomy), carries a five-year survival of 18 per cent for the former and about twice this for ampullary lesions. If these conditions are not resectable, anastomosis of the gall bladder (above the obstruction) to the jejunum allows disappearance of jaundice and distressing pruritis. Carcinoma of the body and tail of the pancreas is usually inoperable and, as a result, prognosis is worse than that described above. On the other hand, a carcinoma of the bile duct may be extremely slow-growing though difficult to resect. Anastomosis of jejunum to the distended extra- or intrahepatic duct sytem above the growth may be possible, as may intubation of the malignant stricture.

CARCINOMA OF THE GALL BLADDER
(c. 600 new cases/year)

This is the commonest tumour of the biliary tract.

Background
Only one certain aetiological factor is recognised, namely, the importance of pre-existing gall bladder disease, particularly gallstones. It is estimated that 5 to 10 per cent of patients with gallstones develop a carcinoma.

Symptoms and Signs

There may be no clear-cut symptoms until spread of growth to the biliary passages produces obstructive jaundice. A preceding history of pain and flatulent dyspepsia may be attributable to previous biliary tract disease. Often, the diagnosis is made for the first time at laparotomy on a patient with obstructive jaundice, while, rarely, it can be identified by its being associated with a right upper abdominal mass or a filling defect on cholecystography in the non-jaundiced patient.

Basis of Treatment

This is surgical excision, where possible, with hepatic lobectomy if the patient's condition is satisfactory and if invasion of the right lobe of the liver has occurred.

OTHER TUMOURS OF THE PANCREAS
ZOLLINGER–ELLISON SYNDROME
Definition
The presence of an ulcerogenic tumour which causes severe intractable peptic ulcer disease due to tumour secretion of gastrin.

Background

The secretion of gastrin by a pancreatic tumour, or by an ectopic tumour in the wall of the duodenum, stomach or hilum of the spleen, produces gastric hypersection, ulceration of the duodenum and jejunum and sometimes diarrhoea. This latter is due to inactivation of enzymes and bile salts and may be associated with steatorrhoea. In two-thirds the tumours are malignant, while in others there may be a history of a familial polyglandular endocrinopathy (hyperparathyroidism, insulinoma, etc.), and in others a history of peptic ulcer.

Symptoms

Chronic ulcer dyspepsia, with attendant complications of repeated haematemeses, perforation, etc. Diarrhoea ± steatorrhoea and symptoms of potassium deficiency. Recurrence of ulcer after surgery.

Signs

Unremarkable.

Investigations

1. Basal and maximal acid levels in the stomach juice are raised, but the ratio of basal/maximal acid is <0.6, e.g. basal hourly acid 20 mEq, maximal hourly acid 40 mEq.
2. Radiology may reveal massive or multiple duodenal and jejunal ulcers.
3. Duodenoscopy may prove to be helpful.
4. It is worthwhile looking for multiple endocrine defects, serum calcium, glucose tolerance curve, etc.
5. Studies of intestinal absorption and serum electrolytes may show malabsorption and potassium or calcium deficiency.
6. A high serum gastrin usually clinches the diagnosis.

Basis of Treatment

It is sometimes possible to remove a single tumour or, should this not be identifiable, to perform a partial pancreatectomy. Even when metastases are present it is important to remove the target organ (total gastrectomy), as otherwise the patient is likely to die from the effects of gastric hypersecretion, perforation, haemorrhage, etc. The early experience with cimetidine suggests that it may be possible now to control this disorder medically – a revolutionary change in approach.

INSULIN-SECRETING ADENOMA OF THE
PANCREAS (*see* page 188)

CARCINOID TUMOURS – THE (MALIGNANT) CARCINOID SYNDROME

Background

These are tumours of argentaffin cells of the intestinal mucosa. They are found anywhere from stomach to rectum, but are most common in the appendix and ileum.

The tumours are relatively common and are usually found as an incidental finding at laparotomy or autopsy. The carcinoid syndrome, on the other hand, is rare. In this case the original tumour is malignant, metastasises to the liver and produces humoral agents including 5 hydroxytryptamine (5 HT: serotonin) and 5 hydroxytryptophan (5 HTP) which are associated with a clinical syndrome characterised by flushing of the skin, abdominal colic and diarrhoea, bronchospasm, peripheral oedema, valvular lesions of the right side of the heart and skin rashes. These are all due to the entry of chemotransmitters directly into the hepatic veins and then the systemic circulation. It is convenient to describe three groups of malignant carcinoid tumours:
(a) The primitive foregut (bronchial, gastric, pancreatic tumours) produces carcinoid syndrome with some unusual features, e.g. 5 HTP production and metastasis to bone and skin.
(b) Midgut. Small bowel, appendix, right colon produces classical carcinoid syndrome.
(c) Hindgut. Descending colon and rectum, no carcinoid syndrome but metastasis to bone and skin.
Note: Rarely, an ovarian tumour may produce a carcinoid syndrome as chemotransmitters enter the ovarian veins and by-pass the liver.

Symptoms (Fig. 4.22)

Flushing of face, neck, extremities, related to the taking of food and alcohol. (These flushes are distressing to the patient.)
Diarrhoea, accompanied by borborygmi.
Oedema, pigmentation and dyspepsia. Rarely, skin rash like pellagra (due to diversion of tryptophan to serotonin production) with resultant deficiency of nicotinic acid.
Attacks of bronchospasm.

Signs

Hepatomegaly.
Abdominal mass usually in the right iliac fossa.
Signs of tricuspid and pulmonary valvular stenosis.

The relationships of these various signs and symptoms with the chemical transmitters involved are shown in Fig. 4.22.
Note: Only the diarrhoea and borborygmi are definitely

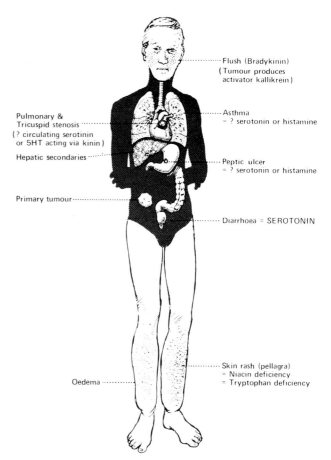

Fig. 4.22 Features of the carcinoid syndrome.

produced by serotonin. The flush results from activation of bradykinin by tumour kinins.

Investigations

1. Detection of increased 5 HIAA in urine.
2. Biopsy of the liver, etc.
3. Production of flushing by 1 to 10 μg of intravenous adrenaline.

Basis of Treatment

Medical:
1. Control diarrhoea with anti-serotonin agents, e.g. methysergide.
2. Give adrenolytic drugs to control flushing (catecholamines are a potent trigger to flushing), e.g. dibenzylene, chlorpromazine. Avoid alcohol, dairy products, and other precipitants.
3. Because bradykinin is inhibited by corticosteroids these may help.
4. Treat heart failure, give vitamin B for pellagra, etc.

Surgical. Remove primary tumour and metastases, e.g. hepatic lobectomy.
Note: Dangerous hypotension a possible complication.

Prognosis

Good – survival for ten or more years is not unusual. A factor to be considered prior to embarking on operations with a considerable risk, for example hepatic resection.

DISEASES OF THE GALL BLADDER

GALLSTONES

Definition

The presence of one or many stones usually containing a mixture of cholesterol, calcium salts and bile pigments either in the gall bladder and/or bile ducts.

Background

Gallstones increase steadily in incidence with age, and about 30 per cent of routine autopsies show their presence. Though commonest in women who have borne children, there is an increasing incidence in both sexes in countries adopting the Western pattern of civilisation and its consequent dietary habits. There is no doubt that the major fault appears to be the production by the liver of a substandard bile, 'lithogenic bile'. The bile shows two abnormalities:
1. A relative deficiency of bile salts.
2. An increased concentration of cholesterol produced by increased hepatic synthesis.

These two render the bile supersaturated with cholesterol and precipitation follows. The contraceptive pill and obesity increase the incidence of gallstones.

Haemolysis by increasing the load of bile pigment is another factor which, though rarer, can be responsible for the presence of gallstones, particularly in young patients and in cirrhosis. Furthermore, the disturbances of bile salt metabolism resulting from ileal disease or resection and chronic liver disease may explain the increased incidence of gallstones in these conditions. Infection is now considered an important aetiological factor.

Pathology

Gallstones may be single or multiple, when they are often faceted. On section they show regular laminations of cholesterol, calcium and bile pigments. Obstruction of the biliary tract may produce inflammatory change in the gall bladder (empyema – chronic cholecytitis) or bile ducts (cholangitis – hepatic abscess formation). Chronic stone formation may be associated with gall bladder carcinoma.

Symptoms

None, or
Pain – either mild and related to food, or severe epigas- tric pain radiating to right upper abdomen and back (angle of right scapula).
    Occasionally left-sided.
    Steady or colicky.
    Accompanied by vomiting.
Pyrexia.
Flatulent dyspepsia.

Signs

Right upper abdominal tenderness.
Right upper abdominal mass (distended gall bladder).
Positive Murphy's sign (catching of the breath due to pain on palpation of the gall bladder area in inspiration).
Icterus (usually mild with itching, dark urine, and pale stools).

Investigations

1. There may be a leucocytosis if there is accompanying cholecystitis.
2. A plain X-ray film may show radio-opaque gall-stones. (*Note:* They are radio-opaque in only 25 per cent of cases.)
3. Intravenous cholangiography is more specific in the diagnosis of gallstones than oral cholecystography. In particular, non-filling of the gall bladder, using the former technique, is always a sign of gall bladder disease, while cholecystography may fail to visualise the gall bladder, though in fact it is later shown to be functionally and structurally normal. In either case the presence of filling defects in an opacified gall bladder is characteristic of gallstones. In acute gallstone disease infusion cholangiography may be the best way of reaching an accurate diagnosis.
4. Liver function tests may show mild obstructive jaundice and/or raised transaminases, and, in patients with severe symptoms, the possibility of pancreatitis must not be forgotten.

Complications (*see* Fig. 4.23)

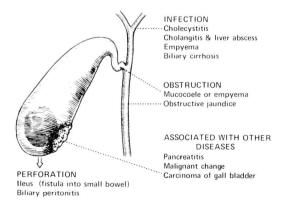

INFECTION
Cholecystitis
Cholangitis & liver abscess
Empyema
Biliary cirrhosis

OBSTRUCTION
Mucocoele or empyema
Obstructive jaundice

ASSOCIATED WITH OTHER DISEASES
Pancreatitis
Malignant change
Carcinoma of gall bladder

PERFORATION
Ileus (fistula into small bowel)
Biliary peritonitis

Fig. 4.23 The complications of gallstones.

Cholangitis. Infection of the biliary tree above an impacted common duct stone causes severe pain, pyrexia with rigors, obstructive jaundice, hepatic tenderness and septicaemic (*E. coli*) shock.

Treatment. With antibiotics (following blood cultures) and later surgery.

Empyema of the Gall Bladder. This is due to infection within a gall bladder with cystic duct obstruction due to an impacted stone. It causes severe pain, pyrexia and right upper abdominal guarding and a mass. It is suspected in any patient with severe or protracted biliary tract pain.

Treatment. Antibiotics followed by emergency or elective surgery.

Pancreatitis. The precise cause is unknown, but gallstones remain the commonest cause of pancreatitis in the United Kingdom (*see* page 90).

Carcinoma of the Gall Bladder (*see* page 88).

Secondary Biliary Cirrhosis. Recurrent infection and prolonged obstruction of the common bile duct may result in permanent liver damage (secondary biliary cirrhosis). This is associated with bouts of cholangitis and with hepatomegaly, and later, the signs of portal hypertension (splenomegaly) and liver failure (oedema, ascites and encephalopathy). Distinction from primary biliary cirrhosis is important, and an antimitochondrial antibody test, cholangiography and liver biopsy are helpful (*see* page 72).

Treatment is of the complications, e.g. bleeding varices, though prophylaxis, thorough treatment of biliary obstruction due to gallstones or to subsequent surgery, is vital.

Gallstone Ileus. A solitary gallstone may ulcerate through the gall bladder wall and enter the small bowel which it obstructs in its narrowest part, the ileum. The disorder may be difficult to diagnose because of the evidence of gall bladder disease and the later pain, vomiting and distension of small bowel obstruction. It is suspect in any patient with intestinal obstruction, particularly the obese, middle-aged female. A plain abdominal X-ray may be helpful in showing gas in the biliary tree, small bowel obstruction and, occasionally, the gallstone itself if it is radio-opaque.

Treatment is surgical following small bowel decompression and intravenous fluids.

Differential Diagnosis

The important conditions to be considered in patients with gallstones include those of the right kidney, e.g. renal stone or tumour, lesions of the right lung base, including pleurisy, and other digestive disorders such as peptic ulcer, hiatus hernia, and pancreatitis. Patients with complicating jaundice must also be considered as having other causes of obstructive jaundice, such as those due to drugs and malignant disease. On occasions the picture may resemble acute hepatitis, though distinction from liver cell jaundice should be possible.

Basis of Treatment

Gallstones are usually removed with the gall bladder surgically and where there is evidence or a suspicion of common duct stones, the opening, examination (if necessary by operative cholangiography), removal of stones, and drainage of the common duct is indicated.

A more difficult decision surrounds the problem of the patient with gallstones and flatulent dyspepsia.

Often, patients are obese, neurotic, and with complicating hiatus hernia, and although many such patients have lost their gall bladders, a significant number retain their symptoms. A low fat diet, though traditional, is of no lasting value. Surgeons often advise cholecystectomy because of the possible complications such as empyema of the gall bladder, cholangitis, etc., which may threaten life, or because of the small though definite risk of gall bladder cancer. Patients must be carefully selected for surgery, and reduction of weight, reassurance and treatment for neurosis and cancerophobia may be all that is reasonable in some, particularly if symptoms are infrequent. A new approach in these older subjects with multiple small (<10 mm) diameter cholesterol, and therefore non-opaque stones, is the use of oral chenodeoxycholic acid. This has to be given over a long period of time and is therefore not sensible treatment in patients with severe symptoms. A functioning gall bladder, a sensible preferably non-obese and virtually asymptomatic patient, are further basic requirements and reformation of stones is a hazard if treatment stops. Life-time therapy may then be required.

DISEASES OF THE PANCREAS

PANCREATITIS

Definition

An acute or chronic inflammatory process associated with destruction of the pancreas.

Background

This is a rare disease in the UK, but it is common in areas where there is a high incidence of alcoholism. The precise cause for the destruction of pancreatic tissue is unknown and possibly variable from case to case. It seems likely that protein-splitting enzymes such as trypsin, either alone or by the activation of other enzymes such as phospholipase A and diastase, can produce substances that either injure cells or cell membranes. Recently, under suspicion have been lysolecithin and lysocephalin formed from lecithin (present in bile) by trypsin activation. There is an important relationship between biliary tract disease and pancreatitis and though reflux of bile into the pancreatic duct is an unlikely cause, the importance of bile as a provider of toxic substrate or of infection cannot be ignored. Vascular factors may be important in various types of pancreatitis, while alcohol not only activates the pancreas but also produces duct spasm, which may partially explain the high incidence of pancreatitis in alcoholics, where recent studies have stressed the importance of plugging of pancreatic ducts by protein material.

There are several other types of pancreatitis whose causes are even more poorly understood. These include 'traumatic' pancreatitis, usually seen postoperatively and perhaps due to vascular injury, while others complicate hyperparathyroidism and certain hyperlipaemias. In certain parts of Africa, a form associated with massive calcification and destruction of the pancreas, perhaps related to previous malnutrition, is seen, while a rare familial (genetic) variety is described and in these instances a renal abnormality (aminoaciduria) is also present. Drugs, for example the Pill, are occasionally causative.

Pathology

The pancreas is acutely inflamed and often haemorrhagic. The microscopy shows acute acinar damage and there is fat necrosis in the mesentery and peritoneal injection. In the chronic phase, fibrosis calcification and duct distortion make the differentiation from carcinoma difficult.

A classification of pancreatitis is complex, but at a conference at Marseilles in 1963 the following types were recognised:

Classification of pancreatitis	
1. Acute pancreatitis	In both of which the gland returns to normal structure and function after the attack(s)
2. Recurrent acute pancreatitis	
3. Recurrent chronic pancreatitis	In both of which the gland is permanently and sometimes (4) progressively damaged.
4. Chronic pancreatitis	

Symptoms

Acute and recurrent acute pancreatitis
Pain:
  Severe, constant, may follow a heavy meal or alcohol.
  Epigastric – radiating to back – shoulder blades right and left.
Vomiting.

Signs

Abdominal guarding.
Tachycardia, low BP (shock).
Rarely – discoloration of loins or round umbilicus (Cullen's sign and Grey Turner's sign).

Investigations

1. Serum and urinary enzyme tests. Serum amylase and lipase are raised, former if >1,000. Somogyi units very suggestive, but elevated levels may occur in many abdominal catastrophes and are also elevated further by renal failure. Urinary enzymes helpful later because levels fall more slowly than blood levels. Some centres stress the value of the ratio of the urinary amylase/creatinine in diagnosis.
2. Aspiration of the abdominal cavity: 'four quarter aspiration' with a fine needle and syringe may yield fluid with a high amylase content, possibly bloodstained.
3. The blood glucose may be low and electrolyte depletion, particularly potassium deficiency, may result from vomiting and paralytic ileus. The serum calcium is lowered and a variety of changes due to electrolyte upsets may cause ECG changes which may be confused with those of myocardial infarction. It has also been shown that tissue anoxia occurs and the PO_2 falls.
4. Radiology may be helpful as it may show:
(a) Opaque gallstones.
(b) Pancreatic calcification (in chronic relapsing cases).
(c) Intestinal distension and changes of paralytic ileus, particularly in loops of gut adjacent to the pancreas, 'sentinal loops'.

It will be helpful in excluding other major abdominal catastrophes, particularly intestinal perforation. Infusion cholangiography can further define biliary tract disease.

Complications (*see* Fig. 4.24)

Differential Diagnosis

1. Other acute abdominal catastrophes:
  Perforation of a peptic ulcer/diverticulitis coli, etc.
  Bowel obstruction due to volvulus, gallstones, mesenteric vascular disease.
  Peritonitis from an appendix abscess, etc.
  Biliary tract disease with gallstones/cholangitis or empyema of the gall bladder.

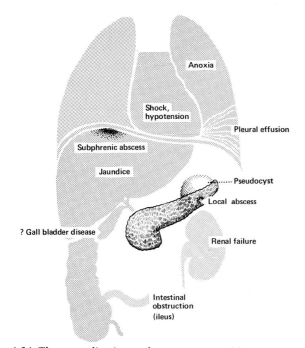

Fig. 4.24 The complications of acute pancreatitis.

2. Other thoracic catastrophes (with radiation of the pain to the epigastrium):
    Pneumonia
    Myocardial infarction
    Dissecting aneurysm.

Basis of Treatment

There are several lines upon which the treatment of this disease, for which there is no specific cure, is based.

1. Restriction of pancreatic secretory activity is effected by ceasing all oral feeding and by the use of antivagal drugs by intramuscular injection, e.g. atropine, poldine, etc. A gastric tube is used for continuous aspiration to maintain an empty (unstimulated) stomach.

2. The relief of pain and shock by adequate fluid and plasma and electrolyte replacement (including Ca and K) supplemented by powerful analgesics which do not cause spasm of the ampulla of Vater. In this respect phenazocine hydrobromide (Narphen) 1 to 3 mg six-hourly is preferable to morphine or pethidine. There may be a place in patients who are severely ill for the use of corticosteroid drugs despite the fact that they have occasionally been implicated in the production of pancreatic necrosis. Shock may require special therapy.

3. Surgery is avoided unless there is diagnostic difficulty, when it seems that a limited diagnostic laparotomy does no harm and on occasions discovery of biliary disease may be followed by biliary drainage. Elective biliary surgery may be required following recovery from the acute attack, as may drainage of a pancreatic pseudocyst or abscess.

4. There is much debate as to whether the antitrypsin agent obtained from bovine parotid gland and presented as Trasylol is of value in this type of pancreatic disease. Experimentally, it can halt the progression of experimentally-produced pancreatitis in animals, if given very early. Though encouraging effects were seen in early trials in man where there was an unusually high mortality in the control subjects, these results have not been verified in later trials. Similarly, the hormone glucagon which has a marked inhibitory effect on pancreatic secretion has apparently no beneficial effect in reducing the mortality of this disease. It seems that the care of a skilled intensive therapy team with attention to electrolytes, blood gases, sepsis etc., is the most rewarding way at the moment of reducing the mortality.

Prognosis

Acute pancreatitis carries a mortality of about 10 per cent. Recovery must be accompanied by a careful appraisal of possible aetiological factors. Alcoholism must be enquired about from the patient and his relatives, while a full radiological examination of the biliary tree is essential. Evidence of hyperparathyroidism and hyperlipidaemia must also be sought.

In 50 per cent of patients no apparent causative factor will be found.

Following recovery, the patient may have no further attacks, but a certain percentage will have recurrent attacks, despite evidence of normal pancreatic function between attacks.

A note on recurrent chronic and chronic pancreatitis.
Some patients will show signs of chronic pancreatic insufficiency (steatorrhoea and diabetes) without, usually, any evidence of other nutritional deficiencies. These patients respond well to replacement therapy with effective pancreatic hormones, for example Cotazym two to three capsules sprinkled on each main meal or taken in a cold drink with each meal. The lipase content of each Cotazym capsule is sufficient to digest 17 g of dietary fat. This measure usually controls diarrhoea if the dietary fat is also restricted. A further preparation, Nutrizym, can be taken as a tablet by mouth and has the possible added advantages of having proteolytic enzymes in its outer shell.

Acute relapses of pancreatitis are treated in a similar way to those described under acute pancreatitis. Alcoholism must be vigorously treated if it is a factor, as relapses often follow a drinking spree. Diabetes, usually mild, may also need treatment, and a further hazard is the possibility of the patient becoming addicted to narcotics used for the treatment of severe pain with relapses.

THE PERITONEUM

TUBERCULOUS PERITONITIS

This is an uncommon disorder in the U.K., but in the tropics it remains common and the student must be alert to the possibility of its existence, for example in the alcoholic and the immigrant. The symptoms are those of abdominal pain, fever, sweating, anorexia and headache, and the signs consist of abdominal distension sometimes with the signs of free intraperitoneal fluid, but in others the abdomen may feel 'doughy' while one or more ill-defined abdominal masses may be present. Diagnosis is aided by evidence of tuberculous disease elsewhere (chest X-ray, etc.), by the presence of fluid with a predominantly lymphocytic cell population and a high protein content on abdominal aspiration, and by a characteristic picture at laparoscopy or laparotomy. Blind peritoneal needle biopsy may occasionally be helpful by providing characteristic histology. The chances of obtaining bacteria on direct microscopy of peritoneal fluid or even culture are not greater than 30 per cent and good circumstantial evidence of its presence must be followed by the speedy administration of antituberculous drugs, i.e. streptomycin 1 g daily for two months with PAS 15 g daily and INAH 100 mg three times a day, the latter two for an eighteen-month course. (For alternatives see page 339.)

Ascites and its cause is dealt with on page 70. Readers are reminded of the relationship of malignant tumours of the peritoneum (mesothelioma) to exposure to asbestos and the fact that they cause bizarre signs and symptoms, including abdominal pain and ascites. The peritoneal cavity may also be involved in the rare condition of periodic disease. This is found in certain Middle Eastern people and consists of recurrent attacks of pleurisy, peritonitis, and arthritis due to sterile inflammation of serous membranes, i.e. the pleura, pericardium, peritoneum, etc. Attacks are accompanied by fever and there is a tendency to develop amyloid infiltration of the kidneys.

SPECIAL TESTS USED IN THE DIAGNOSIS OF ALIMENTARY DISORDERS

BIOPSY

Biopsy of the liver and intestinal tract are most useful procedures in the diagnosis of gastrointestinal disorders. Liver biopsy is usually performed with a needle via the intercostal route. The Menghini technique, using a cutting needle and suction to retain the biopsy in the needle, is the most commonly employed. A bleeding tendency, which is not infrequent in patients with liver disease, precludes the investigation, though vitamin K may be successful in bringing the prothrombin level to an acceptable figure (within three seconds of the control). Liver biopsy is useful:
1. In the diagnosis of jaundice, which cannot be categorised by simpler tests.
2. In the diagnosis of cirrhosis (including the use of special techniques, haemochromatosis, Wilson's disease, etc.)
3. In the diagnosis of hepatomegaly of unknown cause.
4. In the diagnosis of hepatic cancer.

Gastric Biopsy

This is best performed at fibre endoscopy and is valuable in the identification of benign and malignant gastric lesions, while blind gastric biopsy, using a suction apparatus, has been employed for the identification of gastritis.

Small Bowel (Jejunal) Biopsy

This is indicated in most patients with the malabsorption syndrome. A variety of instruments, of which the Crosby capsule is the most convenient, are available. The Crosby capsule is a small capsule containing a suction-released knife which is automatically released when a knuckle of mucosa occludes the biopsy port. Changes found in the mucosa include:
1. Subtotal villous atrophy (see page 77). For all intents and purposes in the UK only found in patients with coeliac disease. Tropical sprue is a rare but further cause.
2. Partial villous atrophy is found in a host of conditions, including malignancy, skin disease, ulcerative colitis, etc.

GASTRIC FUNCTION TESTS

The only important test is the basal and maximal acid output/hour, the latter after stimulation with pentagastrin in a dose of 6 μg/kg intramuscularly.

The patient is fasted, the stomach is intubated, and collections made for fifteen-minute periods, using continuous suction. Acid is best measured as total acid by titration to pH 7.4. (Results of gastric function tests are given in Table 4.9.)

Table 4.9 Results of gastric function tests (approximate values)

	Normal	GU	DU	Z. Ellison	Carcinoma
Vol. ml/hr (basal)	60	60	80	200	60 or less
Vol. ml/hr (stimulated)	240	240	300	360	240 or less
Basal acid output (BAO) mmol/hr	1–2	1–2	1–8	5–65	1–2 or less
Maximal acid output (MAO) mmol/hr	10–25	4–20	20–45	20–65	4–20 or less

Note: Achlorhydria is not a constant feature of gastric carcinoma.

Peak acid output (PAO) is a convenient way of expressing the hourly hypothetical maximal gastric acid secretion and is obtained by doubling the sum of the two highest consecutive 15-minute acid secretions.

SMALL BOWEL FUNCTION

The tests shown in Table 4.10 are useful in the detection of small bowel disease.

Use of Bowel Perfusion

Absorption of any substance may be determined by perfusing a known length of gut simply by using a double lumen intestinal tube which allows entry of the substance at one point and collection of it from a known distance distally. Using a non-absorbable marker in the perfusate, which allows calculation of fluid absorption, one is able, by knowing the concentration of the test substance in the infused and the aspirated fluid, to calculate total absorption. This is currently an important method of investigating bowel function.

LIVER FUNCTION TESTS

The following blood tests are routinely used in the evaluation of liver function:

Serum Bilirubin

Normal: $< 17\ \mu$mol/l (0.2 to 0.8 mg per cent).
Raised in:
   (a) haemolytic,
   (b) liver cell,
   (c) obstructive jaundice.
Bile pigment is unconjugated (i.e. not combined with glucuronide) in haemolytic disease only. This is therefore the only one type of jaundice in which bile pigment is not found in the urine.

Serum Alkaline Phosphatase

Normal 3 to 13 KA units/100 ml. This is raised in liver cell and obstructive biliary disease. However, alkaline phosphatase can also be of bony origin, so that a raised value is not only seen in hepatic disease.

Values over 30 KA units are seen in nearly all patients with biliary obstruction, but they may also occur in liver cell disease. In patients with an elevated alkaline phosphatase of uncertain cause, help can be obtained by estimating 5^1 nucleotidase in the serum. This enzyme is raised only when there is hepatic disease. (Normal 5^1 nucleotidase level is 1.5 to 17 IU/litre.)

Serum Protein Electrophoresis

A low serum albumin is found in patients with chronic liver cell disease. In acute and chronic liver cell disorders serum globulins, particularly γ globulins, are elevated. In chronic liver cell disease the combination of a

Table 4.10 Small bowel function tests

	Method	Normal result	Malabsorption
Fat balance	Estimation of faecal fat over 3 or more days on fixed fat intake.	<23 mmol excreted/24 hrs.	Raised >23 mmol/24 hrs.
Xylose excretion	Urinary and sometimes blood levels of D xylose following 5 g by mouth. *(Note: Figures vary with renal function and age)*	0–2 hr> (23 per cent) in urine. 0–5 hr> (35 per cent) in urine.	Lowered urinary excretion in malabsorption.
Glucose tolerance test	Blood and urine levels of glucose at ½-hourly intervals following 50 g of glucose orally.	Normal rise of 40 mg (2.2 mmol) per cent.	Flat curve in coeliac disease (Bl. glucose rise <40 mg (2.2 mmol) per cent). Diabetic curve in some examples of pancreatic disease.
Lactose tolerance	Blood levels of glucose following 50 g of lactose orally.	Normal rise 20 mg (1.1 mmol) per cent.	Flat curve suggests lactase deficiency.
Vitamin B_{12} absorption	Schilling test. Estimation of 24 hr radioactivity following 1 μg of ^{58}Co labelled. vitamin B_{12}, and a flushing dose of 1,000 μg of non-radioactive vitamin B_{12}.	Normal >10 per cent of labelled dose in 24-hr urine.	Reduced in gastric resection and PA (corrected by repeating test with intrinsic factor). Reduced in blind loop syndrome (corrected by repeating test with effective antibiotics). Reduced in ileal disease or resection. (Not corrected by repeating test with IF or antibiotics unless blind loop present.)

low serum albumin and raised globulin results in reversal of the A/G ratio. Analysis of immunoglobulins (γ globulins) is of little extra value, though high levels of 1gM are found in primary biliary cirrhosis.

Immunological Abnormalities

These are found in the serum of a variety of patients with chronic liver cell disease:

a feto protein found in primary hepatoma is a fetal protein which normally disappears soon after birth. It reappears in 30 to 80 per cent of patients with hepatoma.

Rheumatoid factor ⎫
Serum antinuclear factor (ANF) ⎪ found in chronic
Smooth muscle antibody (SMA) ⎬ active hepatitis, primary
Mitochondrial antibodies (MA) ⎪ biliary cirrhosis,
DNA binding antibodies ⎭ cryptogenic cirrhosis –
in a variable percentage

Note: Mitochondrial antibodies are not found in chronic extrahepatic obstructive jaundice, which is of diagnostic help).

HBsAg (hepatitis B surface antigen) found in acute and chronic serum hepatitis and in carriers of serum hepatitis. Also in some patients with primary liver hepatoma and chronic liver disease, for example cirrhosis.

Serum Enzymes

Certain enzymes are released from damaged liver cells and, thus, elevation of serum levels may be a sign of liver disease.

Examples:
Serum glutamic oxalacetic transaminase, i.e. SGOT or aspartic transaminase. Normal level: <40 units/litre.

Biliary obstruction gives levels up to 300 units/litre (unless there is cholangitis, when higher levels are found).
Liver cell disease gives levels up to 2,000 units/litre.
Serum glutamic pyruvate transaminase, i.e. SGPT or alanine transaminase.

Similar values are seen as with SGOT, despite higher concentration of SGPT in liver.
Isocitric dehydrogenase (ICD). Normal: 1 to 3 units/ml.
Lactic dehydrogenase (LDH). Normal: 150 to 500 units/ml.

Note: Estimation of LDH isoenzymes may be helpful as some are only of hepatic origin (LD_4 and LD_5).

Bromsulphthalein (BSP) Clearance

The dye BSP is largely cleared from blood by the liver. Its rate of removal following intravenous injection is therefore a sensitive test of liver function. A dose of BSP of 5 mg/kg body weight is given intravenously, and 45 minutes later blood is taken from the opposite forearm for estimation of the dye concentration. Normally, less than 5 per cent of the dye is found in the serum at this time. In liver disease and in patients with abnormal vascular communications between the systemic and portal circulations (usually due to liver disease) increased retention is found.

Prothrombin Time, etc.

Factors produced in the liver and responsible for normal blood clotting include prothrombin Factors V, VII, IX (Christmas Factor), X and fibrinogen. Liver disease may thus be associated with a bleeding tendency. Vitamin K deficiency – and hence prothrombin deficiency – is found in obstructive jaundice and is due to malabsorption of vitamin K secondary to bile salt lack. It is corrected by intramuscular vitamin K. A bleeding tendency and a prolonged prothrombin time secondary to liver cell disease is less readily treated. Vitamin K cannot, for example, facilitate production of Factor V, etc., and the prothrombin time may, therefore, not decrease with vitamin K therapy. Increased fibrinolytic activity and a consumptive coagulopathy (disemminated intravascular coagulation – DIC) due to deposition of microthrombi in blood vessels is also recognised as occurring in liver disease (*see* page 420).

Hepatic Scintiscanning

Using a moveable probe or a gamma camera, it is possible, following the intravenous injection of a radioactively labelled substance which is taken up either by the liver cells or the Küpffer cells, to obtain a radioactive 'map' of the liver. In fact, the most usual practice is to give a technetium 99 m labelled sulphur colloid intravenously. This is taken up by Küpffer cells so that cysts, abscesses and tumours appear on the scan as non-functioning (cold) areas. Gallium scanning may also help, though, because of its localisation in inflammatory tissue, liver uptake may represent an abscess or tumour.

PANCREATIC FUNCTION

Loss of pancreatic exocrine function may be detected in the following ways:
1. Evidence of impaired bicarbonate and/or decreased trypsin production following intubation of the duodenum and stimulation of the pancreas. This may be performed following a liquid artificial meal and estimation of duodenal trypsin content (Lundt test meal).
2. An alternative procedure involves intubation of the duodenum and the collection of duodenal juice uncontaminated by acid gastric juice (removed by constant gastric suction). Following secretin or secretin and pancreozymin stimulation, measurement of bicarbonate and enzyme production is made. Specimens are taken

at ten-minute intervals and are kept on ice prior to chemical estimation. Reduced bicarbonate and enzyme production are seen in pancreatic disease and pancreatic duct obstruction.

3. Scanning of the pancreas following intravenous radio-active selenomethionine is also a valuable technique for the recognition of pancreatic disease and pancreatic neoplasms.

4. Endocrine failure is detected by glucose tolerance tests supplemented with serum insulin levels and by estimation of tolbutamide tolerance, etc.

5. A simple way of diagnosing exocrine failure is the estimation of faecal fat excretion for a period on and off a potent pancreatic extract. The patient in whom there is pancreatic deficiency usually notices a lessening of diarrhoea and darkening of the stools. Estimation of sweat sodium is important, as levels over 70 mEq(mmol)/litre are very suggestive of fibrocystic disease of the pancreas.

ENDOSCOPY

Fibre-optic instruments are now available for examination of the oesophagus, stomach and duodenum, jejunum and for all of the colon. These instruments are flexible, cause only moderate discomfort to the patient, and also possess facilities for photography, biopsy and exfoliative cytology. Further, because of their acceptance by patients, the procedure is easily repeated in order to assess the effects of therapy or to repeat biopsies, etc. Patients require bowel preparation even prior to examination of the left colon, so that they are best admitted overnight for this procedure. Because of this, sigmoidoscopy with a rigid instrument is still the first-line investigation for the out-patient with symptoms of colonic or rectal disease. Virtually all cases of ulcerative colitis can be diagnosed by sigmoidoscopy. Examination of the peritoneum, liver and spleen is easily accomplished by means of peritoneoscopy once the peritoneal cavity has been filled with air or carbon dioxide. The available instruments are rigid, but can be used for photography and biopsy of the liver under direct vision. This is particularly important as it allows the diagnosis of cirrhosis and primary and secondary hepatic cancer to be made when deposits of the latter are few and small.

EXAMINATION OF STOOLS FOR OCCULT BLOOD

Stools are tested for occult blood with guaiac. A two per cent solution of guaiac in acetic acid (1 drop) and 40 vol. H_2O_2 (1 drop) produces a blue colour within thirty seconds in patients with blood loss amounting to greater than 10 ml/24 hours. False positive reactions are common and the test is for screening purposes only.

RADIOLOGY OF THE INTESTINAL TRACT

A description of the indications and methods available for examination of the gastrointestinal tract is beyond the scope of this book. Suffice it to say that the co-operation of a skilled radiologist is invaluable in diagnosis, though it must be remembered that negative X-ray investigations are no excuse for assuming that the patient does not have organic disease. Further, co-operation with a department of radiology means taking advice from and providing maximal diagnostic information for the radiologist.

SUGGESTED FURTHER READING

Alcohol and the Liver

Brunt, P. W. (1971) Alcohol and the Liver – progress report. *Gut* **12**: 222.

Bile Salts

Heaton, K. W. (1972) Bile Salts in Health and Disease. London: Churchill Livingstone.

Coeliac Disease

Cooke, W. T. and Asquith, P. (eds.) (1974) *Clinics in Gastroenterology.* **Vol. 3.** No. 1. London: W. B. Saunders.

Crohn's Disease and Ulcerative Colitis

Kirsner, J. B. and Shorter, R. G. (eds.) (1975) *Inflammatory Bowel Disease.* Philadelphia: Lea & Febiger.

Diarrhoea

Low-beer, T. S. and Read, A. E. (1971) Diarrhoea – mechanisms and treatment. *Gut* **12**: 1021.
Cummings, J. H. (1974) Laxative abuse. *Gut* **15**: 758.
Viteri, A. L., Howard, P. H. and Dyck, W. P. (1974) The spectrum of lincomycin-clindamycin colitis. *Gastroenterology* **66**, 1137.

Endoscopy

Salmon, P. R. (1974) Fibre-optic endoscopy. London: Pitman.

Gallstones

Bouchier, I. A. D. (1975) Gallstones. In *Modern Trends in Gastroenterology* (ed. Read, A. E.) **Vol. 5**: 203. London: Butterworth.

Gastritis

Coghill, N. F. (1969) Chronic idiopathic gastritis. In *Fifth Symposium on Advanced Medicine*, Royal College of Physicians. London: Pitman Medical.

Gastrointestinal Bleeding

Jones, Sir F. Avery (1970) Problems of alimentary bleeding. *British Medical Journal* 2: 267.

Forest, J. A., Finlayson, N. D. C. and Shearman, D. J. C. (1974) Endoscopy in gastrointestinal bleeding. *Lancet* **ii**: 394.

General (Pathology)

Morson, B. C. and Dawson, I. M. P. (1972) *Gastrointestinal Pathology*. London: Blackwell.

Hepatitis B

Zuckermann, A. J. (1976) Hepatitis B: Nature of virus and prospects for vaccine development. In *Progress in Liver Disease* (eds. Popper, H. and Schaffner, F.) **Vol. V**: 326. London: Grune & Stratton.

Irritable Bowel

Manning, A. P. and Read, A. E. (1975) *Irritable Colon* (ed. Sauerwein, H. P.) Amsterdam: Excerpta Medica.

Jaundice

Schmid, R. (1972) Bilirubin metabolism in man. *New England Journal of Medicine*, **287**: 703.

Blumgart, L. H., Salmon, P., Cotton, P. B., Davies, G. T., Burwood, R., Beales, J. S. M., Lawrie, B., Skirving, A. and Read, A. E. (1972) Endoscopy and retrograde choledocho-pancreatography in the diagnosis of the jaundiced patient. *Lancet* **ii**: 1269.

Sherlock, S. (1972) The problem of chronic cholestasis. *Journal of the Royal College of Surgeons of England*, **17**: 1.

Liver and Drug Metabolism

Branch, R. A., Nies, A. S. and Read, A. E. (1975) The Liver and Drugs. In *Modern Trends in Gastroenterology* (ed. Read, A. E.), **Vol. 5**: 289. London: Butterworth.

Oesophagus

Earlam, R. (1975) *Clinical Tests of Oesophageal Function*. London: Crosby Lockwood Staples.

Atkinson, M. (1962) Mechanism protecting against oesophageal reflux. A Review. *Gut* **3**: 1.

Pancreatic Cancer

Morgan, R. G. H. and Wormsley, K. G. (1977) Cancer of the Pancreas. *Gut* **18**: 580.

Pancreatitis

Hermon Taylor, J. (1977) An aetiological and therapeutic review of acute pancreatitis. *British Journal of Hospital Medicine* **18**: 546.

Mallinson, C. (1977) Chronic pancreatitis. *British Journal of Hospital Medicine* **18**: 553.

Peptic Ulcer

Wormsley, K. G. (1974) The pathophysiology of duodenal ulceration. *Gut* **15**: 59.

Montgomery, R. D. and Richardson, B. P. (1975) Gastric ulcer and cancer. *Quarterly Journal of Medicine* **44**: 591.

Portal Hypertension

Dawson, J. L. (1975) Treatment of Portal Hypertension. In *Modern Trends in Gastroenterology* (ed. Read, A. E.) **vol. 5**: 149. London: Butterworth.

Skin and Gut

Marks, J. and Schuster, S. (1970) Small intestinal mucosal abnormalities in various skin diseases. *Postgraduate Medical Journal* **11**: 281.

Nutrition 5

K. W. HEATON

This chapter is concerned with the relationship between dietary habits and disease. Disease caused by wrong diet can be called malnutrition. This term is widely taken to mean undernutrition, that is lack of one or more nutrients. However, in industrialised countries it is now far commoner to see overnutrition, especially excess of energy intake over requirements. In such countries, the main deficiency of the diet is its lack of fibre.

In general, malnutrition is due not to lack or excess of food, but to a faulty choice of food. In poor and backward countries, this is due mainly to unwise agricultural practice, with excessive dependence on one crop which provides the staple food, for example maize or cassava. In the lower social classes of rich countries, poor quality food is eaten partly for lack of money (fresh foods costing more than processed ones) and partly from ignorance about the nutritional values of foods. In all classes, people tend to prefer sweetened foods and drinks and convenience foods to their fresh and more nutritious counterparts.

EVOLUTION, CIVILISATION AND MAN'S DIET

Like all animals, man is adapted by evolution to thrive on some foods, but not others (such as leaves). As a hunter-gatherer species, his range of food has been uniquely wide from the earliest times. However, the proportion of animal food was probably high only in colder climates, while plant food predominated in warmer areas. Cooking must have started with the discovery of fire about a million years ago. A mere 10,000 years ago man learnt to grow crops, especially cereals. This allowed storage of food, the development of settled communities and hence civilisation. Civilised man has constantly sought to widen his range of foods by trade, cultivation of new varieties, cross-breeding, and processing in every imaginable way – smoking, salting, grinding, fermenting, etc. The refining of carbohydrate, that is the removal of the fibrous component, began with the sifting of flour to remove bran

more than 2,000 years ago, but became efficient and universal only in the last 100 to 200 years. The mass-production and consumption of refined sugar is also a nineteenth and twentieth century phenomenon. In the last 30 years the rate of change of diet has accelerated, with the introduction of hundreds of food additives and the development of artificial, chemically manipulated foods. The effects on health, if any, are largely unknown. With few of these changes have the long term effects been adequately researched. Recent changes have taken place far too rapidly for evolutionary adaptation to have occurred.

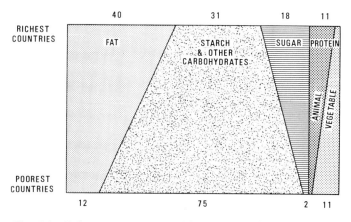

Fig. 5.1 Relative proportions of fat, starch, refined sugar and protein in the diets of countries of differing wealth. Percentage of total energy in the diet.

There are striking differences between the diets of poor and rich countries (Fig. 5.1). In poor countries up to 75 per cent of the energy in the diet comes from starchy foods (wheat, rice, millet, maize, cassava, plantains and yams). Protein is adequate, but this and the little fat come mainly from vegetable sources. With wealth, there is a sharp fall in starch intake, a marked increase in sugar and fat consumption and a swing towards animal fat and animal protein.

MALNUTRITION OF AFFLUENT SOCIETIES

OVERNUTRITION

Overnutrition in the sense of excessive energy (calorie or joule) intake is virtually universal in affluent societies. Few retain their youthful slimness and many spend their lives struggling to control their weight. Those who fail are not necessarily big eaters. They may simply have 'thrifty' metabolism, that is they are efficient at utilising dietary energy and at storing any surplus as fat. This would have survival value in times of food shortage, but renders them susceptible to the high energy value of modern, processed foods.

A consistently high energy intake leads not only to obesity but also to faster growth, earlier puberty, greater fertility and earlier ageing. Overnutrition disturbs metabolism in many ways. Synthesis of cholesterol as well as of triglycerides is increased, and levels of lipids rise in the blood and bile. Insulin secretion is increased, but insulin resistance develops so that glucose tolerance is impaired. Uric acid levels in the blood increase, and blood pressure rises. All these changes are reversible. Unfortunately, the tendency to develop some malignant neoplasms is also increased.

OBESITY

Definition

The excess storage of fat is surprisingly difficult to define and to measure accurately. In practice, an experienced eye is a good judge of the presence of obesity especially in the unclothed patient. To measure it one requires data on weight and height. Life insurance companies have published tables showing the desirable or ideal weights of men and women of different heights, that is the weights associated with the lowest mortality. A person with a body weight 10 per cent greater than this ideal is said to have a relative weight of 110 per cent. Obesity can be defined arbitrarily as a relative weight greater than 110 per cent; some say 120 per cent. Various obesity indices have been invented, the best being W/H^2, where W is the weight in kg and H is the height in metres.

Epidemiology

Prevalence of obesity increases with age but the very old are not often obese because most of their fat contemporaries have already died. There is a well-marked familial tendency. The sex and social class distribution of obesity vary in different countries and at different times. In Britain today obesity is commoner in the lower socio-economic classes. In developing countries it is a disease of the upper classes.

Aetiological factors

Aetiological factors in obesity	
Genetic susceptibility ('thrifty trait').	Refined carbohydrates (high energy, low satiety food).
Physical inactivity. Social pressures (or lack). Sweetness 'addiction'. Failure to breast feed. Eating for solace.	Carbohydrate drinks. Constant availability of palatable, convenient food.

Their relative importance is controversial. Contrary to popular belief, fat people eat no more than average (though of course they have taken in more calories than they need). This emphasises the importance of individual susceptibility and of food quality. Overnutrition often begins in infancy with the use of overconcentrated milk formulae laced with sugar and with too early introduction of solid foods especially cereals. A taste for sweet, refined foods is encouraged through childhood, and may be set for life. Poorer people eat more refined foods and less fresh ones than those who are better off. Physical inactivity is probably only a modifying factor and may even be secondary to the obesity. Psycho-social factors can be important – obesity may be admired, tolerated, shunned or feared. Mass circulation magazines are very influential in determining women's figures. In pregnancy, a woman becomes fatter in physiological preparation for the demands of breast feeding. She may fail to recover her non-pregnant figure if she feeds her baby artificially.

Associated Diseases (Fig. 5.2)

A man of 50 who is 25 lb (11.3 kg) overweight has his life expectancy shortened by 25 per cent. The main reason for the shorter lives of obese subjects is increased coronary and cerebral arterial disease. Cancer is also more likely to develop, especially cancer of the breast, uterus and colon. Gross obesity hinders respiratory movements and can lead to ventilatory insufficiency. Obese people are often depressed by their deformity and have limited social lives. They deserve sympathy, not scorn.

Basis of Treatment

Obesity is a very difficult disease to cure. Early success is quite common with all slimming regimes, but relapse occurs in most cases. The best results are obtained with group therapy where the patient pays (for example, Weight Watchers' clubs). The essence of treatment is a

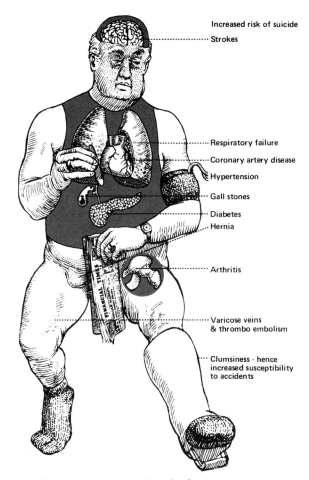

Increased risk of suicide
Strokes
Respiratory failure
Coronary artery disease
Hypertension
Gall stones
Diabetes
Hernia
Arthritis
Varicose veins & thrombo embolism
Clumsiness - hence increased susceptibility to accidents

Fig. 5.2   Disorders associated with obesity.

low calorie intake – 800 to 1,500 calories depending on height and physical activity. Most diets stress restriction of carbohydrate. This gives a quick early fall in weight due to an associated diuresis. Thereafter, progress can be very slow because the body adapts to a lower energy intake by lowering the metabolic rate. This should be countered by increased physical exercise. The patient must expect to feel hungry. Appetite suppressants are sometimes helpful when will-power fails, but should

Treatments in obesity	
First line:	Low calorie diet. Increased exercise.
Second line:	Group therapy, psycho-therapy Anorectic drugs (fenfluramine, chlorphentermine).
Third line:	Supervised starvation.
Fourth line:	Jaw-wiring (dental splint). Small bowel by-pass. Gastric plication.

not be used routinely. In severe and resistant cases it may be necessary to resort to supervised starvation, jaw-wiring or rarely, gastrointestinal by-pass surgery.

UNDERNUTRITION

In a welfare state, chronic undernutrition (a low total food intake) has psychological causes or is secondary to an organic disease. Psychological aversion to food occurs in some teenage girls (anorexia nervosa) (*see* page 446) and in depressed people, especially lonely old people. In the latter, an adequate or even excessive calorie intake may be maintained by an exclusive use of refined carbohydrate foods (white bread, biscuits and sweetened tea), but deficiences of folic acid, ascorbic acid and iron are likely to occur. Addiction to drugs often leads to neglect of food. Alcoholism is especially prone to cause folic acid and thiamine deficiency.

Organic disease may reduce food intake by causing anorexia, premature satiety, or post-prandial pain with consequent fear of eating. Examples of these mechanisms are seen in alcoholism, gastric cancer or resection, and Crohn's disease. All can lead to calorie, protein, mineral and vitamin deficiency.

Acute undernutrition, especially of protein, is liable to occur with any major illness or trauma, including burns and surgical operations. Not only is food intake reduced, but there is a great increase in protein catabolism. This is due, at least in part, to the hormonal response to injury, which includes increased secretion of corticosteroids and catecholamines, and decreased secretion of insulin (or resistance to the action of insulin). Recovery from major illness or trauma is aided by ensuring an adequate diet. Often this involves provision of high protein liquids which can be drunk or delivered down a nasogastric tube. These can be made by homogenising solid meals in an electric blender or, more conveniently, by combining commercial products such as Complan, Caloreen and Prosparol. There is rarely any need for expensive elemental or space diets. Intravenous nutrition is occasionally necessary when there is extensive small intestinal disease, including ileus, or external fistulae, but it is rarely required in a medical ward. It requires special expertise.

FIBRE DEFICIENCY

Recent years have seen the growth and widespread acceptance of the theory, based largely on epidemiological evidence, that the consumption of fibre-depleted or refined foods is responsible for many of the diseases characteristic of urban, technological societies. Dietary fibre is plant cell wall material which is not digested by human enzymes. It is the non-nutritive packaging of plant nutrients. It is plentiful in seeds, hence in unrefined cereal foods (wholemeal flour, brown rice, rolled oats, maize) and in pulses (beans, lentils, peas). Fibre consists of a meshwork of cellulose fibrils embedded in a matrix of non-cellulosic polysaccharides, strengthened by an immensely strong aromatic polymer, lignin. Fibre is largely removed in the production of white flour and completely removed in the extraction of sugar from sugar cane and sugar beet. Diets containing white flour and sugar are low in indigestible residue and satiety, but high in energy in the form of readily absorbed carbohydrate. They are, therefore, blamed for causing disease in two distinct ways – through altered intestinal function, and through increased energy intake and rapid carbohydrate absorption and hence obesity and diabetes.

The disorders most widely accepted as due to intestinal dysfunction are colonic stasis and spasm, hence constipation, spastic colon and diverticular disease. Certainly, a high fibre diet, with or without wheat bran, is effective in the treatment of these chronic disorders. Acute appendicitis has been included in this group, but largely on circumstantial evidence. Constipation leads to straining at stool which raises intra-abdominal pressures. This has been ingeniously linked with hiatus hernia and obstruction to venous return from the legs, hence varicose veins. Carcinoma of the large bowel, which is probably caused by carcinogens in the faeces, has been linked with small, concentrated faeces and slow transit. Direct evidence is lacking but the arguments are plausible.

Research in this field is very active and major advances can be expected in the next few years. Meanwhile sales of bran or wholemeal bread and of other unrefined foods are rising in Britain. Some experts fear this could lead to malabsorption and deficiency of calcium and zinc in vulnerable subjects, but this seems unlikely with a mixed diet. Sales of sugar are falling, but this may be due to rising prices, as well as to increased public concern about obesity.

MALNUTRITION IN POOR COUNTRIES

STARVATION

Crop failures and droughts still lead to famine in the poor countries of Africa and the East. Overpopulation, poverty and civil strife can all play a part.

When food supplies fail, the body draws on its energy reserves (Table 5.1). These are mostly triglycerides in the adipose tissue. Healthy young men and women in the West are about 12 per cent and 26 per cent fat respectively, but many Bangladeshi for instance have much smaller fat stores. Once 25 per cent of body weight has been lost death is increasingly likely to occur, though survival of 50 per cent loss is possible.

Wasting of all tissues occurs, except for the brain. The heart can shrink to half or even a third of its normal weight, and this can lead to irreversible cardiac failure. The small intestine can become paper thin and almost transparent. The resulting loss of absorptive function can negate the effects of re-feeding and prejudice recovery. Up to a point these changes may be considered adaptive. Together with reduced physical activity, they allow most efficient use of limited energy supplies. As further adaptation the brain learns to obtain energy from keto acids instead of the usually obligatory glucose, which reduces the need for gluconeogenesis and so spares protein breakdown in the liver. Famine oedema of the legs is very characteristic of starvation from any cause. It is probably due to loss of elasticity of the connective tissue more than to a fall in serum albumin. It is associated with nocturia.

Other clinical features include dry skin with brown patches, peripheral cyanosis, slow pulse and hypotension. Loss of sexual powers and amenorrhoea are common, and the subject becomes irritable, egocentric and apathetic, even psychopathic. Infections of all kinds are common. Diarrhoea is a terminal sign.

Treatment is simply food, but advanced cases may need to begin with easily digestible skimmed milk feeds.

Infantile Marasmus

This is simply starvation of babies. It is usually caused by early weaning from breast milk on to formula feeds which, through ignorance, are too dilute and often dirty. Maternal deprivation can also cause it. The baby is wasted and weak and often has signs of vitamin deficiencies, anaemia and dehydration. Diarrhoea is common. This disease can overlap with kwashiorkor.

KWASHIORKOR (PROTEIN–ENERGY MALNUTRITION)

In the language of the Ga tribe of Ghana, kwashiorkor means first-second. It is the sickness of a child displaced from the mother's breast because a new baby is expected, and weaned on to gruel which is deficient in protein. It is a very common disease in tropical countries where the population lives on a staple food, such as plantains, cassava or maize, that provides enough energy as carbohydrate, but not enough protein for a growing child. Added factors are poverty, ignorance and taboos against giving milk, eggs, fish or meat to children. It begins usually between 9 months and 2 years and by presentation the child is often desperately

Table 5.1 Energy stores and rates of utilisation in a normal man weighing 65 kg

	Available store			Used daily (g)	Exhaustion time (days)
	(g)	kcal	MJ		
Carbohydrate	150	600	2.5	All used in first 24 hr.	Less than 1
Fat	6,500	58,500	235	150	40
Protein	2,400	9,600	40	60	40

ill. He is stunted, miserable or listless, and anorexic, and usually has diarrhoea (Fig. 5.3). Oedema due to hypoalbuminaemia hides severe muscle wasting. The liver is grossly fatty. Virtually every organ, tissue and biochemical process is abnormal, but all the changes are reversible. One possible exception is that mental development may be permanently retarded. Secondary infections are important because they increase the need for protein and so worsen the deficiency. Overt ill health is often precipitated by an attack of gastroenteritis, measles or pneumonia and may be exacerbated by endemic tropical diseases such as malaria, hookworm and roundworm. Severe cases are often complicated by vitamin and trace element deficiencies. The mortality of cases admitted to hospital varies from 10 to 60 per cent.

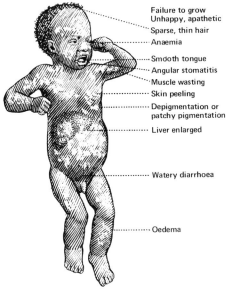

Fig. 5.3 Kwashiorkor – the physical signs.

Labels: Failure to grow / Unhappy, apathetic; Sparse, thin hair; Anaemia; Smooth tongue; Angular stomatitis; Muscle wasting; Skin peeling; Depigmentation or patchy pigmentation; Liver enlarged; Watery diarrhoea; Oedema

Treatment of mild cases is simply provision of adequate food or the addition to the home diet of milk or milk substitutes. Diarrhoea from lactose intolerance may be a problem. Severe cases need electrolyte repletion before beginning small frequent feeds of milk or other protein sources. The mother must then be trained to supplement the family diet with a high protein vegetable such as beans. Prevention requires government action and involves education in good agriculture and good nutrition.

THE CLASSICAL DEFICIENCY DISEASES

The big five – scurvy, beriberi, pellagra, rickets and keratomalacia – all became common in the seventeenth and eighteenth century as a result of major social changes. Their nature as deficiency diseases was not widely recognised until 1912 when Hopkins published his famous paper on vitamins. They have now been largely eradicated, with the exception of keratomalacia, but must still be looked for in certain vulnerable groups.

SCURVY (ASCORBIC ACID DEFICIENCY)

Having been the scourge of sailors for 300 years, scurvy is now seen only in special situations where fruit and vegetables are unobtainable or avoided for many weeks. Tramps, alcoholics, the lonely housebound, and bottle-fed infants are especially at risk. Ascorbic acid or vitamin C is a simple sugar with marked reducing properties. Its function is to maintain the formation of collagen in connective tissue and of the intercellular cement of vascular endothelium.

Of the clinical manifestations of scurvy (Fig. 5.4), the most characteristic is the swollen, offensively infected gums. However, these are found only if natural teeth are present and if there is some underlying periodontal disease (as there usually is in adults in this country). Perifollicular haemorrhages are first seen on the thighs above the knees and are associated with corkscrew hairs. They are followed by petechiae, more extensive purpura and bruising and, in children, painful subperiosteal haemorrhages. Prominent symptoms are lassitude and malaise. In advanced cases, these are contributed to by anaemia, which is normochromic and sometimes macrocytic. By this stage there is danger of sudden death from cardiac failure or cerebral haemorrhage.

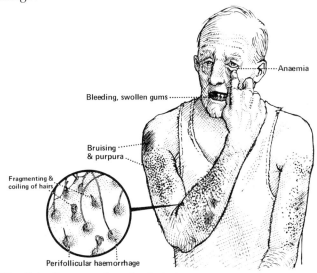

Fig. 5.4 Scurvy – the physical signs.

Labels: Anaemia; Bleeding, swollen gums; Bruising & purpura; Fragmenting & coiling of hairs; Perifollicular haemorrhage

Diagnosis is based on the clinical findings and a compatible dietary history. Laboratory tests are unhelpful except for the leucocyte ascorbic acid concentration. If this is undetectable, the diagnosis of scurvy is practically certain.

Treatment is synthetic ascorbic acid 250 mg four times daily. This saturates the body within a week. Anaemia should be treated with ferrous sulphate. The patient should be educated about healthy eating and cooking, and told to boil vegetables in the minimum of water for the minimum of time to conserve their ascorbic acid. Potatoes are an important source of ascorbic acid in the winter when fruit and vegetables are expensive, especially if they are unpeeled and not mashed.

Claims have been made that huge doses of ascorbic acid prevent and abort the common cold, but these have not been substantiated.

BERIBERI (THIAMINE DEFICIENCY)

This is largely a disease of technology and especially of polished rice. It became common in the rice-eating countries of the East when steel mills were introduced in the nineteenth century. These mills remove the outer layers of the rice grain, which contain most of the grain's thiamine. Latterly, thiamine has been added to polished rice and the disease almost abolished. The only foods rich in thiamine are seeds (wholegrain cereals, pulses and nuts) and yeast, but significant amounts are present in most whole foods. It is added to white flour and many breakfast cereals, but is absent in sugar, butter and oils. In Britain, beriberi is seen rarely, and mainly in alcoholics.

Thiamine pyrophosphate is an essential co-enzyme in a key step in carbohydrate metabolism, the oxidative decarboxylation of pyruvic acid. When thiamine is deficient, the tissues accumulate pyruvate, lactate and α-oxoglutarate. This occurs especially in nervous tissues, which depend heavily on carbohydrate for their energy, and especially on a carbohydrate-rich diet.

There are two main forms of beriberi – wet and dry. Wet beriberi derives its name from its most characteristic symptom, oedema. This occurs because there is extreme vasodilatation and capillary leakage caused by the high tissue levels of pyruvate and lactate. Later cardiomyopathy develops, leading to high output cardiac failure and finally death from circulatory failure. The calf muscles are often tender and there may even be intermittent claudication. In the West, this picture is seen only after prolonged heavy alcohol consumption with very little food.

Dry beriberi is essentially a peripheral, mainly motor polyneuropathy. Even severe wasting and weakness is fully reversible in the East, but less so in alcoholic cases. The latter are prone also to Wernicke's encephalopathy and to Korsakow psychosis.

Diagnosis is confirmed by finding low erythrocyte transketolase levels corrected by adding thiamine pyrophosphate or, less specifically, by raised blood pyruvate levels after an oral load of glucose.

PELLAGRA (NICOTINAMIDE OR NICOTINIC ACID DEFICIENCY)

This occurs wherever maize is the staple food, because in maize nicotinic acid is in a bound form which cannot be digested or absorbed. In addition maize protein is deficient in tryptophan, which can be converted to nicotinic acid by the tissues. Pellagra is endemic only where diets are generally poor, and it is often associated with kwashiorkor. It is occasionally seen in chronic alcoholics in rich countries. Foods rich in nicotinic acid are butcher's meat, especially offals and fish, whole grain cereals, yeast and pulses. Nicotinic acid is part of the NAD molecule.

Pellagra is characterised by erythema progressing to dermatitis in light-exposed areas of skin. There is often a red swollen tongue, angular stomatitis and diarrhoea which is occasionally bloody. Nervous symptoms are prominent, including depression, anxiety, delirium and, in chronic cases, dementia. Pyramidal tract lesions and peripheral neuropathy may also occur. Diagnosis rests on the clinical findings and on the response to treatment with nicotinic acid 100 mg four-hourly by mouth. Deficiencies of riboflavine and protein are common and should also be treated.

VITAMIN A DEFICIENCY

Vitamin A or retinol is a fat-soluble alcohol which can be ingested as such in milk, butter, vitaminised margarine, cheese, egg yolk, liver and fatty fish, but for the most part it is synthesised in the intestinal mucosa from β-carotene, an orange pigment which is abundant in dark green leaves, carrots and other vegetables. Its functions are to take part in:
1. The formation of visual purple (rhodopsin), which is the retinal pigment used in night vision.
2. The metabolism of epithelial tissues.

Clinical deficiency is seen chiefly in hot, dry climates in people whose diet has been deficient for a long time in both dairy produce and vegetables. In practice, it is often found alongside kwashiorkor. It is a major cause of blindness in many poor countries. The first sign of deficiency is night-blindness. Later there is dryness of the conjunctiva and cornea (xerophthalmia), which can lead to corneal ulceration and softening (keratomalacia) and finally perforation of the eyeball and blindness. The skin may show follicular hyperkeratosis in which keratin plugs protrude from the hair follicles, making the skin rough over the buttocks and extensor surfaces. In Europe, mild deficiency is an occasional complication of malabsorption.

Other Fat-soluble Vitamins

Vitamin D is more a hormone than a vitamin and deficiency is due more to deprivation of sunlight than to poor diet. It is discussed in Chapter 11.

Vitamin E deficiency does not occur except rarely in premature infants, when it causes haemolysis.

Vitamin K deficiency is due to malabsorption, not malnutrition (*see* page 75).

Other Water-soluble Vitamins

Riboflavine deficiency does not exist as a pure, isolated condition. It may complicate other deficiency states such as pellagra, when it contributes to angular stomatitis, cheilosis and glossitis. It is surprising that more serious effects do not occur, because riboflavine is an essential part of the flavoproteins as in FAD. The vitamin is widespread in food, especially liver, milk, eggs and green vegetables.

Pyridoxine, pantothenic acid and biotin are essential for the formation of certain co-enzymes, but isolated deficiencies are rare.

Vitamin B_{12} and folic acid, the anaemia-preventing vitamins, are discussed in Chapter 19.

PRINCIPLES OF HEALTHY EATING

Most, probably all, the diseases mentioned in this chapter would be avoided if, like all wild animals, man lived on a variety of fresh, unprocessed foods. In modern civilisation this is often difficult and always expensive (processed foods are cheap because they are mass-produced). Everyone, however, can afford to choose wholegrain cereal products and to eat a helping or two of fruit and raw vegetables daily. Refined bakeries and confectionery are best reserved as occasional treats – cakes were traditionally a feast-day luxury. Sugar is best regarded as a chemical sweetener and used as sparingly as salt. Fatty meat and fried foods should probably be restricted. Lean meat, liver and other offal are good, but not essential. The health of vegetarians is actually better than that of meat-eaters, except that strict vegans can get vitamin B_{12} deficiency. Dairy products are controversial, but probably beneficial in moderation.

SUGGESTED FURTHER READING

General

Davidson, S., Passmore, R., Brock, J. F. and Truswell, A. S. (1975) *Human Nutrition and Dietetics*. Edinburgh: Churchill Livingstone.

McLaren, D. S. (1976) *Nutrition and its Disorders*. 2nd edn. Edinburgh: Churchill Livingstone.

Obesity

Mann, G. V. (1974) The influence of obesity on health. *New England Journal of Medicine*, **291**: 178–185 and 226–232.

Fibre Deficiency

Cleave, T. L. (1974) *The Saccharine Disease*. Bristol: J. Wright and Sons.

Medical Genetics

T. J. DAVID

6

CHROMOSOMES

It was only in 1956 that man was shown to have 46 chromosomes (23 pairs). Methods for studying human chromosomes rapidly improved, and by 1959 patients with Down's syndrome (mongolism) were shown to have 47 chromosomes, the extra chromosome being number 21. This chromosome constitution was described as 'trisomy 21', i.e. the presence of three chromosomes number 21 instead of the normal complement of two.

Each chromosome consists of two identical *chromatids* which are joined together at the *centromere*. Normal chromosomes are divided into three types, according to the site of the centromere (Fig. 6.1). The three types are:
(a) *Metacentric*, where the centromere is approximately central and the arms are of equal length.
(b) *Submetacentric*, where the centromere is nearer one end than the other, resulting in two short arms and two long arms.
(c) *Acrocentric*, where the centromere is near the end so that two arms are very short.

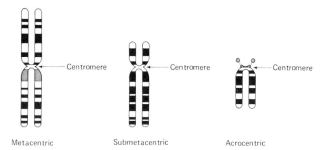

Fig. 6.1 The main features of human chromosomes. The centromere is the point at which the two strands (chromatids) are joined down a longitudinal axis. Chromosomes are classified by the position of the centromere as follows: metacentric, submetacentric, acrocentric.

Chromosomes are grouped by their size and the location of the centromere. Modern techniques show densely staining bands and since each chromosome has a distinctive pattern of light and dark bands (*see* Fig. 6.2) it is now possible to positively identify each chromosome.

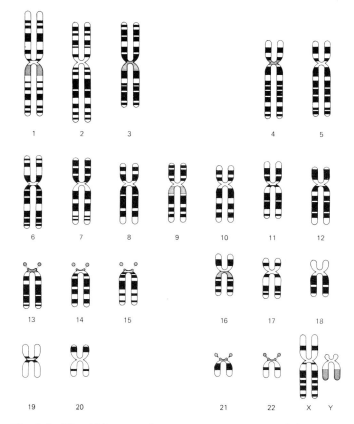

Fig. 6.2 The 46 human chromosomes, represented diagrammatically to show chromosome bands. The methods first used for demonstrating bands used quinacrine mustard or quinacrine dihydrochloride to produce a fluorescent banding pattern. These methods are named Q-staining methods and the resulting bands, Q-bands. Other techniques which demonstrate bands use the Giemsa dye mixture as the stain, and the resulting bands are named G-bands. One technique using the Giemsa dye gives patterns which are opposite in staining intensity to those obtained usually; this technique is called the reverse-staining Giemsa method and the resulting bands, R-bands. A band is defined as a part of a chromosome which is clearly distinguishable from its adjacent segments by appearing darker or lighter with one of the methods above. Bands that stain darkly with one method may stain lightly with other methods. (In this diagram the centromere is representative of Q-staining method only.)
From Paris Conference (1971): Standardisation in Human Cytogenetics. In Bergsma, D. (ed.). White Plains: The National Foundation – March of Dimes, BD:OAS VIII(7), 1972.

CHROMOSOME ANOMALIES AT BIRTH

The incidence of patients with chromosome anomalies is about 4 per 1,000 live births. These anomalies can be divided into those that affect the pair of sex chromosomes and those that involve the other 22 chromosomes (known as *autosomes*). The total load of 4 per 1,000 live births with major chromosome anomalies is almost equally divided between those abnormalities of the sex chromosome pair and those of the autosomes (Table 6.1).

Table 6.1 Incidence of major chromosome anomalies per 1,000 live births

Autosomal anomalies	
Trisomy 21 (Down's syndrome)	1.5
Trisomy 18 (Edwards' syndrome)	0.1
Trisomy 13 (Patau's syndrome)	0.1
Others	0.3
Sex chromosome anomalies	
XYY	0.5
XXY (Klinefelter's syndrome)	0.5
XXX	0.5
45,X (Turner's syndrome)	0.05
Others	0.45
Total	4.0

Autosomal Anomalies

Trisomy 21 (Down's Syndrome). Standard trisomy 21 is found in about 95 per cent of cases. In the rest there is either mosaicism (a mixture of trisomic and normal cells) or a translocation (the extra chromosome 21 is not free in the cell but is attached to another chromosome).

The main features are a characteristic facial appearance, single transverse palmar crease (35 per cent of cases), short incurved little finger (clinodactyly), typical ear shape (small ear lobe with angular overlapping helix), speckled spots in the iris (Brushfield's spots), fissuring of the tongue (not present until about 4 years of age), short broad neck, congenital heart disease (20 per cent of cases – most important lesions are endocardial cushion defects), and severe mental retardation (100 per cent of cases). In the newborn period generalised hypotonia is striking, and there is often marked tongue protrusion.

Trisomy 13 (Patau's Syndrome). If born alive these infants rarely survive more than a few weeks. The fairly characteristic pattern of multiple malformations includes cleft lip and palate, defects of the scalp, microcephaly, arrhinencephaly and other cerebral defects, congenital heart disease, post-axial polydactyly (extra little fingers or extra little toes), and microphthalmos.

Trisomy 18 (Edwards' Syndrome). Death within the first few weeks of life is usual. The fairly characteristic pattern of multiple malformations includes low set ears which are often malformed, absent corpus callosum, small mouth, fixed flexion deformities of the fingers which tend to overlap, 'rocker-bottom' feet, single umbilical artery, cardiac malformations, horseshoe kidney, Meckel's diverticulum, and there is striking intrauterine fetal growth retardation (birth weight considerably less than expected for the period of gestation).

Partial Deletion of the Short Arm of 5 (Cri du Chat Syndrome). The characteristic feature is that the newborn infant has a laryngeal anomaly, giving the baby a cry just like a kitten. Other features include single transverse palmar crease, characteristic facies with hypertelorism (increased interpupillary distance), epicanthic folds, low birth weight, microcephaly, and severe mental retardation. As these babies grow older, the abnormal cry disappears.

Other Chromosome Abnormalities

Translocations. A segment of a chromosome may be transferred from one chromosome to another. Using letters to represent a linear sequence of genes, such a translocation can be represented as follows:

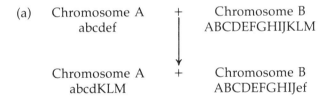

Sometimes fragments of chromosomes are lost in the process:

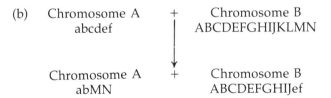

Sometimes genetic material is deleted from one chromosome and transferred to another:

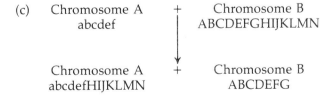

The exchange of genetic material may take place between homologous chromosomes (i.e. chromosomes from the same pair) or between non-homologous chromosomes. A reciprocal translocation (see example (a)) involves exchange of genetic material between two chromsomes, whereas a non-reciprocal translocation (see example (c)) occurs when genetic material is deleted from one chromosome and inserted into another. If a subject carries no more or less genetic material than normal, the translocation is said to be *balanced*. Where there is loss of genetic material to any significant degree (i.e. enough to make the subject in any way abnormal) the translocation is said to be *unbalanced*.

The most clinically important translocations are those which involve chromosome 21. An example is the fusion of a chromosome 14 to a chromosome 21, the two being joined at or near the centromeres. This process is known as *centric fusion* because the chromosomes re-join in regions close to the centromeres. Centric fusion is sometimes called a 'Robertsonian' translocation because it was first described by Robertson, and it is regarded as being a form of reciprocal translocation. The newly constructed chromosome consists of the long arms of the 21 and the long arms of the 14. There is also a *complementary* chromosome formed by the fusion of the short arms of chromosome 21 and chromosome 14. This complementary chromosome seems invariably to disappear after a few cell generations.

14:21 translocation carriers of this sort can produce three types of viable offspring – normal, carriers of the translocation, and Down's syndrome subjects. In theory, there is an expected risk of one in three pregnancies resulting in an affected child, but for reasons which are not clear, the risk is less than this. Where the mother is the 14:21 translocation carrier the risk of having an affected offspring in any particular pregnancy is about 10 per cent, and where the father is the carrier the risk is about 2.5 per cent.

Other translocations can lead to Down's syndrome. Perhaps the most unfortunate of all is the 21:21 translocation, for carriers of this translocation can only produce infants with Down's syndrome.

Clinically, the result of having a pair of long arms of chromosome 21 as extra genetic material is almost the same whether it is attached to another chromosome (as in a translocation) or isolated (as in ordinary trisomy 21).

Deletions. Part of the chromosome is missing:

ABCDEFGHIJKLMN ⟶ ABCDEFG
or
ABCDEFGHIJKLMN ⟶ ABCDEMN

The most important clinical syndromes associated with deletions are the 'cri du chat' syndrome (see above), the syndrome associated with partial deletion of the short arm of chromosome number 4, and the syndromes associated with the deletions of the short or long arms of 18. Note that example (b) in the section on translocations (see above) could also be regarded as a deletion because of the loss of genetic material.

Duplications. Part of the chromosome is duplicated. If the duplicated segment is adjacent to the original piece, it is known as a tandem duplication (as in the example below):

abcdef ⟶ abcdbcdef

Inversions. This is an end-to-end reversal of a segment within a chromosome. When in one arm of a chromosome it is referred to as a paracentric inversion. When the inverted segment includes the centromere, the inversion is called pericentric.

abcdef ⟶ adcbef

Sex Chromosome Anomalies

Monosomy X (45, X). Such patients are females, and have 45 chromosomes with only a single X chromosome. Many (but not all) cases have Turner's syndrome – short stature, dysgenetic ovaries, and somatic abnormalities such as webbed neck, cubitus valgus, short fourth and fifth metacarpals, narrow hyperconvex nails, coarctation of the aorta, congenital lymphoedema. However, some cases have short stature and dysgenetic gonads without any somatic anomalies – the *syndrome of gonadal dysgenesis* – and a few rare cases have dysgenetic gonads with normal stature (and no somatic anomalies) – the so-called *pure gonadal dysgenesis*.

It is important to point out that not all subjects with 45,X have Turner's syndrome (which is a purely clinical description) and that not all subjects with Turner's syndrome have 45,X as their chromosome constitution.

47,XXY (Klinefelter's Syndrome). These patients are male. The main features are tall stature, testicular atrophy (with infertility), gynaecomastia and sparse facial and body hair. Fifteen to twenty per cent have an IQ below 80.

48,XXXY and 49,XXXXY Syndrome. These patients are male. They are mentally deficient. As in Klinefelter's syndrome, there is testicular atrophy and a small penis, but there are often associated minor skeletal deformities, most commonly proximal radio-ulnar synostosis.

47,XYY Syndrome. There is only one certain fact about these males, and that is that they tend to be tall. The suggested association with aggressive and criminal behaviour is controversial.

47,XXX; 48,XXXX; 49,XXXXX. These subjects are female. The mental state varies from normal intelligence (most cases of 47,XXX) to mental deficiency (all cases of 48,XXXX and 49,XXXXX). There is variable amenorrhoea and infertility, and very little in the way of somatic abnormalities.

GENERAL EFFECTS OF THE SEX CHROMOSOMES

The presence of a Y chromosome makes a subject male; the absence of a Y chromosome renders the subject female. This applies however many X chromosomes are present.

When more than one X chromosome is present, the other (or others) largely become inactive from early embryonic development. The inactive X chromosome (or chromosomes if there are three or more X's) becomes condensed, and in this condition is visible as a *Barr body* – a tiny darkly-staining mass lying against the inner surface of the nuclear membrane. The following rule applies:

No of X chromosomes = No. of Barr bodies + 1

In clinical practice Barr bodies are sought in smears of cells from the buccal mucosa, though they can be demonstrated in other tissues too.

If there are two X chromosomes (e.g. in a normal female), then one X chromosome is paternally derived and the other is maternally derived. The Lyon hypothesis states that there is *random* inactivation of one of the X chromosomes, so that in one cell it is the paternally derived X that is inactivated, whereas in another cell it is the maternally derived one that is inactivated. Once this chance selection has been made it is perpetuated by a cell's descendants. Clearly, inactivation is not quite complete, for subjects with the 45,X constitution are not normal females. It is not clear if the inactivated X retains some genic activity, or if the sole function of the inactivated X takes place before inactivation occurs, or if inactivation only takes place in somatic cells and not in germ cells. A further possibility, to explain why subjects with sex chromosome anomalies are not normal, is that the abnormal features of these conditions are possibly not a direct genetic effect of the missing or extra chromosomes, but an indirect effect that these chromosome anomalies have on cell division (and thus influence development). The time taken for cell division becomes progressively longer with an increase in the number of sex chromosomes. This is thought to explain the linear relationship between the number of sex chromosomes and various metrical characteristics. The best examples of this are the inverse linear relationship between the number of X chromosomes and the total finger ridge count (a fingerprint characteristic), the IQ, height and birth weight.

THE ORIGIN OF CHROMOSOME ANOMALIES

Normally, ova or sperms contain only one of a homologous pair of chromosomes. *Meiosis* is the process during the production of ova or sperms by which the diploid chromosome number is reduced to the haploid number. By an error at meiosis, called *nondisjunction*, ova or sperms may be produced in which there are either two chromosomes of a homologous pair or none. In the former case, the resulting zygote will have 47 chromosomes, and in the latter, 45 chromosomes. This is the most common origin of an abnormal chromosome complement. It appears that the risk of nondisjunction increases with increasing maternal age. In addition, there appear to be genes which predispose to nondisjunction, so that once a woman has had an offspring with for example trisomy 21 or trisomy 18, she has a slightly increased chance of having another offspring with a chromosome abnormality (irrespective of her age).

CHROMOSOME ANOMALIES AND SPONTANEOUS ABORTIONS

As a conservative estimate, 25 per cent of all conceptions are lost as spontaneous abortions. Some of these losses occur before implantation, and are not recognised as pregnancies at all. Other losses occur as spontaneous abortions during recognised pregnancies.

It is now established that as many as 40 per cent of these abortuses have major chromosome anomalies. The various types of chromosome anomaly are shown in Table 6.2.

Table 6.2 The frequency of different chromosome anomalies in chromosomally abnormal abortuses

Autosomal trisomy	50%
Triploidy (69 chromosomes)	13%
Tetraploidy (92 chromosomes)	4%
45,X	24%
Others	9%

It appears that the proportion of chromosomally abnormal abortuses is greatest in very early abortions (8 weeks post conception), and becomes less as gestation increases. Whether the proportion of chromosomally abnormal fetuses is even higher in pre-implantation losses is unknown.

How nature achieves such a high rejection rate for chromosome abnormalities is not clear. There is a general relationship between the severity of the abnormality and its prenatal lethality (*see* Table 6.3). However, this is not always the case, and the reasons for the extremely high prenatal loss rate of 45,X (a comparatively 'mild' anomaly) are obscure.

THE GENETIC CODE

Chromosomes consist of a double strand of deoxyribonucleic acid (DNA). Each strand is made of a series of nucleotides attached to one another in a linear sequence. There are four types of nucleotide, which are distinguished from one another by the presence of one of the following bases: cystosine (whose symbol is C), guanine (G), thymine (T) and adenine (A). The two strands contain the same information in complementary form and are paired along their length. The rules are that if in one strand there is a T at a given position, in the other strand there will be an A at that position, and vice versa. The same applies to G and C, and there are therefore only four permitted pairs of nucleotides: TA, AT, GC and CG.

Thus, for example, a strand of DNA could be represented thus:

GATCGGCAATCG

its complementary strand:

CTAGCCGTTAGC

and the double strand thus formed:

G A T C G G C A A T C G
C T A G C C G T T A G C

It appears that normally DNA does not exist as a long thread, but is at least partly coiled up.

A sequence of nucleotides, starting from a given point, is converted into a corresponding sequence of amino acids. The sequence of the nucleotides is critical, for three adjacent nucleotides in a DNA strand code for one amino acid. Three such adjacent nucleotides are called a *triplet*. One triplet codes for one amino acid, but there are only 20 amino acids commonly found and 64 possible combinations of A, T, C and G. Only two

Table 6.3 Prenatal lethality of chromosome abnormalities (i.e. the proportion that are lost as spontaneous abortions or still births)

Abnormality	Proportion lost
Tetraploidy, triploidy	almost 100%
Autosomal monosomies*	almost 100%
45,X	99.9%
Autosomal trisomies	95.0%
Overall	90%

*A *monosomy* occurs when one of a pair of chromosomes is missing, e.g. monosomy 21, when only a single chromosome 21 is present.

amino acids, methionine and tryptophan have a unique coding, and the code in general is, therefore, said to be degenerate. The code is given in Table 6.4.

It can be seen that three triplets, ATT, ATC and ACT, do not code for any amino acids and probably code for the ending of polypeptide chain synthesis.

If there is a change in DNA then this change will be inherited, and such a change is called a *mutation*. The simplest change that can occur in DNA is the substitution of one nucleotide for another, and this is also the most common kind of change:

Example: AAATAAGGA
↓
AGATAAGGA

The original sequence specifies:

phenylalanine-isoleucine-proline

The new sequence specifies:

serine-isoleucine-proline

Table 6.4   The genetic code (for DNA) showing the probable codings for 20 amino acids

1st Base		2nd Base				3rd Base
		Adenine	Guanine	Thymine	Cytosine	
Adenine		Phenylalanine	Serine	Tyrosine	Cysteine	Adenine
		Phenylalanine	Serine	Tyrosine	Cysteine	Guanine
		Leucine	Serine	chain end	chain end	Thymine
		Leucine	Serine	chain end	Tryptophan	Cytosine
Guanine		Leucine	Proline	Histidine	Arginine	Adenine
		Leucine	Proline	Histidine	Arginine	Guanine
		Leucine	Proline	Glutamine	Arginine	Thymine
		Leucine	Proline	Glutamine	Arginine	Cytosine
Thymine		Isoleucine	Threonine	Asparagine	Serine	Adenine
		Isoleucine	Threonine	Asparagine	Serine	Guanine
		Isoleucine	Threonine	Lysine	Arginine	Thymine
		Methionine	Threonine	Lysine	Arginine	Cytosine
Cytosine		Valine	Alanine	Aspartic acid	Glycine	Adenine
		Valine	Alanine	Aspartic acid	Glycine	Guanine
		Valine	Alanine	Glutamic acid	Glycine	Thymine
		Valine	Alanine	Glutamic acid	Glycine	Cytosine

A nucleotide substitution does not necessarily lead to an amino acid substitution because several triplets code for the same amino acid. A single nucleotide substitution is often called a *point* mutation or a *gene* mutation.

Another possible change is the insertion or deletion of one or more nucleotides. This is much more serious because it interferes with the rest of the code.

For example, suppose the original code is:

AAA TAA GGA GAG TTT . . . .

and the fifth nucleotide is deleted, the sequence becomes:

AAA TAG GAG AGT TT . . . .

Such a mutation is a random change in a very complex structure, and it is likely to make the structure either inefficient or totally inoperative – hence most mutations are detrimental. Some mutations have little effect, and a few may turn out to be advantageous. DNA is a very stable substance, and its replication a very precise process; mistakes are rare. Thus the frequency of mutations is low, though there are physical and chemical agents which can increase the frequency of mutations.

DOMINANT, RECESSIVE AND SEX-LINKED INHERITANCE

The fact that the chromosome set is normally double means that nearly all genes are represented twice. Where both *alleles* or genes at a given locus are the same, the subject is said to be *homozygous* for that gene or allele. Individuals who carry two different genes for the same locus are said to be *heterozygous*.

If one of two homologous genes is normal but the other has been affected by a mutation, provided that the remaining normal gene is sufficient for normal function, the subject is protected against the possible harmful effects of the mutation. The amount of protein synthesised as a result of the activity of one normal allele is usually adequate for normal functioning. With a harmful mutation affecting loci for which this is the case, the defect is not expressed in the heterozygote but almost certainly will be expressed in subjects who are homozygous for the harmful mutation. A harmful mutation which only affects the subject if it is present in a double dose is said to be a *recessive* gene.

For a number of loci, the amount of protein synthesised by the activity of a single normal gene is not adequate for normal functioning of the individual. A harmful mutation at such a locus will manifest itself in a single dose, and is known as a *dominant* gene.

DOMINANT GENES

A dominant gene will be transmitted by an affected person to half of his or her offspring. Sometimes an individual is known to possess a dominant gene but does not manifest it in any way – this phenomenon is known as *incomplete penetrance* and is very common. Incomplete penetrance is detected in two ways. One is where skipping of generations occurs (*see* Fig. 6.3). The other way incomplete penetrance is detected is where there is a disturbed ratio of affected to normal offspring in an informative mating. To give an extreme example, if a man with a dominantly inherited deformity had 20 children but only two were affected, one might suspect incomplete penetrance, particularly if this were a feature of other families with the same condition. (There are of course other explanations for this kind of family; dubious paternity is much more common than one might think.)

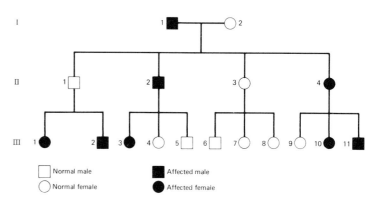

Fig. 6.3 *Family tree of a dominant gene to show generation skipping*. II:1 must have inherited the gene from his father I:1 to have passed it on to his offspring III:1 and 2, yet II:1 is apparently normal and shows no signs of the condition.

Another feature of dominant genes is variable expression. An example of this would be the Holt-Oram syndrome, which consists of:
1. An ostium secundum atrial septal defect.
2. Radial sided upper limb defects, in particular usually involving the thumb.

Some subjects with this condition, which is inherited as a dominant trait, just have the cardiac malformation. Others just have the limb defects, and others have both. This is called *variable expression* and is not the same as incomplete penetrance.

It has been found repeatedly in medical genetics that what was thought to be a single disease entity has proved on close study to consist of two or more distinct entities. *Genetic heterogeneity* is applied to the situation where more than one genetic cause leads to the same or a very similar clinical picture. Sometimes the heterogeneity is *allelic* (i.e. the different genes resulting in the similar clinical disorder are at the same locus), and on other occasions it is *non-allelic*. Genetic heterogeneity has been demonstrated in a large number of genetic disorders, many of which were previously thought to be single diseases, and is almost certainly much more common than generally realised. It is important to remember that a genetic disorder may be mimicked by some environmental agent. This is called a *phenocopy*.

It is thought that the overall incidence of dominantly inherited disorders is about 7 per 1,000 live births, and McKusick's 1975 catalogue of inherited disorders lists 583 as dominant (and another 635 as possibly dominant). The birth frequencies of some common dominant conditions are listed in Table 6.5.

Table 6.5 Birth frequencies of some common dominant conditions†

Condition	Frequency per 1,000 live births
Polycystic disease of the kidneys	0.8
Huntington's chorea	0.5
Diaphyseal aclasia	0.5
Neurofibromatosis	0.4
Myotonic dystrophy	0.2
Congenital spherocytosis	0.2
Polyposis coli	0.1

† These figures apply to the United Kingdom only, and will in certain cases be different in other parts of the world.

RECESSIVE GENES

Recessive traits are only manifest when the gene concerned is present in a double dose, that is in subjects who are homozygous for the abnormal gene. Heterozygous subjects are usually normal (though heterozygotes may be detectable by special testing in some disorders), and are referred to as *carriers*. Homozygotes usually only result from the mating of two carriers (or possibly from the mating of a carrier with an affected subject).

When carriers marry, there is a 1 in 4 chance that any individual offspring is homozygous (and thus affected), a 1 in 2 chance that the offspring is a carrier, and a 1 in 4 chance that the offspring is genetically normal.

The most common recessive gene in the United Kingdom is the gene for cystic fibrosis, and about 1 in 20 people are carriers. The chances that two carriers will meet and marry is 1 in 400, and the incidence of the disease is about 1 in 2,000 live births. However, carriers for other recessive genes are less common, and the chances of carriers of a rare disease meeting one another are clearly low. There is, however, one situation where one might expect carriers of rare recessive genes to meet, and that is the marriage of two related people. There is a general rule that the rarer the recessive disease, the greater are the chances that there will be parental consanguinity.

The overall incidence of recessive disorders is about 2.5 per 1,000 live births, and McKusick's catalogue of inherited disorders lists 466 as recessive (and another

481 as possibly recessive). The birth frequencies of some common recessively inherited conditions are listed in Table 6.6.

Table 6.6 Birth frequencies of some recessively inherited conditions†

Condition	Frequency per 1,000 live births
Cystic fibrosis	0.5
Non-specific severe mental retardation	0.5
Recessive deafness	0.2
Sickle cell anaemia (in Europe)	0.1
Adrenal hyperplasia	0.1
Phenylketonuria	0.1

† These figures apply to the United Kingdom only, and will in certain cases be different in other parts of the world.

SEX-LINKED INHERITANCE

Genes carried on the Y chromosome are said to be *Y-linked*. Genes carried on the X chromosome are said to be *X-linked*. An X-linked recessive trait is determined by a gene carried on the X chromosome and is only manifested in the female when the gene is in a double dose, i.e. when the female is homozygous. In the male

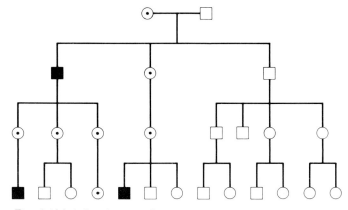

Fig. 6.4(a) A family tree of an X-linked recessive trait in which affected males can reproduce.

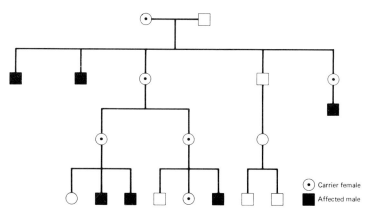

Fig. 6.4(b) A family tree of an X-linked recessive trait in which affected males die before they are old enough to reproduce.

an X-linked recessive gene is always manifested because there is no 'normal' gene at the same locus. An X-linked recessive gene is transmitted by an affected male to all his daughters (who are all heterozygotes), but not to any of his sons (*see* Fig. 6.4).

An X-linked dominant trait is manifested in the heterozygous female as well as in the male having the gene on his X chromosome. An affected male transmits the disease to all his daughters but to none of his sons (*see* Fig. 6.5).

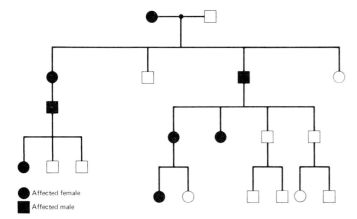

● Affected female
■ Affected male

Fig. 6.5   A family tree of an X-linked dominant trait.

The overall incidence of X-linked conditions at birth is low, being about 0.4 per 1,000 births. McKusick's catalogue of inherited disorders lists 1,142 X-linked disorders (with another 1,194 listed as possibly X-linked). Birth frequencies of some of the more common X-linked disorders are listed in Table 6.7.

Table 6.7   **Birth frequencies of some X-linked conditions**†

Condition	Frequency per 1,000 live births
Duchenne's muscular dystrophy	0.2
Haemophilia	0.1
Non-specific X-linked mental retardation	0.1
Icthyosis	0.1

† These figures apply to the United Kingdom only, and will in certain cases be different in other parts of the world.

POLYGENIC OR MULTIFACTORIAL INHERITANCE

To acquire a disease which has a polygenic or multifactorial aetiology one requires *both* of the following:

1. A genetic predisposition.
2. An environmental factor.

Neither polygenic or multifactorial are particularly good for describing this situation and its implications, but there is no better term at present. The two terms are used interchangeably in this context. This form of inheritance is difficult to prove or disprove. However, a hypothetical model has been produced, and certain assumptions can be derived from the model which can be used to see whether an observed pattern of inheritance within a group of families fits with a polygenic model. For the purposes of explanation, a fictional disease situation will be used.

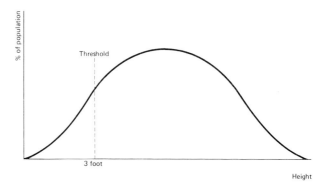

Fig. 6.6   Hypothesised model of polygenic inheritance. The disease: 'The burial of 3 foot dwarfs in snowdrifts'.

The model (*see* Fig. 6.6) assumes the normal distribution of an inherited trait, in this fictional example height. We can make an arbitrary cut-off point (known as the *threshold*) at 3 feet. All subjects to the left of this are 3 foot dwarfs (and even smaller dwarfs). We now have to imagine an environmental factor which will only affect 3 foot dwarfs, and one such factor would be a 4 foot snowdrift. Note that to succumb to the hypothetical disorder one would require both the genetic predisposition (someone 5 foot tall is safe) as well as the environmental factor (even a 1 foot dwarf will be safe if there is no snow).

The model implies that the greater the genetic predisposition the less intense the environmental agent needs to be to produce the disease, and of course vice versa. A one inch dwarf would succumb to 2 inches of snow. (Presumably a 7 foot giant would succumb to an 8 foot snowdrift.)

Some diseases with a supposed polygenic aetiology have a different incidence in the two sexes. For example, infantile pyloric stenosis is about five times as common in males as it is in females. How can this fit with the dwarf-snowdrift model? The answer is that there is no reason why one sex should not be innately protected in some way, or particularly susceptible. Using our model one might respectfully suggest that

113

females, being better insulated against the cold, would be able to withstand snow better than males. If there is such a sex difference, one should be able to make two predictions.

First, the rarer affected sex will on average be genetically more predisposed, and therefore more likely to have an affected relative. For part of the polygenic hypothesis is that the genetic predisposition is due to multiple genes which are additive in their effects, and are derived from both parents. This is exactly the case in infantile pyloric stenosis. The disorder is much more common in males but is more likely to recur in the relatives of affected females (*see* Table 6.8).

Table 6.8 Frequencies of infantile pyloric stenosis in relatives of affected cases

| Sex of index patient | Frequency in relatives | | | |
	Brothers	Sisters	Sons	Daughters
Male	4%	3%	6%	2%
Female	9%	4%	20%	7%

The other prediction which follows from the model is that on average (assuming a constant environment), the more severely affected the individual is, the more genetically predisposed he or she is, and therefore the more likely he or she is to have an affected relative. We cannot use the dwarf in the snowdrift model as an example here, because it is an all-or-none situation as are some polygenic disorders. However, some do vary in their severity, and an example of this is cleft palate. As can be seen from Table 6.9, the more severe the defect the greater the chances are that a sibling or offspring will also be affected.

Table 6.9 Frequency of cleft lip ± palate in relatives of affected cases

Defect in index patient	Frequency in siblings + offspring
Bilateral cleft lip + cleft palate	5.7%
Unilateral cleft lip + cleft palate	4.2%
Cleft lip only	2.5%

Polygenic inheritance has been used to explain the familial incidence of ischaemic heart disease, peptic ulcer, rheumatoid arthritis, diabetes mellitus, schizophrenia, manic depressive psychosis, hypertension, and the common congenital malformations (cardiovascular malformations, neural tube defects, cleft lip and palate, dislocation of the hip, and talipes).

GENETIC COUNSELLING

This is usually done, albeit informally, by general practitioners and by hospital doctors. However, in certain cases patients or their relatives are referred to specialists in regional genetics units. It mainly concerns advising people about the risk that a member of a family will suffer from a disease. The task of the counsellor is to estimate the risk as accurately as possible and try to communicate this as simply and kindly as possible.

The pre-requisites for a correct estimation of risk are an accurate diagnosis and a knowledge either of the mechanisms of inheritance of the disease or availability of data on which to base empirical estimates. A careful family history will be required, and this includes a specific question to elicit consanguinity. It is no use taking the family history in the usual bedside manner, 'Is there anyone else in the family with the disease?'. A full family tree needs to be recorded and this should include live births, stillbirths and abortions in the sibship of the index case and the preceding and succeeding generations.

Genetic counselling

Establish a precise diagnosis.
↓
Discuss prognosis and availability and value of therapy.
↓
Determine risk of recurrence.
Explain genetic implications.
Relieve feelings of guilt.
Help parents to arrive at decision.

When giving the risk in terms of odds it is important to put these odds into perspective. For example, one might point out (if it is appropriate) that the chances of any random pregnancy ending with some serious congenital malformation or that some serious developmental abnormality will manifest itself in early life are about 1 in 30. (This is an approximate figure, and depends partly on what one means by serious.)

PRENATAL DIAGNOSIS

AMNIOCENTESIS

In the past, if a couple had a baby with spina bifida or Down's syndrome or a mucopolysaccharidosis, they had either the option of having no more children or of risking the possibility of having another similarly affected child. However, it is now possible to diagnose antenatally an increasing number of diseases, and such a couple now have the option of availing themselves of these facilities and of having a termination of pregnancy if the fetus is defective or is at high risk of being defective – so-called *selective abortion*. There is very little point performing antenatal diagnosis by amniocentesis if the couple would not agree to a termination, since there is an element of risk to the fetus (*see below*).

Indications for amniocentesis at 14 weeks

1. Previous child with a chromosome abnormality.
2. Family history of a child with a chromosome abnormality.
3. Advanced maternal age (e.g. over 40 years).
4. Parent is a translocation carrier.
5. Parent is a carrier of an X-linked disorder.
6. Previous or family history of a neural tube defect.
7. Family history of biochemical disorder detectable by amniocentesis.
8. Detection of other inherited diseases in the fetus, e.g. thalassaemia.
9. Extreme maternal anxiety.

Technique of Amniocentesis

A small volume of amniotic fluid (5 to 10 ml) can be removed by aspiration through the abdominal wall (*transabdominal amniocentesis*) at about the 14th week of gestation. There is a remote risk of damage to the fetus, and a small but definite risk (1 to 2 per cent) that the procedure will result in loss of the pregnancy within a few days.

The amniotic fluid contains cells which are of fetal origin, being derived from fetal skin and amnion. Some cells are viable and will grow in tissue culture. After 10 to 14 days of cell culture, chromosome studies can be performed, either to look for chromosome abnormalities or to sex the fetus. Sexing can also be done by special direct staining of the cells without culture, but is not entirely reliable. Cell culture for biochemical studies may take a little longer.

Causes of a raised amniotic fluid alpha-fetoprotein level

Anencephaly	Exomphalos
Spina bifida	Intrauterine death of fetus
Oesophageal atresia	Congenital nephrosis
Duodenal atresia	

The fluid itself may be useful, in particular because a high alpha-fetoprotein level strongly suggests the presence of a neural tube defect (anencephaly or spina bifida) in the fetus.

SUGGESTED FURTHER READING
General

Emery, A. E. H. (1975) *Elements of Medical Genetics*, 4th edn. Edinburgh & London: Livingstone.
McKusick, V. A. (1969) *Human Genetics*, 2nd edn. New Jersey: Prentice-Hall.
Roberts, J. A. F. (1973) *An Introduction to Medical Genetics*, 6th edn. London: Oxford University Press.

Catalogue of all Dominant, Recessive and X-linked Diseases

McKusick, V. A. (1975) *Mendelian Inheritance in Man*, 4th edn. Baltimore and London: The Johns Hopkins University Press.

Chromosomes

McDermott, A. (1975) *Cytogenetics of Man and Other Animals*. London: Chapman and Hall.

Clinical Aspects of Chromosome Abnormalities

Smith, G. F. and Berg, J. M. (1976) *Down's Anomaly*, 2nd edn. Edinburgh & London: Churchill Livingstone.
Polani, P. E. (1961) Turner's syndrome and allied conditions. *British Medical Bulletin*, 17(3):200–205.
Warkany, J. (1971) *Congenital Malformations. Notes and Comments*, pp. 296–343. Chicago: Year Book Medical Publishers.

Genetic Counselling

Stevenson, A. C. and Davison, B. C. C. (1976) *Genetic Counselling*, 2nd edn. London: Heinemann.

Clinical Immunology 7

J. VERRIER JONES

The immune mechanism has developed in vertebrates as a protection against the attack of pathogenic viruses, bacteria, fungi, and protozoa. The potential parasite is recognised as foreign, and subjected to an attack combining antibody, which can damage bacteria so that they are readily destroyed by phagocytic cells, and aggressive, cytotoxic lymphocytes, which contribute to the control of viral infections and tuberculosis. The vital importance of the immune defences in man is clear: children in whom the entire immune mechanism fails (Swiss-type agammaglobulinaemia) die within four months, overwhelmed by infection.

Agents that stimulate the immune mechanism (*antigens*) must first be ingested by phagocytic cells (macrophages), which convert antigen into a more immunogenic form. 'Super-antigen' is passed to precommitted lymphocytes, and stimulates them to multiply by repeated cell division. Some lymphocytes differentiate into plasma cells (Fig. 7.1), which secrete antibody, while others may give rise to specialised 'cytotoxic' lymphocytes, capable of destroying foreign cells on contact ('cellular immunity'). Cells that specialise in antibody production are usually descended from bone marrow-derived lymphocytes (B-lymphocytes), while those involved in cellular immunity have usually been modified by a sojourn in the thymus (T-lymphocytes). In many forms of immune response, T and B cells interact. In antibody synthesis, B-cells may require co-operation of 'helper' T-cells, while in some responses 'suppressor' T-cells exert a regulatory and inhibitory effect on B-cells, and on other T-cells. The ability of B-cells and T-cells to interact with each other and with macrophages is determined by the histocompatibility antigens which they carry (*see* page 127).

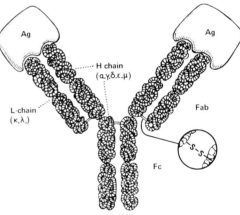

Fig. 7.2 The structure of IgG
H = heavy chain (a, γ, δ, ε, μ); L = light chain (κ, λ); Ag = antigen.
Note: Enzymes cleave molecule into Fab (antibody fraction) and Fc (complement fixing fraction).

Antibodies are found in the plasma proteins among the group known (because of their electrophoretic mobility) as γ-globulins. The majority of antibody molecules belong to the γG (or IgG) class (Fig. 7.2). IgG molecules have a molecular weight of about 160,000 and are built up of four polypeptide chains. IgM molecules consist of five of these 4-chain sub-units linked together, and appear in the primary response. Other immunoglobulin classes have been described in man, and are designated IgA (found mainly in secretions), IgD, and IgE (responsible for reaginic, or allergic antibodies).

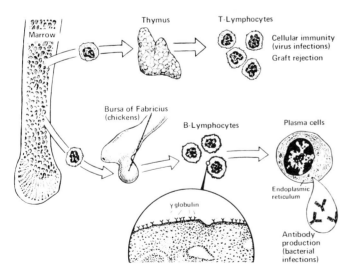

Fig. 7.1 B and T lymphocytes.

Table 7.1 Levels of immunoglobulins in normal serum (mg/100 ml)

IgG	800–1,680
IgA	140–420
IgM	50–190
IgD	0.3–40
IgE	0.0001–0.0007

The immune mechanism may be involved in disease in a number of ways:

1. **Immune Deficiency States.** The system may fail. With its defences crumbling the organism may be overwhelmed by infection.

2. **Monoclonal Gammopathies.** There may be overproduction of a single type of γ-globulin molecule with proliferation of the corresponding plasma cells or lymphocytes.

3. **Autoimmune Disease: Immune Complex Disease.** The immune mechanism may produce antibodies, or develop cellular immunity, which damage the body, either by cross-reacting with autologous tissues, or by forming antigen-antibody complexes.

4. In some individuals, certain antigens (allergens) produce antibodies of a particular type (reagins) which result in the symptoms and signs of *allergy*.

IMMUNE DEFICIENCY STATES

Failure of the immune mechanism may involve mainly antibody production, or mainly cell-mediated immunity, or both. It may be congenital (primary) or acquired (secondary).

CONGENITAL DEFECTS OF IMMUNITY (*see also* page 618).

DEFECTS OF IMMUNOGLOBULIN SYNTHESIS (B-CELL DEFICIENCIES)
X-LINKED INFANTILE HYPOGAMMAGLOBULINAEMIA

The first case of immune deficiency disease was described by Bruton in 1952. Bruton-type agammaglobulinaemia is a congenital, sex-linked recessive condition occurring in boys below the age of ten, and associated with severe depression of the levels of IgG, IgA, and IgM. The lymphoid tissues are depleted and there is a complete absence of plasma cells and of circulating B-lymphocytes. The tonsils and adenoids may be absent. Children with this condition have repeated infections with pyogenic organisms, and may die of a pneumonia produced by *Pneumocystis carinii*. They have normal cell-mediated immunity, however, and can develop a positive Mantoux reaction, and reject skin allografts briskly. They recover normally from virus infections. They can be successfully treated with injections of purified human gammaglobulin.

IMMUNODEFICIENCY WITH HIGH LEVELS OF IgM

A few cases of immunodeficiency have been reported in which levels of IgM are raised, while IgA and IgG are reduced or absent. This may be a congenital, X-linked condition, or may be acquired. It may be due to a failure of maturation of IgM producing cells to IgG and IgA production.

SELECTIVE IgA DEFICIENCY

The most common of all immunodeficiencies (1:600 of the normal population) is a selective deficiency or absence of IgA. B-cells carrying IgA are present in normal numbers in the circulation. The defect is possibly one of IgA synthesis or release. Patients with IgA deficiency may be entirely normal. Some, however, have an increased incidence of allergy, or of gastrointestinal disease such as coeliac disease, while others have an increased tendency to develop autoimmune diseases, including endocrinopathies, pernicious anaemia, systemic lupus erythematosus, and rheumatoid arthritis.

OTHER IMMUNOGLOBULIN DEFICIENCIES

Selective defects of IgM, and of the IgG sub-classes, have also been described and patients are susceptible to infections and to autoimmune diseases.

DEFECTS OF CELL-MEDIATED IMMUNITY

In di George's syndrome (thymic aplasia) there is congenital hypoplasia of the thymus and a depletion of thymus-dependent lymphocytes, with absence of the parathyroid glands. Children with this condition cannot develop a positive tuberculin reaction and fail to show delayed hypersensitivity to chemical allergens such as dinitrochlorobenzene (DNCB). Skin graft rejection is delayed. Antibodies, however, develop normally, and bacterial infections are not a problem. Cellular immunity seems the most important defence against virus infections, and children with this syndrome are particularly susceptible to attack by viruses. The condition has been successfully treated with grafts of fetal thymus-cells. Other forms of T-cell deficiency may occur in combination with chronic mucocutaneous candidiasis. Some of these patients also develop endocrinopathies, including hypoparathyroidism and Addison's disease as well as chronic active hepatitis. Treatment with transfer factor, a soluble product obtained from lymphocytes of normal subjects, sometimes leads to improvement of the candidiasis.

COMBINED DEFICIENCY OF CELLULAR AND HUMORAL IMMUNITY

The disease now known as 'Swiss-type agammaglobulinaemia' (or *severe combined immunodeficiency*) was first described by Glanzman and Riniker in 1950, and subsequently reviewed by Hitzig and his co-workers in 1958. The striking features are severe diarrhoea, thrush, skin rashes, and septicaemia, and the disease is invariably fatal. There is a severe depression of all immunoglobulins, lymphopenia, and absence of plasma cells. All the lymphatic organs are grossly reduced and the thymus is atrophic. The clinical features result from a combined failure of antibody production and cellular immunity. In some families the disease appears to have an autosomal recessive inheritance. A minor form is known as Gitlin's syndrome.

OTHER CONGENITAL IMMUNOLOGICAL DEFICIENCIES

With some sophisticated techniques for measuring humoral and cellular immunity, other less common defects of immunity have been described. Selective deficiencies of one class of immunoglobulin are known. In *Ataxia telangiectasia*, for example, there is often an isolated deficiency of IgA. In the *Wiskott-Aldrich syndrome*, eczema and thrombocytopenia are associated wth recurrent bacterial infections. Levels of IgM are low, while other immunoglobulins may be normal or increased.

In a number of patients with combined immunodeficiency, it has recently been shown that there is a deficiency of the enzyme *adenosine deaminase* (ADA).

ACQUIRED DEFECTS OF IMMUNITY

In normal children, there is a transitory fall in the level of circulating immunoglobulins as the molecules transferred from the mother across the placenta decay and are replaced by those synthesised by the infant. Occasionally, the maturation of the infant's immune system may be delayed and there is a *transient hypogammaglobulinaemia*.

PRIMARY ACQUIRED HYPOGAMMAGLOBULINAEMIA

In adults, repeated infections, especially with Gram-positive cocci, are sometimes found to be associated with a deficiency of circulating immunoglobulins. Replacement therapy with injections of gammaglobulins may be helpful. Although there is no clear inheritance in this condition, other members of the family may show high or low levels of immunoglobulins.

SECONDARY HYPOGAMMAGLOBULINAEMIA

In diseases in which the reticuloendothelial system is affected by a malignant process, there may be a defect in the synthesis of immunoglobulins, presumably because the cells that secrete them are replaced by malignant tissue. Some of the underlying diseases, such as chronic lym-phatic leukaemia or Brill-Symmers disease, are relatively benign, and it may be necessary to consider treatment with gammaglobulin if repeated infections are troublesome.

OTHER ACQUIRED DEFECTS

In Hodgkin's disease there is often complete absence of cellular immunity, and all skin tests for delayed hypersensitivity are negative. This may account 'for the increased incidence of miliary tuberculosis and fungal diseases in patients with Hodgkin's disease. In sarcoidosis, and in Crohn's disease, there is a similar but less profound depression of cellular immunity. In all these conditions, antibody production appears to be normal.

MONOCLONAL GAMMOPATHIES

When an animal responds to an antigen by producing antibodies the gammaglobulin molecules synthesised migrate as a wide band on electrophoresis. Antibody to a single antigen is usually composed of a variety of immunoglobulin molecules differing in their rate of electrophoretic migration. By contrast, in *myelomatosis* and *macroglobulinaemia* there is an over-production of immunoglobulin molecules of a single class and composition (Fig. 7.3) which migrate as a single sharply-defined band on electrophoresis.

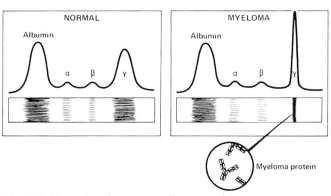

Fig. 7.3 Monoclonal gammopathy – myeloma.
Note: Tall narrow band in electrophoretic pattern of serum.

Disorders of gammaglobulin synthesis have been termed 'gammopathies', and since the disordered cells in myelomatosis and macroglobulinaemia appear to belong to a single family, or clone, the term 'monoclonal gammopathy' has been used to describe them. The term, though etymologically inelegant, is operationally valuable.

MYELOMATOSIS (*see* page 402)

MACROGLOBULINAEMIA (WALDENSTRÖM'S MACROGLOBULINAEMIA) (*see* page 404)

AUTOIMMUNE DISEASES

There are a number of diseases in which the immune mechanism develops antibodies or cellular immunity directed against antigens within the body itself. In many cases, this auto-aggressive immunity may be important in determining the course of the disease. In other cases, autoimmunity may be no more than a harmless side effect of the disease. In some diseases, the auto-aggressive immunity seems to have clearly developed as a reaction against external antigens, which happen to cross-react with normal components of body tissues. These can be described as 'heteroimmune' diseases. Rheumatic fever and some forms of haemolytic anaemia are examples of this.

In other diseases ('immune complex diseases') complexes of antigen and antibody are deposited in the tissues and these produce inflammation and tissue destruction. Post-streptococcal glomerulonephritis, polyarteritis nodosa, and lupus erythematosus are examples of immune complex disease.

Diseases in this group often respond to treatment with cortisone and its derivatives, and to the immuno-suppressive drugs which act by inhibiting cellular protein synthesis and, hence, block cell division. In animals, they reduce or abolish the production of antibodies and the development of cellular immunity. In autoimmune disease they limit the body's ability to harm itself by means of a misdirected immune response.

Disorders of this group can most readily be classified according to the system involved.

AUTOIMMUNE DISEASES OF THE BLOOD

AUTOIMMUNE HAEMOLYTIC ANAEMIAS (*see* page 389)

IDIOPATHIC THROMBOCYTOPENIC PURPURA (ITP) (*see* page 415)

AUTOIMMUNE CONNECTIVE TISSUE DISORDERS

It is convenient to describe under this heading a group of disorders that are neither certainly autoimmune, nor wholly limited to connective tissue. These are *systemic lupus erythematosus, polyarteritis nodosa, systemic sclerosis,* (scleroderma) and *dermatomyositis.* These diseases (sometimes referred to as 'collagen diseases' or 'collagen vascular diseases') are characterised by diffuse vascular inflammation, the deposition of fibrinoid material, and inflammatory changes in connective tissue.

Systemic lupus erythematosus and polyarteritis nodosa belong to a group of disorders referred to as 'immune complex diseases'. Animals injected repeatedly with weak antigens develop 'chronic serum sickness', characterised by joint swelling, an inflammatory arteritis, and glomerulonephritis. These lesions are accompanied by the deposition of antigen-antibody complexes, with attached complement, in small blood vessels, where they trigger an inflammatory response. Chronic serum sickness, produced in humans by repeated injections of horse serum, was originally described by von Pirquet in 1905. It is now recognised that a number of human diseases may be associated with the deposition of immune complexes in the walls of blood vessels, though often the antigen involved is unknown.

In addition to systemic lupus erythematosus and polyarteritis nodosa, immune complex deposition is found in some forms of glomerulonephritis, in a number of skin diseases (including allergic vasculitis) in the arteritis of rheumatoid arthritis, in infective endocarditis, in erythema nodosum, in some forms of purpura, in cryoglobulinaemia (where the complexes are precipitated by cooling), and in the skin manifestations of many infectious diseases.

SYSTEMIC LUPUS ERYTHEMATOSUS (SLE)

DIFFUSE LUPUS ERYTHEMATOSUS (DLE)

Definition

A progressive, generalised disease, with chronic inflammatory changes involving all systems of the body, and characterised by the presence of the LE cell phenomenon, and of antinuclear factor (ANF).

Background

The term 'lupus' (L = wolf) seems to have first been used to describe ulcerating, erosive skin lesions in the thirteenth century. Lupus vulgaris and lupus erythematosus were distinguished in the mid-nineteenth century, and William Osler, about 1900, was among those who recognised that lupus erythematosus could be associated with generalised visceral manifestations. The characterisation of systemic lupus erythematosus was greatly advanced in 1948, when the LE cell phenomenon (Fig. 7.4) was described by Hargraves, Richmond and Morton. It was subsequently shown that the LE cell phenomenon was produced by combination of an antibody to nucleoprotein with DNA in the cell nucleus, and this antibody, now readily recognised by immunofluorescence, has been termed antinuclear factor (ANF) or antinuclear antibody (ANA). There is no convincing explanation of why the immune mechanism should suddenly begin to form antibodies to nucleoproteins. The most favoured theories are:

1. The 'forbidden clone' theory, which suggests that mutation in the system of antibody-forming cells gives rise to cells producing antibody with harmful, self-directed specificity. Those who hold this theory need to show that every manifestation of SLE can be directly attributed to antibody.

2. The 'genetic' theory which suggests that the disease

is caused by an inherited abnormality. There is evidence for abnormally high levels of serum immunoglobulins in the relatives of patients with SLE, and of an increased risk of SLE among close relatives of those with the disease.

3. The 'infective' theory, which suggests SLE is caused by a transmissible agent, perhaps viral, and perhaps transmitted vertically from mother to fetus. There is no direct evidence for the presence of such an agent. A disease clinically similar to SLE and with a positive LE cell test is seen occasionally after exposure to a variety of drugs, including hydrallazine, procaine amide, sulphonamides, penicillin, and phenytoin; mice of the NZB strain (which probably carry a virus) also develop an autoimmune disease resembling SLE.

SLE has an incidence of about one per 100,000 and 80 to 90 per cent of cases are women. The disease is commonest between the ages of twenty and forty.

Pathology

SLE is characterised by the deposition of 'fibrinoid' material in connective tissue and in the walls of blood vessels. Fibrinoid is a homogenous, eosinophilic material with a fibrillar structure, perhaps containing fibrin. 'Haematoxylin bodies', which are spindle-shaped clumps of haematoxylin-stained material, are found in many tissues, including kidney and lymph nodes. They may consist of depolymerised DNA. Granulomas are found less frequently. In the kidney, 'wire-loop' lesions are seen in glomeruli, and electron microscopy shows deposits of DNA, antibody, and complement in clumps on the epithelial surface of the glomerular basement membrane.

Symptoms and Signs (Fig. 7.4)

The clinical picture is highly variable. Skin involvement with erythema in a butterfly pattern over the cheeks, and light-exposed areas of skin, or disseminated over the body, is seen in 80 to 90 per cent of patients. Fever, malaise, arthralgia and weight loss are common, and a deforming joint disease resembling rheumatoid arthritis is sometimes seen. Pleurisy and pleural effusions, and renal involvement occur in about 50 per cent of patients. Antigen-antibody complexes are deposited on the outer surface of the glomerular basement membrane, and produce a patchy, focal glomerulitis. Occasionally, this is associated with the nephrotic syndrome. The prognosis is much worse in cases where the kidney is involved. In the heart, pericarditis, myocarditis and endocarditis occur, and vascular lesions may occur in any tissue as a result of a generalised vasculitis. Involvement of the central nervous system may produce fits or psychiatric changes and mixed sensory and motor peripheral neuropathy is occasionally seen. In the blood, a haemolytic anaemia and lymphopenia are fairly com-

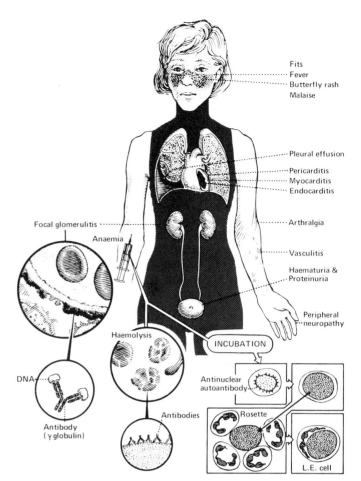

Fig. 7.4 Clinical features of systemic lupus erythematosus and LE cell phenomenon.

mon features. Hair loss, leading to alopecia, is common when the disease is acute.

Investigations

1. The LE cell test (Fig. 7.4) was one of the most reliable ways of making the diagnosis. The LE cell is seen after defibrinated blood or bone marrow has been incubated at 37°C for 2 hours. Initially, antibody to nucleoproteins attacks a leucocyte nucleus, causing it to swell, and lose its chromatin pattern. A ring of normal polymorphs then surrounds the disintegrating cell (rosette-formation). Finally, the swollen mass of nuclear material is ingested by a polymorph, and the resulting structure is an LE cell.

2. Examining films from incubated blood for LE cells is time-consuming, and a more useful screening test for SLE is the detection of antinuclear factor (ANF). Any nucleated tissue (rat liver, or human thyroid is often used) is treated with serum from the patient, followed by a fluoroscein-conjugated antibody to human IgG. If the patient's serum contains antibodies reacting with nuclear antigens, these will become attached to the tissue nuclei, and will fluoresce under ultraviolet light.

Four patterns of nuclear staining can be distinguished, and give an indication of the type and severity of the disease.

The rim pattern. The antinuclear staining is confined to a rim, or circle, associated with the nuclear membrane. The antibodies producing this pattern are directed against ds-DNA, and it is usually associated with active SLE.

The homogenous pattern. The staining is distributed diffusely over the whole nucleus. The antibodies are directed against deoxyribonucleoproteins, and the pattern is seen with SLE in remission, and less commonly, in some of the other collagen vascular diseases.

The speckled pattern. Granules of fluorescence are scattered throughout the target nucleus. The antibodies are directed against extractable nuclear antigens (ENA), and this pattern is seen in SLE, and also in scleroderma, rheumatoid arthritis, and in mixed connective tissue disease.

The nucleolar pattern. Occasionally, only the nucleolus is stained. This pattern is seen in scleroderma, in SLE, and in rheumatoid arthritis. Frequently, more than one staining pattern may be observed with a single serum. This will become apparent when antinuclear staining is observed at various dilutions.

3. Anti-DNA antibodies. These are much more specific. In particular, antibodies to ds native DNA only occur in SLE and some liver diseases. The titre may reflect disease activity.

4. Biopsies of the kidney and liver will show characteristic histological changes if these organs are involved.

Differential Diagnosis

The diagnosis of SLE should be made if the clinical features of the disease are accompanied by a positive LE cell test, or a positive test for ANF. In some cases of rheumatoid arthritis ANF is found; some of these patients proceed to develop a typical clinical picture of SLE.

Basis of Treatment

The skin rash is photosensitive, and exposure to sunlight should be avoided. If joint pains are troublesome, salicylates may be helpful. If there are signs of a systemic illness, treatment with *corticosteroids* is indicated. Initially, doses of prednisone of up to 100 mg/day may be required. When symptoms have begun to improve it may be possible to reduce the dose to 5 to 10 mg daily, or even to discontinue it. Fewer complications of corticosteroid therapy will occur if the daily dose can be replaced by an alternate day schedule. Since the disease is progressive and fatal, careful follow-up is required, and the dose of drugs may need frequent adjustment.

Cytotoxic drugs, especially azathioprine (Imuran) have been found to be of limited value, and should be considered in patients with renal involvement, and in those failing to respond to, or requiring dangerously high doses of prednisone. In some acutely ill patients with high levels of circulating antigen-antibody complexes, there may be a clinical response to plasmaphaeresis.

Prognosis

Some 70 per cent of patients survive for five years after diagnosis, and 50 per cent for ten years. Renal involvement is associated with a poor prognosis.

MIXED CONNECTIVE TISSUE DISEASE

A number of syndromes have been described which overlap between SLE and other connective tissue disease. Mixed connective tissue disease (MCTD) shows a characteristic onset, with Raynaud's phenomenon, myositis of the proximal muscles, mild scleroderma, and some manifestations of SLE. The ANF is typically of the speckled pattern, and the serum contains very high levels of antibody to extractable nuclear antigens (ENA) which are destroyed by treatment with ribonuclease. The disease is usually mild, the kidney is rarely involved, and patients often respond rapidly to treatment with a small dose of corticosteroids.

POLYARTERITIS NODOSA

Definition

A disease characterised by widespread destructive, inflammatory lesions of small and medium-sized arteries with fibrinoid necrosis.

Background

Polyarteritis nodosa belongs to a group of vascular inflammatory diseases known as allergic vasculitis. An allergic vasculitis can be produced in animals by intravenous injection of a foreign protein (such as bovine serum albumin, BSA) into previously immunised animals. The animals pass through a stage in which antigen-antibody complexes are formed in antigen-excess, and deposited in the walls of small arteries, where they give rise to an allergic vasculitis. A similar condition, known as 'serum sickness' was produced in man in the days when immune horse serum was used in the treatment of diphtheria and tetanus. It was due to the development of antibodies to horse serum proteins, followed by the deposition of antigen-antibody complexes in small arteries.

There are resemblances between immune-complex vasculitis and polyarteritis nodosa, and immunofluorescent studies of polyarteritis nodosa have shown the presence of deposits of gammaglobulin in the walls of inflamed arteries. In some cases these deposits have been shown to be associated with the hepatitis B antigen (Australia antigen) (*see* page 67). The disease sometimes follows treatment with penicillin or sulphonamides. Polyarteritis nodosa is a rare condition affecting males more commonly than females, with a peak incidence in young adults. A form is described (Wegener's granuloma) where widespread polyarteritis is accompanied by local destructive changes in the nose, nasal sinuses, ears, and respiratory passages.

Pathology

The histological changes are those of a distinctive inflammatory process affecting initially the media of medium-sized arteries. Oedema and fibrinoid necrosis of the muscle fibres is followed by infiltration with polymorphs, often leading to thrombosis. Chronic inflammation, with scarring and granulation tissue may follow, and is often associated with aneurysmal dilatation of the arteries involved.

Symptoms and Signs

The disease affects many systems, and so may present in a number of ways (Fig. 7.5). The course may be acute and fulminating, leading rapidly to death, or chronic and remittent. Fever and weight loss are common presenting features, often associated with asthma, peripheral neuropathy, and pain and tenderness in muscles. Renal involvement may lead to haematuria and proteinuria, and is often accompanied by hypertension. In the lungs, patchy infiltrative lesions may be seen on X-ray; pleural effusion and lung abscess are rarer complications. Joint pains are common and may resemble rheumatic fever. In the peripheral nervous system a patchy, mainly motor neuropathy is often seen, and in the central nervous system subarachnoid and intracerebral haemorrhage may occur.

Investigations

The plasma viscosity is usually raised, and there is often a polymorphonuclear leucocytosis, sometimes with an increased eosinophil count. Blood and proteins may be found in the urine, together with urinary casts. The diagnosis is clinched by a positive biopsy. A renal biopsy will be helpful if the kidneys are involved, and a biopsy of muscle may show typical changes if the muscle is swollen or tender. Pleural and lung biopsies may be helpful, and skin nodules, if present, should also be biopsied.

Differential Diagnosis

1. Polyarteritis nodosa should be suspected when an

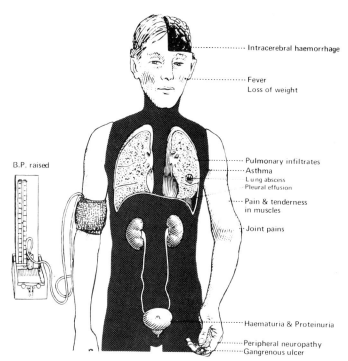

Fig. 7.5 Clinical features of polyarteritis nodosa.

obscure pyrexia is associated with arthralgia, or respiratory or neurological symptoms.
2. Biopsy evidence is necessary to distinguish from sarcoidosis, Hodgkin's disease, and systemic lupus erythematosus, which can often present similarly.

Basis of Treatment

Corticosteroids are used, as in lupus erythematosus, in an attempt to slow down the course of the disease. In individual cases dramatic improvement may be seen. Cytotoxic drugs such as azathioprine and cyclophosphamide may be used in resistant cases.

Prognosis

When the disease is widespread the prognosis is poor; 51 out of 54 untreated patients without lung involvement were dead in six months. Treatment with corticosteroids may produce a dramatic improvement in symptoms, and probably prolongs life. At the Mayo Clinic 110 treated cases had a five-year survival of 48 per cent. Involvement of the lungs and kidneys carries a worse prognosis.

SYSTEMIC SCLEROSIS (SCLERODERMA, GENERALISED MORPHOEA)

Definition

A rare disease in which there is diffuse fibrous thickening of the skin, with involvement of lungs, gut, heart and kidneys.

122

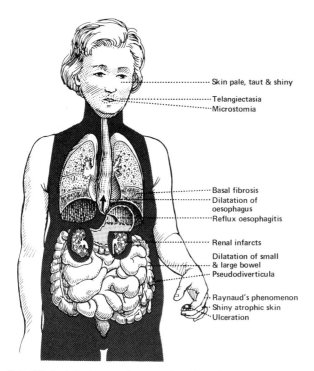

Fig. 7.6 Clinical features of systemic sclerosis.

Labels on figure:
Skin pale, taut & shiny
Telangiectasia
Microstomia
Basal fibrosis
Dilatation of oesophagus
Reflux oesophagitis
Renal infarcts
Dilatation of small & large bowel
Pseudodiverticula
Raynaud's phenomenon
Shiny atrophic skin
Ulceration

Background

Systemic sclerosis is about seven times commoner in women than in men and usually occurs between the ages of 30 and 50. In men, the death rate has been estimated at one per million a year. The aetiology is unknown. There are a few immunological abnormalities. The serum gammaglobulin may be raised, and rheumatoid factor is present in up to 50 per cent of patients. Antinuclear antibodies are often found, often with a speckled pattern. Patients with systemic sclerosis show a higher than normal incidence of rheumatoid arthritis, Sjøgren's syndrome, SLE and Hashimoto's thyroiditis, and the argument of 'guilt by association' has been used to suggest that it is an autoimmune disease. A familial incidence is sometimes recorded in the localised form of scleroderma, but is rare in systemic sclerosis.

Pathology

In areas of involved skin, the epidermis is atrophic, while the dermis shows thickened and hyalinised collagen bundles. There is often widespread obliteration of smaller blood vessels, particularly in the fingers, by endarteritis. Lymphocytic infiltration occurs in affected tissues.

Symptoms and Signs

The disease often presents with symptoms of vascular insufficiency in the fingers (Raynaud's phenomenon,

arterial spasm provoked by exposure to cold, is common). The skin of the hands and later of the face, neck and feet becomes thickened, inelastic and tight. The tips of the fingers may become ulcerated and necrotic, and the mouth is narrowed and fixed. Areas of telangiectasia may occur in affected skin, and calcium deposition is seen deep in affected skin (Fig. 7.6).

The disease often spreads from the skin to involve other systems. Joint pains are frequent, and in severe cases movement of joints, especially in the hands, may be limited by the skin changes. The gastrointestinal tract is frequently involved, dysphagia and reflux oesophagitis are common, due to atrophy of smooth muscles in the oesophagus, with underlying fibrosis. A barium swallow will often show an atonic, non-contractile oesophagus. The small and large intestine can be similarly involved, and steatorrhoea may occur. The heart and pericardium may be affected, and the lungs often show a progressive diffuse fibrosis, more marked at the bases. The kidneys are often affected by the endarteritis seen in this disease, and death from renal failure and hypertension is not uncommon.

Investigations

The appearance of the affected skin is quite characteristic once it has been seen. A skin biopsy may be helpful to clinch the diagnosis in doubtful cases. In general, however, laboratory tests are irrelevant, and this is a disease which is diagnosed by the unaided use of the power of observation.

Differential Diagnosis

1. In localised scleroderma (morphoea) the skin lesions of systemic sclerosis occur in circumscribed areas of skin, but there is no evidence of a progressive or generalised disease.
2. Mixed connective tissue disease is distinguished by the presence of high levels of antibody to extractable nuclear antigens (ENA) and by its responsiveness to corticosteroids.

Basis of Treatment

Corticosteroids may relieve symptoms in the early stages, but are of no ultimate benefit. Physiotherapy is helpful in maintaining movements in the hands. If Raynaud's phenomenon occurs, the patient should avoid cold exposure. Necrosis of digits may require surgical treatment. Aldomet orally, or intra-arterial reserpine may be helpful in the presence of vascular insufficiency. Recently, promising results have been obtained with penicillamine.

123

Prognosis

The disease progresses slowly, with frequent remissions and relapses. In one series of 700 cases, 60 per cent were alive ten years after diagnosis.

DERMATOMYOSITIS

Definition

A rare, usually chronic disease, in which inflammatory changes of proximal muscles are associated with an erythematous rash on the face and upper part of the body. In a number of cases an underlying neoplasm is found.

Background

Dermatomyositis is less common than systemic sclerosis. Women outnumber men by two to one, and it is most often seen between the ages of 40 and 60, though it occasionally occurs in children. The aetiology is unknown. The association with cancer has led to the suggestion that the neoplasm may develop new antigens which cross-react with antigens of normal skin and muscle, so that an immune response directed against the cancer may damage normal tissue. The evidence for this is at present only indirect. Cancer occurs in some 15 to 20 per cent of patients with dermatomyositis; the tumour may be in the breast, stomach, lung, ovary, rectum, kidney, testis or uterus. Dermatomyositis has also been reported in patients with lymphoreticular malignancy. The cancer may precede or follow the development of dermatomyositis. When the cancer is removed, dermatomyositis often improves.

Pathology

Skin. There is oedema of the dermis, with lymphocytic infiltration, and later, atrophy of the epidermis.

Muscles. There is patchy loss of muscle striations, with hyalinisation of the sarcoplasm, followed by breakdown and degeneration of muscle fibres. Areas of lymphocytic infiltration, sometimes massive (lymphorrhages), are found in association with degenerating muscle fibres.

Symptoms and Signs (Fig. 7.7)

The clinical picture will vary, depending on whether skin or muscle are predominantly affected. The polymyositis usually begins with symmetrical involvement of proximal groups of the pectoral and pelvic girdles. Patients may complain of difficulty in rising from a low chair and in climbing stairs. There may be weakness in raising the arms to comb the hair, and in

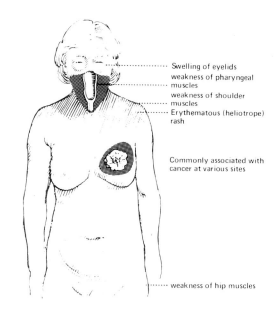

Fig. 7.7 Clinical features of dermatomyositis.

scrubbing. The disease may spread to involve the pharyngeal muscles (giving dysphagia and nasal speech), and, ultimately, the respiratory muscles.

The skin rash, which usually begins on the face, is erythematous, with a purplish ('heliotrope') tinge. Often the shoulders and chest are involved, and eventually the rash may spread to the hands and arms.

In long-standing cases calcinosis may develop in the subcutaneous tissues associated with affected muscles. Arthritis has been described, and gastrointestinal involvement may produce vomiting, constipation and diarrhoea, as well as dysphagia. Involvement of the cardiac muscle occurs occasionally and renal and ocular changes have been described.

Investigations

As in any inflammatory condition, the plasma viscosity will be raised. Destruction of muscle will lead to increased serum levels of muscle enzymes. Estimations of SGOT, SGPT, serum aldolase and serum phosphocreatine kinase may all be helpful. Hypergammaglobulinaemia and rheumatoid factor are sometimes found. In the presence of a suggestive history and skin rash, a muscle biopsy may be necessary to clinch the diagnosis.

Complications

The pharyngeal paralysis may lead to aspiration pneumonia. In severe cases, paralysis of the respiratory muscles may occur. In those cases with an underlying cancer, this may be the cause of death.

124

Differential Diagnosis

Muscular dystrophy and other forms of polymyositis may produce similar symptoms. A muscle biospy may help to make the distinction. The skin changes may be confused with systemic lupus erythematosus (in which, however, the LE cell test is positive) or with scleroderma (in which a skin biopsy will usually show distinctive features).

Basis of Treatment

A search should always be made for an underlying neoplasm. If this can be removed surgically, or destroyed by radiotherapy, the dermatomyositis may improve. In all other cases, corticosteroid drugs should be given in a large initial dose, followed by a maintenance dose sufficiently large to control symptoms and to keep serum enzyme levels within the normal range. About 50 per cent of patients may be expected to improve on corticosteroids. Azathioprine may also be of value.

Prognosis

The course of the disease is very variable. Fifty per cent of children are dead within two years of diagnosis. In adults with a neoplasm, the type and site of the cancer will determine the prognosis.

OTHER AUTOIMMUNE DISEASES

Autoimmune factors are involved in a number of other diseases, which are considered in detail in other sections of the book. In *pernicious anaemia* (*see* page 379), antibodies to intrinsic factor, and to intrinsic factor – B_{12} complex may interfere with the absorption of vitamin B_{12}. In *Hashimoto's thyroiditis* and *myxoedema* (*see* page 173), antibodies occur which react with thyroglobulin and with various components of thyroid cells. There is also evidence of cellular immunity to thyroid antigens. This auto-aggressive response to the thyroid may set up chronic inflammatory changes in the gland. In thyrotoxicosis (*see* page 171), the long-acting thyroid stimulator (LATS) which occurs in most patients, is an antibody to a component of thyroid microsomes. Antibodies to organ-specific antigens are also found in some cases of *Addison's disease* (*see* page 169), *hypoparathyroidism* (*see* page 195), and *ovarian dysgenesis*, and may play an important part in determining the course of the disease. In rheumatoid arthritis, antibodies to altered gamma-globulin are found, but are probably a result, rather than a cause, of the disease.

In many other diseases of the gastrointestinal tract, liver, lungs, heart, central nervous system and skin, autoimmune phenomena have been observed, but much further study will be required to determine their significance.

IMMEDIATE HYPERSENSITIVITY AND ALLERGIC DISORDERS

Definition

The allergic diseases, which include allergic rhinitis (hay fever), allergic (extrinsic) asthma, urticaria and angio-oedema, allergy to insect stings, drug allergy, and anaphylaxis occur in a group of individuals described as atopic. These subjects develop antibodies of the IgE class, on exposure to specific antigens (allergens).

Background

The antibodies responsible for allergic sensitisation are usually of the IgE class. Their molecular weight is higher than that of IgG and the molecules carry an extra domain ($C\varepsilon^4$) in the heavy chain.

IgE molecules are cytotropic: the Fc portion of the molecule has a strong affinity for receptor sites on the surface of mast cells. When these fixed, cell-bound antibodies combine with their specific antigen, the receptors are distorted, and the mast cell degranulates, releasing histamine and related vasoactive substances locally into tissue.

IgE antibodies are found particularly at mucous membranes, and exposure to allergens can lead to either localised or generalised anaphylaxis.

LOCAL ANAPHYLAXIS

Pathology

Individuals who develop local hypersensitivity to grass, flower, or tree pollens in the mucous membranes of the upper respiratory tract will show intense oedema, and an inflammatory reaction, with polymorph infiltration, and eosinophilia, at the site of exposure, associated with the local release of histamine. In allergic *asthma*, exposure to allergens in pollens or dusts leads to histamine release in the bronchioles with wheezing. Similar reactions can take place in the wall of the gut, in response to food allergens, or in the skin, as a result of hypersensitivity to insect stings.

Symptoms and Signs

In *allergic rhinitis* (*hay fever*) there is a typical seasonal incidence, corresponding to the discharge of pollen from anemophilous plants. This may range from late spring to late summer, depending on the area and the type of plant. During the pollen season, sensitive individuals develop painful irritation of the mucous membranes of the eyes and nose, accompanied by the discharge of profuse watery secretions. The onset of symptoms will often correspond to a period of exposure to pollen. Some sensitive individuals may also develop *allergic asthma*, with wheezing and respiratory distress. On examination, there are likely to be widespread expiratory rhonchi.

Investigations

1. In *allergic rhinitis* eosinophils are found in the nasal secretions. Circulating eosinophils are usually normal or slightly elevated. High levels of IgE are found in secretions (though this test is not available in routine laboratories), but IgE levels in the serum are only slightly elevated.
2. In *allergic asthma*, blood and sputum eosinophilia are often found and serum IgE levels are often raised. The chest X-ray may show hyperinflation during an acute episode of bronchospasm, and during intervals between attack may show focal atelectasis.

Pulmonary function studies will show varying degrees of airways obstruction, with decreased ventilatory flow rate and FEV_1.

Testing for Allergens. A careful history will often elicit a story of symptoms related to exposure to allergens. A seasonal incidence will suggest a relation to pollens. Symptoms developing after moving to a new house, or after the acquisition of a pet animal may also be helpful. In some cases it may be useful to carry out skin tests with a battery of test antigens, to determine those to which the individual is allergic. Commercially available test kits include antigens derived from pollens, dusts and mites, which are commonly involved in allergic hypersensitivity. The solutions are placed on the skin in a series of marked areas, and the skin is lightly pricked with a sterile needle through each drop of test solution. The area of test is observed after 20 minutes, and the result is recorded. A positive result will be indicated by the development of erythema alone, or, in stronger reactions, of erythema with a raised wheal.

Complications

Allergic rhinitis may be complicated by the development of *infective sinusitis*, if the mucous membrane swelling obstructs drainage of the paranasal sinuses. Allergic asthma may sometimes be serious enough to lead to irreversible lung damage (*see* bronchial asthma, page 345) or to status asthmaticus (*see* page 350).

Differential Diagnosis

1. Nasal obstruction and mucous discharge may be caused by nasal polyps, which will be seen on examination.
2. Chronic vasomotor rhinitis is a perennial condition without seasonal exacerbations, associated with a post-nasal drip.

3. Intrinsic asthma is not associated with a history of antigenic exposure, and usually shows no clear seasonal history. It may be impossible, however, in some individuals to make a clear distinction between intrinsic and extrinsic asthma.

Basis of Treatment

If a history of exposure to allergens can be elicited, it will be necessary to take steps to prevent exposure as far as possible. This may involve advising subjects with a sensitivity to pollens to remain indoors during the pollen season. When children develop symptoms after acquiring a pet, it may be necessary to dispose of it. *Desensitisation* by repeated injections of small doses of the allergen involved may relieve symptoms in a proportion of subjects.

During an episode of allergic rhinitis, antihistamines may help to reduce the symptoms. In mild asthma, ephedrine may be helpful. More severe cases may need treatment with aerosols of bronchodilator drugs, or parenteral injections of β-adrenergic agents (*see* page 350).

Prognosis

Some children with severe allergic symptoms may become less severely involved in adolescence and adult life, but there is no way of predicting which cases will improve in this way.

GENERALISED ANAPHYLAXIS

When an antigen is injected intravenously or intramuscularly into individuals with reaginic antibodies, generalised anaphylaxis may occur. There is widespread liberation of mast cell products throughout the body, producing generalised vasodilatation and an abrupt fall in blood pressure. This may be rapidly fatal unless treated. Adrenaline, corticosteroids and antihistamines are required urgently and, sometimes, transfusion with blood or plasma may be needed. Severe generalised anaphylaxis may be seen following the administration of anti-tetanus antiserum to individuals previously sensitised to horse serum, or of penicillin to those with reaginic antibodies to the penicillin molecule.

In some individuals, insect bites and stings may lead to localised or generalised anaphylaxis.

COMPLEMENT

This name is given to a series of proteins which, when activated, produce inflammation, cell damage and blood coagulation. The activation process occurs when there is combination of antigen and antibody of the IgG and IgM class and can also be produced by certain proteolytic enzymes. There are two major pathways for complement activation – the classical cascade with sequential activation of all the proteins and an alternative pathway which by-passes the early C_{142} components. The alternative pathway is activated by substances such as endotoxin.

The combination of antibody and antigen may, by fixing and activating complement, result in cell death and in the case of autoimmune haemolytic anaemia it is known that red cell damage actually involves the production of holes in the cell membrane, the cell later being destroyed in the liver and spleen. The combination of antigen and antibody is called an immune complex and these are normally cleared by phagocytosis. The persistence of immune complexes in the body may, however, give rise to systemic disease. Examples of this are serum sickness when fever, skin rashes, arthritis and proteinuria follow the injection of foreign serum. Here the combination of antibody with retained foreign protein results in immune complex deposition in the microcirculation, which is a self-limiting disease. More chronic immune complex disease is a feature of a variety of autoimmune disorders (see page 119).

Immune complexes can be demonstrated in tissues by using immunofluorescent techniques, and the presence of circulating complexes by more indirect means such as binding of the C_{1q} fraction of complement. Reduction in the total complement and/or its fractions may also be of value in the detection and assessment of immune complex disease, particularly where there is renal involvement. Inherited deficiencies of individual complement fractions may render that person susceptible to connective tissue disorders.

HLA ANTIGENS AND DISEASE

These are antigens on the surface of human leucocytes (HLA) which are important in tissue transplantation because they determine histocompatability between donor and recipient, and where a 'match' can be obtained transplantation is likely to be more successful.

Further, it is now well recognised that certain diseases are more common in subjects who have particular HLA types. The diseases are particularly those where there seems to be an immunological cause (see Table 7.2). The major histocompatibility complex is found on part of chromosome 6 and four loci, DBCA, are located there. It is thought that immune responses are somehow controlled by the B locus and this might explain the association between HLA types and immune disease. Certain HLA types may also determine susceptibility or resistance to infection by governing the immune response of the host.

Recent interest also centres around B-lymphocyte antigens which are again coded at this histocompatibility locus, and where further associations with a variety of diseases are being found.

SUGGESTED FURTHER READING

General

Samter, M. (ed.) (1971) *Immunological Diseases*. **Vols. 1 and 2**. New York: Little, Brown.

Fudenberg, H. H., Stites, D. P., Caldwell, J. L. and Wells, J. V. (eds.) (1976) *Basic and Clinical Immunology*. Los Altos, California: Lange Medical Publications.

Table 7.2 HLA antigens and disease

Antigen HLAB8	Chronic active hepatitis
	Addison's disease
	Thyrotoxicosis
	Coeliac disease
	Dermatitis herpetiformis
Antigen HLAB27	*Ankylosing spondylitis*
	Anterior uveitis
	Reiter's syndrome
Antigen HLADW2	Multiple sclerosis
Antigen HLAA10	Pemphigus

The strongest relationships are shown in italics.

Dermatology 8

R. P. WARIN and R. R. M. HARMAN

DISEASES OF THE SKIN

It is impossible in a few thousand words to cover the whole subject of dermatology, or even to mention many diseases familiar to the specialist; or to describe systemic diseases, where the skin is one of the organs attacked in such a characteristic and easily visible way that careful examination enables the physician to arrive at a diagnosis—for example in smallpox, meningococcal septicaemia, porphyria, measles, and Addison's disease. Nevertheless, we hope in this chapter to make plain the nature of some of the more common conditions that affect the skin.

The obscure terminology which has so bedevilled the understanding of disorders of the skin has been avoided as far as possible. Simple descriptive terms include:

Macules – flat lesions.
Papules – small raised lesions.
Nodules – larger, firm lesions deeper in the skin.
Vesicles – small blebs less than 5 mm in diameter, containing fluid.
Bullae – larger blisters filled with fluid.
Pustules – blebs filled with pus.
Weals – transient localised oedematous papules and swellings of the skin.

When confronted by a dermatological problem, a careful history should be taken, including a record of previous treatment, and it should be discovered how this treatment has been applied. Astonishing information is often obtained.

As much of the patient's skin as possible should be examined in bright daylight or under really adequate fluorescent strip lighting. (This is more difficult to arrange than one might suppose.)

Particular attention should be given to the total distribution and character of individual lesions. Never forget that changes in the skin may give priceless information about underlying systemic disease.

THE ECZEMA DERMATITIS REACTIONS

Definition

The term eczema (Gr. zema = 'that which is boiled') refers to an inflammation of the skin which has distinctive clinical and histopathological features. The word dermatitis is used instead where these same changes are caused by external agents, such as detergents or chemicals. However, in every case there are a variety of internal and external factors at work and the phrase 'eczema dermatitis reaction' is more accurate, but is too unwieldy to repeat every time this common process is referred to. Therefore, in general, the word 'eczema' will be used in the pages that follow, when external agents are not playing an important part. 'Dermatitis' will describe precisely the same pathological process when it is provoked largely by external contact factors.

Pathology

The skin involved in this way shows the features demonstrated in Fig. 8.1. The initial change occurs in the epidermis with a swelling and disruption of the epidermal cells. Fluid is attracted from the papillary capillaries, with subsequent development of vesicles and, later, a more general oedema of the epidermis.

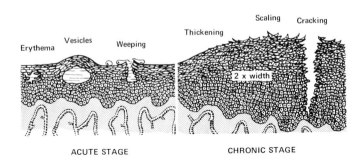

Fig. 8.1 Pathology of the eczema dermatitis reaction.

The reaction is modified by the thickness of the epidermis in the area affected. When this is thick, as on the hands and feet, the vesicles become quite large but in areas where the epidermis is thin, such as the eyelids, vesicles are very rarely seen.

Background

The eczema dermatitis reaction can be evoked in normal skin and is the basis of such common disorders as patches of redness and scaling on the faces of children, scaling and cracking behind the ears, scaling and irritation of the scalp, irritation in the ano-genital area, and isolated vesicles on the fingers in hot weather.

Various factors, internal, external, in the skin itself, or brought to the skin via the bloodstream, may all play a part in provoking the eczema dermatitis reaction and, in most cases, numerous interrelated factors are responsible. These are represented in Fig. 8.2.

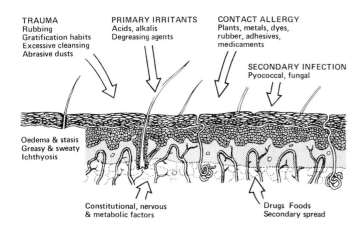

Fig. 8.2 Causative factors in the eczema dermatitis reaction.

Clinical Patterns

Certain common clinical patterns of eczema dermatitis reactions are well recognised and given distinctive labels, although, as would be expected, mixtures of these patterns are common, and in each case the various multiple interrelated factors play a part in aetiology.

INFANTILE ECZEMA (ATOPIC ECZEMA)

Some five per cent of otherwise normal children have eczema of a degree requiring medical attention, and transient minor eczematous changes are so common they merge with normality. The main cause appears to be a constitutional tendency for the eczema dermatitis reaction to be more easily evoked, and there are all degrees of such excessive 'sensitivity of the skin'. General and nervous factors play an important part, and phases when the eczema is worse often coincide with

Classification of eczema

Atopic eczema { infantile eczema
flexural eczema of childhood
atopic eczema of adults

Seborrhoeic eczema
Pompholyx eczema
Discoid eczema
Lichen simplex
Venous (stasis) eczema
Contact dermatitis – due to irritants
due to contact hypersensitivity (Type IV)
Generalised exfoliative dematitis and erythrodermia

periods when the baby or older child is emotionally unsettled or feels insecure, often due to some parent/child stress. In a very few cases food allergy may be responsible and the foods concerned are usually cow's milk, fish, and eggs. Prick tests (immediate hypersensitivity) rarely help the diagnosis in these patients. When food allergy is playing a part, a careful history and accurate observation by the mother are more useful in identifying foods which should be eliminated from the diet. As the child matures such foods can usually be re-introduced without harm.

The condition may start at any age, but often begins at about the third or fourth month. It may occur at first on the scalp and on the cheeks and may develop at any site, but particularly the buttocks, elbow, wrist, knee and ankle creases. There is usually a great deal of itching which promotes scratching and rubbing, and the associated trauma plays an important part in the continuation of the eczema. In some cases there is a tendency for infantile eczema to be worse in cold weather, and more new patients are seen in the early months of the year. However, intense heat may also aggravate the condition.

Many of the mild cases clear in a few weeks or months and the majority have settled down by the time the child is two or three years of age. However, such children may retain a sensitive skin and be more liable to develop eczema in later years. A few children continue to have eczematous eruptions throughout childhood and even into early adult life. In these, the eruption often waxes and wanes, being particularly associated with nervous stress and strain and periods of tension and insecurity. Many of these patients have associated asthma and paroxysmal or seasonal rhinorrhoea. It is difficult to give figures of the incidence of these associated conditions, but in severe infantile eczema of a degree requiring admission to hospital some 50 per cent of the patients will have asthma. In the minor states, the incidence of asthma approaches that of the normal population.

Secondary infection of the eczema is common, most often with streptococci and staphylococci, producing impetigo and boils. Viruses may also infect eczematous skin, and multiple warts and molluscum contagiosum may develop. The virus of herpes simplex may produce a widespread eruption consisting of small vesicles which, if very widespread, can cause a severe general illness (eczema herpeticum). The vaccinia virus may also infect the eczematous sites and may arise from the child being vaccinated or, more commonly, from contact with another person who has been vaccinated. The condition can be very severe or, rarely, fatal and is the main reason why children with infantile eczema should not be vaccinated.

SEBORRHOEIC ECZEMA (INTERTRIGINOUS ECZEMA)

In this type of eczema, patients develop lesions in moist greasy sites, particularly those involving the scalp, behind the ears, the nasolabial furrows, the eyelid margins, the front and back of the mid-chest, the axillae, beneath the breasts, in the ano-genital region, and between the toes. It may be a widespread eruption or involve only one or two areas. In persistent minor states seborrhoeic eczema is an important cause of excessive scaling of the scalp, cracking and scaling round the ears and mouth angles and vulval and anal pruritus. It occurs at any age and may be present in infancy, when it merges with the more usual pattern of infantile eczema.

It readily becomes secondarily infected with pus-forming cocci and seborrhoeic eczema sites may well become reservoirs in which staphylococci build up large numbers which lead to recurrent boils, often in adjacent areas. *Candida albicans* will also readily infect eczema in these moist sites, particularly in the ano-genital area and underneath the breasts.

The tendency may last for many years, with considerable fluctuations in severity, and is often only a minor nuisance. Nervous stress and strain seem to play an important part in the condition and can be responsible for the exacerbations.

POMPHOLYX ECZEMA (pompholyx = blister)

This occurs on the hands and feet. An acute eczema develops and, because of the thick epidermis, fluid cannot escape and vesicles become very large. The condition in which there are only a few scattered vesicles is very common, but widespread, severe pompholyx occurs, in which the vesicles may run together, readily become secondarily infected, and the outer layer of the epidermis may be shed. It is seen commonly in hot humid weather, and is associated with nervous stress and strain. A more chronic stage of eczema which involves the palms and soles and shows as a scaly cracked area is particularly common in middle age. Again, it is largely of constitutional and nervous origin, but the precise causal factors are poorly understood.

DISCOID ECZEMA

A distinctive constitutional pattern of eczema consisting of discrete, intensely itchy round patches which are usually coin-sized is called discoid or nummular eczema (nummulus = coin). The lesions are often so acute that there is serous exudation and crusting.

LICHEN SIMPLEX

This diagnosis refers to patches of chronic thickened eczema, the main cause of which is due to a habit of scratching or rubbing to alleviate irritation, or developed without conscious awareness. These may develop in any area but are common on the nape of the neck, the outer aspects of the forearm and upper arm, the outer aspect of the mid-thigh, on the front of the knees, and on the inner ankle. These are all sites to which the scratching finger can easily stray, and, again, tension and nervous factors may be significant.

The areas may become moist at times, and secondary infection may occur. Habitual scratching may well play a part in the other patterns of eczema.

VENOUS ECZEMA (GRAVITATIONAL ECZEMA)

This occurs at the site of chronic oedema or venous insufficiency and is most commonly seen on the lower legs, often in association with varicose veins. Purpura, pigmentation and ulceration may be present in the same area. If the gravitational eczema is severe, it is commonly associated with eczematous eruptions occurring at other sites (secondary spread), particularly on the face and arms.

CONTACT DERMATITIS

This is a subject of considerable importance because tracking down the particular substance or substances which, by contact with the patient's skin, have caused the inflammatory changes of dermatitis demands much time and effort by the dermatologist. Such substances are divided, according to the mechanism by which they can be shown to provoke dermatitis, into:
1. Primary irritants.
2. Sensitisers.

Primary irritants exert a direct effect on the skin and, in general, are not too difficult to identify. Examples are sodium hydroxide and sulphuric acid. Sensitisers, on the other hand, cause allergic response of the delayed type through the mechanism of cellular immunity.

Certain substances are known to cause such an allergic response more readily than others. For example,

130

among the metals, nickel is a common sensitiser, which is met with in the form of an allergic response to common metal objects in contact with the skin. Particularly in industry, chrome, too, is a potent sensitiser, the source of which can be quite difficult to trace; for example, cement dermatitis is often caused by the chrome contained in the cement, and shoe dermatitis is sometimes caused by chrome in leather. Other metals, for example, mercury, are less commonly the cause of contact dermatitis. At the other extreme, zinc is an uncommon sensitiser, which is one of the reasons why so many applications contain as a base, zinc oxide or zinc carbonate (calamine). Similarly, chrysanthemums and primulas are common causes of contact dermatitis, but some other flowers virtually never produce such sensitivity. Among dyes, the black dye paraphenyline diamine found in fabrics or in hair dyes will readily sensitise, but other dyes such as gentian violet very rarely do so. Various vulcanising chemicals used in rubber may produce this allergic contact response and may be difficult to discover. For example, a housewife with an eczematous dermatitis reaction due partly to household irritants may later develop a rubber sensitivity from the rubber gloves she is using to protect her hands. Important causes of contact dermatitis are medicaments, and certain preparations quite commonly produce an allergic sensitivity, as for example, the antibiotics. It is for this reason that certain antibiotic preparations such as penicillin and the sulphonamides are very rarely used as local applications, and some of the newer topical antibiotic agents, particularly neomycin and soframycin are now causing similar reactions. The cocaine derivatives, for example amethocaine, and the antihistamines when used as local applications very readily sensitise and are best not prescribed.

The type of eruption that develops depends on the substance responsible and the site of contact. Exposed areas of skin are usually involved (Fig. 8.3) unless the substance is in clothing or there is some special contact, for example a rubber condom. The cause may be obvious, or a very careful history may suggest one or two possibilities.

Patch Testing

The aim of patch testing is to demonstrate the presence of delayed type hypersensitivity to certain previously encountered antigens. The mechanism relies on the presence in the skin of sensitised lymphocytes which recognise the antigen and excite an inflammatory response in its presence. This response can be seen as a neat red, swollen area varying in intensity which can be recorded on a visual + to ++++ scale.

The test substance, which must be in a proper dilution known not to be irritant to normal skin, is applied on specially prepared aluminium foil tapes devised for simplicity and accuracy. Readings are taken at 2 and 4 days and are charted.

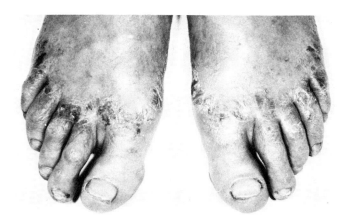

Fig. 8.3 Contact dermatitis showing eczema in area of main pressure contact with upper of lady's shoe.

The term *occupational dermatitis* is used when a contact dermatitis reaction occurs largely due to an irritant or sensitiser encountered at the patient's work. In many cases the substance concerned is a primary irritant such as an acid, an alkali, or a degreasing agent like trichlorethylene. Constant maceration with mechanical trauma, abrasive dusts such as fibre glass, fine particles of ragged metal (swarf) in oil, and extremes of temperature may also be responsible.

In other cases a substance that is acting as a sensitiser can be traced and a true allergic hypersensitivity can be demonstrated by patch testing. Examples are nickel in electroplating, chromate occurring in cement and paint primers, epoxy resins very widely used in the aircraft and other industries, chlorpromazine and its derivatives in the pharmaceutical industry, certain amines in soldering fluxes and so on. The list is enormous and constantly expanding with technological advances in industry. There are often important medico-legal considerations in these cases and the patient may receive industrial injury or disablement benefit of a higher scale than unemployment benefit. Also, compensation may be sought if it is considered that the employers have been negligent in exposing the workman to a particular substance in adverse conditions. As with the other common clinical patterns of eczema dermatitis reactions, other factors will play a part in these cases, particularly nervous stress and strain which, of course, can be increased if the patient becomes unemployed because of the skin disorder. Well-designed protective clothing, or special working areas designed to minimise contact with sensitisers, and sensible and cleanly working habits will keep cases of occupational dermatitis to a minimum. So-called barrier creams, though widely provided in industry, are of little value, though they do make cleansing the hands easier. If, however, the condition continues, particularly if there is a contact allergic cause discovered, the patient may well have to change his job.

GENERALISED EXFOLIATIVE DERMATITIS AND ERYTHRODERMIA

The term is applied when eczema dermatitis affects the whole skin surface, and the patient presents with complete redness and scaling. There may also be involvement of the hair follicles, with falling hair, and the nail beds which may lead to loosening and shedding of nails. It sometimes occurs following an allergic response to a topical medicament, or it may develop as a drug eruption due to gold or penicillin or sulphonamide or butazolidine. An almost identical clinical picture is seen if psoriasis merges over the whole skin surface. The condition can also occur in association with various reticuloses. It is serious, since the demands on the cardiac output are increased, the temperature-regulating function of the skin is grossly impaired, and there is fluid and protein loss.

Basis of Treatment

The management of eczema depends on

1. Unravelling the causal factors.
2. Eliminating these factors where possible.
3. Local and systemic treatment of the eczematous skin.

Explanation and reassurance and help with any nervous aspects is important. Sedation may be indicated in the face of tension and anxiety, particularly if sleep is adversely affected by itching and scratching during the night. Antihistamines by mouth have no specific effect on the eczema reaction but are sometimes used for their sedative side effects, particularly in children, when promethazine or trimeprazine at night often helps. Steroids by mouth or in the form of ACTH or Synacthen by injection will rapidly clear up an eczematous dermatitis reaction and are of great value in acute widespread eruptions, particularly if the cause can be removed. However, prolonged steroid therapy is very rarely employed in the persistent type of eczema because of the serious side effects and the difficulty of withdrawing the drug.

There is still a place for simple bland local applications such as calamine and zinc creams, and the more protective zinc pastes. Tar preparations, often in a paste base, are still employed in the more chronic forms of eczema, having among other effects an antipruritic action. However, the most commonly used and effective local applications are steroid preparations. These range from 1 per cent hydrocortisone to the more powerful fluorinated preparations such as fluocinolone and betamethazone. The latter are more effective, but are liable to cause complications when applied for a long period. The preparation should be applied gently with sufficient friction to spread only a very thin film, and the optimal frequency of application is four times a day. As the condition improves, this can be reduced to twice a day and, later, once at night. There is a very large range of steroid applications, creams, ointments, and lotions with various added medicaments available, some of which have an important place in therapy. For example, the addition of an antibiotic or bactericidal chemical may be indicated if infection is present, but it is important to remember the sensitising potential of such chemicals. Nystatin can be added to the steroid if a secondary candida infection is present. In some cases the effect of the steroid is increased by use of polythene occlusion overnight, but care is required as this will also increase the risk of secondary infection, and if used persistently causes atrophy of the skin.

Steroid absorption and general effects may occur, particularly when the more potent preparations are used over very large areas and in warm moist sites; for example in the napkin area of infants. There is no significant absorption from the more dilute preparations, in particular hydrocortisone. Steroids will increase secondary infection and may cause a rapid extension of an ulcerated area. Local atrophy of the skin will occur if the treatment is prolonged. This is seen particularly on the face, where the skin may become thin and the underlying vessels show through if one of the more potent steroids is used for many months for the treatment of rosacea or eczema. Atrophic striae will also occur at the site of continued steroid therapy, particularly when it has been used in the flexures. In spite of these complications, local steroid therapy has transformed the management of eczema dermatitis reactions and their proper careful use has produced a great deal of relief in patients with these conditions.

There are many other general and local treatments that can be employed in resistant cases. Fractional doses of X-rays were often employed in the past, but are now not used so commonly.

PSORIASIS, LICHEN PLANUS AND PITYRIASIS ROSEA

PSORIASIS

Definition

A common constitutional disorder of turnover of epidermal cells leading to the formation of sharply defined scaly red patches.

Background

About 1 to 2 per cent of the general population will have psoriasis at some time in their lives, and 5 to 10 per cent of all patients presenting in a dermatology department have psoriasis. It may start at any age, but commonly it develops between the age of 5 and 25 with an increased incidence in the 45 to 55 age group, particularly in women. It is much less common in the dark-skinned races. Among white populations it is more prevalent in the northern countries, and tends to improve in sunny climates and during the summer months.

About one-third of psoriatic patients have a family history, and the risk of psoriasis in children with one affected parent is 25 per cent. It is essentially a constitutional disorder, and psoriatic patients, even when clinically clear, carry through life a potential to develop psoriasis. In such a patient it is precipitated, or increased by various factors. Local trauma in the form of cuts, scratches, infections and other eruptions, can lead to patches of psoriasis which may be linear in pattern. Infection, particularly streptococcal tonsillitis, sometimes plays a part in attacks. This is particularly so in children, when, about two weeks after such an infection a widespread papular form of psoriasis develops (guttate psoriasis). Nervous stress and strain are important factors, particularly in exacerbations of established psoriasis.

Pathology

The change is probably due to the rapidity of growth of epidermal cells which, from development in the basal layer to the time they are shed (epidermal turnover time) is, in psoriasis areas, 3 to 4 days compared with the normal of 25 to 30 days. The cells do not lose their nuclei, remain clumped together, and are, therefore, shed as a perceptible scale.

Symptoms and Signs

The most characteristic finding is the well-demarcated edge. The patches may be any size, but the larger ones quite often take on curious patterns with polycyclic margins. The silvery white scale may be pronounced, but after treatment it is sometimes not obvious unless the surface of the skin is scratched. This will readily increase the silvery white appearance by pushing air pockets between the layers of scales. The common sites involved are the elbow tips, fronts of the knees, scalp and sacral area. Usually, psoriasis occurs as a widespread eruption, but isolated areas alone can be involved when, for example, patients may present with a single patch, or perhaps just the scalp is affected. Acute attacks of widespread papular psoriasis may occur and patches may also involve the sites commonly affected in intertriginous eczema dermatitis. In such cases, the well-demarcated edge may distinguish psoriasis, but the differential diagnosis can be difficult and, indeed, the two reactions tend to merge. Patches of psoriasis may occur on the hands and feet, but are again distinguished by the well-defined edge. Sometimes, pustules appear on the palms and soles (pustular psoriasis); they are sterile, and appear to be part of the psoriatic reaction. There is also a widespread serious form of pustular psoriasis – generalised pustular

psoriasis. Nail changes are usually associated with lesions elsewhere, but may occur as a sole manifestation of psoriasis. Pinpoint pits are the characteristic feature, but there may be plaques beneath the nail, or the whole nail may become thickened and irregular. The differential diagnosis from ringworm (a fungus infection) of the nails can be very difficult and mycological examination is likely to be important unless there is obvious psoriasis elsewhere. In a few cases the patches of psoriasis can all merge and involve the whole skin surface. This will present as a general exfoliative dermatitis. Itching is not a frequent feature of psoriasis, but it may occur, particularly in the flexural pattern, or when psoriatic areas become the focus of a scratching habit.

Complications

Psoriasis may be complicated by arthritis. This psoriatic arthropathy occurs in about seven per cent of hospital patients with psoriasis. Any joints may be affected, but commonly they are the interphalangeal joints, particularly the terminal one, and X-rays may show typical erosive changes.

Basis of Treatment

The effect of treatment in psoriasis is difficult to assess, as 'suggestion' may play a part in the treatment applied. Help may well be required from the nervous aspect, and small doses of sedatives often help. A holiday will sometimes clear up psoriasis, or a period of living in a sunny climate. Explanation and reassurance is important and it is helpful to maintain an optimistic approach to treatment, although obviously a permanent cure cannot be looked for. Steroid therapy by mouth will usually clear psoriasis, but in view of the difficulties of discontinuing treatment such systemic steroid therapy is reserved for very exceptional cases and circumstances. In recent years various cytotoxic agents have been used, and these probably have a direct effect on the rapidity of growth of the cells in the psoriatic patch. Methotrexate and azathioprine are the drugs most commonly used. Methotrexate is usually given in intermittent doses of, for example, 25 mg every one or two weeks. Gastrointestinal ulceration, granulocytopenia and hepatic cirrhosis may occur. It is probably as well to keep such treatments for those patients regularly attending a hospital out-patient department, and only for very severe cases, but they may dramatically alter the outlook for incapacitated patients. It is interesting that inorganic arsenic is a very old treatment for psoriasis but it has been discontinued because chronic arsenical poisoning and neoplasia may develop.

Tar and salicylic acid ointments are commonly used for simple patches of psoriasis, and form the basis of many proprietary preparations. Baths containing tar preparations may also help and are often taken before exposure to ultraviolet light. Dithranol is more effective, but it is an irritant preparation and care is required in its use. It is usual to employ dithranol in 0.1 to 0.5 per cent preparation in Lassar's paste. This can be applied at night to the patches of psoriasis and the areas then powdered over with a dusting power, and covered with tube gauze. It has a slight staining effect on clothing and the surrounding skin. The fluorinated steroids have an effect in psoriasis but this may not be sufficient unless polythene occlusion is also used. The different patterns of psoriasis require different applications. For example, flexural psoriasis will usually improve well with topical steroids but would be irritated by dithranol. On the scalp, scales tend to build up and patients often attempt removal by scratching, combing, brushing, excessive massage, and washing. Such trauma may well increase the psoriasis. Coal Tar and Salicylic Acid Ointment, NF, applied in a trace night and morning, and the scalp washed gently every three to four days with 10 to 15 per cent Cetrimide or a simple shampoo will often clear the lesions. A fluorinated steroid cream or lotion may be preferable in some cases. A newly introduced treatment PUVA based on the production of photosensitivity in the skin by Psoralen (taken by mouth or applied topically) and irradiation with that part of the UVR spectrum called UVA is strikingly effective in some severe cases. The UVA range lies between the middle part of the UVR spectrum (burning effect) and visible light. Special equipment is needed and the treatment is time consuming. The long term toxicities of Psoralen and intense UVA irradiation are unknown, and a cautious approach is advisable.

Prognosis

Many cases of psoriasis drag on for many years with remissions and exacerbations, and in some patients it can be a very severe and crippling condition, and have a disastrous effect on the quality of life. In others, it may be just a mild nuisance. The prognosis in any individual case is unpredictable, but it must be remembered that in many it will clear up completely and remain so for substantial periods, or permanently. In acute attacks or when there is some obvious precipitating factor that can be removed, the outlook is better.

LICHEN PLANUS

Definition

An acute or chronic condition of the skin and mucous membranes with characteristic shiny flat-topped papules often violaceous in colour.

Background

Although the aetiology of this condition is not known, it has many features in common with the other constitu-

tional reactions involving the skin, such as eczema and psoriasis, in that the patients may have attacks at different times in their lives; nervous stress and strain seem to play an important part. Certain drugs, including gold, mepacrine, and chloroquine can produce a lichen planus-like eruption which will gradually fade when the drugs are discontinued.

Pathology

There is a band of mononuclear cells lying just below the epidermis. The latter is thickened, the papillary ridges splayed out, and the granular layer is increased. This gives rise to white streaks which are apparent in some larger papules.

Clinical Features

The eruption, which often tends to itch, consists of distinct papules which have a shiny surface and a characteristic violaceous colour due to horizontal capillary proliferation. It may occur as a widespread eruption or be localised to sites such as the front of the wrists or over the lower back. At times the papules appear in rows, where there has presumably been a scratch. In some cases the lesions persist for months or years and, particularly on the lower legs, the epidermis may become hyperkeratotic (warty lichen planus). Sixty to seventy per cent of patients with lichen planus have involvement of the buccal mucosa, which takes the form of white dots or streaks and, sometimes, figurate lesions like Chinese letters. The tongue may also be involved, with bluish-white patches. In persistent cases, superficial chronic ulcerations may develop, often at the site of trauma from teeth or dentures. The condition in the mouth may develop without obvious lichen planus elsewhere or may persist after skin lesions have cleared.

Basis of Treatment

A period of rest or a holiday will often settle an attack, and sometimes small doses of sedatives help. In a very widespread eruption, steroid therapy by mouth is advisable. Locally, simple antipruritic agents help in the mild cases and topical steroids will also give some symptomatic relief. The more persistent localised lesions may respond to a local steroid together with polythene occlusion overnight.

Prognosis

Lichen planus will often persist for some months or even one to two years, but most cases clear in six to nine months. When the lesions start to disappear they become flat and the area of skin involved is pigmented.

PITYRIASIS ROSEA

Definition

This is a disease of unknown aetiology with a widespread eruption bearing characteristic features. It lasts approximately six weeks.

Clinical Features

It is a common disorder chiefly affecting the young adult. There is usually a 'herald spot' which precedes the main eruption. Usually, it consists of a red scaling area a few cm in diameter, which may be anywhere on the body, but it may also be absent or overlooked. A few days, or more rarely, two to three weeks, later a mild, itching, general eruption becomes apparent. This is visible over the trunk and the upper part of the limbs and lower neck, this characteristic distribution often being described as the 'bathing suit' area, of Victorian times. It consists of patches, 1 to 4 cm in diameter, of rosy pink, scaly skin, sometimes slightly raised. The scales tend to be less marked in the centre of the lesions and the free edge of the scale points towards the centre. Between these patches there is often a fine papular eruption. After about a week the eruption begins to fade, the whole disease lasting three to six weeks, occasionally persisting for a week or two longer.

Differential Diagnosis

This is often difficult.
1. Ringworm may give rise to red, scaling, widespread patches, but they are usually better defined and would be very unlikely to simulate the whole distribution of the pityriasis rosea eruption.
2. The rash of early syphilis can also cause confusion in diagnosis.
3. Nummular eczema may cause a widespread eruption with scaly, red areas, but there are usually some eczematous patches in other sites and the eruption has not the regular pattern and distribution of pityriasis rosea.
4. Guttate psoriasis causes more circumscribed raised areas, and more obvious psoriasis patches are often present elsewhere.

In atypical cases the diagnosis may have to be made after a period of observation as pityriasis rosea will clear up spontaneously whereas the other conditions tend to persist for much longer periods.

Basis of Treatment

The course of the condition is not affected by treatment, but symptomatic relief of the itching is often necessary.

THE URTICARIAL ERUPTIONS

URTICARIA

Definition

Urticaria is characterised by the production of weals and is sometimes referred to as 'nettle rash'. The production of these weals is by a similar mechanism to that seen in the 'triple' response and, although other substances are involved, liberation of histamine from mast cells plays an important part.

There are several different patterns of urticarial wealing varying from small weals to very large patches which often have a figurate or annular pattern. At times they develop in the subcutaneous tissues, giving rise to a very large deep weal (angio-oedema).

Background

Weals are due to a collection of oedema in the dermis arising from dilated vessels. When the oedema later compresses these vessels the weal becomes pale.

Pathology

The epidermis is not affected, there is no weeping, and when the oedema is reabsorbed there is no scaling or other change apparent. Occasionally, purpuric staining is left at the site of the weal, but apart from this, it is a feature of urticaria for the eruption to last a few hours and then clear away, leaving normal skin.

Acute Urticaria. Acute urticaria occurs in attacks usually lasting a few days or weeks. Very often a cause cannot be discovered, but some cases are due to an allergic response to certain drugs, food, or parasites. The commonest drug to cause an acute attack of urticaria is penicillin. It needs to be recognised that the wealing may develop up to three to four weeks after penicillin has been discontinued. The radicals causing the allergy vary, and prick testing to penicillin is rarely carried out because negative tests do not exclude an allergy.

Salicylates, morphia and other drugs sometimes cause acute urticaria. Various sera and other preparations from animal sources, particularly those in which horse serum is present, have been an important cause. Of the foods, certain fish, particularly shell-fish, crabs, lobsters and salmon, are well-recognised causes, the fish concerned often having been tinned or preserved in other ways. Occasionally, eggs, oranges and other foods have been shown to be responsible. Food additives, particularly azo dyes may be a cause. Parasitic infections with liver fluke, various intestinal worms, *Trichinella spiralis* and *loiasis* (*see* pages 594 and 600) may present as an urticaria. Acute attacks may be associated with fever, a general lymphadenopathy, and swelling and pain in the joints.

Chronic Urticaria. Chronic urticaria gives rise to recurring weals present over periods of a few months or sometimes years. There are phases when the wealing tendency is severe and remissions which may last for long periods or indefinitely. The weals may have a diurnal variation and occur in the early morning or in the evening, dying away in a few hours. There may be associated deep urticarial swellings (angio-oedema) or, in a few cases, the latter swellings occur without coincidental dermal weals. These angio-oedema swellings occur most commonly around the eyelids and on the lips but they may appear anywhere and, very rarely, involve the tongue and larynx. In most cases of chronic urticaria the cause is unknown. Nervous stress and strain may well play an important part, and patients are seen who have some obvious worry or anxiety associated with the phase of wealing, the condition tending to recur in association with unsettled or difficult phases in their lives. It is uncommon to find some specific allergic sensitivity. Recently, it has been shown that in about twenty per cent of patients with chronic urticaria there is an association with *Candida albicans* infection and, also, brewers' yeast in the diet. Salicylates cause exacerbations of chronic urticaria in half the cases and the attacks so produced will often take a week or two to settle down. Many cases of chronic urticaria improve considerably after stopping all salicylates.

A rare type of angio-oedema, which is familial, has been shown to be due to the absence of, or reduction in, C1 esterase inhibitor component of complement. Rare cases have recently been described associated with other abnormalities of complement.

Physical Urticaria. Physical urticaria refers to wealing in response to certain physical agents. The commonest condition is dermographism which is due to an increased wealing response to simple trauma. There are all degrees of response to such trauma, but if a pressure of 5,000 g/cm^2 is applied to the skin (about the pressure of a thumb nail drawn firmly over the skin) it has been found that between four and five per cent of the normal population will weal. For most of them this may be just a curious fact, but for others it may set up considerable irritation, and they may present for treatment. Although the incidence of dermographism is constant throughout life, it is nearly always patients in the second and third decade who complain of irritation. The incidence of dermographism in the other urticarial disorders is that of the normal population. Cold also, may cause wealing. This is most often seen after bathing in cold water, weals then coming up in those areas of skin in contact with the water. It may also occur in winter, particularly if there has been a movement of air across the skin. In minor degrees it is quite common, but when it is severe it can be a considerable disability and may even occasion fainting when bathing in cold water for a long time. Exertion urticaria (cholinergic) occurs when the patient has exercised to the point of sweating. The weals characteristically are very small, 1 to 3 mm in diameter, are widely scattered, chiefly over the trunk, and clear in half to one hour. Actinic urticaria is a weal response to certain wavelengths of ultraviolet light. Pressure urticaria occurs at sites where there has been prolonged pressure, a subcutaneous weal developing some three to four hours later.

Papular urticaria refers to urticarial weals which, after a day or two, die back to an itching papule which then lasts for a few more days. These used to be referred to as 'heat spots', but it is now known that the complaint is due to insect bites, commonly by fleas, usually from the cat or dog. Occasionally, various species of animal mites will produce similar lesions.

Basis of Treatment

Treatment of the urticarias will obviously depend on the cause and whether or not this can be eliminated. In chronic urticaria the physician may well be able to help from the nervous aspect. For example, if a yeast allergy can be demonstrated a low-yeast diet and anti-candida treatment may well help. It is, of course, important to avoid all salicylates. Antihistamines will reduce the wealing tendency in all the urticarial disorders, but in the severe attacks this may be so great that the effect of the antihistamine appears to be very slight. Most cases of chronic urticaria can be kept comfortable by the regular use of antihistamines. Chlorpheniramine 4 mg three times a day is one of the most commonly used antihistamines; the dose may be increased and the frequency of administration altered to get a maximum effect when the wealing tendency is greatest. There are some long-acting antihistamines which can be given just at night; brompheniramine maleate LA 12 mg in a single dose at night is often helpful. With all antihistamines some sedative side effects occur, but in most patients an adequate dose can be taken without undue drowsiness.

ACNE VULGARIS AND ROSACEA

ACNE VULGARIS

Definition

A chronic inflammatory condition of the pilosebaceous follicles chiefly of the face and upper trunk and common in teenagers.

Background

This condition is very common and minor degrees merge with normality. It coincides with the phase of overactivity of the sebaceous glands shortly after the onset of puberty. The phase of acne often lasts a few years in the 'teens' but may drag on into the early twenties or beyond. The period of overactivity of the sebaceous glands is related to an increased androgen/oestrogen ratio and, rarely, can develop in association with increased androgen production from suprarenal and gonadal hyperplasia or tumour formation, other steroid producing tumours, and testosterone or cortisone therapy. Similarly, it can be reduced by oestrogen administration. Apart from the endocrine balance other factors may play a part, such as emotional tension and introspective worry over the acne. Warm dry climates are beneficial, and humid and relatively sunless areas are associated with an increase in the acne. Too much chocolate and, possibly, pig fat may occasionally aggravate the condition, but diet factors have been overstressed in the past and controlled trials have not confirmed the value of dietary omissions. A habit of squeezing, fiddling, and repeatedly touching the lesions may aggravate the condition.

Pathology

The lesions are due to blocking of the pilosebaceous follicles with a plug of inspissated sebum and keratin scales, which become black due to the deposition of melanin (comedo). The sebaceous follicles then become distended and inflamed and may develop into a pustule. This may rupture either onto the surface or into the dermis. Scars occur at the sites of the larger lesions and, later, cysts may develop which can become recurrently infected before eventually sclerosing. The part played by bacteria including corynebacteria, and the presence of free fatty acids and fibrin in the production of the acne lesions is complex.

Clinical Features

Acne lesions are present over the face, upper chest, and back. Comedos are more likely to be present in the earlier age group, and recurrently infected cysts in the older person. A similar pustular eruption can occur from the administration of iodides or bromides or from the application of certain oils. Rosacea is usually present in the older person and is associated with erythema and pustules in flushed patches on the face. Seborrhoeic eczema may give rise to scaling and secondary pustules in the naso-labial furrows and round the mouth. Mixtures of acne vulgaris, rosacea, and seborrhoeic eczema occur.

Basis of Treatment

From the general aspect this largely consists of reassurance and careful explanation of the various factors that may play a part in the condition. In recent years, the use of small doses of an antibiotic, usually tetracycline, over a prolonged period has become a popular treatment. The usual dose of tetracycline is 250 mg twice a day taken before meals, but after three to four weeks the dose can often be reduced to 250 mg daily, then continued for another two to three months. The mode of action is not fully understood, but is probably *not* due to a simple antibiotic effect on secondary staphylococcal infection. In tense, agitated acne sufferers a small dose of sedative will sometimes help. The contraceptive pill, particularly one with a relatively high dose of oestrogen, may help some women with acne.

There are many agents available for use as local applications. The main effect of these is to cause an exfoliation of the top layer of the epidermis and so help to bring out the plugging comedos. Sulphur has been used for this purpose and is available in commercial preparations, which may also help to mask the acne lesions. In minor cases, Sulphur Compound Lotion, NF or 1 per cent sulphur in calamine lotion dabbed on at night or twice a day will probably be enough. In the more severe cases, Resorcinol and Sulphur Paste, BPC may be used. Benzoyl peroxide applications are now very widely prescribed. Washing should be carried out regularly night and morning with soap and hot water. Particularly in the older acne sufferer it is important not to use too much friction when washing, and if camouflaging cosmetics are used they should be removed at night with the least trauma possible. Ultraviolet light treatment is helpful, particularly in the more severe cases, and mild peeling doses are aimed at, usually twice a week for six weeks. Recurrently infected large cysts are sometimes helped by surface cryotherapy or by injecting the area with small amounts of corticosteroids.

Oil acne is a related condition due to the effect of certain oils repeatedly covering the skin, particularly in association with oil-contaminated clothing. The pilosebaceous follicles become blocked, and pustules develop. Occupations in which a repeated covering of oil is hard to avoid may adversely affect an acne vulgaris sufferer. Chlor-acne occurs when certain chlorinated hydrocarbons are absorbed and have a general effect on sebaceous glands, the resulting eruption being very like a severe acne vulgaris.

ROSACEA

Definition

A persistent flush of the face with secondary hyperplasia of sebaceous glands and the development of papules and pustules.

Background

This condition frequently occurs in middle age and is very common in minor degrees. It is due largely to a persistent flush, the hyperaemia from this leading to hyperplasia of the sebaceous glands which then may become pustular. Particularly on the nose, the hyperplasia leads to the development of a bulbous condition known as rhinophyma.

The flush tendency may be familial and is often related to emotional tension and stress. Other factors may play a part such as menopausal flushes, climatic conditions, and a gastric flush mechanism due either to a constitutional tendency or to excessive gastric stimulation from irritant foods and drinks, including alcohol.

The eruption develops on one or more of the flush areas of the face, namely the cheeks, nose, centre forehead and chin, and consists of a red area with papules and pustules (Fig. 8.4).

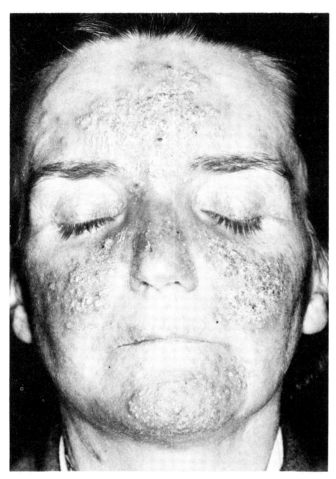

Fig. 8.4 Rosacea.

Basis of Treatment

This largely consists of considering the underlying causes of the persistent flush and reducing their effect as much as possible. Small doses of sedatives will sometimes be of help, and explanation and reassurance are important. It is as well to avoid gastric irritants, but in view of the emotional factor, it is perhaps a mistake to over-restrict the diet. Locally, sulphur 1 per cent in calamine lotion or Salicyclic Acid and Sulphur Cream, BPC applied in a trace once or twice a day will often help. Topical steroids such as 1 per cent hydrocortisone cream will often improve the condition, but it is important to avoid the more potent steroids since, if they are used for long periods, there is a tendency to develop atrophy of the epidermis and, subsequently, an increase in the prominence of the dilated small vessels. In recent years, a prolonged course of a small dose of an antibiotic has been found effective in a number of the more severe cases of rosacea, much more efficient than when used in acne. It is usual to give tetracycline 250 mg twice a day before meals for three to four weeks and then to reduce the dose to 250 mg daily and continue for some months. The mechanism of this treatment is not completely understood. Severe degrees of rhinophyma can be helped by planing off the excessive tissue under a general anaesthetic after which the area will quickly re-epithelialise (dermabrasion).

Complications

An important complication is rosaceous conjunctivitis and, in some cases, keratitis.

Prognosis

The condition may persist for many years with considerable fluctuations in severity and periods of remission.

BLISTERING DISEASES

PEMPHIGUS AND PEMPHIGOID

Definition

Widespread spontaneous blisters appear in both these conditions, pemphigus being situated in the epidermis, and pemphigoid just below the epidermis.

Background

Although the aetiology is not fully understood, it seems likely that both conditions are due to autoimmune processes. Pemphigus occurs in any age in adult life and may initially involve the mucous membranes of the mouth, conjunctiva or, sometimes, the vulva. Pemphigoid tends to occur over the age of 65 and there is often a pre-existing urticarial or eczematous eruption for a few weeks before the bullae develop.

Clinical Features (Fig. 8.5)

The position of the blister gives rise to certain differences between the two conditions. In pemphigus the blisters are fragile and can be pushed along in the epidermis by gentle pressure, whereas in pemphigoid the blisters do not show this feature and tend to be larger, are more likely to be haemorrhagic, remain intact for a longer period, and may leave scarring. Although

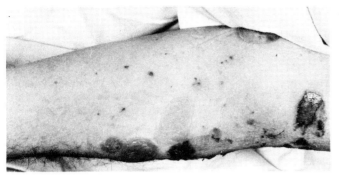
Fig. 8.5 Pemphigus.

the conditions are clinically and histologically distinct it can be difficult in some cases to distinguish them.

There are a number of variants of these conditions and so-called benign mucous membrane pemphigoid is a very persistent eruption involving the conjunctivae, nose, mouth, anus and vulva, with at times cutaneous bullae; mutilating scarring of conjunctivae and vulva often develops.

Basis of Treatment

Pemphigus and pemphigoid respond to steroids by mouth, but initially they may need to be given in quite large doses such as prednisone 40 to 60 mg daily. This dose can then be reduced, but the patient usually needs to be maintained on a small dose of steroids for many years. Recently the combination of azathioprine with systemic steroids has been shown to be safer and more effective than steroids alone.

Prognosis

Patients continue to develop new blisters over a period of weeks, months, or years. In pemphigus, with its severe involvement of mucous membranes and persistence, the complaint may be fatal due to intercurrent infection. The formation of blisters may be impossible to control even with very large doses of steroids. In pemphigoid, however, remission after a period is likely, and steroid dosage may be reduced to a very low level or abandoned altogether.

DERMATITIS HERPETIFORMIS

Definition

A widespread eruption consisting of groups of vesicles arising on weals, particularly over bony prominences.

Background

This may start at any age and usually persists for a few years with fluctuations in severity. The aetiology is unknown, but it is now thought to be due to an immunological disorder since immunoglobulin A deposits are found on the basement membrane of the epidermis. It is closely associated with coeliac disease (see page 76), for it has been observed that at least two-thirds of patients with dermatitis herpetiformis have the type of intestinal changes seen in coeliac disease, and in some patients the skin improves on a gluten-free diet.

Clinical Features

The eruption is characterised by considerable itching and the development of papules which later show a small central vesicle. Occasionally, bullae develop. The eruption develops in patches, commonly on the backs of the elbows, over the back, round the buttocks, and on the front of the knees. The affected area of skin usually becomes pigmented.

Basis of Treatment

Small doses of certain sulphonamide preparations usually keep the eruption in check but need to be continued for prolonged periods. That most usually employed is diamino-diphenylsulphone (Dapsone) 25 to 100 mg twice daily. The response to treatment is often dramatic and can be used as a diagnostic test.

Prognosis

The condition usually persists for many months or years, but may be kept under almost perfect control by continued treatment.

INFECTIONS OF THE SKIN

FUNGUS INFECTIONS

There are two main types of fungus infections involving the skin, namely those due to species of candida, which is a yeast-like fungus, and those due to the ringworm fungi (dermatophytes), which have a spreading mycelium in the skin and cause the various patterns of tinea.

CANDIDIASIS

Background

Various species of candida may cause disease, but the commonest with which we are concerned is *Candida albicans*. This is very widespread in nature, being a normal inhabitant of the gut of warm-blooded animals. It so commonly involves man that small numbers of candida can be regarded as normal components of the flora of the human skin, vagina and intestinal tract. It will grow excessively and lead to disease only if there are either general or local changes that favour the development of the fungus. From the general aspect,

139

debility in the form of under-nutrition, malignant disease, immunological deficiency states, diabetes, and therapy with antibiotics, steroids and antimitotic agents may play a part. Local factors favouring excessive growth include moisture, the presence of other eruptions, chiefly eczema of the intertriginous sites, pockets between the nail fold and nail plate, glycosuria, and the use of antibiotics.

Clinical Features

In the mouth, candidiasis takes the form of white spots and patches over the buccal mucous membrane and tongue. The surrounding skin is red, and the white patches can be partially scraped off with a spatula. Chronic oral candidiasis persisting for many months is often related to wearing a denture overnight, and associated lack of oral hygiene. Candida will often secondarily invade mouth angle cracks. These are commonly due primarily to faulty denture mechanics giving rise to an overlap of the mouth angles, a general eczematous state, an iron deficiency anaemia, or, very rarely in the UK, a vitamin B deficiency. On the skin, candida is present in moist sites, and for example, in the finger clefts in patients with an underlying disorder such as rheumatoid arthritis, when the fingers are kept close together or dragged over into the palm. It readily involves the groins and ano-genital region, and also appears beneath the breasts. It is often present in persistent napkin rashes in infants from whatever cause.

The appearance of the skin infected with candida is quite typical, a well-marked edge is present, sometimes with a raised line of epidermis. Beyond the well-defined edge are small grey white flaccid vesicles which readily rupture and leave circular areas with a defined edge of scale raised towards the centre of the lesions.

Chronic paronychia is due to a gap developing between the nail fold skin and nail plate. This is usually due to a persistent maceration, but faulty manicuring, or a habit of pushing back the cuticle may lead to the development of such a gap. Once formed, it is then secondarily infected with candida and various bacteria. The nail fold becomes red and swollen, which helps to keep the gap open. The nail plate may grow out irregularly due to the inflammatory change round the nail bed and, rarely, candida will grow in the nail plate itself. Chronic paronychia is *not* due to dermatophyte fungi – an important point in treatment.

Basis of Treatment

Attention must obviously be directed to the underlying causes, but candida responds very well to nystatin and to amphotericin B and these two preparations have largely superseded the various chemicals used in the past. Neither nystatin nor amphotericin B are absorbed to any extent and must therefore be used as local applications. When tablets are given by mouth, it is only to reduce any coincidental excessive intestinal candida infection. These agents have no effect at all on the ringworm fungi.

RINGWORM

Background

There are a number of different types of ringworm fungi involving the skin, but in the UK there are only six common fungi causing such infections. Three of these are of animal origin, and three involve the human species only. In all cases the diagnosis can be checked by examining scrapings of the skin direct under the microscope, and by culture.

Clinical Features

Animal Ringworm. Of the three animal ringworm fungi, the commonest is cattle ringworm, which, particularly in hairy parts causes an inflamed raised pustular area, usually with shedding of the hair (kerion). Such lesions are often mis-diagnosed as boils or carbuncles due to pyogenic bacteria, and usually they persist for some six to twelve weeks. The disease is, of course, commoner in farmers and other people handling cattle, particularly calves, and its infectivity to other humans is low.

Small mammal ringworm is acquired from rats, mice, voles, hedgehogs, etc., and each species of fungus has separate cultural characteristics depending on the particular animal source. The patches of such ringworm show a red scaling area with a well-defined edge and a tendency to clear towards the centre of the lesion.

The third type of animal ringworm is that acquired from the cat and dog, and in addition to the red, scaling, ringed lesions present in the other patterns of ringworm, this fungus may involve the scalp and cause

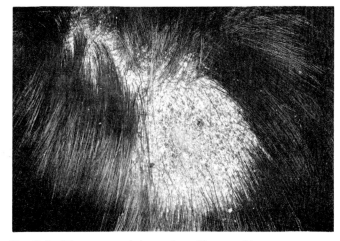

Fig. 8.6　Ringworm of the scalp – *Tinea capitis*.

patches of scaling and broken hairs. This type of ring-worm in the scalp fluoresces under a particular wavelength of ultraviolet light (Wood's light) and clears spontaneously at puberty. The appearance is very similar to that given by a species of human ringworm seen on the scalps of children, which is now uncommon, but which used to give rise to many problems of management.

Human Ringworm. The three types of fungi involving man all tend to infect between the toes and in the groins, with occasional involvement of the nails or other sites. One of the three, however, namely *Trichophyton rubrum*, which has a red colour on culture, has a tendency to spread to other sites, and large scaly red patches may develop in any area. These may be very persistent and lead to difficulties in diagnosis. However, it is usual to discover some well-defined active edge that would suggest a ringworm infection.

Toe ringworm leads to scaling and cracking between the toes, particularly the fourth and fifth toes, but it must be remembered that in less than one-third of patients with such lesions is the complaint due to ringworm fungi. The more common causes of such changes are maceration, intertriginous eczema, and secondary infection with a wide range of bacteria, including diphtheriods. In the groins, ringworm infection is characterised by involvement of the inner thigh away from the groin crease, and the edge is usually well-defined with a polycyclic edge.

Basis of Treatment

The ringworm fungi are all affected by griseofulvin taken by mouth. Keratin laid down while a patient is taking griseofulvin appears to be resistant to the invasion of the ringworm fungus. The length of treatment will therefore depend on the rate of turnover of the keratin in the particular structure involved. In skin, about four weeks will usually be sufficient; in hair, two to three months, until the new hair is long enough to allow removal of the infected hair. For the nails, treatment will have to continue for six to eighteen months. Griseofulvin is absorbed better after meals, and its effect is reduced if the patient is receiving barbiturates at the same time. It has no action on *Candida albicans* infections, and, for example, has no effect in chronic paronychia. Various local fungicides are used and there is a whole range of preparations available. Whereas they will show activity against the ringworm fungi *in vitro*, they are often ineffective in treating skin lesions, presumably because they are unable to get through the keratin to the site of the fungi. Benzoic Acid Compound Ointment, NF is the preparation still often employed, but tolnaftate and miconazole preparations are also in common use.

There are a number of other fungus infections involving the skin and some are usually met in tropical climates. Pityriasis versicolor is quite common and is due to a specific fungus which involves particularly the skin of the upper trunk, causing diagnostic well-defined patches of scaling skin that tend to appear brown in the winter time, and in covered areas, but pale in the summer time when the surrounding skin becomes more pigmented. It responds quickly to local treatment with Benzoic Acid Compound Ointment, NF, tolnaftate cream or selenium sulphide, but it is necessary to continue with local applications for a few weeks after it is apparently clear.

VIRUS INFECTIONS

VIRUS WARTS (VERRUCAE)

Perhaps the commonest virus to involve the skin is the common wart virus. This will produce the type of wart usually seen on the fingers of children, but may also produce filiform warts (thread-like), particularly round the neck and axillary folds, or digitate warts (finger-like processes), particularly in the scalp. Plantar warts occur when the virus involves a pressure area of the foot, and the surface then becomes level with the rest of the skin. Plane (flat) warts often occur in patches, particularly over the face and backs of the hands. In the genital area the wart virus will produce a papillomatous lesion with very little hyperkeratosis (condyloma acuminata). In all cases the warts may be single or multiple and discomfort is largely related to the site involved. Warts may disappear spontaneously after a few weeks or months, and may clear in some cases in response to treatment by various methods of 'suggestion'. There are a large number of ways in which warts can be destroyed, ranging from freezing with liquid nitrogen to curetting out under a local anaesthetic. Genital warts will often respond to painting with 5 to 20 per cent podophyllin resin in spirit or propylene glycol at weekly intervals.

MOLLUSCUM CONTAGIOSUM

Caused by one of the largest viruses infecting man, molluscum contagiosum has many clinical features in common with virus warts. The lesions appear as tiny pearly papules with a central hyperkeratotic area which may be slightly depressed. They commonly develop in a group of 10 to 20 lesions but may be single, or form a widespread eruption. They may disappear spontaneously but can be treated by cryotherapy or by spiking the centre of the lesion with an applicator dipped in carbolic acid (Fig. 8.7).

HERPES SIMPLEX (COLD SORES) (*see also* page 19)

This is another very common virus infection, which most of the population carry in a dormant state. The

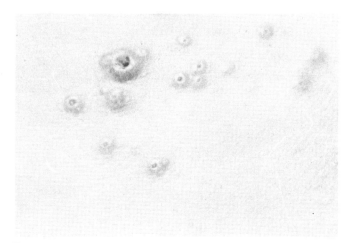

Fig. 8.7 Molluscum contagiosum.

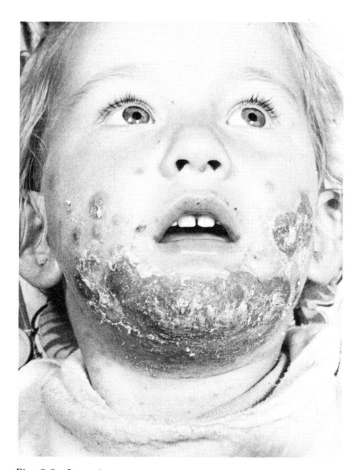

Fig. 8.8 Impetigo.

initial infection sometimes takes the form of an ulcerative stomatitis, but after this skin lesions will develop recurrently, usually being precipitated by some general illness which may include fevers, emotional upsets, exposure to cold winds, excessive ultraviolet light, and the menses. Lesions most commonly occur on the lips as small blisters which then dry up and become crusted in a few days. Groups of the vesicles may occur elsewhere, particularly round the face, but also on the fingers and the genitalia and they readily become secondarily infected. There is usually a well-marked regional lymphadenitis.

Cow-pox. Still occasionally seen in people who are in contact with cattle, the lesion looks very much like that produced by smallpox vaccination.

Contagious Pustular Dermatitis of Sheep (Orf) and milker's nodes are caused by a specific virus and lead to a development of persistent papules, sometimes surmounted by a pustule. These will last for two to three months and are most commonly seen in farmers or veterinary surgeons.

BACTERIAL INFECTIONS

Staphylococci

One of the commonest of bacteria to cause skin lesions is the staphylococcus. The effect will depend to some extent on the phage type of the organism.

IMPETIGO (Fig. 8.8)

When staphylococcal infection involves the surface of the skin (impetigo) it gives rise to blisters which last one or two days and then dry up, leaving a crust. It is likely to occur in patients who have breaks in the surface of the skin and particularly in conditions leading to itching and scratching, such as eczema or parasitic infestations. Streptococci may also play a part in impetigo.

BOILS

When staphylococci involve hair follicles they cause pustules, boils or carbuncles, depending on the depth, size and involvement of adjacent follicles. There is sometimes an external source of infection from some close contact, but very often general factors and local skin changes play an important part. General factors include debilitating illnesses and nervous stress and strain. Diabetes is often mentioned as a cause, but the incidence of recurrent boils in diabetes is probably that of the normal population. However, severe boils may well increase glycosuria or lead to its appearance if there is a latent tendency. Locally, eczematous eruptions or any lesion that leads to scratching and picking, and blocked follicles, as in acne or oil acne, will favour the development of boils, Small numbers of staphylococci occur normally on the skin, but recurrent boils are associated with the building up of large numbers of staphylococci in reservoir sites. These are commonly in the nasal vestibule and on various minor eczematous areas round the eyelids, ears, scalp, and ano-genital cleft. In the management of recurrent boils, the discovery and treatment of these reservoir sites is important.

TUBERCULOUS INFECTION (LUPUS VULGARIS)

The main chronic bacterial diseases involving the skin are leprosy and tuberculosis. Only the latter will be considered here. At one time it was a common and important skin disease, although in the past 20 years the incidence has become much less. Primary tuberculosis of the skin causes a small persistent ulcerated area with marked regional lymphadenopathy. The commonest post primary tuberculosis of the skin is lupus vulgaris. This usually develops in children giving rise to patches of slowly extending lesions, commonly on the face and neck. These consist of thickened skin with a very characteristic brown yellow colour (apple jelly). Scarring usually occurs, and if untreated the condition persists for many years and will gradually destroy the tissues. Treatment with isoniazid is effective.

Syphilis due to *Treponema pallidum* is described elsewhere (*see* page 158).

PARASITIC INFESTATIONS

SCABIES

Definition

An intensely itchy contagious disease due to the invasion of the epidermis by a mite.

Background

The mite is just visible to the naked eye and is acquired from another human subject infected with scabies; contact needs to be prolonged. The mite dies in a few hours if away from the skin surface and therefore infestation from clothing and bedding is not common.

Clinical Features

Itching, which is always worse at night, will begin some four to six weeks after infestation, the time it takes for sensitivity to develop to mite protein. The female mite lays eggs in small burrows varying in length from 5 to 20 mm, and it is the discovery of these burrows that confirms the diagnosis. Burrows are most commonly found on fingers, hands, fronts of the wrists, feet, penis, round the nipples of the female, and in other sites such as the axillary folds, round the umbilicus, and in the buttock creases. In babies, the commonest sites for burrows are the palms and soles. A general eruption consisting of a widespread follicular papular rash, and, sometimes, urticarial weals may be present. Scratch marks are often seen and the skin may become eczematised. Secondary infection commonly develops with the appearance of impetigo and boils.

Basis of Treatment

The principle of treatment is to keep the patient coated over the whole body surface, below the neck, for forty-eight hours with an appropriate preparation lethal to the mite. Benzyl benzoate application has been used for many years for this purpose, but has recently largely been superseded by gamma BHC (Lorexane), which is applied on two consecutive nights before going to bed, making certain that every area of skin has a thin coating of the cream. On the third night fresh clothing and bed linen are used and the discarded linen is washed in the normal way and stored for two to three days. It is essential to treat any close contacts whether they are itching or not. The incidence of scabies varies over the years. It was a very common condition during and immediately after the Second World War, and there has been a further wave of scabies in the last three to four years.

Whereas the human scabies mite will involve only humans, other mites can be present on various animals such as dogs and cats, and migrate to individuals who are in close contact with them. These mites are unable to live for long periods on human skin, do not produce burrows, but cause a widespread papular eruption that often causes difficulty in diagnosis.

PEDICULOSIS (INFESTATION WITH LICE)

Background

There are three distinct species of pediculi which are in each case confined to certain areas, namely, the head, the pubic area, and the body. The adult louse is 4 to 5 mm long and has a thin diamond-shaped body, with the exception of the pubic louse (crabs) which is much shorter and broader. They are blood-sucking insects and lay small shiny eggs in capsules (nits) which head and pubic lice cement on to hair, and body lice on to the seams of clothing.

HEAD LOUSE

The head louse is now not so common in Britain, but still occurs, mostly in children. It leads to itching and scratching and, subsequently, to secondary impetigo.

DDT, gamma BHC and Malathion are effective, the commonest treatment for head lice perhaps being gamma BHC shampoo, which will kill the adults and, if repeated a week later, will destroy any lice that have emerged from eggs in the meantime. When treatment is repeated in this way there is no need to comb out nits except for cosmetic reasons.

BODY LOUSE

The body louse is now a rarity in Britain. Its presence on the human body may be revealed by scratch marks on the trunk, and adult lice may be found on the patient's clothing, and eggs in the seams of underclothes. However, the seriousness of infestation by body lice lies in the fact that it transmits typhus fever and, in Asia, can be the cause of epidemics. Treatment consists of disinfesting the clothing by steam heat or by chemical methods. Treating clothing with DDT or gamma BHC powder will often suffice to control body lice and is a quick, simple way of dealing with a large number of infested people.

PUBIC LOUSE

The pubic louse may also spread to the axillary hair and sometimes to other sites. It is often acquired during sexual intercourse. Considerable irritation occurs and secondary infection may develop. The area involved is readily treated with DDT or gamma BHC powder or shampoo.

TOXIC ERUPTIONS

ERYTHEMA MULTIFORME

Definition

A widespread eruption of characteristic morphology which is an uncommon reaction to either drugs or infective agents.

Background

The commonest underlying cause is a virus infection which in most cases is *Herpes simplex*. The eruption usually develops one to two weeks after such an infection. Other viruses and bacteria may be responsible. Of the drugs, barbiturates and sulphonamides are the two that most commonly cause this condition, particularly the long-acting sulphonamides. Further attacks may occur and can be responsible for recurrent episodes of ulceration in the mouth with or without lesions in other sites.

Clinical Features (Fig. 8.9)

The eruption is acute in onset and commonly involves the forearms, hands, and lower parts of the legs, but it may be more widespread and affect the mouth and lips. It consists of discrete papules varying in size from a few mm up to 2 to 3 cm, many of them running together. Distinct lesions surrounded by a red halo are often present, and in the centre of the raised area there is a small vesicle or crust. This gives the appearance of concentric rings which are often referred to as target lesions. There are mouth ulcers, and the lips become covered with a blood crust. In the severe form, when the mouth and other mucous membrane orifices are involved, it is sometimes referred to as the Stevens-

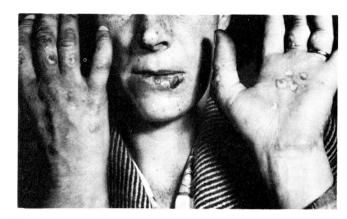

Fig. 8.9 Erythema multiforme (iris).

Johnson syndrome. The whole condition clears in seven to fourteen days. There is no specific treatment, but steroids by mouth in very severe attacks will reduce the severity and shorten the course.

ERYTHEMA NODOSUM

Definition

A nodular erythematous eruption, usually affecting the extensor aspects of the legs, running a course of a few weeks, and associated with a number of systemic diseases.

Background

The complaint is most common in women in their twenties, though it can occur at any age. It is a form of vasculitis starting with an intense inflammatory reaction which is followed by a granulomatous phase and eventual resolution, the whole process taking from three to six weeks. The vasculitis is due to a sensitivity reaction to certain systemic diseases. Sarcoidosis and streptococcal infections of the tonsils and pharynx are the commonest. Tuberculosis, drugs such as sulphonamides, fungus infections, diseases of the intestine such as ulcerative colitis, viral diseases and, occasionally, malignant disease may less commonly be responsible.

Clinical Features

The eruption may have been preceded by a well-defined streptococcal infection a week or a fortnight previously, or by a period of poor general health and variable symptoms of malaise as is found in sarcoidosis. There may also be arthralgia and unexplained pyrexia. The eruption begins with a low fever, and erythematous nodules appear on the shins, or near the knees and ankles. They vary in number, but usually there are about a dozen of variable size; the commonest is about 3 cm across. They are elevated from the surface and are of different sizes one from another. They are hot and painful, bright red in colour at the onset, but change within a few days to a blue or purplish tint, rather like a bruise. New lesions may continue to arise after the first crop and there is oedema of the legs and ankles, and considerable discomfort.

In three to six weeks there is normally spontaneous resolution, though residual oedema may persist for longer.

Investigations

A full blood count, ESR, chest X-ray and ASO titres may help to discover the underlying cause.

Basis of Treatment

In the presence of a streptococcal infection this should be fully treated with penicillin. The patient should be at rest in bed, and in the resolving stage a firm supporting bandage should be worn on the legs to prevent oedema and to reduce aching.

DRUG ERUPTIONS

Definition

These eruptions are due to a toxic or allergic response to drugs absorbed from the alimentary tract, injections or, less commonly, through other mucous membranes or the skin. Contact dermatitis of the allergic type, in which an eczema dermatitis reaction results from the application of a substance to the skin itself, is not included under this heading.

Background

An eruption may develop shortly after the drug has been administered, or there may be an interval of two to three weeks or longer before the rash develops. Almost any kind of eruption can develop from different drugs, but a few drugs are commonly associated with fairly distinctive patterns of rash.

Clinical Features

One of the commonest types of drug eruption is the one that causes a measles-like (morbilliform) rash. Barbiturates and sulphonamides commonly produce this kind of rash, but it is seen with many other drugs including some of the non-barbiturate hypnotics such as glutethimide. Urticarial weals are seen, particularly with penicillin and salicylates. Penicillin urticaria may persist for weeks or months after stopping the penicillin. Ampicillin quite commonly produces rashes, but these are more commonly of a fine morbilliform pattern often with purpura, and occur very commonly when the drug has been used in the treatment of glandular fever. A widespread punctate erythema (scarlatiniform) and an

eczematous eruption can result from the use of many drugs, for example, gold. A general pruritus unaccompanied by any rash can be caused by barbiturates.

Drug-induced purpura may be due to thrombocytopenia as in the case of Sedormid, in which an antigen-antibody reaction can be demonstrated. Purpura is also commonly due to damage to capillary walls and is the common type of eruption with phenylbutazone, chlorothiazide, and Carbromal. The last-named drug produces a characteristic eruption as, apart from the purpura, there is also some scaling and the rash commonly starts round the legs and spreads up to the buttocks and other sites.

A fixed drug eruption is so-called because on each administration of the causative drug, lesions recur on the same site. These are commonly raised, red areas, often of a purple hue, and sometimes with bullae. Phenolphthalein is the commonest cause of a fixed drug eruption.

Acneform papules and pustules, especially on the face, can be produced by the halogens, particularly bromides and iodides. A lichen planus-like eruption may be caused by some antimalarial drugs, namely mepacrine, chloroquine, and by gold salts and other drugs.

Chronic poisoning with inorganic arsenic is still seen, although arsenic is seldom administered today. It was commonly given in certain chronic skin disorders, with bromides in epilepsy, and with iron in anaemia. When taken for months or years it leads to changes in the skin which are often visible many years later. These consist of a general pigmentation of the skin, which has a dappled appearance, and hyperkeratotic lesions, particularly on the palms and soles, and, in some cases, cutaneous and internal malignant lesions develop.

A generalised exfoliative dermatitis can be produced by any drug, but particularly when administration is continued after an eruption has started to develop. Gold, penicillin, and organic arsenicals are three drugs commonly causing an exfoliative dermatitis.

Other curious effects are produced by drugs, including patches of white hair, from chloroquine; pink disease from taking mercury, particularly in the form of teething powders; and hypertrophic gingivitis, due to phenytoin. A light sensitivity may also develop with some drugs, particularly the sulphonamides, chlorpromazine, and some tetracyclines.

Confirmation of the diagnosis by patch or prick testing is possible with only a few drugs, and as test doses may be dangerous in some cases, the diagnosis can often only be presumed.

Basis of Treatment

The treatment of drug eruptions largely consists of stopping administration of the drug, which may be enough for the whole condition to settle down. If, however, there has been a widespread eruption associated with severe constitutional symptoms, steroid therapy by mouth may be necessary. Urticarial eruptions will be helped by antihistamines.

Desensitisation is sometimes undertaken if it is essential that the drug be continued, but it is not always possible to desensitise, and severe reactions may develop. Once a drug sensitivity is established the patient will remain in this sensitive state for the rest of his life and he must be warned not to take that particular drug again.

TUMOURS

Diseases of the skin include a very large number of tumours.

EPITHELIAL TUMOURS

Classification of epithelial tumours

Benign:

Seborrhoeic keratoses
   (seborrhoeic warts)
   (basal cell papilloma)
Kerato-acanthoma
Skin tags

Pre-malignant:

Actinic keratoses
Arsenical keratoses
Tar and oil keratoses
   (especially on scrotum)

Malignant:

Intraepidermal epithelioma
   (Bowen's disease)
Basal cell carcinoma
Squamous carcinoma
Malignant melanoma

A wide variety of benign and malignant tumours of the other structures of the skin (hair follicles, sebaceous glands, apocrine and eccrine sweat glands, blood vessels, nerves, fibrocytes, lymphoid tissue, etc.) also occur, though not very frequently, and are discussed in larger volumes. They provide intense interest to histopathologists and biopsy can give a very precise diagnosis often of value where systemic disease is associated, e.g. Hodgkin's disease.

Benign

Seborrhoeic Keratoses. These are raised, rough with a colour ranging from normal skin to dark brown and occurring in areas rich in pilosebaceous follicles (face, chest and back). They tend to erupt in the fifth decade of life and affect both sexes equally. They cause anxiety to the doctor because of their pigmentation, and distress to the patient because of unsightliness. They are easily removed with curette and cautery or cryotherapy. Malignant change does not occur.

Kerato-acanthoma. A painful tumour growing in a few weeks, shaped like a volcano with a central crater and overhanging lip. Usually 1 to 2 cm in diameter. Although benign, it closely mimics a squamous carcinoma. Unless the whole lesion is excised, even the histopathologist has difficulty in making the distinction from squamous carcinoma.

Skin Tags. The name is apt and describes common fibro-epithelial polyps which develop on the eyelids, neck, axillary folds and intertriginous sites. A special type of skin tag associated with darkly pigmented thickened skin in flexures is called *acanthosis nigricans* and is usually associated with internal malignancy.

Pre-malignant

Actinic Keratoses. These are small localised thickenings of horn and disorganised epidermal cells which have the appearance of being stuck on to sun-exposed skin. They often resemble tiny barnacles 3 to 5 mm in diameter. They are common in white races in patients with outdoor occupations, for example farmers, road workers, elderly sailors and especially where the individual has lived in tropical climates. The face, bald head, backs of hands and tips of pinnae are most affected and most patients are men. Malignant change is not frequent and if it occurs the degree of invasiveness is low. Treatment with 5-fluorouracil topically can be very effective.

Arsenical Keratoses. These look like the actinic variety but occur on skin not subject to ultraviolet radiation. They occur in the elderly who have ingested arsenic in tonics in youth or who have had it prescribed for the treatment of psoriasis decades ago. They may accompany internal malignancy which is also due to arsenic ingestion.

Tar and Oil Keratoses. These are similar and occur on skin surfaces where there has been long occupational contact with the substance, for example tar on the forearms in road workers, oil on thighs and scrotum in drillers and turners. Scrotal keratoses may change into squamous carcinoma and are to be regarded seriously.

Malignant

Intraepidermal Epithelioma (Bowen's Disease). This is a very slowly progressive tumour of squamous cells confined to the epidermis. It forms a perfectly demarcated slightly scaly plaque and can mimic psoriasis.

Basal Cell Carcinoma. This is common in white races on the sun-exposed face. The melanin pigmentation of negroes protects them from this tumour, even though sunlight exposure may be prolonged and intense. The tumour is usually close to the eyes or nose. It is flesh-coloured, painless and has a pearly border. Tiny capillaries can be seen running close to the surface in the pearly tissue and often there are a few flecks of pigment, too. When first seen the lesion is commonly 0.5 to 1.0 cm in diameter, but with neglect it can spread to any size, for example the entire scalp. Ulceration occurs late (rodent ulcer) and metastasis to glands does not occur. Careful complete removal by excision, thorough curetting and cauterisation or radiotherapy all give good results.

Squamous Carcinoma. This usually arises in skin damaged by ultraviolet, heat energy, chronic infection, for example lupus vulgaris (*see* page 143) and rarely in venous ulcers. The tumour is invasive, ulcerates early, is soft, vascular and friable and metastasises to lymph nodes. Radical excision and skin grafting are usually essential.

Malignant Melanoma. This is an exceedingly important soft, dark skin tumour which bleeds readily.

NAEVI

A naevus is a developmental defect of the skin of limited extent. The word is derived from the Latin meaning 'a birthmark'. Everybody's skin contains some naevi of which the most common are moles (melanocytic naevi). Naevi are usually predominantly composed of one tissue type and are classed thus:

Classification of naevi

Epithelial naevi:

    Epidermal verrucous naevus
    Sebaceous naevus
    Apocrine naevus

Melanocytic naevi:

    Cellular naevi (moles)
    Lentigines

Dermal naevi:

    Vascular (strawberry naevus)
         (port wine stain)
    Lymphangioma
    Connective tissue naevi
    Fatty tissue naevi.

Melanocytic Naevi

Cellular Naevi (Moles). These are rare in infancy and usually increase in number in adolescence. They are soft raised lesions which may be pigmented or non-pigmented, hairy or non-hairy. They are common and harmless.

Lentigines. These are flat, dark brown macules due to melanocytic proliferation. A dark, extending, thickening patch of lentigo with a red edge must be treated very seriously as it is showing signs of changing into a malignant melanoma.

Dermal Naevi

Strawberry Naevi. These raised bright red naevi usually erupt in the first week of life and enlarge during the first year. They gradually shrivel during the next few years. Resolution may be delayed if a deep (subcutaneous) extension is present and a fibro-fatty pad left at the site.

Port Wine Stains. These are flat or irregularly slightly raised patches of dilated capillaries and larger vessels. They are present at birth, can be highly disfiguring and unfortunately do not fade with age.

Paler vascular lesions called 'salmon patches' are commonly present at birth between the eyebrows, on the eyelids and nape of the neck and are transient blemishes.

CONNECTIVE TISSUE DISEASES

This group of diseases includes disorders sometimes confined to the skin, but frequently systemic in extent. Understanding of the aetiology is incomplete and classification remains a problem, but extensive change in the connective tissue is a feature common to all.

Definition

Lupus erythematosus, scleroderma, and dermatomyositis are widespread or localised eruptions with systemic changes having certain features in common, probably due to autoimmune mechanisms.

LUPUS ERYTHEMATOSUS (*see* page 122)

This may occur in a chronic localised cutaneous form, in an acute widespread cutaneous form, and as a systemic disorder. The chronic localised condition is more commonly found in the adult, and is more frequent in women. The lesions are usually on light-exposed sites and may vary from a single patch to numerous areas. The involved skin is red, slightly thickened, often puckered, and with adherent scale on the surface. There is often follicular hyperkeratosis and this feature may be

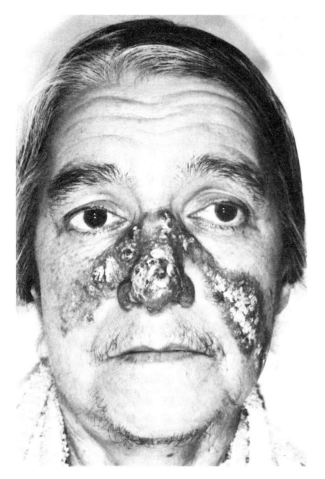

Fig. 8.10   Chronic discoid lupus erythematosus.

more apparent when a scale is removed and the follicular projections are seen adhering to the underside of the scale. The patches persist for months or years and gradually extend, new lesions also developing. The condition is often worse after exposure to sunlight.

Widespread cutaneous lupus erythematosus develops more quickly and involves larger areas, but, again, is commonly in light-exposed sites, and, characteristically, involves the cheeks and the bridge of the nose in the so-called 'butterfly' distribution (Fig. 8.10). The aetiology of lupus erythematosus is unknown, but there is mounting evidence that it is an autoimmune disease. Blood investigations in cases of chronic cutaneous lupus erythematosus may show a raised ESR and in a very few of the cases the presence of LE cells, antinuclear and anti-DNA antibodies. However, it is rare for cutaneous lupus erythematosus to develop into systemic lupus erythematosus and, indeed, it is still possible that the two conditions are entirely separate diseases.

SCLERODERMA (see page 122)

The commonest pattern of this disease consists of patches of hardened white skin with, often, a violaceous

border (morphoea). The patches may be single or multiple, or large areas of the skin surface can be involved. Progressive symmetrical scleroderma (systemic sclerosis) is a different disorder in which the sclerodermatous process affects the finger and toe tips and gradually involves other areas. It is associated with Raynaud's phenomenon and a thinning and rigidity of the facial skin with telangiectasia. Systemic involvement is common.

DERMATOMYOSITIS (see page 124)

This may be associated with various non-specific eruptions, but there is a characteristic swelling of the face and the muscles become painful, swollen, and weak. Over one-quarter of adult patients with dermatomyositis have underlying visceral malignant disease.

DISORDERS OF THE HAIR

The number of hairs on the human scalp is approximately one hundred thousand. There is a daily loss of 20 to 100 scalp hairs. Scalp hair grows about 2 mm a week; each hair has a long growing phase of two to three years, followed by a resting stage during which the hairs are retained in the follicles. This lasts for a few months before the hairs are finally shed. Hairs in the resting stage make up to 5 to 15 per cent of the total scalp hair. If there is a major illness, more hairs tend to pass to the resting stage, and so a few months afterwards there is considerable general hair fall, which is followed a few months later by regrowth.

ALOPECIA AREATA

Apart from male pattern baldness, one of the commonest complaints of the scalp is alopecia areata, a condition that involves any age group. There is a family history in one-third of the cases, and some patients have attacks at different times during their life, suggesting some constitutional tendency.

Commonly, the hair is lost in patches and the scalp skin appears normal. Often, at the margins of the patch involved, there are short hairs which taper at the skin surface and are referred to as exclamation mark hairs. Such patches of alopecia areata will remain for months, but regrowth then occurs and the new hair is often white, gradually becoming pigmented as regrowth progresses. In some cases the patches spread and there is complete baldness over the whole scalp. Occasionally, there is loss of hair in other sites, including the eyebrows, eyelashes, beard, trunk and limb hair. In some cases the areas of baldness persist for many months or years. Apart from the inborn constitutional tendency, nervous stress and strain seem to play a part in many cases. The condition is probably an autoimmune disorder. Explanation and reassurance is probably the most important aspect of treatment, but it is interesting that steroids injected into the site will usually cause regrowth. Local applications of steroids are often prescribed and these may help to some extent.

SCURF

Excessive scaling of the scalp occurs mechanically when the scalp is very greasy, and in any condition such as eczema and psoriasis in which the skin tends to scale this feature will be exaggerated in the scalp as the scales are held to the scalp by the surrounding hairs. In patients who have developed excessive scaling, particularly when the scalp is greasy, a fungus (*Pityrosporum ovale*) readily colonises the scalp. This fungus is present in normal scalps and merely grows if the conditions favour its development. Its presence has, however, led to the popular misconception that scurf is an infectious condition. In many cases of mild eczema of the scalp, a habit of scratching and picking will increase the condition, as will excessive washing, brushing, and combing. In such a condition the gentle application of a steroid cream or tar salicylic acid cream once a day, and the gentle washing every four to five days with a simple shampoo will usually suffice to settle it down.

GENERAL HAIR LOSS

The scalp hair can fall or become thin from many causes and often in each case a number of factors are present, including a constitutional inborn tendency, endocrine factors, emotional stress and strain, general illnesses, and local trauma from excessive brushing, and other manipulations of the hair. Drugs may cause general alopecia, and steroids, antimitotic drugs and heparin are among those commonly leading to this condition.

SUGGESTED FURTHER READING

Baker, H. (1977) Psoriasis, in *Dermatology*, p. 152. (Marks, R. and Samman, P. D. eds.). London: W. Heinemann.

Calnan, C. D. (1977) Eczema, in *Dermatology*, p. 116. (Marks, R. and Samman, P. D., eds.). London: W. Heinemann.

Cunliffe, W. J. and Cotterill, J. A. (1975) *The Acnes, Clinical Features, Pathogenesis and Treatment*. W. B. Saunders & Co.

Harman, R. R. M. (1977) Tropical skin diseases in temperate climates in *Recent Advances in Dermatology* (Rook, A. ed.). London: Churchill Livingstone.

Meara, R. H. (1977) Epithelial and melanocytic tumours of the skin, in *Dermatology*, (Marks, R. and Samman, P. D. eds.). London: W. Heinemann.

Peachey, R. D. G. (1977) Leg Ulcers, in *Recent Advances in Dermatology*, p. 199. (Rook, A., ed.). London: Churchill Livingstone.

Warin, R. P. and Champion, R. H. (1974) *Urticaria*, W. B. Saunders & Co.

Venereology

9

A. E. TINKLER

The venereal diseases are a group of conditions transmitted during sexual intercourse or close sexual contact with an infected person. The 1917 Public Health Act lists only syphilis, gonorrhoea and chancroid as venereal, but other sexually transmitted diseases include non-gonococcal urethritis in the male, trichomonal vaginitis in the female, and conditions which are now very rare in Britain such as lymphogranuloma venereum and granuloma inguinale. Other conditions, not generally regarded as venereal, but which are commonly associated with sexual contact include herpes genitalis, condylomata accuminata, molluscum contagiosum, scabies, and pediculosis pubis.

GONORRHOEA

Definition

A sexually transmitted infection due to *Neisseria gonorrhoea* (the gonococcus) which affects primarily the anterior urethra in the male and the urethra and cervix in the female.

Background

In recent years there has been a great increase in the incidence of gonorrhoea throughout the world. Approximately, 60,000 cases are seen annually in the clinics of England and Wales (Fig. 9.1).

GONORRHOEA IN THE MALE

Symptoms

After three to five days incubation period:
Dysuria – scalding on micturition.
Urethral discharge – seropurulent becoming purulent and yellowish.

Signs

A yellow purulent urethral discharge.
Reddening of urethral meatus.

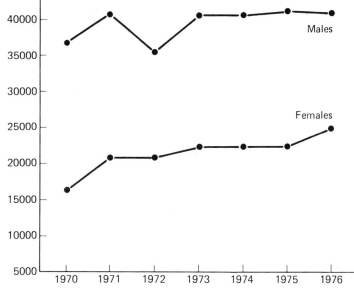

Fig. 9.1   Gonorrhoea, England 1970–76.

Two-glass urine test: urine passed into two glasses shows haze and threads in the first glass. If treatment is delayed and the posterior urethra has become involved both glasses will be hazy and contain threads.

In male carriers (five per cent of total), and in chronic cases, a slight purulent urethral discharge is seen occasionally or in the morning only, with some yellow staining of the underclothes.

Gonococcal proctitis is common in male homosexuals, and is often symptomless.

Investigations

Urethral Smear. The Gram-stained urethral smear will show numerous pus cells and both intra- and extracellular Gram-negative diplococci (Fig. 9.2). In smears from carriers and chronic cases the gonococci may be scanty and predominantly extracellular and the organism may not be found in a smear taken soon after micturition. An early morning smear before the patient urinates may be necessary to establish the diagnosis in such cases.

Urethral Cultures. These should always be taken if possible, but treatment need not await the result when the smear and history are typical. When these are atypical, confirmation by culture is essential, and this is particularly important where marital problems are involved.

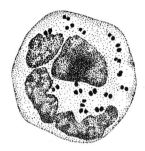

Fig. 9.2 A pus cell showing intracellular diplococci (gonococcus).

Complications

Local complications are comparatively rare, and systemic complications very rare. All can be prevented by effective early treatment followed by full tests of cure.

Local. Posterior urethritis.
Prostatis – acute and chronic.
Vesiculitis.
Acute epididymitis.
Peri-urethral abscess.
Urethral stricture.

Systemic. Gonococcal arthritis.
Gonococcal septicaemia.
Gonococcal endocarditis.

GONORRHOEA IN THE FEMALE

1. *Gonorrhoea is frequently asymptomatic in the female.*
2. It can never be diagnosed on clinical grounds. Almost three-quarters of all female patients attend initially as contacts of male cases and not because of their signs or symptoms.

Symptoms

None.
Slight dysuria.
Slight or moderate vaginal discharge, often unnoticed by the patient.

Signs

May be none.
Inflamed meatal orifice.
Reddening or acute erosion of the cervix.
Mucopurulent cervical plug.
Copious vaginal discharge is more likely to be due to a concomitant trichomonal vaginitis.

Investigations

1. Gram-stained smears of urethral and cervical secretions.
2. Culture of these secretions is essential.
3. Wet film and culture for trichomonads from the vaginal secretion.

In cases diagnosed at special clinics it is found that about 40 per cent of females with gonorrhoea also have vaginal trichomoniasis.

These investigations must be repeated three times with negative results as tests of cure after treatment, or to exclude the diagnosis in suspected cases.

The gonococcal complement fixation test (GCFT) is of limited diagnostic value. It is useless in early uncomplicated gonorrhoea, it may be negative in chronic or complicated cases, or positive in the absence of any gonococcal infection past or present.

Complications

Local:
Gonococcal proctitis, occurs in 40 per cent of cases. It is spread from the vaginal discharge and is often symptomless.
Salpingitis. Ten per cent of cases will present evidence of involvement of one or both tubes, acute or subacute, usually the latter. Lower abdominal pain and tenderness is present, with thickening and tenderness of the affected tube on bimanual palpation.
Infertility following bilateral gonococcal salpingitis is now uncommon.
Bartholinitis.

Systemic:
As in the male – Rare.

Basis of Treatment

Increased resistance of the gonococcus to penicillin is being reported from many parts of the world, but the organism is sensitive to a variety of antibiotics. Treatment schedules for which over 90 per cent cure rates are claimed include:

Ampicillin 3g stat, with 2g probenecid to delay excretion
Procaine penicillin IM. 1.2 to 2.4 mega units with probenecid

Septrin 4 tablets twice daily for two days.
Kanamycin 2g stat.
Spectinomycin 2 to 3g stat.

Both Septrin and kanamycin are non-treponemicidal and will not mask a concomitantly acquired syphilitic infection and can be given to patients allergic to penicillin.

TRICHOMONIASIS

TRICHOMONAL VAGINITIS

Definition

An acute, subacute, or chronic vaginitis due to the protozoon *Trichomonas vaginalis*. It is transmitted sexually in the great majority of cases but, in a minority, the mode of transmission is uncertain.

Symptoms

Acute. A profuse malodorous vaginal discharge. Intravaginal pain or discomfort.

Subacute or Chronic. Persistent moderate or slight discharge.

Signs

Acute. Copious frothy yellowish vaginal discharge. Acutely inflamed vaginal mucosa with punctate erythema, and 'strawberry' cervix.
Possibly vulval oedema and adjacent intertrigo.

Subacute or Chronic. Moderate to slight frothy vaginal discharge with some reddening of the vaginal mucosa.

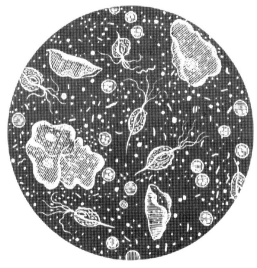

Fig. 9.3 *Trichomonas vaginalis* with epithelial cells and leucocytes (drawing from dark field microscopy).

Investigations

1. A smear and culture of the vaginal secretion. The smear is usually examined wet, by hanging drop, dark field (Fig. 9.3) or phase contrast microscopy and the protozoon is recognised by its characteristic jerky movement.
2. Smears and culture of urethra and cervix to exclude a concomitant gonococcal infection. Gonorrhoea in the female is frequently associated with trichomoniasis in patients attending venereal disease clinics.

Complications

None.

Basis of Treatment

Metronidazole (Flagyl) 200 mg three times daily for seven days, or 400 mg twice daily for five days is effective in over 95 per cent of cases where reinfection can be excluded. Equally good results are claimed for nimorazole (Naxogin).

Simultaneous treatment of the sexual partner is important.

TRICHOMONIASIS IN THE MALE

This is much rarer, but the protozoon is responsible for five per cent or more of all cases of non-gonococcal urethritis. Balanitis and prostatitis may also occur.

NON-GONOCOCCAL URETHRITIS (NGU) OR NON-SPECIFIC URETHRITIS (NSU)

Definition

An acute or subacute inflammation of the urethral mucosa in the male, uncertain in origin but related to sexual activity and with a tendency to relapse.

Background

This is a very common condition in which the cause remains undetermined in over 90 per cent of the 70,000 cases seen annually in the clinics of England and Wales. Of the known causes *Trichomonas vaginalis* accounts for five to ten per cent of all cases. Urethritis due to *Candida albicans*, or secondary to upper urinary tract infection, together with chemical or traumatic causes account for less than five per cent of cases.

Bacterial Causes. The only bacterium which can be incriminated with certainty as a primary pathogen in urethritis in the male is the gonococcus. Other bacteria, e.g. staphylococci, streptococci, coliforms, diphtheroids, *Corynebacterium vaginale* may sometimes be found in the discharge in cases of non-gonococcal urethritis but their role as primary pathogens is by no means proven.

Pleuropneumonia-like organisms (PPLO: mycoplasma) can be isolated from the discharge in 15 to 70 per cent of cases and also from the vaginal discharge in non-specific genital infection in women, but since they can be found in apparently normal individuals their pathogenicity is in doubt.

Chlamydia trachomatis is a virus-like particle possibly pathogenic in the eye, urethra and cervix. Positive cell cultures are reported from urethral swabs in 30 to 70 per cent of cases of non-gonococcal urethritis and from cervical swabs in a significant proportion of the sexual partners of such patients. Positive isolates from these sites can usually be obtained from the parents of an infant which develops neonatal inclusion conjunctivitis.

Symptoms

A mucopurulent or purulent urethral discharge ten to fourteen days after risk.

Slight discomfort on micturition or, rarely, marked dysuria with urgency and frequency. Sometimes symptomless or a slight seropurulent morning discharge.

Signs

A urethral discharge varying from persistent, copious and purulent to occasional, slight and seropurulent.

Investigations

1. Urethral smear, Gram-stained, shows pus cells but no gonococci.
2. Urethral culture – negative for gonococci.
3. Urine is hazy with threads in the first glass.

Prognosis

Relapse and reinfection are common and these recurrences can be very distressing, particularly in the married man, where there is sometimes no question of extra-marital intercourse by either partner.

Complications

Chronic prostatitis.
Reiter's Syndrome (1 per cent) (*see* page 39).

Basis of Treatment

The tetracyclines provide the cheapest and most effective treatment. The discharge rapidly clears in about 80 per cent of cases after 500 mg three times daily for five to seven days, or 250 mg four times daily for ten to fourteen days.

SYPHILIS

Definition

A venereal infection caused by *Treponema pallidum*.

Background

Following a dramatic decline in incidence after the second world war, there has been a gradual increase in early infectious syphilis since 1955, especially amongst male homosexuals, but late and congenital syphilis are gradually being eradicated (Table 9.1).

Table 9.1 Syphilis, England 1970–76

Year	Early		Late	
	Male	*Female*	*Male*	*Female*
1970	1,277	268	883	489
1971	1,264	336	849	368
1972	1,350	297	765	394
1973	1,802	331	795	377
1974	1,906	374	822	378
1975	1,928	335	801	398
1976	2,075	371	876	426

Treponema pallidum (Fig. 9.5), a delicate slender spirochaete 6 to 15 microns in length is the causative organism.

Acquired syphilis has four stages, primary, secondary, latent and late (tertiary).

Transmission

The disease is acquired when, on direct contact with an early lesion, treponemes pass from the lesion through the mucosa or an abrasion of the skin at the point of contact. Since treponemes are present only in the surface lesions of *early* syphilis, i.e. primary, secondary and possibly in the first year or two of latency, and as they favour moist sites, e.g. the genitalia or mouth, the disease is infectious only in its early stages and almost always takes place during close sexual contact.

PRIMARY SYPHILIS

A primary sore or chancre develops at the site of entry of the treponemes in about three to four weeks and heals spontaneously about six weeks later. Starting as an indurated papule, it becomes eroded and if it develops fully will present as a classical *Hunterian chancre*. It may resolve at any stage in its development, thus atypical chancres are common and any papular, erosive or ulcerative lesion of the genitals, or of the ano-genital area in a homosexual, must be regarded with suspicion.

Extra-genital chancres are rare, e.g. lip, mouth, etc.,

but in homosexuals perianal and rectal chancres are common and frequently atypical, e.g. anal fissures.

Symptoms

The appearance of an indurated papule which becomes eroded and develops the following signs.

Signs of the Typical Hunterian Chancre (Fig. 9.4)

A shallow ulcer.
Indurated.
Painless.
Non-bleeding.
Usually single.
Rounded or oval.
Slightly raised hyperaemic margin.
Painless enlargement of the local lymph nodes.
Note: A female patient will be unaware of the presence of an intravaginal chancre.

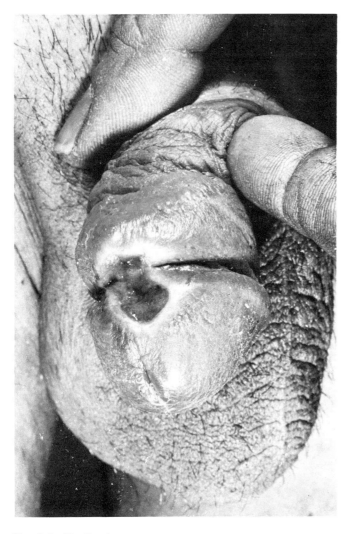

Fig. 9.4 Penile chancre.

Investigations

1. Serum tests for syphilis do not usually become positive for one or two weeks after the appearance of the chancre. Diagnosis thus depends on the demonstration of *Treponema pallidum* by –
2. Dark field microscopy of the exudate from the lesion (Fig. 9.5). If negative, the test should be repeated on three successive days and be followed by serum tests for three to six months if doubt still persists.

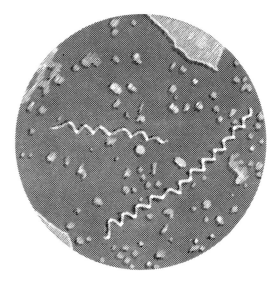

Fig. 9.5 *Treponema pallidum* (drawing from dark field microscopy).

Differential Diagnosis

Chancres must be distinguished from genital herpes, traumatic ulceration, chancroid, granuloma inguinale, and early carcinoma.

SECONDARY SYPHILIS

This may become manifest before the chancre heals, or be delayed some months.

Symptoms

Skin rash – common.
Sore throat, hoarseness of voice.
Headache, malaise, pyrexia – mild or absent.
Loss of hair – infrequent.
Bone and joint pains – infrequent.
Jaundice.

Signs

The Skin. A dull red or coppery macular or maculo-papular rash, symmetrical, indolent, and non-irritant.

More rarely, papular, papulosquamous, follicular, psoriasiform, or pustular. Never vesicular.

Ano-genital condylomata lata. Fleshy wart-like lesions, highly contagious, but uncommon.

The Mucous Surfaces of Mouth or Genitals. Small superficial oval or serpiginous erosions (mucous patches) causing bald patches on the tongue or 'snail track' ulcers on the palate or pharynx.
Generalised painless lymphadenitis.
'Moth-eaten' alopecia.

Investigations

1. Dark field microscopy. Demonstration of *Treponema pallidum* in the exudate from the moist lesions.
2. The serum tests for syphilis are always strongly positive at this stage.

LATENT SYPHILIS

This follows the untreated secondary stage and lasts anything between two years and a life-time (average ten to fifteen years). Mucocutaneous relapses may occur in the genital area or in the mouth in the first year or so of latency – small transient erosive lesions similar to the mucous patches of the secondary stage. Apart from this there are no clinical signs and in the absence of surface lesions the patient is non-infectious.

Diagnosis can only be made on serological grounds. Ultimately, routine serum tests may be only weakly positive, doubtful, or even negative.

LATE SYPHILIS (TERTIARY)

The extraordinary variety of clinical manifestations prompted Sir William Osler's remark – 'He who knows syphilis knows medicine'. The disease is as unpredictable as it is varied, and only about 40 per cent of untreated syphilitics will develop clinical signs of late syphilis some five to fifteen years after infection. About 10 per cent will develop neurosyphilis (page 550), 10 to 12 per cent cardiovascular syphilis (page 299), and 15 to 20 per cent late benign syphilis where less vital structures are involved. The three types are not mutually exclusive, and wherever the lesion the pathology is the same – an obliterative endarteritis of terminal vessels leading to necrosis and subsequent fibrosis. This process may be circumscribed or diffuse and take place almost anywhere in the body. Clinical signs and prognosis will therefore depend on the site and system involved and the extent of the lesions.

LATE BENIGN SYPHILIS

The *gumma*, a syphilitic hypersensitivity tissue reaction, is the essential lesion. Gummatous lesions are not infectious.

Visceral Gummata. A circumscribed gumma of an internal organ, e.g. liver, brain, will present as any other space-occupying lesion. Differentiation is by positive serology and response to treatment.

Bones. Periostitis with new bone formation; gummatous osteitis with destruction of bone.

Symptoms

Nocturnal pain, tenderness and swelling.

Cutaneous and subcutaneous gummatous lesions are extremely varied in clinical manifestations, 27 skin diseases are listed in the differential diagnosis.
Basically there are three types:
1. Nodular.
2. Nodular ulcerative (Fig. 9.6).
3. Ulcerative – the simple gummatous ulcer (Fig. 9.7).

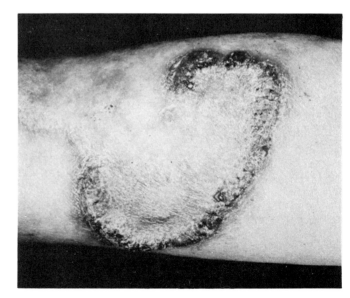

Fig. 9.6 Nodular gumma of forearm.

All cutaneous gummatous lesions show some of the following basic characteristics:
Solitary, or grouped in one area of the body.
Asymmetry.
Induration.
Indolence.
Sharply defined margins. 'Punched out' if ulcerated.
Peripheral hyperpigmentation.

Individual lesions circular or oval. Grouped lesions arciform in general outline.
Central healing, peripheral spread.
Silvery, non-contractile 'tissue paper' scar on healing.
Excellent response to anti-syphilitic treatment.

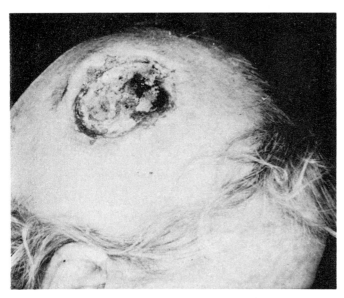

Fig. 9.7 Ulcerative gumma of skull (the patient died of pyogenic meningitis).

CONGENITAL SYPHILIS

This is a preventable disease. Each case represents a missed case of maternal syphilis. The vast number of circulating treponemes present in the bloodstream in *early* syphilis are progressively reduced as time goes on. Thus treponemes from an expectant mother with primary or secondary syphilis are almost certain to be blood-borne across the placenta to the fetal circulation, whereas the fetus may escape infection if the mother is in the latent stage. The older the disease in the mother the less likely is fetal infection, but the outcome of any particular pregnancy is unpredictable as long as the mother remains untreated. Infection of the fetus may result in:
1. Abortion after the fourth month.
2. A stillborn macerated fetus.
3. A live child who develops signs of early congenital syphilis at or soon after birth and, if it survives, signs of late congenital syphilis in later years.
4. An apparently healthy child who in later years shows evidence of late congenital syphilis. With the exception of the primary chancre all the manifestations of acquired syphilis can occur in congenital syphilis although some, e.g. cardiovascular congenital syphilis, are very rare. On the other hand, certain manifestations of congenital syphilis never occur in acquired syphilis.

EARLY CONGENITAL SYPHILIS

Signs

These usually appear some weeks after birth. Their presence at birth indicates a severe infection.

The Skin. (a) Generalised, macular, papular or maculopapular rash, most marked in napkin and circumoral areas.
(b) A bullous eruption on palms and soles indicates a severe infection.
(c) Condylomata lata in moist areas, infrequent.

Mucous Surfaces. (a) The snuffles. A syphilitic rhinitis with nasal discharge interferes with suckling, hence failure to gain weight.
(b) Mucous patches in mouth or on lips.

Bones and Joints. Epiphysitis, osteochondritis, periostitis.

Hepatosplenomegaly

Syphilitic Basal Meningitis. Causing irritability, aphonic cry.
Note: Early signs may be so slight as to escape notice. In general, the older the disease in the mother the less serious is the infection in the child.

LATE CONGENITAL SYPHILIS

Hutchinson's classical triad consists of:
Interstitial keratitis.
Eighth nerve deafness.
Hutchinson's teeth.

Interstitial Keratitis

A syphilitic hypersensitivity reaction of the cornea.
Onset usually between five to fifteen years.
Bilateral, but intervals between attacks in both eyes variable.
Tendency to recur.
Uninfluenced by anti-syphilitic treatment.

Symptoms. Pain, lachrymation, photophobia.

Signs. Marked circum-corneal injection.
Opacity of cornea – ground glass appearance after prolonged, severe, or recurrent attacks.
Salmon patch. Yellowish-red corneal patches in severe cases.
Slow spontaneous resolution.
Lesions in deeper structures of eye common, e.g. iritis, choroiditis.

Eighth Nerve Deafness

A progressive bilateral perceptive deafness.
Onset usually about puberty or later.
Uninfluenced by treatment.
Precise pathology obscure.

Dental Stigmata

Hutchinson's teeth – a peg-shaped deformity of the upper central incisors, second dentition. Moon's teeth (mulberry molars). The six year molars erupt with dwarfed cusps.
Other late manifestations include:
Saddle nose. A gummatous collapse of the nasal ridge. (Fig. 9.8).
Gummatous perforation of the palate.
Sabre tibia; due to syphilitic periostitis.
Clutton's joints. A painless hydrarthrosis.
Rhagades. Linear fissures radiating from the lips.
Congenital neurosyphilis – as in acquired syphilis.
Gummata – cutaneous, visceral or skeletal.
Congenital cardiovascular syphilis is extremely rare.

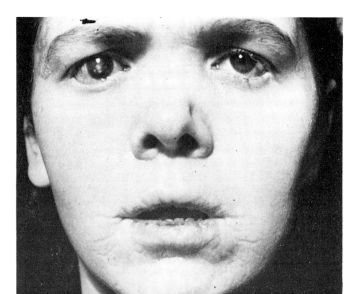

Fig. 9.8 Some stigmata of congenital syphilis. Saddle nose, rhagades, and interstitial keratitis.

Prevention

Congenital syphilis is now a very rare disease in Great Britain due to:
1. Routine serum testing of all mothers early in pregnancy.
2. Penicillin treatment of maternal syphilis which can prevent fetal infection if given in the first trimester, or cure an already infected fetus if given later in the pregnancy.
Note: The longer treatment of the mother is delayed, the less certain is the outcome for the child. The slightest doubt about the antenatal serology calls for the immediate and detailed clinical and serological re-examination of the mother.

SEROLOGICAL TESTS FOR SYPHILIS

There are two types of tests:
1. Non-specific (lipoidal antigen reagin) tests.
2. Specific (treponemal antigen) tests.

Non-specific (Reagin) Tests

Examples
(a) Cardiolipin Wassermann test (C/WR).
(b) Venereal Disease Reference Laboratory slide test (VDRL).
(c) Kahn.

These are simple, reproducible tests which demonstrate the presence or absence of an antibody *reagin* which is present in the serum of patients with treponemal disease, e.g. syphilis, yaws, bejel, pinta.

False positive reactions occur because reagin may also be present in the serum of patients with malaria, glandular fever, vaccinia, typhus or Weil's disease. In such cases the positive reaction is usually weak and of short duration. Auto-immune conditions, e.g. SLE and lepromatous leprosy, may give stronger and more persistent positive reactions.

Specific (Treponemal Antigen) Tests

One or more of these tests should always be included in routine screening.
Examples:
(a) Reiter's protein complement fixation test (RPCFT).
(b) Fluorescent treponemal antibody test (FTA).
(c) *Treponema pallidum* haemagglutination assay (TPHA).
(d) Treponemal immobilisation test (TPI).

In primary syphilis the VDRL and C/WR usually become positive first. In the secondary stage all tests are strongly positive. After successful treatment of primary or secondary syphilis the reagin tests should become negative in about six to eighteen months respectively, but the specific tests may remain weakly positive for life. All tests may remain positive indefinitely after treatment of late or latent syphilis due to continued production of IgG antibodies, but it is claimed that IgM class antibodies cease to be produced a few months after successful treatment, hence negative serum tests on the IgM fraction indicate arrest of the disease.

157

Basis of Treatment of Syphilis

Apart from saline compresses no local treatment should be applied to a suspected chancre until the exudate has been examined and found negative by dark field microscopy for three successive days.

Penicillin has now supplanted all other forms of treatment and the organism has shown no signs of increasing resistance. It is essential to maintain a treponemicidal serum concentration throughout the whole duration of treatment. Daily intramuscular doses of 900,000 units of procain penicillin G will achieve this. Treatment must continue for seven to fourteen days in early syphilis and is often prolonged to fourteen to twenty-one days in cases of late syphilis. Observation, including serum tests, should be continued for two years after treatment.

Other treponemicidal antibiotics include cephaloridine, tetracycline, erythromycin and chloramphenicol, but none are as effective as penicillin, and experience with them in the treatment of syphilis is limited. When they are used in the treatment of penicillin-sensitive patients the usual two year follow-up should be prolonged.

Herxheimer Reaction. About 40 per cent of early syphilitics develop a reaction of uncertain origin about six hours after the first injection. It consists of fever, malaise, headache and possibly rigors, lasting a few hours only. It is less frequent, but may be more serious, in late syphilis.

Prognosis

Early Syphilis. In patients who soon become seronegative after treatment and remain so for two years, the cure rate approaches 100 per cent.

Late Syphilis. Treatment at this stage will arrest the progress of the disease, but may only marginally improve the prognosis or expectation of life of the patient, since this largely depends on the structures involved and the duration and severity of the signs at the onset of the treatment. In general terms it can be said that gummatous lesions heal rapidly, but may leave mutilating or incapacitating scars. Patients with neurosyphilis are likely to be left with the degree of mental or physical incapacity found at the onset of treatment.

Cardiovascular syphilis has the worst prognosis and is least influenced by the arrest of the underlying disease, but in selected cases cardiovascular surgery may completely change this otherwise poor prognosis.

Persistently positive serum tests are common after treatment for late or latent syphilis and, if constant at low titre, are of no prognostic importance.

CHANCROID, LYMPHOGRANULOMA VENEREUM, AND GRANULOMA INGUINALE

Less than 100 cases per annum of these three conditions together are seen in the clinics of England and Wales. For details, reference should be made to a textbook on Venereal Disease.

SUGGESTED FURTHER READING

General

Wisdom, A. (1973) *Colour Atlas of Venereology.* London: Wolfe Medical Books.
Schofield, C. B. S. (1974) *Sexually Transmitted Diseases.* Edinburgh & London: Churchill Livingstone.

Epidemiology

Willcox, R. R. (1972) Epidemiological treatment of venereal disease other than syphilis. Geneva: WHO.

Non-specific Urethritis

Richmond, S. and Oriel, J. D. (1978) Recognition and management of genital chlamydial infection. *British Medical Journal* 2: 480–482.

Syphilis

Wilkinson, A. E. (1972) Serology of syphilis. *British Medical Journal*, 2: 573–575.

Endocrinology and Diabetes 10

M. HARTOG

Substances secreted by exocrine glands are carried by ducts to nearby organs where they are active. In contrast, the endocrine (ductless) glands discharge their secretions (hormones) into the bloodstream to act upon tissues which are often far distant from their site of synthesis. In addition, the importance of the local action of some hormones, particularly those of the gastrointestinal tract, has become recognised recently.

Origin of Hormone Secreting Cells

A considerable number of polypeptide hormone secreting cells arise from neural crest tissue. They subsequently migrate to their ultimate sites in the anterior pituitary (to form the cells that secrete growth hormone, prolactin and ACTH), the neck and upper mediastinum (to form the cells that secrete calcitonin), the bronchial mucosa, the gastrointestinal tract (to form the cells that secrete the gastrointestinal hormones) and the pancreas (to form the islets of Langerhans). Furthermore, the cells contain similar enzymes from which their name of APUD (amine precursor uptake and the presence of amino acid decarboxylase) cells has been derived.

Structure and Mechanism of Action of Hormones

A large number of hormones are polypeptides, consisting of sequences of amino acids of different length and configuration. Other hormones, however, notably the steroids produced by the adrenal cortices and the gonads, are quite different in structure.

The specificity of the effects of hormones on different tissues is thought to depend upon the presence of receptors within those tissues that are only sensitive to the action of the particular hormone, although the exact nature of such receptors is still unknown. It has been clearly demonstrated that a system of 'two messengers' subserves the action of many of the polypeptide hormones. The interaction between the hormone (the first messenger) and its receptor, which is located on the cell membrane, results in the formation of the nucleotide cyclic AMP from its precursor ATP. Cyclic AMP (the second messenger), by its effects upon different enzymes within the cell, is thought to mediate the action of the hormone. Steroid hormones have an entirely different mode of action. They enter the target cells and become attached to specific receptors in the cytoplasm. The hormone-receptor complex then enters the nucleus where it affects the synthesis of ribonucleic acid.

Factors Controlling Hormone Secretion

Some of the endocrine glands are controlled by hormones produced by other glands. In addition, their secretion rate may be affected by the circulating levels of hormone produced by the target gland itself. Thus an increase in the concentration of the hormone in the blood may, directly or indirectly, inhibit further secretion by the gland which helps to maintain a constant level of circulating hormone (a 'negative feed-back' system).

The Transport of Hormones in the Blood

The steroid and thyroid hormones circulate in blood in combination with specific binding plasma proteins, whilst others, such as polypeptide hormones, appear to have no such transport mechanism. Much of the knowledge of the physiology of individual hormones has been derived from the measurement of their blood levels under different circumstances. Hormones, however, circulate in very low concentrations and such measurements present considerable difficulties. Some assays are based on the biological effects of the hormone (bioassays) although these methods are often laborious, insensitive and not suitable for numerous samples. A variety of other techniques of assay are also available. Radioimmunoassays, for example, have been widely applied to the measurement of hormones. These assays depend on the binding of a hormone by an antibody prepared to that hormone. A minute (trace) amount of the hormone labelled with a radioactive isotope is incubated *in vitro* with an aliquot of antibody, and the amount bound to the antibody is determined (Fig.

159

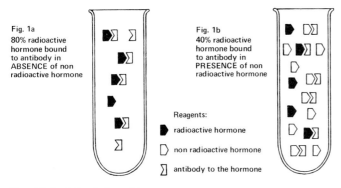

Fig. 1a
80% radioactive
hormone bound
to antibody in
ABSENCE of non
radioactive hormone

Fig. 1b
40% radioactive
hormone bound
to antibody in
PRESENCE of non
radioactive hormone

Reagents:

◗ radioactive hormone

◻ non radioactive hormone

Σ antibody to the hormone

Fig. 10.1   Principles of immunoassay.

10.1a). In other tubes, unlabelled hormone is also added to the incubates, that, by competition, reduces the amount of labelled material bound to antibody (Fig. 10.1b). The assay is performed by comparing the binding of labelled hormone in incubates containing the unknown sample, such as serum, with that in incubates containing standard solutions of the unlabelled hormone of known strength.

THE PITUITARY GLAND

The pituitary gland is situated at the base of the brain, to which it is joined by the pituitary stalk. It is partially enclosed by the bony sella turcica and normally weighs about 500 mg. It is composed of two parts, the anterior and posterior lobes. The anterior lobe develops from an upward extension (the pouch of Rathke) of the primitive buccal cavity. The posterior lobe is derived from neural tissue and is formed from a downgrowth of the floor of the brain. These two parts have different functions, and will be considered separately.

THE ANTERIOR LOBE – NORMAL

The hormones produced by the anterior lobe are polypeptides and comprise the following:

Growth Hormone (GH, Somatotrophin). Growth hormone has widespread metabolic effects resulting in the stimulation of protein anabolism and the breakdown of adipose tissue. It also antagonises some of the actions of insulin and, if secreted in excess, causes impairment of carbohydrate tolerance.

Prolactin. Prolactin is very similar in structure to GH and, in fact, its independent existence in man has been doubted, but is now certain. It plays an essential role in the initiation and maintenance of lactation. It also affects the response of the gonads to the gonadotrophins and, in some animal species, is concerned with the maintenance of the corpus luteum.

Adrenocorticotrophic hormone (ACTH). ACTH is a polypeptide consisting of 39 amino acids of which the first 24 are necessary for biological activity. It has a number of actions on the adrenal cortex, but in particular controls the secretion of cortisol. Two other polypeptides, a-MSH and corticotrophin-like intermediate lobe peptide (CLIP) have the same amino acid sequences as part of the ACTH molecule. They are produced by the pars intermedia of the pituitary. In man they are apparently only secreted in fetal life and during pregnancy, these being the only times that this zone of the pituitary is distinct.

Lipotrophin. This hormone was first detected by its effects upon adipose tissue. It is now recognised, however, that shorter sequences of amino acids, probably derived from the parent molecule, have a variety of metabolic effects some of which are likely to be of profound importance. Lipotrophin probably stimulates the activity of melanin-producing cells of the skin (the melanocytes). Formerly β-MSH was thought to control the activity of these cells. It now appears, however, that in man this substance is an artefact of the extraction procedures used for the study of pituitary and circulating polypeptides. A number of other polypeptides (the endorphins), similarly with identical amino acid sequences to part of the lipotrophin molecule, have been described. Some of them have analgesic properties and appear to bind to the same receptors within the central nervous system as the analgesic morphine.

Thyroid Stimulating Hormone (TSH). TSH stimulates the synthesis and release of thyroid hormones. TSH, FSH, LH and human chorionic gonadotrophin (*see below*) are glycoproteins. They share a common a subunit, but differ in the composition of the β subunit.

Gonadotrophins. There are two of these:
(a) *Follicle-stimulating hormone (FSH).* In women, FSH is concerned with the development of the ovarian follicle. In men, in whom the hormone is inappropriately named, it controls the development of the seminiferous tubules of the testis and spermatogenesis.

(b) *Luteinising hormone (LH).* In women, LH acts synergistically with FSH in controlling the development of the ovarian follicle and the formation of the corpus luteum. A mid-cycle peak of LH secretion is, in fact, necessary for ovulation to occur. In men, it is known as the interstitial cell stimulating hormone (ICSH), and stimulates the growth of the interstitial (Leydig) cells of the testis that secrete testosterone.

The hormones are secreted by different cells of the pituitary that are distinguished by their staining properties. The acidophil cells produce GH and prolactin, while the basophil cells, of which several different types can be recognised histologically, secrete ACTH, lipotrophin, TSH, FSH and LH. The third type of cell, the chromophobe, was formerly thought to be inactive. It is now known, however, that granules can be demonstrated in the cytoplasm of most chromophobe cells by electron microscopy, and the majority, if not all of them, appear to actively secrete hormones.

The anterior pituitary has virtually no nervous connections and its activities are controlled by chemical factors secreted by cells of the hypothalamus. This forms part of the floor of the third ventricle where it receives nerve fibres from many other parts of the brain. These factors are secreted into capillaries of the hypophyseal portal system, whence they are carried in larger vessels surrounding the pituitary stalk to be distributed to the cells of the anterior lobe by another capillary network (Fig. 10.2). Here they either stimulate

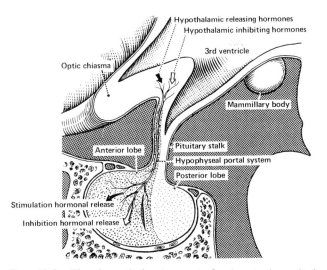

Fig. 10.2 The hypothalamic control of anterior pituitary function.

or inhibit the release of anterior pituitary hormones. These substances appear to be small polypeptides and the amino acid sequences of releasing factors for TSH (called TSH releasing hormone or TRH) and for LH and FSH (called LH releasing hormone, LHRH or LRH, LH/FSH releasing hormone, or gonadotrophin releasing hormone or GnRH) are known. Similarly, the structure of a hormone that inhibits the secretion of GH (called growth hormone-release inhibiting hormone or GHRIH, somatotrophin-release inhibiting factor or SRIF, or somatostatin) has also been established. Most interestingly, GHRIH has been shown to be widely distributed throughout different regions of the nervous system and also in the gastrointestinal system, in particular within specific cells (the D cells) of the islets of Langerhans in the pancreas. The hormone has widespread inhibitory actions both on the pituitary, where it inhibits the release not only of GH but also of TSH and prolactin, and on the stomach and pancreas where it

inhibits the secretion of gastrin, pepsin, gastric acid, insulin and glucagon.

In addition to the system of releasing and inhibiting hormones, the function of the anterior pituitary is known to be markedly affected by three classical central nervous system neurotransmitters, dopamine, noradrenaline, and serotonin (5-hydroxytryptamine). These substances usually exert their effects by altering the secretion of the different releasing and inhibiting hormones. In the case of prolactin, however, dopamine itself appears to be the major inhibitory factor produced by the hypothalamus and acts directly upon the anterior pituitary. The recognition of the widespread distribution of GHRIH, the endorphins and some of the gastro-intestinal hormones throughout the nervous system, has led to the realisation that the former distinction of neurotransmitters, with actions upon many diverse cells, and the polypeptide hormones with more limited specific effects, is probably incorrect, and many of these polypeptides may also act as neurotransmitters within the central and peripheral nervous systems.

Function Tests

Direct Tests. Until recently the measurement of pituitary hormones was by bioassay. Radioimmunoassays (*see* page 159), however, are now in routine use for most of them.

Indirect Tests. These depend on the assessment of the function of the target endocrine gland by appropriate tests. Thus, for example, circumstantial evidence as to TSH secretion can be obtained from conventional tests of thyroid function. If subnormal function is found, the response to administered TSH can be determined. If the test result remains unchanged, the patient has a primary abnormality of the thyroid. If, however, thyroid function is improved, TSH deficiency can be diagnosed. The secretion of ACTH and, to some extent, of FSH and LH can be assessed in this way. With the development of direct assays of pituitary hormones these indirect tests are now hardly ever used.

THE ANTERIOR LOBE – ABNORMAL

Clinical disorders of two types may be produced by lesions of the pituitary gland.

Local Pressure Effects. These are caused by expanding pituitary lesions, usually tumours, producing headaches and damage to surrounding structures. The optic chiasma is situated just above the pituitary fossa and is commonly affected by such lesions. The classical visual field defect found with pituitary tumours is a bitemporal hemianopia from pressure on the decussating nerve fibres from the nasal parts of the retina. Other cranial nerves such as the oculomotor and trigeminal nerves may also be involved.

Endocrine Effects. These result from either excessive or diminished secretion of the anterior pituitary hormones and are discussed below.

1. HYPERFUNCTION OF THE ANTERIOR LOBE

The conditions caused by excessive secretion of the pituitary are shown in Table 10.1.

Table 10.1 Conditions caused by hypersecretion of pituitary hormones

Hormone	Condition
Anterior lobe	
Growth hormone	Acromegaly
	Gigantism
ACTH	Cushing's syndrome
Lipotrophin	Excessive pigmentation of the skin
FSH	Precocious puberty
LH	
Prolactin	Amenorrhoea, infertility, galactorrhoea, impotence
Posterior lobe	
Vasopressin	Water intoxication

ACROMEGALY

Definition

Acromegaly is a disease caused by persistent oversecretion of GH by eosinophil or chromophobe pituitary tumours.

Symptoms and Signs (Table 10.2, Fig. 10.3)

The condition is characterised by soft tissue overgrowth causing coarsening of the features and enlargement of the hands and feet. The process is often slow and the changes may pass unnoticed by the patient and his close relatives. Comparison of the patient's appearance with that seen in old photographs is of help in diagnosis.

Impairment of carbohydrate tolerance, with or without frank diabetes mellitus, occurs in about 25 per cent of patients. Hypertension is common and heart failure may be caused by a specific acromegalic cardiomyopathy associated with massive enlargement of the heart. In children, with the onset of the condition before cessation of growth, excessive growth promotion results in gigantism.

Investigations

1. There are characteristic radiological changes showing soft tissue overgrowth and periosteal new bone formation.
2. Serum GH levels are elevated and do not show a

decrease following the administration of glucose which, in normal subjects, suppresses GH secretion. This is due to autonomous secretion of GH by the pituitary tumour.

Table 10.2 Acromegaly

Symptoms	Signs
Effects of excess GH secretion	
Enlargement of hands and feet	Soft tissue overgrowth – particularly of face and extremities
Change of appearance	Thickened skin
Excessive growth (children)	Gigantism
Paraesthesiae	Evidence of carpal tunnel syndrome
Thirst and polyuria	Evidence of diabetes mellitus
Joint symptoms	Evidence of arthritis
	Weakness, sweating
	Goitre (non-toxic)
	Hypertension
	Enlargement of lower jaw producing malocclusion of teeth (prognathism).
Local pressure effects of pituitary tumour	
Impairment of vision	Visual field defects
Headache	

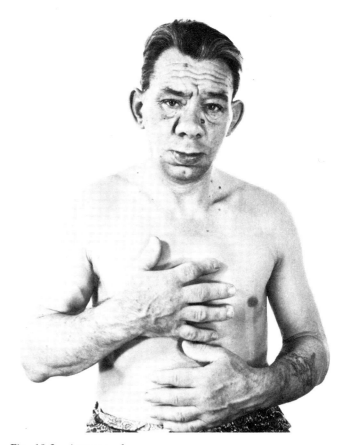

Fig. 10.3 Acromegaly.

Basis of Treatment

Until recently, treatment has been reserved for patients with severe symptoms or evidence of complications such as impairment of vision. With the realisation that even apparently mild cases may have a reduced life expectancy, nowadays treatment is usually recommended, unless there is some contraindication such as the age of the patient.

There is considerable controversy as to the most satisfactory form of therapy. External irradiation of the pituitary often does not relieve the endocrine syndrome sufficiently. Patients are therefore usually treated either by surgical removal of the pituitary tumour, or total or partial ablation of the pituitary by other means such as freezing (cryohypophysectomy) or implantation of radioactive sources. These techniques involve the introduction of a probe or cannula into the substance of the gland by the transethmoidal route.

Recently, the dopamine agonist bromocriptine has been shown to produce a fall of serum GH in some acromegalics, in contrast to its effect in normal subjects in whom it produces a rise, and is sometimes used in the treatment of acromegaly.

Prognosis

Patients with acromegaly have a reduced life expectancy due to several factors such as cardiovascular complications, local effects of the tumour, and complications of diabetes mellitus.

HYPERPROLACTINAEMIA

Definition

Hyperprolactinaemia is a consequence of excessive prolactin secretion by the pituitary. This is sometimes due to drugs (such as phenothiazines), hormones (such as oestrogens) or thyroid deficiency. Commonly, however, it is due to a prolactin producing pituitary tumour.

Symptoms and Signs

The condition is most commonly recognised in women who present with amenorrhoea and infertility. Abnormal lactation (galactorrhoea) is not uniformly found and only occurs in about one-third of such patients. Hyperprolactinaemia in men usually results in impotence. On examination, the only abnormal signs that may be found are those of galactorrhoea and evidence in women of oestrogen deficiency, such as dryness of the vagina. Occasionally, there are local pressure effects of a pituitary tumour, such as a visual field defect (*see* page 489).

Investigations

1. The diagnosis is made by finding an elevated level of serum prolactin.

2. X-rays of the pituitary fossa show evidence of a pituitary tumour in about one-third of patients in whom no other cause for the hyperprolactinaemia can be found. However, these tumours are often quite small (microadenomata), and the presence of an underlying tumour cannot therefore be excluded by finding a radiologically normal pituitary fossa.

Basis of Treatment

An ergotamine derivative, bromocriptine, has proved to be a potent dopamine agonist which effectively reduces elevated serum prolactin levels to normal. The drug is therefore widely used in the treatment of patients with hyperprolactinaemia. If, as only occurs rarely, the pituitary tumour is causing local pressure effects, some form of ablative treatment to the tumour is indicated, as with external irradiation or surgery. Pituitary tumours can enlarge further during pregnancy and give rise to these pressure effects. In patients with hyperprolactinaemia whose fertility can usually be restored with bromocriptine, this is a serious cause for concern. Hence such patients are usually treated first with an ablative procedure to the pituitary, ideally a selective surgical removal of the tumour, before beginning treatment with the drug if they have an overt pituitary tumour as detected radiologically.

CUSHING'S SYNDROME

This is considered in the section on the adrenal cortex (*see* page 167).

PRECOCIOUS PUBERTY

This condition is also discussed in the section on the gonads (*see* page 179). Among its causes are hypothalamic lesions such as encephalitis, granulomata and tumours resulting in premature secretion of the gonadotrophins. In some patients, particularly in girls, no organic lesion can be detected, and the defect is presumably a functional abnormality of the hypothalamus.

2. HYPOFUNCTION OF THE ANTERIOR LOBE

The anterior pituitary has a large reserve of function so that more than 85 to 90 per cent of gland tissue must be destroyed before any hormonal deficiency becomes clinically apparent. Such a deficiency may be partial, affecting some hormones more than others, or total. Partial hypopituitarism occurs, for example, at an early stage of damage to the pituitary by a tumour. Isolated defects of hormone secretion, in the absence of any recognisable lesion of the pituitary or hypothalamus, are also known, possibly due to a congenital deficiency of an enzyme required for synthesis of the hormone.

Hypopituitarism also occurs after surgery to the pituitary and as a complication of severe postpartum haemorrhage from infarction of the gland (Sheehan's syndrome). In this latter condition patients fail to lactate and develop persistent amenorrhoea.

The effects of the loss of individual pituitary hormones are shown in Table 10.3. Growth hormone

Table 10.3 Conditions caused by hyposecretion of pituitary hormones and their treatment

Hormone	Condition	Treatment
Anterior lobe		
GH	Dwarfism	Human growth hormone
ACTH	Adrenocortical insufficiency	Glucocorticoids
Lipotrophin	Pallor skin	None required
TSH	Hypothyroidism	Thyroxine
FSH	Hypogonadism	Androgens or oestrogens as required
LH		
	Infertility	Gonadotrophins
Posterior lobe		
Vasopressin	Diabetes insipidus	Vasopressin
		Chlorpropamide
		Carbamazepine
		Clofibrate

deficiency in children results in dwarfism, but in adults does not produce any ill effects. The administration of GH to such children produces an acceleration of growth, but supplies of the hormone are limited as it has to be extracted from human pituitaries. Deficiency of ACTH causes diminished secretion of cortisol by the adrenal cortex, the production of mineralocorticoid being largely unimpaired. Diminished secretion of the gonadotrophins in children results in failure of development of secondary sexual characteristics. In adults, infertility occurs with impotence and failure of spermatogenesis in men and amenorrhoea in women. Preparations of gonadotrophins are available for the treatment of infertility due to hypopituitarism, but this requires careful monitoring, and is only performed in specialised centres.

PITUITARY TUMOURS (Table 10.4)

The most common pituitary tumour in the adult is the prolactin secreting adenoma and, in children, the

Table 10.4 Types of pituitary tumours

	Type of tumour	Endocrine syndrome (if any)
Primary	Eosinophil	Hyperprolactinaemia
		Acromegaly
	Basophil	Cushing's syndrome
	Chromophobe	Hyperprolactinaemia
		Acromegaly
		Cushing's syndrome
		Hypopituitarism
	Craniopharyngioma	Hypopituitarism
Secondary	(Rare in anterior lobe)	Diabetes insipidus

craniopharyngioma which arises from remnants of the pouch of Rathke. Symptoms are caused by local pressure producing headaches or damage to nearby cranial nerves, or by endocrine effects of the tumour. Treatment of pituitary tumours is by deep X-ray therapy, surgical removal, or destruction of the gland by measures such as freezing or implantation of radioactive sources.

THE POSTERIOR LOBE – NORMAL

Two hormones are produced by the posterior lobe. They are small polypeptides, similar in structure and composed of eight amino acids.

Vasopressin (Antidiuretic Hormone, ADH). Vasopressin causes contraction of smooth muscle and a rise of blood pressure. In man, however, these effects are of little significance and its most important action is to cause the secretion of hypertonic urine by rendering the distal and collecting tubules of the kidney permeable to water.

Oxytocin. Oxytocin also produces contraction of smooth muscle. Its effects, however, are largely restricted to the smooth muscle of the uterus, where it plays a part in the delivery of the fetus and the smooth muscle surrounding the larger ducts in the breast, where it is of importance in milk ejection during suckling.

Both hormones are manufactured in specialised neurones of the hypothalamus by a process known as neurosecretion. The hormones are transported along the axons of these neurones to the posterior lobe where they are stored in the terminations of the nerve fibres. The release of vasopressin is controlled by changes in osmotic pressure of the extracellular fluid and in circulating plasma volume. There is thought to be an 'osmoreceptor', probably within the hypothalamus, that is sensitive to changes of osmotic pressure of the surrounding fluid. A fall of osmotic pressure, as after drinking water, will cause suppression of vasopressin release, with subsequent secretion of hypotonic urine and preservation of plasma osmolarity. The converse changes occur with water depletion. The stimulus for the release of oxytocin at delivery is not known. During lactation, the infant's sucking of the nipple excites a 'milk ejection reflex', whereby the release of oxytocin occurs.

Function Tests

Bioassays of vasopressin and oxytocin can be performed, but are time-consuming and difficult. However, radioimmunoassays of these hormones have been developed. Circumstantial evidence as to the secretion of vasopressin can be obtained from measurements of plasma and urine osmolarity during fluid deprivation.

Persistent hypotonicity of urine with respect to plasma under such circumstances constitutes strong evidence of vasopressin deficiency.

THE POSTERIOR LOBE – ABNORMAL

1. HYPERFUNCTION OF THE POSTERIOR LOBE

Excessive secretion of vasopressin has been reported in some conditions affecting the base of the brain, such as tuberculous meningitis. A vasopressin-like peptide has also been shown to be secreted by certain carcinomas, notably of the bronchus. The syndrome of water intoxication occurs in such patients, characterised by weight gain, mental confusion, fits, and eventually coma and death. Despite marked reduction in the levels of serum sodium and chloride, the urine is persistently hypertonic indicating 'inappropriate antidiuretic hormone secretion'. Treatment is by water restriction as well as of the underlying condition; occasionally hypertonic saline is given.

2. HYPOFUNCTION OF THE POSTERIOR LOBE

Oxytocin deficiency has not yet been described as a clinical entity. Such patients would presumably experience difficulty during labour and, in fact, synthetic oxytocin is widely used in obstetrics when spontaneous uterine contractions during labour are inadequate.

DIABETES INSIPIDUS

Definition

Diabetes insipidus is a condition caused by ADH deficiency, characterised by the passage of large volumes of dilute urine.

Pathology

The condition may be due to tumours, infections, granulomata and operations that interfere with the function of the posterior lobe and pituitary stalk. Sometimes no underlying cause can be detected (idiopathic diabetes insipidus).

Symptoms and Signs

Patients complain of passing excessive amounts of urine (polyuria), extreme thirst (polydipsia) and weakness.

Investigations

1. During a fluid deprivation test the urine fails to become normally concentrated; patients continue to pass large amounts of hypotonic urine and may not be able to tolerate the test for long.
2. Other investigations such as skull X-rays are performed to try and detect an underlying condition.

Differential Diagnosis

The condition must be distinguished from polyuria caused by other disorders such as chronic renal disease, hypokalaemia and hypercalcaemia. There is also a rare anomaly of the renal tubules of lack of responsiveness to ADH, kidney function being otherwise normal ('nephrogenic diabetes insipidus'). This is inherited as a sex-linked characteristic and is characterised by intense craving for fluids in male infants.

The distinction of diabetes insipidus from compulsive water drinking may be difficult. This latter disorder is a psychiatric abnormality in which the patient drinks excessively, although there is no primary defect of urine concentration.

Basis of Treatment

Preparations of vasopressin are available for the treatment of diabetes insipidus. Thus DDAVP (desmopressin) is a synthetic analogue of vasopressin that is administered intranasally twice daily. Similarly, lysine vasopressin is administered by the intranasal route, but is somewhat less potent than DDAVP and has to be given three or four times daily. Several drugs, in particular chlorpropamide, carbamazepine and clofibrate are also of therapeutic value in diabetes insipidus. They appear to act in the presence of some residual vasopressin by potentiating the action of the hormone on the renal tubules. Paradoxically, thiazide diuretics may also be effective in diabetes insipidus and are, in fact, the only treatment available for the nephrogenic form of the condition, although the mechanism of their action is still uncertain.

THE ADRENAL GLANDS

The adrenals are two small glands each weighing approximately 5 g, situated around the upper poles of the kidneys. They consist of an outer cortex, surrounding an inner medulla. These two zones have different functions, and will therefore be considered separately.

THE ADRENAL CORTEX – NORMAL

The hormones produced by the adrenal cortex are steroids with the same basic structure – the cyclopentenophenanthrene nucleus (Fig. 10.4). Modifications of this structure result in the production of steroid hormones with different biological effects.

Glucocorticoids. These are produced by the middle and inner zones of the adrenal cortex, the zona fasciculata and reticularis. The most important steroid of this group secreted in man is cortisol, formerly called hydrocortisone, approximately 15 mg of which is secreted daily. Glucocorticoids have numerous actions including stimulation of protein catabolism and gluconeogenesis,

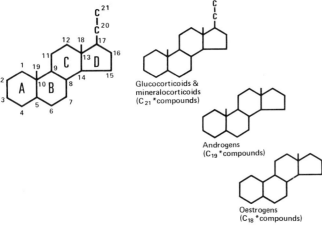

Fig. 10.4 The cyclopentenophenanthrene nucleus and its derivatives.

promotion of resistance to stress, inhibition of the tissue response to inflammation and suppression of antibody formation; they also antagonise the action of insulin. A large number of compounds of this group have been synthesised that differ in their potency and amount of mineralocorticoid activity. They are used for the treatment of a variety of conditions, in many of which the exact mechanism of their action is not fully understood. In some, such as rheumatoid arthritis, their usefulness may depend on the suppression of an inflammatory response.

Mineralocorticoids. These substances stimulate the exchange of sodium for potassium and hydrogen ions in cells of the distal kidney tubules and some other tissues. Their administration therefore results in a reduced amount of sodium and an increased amount of potassium and hydrogen ion in the urine. In man, the predominant mineralocorticoid is aldosterone which is secreted by the outermost zone of cells, the zona glomerulosa, in amounts of approximately 150 μg daily.

Androgens. These steroids promote the development of male secondary sexual characteristics and stimulate protein anabolism in muscle. A variety of androgenic steroids are produced by the adrenal cortex. They are considerably less active than testosterone but, when produced in excess, can result in virilisation.

The secretion of cortisol and adrenal androgens is largely dependent on the production of adrenocorticotrophic hormone (ACTH) by the pituitary, the release of which is controlled by a specific releasing factor secreted by cells of the hypothalamus (*see* page 160). As with some other functions of the body, the secretion of ACTH varies rhythmically throughout the 24 hours (the circadian rhythm), being at its maximum at about 0700 hours, the usual time of awakening, and at its lowest about 2400 hours. The levels of plasma cortisol show a corresponding circadian rhythm. An increase in the

level of circulating cortisol acts on the hypothalamus to reduce the secretion of ACTH releasing factor and hence of ACTH, thus attempting to maintain normal levels of plasma cortisol. As with thyroid hormones, the majority (about 95 per cent) of circulating cortisol is bound to plasma proteins, leaving only a small proportion of biologically active free hormone.

The mechanism of control of aldosterone secretion is quite different. It is largely independent of ACTH secretion, but is affected by changes of sodium balance, extracellular fluid volume, and the level of serum potassium. Sodium depletion and a fall of extracellular fluid volume results in a rise of aldosterone secretion which, by increasing sodium reabsorption by the renal tubules, helps to repair the deficit.

The increased secretion of aldosterone under such circumstances is effected by the 'renin-angiotensin' system (Fig. 10.5) in which renin is released from its site of

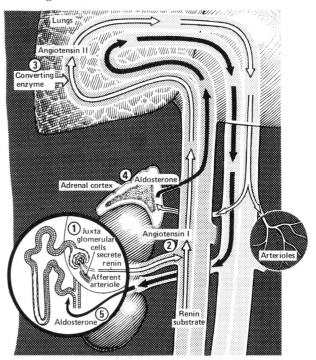

Fig. 10.5 The renin-angiotensin system.

formation in specialised cells situated close to the renal glomeruli in response to a fall in renal blood flow. Renin is an enzyme that acts on a circulating globulin with the ultimate formation of angiotensin II. This is a polypeptide that stimulates the secretion of aldosterone and also has a direct effect on blood vessels, causing a rise of blood pressure. A rise of plasma potassium will also increase aldosterone secretion directly.

Adrenocortical Function Tests

Glucocorticoids. Methods are generally available for measuring circulating levels of cortisol. The urinary excretion of products of cortisol metabolism can also be determined as 17-oxogenic steroids or 17-hydroxy-corticosteroids, depending on the method of assay. The actual secretion rate of cortisol can be measured, but only in specialised centres. In the investigation of adrenocortical disorders, levels of plasma and urinary corticosteroids are determined in the 'basal' state and also after various procedures designed to stimulate or suppress different parts of the hypothalamic-pituitary-adrenocortical axis. Thus ACTH can be used in an attempt to stimulate the gland directly in suspected Addison's disease (*see below*). When a disorder of ACTH secretion is suspected, the whole axis can be tested by measuring plasma cortisol levels during a 'stress' test such as insulin induced hypoglycaemia, or by administering the drug metyrapone that blocks 11β-hydroxylation by the adrenal cortex and thereby lowers the plasma cortisol.

Mineralocorticoids. Measurements of plasma and urinary levels of aldosterone and of plasma levels of renin and angiotensin can be undertaken, but are technically difficult. Circumstantial evidence of mineralocorticoid secretion can be obtained by measuring the urinary content of sodium and potassium and observing any changes after the administration of spironolactone, a drug that inhibits the action of aldosterone on the renal tubule.

Androgens. These can be crudely assessed by measurement of the urinary 17-oxosteroids. These are steroids with an oxo (keto) group attached to the 17 carbon atom (Fig. 10.4). This measurement, however, is non-specific and other techniques are available for the isolation of individual androgens and their metabolic products.

THE ADRENAL CORTEX – ABNORMAL

1. HYPERFUNCTION OF THE ADRENAL CORTEX

CUSHING'S SYNDROME

Definition

Cushing's syndrome is a condition of excessive glucocorticoid secretion.

Background

The underlying pathology is usually bilateral adrenocortical hyperplasia (70 per cent of cases), the exact cause of which is unknown. It is probable that the basic defect lies in the hypothalamus or the anterior pituitary, and a considerable number of such patients have an associated pituitary tumour. Other causes of the condition are adenomas (15 per cent) and carcinomas (5 per cent) of the adrenal cortex. The remaining 10 per cent are due to extra-adrenal carcinomas, notably undifferentiated carcinomas of the bronchus, that secrete an ACTH-like peptide (the 'ectopic ACTH syndrome'). Although Cushing's syndrome is rare, it is of particular importance as it has to be considered in the differential diagnosis of such common conditions as obesity and hypertension, and because the same clinical features are found in patients requiring treatment with glucocorticoids in high dosage (iatrogenic Cushing's syndrome).

Symptoms and Signs (Table 10.5, Fig. 10.6)

Table 10.5   Clinical features of Cushing's syndrome

Due to protein wasting and anti-insulin effects of glucocorticoids	Muscles: Weakness, wasting, (myopathy) Skin: Thin, purple striae, easy bruising Bones: Osteoporosis, fractures Evidence of diabetes mellitus
Others	Central obesity. Moon shaped, plethoric face. Hirsutism. Acne. Amenorrhoea. Hypertension. Oedema. Mental changes (sometimes frank psychosis).

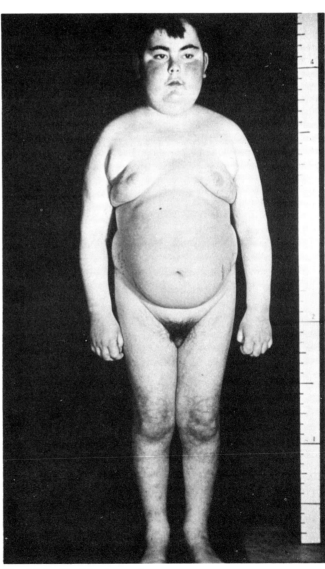

Fig. 10.6 Cushing's syndrome.

The change in appearance of the patient can be striking, especially when compared with that seen in old photographs. The obesity is characteristically central in distribution, with sparing of the limbs. Muscle weakness is almost invariably present and may be profound. Frank diabetes mellitus is found in about 25 per cent of patients. In children, arrest of growth always occurs. Patients with bilateral adrenal hyperplasia often show brown pigmentation of the skin, due to the effect of elevated levels of circulating ACTH and lipotrophin and this may be a useful clue to the nature of the underlying lesion.

Investigations

These are designed initially to establish the diagnosis and subsequently to try to identify the source of the condition. Plasma and urinary corticosteroid levels are raised and, in particular, there is a loss of the normal circadian rhythm of plasma cortisol. A glucose tolerance test may also be helpful.

The distinction between pituitary dependent Cushing's syndrome (bilateral adrenal hyperplasia) and other causes of the condition can usually be made by measuring plasma ACTH levels and by measuring any changes in the patient's corticosteroid levels after the administration of dexamethasone, in large dosage, or metyrapone. In addition, X-rays of the pituitary fossa will reveal an overt pituitary tumour and a variety of radiographic procedures can be undertaken to try and locate the site of an adrenal tumour.

Basis of Treatment

Patients with adrenal or extra-adrenal tumours require surgical treatment or, as in the case of malignant tumours where this might not be possible, irradiation or chemotherapy. The treatment of patients with bilateral adrenal hyperplasia is controversial. The most usual method is by total adrenalectomy, which will clearly relieve the condition. This, however, is a considerable undertaking in seriously ill patients and life-long therapy with gluco- and mineralocorticoids is subsequently required. Furthermore, a pituitary tumour may become clinically apparent in patients treated in this way, possibly because the restraining effect of elevated circulating cortisol levels has been removed. Such patients become deeply pigmented (Nelson's syndrome). For these reasons, therefore, many centres treat patients with this form of Cushing's syndrome by one of the techniques available for partial or total destruction of the pituitary gland.

Prognosis

The prognosis of the untreated condition is poor and a 50 per cent mortality within five years has been reported. Death is often due to ischaemic heart disease.

PRIMARY HYPERALDOSTERONISM

Definition

Primary hyperaldosteronism is a condition of excessive aldosterone secretion.

Background

The condition is usually due to an adenoma but may occasionally be caused by bilateral hyperplasia or a carcinoma of the adrenal cortex. As with Cushing's syndrome it has to be considered in the differential diagnosis of hypertension, but only accounts for less than one per cent of patients presenting with raised blood pressure. Increased aldosterone production also occurs in the absence of a primary abnormality of the adrenal cortex in patients with renal artery stenosis and malignant hypertension, probably because renal ischaemia stimulates renin release. This 'secondary hyperaldosteronism' is also found in patients with disturbed sodium metabolism, such as cirrhosis of the liver and the nephrotic syndrome, when it plays a part in maintaining the oedema that is a characteristic of these conditions.

Symptoms and Signs (Table 10.6)

Table 10.6 Clinical features of primary hyperaldosteronism

Due to potassium depletion	Muscle weakness (sometimes episodic paralysis) Polyuria, polydipsia Impairment of carbohydrate tolerance
Due to sodium retention	Hypertension (only rarely 'malignant')
Others	Paraesthesiae, tetany (possibly from magnesium deficiency)

Oedema does not occur as there appears to be an 'escape' mechanism whereby the amount of retained sodium is kept at a level below that at which oedema is clinically detectable.

Investigations

Plasma sodium and bicarbonate concentrations are raised and the plasma potassium is low. Plasma levels of renin and angiotensin are subnormal, due to the sodium retention and increased extracellular fluid volume. In contrast, in secondary aldosteronism plasma renin and angiotensin concentrations are elevated.

Basis of Treatment

Most cases of primary hyperaldosteronism are treated surgically. The actions of aldosterone can be blocked by spironolactone which is often used in the diagnosis of the condition and sometimes as long term therapy.

ADRENAL VIRILISM

Definition

Adrenal virilisation is a condition of excessive secretion of androgens by the adrenal cortex.

Background

In infants and children it is usually due to a congenital deficiency of one of the enzymes concerned with the synthesis of cortisol. This results in an increased secretion of ACTH that is often able to compensate for the defect and maintain normal or near normal levels of plasma cortisol, but only at the expense of simultaneously causing an excessive production of other steroids, some of which are androgenic. The condition is known as the adrenogenital syndrome or congenital adrenal hyperplasia. In adults, excessive adrenal androgen production is usually caused by an adrenal tumour.

Symptoms and Signs

The syndrome of virilisation occurs (*see* page 179).

Basis of Treatment

Patients with the adrenogenital syndrome require treatment with physiological doses of cortisol, or some other glucocorticoid, that suppresses the excessive secretion of ACTH by the pituitary. Where there is an underlying adrenal tumour, surgical therapy is indicated.

2. HYPOFUNCTION OF THE ADRENAL CORTEX

Hypopituitarism causes secondary adrenocortical insufficiency with cortisol and androgen deficiency, but aldosterone secretion is usually preserved.

ADDISON'S DISEASE

Definition

Addison's disease is a condition of generalised adrenocortical hormone deficiency.

Background

Formerly, the disease was usually due to disseminated tuberculosis causing destruction of the adrenals. Nowadays, however, in about 60 per cent of cases there is atrophy of the adrenal cortex associated with lymphocytic infiltration. This is thought to be an autoimmune condition and antibodies to cells of the adrenal cortex have been demonstrated in the sera of such patients. Furthermore, some of them have associated conditions such as Hashimoto's thyroiditis and pernicious anaemia that are also thought to be autoimmune in origin.

Most of the remaining 40 per cent of cases are due to destruction of the glands by tuberculosis, although this may be produced by other conditions such as secondary neoplasms and amyloidosis. Although Addison's disease is rare, suppression of adrenocortical function commonly occurs after treatment with high doses of glucocorticoids and abrupt cessation of such treatment can precipitate acute adrenocortical insufficiency. This suppression is usually transient but may be permanent, depending on the dose of glucocorticoids and the duration of treatment.

Symptoms

Acute:
Collapse with shock, hypotension and vomiting.

Chronic:
Weakness.
Anorexia.
Nausea.
Vomiting.
Fainting on standing (due to postural hypotension).
Loss of weight.

Signs

Brown pigmentation, especially affecting palmar creases, nipples, pressure areas and the buccal mucous membrane.
Hypotension, made worse on standing (postural hypotension).

Investigations

The condition is characterised by low levels of urinary and plasma corticosteroids. In an adrenal crisis, however, there is no time to wait for the results of such measurements as therapy is needed urgently. Fortunately, treatment for a short period does not invalidate the results of a subsequent ACTH stimulation test. This is the definitive test of adrenocortical hypofunction and demonstrates an absent or subnormal rise of urinary and plasma corticosteroids. Aldosterone deficiency results in a raised level of plasma potassium, a reduced level of plasma sodium and uraemia. In cases due to tuberculosis, X-ray of the abdomen often shows adrenal calcification.

Basis of Treatment

In acute adrenocortical insufficiency, large doses of cortisol of 200 to 400 mg in 24 hours are required, together with intensive fluid and glucose repletion. For chronic replacement therapy, 20 to 30 mg of cortisol daily in two divided doses is adequate.

Additional mineralocorticoid is necessary and is conveniently given by mouth as 9-*a* fluorohydrocortisone 0.05 to 0.2 mg daily. Patients with Addison's disease are unable to increase their own production of cortisol in the event of an intercurrent illness or accident and they must be given additional glucocorticoid therapy.

THE ADRENAL MEDULLA

The adrenal medulla is derived from neural crest tissue and is richly supplied with preganglionic sympathetic nerve fibres. Its cells stain brown with chromic acid – the chromaffin reaction. Similar tissue is found elsewhere throughout the body, particularly in the retroperitoneum along the course of the aorta. The adrenal medulla secretes the catecholamines adrenaline and nor-adrenaline; whereas it is almost the sole source of adrenaline, nor-adrenaline is also secreted by post-ganglionic sympathetic nerve endings. The catecholamines have widespread actions, affecting particularly the heart and blood vessels. These have been classified as alpha and beta effects depending upon two different types of tissue receptor that have been postulated to exist. The control of the secretion of the adrenal medulla is exclusively through its sympathetic innervation, which affords the possibility of rapid catecholamine response to situations of danger and stress.

THE ADRENAL MEDULLA – ABNORMAL

1. HYPERFUNCTION OF THE ADRENAL MEDULLA

PHAEOCHROMOCYTOMA

Definition

Phaeochromocytomas are catecholamine producing tumours. They usually arise from the adrenal medulla, but may develop in chromaffin tissue situated elsewhere.

Symptoms

Sweating
Headache
Palpitations   } in attacks.
Chest and abdominal pain
Tremor

Signs

In attacks:
Hypertension.
Tachycardia or bradycardia.
Pallor.
Sweating.
Anxiety.

In between attacks:
There may be none. Sometimes:
    Sustained hypertension.
    Retinal haemorrhages.
    Diabetes mellitus.

Investigations

The urinary excretion of catecholamines and their metabolites is elevated, although sometimes only in an attack. Patients who are hypertensive show a fall of blood pressure when given the drug phentolamine, that blocks alpha sympathetic effects of catecholamines. Provocative tests are used in patients who are normotensive at the time of investigation, using glucagon or tyramine. These stimulate the release of catecholamines from a phaeochromocytoma and cause a rise of blood pressure. Impairment of carbohydrate tolerance and sometimes frank diabetes may be found.

Basis of Treatment

Surgical excision of the tumour is indicated. This may be hazardous owing to the release of catecholamines during the operation. The use of sympathetic blocking drugs, however, such as phenoxybenzamine (alpha blocker) and propranolol (beta blocker) before and during operation has considerably eased the management of these patients.

2. HYPOFUNCTION OF THE ADRENAL MEDULLA

No clinical condition has, as yet, been ascribed definitely to hypofunction of the adrenal medulla.

THE THYROID GLAND

THYROID GLAND – NORMAL

The thyroid gland is a bilobed structure overlying the trachea, and normally weighs about 20 g. The gland develops from an outgrowth of the inferior aspect of the primitive foregut. It is composed of cells forming follicles which enclose a homogenous substance, the thyroid 'colloid', consisting of a protein of high molecular weight, thyroglobulin. Interspersed between the follicles are the parafollicular cells that are one of the sites of formation of the hormone calcitonin (*see* Chapter 11). The follicles and the enclosed colloid are concerned with the synthesis of the two thyroid hormones thyroxine (T4) and triiodothyronine (T3). These are both formed by the iodination of tyrosine, and the processes leading to their synthesis are depicted in Fig. 10.7. The thyroid hormones circulate in the blood largely (over 99.9 per cent) in combination with certain plasma proteins. It is, however, the very small proportion that

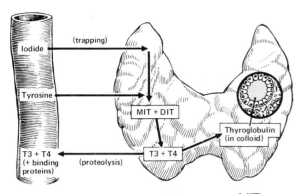

Fig. 10.7 Synthesis of thyroid hormones. MIT = mono-iodotyrosine; DIT = diiodotyrosine; T3 = triiodothyronine; T4 = thyroxine.

circulates in the free or unbound state that determines the thyroid state of the individual.

The functional activity of the gland is controlled by the thyroid stimulating hormone (TSH) secreted by the pituitary, the release of which is stimulated by TSH releasing hormone (TRH) manufactured by cells of the hypothalamus (see page 161). An increase in the level of circulating thyroid hormones depresses the activity of the thyroid gland by suppressing the secretion of TRH and of TSH, thereby attempting to maintain a constant level of circulating hormone.

The activities of the thyroid hormones affect most tissues. These include control of oxygen consumption and of heat production, and a role in promoting growth and development. The action of thyroxine is slow, with a peak effect nine days after a single dose, while triiodothyronine acts more rapidly, probably because it is less strongly bound to plasma proteins, and has a maximum effect two days after administration. The metabolic effect of 80 μg of thyroxine by mouth is approximately equivalent to that of 20 μg of triiodothyronine.

Function Tests

Three main types of test are used:

1. Measurement of circulating thyroid hormone. This was formerly done by measuring the amount of protein-bound iodine (PBI) in the blood. Nowadays, however, the direct measurement of serum thyroxine is widely available. The level of serum thyroxine (and PBI) is affected not only by the rate of secretion of thyroxine by the thyroid, but also by the level of thyroxine binding plasma proteins in the blood. For this reason another technique that involves the addition of radio-iodine labelled triiodothyronine to an aliquot of the patient's plasma *in vitro* and determining the proportion bound to plasma proteins, is often undertaken. A simple calculation based upon this measurement and that of the serum thyroxine gives an index of the level of circulating free thyroxine. In the last few years, methods

for the measurement of serum triiodothyronine and TSH (both by radioimmunoassay) have also been developed.

2. Measurement of the metabolic effect on thyroid hormones. These are summarised in Table 10.7.

Table 10.7 Metabolic effects of thyroid hormones used as tests of thyroid function

Metabolic effect	Findings in	
	Hyperthyroidism	Hypothyroidism
Relaxation tendon reflexes	(Shortened)*	Prolonged
Electrocardiogram	(Sinus tachycardia)* Atrial fibrillation	(Sinus bradycardia)* Low voltage Flat T waves
Basal metabolic rate†	Increased	Decreased

*Too much overlap with normal subjects to be useful as test of thyroid function.
†Seldom done as technically difficult.

3. Measurement of the uptake of radioactive isotopes by the thyroid. These tests involve the administration of tracer amounts of radioactive isotopes (usually ^{131}I or ^{99}Tc) and measurement of their uptake by the thyroid. As tests of thyroid function they have been superseded by measurements of circulating thyroid hormone. However, thyroid scans are still in use, particularly in the investigation of thyroid nodules.

THYROID GLAND – ABNORMAL

HYPERTHYROIDISM (THYROTOXICOSIS)

Definition

Hyperthyroidism is a condition of excessive thyroid hormone secretion.

Background

The normal homeostatic mechanism for the maintenance of a normal level of circulating free thyroid hormone is disturbed. A goitre is found in the majority of cases that may be due to diffuse enlargement of the gland, multiple nodules or, occasionally, a single 'hot' nodule. Thyrotoxicosis in the latter group and in some of the cases with multinodular glands is due to a primary thyroid disorder, in which one or more nodules become autonomously overactive. The aetiology of the remainder is quite different. Early suggestions that excessive secretion of TSH is responsible have not been substantiated.

Another substance capable of stimulating thyroid activity has been found in the serum of patients with thyrotoxicosis and called the 'long acting thyroid stimulator' (LATS) from its behaviour in a bioassay system. It is not secreted by the pituitary gland and, unexpectedly, has been found to be an IgG immuno-globulin.

It is now known that a group of thyroid stimulating antibodies (TSAbs) can be demonstrated in the serum of thyrotoxic patients with diffuse goitres or, sometimes, multinodular goitres and the condition is thought to be autoimmune in origin. It appears that TSAbs are antibodies to receptors for TSH in the membrane of thyroid cells that are capable of stimulating the activity of the cell, in addition to blocking the action of TSH. Furthermore, it has been suggested that the ophthalmic and possibly the cutaneous complications of Graves' disease (*see below*) are also autoimmune in origin.

Symptoms and Signs

1. Clinical features of excessive thyroid hormone secretion (Table 10.8). The condition is characterised by a 'hypermetabolic state'. Some of the clinical features are similar to the metabolic effects of catecholamines and there does seem to be increased sensitivity to circulating catecholamines in thyrotoxicosis.

Table 10.8 Clinical features resulting from excessive thyroid hormone secretion

	Symptoms	*Signs*
General	Loss of weight (despite good appetite)	Evidence of weight loss
	Heat intolerance Increased sweating	Warm, moist skin
Cardiovascular system	Shortness of breath Palpitations	Tachycardia Peripheral vasodilation Increased pulse pressure Atrial fibrillation Cardiac failure (particularly in the elderly)
Muscles	Weakness	Muscle weakness and wasting (thyrotoxic myopathy)
Nervous system	Anxiety state Irritability Nervousness Sometimes frank psychosis	Fine tremor Brisk tendon jerks
Gastrointestinal system	Diarrhoea	

2. *Goitre.* This may be diffuse, multinodular or uninodular and there is frequently an overlying bruit from increased vasculature of the gland.

3. *Eye signs.* The eyes are commonly involved, particularly in younger patients, and the association of thyrotoxicosis, goitre and eye signs is known as Graves' disease (Fig. 10.8). There may be exophthalmos (protrusion of the eyes), impaired movement of the oculomotor muscles (particularly affecting upward gaze) which sometimes causes double vision (exophthalmic ophthalmoplegia), and retraction of the upper eyelids so that

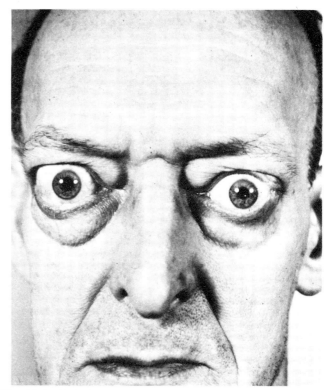

Fig. 10.8 Ophthalmic Graves' disease.
Note: exophthalmos and retraction of upper eyelids.

the white sclera is visible between the eyelid and the upper margin of the cornea. Lid retraction often becomes more obvious if the patient is asked to look at the examiner's finger as it moves slowly downwards (lid lag). Oedema of the conjunctiva (chemosis) and periorbital oedema may also occur. The exophthalmos and chemosis are occasionally so severe that corneal ulceration occurs and sight is threatened ('malignant exophthalmos'). The eye signs are sometimes assymetrical and may occur in the absence of other features of thyrotoxicosis (ophthalmic Graves' disease).

4. *Pretibial myxoedema.* This occurs less commonly than the eye signs. There is an infiltration of the skin overlying the tibiae with a mucopolysaccharide material, that results in the appearance of dark red, thickened, raised areas of skin.

5. *Thyroid acropathy.* This is a rare condition in which finger changes resembling clubbing, and radiological changes similar to those of hypertrophic pulmonary osteoarthropathy occur in association with the eye changes of Graves' disease and pretibial myxoedema.

Investigations (*see* page 171)

The serum thyroxine and free thyroxine index are raised. Occasionally, they are within normal limits in patients suspected on clinical grounds of having thyrotoxicosis and the diagnosis is confirmed by finding an increased level of serum triiodothyronine ('T3 toxicosis'). In patients in whom there is still doubt as to the diagnosis a TRH test may be helpful. This test consists of measuring serum TSH levels at 0, 20 and 60 minutes after an injection of TRH. A normal rise of serum TSH excludes the diagnosis as the normal pituitary response to TRH is inhibited in the presence of even mild thyrotoxicosis.

Differential Diagnosis

Thyrotoxicosis has often to be distinguished from an anxiety state, which it may clearly resemble and with which it sometimes coexists. In the elderly, many of the usual features of the condition are often absent and thyrotoxicosis can present solely with atrial fibrillation and cardiac failure.

Complications

Severe uncontrolled thyrotoxicosis may result in a 'thyroid crisis' with hyperpyrexia, extreme muscle weakness and cardiac failure. This complication is now fortunately rare.

Basis of Treatment

Hyperthyroidism. There are three types of treatment:

1. **Drug Therapy.** A variety of drugs inhibit the synthesis of thyroid hormones. The drugs most commonly used for the medical treatment of thryotoxicosis are the thionamides, that block the stages of iodination of tyrosine and the coupling of iodinated tyrosine to form triiodothyronine and thyroxine.

These drugs control the disease during the period of their administration, but only about 50 per cent of patients sustain a permanent remission, even when therapy is maintained for eighteen months which is thought to be the optimum period. At present, it is not possible to predict for certain those patients who will be cured with drug treatment, but the most satisfactory results are obtained in young women with small diffuse goitres. In the UK the drug most commonly used is carbimazole, in an initial dose of 10 to 15 mg eight-hourly which is reduced in about ten weeks once the patient is euthyroid. Carbimazole carries a small risk of side effects of which the most dangerous is agranulocytosis. It is, therefore, essential that patients taking the drug should be warned to stop taking it at once should they notice any unusual fever, rash, or sore throat and have a full blood count performed.

Other drugs are also used in the management of thyrotoxicosis. Thus beta sympathetic blocking drugs often produce a rapid symptomatic improvement of the cardiovascular manifestations. Their action, however, is a peripheral one and they do not affect thyroid function.

Iodine rapidly reduces the rate of secretion of thyroid hormone and also makes the gland less vascular; it is thus widely used prior to surgery.

2. **Surgery.** Partial thyroidectomy is performed once the patient is euthyroid on medical treatment. The immediate results are good in over 90 per cent of patients and the mortality of the operation is low. There is a small incidence of serious complications such as paralysis of the recurrent laryngeal nerve and hypoparathyroidism from damage to the parathyroid glands. On follow-up, thyrotoxicosis recurs in 5 to 10 per cent of patients. The risk of subsequent hypothyroidism is at present uncertain as the reported incidence varies widely from 5 to 40 per cent.

3. **Radio-iodine Treatment.** This is a very convenient form of treatment as it consists solely of a drink of water containing radioactive iodine (usually ^{131}I) in a dose estimated to be adequate to restore normal thyroid function. About two-thirds of patients so treated become euthyroid after a single dose, and further doses can be given as necessary. The disadvantage of this treatment is the high incidence of hypothyroidism in subsequent years. Thus, 3 to 4 per cent of patients develop thyroid deficiency each year and this incidence shows no sign of declining even with prolonged follow-up. Radio-iodine is contraindicated in children and during pregnancy, as there is a risk of producing thyroid carcinomas in the young. In adults there appears to be no such risk. Nevertheless, in many centres this form of treatment is confined to patients over the age of 45 to avoid any possible genetic hazard.

Ophthalmic Graves' Disease. The management of this condition is unsatisfactory. Any associated hyperthyroidism should be treated and thyroxine given once the patient is becoming euthyroid, as rapid swings of thyroid state are known to make the eye symptoms worse. Patients with mild symptoms are given diuretics and advised to sleep propped up to try to prevent the conjunctival oedema that is often most troublesome on waking. Guanethidine eye drops often improve lid retraction. In severe cases, corticosteroids in high doses are of value, but it may be difficult to reduce the dose subsequently without an exacerbation of symptoms. In those cases where the proptosis and exposure of the cornea constitute a threat to vision, the eyelids are sometimes completely or partially sewn together (tarsorraphy) as a protective measure, or surgical decompression of the orbit by removal of some of its bony wall may be required.

HYPOTHYROIDISM (MYXOEDEMA)

Definition

Hypothyroidism is a condition of deficient thyroid hormone secretion.

Background

Hypofunction of the thyroid is usually the result of a primary thyroid disorder (primary hypothyroidism), although it is sometimes caused by reduced TSH production by the pituitary (secondary hypothyroidism). Primary hypothyroidism may occur for the following reasons:

1. **Failure of Development of the Thyroid.** If severe, this results in hypothyroidism at birth or in early infancy (cretinism).
2. **Removal at Operation, Destruction by Radio-iodine Therapy, or Replacement of the Normal Gland by Infiltrative Lesions.**
3. **Iodine Deficiency.** This occurs particularly in mountainous areas, as seafish and edible seaweeds are rich sources of iodine. The incidence of iodine deficiency in such areas is markedly reduced by adding iodide to table salt or drinking water.
4. **Autoimmune Thyroiditis (Hashimoto's Disease or Hashimoto's Thyroiditis).** This condition most often affects middle-aged women. The histology of the thyroid shows lymphocyte infiltration and, in the later stages, fibrosis. It may present in a subacute form with pain and tenderness of the gland. Circulating antibodies to different constituents of thyroid tissue can be demonstrated in the patient's serum, and are of value diagnostically. It is thought that the thyroid follicles are destroyed by an autoimmune process, although the circulating auto-antibodies are probably not themselves solely responsible. An association between this condition and other 'organ specific' autoimmune diseases, such as pernicious anaemia (*see* page 379), is found in patients with autoimmune thyroiditis and their close relatives.
5. **'Idiopathic Atrophy' of the Thyroid.** In many cases this probably represents an end stage of autoimmune thyroiditis.
6. **Congenital Enzyme Defects of Thyroid Hormone Synthesis.** These abnormalities are usually familial and inherited as recessive characteristics. Defects involving all the stages of thyroid hormone synthesis have been described and one form is associated with congenital nerve deafness (Pendred's syndrome). Patients usually manifest their disease in childhood.
7. **Drug Induced.** Hypothyroidism may be caused by the antithyroid drugs and other compounds that inhibit thyroid hormone synthesis such as iodine (used in many cough medicines). Natural goitrogens also exist and may occasionally produce hypothyroidism.

Symptoms and Signs (Table 10.9, Fig. 10.9)

The term myxoedema is derived from subcutaneous deposits of a mucopolysaccharide material that produces non-pitting oedema ('mucoid oedema'). The condition is one that tends either to be diagnosed on sight or overlooked. In infants, early diagnosis is critical otherwise the child is likely to sustain permanent mental impairment.

Table 10.9 Clinical features of hypothyroidism

	Symptoms	Signs
General	Cold intolerance Weight gain	Dry, coarse skin Dry, coarse, sparse hair Pallor
From infiltration with myxoedematous tissue	Change in appearance Hoarseness of voice Paraesthesiae of hands	Puffiness of face and extremities Involvement of larynx Evidence of carpal tunnel syndrome
Muscles	Aches and pains	Rarely, stiff swollen muscles
Nervous system	Slowness of thought Lethargy Poor memory Drowsiness Ataxia Sometimes frank psychosis ('myxoedema madness')	Slowness of speech and thought Delayed relaxation tendon jerks Sometimes cerebellar ataxia
Cardiovascular	Angina of effort	Bradycardia Evidence of ischaemic heart disease Sometimes pericardial effusion
Gastrointestinal system	Constipation	May be distended abdomen Rarely, frank ileus
Also: Children (juvenile hypothyroidism) Infants (cretinism)	Retardation of growth Mental deficiency (if treatment delayed)	Dwarfism Characteristic appearance

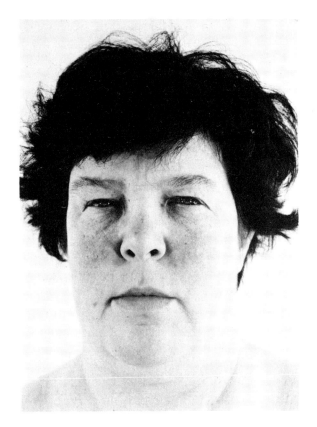

Fig. 10.9 Myxoedema.

Investigations (*see* page 171)

The diagnosis is usually confirmed or denied by measuring the serum thyroxine and free thyroxine index. When the results are borderline, or disagree with the clinical diagnosis, measurement of the serum TSH is of great value. An elevated serum TSH is found in primary hypothyroidism and a normal level excludes this diagnosis.

Complications

Profound hypothyroidism may lead to myxoedema coma which is characterised by hypothermia and must be distinguished from spontaneous hypothermia in an elderly person not suffering from hypothyroidism. Ischaemic heart disease is common, probably because of the associated hyperlipidaemia.

Basis of Treatment

Treatment is with thyroxine. A usual adult replacement dose is 0.2 mg per day that, in view of its long duration of action, need only be given once daily. In elderly subjects and patients with long-standing hypothyroidism, there is a risk of precipitating ischaemic heart disease on starting treatment. It is, therefore, essential to begin with a small dose of thyroxine, such as 0.025 mg daily, which is then gradually increased every two or three weeks so long as there are no side effects. When there is need for a quick response, as in myxoedema coma, the rapidly acting thyroid hormone triiodothyronine is indicated and can, if necessary, be given parenterally.

GOITRE

Definition

The term goitre is used for any enlargement of the thyroid gland.

Background

With the exceptions of neoplastic and inflammatory diseases, goitres are due to thyroid disorders that diminish thyroid hormone production. TSH secretion by the pituitary is secondarily increased and causes hypertrophy of the gland. If the response from the thyroid is adequate the patient remains euthyroid, otherwise hypothyroidism ensues. The majority of goitres do not give rise to any local pressure effects and are asymptomatic, other than the disturbance caused by their cosmetic appearance. Treatment with thyroxine is often successful in reducing the size of the gland especially when the enlargement is diffuse rather than nodular.

Goitres occur under the following circumstances (*see also* under hypothyroidism):

1. **Physiological.** Moderate enlargement of the thyroid is common at puberty and during pregnancy.
2. **Iodine Deficiency.** Goitres are endemic in regions of iodine deficiency (hence the term 'Derbyshire neck').
3. **Congenital Enzyme Defects.** Partial forms of enzyme defects are commonly responsible for sporadic goitres.
4. **Autoimmune Thyroiditis.** The goitre is characteristically firm or, if there is much fibrosis, hard.
5. **Drug Induced** (as with lithium, PAS, resorcinol and excessive doses of iodides).
6. **Inflammatory Conditions of the Thyroid:**

Acute thyroiditis. This occurs from bacterial infection of the gland, usually as a result of blood-borne infection, and is very uncommon.

Subacute thyroiditis (de Quervain's thyroiditis). This disease is probably due to a virus infection – sometimes by the mumps virus. The patient complains of severe pain in the neck and the thyroid is tender. The condition may follow a prolonged fluctuating course, but resolution usually finally occurs without any permanent impairment of thyroid function. Treatment with thyroxine may be effective and in severe cases corticosteroid therapy is indicated.

Fibrous thyroiditis (Riedel's thyroiditis). A very rare condition with massive fibrous infiltration of the thyroid and surrounding structures.

7. Neoplasms of the Thyroid:

Benign. Adenomas of the thyroid are common and may be single or multiple. They occur particularly in regions of endemic goitre.

Malignant. This is an unusual form of carcinoma in that differentiated tumours, that have the best prognosis, are more common in the young than the elderly. In children, thyroid carcinomas may arise from irradiation involving the thyroid gland. Thyroid carcinomas should be suspected in patients (particularly men) with a single thyroid nodule that, on scanning of the gland after the administration of radio-iodine, does not take up any isotope (a 'cold nodule'). The nodule is usually hard and may be fixed to surrounding structures in the neck causing symptoms such as dysphagia and dysarthria. The following types of malignant tumour occur:

(a) Differentiated tumours. These are distinguished as papillary, follicular, or medullary depending on their histological appearance. Medullary carcinomas are derived from parafollicular cells and secrete calcitonin (*see* page 191). Papillary and follicular tumours tend to grow slowly and metastasise locally causing cervical lymphadenopathy. Their prognosis is fairly good and ten-year survivals of the papillary type of 80 per cent have been reported. Many of these tumours concentrate radio-iodine which can be used in their treatment. Some are partially under TSH control and respond to treatment with thyroid hormone.

(b) Undifferentiated tumours. These anaplastic tumours are highly malignant and have a bad prognosis. Deep X-ray therapy may produce a short-lived improvement.

THE GONADS

The gonads comprise the testes, responsible for the production of spermatozoa and the secretion of testosterone, and the ovaries that produce ova and secrete oestrogens and progesterone.

THE GONADS – NORMAL

Differentiation of Sex

Sex differentiation in the embryo is ultimately determined by the chromosomal composition (karyotype). The normal human cell contains 22 pairs of autosomes and one pair of sex chromosomes. In the female this consists of two X chromosomes and in the male an X and a smaller Y chromosome (*see* page 106). One of each pair of chromosomes is derived from each of the parents.

The gonads develop from the embryonic genital ridges. The factors that determine the development of an ovary in an embryo of XX constitution and of a testis in one of XY constitution are not fully understood. The early embryo has both Müllerian and Wolffian duct systems. From the eighth week of fetal life, the primitive testis secretes a substance that acts locally (i.e. on the same side) to cause suppression of the Müllerian duct system. The Wolffian duct system thereafter develops with the formation of the vas deferens and the epididymis. Later, the testis secretes androgens, that results in the further development of male sex organs such as the prostate and the seminal vesicles. In the female fetus the Müllerian duct system prevails to form the uterus, Fallopian tubes and part of the vagina. This appears to be an automatic process that also occurs if the primitive testis is unable to secrete the factors necessary to promote masculinisation. The fetal testes migrate down the posterior abdominal wall, through the inguinal canals and are usually within the scrotum at birth.

The Testes

The testes are composed of seminiferous tubules and interstitial (Leydig) cells. The seminiferous tubules provide most of the bulk of the organ and are the site of manufacture of spermatozoa. In addition to spermatogonia, they contain the Sertoli cells that may play a part in the nutrition of the tubules. The interstitial cells secrete the potent androgen testosterone (for basic structure *see* page 166). The activity of the testes is controlled by the gonadotrophins, FSH and ICSH, secreted by the anterior pituitary. These are responsible for the initiation of puberty, although the stimulus for their increased secretion at this time is not known. FSH promotes the production of spermatozoa by the germinal cells of the seminiferous tubules, while ICSH stimulates testosterone production. Discharge of the gonadotrophins is controlled by a releasing hormone produced by cells of the hypothalamus (*see* page 161) and is affected by the level of plasma testosterone, a rise of which inhibits the release of ICSH and, to a lesser extent, FSH. In addition there appears to be another hormone called *inhibin*, probably secreted by the Sertoli cells, that has a feed-back effect upon the secretion of FSH. Testosterone undergoes reduction in some tissues to 5 α-dihydrotestosterone. These two highly potent androgens stimulate the development of male secondary sexual characteristics such as hair growth on the face, chest and pubis (in the characteristic distribution extending towards the umbilicus), laryngeal changes (causing deepening of the voice), growth of the penis, scrotum and testes and psychological changes. They also promote protein anabolism, causing an increase in musculature and stimulation of maturation of the bones. This produces the pubertal growth spurt but also causes the fusion of the epiphyses that brings growth to an end.

Assessment of Testicular Function. The function of the seminiferous tubules can be assessed from examination of seminal fluid, usually obtained by masturbation. The number of sperms is counted and their motility and proportion of abnormal forms are determined. Testicular biopsy may also be necessary to examine the histological appearance of the tubules. Androgen production can be crudely assessed by measurement of the urinary 17-oxosteroids (see page 167), one-third of which are derived from testicular androgens and the remainder from the adrenal cortex. Measurement of plasma testosterone is now widely available and is much more informative.

The Ovaries

The ovaries are composed of a stroma of connective tissue enclosed by a capsule and contain large numbers of primordial follicles embedded within them. From puberty until the end of menstruation (the menopause), several ovarian follicles mature each month to form Graafian follicles. These consist of a centrally placed ovum surrounded by granulosa cells and the theca interna and externa. At mid-cycle, one (or occasionally more than one) follicle ruptures with release of the ovum (ovulation) that may become fertilised by a sperm. The other follicles then atrophy and the cells lining the ruptured follicle form the corpus luteum. This persists until menstruation (unless fertilisation occurs), when the cycle begins again.

The ovaries secrete oestrogens (for basic structure see page 166), small amounts of androgens and progesterone. Their cyclical activity is controlled by changes in the circulating levels of FSH and LH, and a mid-cycle peak of LH secretion is essential for the initiation of ovulation. This LH peak appears to be triggered off by the rising levels of plasma oestrogens immediately preceding it (a 'positive feed-back' effect). The production of the gonadotrophins is controlled by a hypothalamic releasing hormone (see page 161). Changes in the levels of circulating oestrogens and progesterone affect the release of LH and FSH by direct actions upon the pituitary and the hypothalamus.

Oestrogens cause development of the breasts and external genitalia, deposition of fat to produce the feminine contour and psychological changes. They also have similar effects to those of androgens in promoting protein anabolism and the maturation of bones. Cyclical secretion of oestrogens and progesterone causes changes in the endometrium of the uterus that result in menstruation. Oestrogen activity in the first half of the cycle produces a proliferative response, while the combined effects of oestrogens and progesterone in the second half produce a secretory endometrium suitable for the early nourishment of a fertilised ovum. If fertilisation does not occur, a fall in the levels of circulating progesterone and oestrogens results in desquamation of the superficial layers of the endometrium and menstrual bleeding.

Assessment of Ovarian Function. Plasma and urinary levels of oestrogens and their metabolic products can be determined. In addition, an assessment of oestrogen secretion can be obtained from examination of vaginal cytology and cervical mucus, and curettings of uterine endometrium. As progesterone is mainly produced by the corpus luteum, evidence of progesterone secretion provides circumstantial evidence of ovulation. Serum progesterone and urinary pregnanediol, a product of progesterone metabolism, can be measured. In addition the basal body temperature can be measured daily by the patient as progesterone causes it to rise, and secretory changes of the uterine endometrium can be detected on biopsy. It is sometimes necessary to inspect and biopsy the ovary and this can be performed by culdoscopy, laparoscopy, or laparotomy.

Pregnancy. The fertilised ovum becomes embedded within the uterine endometrium and undergoes division to form the fetus, while further ovulation and menstruation are inhibited by the persistence of high levels of circulating progesterone and oestrogens. Initially, these are secreted by the corpus luteum and this is maintained by an LH-like substance, human chorionic gonadotrophin (HCG), produced soon after fertilisation by cells of the developing placenta. Later, the placenta itself manufactures oestrogens and progesterone, in addition to other hormones and the corpus luteum degenerates.

Pregnancy Tests. These are based on measurements of the urinary content of HCG and become positive as early as 14 to 28 days after conception. Formerly, assays depended on the biological effect of HCG in a test animal. Nowadays immunological methods of assay are available and the result is known within a few hours.

THE GONADS – ABNORMAL

1. HYPOGONADISM

Definition

Reduced function of the gonads is known as hypogonadism.

MALE HYPOGONADISM

Background

There is a large reserve of testicular function so that unilateral disease does not produce any clinically detectable defect. The seminiferous tubules, interstitial cells or both, may be affected. The condition may be due to primary disease of the testes or be secondary to complete or partial hypopituitarism. Primary disorders of the testes include trauma, torsion, orchitis (usually due to mumps), undescended testes (cryptorchidism) and disorders of differentiation of sex such as Klinefelter's syndrome (*see below*). Functional disturbances of the seminiferous tubules are common and result in abnormalities of spermatogenesis alone, the subject having otherwise quite normal testicular function.

Symptoms

Onset before puberty:
Lack of normal pubertal changes.

Onset after puberty:
Infertility.
Loss of libido and potency.

Signs

Onset before puberty:
Failure of male pattern of body hair to develop.
Infantile genitalia.
Relatively long arms and legs (from delayed epiphyseal closure).
High pitched voice.
Lack of adult musculature.
Deficiency of body hair.

Onset (or recognition) after puberty:
Often none (as in functional disorders of spermatogenesis).
If associated androgen deficiency, some loss of body hair.

Investigations

Measurement of plasma testosterone is helpful in confirming the diagnosis. Measurement of serum gonadtrophins distinguishes between primary testicular disease when the levels are high, and hypothalamic or pituitary disorders when they are low.

Differential Diagnosis

Male hypogonadism must be distinguished from impotence due to psychiatric causes when clinical examination and investigations are normal.

Basis of Treatment

A variety of preparations of androgen are available for the treatment of patients with testosterone deficiency. Some, such as methyltestosterone and fluoxymesterone, are given by mouth but may cause cholestatic jaundice and possibly hepatoma of the liver. Others are given by intramuscular injection and long-acting preparations of testosterone esters are active for three to four weeks.

The treatment of infertility is unsatisfactory. An associated varicocoele should be operated on as this sometimes improves fertility and, rarely, an obstructive lesion of the vas deferens can also be treated surgically. Sometimes spermatogenesis can be transiently restored in patients with hypopituitarism by treatment with gonadotrophins, but supplies of FSH for such therapy are limited.

Cryptorchid testes usually require surgical fixation in the scrotum (orchidopexy), although they sometimes descend after a course of human chorionic gonadotrophin. Operation must be undertaken before the age of ten for fear of irreversible damage to the testis. It must, however, be remembered that testes are often undescended because of some primary abnormality. There is an increased incidence of malignancy in undescended testes.

FEMALE HYPOGONADISM

Background

There is failure of ovum production with or without diminished hormone secretion by the ovary. The condition is due to a primary ovarian disorder, impaired gonadotrophin secretion or increased prolactin secretion by the pituitary (*see* page 160). Primary loss of ovarian function may be caused by ovarian tumours, surgical excision, radiation damage, infections such as tuberculosis, disorders of sex differentiation such as gonadal dysgenesis (*see below*) and spontaneous ovarian failure (premature menopause). Disturbances of gonadotrophin production are produced by organic lesions of the pituitary or hypothalamus, but more commonly occur after an emotional disturbance or a chronic debilitating condition because of a functional abnormality at the hypothalamic level.

Symptoms

Onset before puberty:
Failure to menstruate (primary amenorrhoea).

Onset after puberty:
Irregular scanty menses and, later, (secondary) amenorrhoea.
Infertility.
Reduction in breast size.
Sometimes galactorrhoea (if underlying hyperprolactinaemia).
Hot flushes.

Signs

Onset before puberty:
Lack of development of breasts and external genitalia.
Relatively long arms and legs (from delayed epiphyseal closure).

Onset after puberty:
Partial breast atrophy.
Sometimes galactorrhoea (if underlying hyperprolactinaemia).

Investigations

An organic cause is usually found in patients with primary amenorrhoea. In patients with secondary amenorrhoea, pregnancy must first be excluded. Subsequently, an X-ray of the skull (for the appearance of the pituitary fossa) and measurements of serum gonadotrophins and prolactin are necessary, to decide whether the lesion is in the hypothalamus or pituitary (when the gonadotrophin levels are low), or in the ovary (when these are high), or whether there is hyperprolactinaemia. Frequently, no underlying lesion is found and a functional abnormality has to be postulated.

Women with infertility must be investigated to determine, in particular, whether they are ovulating and whether the Fallopian tubes are blocked.

Basis of Treatment

The underlying lesion must first be treated. When no lesion can be detected, or if it cannot be treated, oestrogens can be given to promote development of female secondary sexual characteristics, restore menstruation and for their psychological effects. Synthetic oestrogens such as ethinyloestradiol are commonly used. It is usual to give compounds with a progesterone-like action towards the end of each treatment cycle to produce a more normal menstrual loss. Progesterone itself cannot be given by mouth, but a number of orally active synthetic progestogens are available. Combined oestrogen and progestogen therapy is conveniently given as one of the oral contraceptive preparations.

Some forms of infertility can be treated with the drug clomiphene that stimulates gonadotrophin secretion. Resistant infertility is treated with gonadotrophins, but this carries a particular risk of multiple pregnancies and is only undertaken in specialised centres.

2. EXCESSIVE PRODUCTION OF HORMONES

PRECOCIOUS PUBERTY

Background

Sexual development before the age of ten in boys and eight in girls is commonly accepted as abnormal. Precocious puberty may be due to lesions of:
1. The hypothalamus or pituitary, producing premature secretion of the gonadotrophins.
2. The gonads or the adrenal cortex, producing excessive amounts of androgens or oestrogens.

Sometimes, particularly in girls, no underlying lesion can be detected and the disorder is thought to be a functional abnormality of the hypothalamus.

The condition known as Albright's syndrome consists of a bony lesion – fibrous dysplasia – which may involve one or several bones, together with skin pigmentation and sexual precocity.

Symptoms and Signs

There is premature development of pubertal changes with growth of the breasts and onset of menstruation in girls and deepening of the voice and development of the external genitalia in boys. Furthermore, owing to the action of sex hormones on muscle and bone, patients grow excessively in their early years, but ultimately become dwarfed from premature fusion of the epiphyses.

Basis of Treatment

This is of the underlying condition if possible. In those patients in whom no underlying abnormality can be detected, or where this is untreatable, certain progestational agents can be used to try and inhibit gonadotrophin secretion. In boys, the drug cyproterone acetate, that antagonises the peripheral action of androgens, is the treatment of choice.

HIRSUTISM AND VIRILISM

Definition

Hirsutism is excessive body hair and virilism constitutes the syndrome of masculinisation of females.

Background

No frank endocrine abnormality can be detected in the majority of women with hirsutism (idiopathic hirsutism). It is often familial and there are considerable racial differences in the amount of hirsutism normally found in women. In some patients it appears to be due to mild over-production of androgens by the ovaries or the adrenal cortex, while in others there may be an increased sensitivity of the hair follicles to normal amounts of circulating androgen.

Hirsutism is also a feature of the Stein-Leventhal syndrome. This is an ill-defined condition characterised by thickening of the ovarian capsule and multiple ovarian cysts, hence the alternative name of polycystic disease of the ovaries.

Virilism is caused by androgen-secreting ovarian tumours, such as hilus cell tumours and arrhenoblastomas, adrenal tumours or congenital adrenal hyperplasia (*see* page 169).

Symptoms and Signs

Excessive hair is found on the face, extremities, breasts and abdomen, where it has the male distribution extending in the midline to the umbilicus. Patients with idiopathic hirsutism often have irregular periods but may be normally fertile. Patients with the Stein-Leventhal syndrome are usually obese, infertile and have scanty periods or complete amenorrhoea. In virilism, there are additional features of excessive muscularity, deepening of the voice, temporal recession of hair and enlargement of the clitoris; amenorrhoea is invariable.

Investigations

Patients with virilism require full investigation to find the underlying cause. Measurements of plasma or urinary androgen levels are essential, but sometimes no definite diagnosis can be made without an exploratory laparotomy.

Basis of Treatment

Idiopathic Hirsutism. The administration of glucocorticoids or oestrogens are sometimes of value, but usually treatment is restricted to cosmetic measures.

Stein-Leventhal Syndrome. Normal menstruation, ovulation and fertility can often be restored by excision of small amounts of ovarian tissue (wedge resection), but this does not improve the hirsutism.

Virilism. The rare cases of adults with congenital adrenal hyperplasia require treatment with glucocorticoids in replacement dosage. Other patients with virilism are treated by surgical excision of the underlying lesion.

3. DISORDERS OF SEX DIFFERENTIATION

These can be classified on the basis of the patient's body shape and external genitalia (the phenotype).

PATIENTS WITH A MALE PHENOTYPE. SEMINIFEROUS TUBULE DYSGENESIS (KLINEFELTER'S SYNDROME) (*see also* page 108)

Background

There is usually an abnormal karyotype that is most often XXY. The testes are very small (microorchidism) and the seminiferous tubules are grossly abnormal and hyalinised. The interstitial cells, however, may appear normal or even increased in number, but their function is often defective. The condition is relatively common and has been estimated to occur about once in 500 male births.

Symptoms and Signs

Patients are infertile, often have gynaecomastia (enlargement of the breasts) and are sometimes of low intelligence. The degree of androgen deficiency is variable. Some patients have marked eunuchoidism, while others are fully masculinised and their only symptom is infertility.

Basis of Treatment

Androgen deficiency is treated with testosterone. There is no effective treatment for the infertility.

PATIENTS WITH A FEMALE PHENOTYPE. GONADAL DYSGENESIS (TURNER'S SYNDROME) (*see also* page 108).

Background

The gonads fail to develop and remain rudimentary structures mainly composed of connective tissue ('streak gonads'). Most patients have an XO karyotype, although other chromosomal abnormalities are also found.

Symptoms and Signs

There is hypogonadism of the prepubertal type with primary amenorrhoea. In addition, most patients are dwarfed and show a number of other associated features such as a short webbed neck, shortness of one or more metacarpal bones and other skeletal abnormalities, an increased carrying angle at the elbow, osteoporosis and skin naevi.

Basis of Treatment

Cyclical oestrogen therapy is required to promote the development of female secondary sexual characteristics. However, the prognosis for growth is poor and patients are infertile. Some forms of chromosomal abnormality have a tendency to malignant change of the gonads and these have to be removed as a prophylactic measure.

TESTICULAR FEMINISATION

This is a rare condition characterised by patients of female phenotype with absent pubic and axillary hair. Testes are present, but there appears to be tissue insensitivity to the action of androgens.

PATIENTS WITH AN INDETERMINATE PHENOTYPE

Hormonal Abnormalities. Varying degrees of masculinisation of the genitalia occur in female infants with congenital adrenal hyperplasia (*see* page 169) and after treatment of the mother with certain progestational agents during pregnancy.

Others. A variety of other types of intersex are also known, such as true hermaphroditism. This is a rare condition in which the patient has both testicular and ovarian tissue.

Assessment of Sex Differentiation

Chromosome counts are usually done on cultures of lymphocytes although other tissues can also be used. Cells of different chromosomal composition may be found in one individual (mosaicism). Information as to the number of X chromosomes can more easily be obtained from examination of cells taken from a scraping of the buccal mucosa. A mass of deeply staining material ('Barr body') is seen lying against the nuclear membrane in normal women that represents one of the X chromosomes. Normal males are 'chromatin negative'.

GROWTH

Growth is a complex process affecting all tissues. Increase in length occurs at the epiphyseal cartilages of the long bones and the vertebrae. As children get older, the growth of the limbs is relatively greater than that of the trunk, so that the ratio of the 'upper segment' (from the top of the head to the pubis) to the 'lower segment' (from the pubis to the soles of the feet) gradually decreases, to reach the adult figure of just under one by the age of 12. Growth is affected by the following factors:

1. **Genetic.** The growth potential of an individual is ultimately determined by his genetic constitution.
2. **Nutrition.** Malnutrition is associated with stunting of growth. Conversely, growth is accelerated in obese children. However, their ultimate height is usually no greater than that of children of normal weight as their growth ceases earlier.
3. **Endocrine.**
(a) Thyroid hormone.
(b) Growth hormone.
(c) Sex hormones. These are largely responsible for the pubertal growth spurt and, later, for the fusion of the epiphyses that stops further growth.
4. **Psychological.** The importance of psychological factors is difficult to assess, nevertheless severe disorders of behaviour can undoubtedly impair growth.

DISORDERS OF GROWTH

Charts are available that show the ranges of heights and weights of normal children of different ages. These can be used to assess the degree of abnormality of an individual patient.

Assessment of Growth Disorders

The history must include the birth weight of the patient, his feeding habits and the heights of his close relatives. Investigations include an X-ray of the skull for the appearance of the pituitary fossa, and of the left hand for estimation of bone maturity ('bone age'). It may also be necessary to investigate endocrine and intestinal function.

SHORT STATURE

Background

Shortness occurs under the following circumstances:

Constitutional Shortness. Shortness also occurs in other members of the family and is genetically determined.

Primordial Dwarfism. There is no family history of shortness. The birth weight is sometimes low in relation to the period of gestation (the 'light-for-dates' baby), suggesting impairment of placental function *in utero*. With increased awareness of the importance of nutritional and psychological factors for normal growth and the increased sophistication of hormone assays, fewer and fewer patients are likely to be given this diagnosis.

Delayed Development. Delayed development affects not only growth but also the onset of puberty; X-rays show the 'bone age' to be correspondingly delayed. Patients' ultimate height is usually normal.

Endocrine Disorders.
(a) *Hypothyroidism*. This is associated with markedly delayed maturation so that the child retains the body proportions of far younger children.

(b) *Growth hormone deficiency*. This may be associated with generalised hypopituitarism, as with pituitary tumours. However, isolated growth hormone deficiency also occurs and is sometimes familial. Peripheral resistance to the action of growth hormone and abnormal forms of circulating growth hormone have also been reported.

(c) *Sex hormone excess*. Children with syndromes of androgen or oestrogen excess show early acceleration of growth, but ultimate dwarfism from premature fusion of the epiphyses.

Associated Organic Disease. Many chronic disorders may interfere with growth, in particular cyanotic congenital heart disease and renal disease.

Malnutrition. This may be due to food deprivation or a malabsorption syndrome.

Skeletal Disease. A variety of skeletal diseases are associated with shortness. These are usually obvious from clinical and radiological examination.

Chromosomal Abnormalities. Shortness is a feature of patients with some types of chromosomal abnormality such as gonadal dysgenesis (*see* page 108) and Down's syndrome (*see* page 107).

Psychological Disorders. Severe emotional deprivation and other psychological disorders may retard growth, possibly by reducing food intake or impairing growth hormone secretion.

Basis of Treatment

Treatment is of the underlying condition, when this is possible.

Children with delayed development usually ultimately show normal growth and pubertal changes. Many boys, however, become seriously embarrassed by their relative immaturity as compared with other boys of their age. It is sometimes helpful to give them a six-week course of human chorionic gonadotrophin. This stimulates the interstitial cells of the testis to produce testosterone and often seems to initiate puberty. Growth hormone has to be extracted from human pituitaries and is thus available in only limited supplies. Its use is virtually restricted to children with growth hormone deficiency in whom it causes striking stimulation of growth.

TALL STATURE

Background

Tallness of stature occurs for the following reasons:

Constitutional Tallness. Other members of the family are also unusually tall and the condition is genetically determined.

Endocrine Disorders
(a) *Growth hormone excess (gigantism).* This rare condition is due to a growth hormone secreting pituitary tumour.
(b) *Sex hormone deficiency.* Patients with hypogonadism may ultimately become tall. This is due to delayed fusion of the epiphyses resulting in disproportionately long arms and legs.
(c) *Marfan's syndrome (see* page 627).

Basis of Treatment

Sex hormones in large doses are sometimes given to children who seem likely to develop constitutional tallness, in the hope of producing early fusion of the epiphyses and thereby reducing ultimate height.

THE PANCREAS

The pancreas is an elongated structure weighing approximately 60 g situated retroperitoneally at the level of the second and third lumbar vertebrae. The majority of the organ is made up of exocrine glandular tissue that secretes pancreatic juice into the duodenum. About one per cent of the gland is composed of the islets of Langerhans. These contain different types of cell distinguished by their staining characteristics. The alpha cells secrete the hormone glucagon, while the beta cells produce insulin. These hormones, and the clinical disorders associated with abnormalities of their secretion, will be considered separately.

INSULIN

Insulin is a polypeptide of molecular weight 6,000. It is composed of an A-chain made up of 21 amino acids and a B-chain of 30 amino acids, joined by two sulphydryl bonds. The immediate precursor of insulin within the beta cell is pro-insulin in which the A and the B chains are joined by a connector piece (C-peptide) composed, in man, of 31 amino acids. Insulins derived from different animal sources show certain differences in their amino acid sequences, but are active in almost all species with a biological activity of approximately 25

Table 10.10 Actions of insulin

Substrate	Action	Site
Carbohydrate	Stimulation of glucose utilisation	Muscle, adipose tissue, liver
	Stimulation of glycogen synthesis	Muscle, adipose tissue, liver
	Inhibition of glycogen breakdown	Liver
	Inhibition of gluconeogenesis	Liver
Fat	Stimulation of fatty acid and triglyceride synthesis	Adipose tissue, liver
	Inhibition of triglyceride breakdown	Adipose tissue
Protein	Stimulation of incorporation of amino acids into protein	Muscle, adipose tissue, liver
Electrolytes	Stimulation of potassium entry into cells	Muscle, adipose tissue, liver

units per mg. The unit is a standard based on the fall of blood sugar produced in rabbits. The normal human pancreas produces about 40 units of insulin daily.

Actions of Insulin (Table 10.10)

The overall effect of insulin on carbohydrate metabolism results in a fall of blood glucose, while inhibition of fat breakdown in adipose tissue produces a fall of plasma free fatty acids. At the time of peak insulin action the main metabolic fuel of the body is carbohydrate, the utilisation of fat is reduced and the incorporation of amino acids into muscle protein is stimulated.

Factors Controlling Insulin Secretion (Table 10.11)

The most important factor controlling insulin secretion is glucose. In perfusion studies, this produces an almost instantaneous rise of insulin in the effluent, presumably from release of preformed hormone. More prolonged exposure to glucose results in increased insulin synthesis. Conversely, a fall of blood glucose inhibits insulin secretion. Although the rise of blood glucose and amino acids, after a carbohydrate and protein meal respectively, directly stimulate insulin release, much of the early response to carbohydrate or protein ingestion is due to the stimulation of insulin release by hormones produced in the upper intestine. There is still uncertainty as to which hormone(s) is responsible for this effect, but it appears that gastric inhibitory polypeptide (GIP) is important in this respect.

Table 10.11   Some factors affecting insulin release

Stimulation of release	Inhibition of release
Glucose and certain other monosaccharides	Catecholamines
	Diazoxide
Leucine and certain other amino acids	Potassium deficiency
Hormone(s) from upper intestinal tract (in particular gastric inhibitory polypeptide)	
Glucagon	
Sulphonylureas	
Cyclic AMP	

Assessment of Insulin Secretion

Assays of circulating insulin are widely available. Formerly, the methods depended on the biological effects of the hormone; nowadays, radioimmunoassays (see page 160) have been developed and have enormously facilitated studies of insulin secretion.

Disorders of Insulin Secretion

Over-production of insulin is one of the causes of hypoglycaemia and will be discussed under that heading (see page 188). Insulin deficiency is considered below.

DIABETES MELLITUS

Definition

Diabetes mellitus is a condition of impaired carbohydrate utilisation caused by an absolute or relative deficiency of insulin.

Background

The disease has been recognised since antiquity, and is of particular importance because of its prevalence. The name is derived from the sweet taste of urine from patients with the disorder (mellitus = honey) due to the glycosuria resulting from elevated levels of blood glucose. The condition is defined on the basis of raised blood glucose levels, although a large number of other metabolic abnormalities can be demonstrated. Some patients have clearly elevated levels of glucose in random blood samples, whereas others, with lesser degrees of hyperglycaemia, require special tests of glucose tolerance for diagnosis (see below). Different groups of patients with abnormalities of glucose tolerance are recognised as follows:*

1. **Clinical Diabetes.** A person with a diabetic response with the symptoms or complications of diabetes.
2. **Asymptomatic or Chemical Diabetes.** A person with a diabetic response who has no clinical abnormalities.
3. **Latent Diabetes.** A person with a normal response at the time of testing, but who is known to have had a diabetic response at some time during pregnancy, infection or other stress, or when obese.
4. **Potential Diabetes.** A person with a normal response, but with an increased potential risk of developing diabetes, such as an identical twin, the other twin being diabetic, a person with both parents diabetic, or a woman who has given birth to a live or stillborn child weighing 4.5 kg (10 lb) or more at birth.
5. **Prediabetes.** A diagnosis that can only be made retrospectively to cover the period of life before the diagnosis is made.

Incidence

Many surveys have been undertaken to establish the incidence of the disease. There is considerable variation between communities, but in the UK and North

* From Fitzgerald, M. G. and Keen, H. (1964) British Medical Journal **1**: 1568.

America at least 2 per cent of the population has clinical or chemical diabetes. There is a marked rise in the proportion of subjects with impaired glucose tolerance with increasing age, so that over the age of 70 more than 40 per cent show a diabetic response.

Clinical Types

Patients can be divided into two main groups:

Juvenile Onset Type (Type I Diabetes).

As implied by the name, these patients usually develop diabetes when young, but not necessarily so. They are grossly insulin deficient and require insulin treatment. The severity of the insulin deficiency is shown by their tendency to develop ketosis. The onset of this type is often sudden and usually associated with loss of weight.

Maturity Onset Type (Type II Diabetes).

These patients are usually middle-aged or elderly and are frequently obese. The condition is often detected on routine examination of the urine, or because of the onset of diabetic complications. Such patients are not severely insulin deficient and, hence, are not prone to ketosis. They do not usually require insulin treatment. Maturity onset diabetics are approximately four times more common than those of the juvenile onset type.

Aetiology

The disease appears to be determined by several different factors rather than by a single cause. A number of these factors are now recognised.

Inadequate Insulin Production:

(a) *Pancreatic disease (acute and chronic pancreatitis, pancreatic carcinoma, surgical pancreatectomy)*. Such patients do not usually require treatment with more than 40 units of insulin daily, whereas many other insulin dependent patients need larger doses than this.

(b) *Genetic factors*. Diabetes is clearly recognised as having a familial tendency, and the risk of developing the disease is increased the more relatives who are diabetic and the closer their relationship. The exact mode of inheritance is uncertain and there appear to be several genes involved. These genetic factors probably determine whether or not an individual can continue to secrete sufficient insulin to overcome states of insulin antagonism such as those described below. If the genetic constitution is sound, the subject retains normal carbohydrate tolerance, otherwise such factors precipitate diabetes.

(c) *Histocompatibility antigens*. The juvenile onset type of diabetes is commoner in subjects possessing the histocompatibility antigens B8, BW15, DW3 and DW4.

(d) *Autoimmunity*. Circulating antibodies to islet cells can be demonstrated in the majority of juvenile onset type diabetics within a short time of diagnosis. Such antibodies are also found in a few patients apparently with the maturity onset form of the disease, some of whom later become insulin dependent. These and other findings strongly suggest that, in some diabetics, the condition is induced by an autoimmune process.

(e) *Viruses*. There is evidence that infection with certain viruses, notably of the Coxsackie group, plays a part in the development of juvenile onset type diabetes in some patients.

(f) *Drugs*. Certain drugs such as the thiazide diuretics reduce insulin secretion, although their effect is usually reversible once the drug is withdrawn.

Insulin Antagonism:

(a) *Endocrine conditions*. Diabetes mellitus may develop when the following hormones are produced in excess:
(i) Growth hormone (as in acromegaly).
(ii) Glucocorticoids (as in Cushing's syndrome). Similarly diabetes may occur in patients requiring treatment with high doses of glucocorticoids.
(iii) Catecholamines (as in phaeochromocytoma).
(iv) Glucagon. Patients with glucagon secreting tumours have mild diabetes. In addition, it has been suggested that 'inappropriate' glucagon secretion plays a part in the development of diabetes even in patients who do not have such tumours.

(b) *Obesity*. Obesity is associated with insulin resistance, the exact cause of which is unknown.

(c) *Pregnancy*. Diabetes may present during pregnancy, or established diabetes may become worse. Furthermore, there is an increased incidence of the condition in multiparous women as compared with those who have had no children. Among the insulin antagonists produced in pregnancy is one of the hormones synthesised by the placenta, human placental lactogen, that is similar in many respects to growth hormone.

(d) *Others*. Several other insulin antagonists have been described. The most important of these are fatty acids and a factor associated with serum albumin known as the synalbumin antagonist. The importance of these factors in the aetiology of diabetes is unknown.

Pathology

The changes within the pancreas may not be particularly striking, but there is usually degranulation or loss of beta cells and hyalinisation or fibrosis of islet cell tissue. There is an increased incidence of atherosclerosis of large arteries (macroangiopathy), while the small vessels show thickening of the basement membrane with deposition of a mucopolysaccharide material (microangiopathy). The renal glomeruli show similar changes that may be either diffuse or nodular (the Kimmelstiel-Wilson lesion).

Chemical Pathology. In extreme insulin deficiency, the normal restraining influence of insulin on the breakdown of fats within adipose tissue is lost, and there is massive liberation of fatty acids into the circulation. Metabolism of these substances in the liver produces aceto-acetic acid, beta-hydroxybutyric acid and acetone. These 'ketone bodies' are released into the bloodstream in large amounts, causing diabetic ketosis (*see below*). Poorly controlled diabetes is characterised not only by raised levels of blood glucose, but also by elevated levels of a number of other substances such as ketone bodies, triglycerides and cholesterol, that may be of importance in the development of diabetic complications.

Symptoms and Signs

Due to glycosuria. This leads to polyuria (from an osmotic diuresis) and increased thirst (polydipsia). It may give rise to pruritus (itching) of the vulva in women and balanitis (inflammation of the glans penis) in men.

Due to severe insulin deficiency:
Loss of weight. This may occur despite a normal or even increased appetite.
Ketosis (also called keto-acidosis). Minor degrees of ketosis are not uncommon in poorly controlled juvenile onset diabetics. Severe ketosis, however, is of immediate serious significance. It may develop as the present-

ing syndrome in a patient not previously known to be diabetic. More often, however, it arises in known insulin requiring patients whose control has deteriorated. This commonly occurs because of some intercurrent illness resulting in an increase of insulin requirements. Patients with severe ketosis feel unwell with nausea and vomiting and occasionally severe abdominal pain. Later, they become drowsy and lapse into coma. The condition is fatal if left untreated. Patients in precoma or coma due to diabetic acidosis present a striking appearance with dehydration, hypotension, deep acidotic breathing and a sweet 'fruity' smell of ketone bodies on the breath. It is essential to realise that life-threatening ketosis may arise within hours and the condition must be treated as a medical emergency.

Other symptoms and signs:
Diabetics show a susceptibility to a variety of infections; these include tuberculosis, pyelonephritis, and boils and carbuncles of the skin.
Amenorrhoea.
Complications of pregnancy. There is a considerably increased incidence of stillbirths and neonatal (within the first 28 days of life) deaths in pregnancies of women with untreated or poorly controlled diabetes. Furthermore, the babies of diabetic mothers are sometimes grossly overweight. This is due to hyperplastic islets and the secretion of excessive amounts of insulin that may be caused by the maternal hyperglycaemia. Both the increased mortality rate and the incidence of big babies can be reduced with effective control of the mothers' diabetes during pregnancy. Big babies are also born to mothers many years before they develop diabetes. Thus, a woman with a baby of birthweight over

Table 10.12 Complications of diabetes mellitus

Organ	Complications	Clinical effects
Arteries	Atherosclerosis (macroangiopathy)	Ischaemic heart disease
Arterioles	Microangiopathy	Cerebrovascular disease
		Peripheral vascular disease
Kidneys	Glomerulosclerosis	Nephrotic syndrome Hypertension Renal failure
Eyes Diabetic retinopathy	(a) *'Background'* retinopathy: microaneurysms, haemorrhages, exudates	Usually do not impair vision

	(b) *Proliferative'* retinopathy:
	  new vessel formation, vitreous haemorrhages,
	  fibrous tissue proliferation
		Impairment of vision leading to blindness

	Cataracts	Impairment of vision
Nervous system	Peripheral neuropathy	*Sensory:* Paraesthesiae, analgesia, ulceration, arthropathy (diabetic pseudo-tabes) *Motor:* Weakness, muscle wasting *Autonomic:* Impotence, diarrhoea, postural hypotension
Skin	Necrobiosis lipoidica	Discoloured areas fading to white atrophic patches usually on front of legs

4.5 kg (10 lb) has about a 33 per cent chance of later developing the disease and is, thus, a potential diabetic.

Complications (Table 10.12)

The causes of these complications are still poorly understood. It has been suggested that they are due to independent defects inherited in association with those resulting in insulin deficiency. However, the incidence of diabetic complications increases strikingly with the duration of the disease and it is now widely held that the complications are due to metabolic abnormalities that occur as part of the condition.

Investigations

A level of blood glucose over 11 mmol/litre (198 mg/100 ml) is abnormal under most circumstances and establishes the diagnosis. With lesser degrees of hyperglycaemia, glucose tolerance must be specially tested. This is done with the patient at rest after an overnight fast. A dose of 50 g or 100 g of glucose, or an amount related to the patient's body size, is given by mouth. Blood samples are taken before the glucose load and at half-hourly intervals for two-and-a-half hours thereafter. Normal blood glucose values (Table 10.13)

Table 10.13 Commonly accepted normal limits of blood glucose during a 50 g oral glucose tolerance test (values for individual laboratories will depend on method of estimation and whether venous or capillary blood used)

Time (min)	Blood glucose in mmol/l (mg/100 ml)
0	<5.0 (90)
60	<8.9 (160)
90	<7.8 (140)
120	<6.7 (120)
150	<5.5 (100)

vary somewhat with the method of estimation used and according to whether capillary or venous blood samples are taken. An intravenous glucose tolerance test is sometimes performed instead of the oral test, in which repeated blood samples are taken after an intravenous injection of glucose and the rate of fall of blood glucose calculated.

Basis of Treatment

Since the discovery of insulin, patients have been largely preserved from severe ketosis and can lead a normal life. The critical issue, however, concerns whether or not strict diabetic control reduces the incidence of complications and there is now clear evidence that good control is, to some extent, effective in this respect. There are three main types of treatment:

Diet. All diabetics should be on a diet (*see* page 630). In the obese, a reducing diet is essential and weight reduction may even be associated with a return to normal glucose tolerance (the patient then becoming a latent diabetic). For those who are not overweight, a diet of modest carbohydrate restriction is usually advocated. This is conveniently prescribed as the number of grams of carbohydrate per day in units of 10 grams. The patient is then given a list of equivalent amounts of food that contain 10 g carbohydrate. The maintenance of a constant carbohydrate intake is as important as the composition of the diet, as this helps to reduce wide fluctuations of blood glucose.

Hypoglycaemic Drugs. These are used for maturity onset diabetics whose disease is not adequately controlled with dietary measures. There are two groups of such drugs (Table 10.14) and they may be used in combination. The sulphonylurea drugs act largely, if not exclusively, by stimulating the release of insulin from the pancreas. The mode of action of the biguanide groups is different. They act, at least in part, by reducing glucose absorption from the gut and by increasing the peripheral effectiveness of insulin. They also have the property *in vitro* of inhibiting aerobic glycolysis and have a tendency to cause a rise of blood lactic acid. Occasionally, they produce the serious clinical condition of lactic acidosis. The use of oral hypoglycaemic drugs has been questioned by a large American study, the results of which suggested that treatment with tolbutamide and phenformin not only failed to improve the patient's prognosis, but may even have made it worse due to an increase in deaths from cardiovascular causes.

Table 10.14 Some oral hypoglycaemic drugs

Group	Side effects*	Drug	Daily dose
Sulphonylureas	Hypoglycaemia	Tolbutamide	1 to 2 g
	Skin rashes	Chlorpropamide	100 to 350 mg
	Cholestatic jaundice	Glibenclamide	2.5 to 20 mg
	Facial flushing with alcohol	Glipizide	2.5 to 30 mg
	Blood dyscrasias	Glibornuride	12.5 to 75 mg
Biguanides	Anorexia	Metformin	1 to 2.5 g
	Nausea, vomiting, diarrhoea	(Phenformin)	(50 to 100 mg)†
	Lactic acidosis		

*These have not all been reported with each of the compounds listed.
†Use severely restricted because of particular risk of lactic acidosis.

186

Table 10.15 Preparations of insulin and their properties

Preparation	Peak action (hrs)	Duration of action (hrs)
Soluble*	2–4	6–10
'Actrapid' (highly purified porcine)	2–4	6–10
Isophane (NPH)†	4–10	18–24
Insulin zinc suspension		
Semilente‡	3–6	8–12
Ultralente	12–20	24–36
Lente§	4–10	18–24
Biphasic	4–10	18–24
Protamine zinc	12–20	24–36

*Available in highly purified porcine form as 'Leo-Neutral'.
†Available in highly purified porcine form as 'Leo-Retard'.
‡Available in highly purified porcine form as 'Semitard MC'.
§ (i) Made up of 3 parts semilente and 7 parts ultralente;
  (ii) Available in highly purified porcine form as 'Monotard MC'.

Insulin. Insulin has to be given subcutaneously as it is destroyed in the gastrointestinal tract, but patients soon become adept at giving their own injections. A variety of different types of insulin are available (Table 10.15), some of which can be given together in a mixture in the same syringe. Some patients can be controlled on a single daily injection of preparations such as insulin zinc suspension lente. If diabetic control remains unsatisfactory despite increasing the dose of insulin to more than 52 units, twice daily injections are usually needed and this is practically always required during pregnancy and in children and young adults. Thus, for example, a twice daily mixture of soluble and isophane insulin provides a good flexible regimen. Most insulin preparations are bovine in origin and contain some impurities (such as pro-insulin). Antibodies to these preparations can be found in virtually all patients after a few weeks of treatment, although it is still not clear whether or not these antibodies are harmful to the patient. Recently, highly purified porcine insulins have become available from Danish manufacturers that result in little or no antibody formation. The carbohydrate content of meals throughout the day must be related to the type of insulin treatment. Furthermore, exercise reduces insulin requirements and any marked variation in the patient's activity must be remembered when planning their insulin regimen.

Side effects of insulin treatment:
Hypoglycaemic reactions. These may occur in any insulin requiring diabetic, usually because of a missed meal, an error of insulin injection, or unaccustomed exertion. All insulin treated patients should carry sugar lumps or biscuits in case of hypoglycaemia. The clinical features of hypoglycaemia are discussed below.
Insulin allergy. Skin reactions and other manifestations of allergy sometimes occur. They usually respond to a change to one of the highly purified insulins.
Lipodystrophy at sites of injection. This is not uncommon and may be very unsightly. It can, to a considerable extent, be avoided by repeated changes of the site of injection. If it does occur, it can be treated by changing the patient to one of the highly purified insulins and injecting the insulin into the edges of the lesions.

Assessment of Diabetic Control

The most certain way of assessing diabetic control is by serial measurements of blood glucose levels throughout the day, but this is difficult to arrange for the majority of out-patients. Great reliance is therefore placed on patients testing their urine at home and recording the degree of glycosuria; this has become easy since the introduction of 'Clinitest' tablets. It must be remembered, however, that glycosuria when tested in this relatively crude way does not usually become detectable until the blood sugar level is above 10 mmol/l, which already represents a considerable degree of hyperglycaemia. It is important to assess the renal glucose threshold to ensure that the measurement of glycosuria is not misleading as to blood glucose levels. This can be roughly estimated by comparing simultaneous urine and blood sugar concentrations. The degree of ketosis can be rapidly asessed with 'Acetest' tablets. A small amount of ketonuria as shown by this test is usually of no importance. A strongly positive test, however, especially if confirmed by a positive ferric chloride reaction (Gerhardt's test) indicates a serious degree of ketosis and the need for urgent treatment. Confirmation is obtained by finding a low serum bicarbonate concentration.

Treatment of Severe Diabetic Ketosis

The essential features of therapy are:

Insulin Treatment. Only soluble insulin or 'Actrapid' should be used as they are the most rapidly effective forms of insulin. Formerly, it was common to give large doses of insulin during the treatment of severe diabetic ketosis. Nowadays, however, smaller doses are used such as 10 units hourly given either by the intravenous route or deep intramuscular injection.

Fluid Repletion. Patients are always severely dehydrated. In mild cases it may be possible to restore fluids by mouth, but this is often prevented by vomiting and the intravenous route is required. Large amounts of saline must be given and sodium bicarbonate is sometimes added if there is very severe acidosis.

Potassium Repletion. Although the level of serum potassium is often raised initially, due to the acidosis and dehydration, it falls rapidly with insulin treatment and intravenous potassium must always be given, often in large amounts.

Treatment is monitored by repeated measurements of blood glucose and electrolytes. A cause of the episode, such as an infection or myocardial infarction, must be sought and treated appropriately.

Treatment of Complications

There is no specific treatment for most diabetic complications and they are managed as they would be in a non-diabetic, together with efforts to improve diabetic control. The technique of photocoagulation, in which new vessel systems in the retina and areas of abnormal capillary permeability are destroyed by either light or laser beams, has been shown to be effective treatment for some forms of diabetic retinopathy. Total hypophysectomy also produces regression of retinal new vessels for reasons that are still unknown. It is a serious undertaking, but is indicated in a few patients with very severe retinopathy.

Prognosis

The discovery of insulin has greatly reduced the incidence of deaths due to diabetic ketosis. Despite this, however, diabetics still show a considerably increased mortality rate. In one study the mortality rate in diabetics was 154 per cent as compared with the general population over a 15-year period. The commonest causes of death are ischaemic heart disease and cerebrovascular disease.

HYPOGLYCAEMIA

Hypoglycaemia is said to exist when the level of blood glucose is less than 2.2 mmol/l (40 mg/100 ml). The nervous system is one of the few organs whose metabolism, under most circumstances, depends exclusively on glucose as a source of energy and is at particular risk during hypoglycaemic episodes. Patients, however, vary greatly in the levels of blood glucose at which they develop symptoms. Similarly, the clinical syndrome is variable, although a patient subject to repeated attacks tends to develop the same symptoms each time. Sometimes consciousness is lost without warning. More often, however, there are early symptoms such as weakness, faintness, hunger, anxiety, palpitations and excessive sweating. Later, patients become unconscious and may have convulsions; if untreated, the condition may be fatal. Repeated attacks of hypoglycaemia can cause psychiatric abnormalities and intellectual impairment.

Treatment is a matter of urgency and consists of the administration of 20 to 50 g of glucose. In the early stages this can be given by mouth, but must be given intravenously to the unconscious patient. Intramuscular glucagon is sometimes used, especially in children, to produce a sufficient rise of blood glucose and improvement of the level of consciousness for the patient to be able to take sugar by mouth. The response to intravenous glucose usually occurs within seconds, although the patient may be confused for a short time afterwards. With profound or prolonged hypoglycaemia, consciousness may be slow to return and, in very severe cases, patients may be left with mental deterioration from neuronal degeneration.

Causes of Hypoglycaemia (Table 10.16)

Table 10.16 Some causes of hypoglycaemia

Type	Condition
Fasting hypoglycaemia	Islet cell tumours of the pancreas
	Non-pancreatic tumours
	Liver disease
	Endocrine disease (Addison's disease, hypopituitarism)
	Glycogen storage disease
	Idiopathic hypoglycaemia of childhood
Stimulative hypoglycaemia	Exogenous hypoglycaemic agents (e.g. insulin)
	Essential reactive hypoglycaemia
	Hereditary fructose intolerance
	Galactosaemia
	Alcohol-induced hypoglycaemia

These are conveniently considered in two groups:

Fasting Hypoglycaemia. The blood glucose level is low in the fasting state.

Stimulative Hypoglycaemia. Hypoglycaemia occurs in response to some preceding stimulus. The most common form of hypoglycaemia is that produced by insulin in insulin dependent diabetics and therefore falls in this group.

In adults the most difficult differential diagnosis of fasting hypoglycaemia is between an islet cell adenoma and a non-pancreatic tumour. The latter are usually large fibrosarcomas lying within the abdomen or thorax. The mechanism of the associated hypoglycaemia is still uncertain. In islet cell tumours, hypoglycaemia is characteristically associated with inappropriately high levels of serum insulin, whereas this is not found in patients with non-pancreatic tumours. The treatment of islet cell tumours is usually surgical. The drug diazoxide, however, directly inhibits insulin secretion and can be used in the treatment of this and other forms of hypoglycaemia.

GLUCAGON

Glucagon is a hormone of molecular weight 3,500 and consists of 29 amino acids. It is produced by the alpha cells of the islets of Langerhans. A very similar hormone is manufactured throughout the mucous membrane of the small intestine and is called 'gut glucagon'. Until recently it has not been possible to measure these different forms separately, but radioimmunoassays have now been developed that achieve this. The main actions of pancreatic glucagon are stimulation of the breakdown of hepatic glycogen, by activating the enzyme phosphorylase, with a resulting rise of blood glucose and stimulation of lipolysis and gluconeogenesis. Interestingly, it also produces a rise of serum insulin. The release of pancreatic glucagon is stimulated by a fall of blood glucose and by the administration of amino acids. Glucagon secreting carcinomas of the alpha cells of the pancreas have been reported. The clinical syndrome is that of mild diabetes mellitus, extreme muscle wasting and weight loss and a characteristic skin rash.

SUGGESTED FURTHER READING

General

Hall, R., Anderson, J., Smart, G. A. and Besser, M. (1974) *Fundamentals of Clinical Endocrinology*. London: Pitman Medical.

Hamilton, W. (1972) *Clinical Paediatric Endocrinology*. London: Butterworths.

Loraine, J. A. and Bell, E. T. (eds) (1976) *Hormone Assays and their Clinical Applications*. London and Edinburgh: Livingstone.

Rimoin, D. L. and Schimke, R. W. (1971) *Genetic Disorders of the Endocrine Glands*. St Louis: C. V. Mosby.

Williams, R. H. (ed) (1974) *Textbook of Endocrinology*. London: W. B. Saunders.

The Pituitary

Besser, G. M. (ed) (1977) The hypothalamus and pituitary. *Clinics in Endocrinology and Metabolism* **6**, No. 1. London: W. B. Saunders.

Jenkins, J. S. (1973) *Pituitary Tumours*. London: Butterworths.

The Adrenals

Burke, C. W. (1973) *The Adrenal Cortex in Practical Medicine*. London: Gray Mills.

Cope, C. L. (1972) *Adrenal Steroids and Disease*. London: Pitman Medical.

The Thyroid

Evered, D. C. (1976) *Diseases of the Thyroid*. London: Pitman Medical.

Werner, S. C. and Ingbar, S. H. (eds) (1971) *The Thyroid: A Fundamental and Clinical Text*. New York: Harper-Row.

The Gonads

Butt, W. R. and London, D. R. (eds) (1975) The testis. *Clinics in Endocrinology and Metabolism* **4** No. 3. London: W. B. Saunders.

Cooke, I. D. (ed) (1974) The management of infertility. *Clinics in Obstetrics and Gynaecology* **1** No. 2. London: W. B. Saunders.

Shearman, R. P. (ed) (1972) *Human Reproductive Physiology*. Oxford: Blackwell.

Growth

Tanner, J. M. (1962) *Growth at Adolescence*. Oxford: Blackwell.

Diabetes

Malins, J. M. (1968) *Clinical Diabetes Mellitus*. London: Eyre and Spottiswoode.

Oakley, W. G., Pyke, D. A. and Taylor, K. W. (1975) *Diabetes and its Management*. Oxford: Blackwell.

Tattersall, R. (ed) (1977) Diabetes. *Clinics in Endocrinology and Metabolism* **6**, No. 2. London: W. B. Saunders.

Disorders of Calcium Metabolism and Bone

11

D. A. HEATH

The body contains over 25 mol (1,000 g) of calcium of which only one per cent is found outside the skeleton. Apart from its obvious mechanical role, part of the bone calcium acts as a pool of calcium that can be mobilised to counteract changes in the serum calcium. Outside the skeleton, calcium plays essential roles in many body functions which include nerve conduction, muscle contraction, blood coagulation, and hormone secretion.

BONE

The inorganic component of bone consists predominantly of crystals of a complex salt of calcium and phosphate called hydroxyapatite. These crystals are deposited in and around collagen fibres which themselves are embedded in the ground substance of bone that is rich in mucopolysaccharides. The collagen and ground substance constitute the organic component of bone known as the osteoid. Within the bone are to be found three major types of cells – osteoblasts, osteoclasts and osteocytes. Osteoblasts are associated with bone formation and are rich in the enzyme alkaline phosphatase. They secrete the collagen fibres on to which the bone salts are deposited. Both the osteocyte and the multinucleated osteoclast are capable of causing bone resorption, and both cells are stimulated by parathyroid hormone. The different roles of these two cells are at present not completely resolved, but it appears that the osteocyte can cause the rapid release of calcium from bone, while the osteoclast is more concerned with remodelling of bone.

The mechanism of calcification remains unclear, but there is little doubt that the phosphatase enzymes are involved. In conditions of increased bone formation and remodelling, there is a rise in the total serum alkaline phosphatase due to an increase in the alkaline phosphatase isoenzyme of bony origin. (The other major alkaline phosphatase isoenzyme found in plasma is of hepatic origin.)

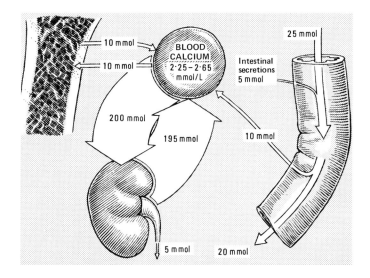

Fig. 11.1 The major compartments of calcium metabolism.

CALCIUM (Fig. 11.1)

Most adults ingest approximately 25 mmol (1,000 mg) of calcium each day. In addition to this dietary source, about 5 mmol (200 mg) of calcium pass into the intestine in the intestinal secretions, making a total entry of calcium into the intestine of 30 mmol (1,200 mg). Of this, about 20 mmol (800 mg) appears in the faeces, and the other 10 mmol (400 mg) is absorbed chiefly in the upper small intestine. If calcium intake is reduced, or if calcium requirements are increased, e.g. during pregnancy, lactation and infancy, then a greater amount of calcium is absorbed from the intestine. This adaptive mechanism whereby absorption is regulated by the body's requirements is dependent on the presence of adequate amounts of vitamin D.

The normal serum calcium concentration ranges between 2.25 and 2.65 mmol/l (9.0 and 10.6 mg/100 ml). (Due to differing analytical techniques the normal range

190

may vary considerably from one laboratory to another.) Of the total serum calcium, only about half is present as the physiologically active, ionised form. The other major form is the protein-bound fraction, while a small amount is complexed to compounds such as citrate and phosphate. Most of the protein-bound fraction is associated with the serum albumin. Variations in the total plasma proteins, and particularly in the albumin fraction, alter the amounts of calcium bound to protein. These changes are reflected in the total serum calcium. Conditions causing hypoproteinaemia will, therefore, tend to cause a lowering of the total calcium, while prolonged venous occlusion by raising the plasma protein concentration may produce an apparently elevated total calcium (Fig. 11.2).

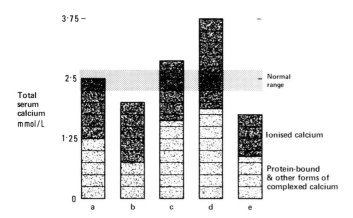

Fig. 11.2 Some factors affecting the serum calcium. a = normal, b = hypoproteinaemia, c = venostasis, d = hyperparathyroidism, e = hypoparathyroidism.

In b and c, despite an abnormal total calcium, the physiological ionised fraction is normal. In d and e both fractions are altered.

Kinetic studies of bone have shown that calcium is constantly being deposited and released from bone, and that calcium can readily be mobilised from the skeleton. Radioactive tracer studies suggest that between 7.5 and 15 mmol (300 and 600 mg) of calcium are deposited and released from bone daily.

The kidneys also play an important role in calcium homeostasis. Of the total calcium passing through the kidney, only the ionised and complexed fractions are filtered. The concentration of calcium in these fractions is about 1.25 mmol/l (5 mg/100 ml), so that with normal renal function, quantities of calcium ranging from 175 to 250 mmol (7 to 10 g) may be filtered each day, of which less than 7.5 mmol (300 mg) is excreted in the urine, the remainder being reabsorbed by the renal tubules.

These features of calcium balance are represented in Fig. 11.1.

REGULATION OF CALCIUM METABOLISM

Although many hormones are known to affect calcium metabolism, the major controlling factors are parathyroid hormone, vitamin D and, possibly, calcitonin.

Parathyroid Hormone

The secretion of this polypeptide hormone is inversely related to the serum calcium levels so that hypocalcaemia leads to rapid release of hormone. The hormone acts on the bone, kidney and intestine.

Bone. To increase the resorption of bone with passage of calcium from bone into the extracellular fluid.

Kidney. (a) To increase the renal tubular reabsorption of calcium; (b) To decrease the renal tubular reabsorption of phosphorus.

Intestine. To increase absorption of calcium from the gut.

Calcitonin

The main source of this polypeptide hormone in man is the parafollicular or 'C' cells of the thyroid. The hormone is secreted in response to elevation of the serum calcium. In animals, injections of the hormone produce hypocalcaemia by suppressing bone resorption. However, in man a significant hypocalcaemic effect is seen only when the rate of bone turnover is pathologically increased, e.g. in Paget's disease and hypercalcaemic states. At present, it is not known conclusively whether calcitonin plays a physiological role in man. Pathologically, high circulating levels are found in cases of medullary carcinoma of the thyroid, a malignant tumour of thyroid 'C' cells. Despite very high calcitonin levels the serum calcium is usually normal in such cases.

Vitamin D

Vitamin D is a fat-soluble vitamin available in several natural and synthetic forms. The vitamin of natural sources is cholecalciferol, or Vit.D_3, found particularly in certain fish oils and egg yolks. In animals, vitamin D is produced in the skin by the action of ultra-violet light on its precursor – 7-dehydrocholesterol. Synthetic forms of vitamin D are produced by the irradiation of plant sterols and are known as ergocalciferol (Vit.D_2) and dihydrotachysterol. Human sources of vitamin D come from the action of ultraviolet light on the skin, from foods naturally rich in vitamin D, and the addition of synthetic forms of the vitamin to various products, e.g. margarine and baby foods.

Vitamin D is essential for the normal absorption of calcium by the gut and is more potent than parathyroid hormone in this respect. Normal calcification of bone requires the presence of vitamin D, but increased amounts cause bone resorption and, hence, hypercalcaemia.

It has been known for a long time that following the administration of vitamin D there is a time lag before the physiological actions of the vitamin are seen. The reason for this delay is now known to be due to the need to metabolise the vitamin to an active form. The first stage occurs in the liver with the conversion of the native vitamin to 25-hydroxy vitamin D. This compound is then further metabolised in the kidney to 1,25-dihydroxy vitamin D. It is this latter compound that now appears to be the physiologically active form of the vitamin. The kidney also produces a relatively inactive metabolite 24,25-dihydroxy vitamin D; its production is inversely related to the production of 1,25-dihydroxy vitamin D. This means that depending on its physiological needs the kidney can either make a very active vitamin D metabolite or an inactive one.

To add further to the finesse of calcium regulation, it has now been shown that parathyroid hormone helps to regulate vitamin D metabolism in the kidneys and that the vitamin D metabolites influence parathyroid hormone secretion. Hence, there is a delicate interrelationship between parathyroid hormone and vitamin D at numerous sites – namely, intestine, bone, kidney and parathyroid gland.

Alterations and defects of the metabolism of vitamin D are important in several conditions. Anti-epileptic drugs (e.g. phenobarbitone, phenytoin) stimulate a variety of hepatic enzymes that are concerned with the metabolism of drugs within the liver. This may explain why some patients on long term anticonvulsant therapy develop osteomalacia. In kidney failure there is impaired production of the active metabolite, 1,25-dihydroxy vitamin D and severe osteomalacia may occur in cases of long-standing renal failure. Finally, one of the rare inherited forms of rickets – vitamin D dependent rickets – is due to a deficiency of the kidney enzyme necessary to convert 25-hydroxy vitamin D to the 1,25-dihydroxy form of the vitamin.

The overall control of calcium metabolism probably involves an intricate interrelationship among these three substances. The opposing actions of parathyroid hormone and calcitonin may help to explain the precision with which the serum calcium is maintained in the normal individual.

HYPERCALCAEMIA

The symptoms and signs of hypercalcaemia are non-specific and varied. Many systems may be affected:

Kidneys. Hypercalcaemia may be associated with hypercalcuria. This may lead to renal stone formation, nephrocalcinosis, or renal failure and uraemia. In addi-tion, hypercalcaemia interferes with tubular concentrating ability causing polyuria and, hence, increased thirst.

Gastrointestinal Tract. Epigastric pain, nausea, vomiting and constipation are common features. Pancreatitis may occasionally be seen.

Muscle. Muscle weakness is frequently seen in hypercalcaemia, with the proximal muscles in particular being affected.

Metastatic Calcification. This may occur in the conjunctiva of the eyes, causing discomfort and redness of the eye. Deposits in the cornea cause a band keratopathy. Nephrocalcinosis has been mentioned already and other organs may be affected.

Psychiatric and Neurological. A variety of psychiatric conditions may be produced, ranging from depression to psychotic states. With levels of calcium above 4 mmol/1 (16 mg/100 ml) impaired consciousness and, eventually, coma may occur.

Despite the many possible symptoms of hypercalcaemia, it is becoming increasingly common to find, by chance, elevated calcium levels in patients who are symptom-free.

Causes of hypercalcaemia

1. Hyperparathyroidism.
2. Malignancy.
3. Sarcoidosis.
4. Multiple myeloma.
5. Hypervitaminosis D.
6. Thyrotoxicosis.
7. Milk-alkali syndrome.

HYPERPARATHYROIDISM

Definition

Primary hyperparathyroidism (Fig. 11.3) is a condition resulting from the primary over-production of parathyroid hormone.

Background

The incidence of the condition is hard to ascertain at present. Surveys of patients presenting to medical clinics suggest an incidence of about 1 in 850 patients. Eighty per cent of cases are due to a single parathyroid adenoma. Multiple adenomas and diffuse hyperplasia of the parathyroid glands may occur, while parathyroid carcinoma is rare. The manifestations of hypercalcaemia mentioned above may be present and there is also an increased incidence of peptic ulceration. Occasionally, patients with hyperparathyroidism have functional tumours of other glands. These include insulinomas, phaeochromocytomas, pituitary adenomas, gastrin-secreting pancreatic tumours and calcitonin-producing thyroid medullary carcinomas.

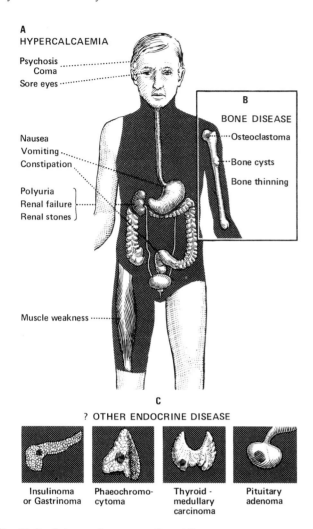

Fig. 11.3 Primary hyperparathyroidism.

Hyperparathyroidism may occur at any age but two-thirds of cases present over the age of 40, women being affected at least twice as frequently as men.

Symptoms and Signs

With the introduction of the multi-channel auto-analyser, serum calcium is being measured in many patients in whom previously no such measurement would have been made. As a result, many more cases of hyperparathyroidism are being diagnosed, many of whom do not have the previously considered classical symptoms of the disease. A number of cases of hyper-parathyroidism seen today have no symptoms of the disease and its discovery is a chance finding. The commonest symptoms of the disease are tiredness, muscle weakness and vague ill-health. Increased thirst,

polyuria, epigastric discomfort, nausea and vomiting may also occur. Except in specialist clinics, the majority of cases seen today do not have renal stones. Of patients presenting with renal stones, only about one per cent will be shown to have hyperparathyroidism, but in cases of multiple renal stones this rises to around five per cent. Clinical bone disease is now rare in Britain except in patients with renal failure. When present the symptoms include bone pain, deformity or fracture.

Investigations

1. The typical serum biochemical changes consist of hypercalcaemia with a lowered serum phosphate (due to the phosphaturic effect of parathyroid hormone). In the presence of clinical bone disease the serum alkaline phosphatase is usually elevated.
2. Radiologically, in cases with bone disease, there may be subperiosteal erosions especially affecting the phalanges, loss of the lamina dura around the teeth, generalised bone demineralisation and, rarely, localised bony tumours, namely, osteoclastomas or bone cysts. Histologically, the classical bone changes are those of osteitis fibrosa cystica.
3. The hypercalcaemia of hyperparathyroidism is not corrected by the administration of cortisone or hydro-cortisone.
4. When the diagnosis is not clear measurement of serum parathyroid hormone concentration may be help-ful. It is elevated in most cases of hyperparathyroidism, but rarely increased in hypercalcaemia due to other causes.

Basis of Treatment

In patients who are symptomatic, parathyroidectomy is indicated. Asymptomatic patients with mild hypercal-caemia and no complications of the disease are in some centres being left untreated. Further follow-up will be needed before knowing whether such a policy is correct.

SECONDARY HYPERPARATHYROIDISM

Hypocalcaemia is a potent stimulus to parathyroid hor-mone secretion. Conditions causing hypocalcaemia, other than hypoparathyroidism, should therefore be associated with a compensatory increase in parathyroid function. The commonest causes of such an increase are renal failure and osteomalacia. The excess parathyroid hormone causes increased bone resorption. Clinical and radiological bone disease may follow. The serum cal-cium is low or normal in such cases, and the alkaline phosphatase is frequently elevated. In renal failure the serum phosphate is high, while in osteomalacia it is usually low. When the underlying condition cannot be treated, vitamin D therapy may be necessary to correct the hypocalcaemia and heal the bone lesions.

TERTIARY HYPERPARATHYROIDISM

Occasionally, after long-standing secondary hyperparathyroidism, the serum calcium may become abnormally high. In such instances it would appear that the chronically stimulated parathyroid glands have become autonomous and are no longer suppressed by hypercalcaemia. Parathyroidectomy may then be necessary to control the hypercalcaemia.

HYPERCALCAEMIA OF MALIGNANCY

Widespread metastases to bone may be associated with hypercalcaemia and this is particularly true with carcinoma of the breast, bronchus, kidney, and prostate. Occasionally, however, hypercalcaemia may be seen in the apparent absence of bone secondaries. This is most frequently seen with hypernephromas and squamous cell carcinoma of the bronchus. In some of these cases, the primary tumour has been shown to produce a substance biologically and immunologically similar to parathyroid hormone. In the majority of cases, however, it appears as though the tumour is secreting compounds completely distinct from parathyroid hormone. The exact nature of these compounds has not been fully elucidated, but in some instances prostaglandins may be involved. The hypercalcaemia is often associated with a raised serum alkaline phosphatase, a reduced serum albumin and elevated serum globulin. Occasionally, the hypercalcaemia is corrected by steroids.

SARCOIDOSIS

The incidence of hypercalcaemia in sarcoidosis has probably been over-estimated in the past and recent surveys have put the incidence at less than five per cent of cases. The hypercalcaemia is readily corrected by corticosteroid administration (*see below*, the hypercalcaemia of hyperparathyroidism). The mechanism of the hypercalcaemia is thought to be due to an increased sensitivity to vitamin D, leading to excessive intestinal absorption of calcium and increased release of calcium from bone.

MULTIPLE MYELOMA (*see* page 402)

In about 20 per cent of cases of myeloma, hypercalcaemia is found. Unlike secondary osseous malignancy, the serum alkaline phosphatase is usually normal. In many cases the hypercalcaemia is corrected by steroid therapy.

HYPERVITAMINOSIS D

Excess vitamin D causes increased bone resorption and, hence, hypercalcaemia. Treatment with large doses of this vitamin is not infrequently complicated by the development of hypercalcaemia, and this danger should be constantly kept in mind when large doses of the vitamin are given, usually in the management of hypoparathyroidism.

THYROTOXICOSIS

Rare cases of thyrotoxicosis have an elevated serum calcium, usually of a mild degree. This is probably related to the action of thyroxine which increases the rate of bone turnover. With control of the hyperthyroidism, the calcium returns to normal.

MILK-ALKALI SYNDROME

This is a very rare cause of hypercalcaemia and is usually associated with progressive renal impairment. It occurs in some cases of peptic ulceration receiving large amounts of milk and alkalis.

Management of the Hypercalcaemic Patient

When a patient is reported to have hypercalcaemia it is advisable to check the serum calcium again before embarking on extensive investigations. If the level is repeatedly high, then a variety of investigations should be performed. The patient should be closely questioned regarding any vitamin D-containing preparations. Radiological studies of the chest and skeleton may bring to light evidence of sarcoidosis, carcinoma of the bronchus, myeloma, or bony secondaries. In females, it is imperative to check carefully for evidence of a primary carcinoma of the breast. The plasma proteins and urine should be examined for evidence of myeloma. Thyroid function studies should be performed when indicated. The presence of renal stones or radiological evidence of subperiosteal erosions almost invariably indicates that the underlying disease is hyperparathyroidism. Should the diagnosis remain uncertain the measurement of the serum parathyroid hormone concentration may be very helpful, being elevated only in hyperparathyroidism (apart from the rare non-parathyroid malignancy which ectopically secretes the hormone). If such hormone assays are unavailable, a hydrocortisone suppression test – 40 mg of hydrocortisone, given eight-hourly for ten days – may occasionally be of use. Should the serum calcium fall to normal values during such a test a diagnosis of hyperparathyroidism is very unlikely. Unfortunately, many cases of hypercalcaemia due to malignancy fail to suppress. Once a diagnosis of hyperparathyroidism has been confirmed, symptomatic cases should be referred for parathyroidectomy.

Corticosteroids are usually effective in controlling the hypercalcaemia of sarcoidosis, hypervitaminosis D, and sometimes of myeloma and other cases of malignancy. The mode of action is not really understood and the minimum dose required to control the hypercalcaemia should be used.

Administration of phosphate readily corrects hypercalcaemia, probably by promoting the formation of calcium phosphate salts in bone. Where specific treatment of the underlying condition is not possible, oral phosphate therapy can be very helpful in relieving the symptoms of hypercalcaemia. A dose of 1 to 2 g of elemental phosphorus per day is usually required. Such doses may cause diarrhoea and epigastric discomfort.

The management of the case of acute, severe hypercalcaemia consists initially of fluid replacement, which in itself causes a fall in the calcium level. Phosphate therapy orally, or when necessary intravenously, will cause a rapid fall in the calcium levels. Once the acute events have been controlled, the patient can be investigated and the underlying condition evaluated.

HYPOCALCAEMIA

The most prominent feature of hypocalcaemia is tetany, which usually occurs when the serum calcium falls below 1.75 mmol/1 (7 mg/100 ml). This causes paraesthesia and numbness in the limbs and face. Muscle cramps are often prominent, carpo-pedal spasm may occur, and in the hands this produces the 'main d'accoucher' with extension of the fingers, flexion at the metacarpo-phalangeal joints and adduction of the thumbs.

Latent tetany may be elicited by Chvostek's and Trousseau's signs. Chvostek's sign consists of a twitching of the face following tapping on the facial nerve in front of the ear. Trousseau's sign is the production of carpal spasm when a sphygmomanometer cuff applied to the upper arm is inflated above systolic pressure for three minutes.

In addition to hypocalcaemia, tetany may be seen in alkalotic conditions such as that produced by hyperventilation and, occasionally, in hypokalaemia and hypomagnesaemia.

Other features of hypocalcaemia include coarse, dry skin, alopecia, brittle nails, cataracts, depression, weakness, calcification of the basal ganglia and prolongation of the Q-T interval of the electrocardiograph.

Causes of hypocalcaemia

1. Hypoparathyroidism and pseudo-hypoparathyroidism.
2. Renal failure.
3. Osteomalacia or rickets.
4. Acute pancreatitis.
5. Low serum proteins – in this circumstance the ionised calcium is normal.

HYPOPARATHYROIDISM

Definition

A condition of undersecretion of parathyroid hormone by the parathyroid glands.

Background

The commonest form of hypoparathyroidism is seen following surgical removal of the thyroid gland. The incidence is hard to ascertain, but overt hypoparathyroidism is probably seen in less than one per cent of patients after thyroidectomy. As well as actual removal of parathyroid glands, interference with the blood supply of the parathyroid glands during the operation is probably of importance. Symptoms of tetany usually occur within the first week or two after the operation. Occasionally, a long period may elapse before the hypoparathyroidism becomes manifest.

Idiopathic hypoparathyroidism is a rare condition. Occasionally in this condition, there is associated hypoadrenalism and hypothyroidism. In such cases antibodies to adrenal, thyroid, and parathyroid tissue may be found. In addition to the features of hypocalcaemia mentioned above, there may also be widespread cutaneous moniliasis.

Cases of hypoparathyroidism respond to injected parathyroid hormone with an increased excretion of phosphate and cyclic adenosine monophosphate in the urine. Treatment is with calcium supplements and vitamin D – 50,000 to 100,000 units usually being required daily. (At present long term therapy with parathyroid hormone is not possible.)

In pseudo-hypoparathyroidism the biochemical changes are similar to those seen in hypoparathyroidism in that the serum calcium is low and the phosphate high. These patients, however, do not show any significant response to injected parathyroid hormone and, in fact, show high concentrations of parathyroid hormone in the blood. This condition has been attributed to a defect in the receptor tissues for parathyroid hormone, so that the tissues are unable to respond to the hormone. Clinical features frequently seen in this disorder are short stature, round faces, skeletal abnormalities, especially short metacarpal and metatarsal bones, ectopic calcification, and mild mental deficiency.

RENAL FAILURE (*see* page 198)

RICKETS AND OSTEOMALACIA (*see* page 197)

ACUTE PANCREATITIS

Transient hypocalcaemia may be seen in cases of acute pancreatitis. The calcium becomes complexed to the products of enzymic fat digestion. Severe hypocalcaemia is a bad prognostic sign.

DISEASES OF THE BONE

OSTEOPOROSIS

Definition

Osteoporosis is a condition in which there is a reduction of the amount of otherwise normal bone.

Background

Investigation of normal subjects shows that with increasing age there is a gradual reduction in bone density, which tends to be accelerated in women following the menopause. In some patients there seems to be an increase in this apparently natural loss of bone, leading to clinical symptoms, particularly in later life; hence the terms post-menopausal and senile osteoporosis. The condition is unusual in children and young adults.

In the majority of cases there seems to be no underlying cause for the osteoporosis, but a variety of conditions may be associated with the disorder. These include:
1. Cushing's syndrome or steroid administration.
2. Immobilisation.
3. Rheumatoid arthritis.
4. Thyrotoxicosis.

Symptoms

None.
Episodes of sudden severe backache (often associated with pathological fracture).
Chronic backache.

Signs

Loss of height.
Kyphosis and other spinal deformity.

Investigations

The exact cause of osteoporosis remains unclear. Studies of bone kinetics have brought conflicting results, but the majority suggest that bone formation is normal whereas bone resorption is increased.
1. Biochemical investigations are unrewarding as the serum calcium, phosphate and alkaline phosphatase are normal.

2. Radiologically, in addition to decreased bone density, there may be changes due to vertebral collapse, with wedging of the vertebrae.

Basis of Treatment

Many treatments for osteoporosis have been suggested, but to date none has been proven to cure or correct the disease. It is possible that in some cases progression of the disease has been prevented, but even this claim is uncertain. It should be remembered that the clinical manifestations of the disease are often intermittent and that there may be severe disease detectable by X-rays without clinical symptoms. The most common forms of treatment at present used include calcium or phosphate supplements and treatment with sex hormones. Calcium and vitamin D supplements certainly should be given if there is any evidence of a dietary deficiency.

Immobilisation, except during periods of acute exacerbations, should be avoided and the use of spinal supports discouraged.

PAGET'S DISEASE OF BONE (OSTEITIS DEFORMANS) (Fig. 11.4)

Definition

A condition of localised or generalised formation of excessive spongy bone with simultaneous reabsorption of bone of normal architecture.

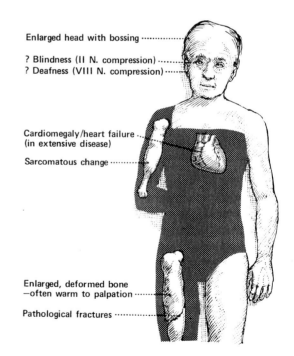

Fig. 11.4 Paget's disease of bone.

Background

In many countries Paget's disease is the most common generalised bone disease, other than osteoporosis, and autopsy studies in patients over the age of 40 have shown it to be present in up to three per cent of the population. However, many cases are subclinical, so that clinical manifestations of the disease are rare.

In Paget's disease there is an increased production and reabsorption of bone, producing an abnormal, spongy type of bone with coarse trabeculae. Within this there are often areas of very dense bone. There is also a marked increase in bone vascularity. The disease is usually localised to one or several areas of the skeleton, but, occasionally, may be quite widespread. The bones most commonly affected are the tibia, femur, pelvis, spine, clavicle, and the skull.

Symptoms and Signs

The commonest symptom is pain in the areas of bony involvement. With extensive involvement, bones become enlarged and deformed and this is seen most prominently in the tibiae and femora. When the skull is affected it may lead to a marked enlargement in head circumference, while the facial bones are often unaffected.

Investigations

Biochemically, the serum calcium and phosphate are normal, but there is usually a marked elevation of the serum alkaline phosphatase.

Complications

Various complications may occur of which the commonest is fracture occurring through the abnormal bone.
The increased vascularity of the affected area may lead to the development of 'high-output' cardiac failure.
Cranial nerve lesions especially of the eighth nerve occur.
The most serious complication is the development of an osteogenic sarcoma, which occurs in less than one per cent of cases and which occurs most frequently in the skull and humerus. Such a change is usually associated with the development of persistent, severe, localised pain.
Hypercalcaemia may occur with immobilisation.

Basis of Treatment

Treatment of the condition until recently was unsatisfactory. Little can be done to prevent bony deformity. Bone pain should be treated with simple analgesics. Trials with calcitonin have produced very promising improvements in symptoms, together with return of the biochemical changes towards normal. It is costly and should be reserved for those with severe symptoms. Calcitonin has to be given as daily subcutaneous injections.

RICKETS AND OSTEOMALACIA

Definition

Rickets and osteomalacia are identical conditions associated with an increase in the amount of osteoid tissue which fails to calcify at a normal rate.

Background

Changes are produced by a variety of disorders, particularly by a deficiency of vitamin D or a resistance to its action. In children, this results in the clinical disorder of rickets, while in adults osteomalacia is produced. Because significant amounts of vitamin D are produced in the skin, a vitamin D-deficient diet probably needs to be supplemented by a lack of exposure to sunlight before clinical rickets is produced. Rickets as a dietary deficiency disease is, therefore, virtually confined to the inhabitants of overcrowded slum areas, where the combination of poor diet and inadequate sunlight operates. The commonest group of people in Britain with osteomalacia are the Asians, there being a high incidence of clinical disease in neonates, growing children and pregnant women. The incidence of clinical rickets in Asian school children may be as high as fifteen per cent. The reason for such a high incidence is probably due to a combination of a diet low in vitamin D and high in phytate, and avoidance of the sun. Poor diet, together with little exposure to sunlight, is seen also in elderly and infirm patients and there is an increased incidence of osteomalacia in such people.

People with intestinal malabsorption due to any cause usually have an impaired absorption of both vitamin D and calcium and are consequently very prone to develop osteomalacia unless adequate supplements are given. In all the above circumstances the condition can be explained by a deficiency of normal amounts of vitamin D. Biochemically, such patients usually have a lowered serum calcium and phosphate and an elevated serum alkaline phosphatase.

In addition to osteomalacia or rickets due to a deficiency of vitamin D, there are a group of disorders causing rickets in which the condition cannot be healed by the administration of physiological amounts of vitamin D. Previously, such conditions were grouped together under the title of vitamin D-resistant rickets. Recent advances allow a more rational nomenclature. Vitamin D-dependent rickets is a rare condition usually transmitted by a recessive gene. The biochemistry and clinical presentation is similar to nutritional rickets. The disease, however, can only be healed with doses of vitamin D around 50,000 units daily. On such doses *complete* healing occurs. The disorder appears to be due to a renal deficiency of the enzyme converting 25-hydroxy vitamin D to 1,25-hydroxy vitamin D. The other group of resistant rickets is hypophosphataemic rickets in which there is a defect in renal phosphate handling. This results in the loss of large amounts of phosphate in the urine and a marked fall in the serum phosphate. In other cases there are multiple renal tubular defects leading to combinations of phosphaturia, glycosuria and adminoaciduria (Fanconi's syndrome). A third type of tubular defect that may cause rickets is renal tubular acidosis. These hypophosphataemic forms of rickets are often familial and are usually associated with a normal serum calcium, a very low serum phosphate and an elevated alkaline phosphatase. Unlike vitamin D-dependent rickets complete healing seldom occurs even on massive doses of vitamin D.

Other conditions causing rickets or osteomalacia are chronic renal disease, which is considered later, and hypophosphatasia. This latter condition is a rare disorder characterised by defective mineralisation of bone and a deficiency of bone alkaline phosphatase and, hence, low serum alkaline phosphatase. The disease may present in childhood or in adult life and is further characterised by the excretion of phosphoethanolamine in the urine.

RICKETS

Symptoms and Signs

Bowing of legs.
Waddling gait due to coxa vara deformity of femoral neck and muscle hypotonia.
Misery.
Tetany, fits, and laryngeal spasm.
Widening of epiphyses.
Rickety rosary due to expanded costochondral junctions of ribs.
Softening of the cranial bones (craniotabes).
A Harrison's sulcus (depression of the chest wall in the region of the sixth rib).

OSTEOMALACIA

Symptoms and Signs

Waddling gait.
Generalised bone pains.
Bone deformity due to bending and fracture.

Investigations

Radiologically, the bones have an increased translucency, and deformity of the spine, pelvis and leg bones may be apparent.

Looser's zones may be seen. These consist of perpendicular bands of decalcification running in from the surface of the bone, surrounded by a denser area of callus formation. These zones occur at areas of increased stress, or at the site of nutrient arteries, and are most commonly seen around the neck of the femur, humerus, pelvic rami, ribs, and borders of the scapulae.

Basis of Treatment

Simple vitamin D-deficiency rickets is treated with 2,000 to 4,000 units of vitamin D daily for up to six months, followed by maintenance doses of 400 units a day.

Vitamin D-dependent rickets requires daily doses of vitamin D of around 50,000 units per day. Hypophosphataemic rickets may require doses of up to 100,000 to 400,000 units a day. In addition, phosphate supplements are often beneficial and may allow healing with smaller doses of vitamin D.

Close laboratory monitoring is required as the risk of hypercalcaemia is very real. When underlying malabsorption is present this should, wherever possible, be treated, e.g. by a gluten-free diet in coeliac disease, but vitamin D supplements may also be required.

RENAL OSTEODYSTROPHY (*see also* page 232)

Definition

The various forms of metabolic bone disease which complicate renal failure are collectively known as renal osteodystrophy.

Background

The recent successful management of chronic renal failure with diet, dialysis, and renal transplanation has emphasised the severe disturbances of calcium metabolism seen in renal failure.

In both acute and chronic renal failure there is a fall in the serum calcium. In acute renal disease this may be consequent on the sudden rapid rise in the serum phosphate, while in chronic renal failure there seems to be a resistance to the action of vitamin D. This, therefore, leads eventually, in some cases, to the development of rickets or osteomalacia, with similar features to those mentioned above. The occurrence of hypocalcaemia, however, causes increased secretion of parathyroid hormone in an attempt to correct the low calcium levels (secondary hyperparathyroidism). Despite this, the serum calcium often remains low in renal failure. The prolonged stimulus to the parathyroid glands, however, may lead to the development of overt bony changes of hyperparathyroidism. Eventually, sufficient parathyroid hormone may be produced to correct completely the hypocalcaemia. Rarely, this may be followed by an increase in the serum calcium to abnormally high levels, due presumably to the grossly overactive parathyroid glands becoming autonomous (tertiary hyperparathyroidism).

Symptoms and Signs

May be none.
Bone pains.
Sore eyes, conjunctivitis (metastatic calcification in the conjunctiva).
Bone deformity.

Basis of Treatment

Vitamin D therapy requires very careful monitoring because of the risk of hypercalcaemia and metastatic calcification. The risk of the latter may be reduced by lowering the serum phosphorus with oral aluminium hydroxide which binds phosphate in the gut.

Recently the synthetic vitamin D metabolite 1-a-cholecalciferol has become available. This compound is fully active in patients with renal failure and may be more useful than conventional vitamin D therapy. Its exact role in renal osteodystrophy has yet to be decided, and its extreme potency necessitates marked caution in its use. Daily requirements appear to be between 1 and 2 μg a day.

OSTEOPETROSIS

Definition

This is a rare condition of greatly increased bone density, probably due to impaired resorption of bone.

Background

The condition may be transmitted by either recessive or dominant inheritance, but the former is more common. Despite the increased bone density, the bones have an increased tendency to fracture. Some cases are associated with anaemia and hepatosplenomegaly. Part of the anaemia may be due to encroachment on the marrow by the bone but, in addition, extravascular haemolysis often plays an important role in the genesis of the anaemia. The disease tends to be more severe in children.

Biochemically, the serum calcium, phosphate and alkaline phosphatase are normal.

Treatment is unsatisfactory, but severe restriction of dietary calcium occasionally appears to limit the progress of the condition.

OSTEOGENESIS IMPERFECTA

Definition

This is a condition in which there is an increased tendency for the bones to fracture when exposed to minor trauma.

Background

This is often associated with a definite blue colour of the sclera of the eyes and, rarely, with deafness from otosclerosis. Transmission is usually by a dominant gene, although a recessive inheritance may be seen.

A whole range of severity may be seen with the most severe cases presenting with multiple fractures *in utero*, while in the milder cases the increased liability to fracture may not occur until adulthood. Because of the multiple fractures, bony deformity is common in severely affected patients. It is not unusual for the condition to improve after puberty.

The serum calcium and phosphorus are normal as is the alkaline phosphatase, except when it is raised at the time of a new fracture.

ACHONDROPLASIA

This condition, which has an incidence of about 1 in 10,000, is due to an inherited disorder of cartilage growth and endochondral bone formation. Clinically, this leads to a characteristic picture of severe dwarfism, due predominantly to shortening of the extremities. The arms and legs, in addition to being short, are often bowed. The spine is often kyphotic and is associated with a marked backward rotation of the sacrum, thus making the buttocks prominent. The skull is less obviously affected, but there is usually a marked depression of the bridge of the nose and, because of the severe dwarfism, the head often appears disproportionately large. Many cases die *in utero*, but those surviving often have a normal life expectancy. Mental development is normal, as is physical strength.

Biochemical studies are normal and no treatment is available.

SUGGESTED FURTHER READING

General

Paterson, C. R. (1974) *Metabolic Disorders of Bone*. London: Blackwell.
Potts, J. T. jnr. and Deftos, L. J. (1974) Parathyroid hormone, thyrocalcitonin, vitamin D, bone and bone mineral metabolism. In *Duncan's Diseases of Metabolism*. Philadelphia: W. B. Saunders.

Bone

Wadkins, C. L., Luben, R., Thomas, M. and Humphreys, R. (1974) Physical biochemistry of calcification. *Clinical Orthopaedics*, **99**: 246–266.

Control of Calcium Metabolism

Rasmussen, H., Bordier, P., Kurokawa, K., Nagata, N. and Ogata, E. (1974) Hormonal control of skeletal and mineral metabolism. *American Journal of Medicine*, **56**: 751–758.

Deluca, H. F. and Schnoes, H. K. (1976) Metabolism and mechanism of action of vitamin D. *Annual Review of Biochemistry*, **45**: 631–666.

Hyperparathyroidism

Mallette, L. E., Bilezikian, J. P., Heath, D. A. and Aurbach, G. D. (1974) Primary hyperparathyroidism. *Medicine*, **53**: 291–294.

Pyrah, L. N., Hodgkinson, A. and Anderson, C. K. (1966) Primary hyperparathyroidism. *British Journal of Surgery*, **53**: 245–316.

Hypoparathyroidism

Dimich, A., Bedrossian, P. B. and Wallach, S. (1967) Hypoparathyroidism. *Archives of Internal Medicine*, **120**: 449–458.

Osteoporosis

Thompson, D. L. and Frame, B. (1976) Involutional osteopenia – current concepts. *Annals of Internal Medicine*, **85**: 789–803.

Dent, C. E. and Watson, L. (1966) Osteoporosis. *Postgraduate Medical Journal*, October suppl. 1–28.

Paget's disease

Barry, H. C. (1969) *Paget's Disease of Bone*. Edinburgh: Livingstone.

Galbraith, H-J. B., Evans, E. C. and Lacey, J. (1977) Paget's disease of bone – a clinical and genetic study. *Postgraduate Medical Journal*, **53**: 33–39.

Rickets and Osteomalacia

Holmes, A. M., Enoch, B. A., Taylor, J. L. and Jones, M. E. (1973) Occult rickets and osteomalacia amongst the Asian immigrant population. *Quarterly Journal of Medicine*, **42**: 125–149.

Goel, K. M., Logan, R. W., Arneil, G. C., Sweet, E. M., Warren, J. M., and Shanks, R. A. (1976) Florid and subclinical rickets among immigrant children in Glasgow. *Lancet* **i**: 1141–1145.

Walton, J. (1976) Familial hypophosphataemic rickets – a delineation of its subdivision and pathogenesis. *Clinical Paediatrics*, **15**: 1007–1012.

Poisoning

12

A. J. MARSHALL

Definition

Poison. A substance which kills or impairs health if introduced into the body. Some substances, for example cyanide, are always poisonous. Others, for example iron, only become so if taken in high dosage (overdose).

Classification of poisoning

Intentional self poisoning
Accidental poisoning
Iatrogenic (doctor induced) poisoning
Homicidal poisoning

INTENTIONAL SELF POISONING

'Gun's aren't lawful,
Nooses give,
Gas smells awful,
You may as well live.'   (Dorothy Parker)

This is wise advice, yet in developed countries self poisoning has become a modern epidemic. One in six patients admitted as a medical emergency to a British hospital has deliberately taken an overdose. The number has doubled in the last decade. Women outnumber men 2:1. The peak age is between 20 and 30 years and 75 per cent are under 40. A wide range of people poison themselves (1 in 50 doctors commits suicide). Some patients are depressed and others are psychopaths. Many take an overdose on sudden impulse as a reaction to some social or psychological stress. Twenty-five per cent have a history of repeated self poisoning.

The majority do not actually intend to die. In Britain about 2,500 men and 1,500 women kill themselves each year. The incidence of suicide increases with age. It is usually achieved by poisoning. Hanging, shooting, jumping and cutting are now unfashionable. The drugs used for self poisoning change with current prescribing

habits and availability. The most common taken at present are listed below:

Type of drug	Examples
Tranquillisers and non-barbiturate hypnotics	Benzodiazepines: Nitrazepam Diazepam Flurazepam Phenothiazines: Chlorpromazine Thioridazine
Analgesics	Aspirin Paracetamol Dextropropoxyphene
Antidepressants	Tricyclics: Amitriptyline Imipramine Monoamine oxidase inhibitors
Barbiturates	Phenobarbitone Amylobarbitone

Cocktails

Thirty per cent of patients admitted have taken mixtures of drugs and alcohol. Drug interactions can then be important. For instance alcohol potentiates the effect of the hypnotic, chloral hydrate. This interaction when popularly realised resulted in the 'Mickey Finn' cocktail for rapid induction of unconsciousness.

ACCIDENTAL POISONING

This only usually occurs in children under 10 years of age. In adults, the explanation that a self poisoning is accidental should not be accepted without a searching enquiry. Exposure to poison is sometimes an occupational hazard and industrial and agricultural workers may unintentionally ingest or inhale poison at work.

IATROGENIC POISONING

This may be due to a relative overdose due to an underlying abnormality in the patient. An example of this is digoxin poisoning in a patient with renal failure. The rate of excretion is reduced. Despite being taken in normal dosage high and harmful blood levels result.

Adverse reactions to drugs are quite common. They take many forms (*see* Chapter 13). All cases should be reported to the Committee on Safety of Medicines (on yellow cards).

HOMICIDAL POISONING

Although rare, the possibility should not be forgotten.

Poison Information Centres

Information on the toxicity of a drug and the treatment of poisoning is available at any time from one of the specialist centres.

Poison centre		Telephone
London	Guy's Hospital	01-407 7600
Edinburgh	Royal Infirmary	031-229 2477
Cardiff	Royal Infirmary	0222-33101
Belfast	Royal Victoria Hospital	0232-40503
Manchester	Booth Hall Children's Hospital	061-740 225
Newcastle	Royal Victoria Infirmary	0632-25131
Leeds	General Infirmary	0533-32799

Medico-Legal Aspects

All deaths from poisoning from any cause, intentional, accidental, occupational, therapeutic or homicidal must be reported to the coroner. Accurate documentation is vital not only for the clinical management of a poisoned patient but also for legal reasons. Tablets, gastric washings and a heparinised sample of venous blood should be kept for examination in case the patient dies.

Sometimes patients who take poison are in physical danger but are unwilling to accept treatment. An order under the *Mental Health Act*, 1959 can then be made. Section 29 allows for emergency admission, Section 25 detention in a mental hospital for observation, and Section 30 retention in hospital.

Principles of Management

Medical. To save the patient's life. Transfer to hospital is recommended for all cases.

Psychiatric. Patients who intentionally poison themselves should have a psychiatric assessment. This should be done as soon as possible and *before* discharge from hospital.

The size of the overdose does not correlate with the severity of the underlying psychiatric or social upset. (Patients are not pharmacologists.)

History

Poisoning is the most likely reason for a young or middle-aged patient presenting in coma. However, other causes must always be considered. The diagnostic clues come from a complete history and examination (Fig. 12.1).

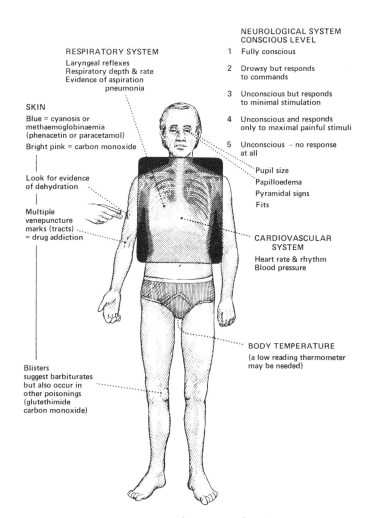

RESPIRATORY SYSTEM
Laryngeal reflexes
Respiratory depth & rate
Evidence of aspiration pneumonia

SKIN
Blue = cyanosis or methaemoglobinaemia (phenacetin or paracetamol)
Bright pink = carbon monoxide

Look for evidence of dehydration

Multiple venepuncture marks (tracts) = drug addiction

Blisters suggest barbiturates but also occur in other poisonings (glutethimide carbon monoxide)

NEUROLOGICAL SYSTEM CONSCIOUS LEVEL
1 Fully conscious
2 Drowsy but responds to commands
3 Unconscious but responds to minimal stimulation
4 Unconscious and responds only to maximal painful stimuli
5 Unconscious – no response at all

Pupil size
Papilloedema
Pyramidal signs
Fits

CARDIOVASCULAR SYSTEM
Heart rate & rhythm
Blood pressure

BODY TEMPERATURE
(a low reading thermometer may be needed)

Fig. 12.1   The examination of a poisoned patient.

Differential Diagnosis (*see also* page 515)

1. Head injury.
2. Epileptic fit.
3. Stroke.
4. Meningitis.
5. Metabolic coma:
   Diabetes (hypo- or hyperglycaemia).
   Uraemia.
   Hepatic failure.
   Pituitary or adrenal insufficiency.
6. Respiratory failure.

In poisoning find out:
(a) When the poison was taken.
(b) The time of onset of symptoms.
(c) The patient's previous physical and psychiatric illnesses.
(d) If possible, identify the poison. Tablet identification charts are available.

Patients are often unreliable. Better information may be obtained from relatives, the family doctor, ambulance men or police. They might have found tablets, drug bottles or a suicide note with the patient.

Investigations

The tests and indications for common investigations of poisoning are shown in Table 12.1.

Table 12.1 Investigations of poisoning

Test	Indications
Toxicology	
Plasma levels	Salicylate
	Paracetamol
Spectroscopy	Carbon monoxide (carboxyhaemoglobin)
Urine	Phenistix (+ if salicylate)
	Paraquat test (specific poisons)
	Save samples for legal reasons
Urea and electrolytes	Forced diuresis
	Salicylate poisoning
	Dehydration
	Hypotension
	Renal failure
Blood sugar	Differential diagnosis
	Paracetamol (low in liver failure)
Blood gases	Respiratory depression
Chest X-ray	Respiratory depression
	Aspiration
Electrocardiogram	Tricyclic antidepressants
	Phenothiazines (arrhythmias occur)

Basis of Treatment

1. Treat special complications of poisoning.
2. Eliminate poison.
3. Care of the comatose patient (*see* page 515).

Complications

Respiratory failure.
Arrhythmias.
Hypothermia.
Hypotension.

Respiratory Depression. Five to ten per cent of poisoned patients need endotracheal intubation at some time. Two to five per cent have to be mechanically ventilated.

Poisoning causes some depression of consciousness in one-quarter of cases and it is essential that the airway and lungs should be protected in these. To prevent aspiration of vomit the patient should be transferred to hospital and nursed in a lateral position with an airway inserted if necessary. Endotracheal intubation should be carried out before gastric lavage if the laryngeal and pharyngeal reflexes are absent.

When there is any doubt about the adequacy of breathing the opinion of an anaesthetist should be sought. The signs of respiratory depression are reduced depth and rate of breathing, and cyanosis. The decision to ventilate the unconscious patient is based on blood gases and the presence of respiratory complications such as retention of lung secretions. When the Po_2 is reduced but Pco_2 is normal, artificial ventilation may not be needed. The patient should breathe 24 to 28 per cent oxygen through a Ventimask and be closely observed for any signs of deterioration. Respiratory failure is present when the Po_2 is below 8.0 kPa (60 mmHg) and the Pco_2 more than 6.7 kPa (50 mmHg).

Respiratory depression due to opiate or dextropropoxyphene poisoning is improved by giving the antagonist naloxone (preferable to nalorphine which has some agonist activity).

Arrhythmias. A serious cardiac arrhythmia can occur after poisoning with a tricyclic antidepressant or phenothiazine. It may start at any time during the first twenty-four hours. Continuous electrocardiographic monitoring throughout this time is recommended after a large overdose of these drugs. Conduction abnormalities, a prolonged Q-T interval, S-T segment changes, supraventricular and ventricular tachyarrhythmias are described. Treatment with an antiarrhythmic agent or cardiac pacing depends on the type of cardiac disturbance.

Hypothermia. This is particularly common after barbiturate or phenothiazine poisoning. It is diagnosed using a low reading thermometer and is both prevented and treated by covering with adequate blankets.

Hypotension (Fig. 12.2). This usually results from hypovolaemia. The signs are a falling systolic blood pressure to below 10.6 kPa (80 mmHg) and evidence of poor tissue perfusion (pallor, cold extremities and little

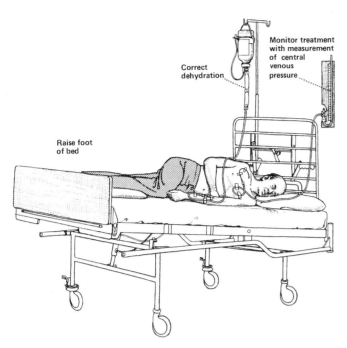

Fig. 12.2 The management of hypotension.

urine). The aim of treatment is to increase cardiac filling pressure so that the output from the left ventricle is adequate to perfuse the vital organs. Venous return to the heart is enhanced by raising the legs. Dehydration is corrected with intravenous 5 per cent dextrose and plasma volume increased with plasma protein fraction or dextran. The infusion of all fluids should be carefully monitored with a central venous pressure line. Respiratory failure, hypothermia and arrhythmias, if present, should be treated. If these measures fail and hypotension is life-threatening, then a pressor agent like metaraminol can be used. This is the last resort because the rise in blood pressure it causes is only obtained at the expense of a further drop in tissue perfusion due to vasoconstriction.

Elimination of Poison

Possible methods for the elimination of poison are:
1. Gastric aspiration and lavage.
2. Forced diuresis.
3. Dialysis.
4. Specific antidotes.

Gastric Aspiration and Lavage (Fig. 12.3). This is worthwhile provided that the patient has not swallowed paraffin, corrosives or caustics and that the drug has been taken by mouth within the last four hours. The time period is less important with salicylates which cause pylorospasm and can remain in the stomach for twenty-four hours. A wide bore, lubricated Jacques tube is used (size 30 in adults). To ensure that it is in the stomach and not the lungs the aspirate should be tested

with blue litmus paper. Stomach contents produce an acid reaction. Aspiration is advisable before lavage, as otherwise, more of the drug may be driven into the small bowel and absorbed. Lavage is usually carried out with tepid tap water, 300 ml on each occasion, until the siphoned washings are clear. (*For glutethimide* – water and castor oil in equal quantities, *for cyanide* – 25 per cent sodium thiosulphate.) Gastric lavage should not be performed just as a punishment. It must never be done when a patient is deeply unconscious until a cuffed endotracheal tube is inserted, because of the risk of aspiration pneumonia.

Producing vomiting with ipecacuanha is only preferred as the method of emptying the stomach in children. For them it is safer and less frightening. Stomach intubation is necessary to leave substances in the stomach, for example desferrioxamine after iron poisoning. Ipecacuanha syrup, 15 ml, followed by a large drink induces vomiting within twenty minutes. Saline emetics should never be used. Fatal salt poisoning as a result has been described.

Forced Diuresis (Fig. 12.4). Some poisons which are excreted in the urine can be removed more rapidly by increasing diuresis. When a drug is ionised it is less lipid-soluble and is less likely to be reabsorbed when passing through the renal tubules. The value of altering the pH of the urine is that acid drugs (e.g. salicylates) are more ionised in a basic medium and bases (e.g. amphetamine) in acid. Urinary excretion is therefore increased by maintaining a urinary pH which renders the drug ionised.

Forced diuresis carries the risk of causing fluid overload and electrolyte abnormalities (the dangers are small

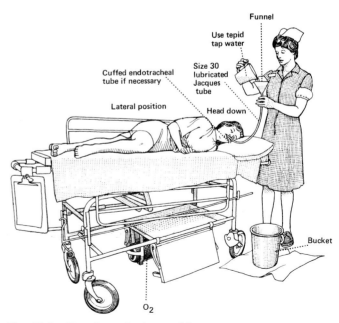

Fig. 12.3 Gastric aspiration and lavage.

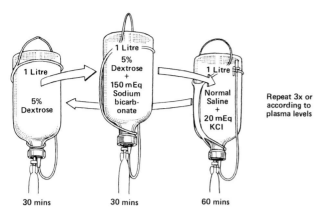

Fig. 12.4 Forced alkaline diuresis: IV fluid requirements.

in young healthy adults). An alkaline diuresis accelerates the excretion of salicylate and the long-acting barbiturates (barbitone; phenobarbitone).

A forced acid diuresis for amphetamine poisoning is similar to that above with the substitution of 1.5 g of ammonium chloride in 5 per cent dextrose for bicarbonate.

Dialysis. Both peritoneal and haemodialysis have been used to treat severe poisoning. It is usually unnecessary to consider either unless a patient is clearly not responding to other treatment. A poison centre should be consulted to ensure that the poison is dialysable. Occasionally, dialysis is used when it is impossible to give a forced intravenous diuresis (due to cardiac or renal failure).

Specific Antidotes. There are few real antidotes, but some that are of use are listed below. A chelating agent (e.g. desferrioxamine, dimercaprol) is a substance which forms a stable complex with a metal ion (chele = claw).

Poison	Antidote
Iron	Desferrioxamine
Arsenic	Dimercaprol
Mercury	(BAL British
Gold	Anti-Lewisite)
Lead	Sodium calcium edetate
Cyanide	Amyl nitrite and sodium thiosulphate
Opiates	Naloxone
Carbon monoxide	Oxygen
Methanol	Ethanol
Organo-phosphorus insecticides	Pralidoxime and atropine
Paracetamol	Cysteamine or methionine

SPECIFIC POISONS

TRANQUILLISERS AND NON-BARBITURATE HYPNOTICS

BENZODIAZEPINES (e.g. chlordazepoxide (Librium), diazepam (Valium), nitrazepam (Mogadon), flurazepam (Dalmane))

Dose causing severe poisoning, 10 to 20 g.
(*See* Table 12.2 for clinical features etc.).
These are now the most frequently used drugs for self poisoning. Fortunately most patients recover without specific therapy.

PHENOTHIAZINES
(e.g. chlorpromazine (Largactil), thioridazine (Melleril))

Dose causing severe poisoning, 1 g (20 × 50 mg tablets chlorpromazine).
(*See* Table 12.3 for clinical features etc.)

GLUTETHIMIDE (Doriden)

Dose causing severe poisoning, 10 g (40 tablets).
(*See* Table 12.4 for clinical features etc.)

ANALGESICS

SALICYLATE (Table 12.5)

There are over 50 pharmaceutical preparations which contain salicylate. Many can be bought without prescription. (Examples: Anadin, Alka Seltzer, Beechams Powders, Disprin, Phensic, Hypon.)

The dose causing severe poisoning is 15 g (50 × 300 mg tablets aspirin). The patient may look well despite taking a serious overdose of salicylate (Fig. 12.5).

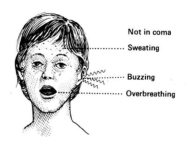

Fig. 12.5 Serious salicylate poisoning.

Table 12.2 Poisoning with benzodiazepines

Clinical features	Cause	Biochemistry	Clinical care
Coma	Sedative effect on brain	Serum levels not helpful and low	1. Intensive supportive therapy
Occasionally excited, euphoric			2. Gastric lavage within 4 hours
Bradycardia			3. Psychiatric opinion
Hypotension			
Respiratory depression			

Table 12.3 Poisoning with phenothiazines

Clinical features	Cause	Biochemistry	Clinical care
Coma	Sedative effect on brain	Serum levels (i) Not routine	1. Intensive supportive therapy
Muscle rigidity	Stimulant effect on basal ganglia	(ii) Not helpful (low serum levels)	2. Gastric lavage within 4 hours
Tremor			3. Treat cardiac arrhythmias.
Dyskinesia			4. Treat convulsions
Convulsions	Lowering of seizure threshold		5. Psychiatric opinion
Hypotension	Adrenergic blockade		
Tachycardia and cardiac arrhythmias			
Respiratory depression	Sedative effect on brain		
Hypothermia			

Table 12.4 Glutethimide poisoning

Clinical features	Cause	Biochemistry	Clinical care
Fluctuating conscious state	Sedative effect on brain	Acidosis common	1. Intensive supportive therapy
Coma (intermittent)			2. Gastric lavage within 4 hours:
Aggressive when conscious			Use water and caster oil in equal quantities
Apnoea	Raised intracranial pressure		3. Treat acidosis
Papilloedema	Cerebral oedema		4. Treat cerebral oedema (mannitol I.V.)
Dilated pupils			5. Psychiatric opinion
Severe hypotension			
Myocardial damage			
Convulsions (during recovery)			

Table 12.5 Salicylate poisoning

Clinical features	Cause	Biochemistry	Clinical care
Not initially in coma		Routine serum salicylate level	1. Gastric lavage
Tinnitus	Direct effect of drug		2. Forced alkaline diuresis
Overbreathing	Direct effect on respiratory centre	Severe case if level is greater than 50 mg/100 ml	3. I.V. fluids to correct dehydration and hypokalaemia
Hyperpyrexia	Increased metabolic rate	Beware in an untreated case the level may later increase	
Vomiting ?haematemesis	Gastric irritation	Initially, respiratory alkalosis from overbreathing, i.e. $pH\uparrow$, $PCO_2\downarrow$	4. I.M. vit.K (hypoprothrombinaemia)
Sweating	Direct effect on sweat glands		5. Psychiatric opinion
Dehydration and K^+ loss	Vomiting, sweating, overbreathing		
Coma	1. Acid/base disturbance uraemia and dehydration	Then metabolic acidosis i.e. $pH\downarrow$, $PCO_2\downarrow$	
	2. Direct effect on brain		

PARACETAMOL (e.g. Panadol, Distalgesic, Safapryn, Veganin)

It is a commonly used analgesic and is readily available without prescription. Self poisoning is increasing.
The dose causing liver damage can be as little as 6 g (12 × 500 mg tablets paracetamol). Death can occur after 15 g.

The great danger of paracetamol overdosage is of liver failure due to centrilobular hepatic necrosis. A small proportion of paracetamol is converted by a liver mixed function oxidase to a toxic metabolite. This binds to vital liver cell macromolecules. After a normal dose, the harmful metabolite is detoxified within the liver cells by conjugation with glutathione (a source of SH groups). When an overdose is taken this mechanism may be overwhelmed and liver cell damage result.

The place of antidotes in treatment has yet to be established. The most tried are intravenous cysteamine and oral methionine. These are precursors of glutathione and may prevent or lessen hepatotoxicity. Cysteamine does not have a product licence, but is available for use on the clinician's own responsibility. It makes the patient feel ill, causing vomiting, abdominal pain, drowsiness and flushing. Methionine is less unpleasant. There is a danger of precipitating hepatic coma if either antidote is given more than ten hours after the overdose. By then the liver is damaged and may be unable to metabolise them.
Paracetamol levels are of some therapeutic value.

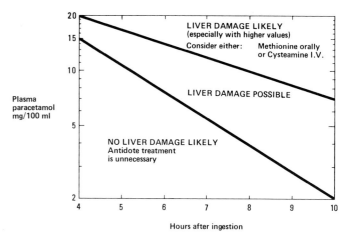

Fig. 12.6 Paracetamol overdose: therapeutic possibilities are determined by blood drug concentrations.

Antidote should only be given to patients who are seen early and in whom liver toxicity is likely (Fig. 12.6).
Further details of paracetamol poisoning are given in Table 12.6.

DEXTROPROPOXYPHENE (e.g. Distalgesic, Depronal S.A.) (Table 12.7)

Prescriptions for this drug are rapidly increasing and so it is becoming an important cause of self poisoning.
The dose causing serious poisoning is 6 g (20 tablets Distalgesic). Alcohol increases the risks. A serious

Table 12.6 Paracetamol poisoning

Clinical features	Biochemistry	Clinical care
12 to 24 hours Patient well Pallor Nausea 24 hours to 6 days Liver failure may develop Upper abdominal pain Tenderness right hypochondrium	Paracetamol level Elevated prothrombin time* Bilirubin↑* A.S.T.↑* Metabolic acidosis Hypoglycaemia	1. Gastric lavage and oral charcoal within 4 hours 2. ?antidote within 10 hours 3. Intensive supportive care 4. Treatment of liver failure if it occurs (prognosis poor) 5. Psychiatric opinion

*Note: The sooner these changes occur, the worse the prognosis.

Table 12.7 Dextropropoxyphene poisoning

Clinical features	Biochemistry	Clinical care
Constricted pupils Respiratory depression Coma Convulsions Circulatory collapse (Like opiate poisoning)	Not routine	1. Intensive supportive care 2. Gastric lavage within 4 hours 3. Nalorphine for respiratory depression 4. Treat fits (Valium) 5. Psychiatric opinion

feature is the marked fluctuation in the patient's condition. Death may suddenly occur at any time during the first twenty-four hours even after apparently satisfactory progress.

Distalgesic is a combination tablet of dextropropoxyphene (32.5 mg) and paracetamol (325 mg). The toxic effects of paracetamol may develop after overdosage.

BARBITURATES (Table 12.10)

The dose causing severe poisoning is 2 g. They are less often the cause of poisoning as the prescribing of barbiturates as hypnotics is now discouraged. (They are drugs of dependence.) In 1966, 91 of the 275 patients admitted for poisoning to the Bristol Royal Infirmary had taken a barbiturate. In 1976 the number had fallen to 44 of 560 admissions. Epileptics take phenobarbitone in overdosage.

TRICYCLIC COMPOUNDS (i.e. amitriptyline, imipramine, nortriptyline) (Table 12.8)

Dose causing severe poisoning, 1 g (40 tablets, 25 mg amitriptyline).

MONOAMINE OXIDASE INHIBITORS (Table 12.9)

Dose causing severe poisoning, 1.5 g (40 tablets phenelzine (Nardil)).

ALCOHOLS

ETHYL ALCOHOL

The fatal dose of ethyl alcohol for an average adult is 300 to 400 ml of the pure substance consumed over a short period of time. This is over two pints of spirit, i.e. whisky, gin, etc. Alcohol is oxidised in the liver, principally by alcohol dehydrogenase, which is present in the cytoplasm of hepatocytes, and to a much smaller extent by a microsomal (smooth endoplasmic reticulum) enzyme system. This latter system explains some of the known interactions of drugs and alcohol. Severe poisoning occurs when both enzyme systems are saturated, and if at this time a barbiturate or other sedative drug is taken it is then only slowly broken down and severe fatal poisoning from the mixture can occur. On the other hand, the chronic alcoholic whose microsomal enzyme

Table 12.8 Tricyclic compound poisoning

Clinical features	Cause	Biochemistry	Clinical care
Varying coma Hyperactivity Convulsions Dry mouth Dilated pupils Cardiac arrhythmias Hypotension Tachycardia Urinary retention	Atropine-like effect of drugs	Serum levels not routine and unhelpful	1. Intensive supportive therapy 2. Gastric lavage within 4 hours 3. Treat cardiac arrhythmias 4. Sedation (Valium) for convulsions 5. Psychiatric opinion

Table 12.9 Monoamine oxidase inhibitor poisoning

Clinical features	Cause	Biochemistry	Clinical care

Excitability then coma
Hyperthermia
Hypo or hypertension
Convulsions
	Due to potentiation
	of other drugs, e.g.
	morphine, alcohol or
	other amines, e.g.
	tyramine, amphetamine,
	noradrenaline,
	serotonin. These are
	found in foods,
	especially cheese and
	self medications like
	cough mixtures
		Serum levels not
		routine and unhelpful
			1. Intensive supportive therapy
			2. Avoid sympathomimetic
			   agents for hypotension,
			   i.e. no aramine,
			   noradrenaline, etc.
			3. Possibly hypotensive
			   agents
			4. Treatment of
			   hyperthermia
			5. Psychiatric opinion

Table 12.10 Barbiturate poisoning

Clinical features	Cause	Biochemistry	Clinical care

Coma
Respiratory failure
Hypotension
Hypovolaemia
Renal failure
	Depression of
	cerebral and brain
	stem function
	Venous pooling
	Hypotension
	Low cardiac output
		Serum levels of
		barbiturate. In
		severe cases medium
		and short acting
		>3.5 mg per cent
		Long acting >10 mg per cent
		Acidosis
		Uraemia
			1. Intensive supportive therapy
			2. Gastric lavage if less
			   than 4 hours
			3. Forced alkaline diuresis
			   for phenobarbitone
			4. Psychiatric opinion

system is hypertrophied from chronic (alcoholic) induction metabolises sedative drugs rapidly and is particularly insensitive to them.

Commonly taken alcoholic drinks contain the following amounts of alcohol:

Beer, 3 g/100 ml.
Cider, up to 10 g/100 ml.
Wine, 10 to 15 g/100 ml.
Spirits, 30 g/100 ml.

Clinical Effects

Alcohol depresses the central nervous system from the cortex to the brain stem, and the blood levels usually associated with various grades of poisoning are:

Mild: 0.05 to 0.15 per cent
Moderate: 0.15 to 0.3 per cent
Severe: 0.3 to 0.5 per cent
Coma: 0.5   per cent

The breathalyser test becomes positive at 80 mg per cent (0.08 per cent) and at this level, by legal definition, it leads to driving disqualification in the UK. The maximum blood alcohol level reached depends on a number of factors, including the amount taken, whether this is accompanied by food, and whether the patient vomits.

Physical signs of acute alcoholism include sweating, tachycardia and an alcoholic foetor, slurred speech, ataxia and loss of finer control of behaviour. Coma and respiratory depression are features of severe poisoning.

Coma in the alcoholic is of importance because of the numerous possibilities. The alcoholic suffers from all the usual causes of coma, but is particularly prone to that due to head injury, the taking of other drugs, alcoholic hypoglycaemia and coma following 'alcoholic' fits. One clinical catch is that alcohol may be given as first aid to an ill patient who later becomes comatose. Coma may be wrongly attributed to it.

Table 12.11   Methanol poisoning

Clinical features	Cause	Biochemistry	Clinical care
Similar to ethyl alcohol *After 12 to 24 hours* Headache Photophobia Dilatation of pupils Papilloedema, leading to optic atrophy (blindness) Coma	Direct effect of metabolites: methanol is distributed in tissues according to water content, therefore high concentration in optic nerve	Severe metabolic acidosis	1. Intensive supportive care 2. Gastric lavage within 4 hours 3. Treat acidosis with I.V. bicarbonate 50 per cent 4. Ethyl alcohol (slow rate of accumulation of toxic products), 1 ml/kg orally at once. 0.5 ml/kg every 2 hours for 5 days 5. Haemodialysis in severe case

Table 12.12   Carbon monoxide poisoning

Clinical features	Cause	Biochemistry	Clinical care
0 to 10 % No symptoms *10 to 30%* Headache Yawning Insidious impairment of mental faculties Dizziness Palpitations *>30%* Coma, incoordination/ agitation Papilloedema Resultant permanent brain damage, e.g. cerebellar or Parkinsonism Myocardial damage Hypotension Nausea and vomiting Respiratory distress Skin bright pink colour	 Cerebral oedema Myocardial anoxia Inhalation Carboxyhaemoglobin	Spectroscopy for carboxyhaemoglobin	1. Remove from source 2. Give artificial respiration and 90% oxygen, 5% CO_2 Hyperbaric oxygen* 3. Mannitol 500 ml 20% I.V. for cerebral oedema 4. Rest in bed (myocardial necrosis) 5. Psychiatric opinion

*Note: Potential danger of hyperbaric oxygen is cerebral spasm with resultant brain oedema.

Basis of Treatment

1. Intensive supportive care.
2. Gastric lavage within four hours.
3. The rate of metabolism of alcohol may be increased by giving intravenous fructose (1 litre of 10 per cent IV).

METHANOL (Methylated spirits, antifreeze) (Table 12.11)

Methanol has foolishly been sometimes added to party drinks.

The dose causing serious poisoning is 15 ml. It is more toxic than ethanol because it is metabolised to formic acid or formaldehyde which inhibit all metabolism.

CARBON MONOXIDE (Table 12.12)

(*Note:* At present, conversion to natural gas for domestic use is complete in England, Scotland and Wales but not in Northern Ireland or Eire.)

Natural gas consists essentially of methane. It is non-toxic unless it is present in such a large amount that the oxygen pressure in the air is lowered sufficiently to cause the effects of oxygen deprivation – asphyxia. In Bristol in 1966, 10 per cent of poisonings were due to carbon monoxide, in 1976, 0.5 per cent.

Carbon monoxide is present in mains supply manufactured gas in areas not converted to natural gas. There is a high concentration in exhaust fumes from car engines. Its extreme toxicity is due to its great affinity for haemoglobin (300 times that of oxygen). Carboxyhaemoglobin is formed and this is unable to carry oxygen. A concentration of 1 part per 10,000 produces 80 per cent saturation of haemoglobin in twenty minutes. This level is fatal. The combination of carbon monoxide and haemoglobin is reversible, and is speeded by breathing a high concentration of oxygen particularly under increased atmospheric pressure.

METALS

IRON

The lethal dose in children is 0.3 g/kg. Severe toxicity may occur with smaller doses.

Clinical Features

1 to 2 hours: Vomiting and bloody diarrhoea.
6 to 8 hours: Profound cardiovascular collapse (direct effect of free iron causing peripheral dilatation).
Days to weeks: Liver necrosis, renal failure, gut strictures.

Basis of Treatment

Gastric aspiration and lavage. Then 6 g of desferrioxamine should be put into the stomach to chelate any remaining unabsorbed iron and 2 g of desferrioxamine injected intramuscularly. If the plasma iron in a child is greater than 500 μg or in adult 800 μg, desferrioxamine should be infused intravenously at a dose of 15 mg/kg/hour.

LEAD

This type of poisoning is important because of the difficulty in diagnosis. It is the result of ingestion of lead by those engaged in smelting and refining it (lead is then absorbed from the respiratory tract), as well as by painters using lead-based paints and children who chew toys or cot rails painted with lead paint. Accidental poisoning has resulted from burning old car batteries and from ingesting tetra-ethyl lead (anti-knock). Some patients have been poisoned by drinking cider or home made wine allowed to stand in old fashioned earthenware pots (lead comes out in solution). The results are variable but usually include a haemolytic anaemia. This is the result of a direct effect of lead on red cell membranes and there seems also to be inhibition of haemesynthesis at the level of delta-aminolaevulinic acid (δ ALA). Lead intoxication results in an increased stippling of normoblasts associated with abnormal haemoglobinisation and this sign is of diagnostic importance. The stipple cell seems in fact to be a reticulocyte altered in appearance by the presence of lead.

Other features are (Fig. 12.7):

Lead colic: Gripping abdominal pain and rigidity sometimes accompanied by constipation. This is due to intestinal spasm.

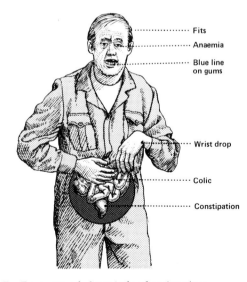

Fig. 12.7 Features of chronic lead poisoning.

210

Lead encephalopathy. Usually confined to organic lead poisoning, when there is agitation, restlessness, trembling, etc. leading to convulsions and coma. This may resemble acute prophyria.
Note: There is, as in porphyria, increased porphyrins in the urine.

A blue line on the gums. Due to lead sulphide deposition – not found in the edentulous.

Peripheral neuritis. Maximal sometimes in the muscles supplied by the radial or lateral popliteal nerve. This suggests a muscular action, and muscle fatigue may play a part in painters' paralysis (paralysis of wrist extensors).

Chronic nephritis and hypertension. Occasionally.

Investigations

1. A raised blood ($>100\ \mu g/100$ ml) or urine (>1 mg/24 hr) level.
2. An increased stipple cell count and evidence of mild haemolytic anaemia.
3. X-ray of bones (particularly in children) may show a line of deposited lead in the growing end of the bones.

Basis of Treatment

This is removal of lead using a chelating agent, e.g. EDTA (calcium disodium edete), which exchanges lead for calcium. Administration is by intravenous drip over two-day periods using 1 to 2 g on each occasion. Lead excretion in the urine is monitored, and treatment ceases when it falls to 1.5 mg/24 hr after the second 24 hours of the two-day period. Up to about 700 g may be given in repeated courses.

ARSENIC

White arsenic is a gritty powder. It is tasteless – hence its past popularity for murder.

Clinical Features

Intense thirst, abdominal pain and vomiting. Severe gastroenteritis and circulatory collapse may occur.

Basis of Treatment

1. Gastric lavage with a 1 per cent solution of sodium thiocyanate.
2. Dimercaprol.
3. Intensive supportive care.
4. Correction of dehydration and electrolyte loss.
   Chronic poisoning causes anorexia, salivation, polyneuritis and weakness and wasting of the muscles.

There may be raindrop pigmentation of the skin, hyperkeratosis of the palms and soles, skin cancer and hepatic fibrosis. Ridging of the nails is a physical sign. (Forensic scientists can detect arsenic long after poisoning, in the nails and hair.)

MERCURY

The risk is to people exposed to mercury or its salts for more than a short period. Laboratory workers, scientific instrument and thermometer makers, mirror silverers and hat makers (they paint mercury nitrate on to felt) are among those who have been poisoned.

Clinical Features

Tremor affecting the corners of the mouth, face and limbs (hatter's shakes).
Scanning speech, ataxia. Excessive salivation. Blushing of the skin due to vasomotor disturbance.
Erythism. This is a psychological disorder of shyness, anxiety and depression caused by mercury ('mad as a hatter').

Basis of Treatment

The most important treatment is to remove the patient from exposure. Dimercaprol (BAL) and other chelating agents have been used but their efficacy remains to be proven.

AGRICULTURAL POISONS

PARAQUAT (Table 12.13)

There are two main commercial preparations:
   20 per cent aqueous solution (Gramoxone).
   2.5 per cent granular preparation (Weedol).

OTHER WEEDKILLERS

(a) Dinitro-ortho-Cresol
(b) Dinitrophenol
   These poison by increasing cellular metabolism. The concentrated form of each has to be diluted and may then come in contact with the skin causing a yellow staining. They may be inhaled during spraying of crops.

Clinical Features

These resemble a thyrotoxic crisis. Tachycardia, sweating, hyperpyrexia, convulsions and coma occur.

Basis of Treatment

1. Wash off from the skin.
2. Supportive treatment of hypopyrexia.
3. Sedation with chlorpromazine.
4. Correction of dehydration and cardiac arrhythmias.

Table 12.13 Paraquat poisoning

Clinical features	Cause	Biochemistry	Clinical care

Skin blistering
Inflammation of eyes
Nose bleeding
Ulcers in mouth and
  oesophagus
Diarrhoea and vomiting
	Local effects	10 ml urine +
		  2 ml 1% alk.
		  sodium dithionite
		Blue colour develops if
		  paraquat present
			1. Local effects.
			  Wash skin, irrigate
			  eyes at once
			2. Gastric lavage
			  Then Fullers earth,

Pulmonary oedema
  (within hours)
Pulmonary fibrosis and
  respiratory failure
  (up to 6 weeks)
Acute tubular necrosis
Circulatory failure
	Direct effect of
	paraquat in tissues
			(removes paraquat from
			  gut) + magnesium sulphate
			  (to increase elimination of
			  Fullers earth and
			  paraquat)
			3. Fluid and electrolyte
			  replacement.
			4. ?low O$_2$ therapy
			  (oxygen enhances toxicity)
			5. ?d:propranolol and
			  superoxide dismutase
			  (experimental)
			6. Psychiatric opinion

ORGANO-PHOSPHORUS PESTICIDES

These are very poisonous. They produce profound parasympathetic overactivity by inhibition of cholinesterase. They may be absorbed through the skin.

Clinical Features

The presentation is often of severe respiratory or abdominal disease with bronchospasm, pulmonary oedema and respiratory failure, abdominal cramps, profuse diarrhoea and vomiting. Marked salivation, blurred vision, muscle weakness and convulsions occur.

Diagnosis

Estimate plasma cholinesterase which is usually less than 30 per cent of normal.

Basis of Treatment

1. Thoroughly wash the skin or gastric lavage.
2. Treat respiratory failure with oxygen. When the cyanosis is corrected give atropine sulphate 2 mg intravenously and repeat at five-minute intervals until the patient is atropinised. Continue for two days.

   Pralidoxime (PAM) is a specific reactivator of cholinesterase. It can be obtained from the Poisons Information Service. The dose is 1 g intravenously, repeated.

FUNGI

The most important is *Amanita phalloides* (Death Cap) for it can be easily mistaken for an edible mushroom (Fig. 12.8). The dose causing fatal poisoning is 1 to 2 g.

Clinical Features

There is often a delay before any symptoms. These are violent vomiting, diarrhoea and colic. Circulatory collapse may result and within a few days renal and liver failure occur.

Basis of Treatment

1. Intensive supportive care.
2. Correct dehydration and electrolyte loss.
3. Atropine sulphate to control parasympathetic effects of muscarine.
4. The treatment of acute renal and hepatic failure may be required (*see* pages 231 and 71).

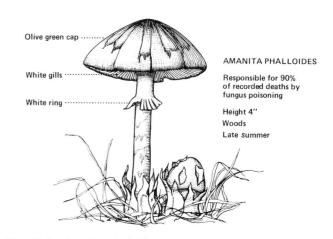

Olive green cap
White gills
White ring

AMANITA PHALLOIDES

Responsible for 90% of recorded deaths by fungus poisoning

Height 4''
Woods
Late summer

Fig. 12.8 *Amanita phalloides.*

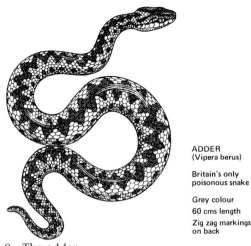

ADDER
(Vipera berus)

Britain's only
poisonous snake

Grey colour
60 cms length
Zig zag markings
on back

Fig. 12.9   The adder.

SNAKEBITE (Fig. 12.9)

Lie the patient down and immobilise the part. Reassurance is necessary. The majority of deaths from snake bite are said to owe more to fear than toxin. Adder bites are very rarely fatal. Even the most dangerous snake bites have a mortality of only about 50 per cent.

The value of a tourniquet is controversial but it may help to delay the dissemination of venom until antiserum is available. It may be applied about two inches above the bite, tight enough to distend the veins without impeding arterial blood flow. It should be released for a minute at the end of each half hour and removed after four hours since longer use may increase local tissue damage.

Do *not* cut or suck or burn. Cleanse the bite with saline, water or dilute antiseptic solution. Relieve pain, but avoid opiates.

The value of antisera, if available, must be weighed against the dangers of anaphylaxis. It is very doubtful whether the use of viper antiserum is justified in ordinary circumstances.

Antibiotics and tetanus prophylaxis are advisable.

Steroids, for example intravenous hydrocortisone, may give some protection against allergic reactions to the snake venom.

It is usual to recommend that the snake be kept for identification of the correct antiserum. However, more men than snakes are killed in snake hunts.

INSECT STING

About five people each year in Britain die following a bee or wasp sting. The venom contains active polypeptides and phospholipases. These cause pain and swelling at the site of the sting. The danger is that the venom acting as an allergen may produce anaphylactic shock. The signs are a fall in blood pressure, bronchoconstriction and angioneurotic oedema. Treatment is urgent (0.25 ml intramuscular 1:1,000 adrenaline, antihistamine and intubation and tracheostomy if necessary).

Bee sting is a rare cause of the nephrotic syndrome.

SUGGESTED FURTHER READING

General

Breckenridge, A. M. (1975) *Advanced Medicine. Topics in Therapeutics. Problems of Poisoning and Drug Overdosage.* London: Pitman Medical.

Matthew, H. and Lawson, A. A. H. (1975) *Treatment of Common Acute Poisonings.* Edinburgh: Churchill Livingstone.

Standing Medical Advisory Committees: Report of Joint Sub-Committee (1968) *Hospital Treatment of Acute Poisoning.* London: HMSO.

Children

Craft, A. W. and Sibert, J. R. (1977) Accidental poisoning in children. *British Journal of Hospital Medicine* **17:** 469.

Glutethimide

Leading Article (1976) Glutethimide – an unsafe alternative to barbiturate hypnotics. *British Medical Journal* **1:** 1424.

Paracetamol

Leading Article (1977) Treatment of acute paracetamol poisoning. *British Medical Journal* **2:** 481.

Dextropropoxyphene

Carson, D. J. L. and Carson, E. D. (1977) Fatal dextropropoxyphene poisoning in Northern Ireland. *Lancet* **i:** 894.

Tricyclic Antidepressants

Freeman, J. W., Mundy, G. R., Beattie, R. R. and Ryan, C. (1969) Cardiac abnormalities in poisoning with tricyclic antidepressants. *British Medical Journal* **2:** 610.

Barbiturates

Matthew, H. (1971) Acute barbiturate poisoning. *Excerpta Medica Monograph.* Amsterdam: Excerpta Medica.

Industrial and Agricultural Poisoning

Department of Health and Social Security (1969) *Poisonous Chemicals used on Farms and Gardens.* London: HMSO.

Hunter, D. (1969) *Diseases of Occupations.* London: English Universities Press.

Lead Symposium (1975) *Postgraduate Medical Journal* **5:** 743.

Poisonous Plants

North, P. (1967) *Poisonous Plants and Fungi in Colour.* London: Blandford Press.

Poisonous Animals

George, C. F. (1975) Poisoning by Animals. *Medicine 2nd Series* **5:** 228.

Adverse Drug Reactions 13

C. J. C. ROBERTS

Ten to twenty per cent of patients in hospital suffer an adverse reaction to a drug and about five per cent of hospital admissions are precipitated by drug reactions. The drugs most commonly responsible are antimicrobials, aspirin, digitalis, diuretics, corticosteroids, anticoagulants and insulin. Adverse drug reactions can be broadly classified into two types.

PREDICTABLE REACTIONS

1. The reaction can be predicted from the known pharmacology of the drug and may be either an exaggeration of the therapeutic effect, e.g. excessive anticoagulation with warfarin leading to bleeding, or the effect of the drug on receptors other than the target receptor, e.g. bronchoconstriction caused by beta receptor blockade with propranolol.
2. The effect is directly related to the amount of drug presented to the receptor. Factors which cause variability in drug tissue concentration (pharmacokinetic factors) and factors which alter the sensitivity of that receptor to the drug (pharmacodynamic factors) will increase the likelihood of this type of reaction.
3. These reactions are largely avoidable with skilful use of the drugs.

UNPREDICTABLE REACTIONS

1. The reaction is unrelated to the known pharmacology of the drug, e.g. oculomucocutaneous syndrome, caused by the beta blocker, practolol, and aplastic anaemia, caused by phenylbutazone.
2. The effect is not directly related to drug tissue concentrations, although some dependence on dose is usual.
3. The reaction constitutes a known risk associated with the use of the drug and influences choice of drug.

For examples of both types of drug reaction *see* Table 13.1.

PHARMACOKINETIC MECHANISMS

The blood level of a drug is determined by the effects of factors within the patient on absorption, distribution

Table 13.1   Drug reactions with some commonly used drugs

Drug	Predictable	Unpredictable
Methyldopa	Postural hypotension Nasal obstruction Drowsiness Depression Ejaculatory failure Galactorrhoea	Haemolytic anaemia Hepatitis
Phenytoin	Ataxia Choreoathetosis Cerebellar syndrome Dementia Cardiac arrhythmias Enzyme induction Osteomalacia	Lymphadenopathy Folate deficiency Lupus syndrome Erythema multiforme Gingival hyperplasia Granulomatous hepatitis
Digoxin	Nausea and vomiting Cardiac arrhythmias Delirium Visual disturbance	Gynaecomastia
Chlorpromazine	Drowsiness Confusion Parkinsonism Postural hypotension Cardiac arrhythmias Galactorrhoea Enzyme induction	Cholestatic jaundice Aplastic anaemia Photosensitivity Retinal damage Lupus syndrome
Chlorothiazide	Sodium depletion Hypokalaemia Hyperuricaemia Hyperglycaemia	Agranulocytosis Thrombocytopenia Erythema multiforme Cholestatic jaundice

and elimination. Pharmacokinetic behaviour depends on physico-chemical properties (water solubility, lipid solubility, pKa and affinity for body proteins).

> **Expectations of high lipid solubility**
>
> 1. Rapid and complete absorption.
> 2. Wide distribution with penetration of CNS.
> 3. Metabolism to water-soluble products is required before excretion is possible.

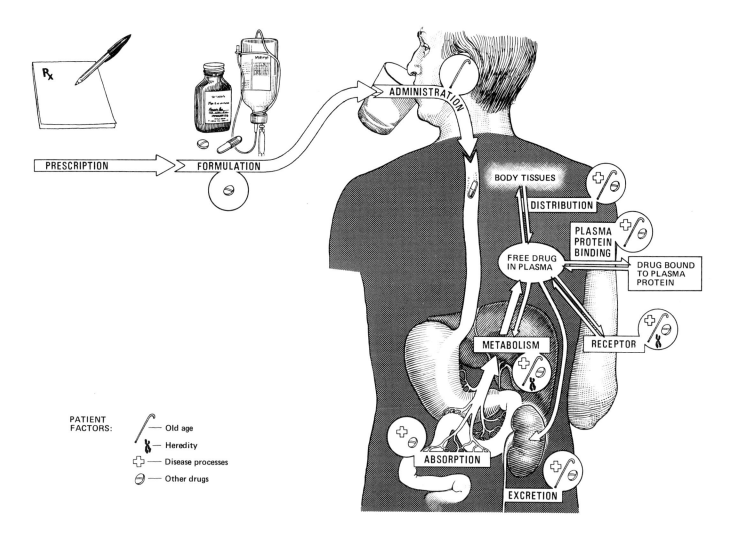

PATIENT
FACTORS:
— Old age
— Heredity
— Disease processes
— Other drugs

ADMINISTRATION

PRESCRIPTION

FORMULATION

BODY TISSUES

DISTRIBUTION

PLASMA
PROTEIN
BINDING

FREE DRUG
IN PLASMA

DRUG BOUND
TO PLASMA
PROTEIN

METABOLISM

RECEPTOR

ABSORPTION

EXCRETION

Fig. 13.1   The site and nature of factors causing adverse drug reactions.

Weakly acidic drugs become less ionised and more lipid-soluble in an acid medium.

Factors within the patient and the sites at which they operate to cause variability are shown in Fig. 13.1. Variability in drug levels predisposes to the development of predictable reactions.

Errors of prescription and administration

These result from:
1. Illegible and inadequate instructions.
2. The use of proprietary drug combinations.
3. Poor patient compliance (common in the elderly and the socially isolated; worsened by complexity of drug therapy and poor doctor–patient relationship)

The formulation term 'bioavailability' implies the fraction of drug which is available for absorption from the tablet. It may vary from one product to another. The product with the highest bioavailability should always be used.

Factors influencing bioavailability

1. Particle size.
2. Tablet dissolution rate.
3. Presence of substances within the tablet which may bind active drug.
4. Water solubility of drug.

Absorption

Absorption from the gastrointestinal tract is usually by passive diffusion of drug in its lipid-soluble, unionised form. Changes in gastrointestinal motility, mucosal surface and pH may influence either the rate or extent of drug absorption. Thus, diseases in which there is intestinal hurry may be expected to decrease absorption of poorly soluble drugs (Table 13.2). Drugs which increase gut motility, e.g. metaclopramide, may have a similar effect, and those which delay gastric emptying and decrease motility may increase the extent of absorption of poorly soluble drugs whilst delaying the absorption of others. Certain drugs may bind chemically with others in the gut lumen and thus prevent their absorption.

'First Pass Metabolism'. Drug absorbed from the gastrointestinal tract must pass through the liver via the portal vein before reaching the systemic circulation. If there is an avid metabolising system within the liver for the drug, a substantial proportion will be metabolised during that first pass through the liver. Some examples of drugs which suffer significant 'first pass metabolism' are propranolol, nortriptyline, isoprenaline and glyceryl trinitrate. Genetically determined variation in the extent of 'first pass metabolism' accounts for the wide range of dosage requirements for propranolol. Decreased 'first pass metabolism' in the elderly and in patients with liver disease accounts for the higher drug levels obtained in those patients.

Plasma Protein Binding

In the circulation a proportion of many drugs is transported loosely chemically bound to plasma proteins (usually albumin). Only the free drug is available for distribution to other tissues, including the target organ and organs of elimination. A state of equilibrium exists between the protein-bound and free drug. Thus factors which influence protein binding may have a profound effect on the behaviour of those drugs which are normally transported protein-bound.

Diminution in protein binding sites occurs in hypoalbuminaemic states such as liver cell failure and the nephrotic syndrome. In old age and uraemia, phenytoin binding is decreased so that it is effective at lower blood levels. Warfarin, which is usually 99 per cent protein-bound, can be displaced from binding sites by other drugs, e.g. salicylates, and thus potentiated (Table 13.2).

Tissue Distribution

The distribution of a drug into body tissues is dependent on its physico-chemical characteristics. Many drugs are concentrated in tissues outside the blood and therefore have a high 'apparent volume of distribution' (the volume into which the total dose would have to be diluted to achieve the plasma concentration). Some drugs bind body tissues irreversibly. For example, tetracyclines chelate newly formed bone. The binding of chlorpromazine and chloroquine to melanin-containing tissues is responsible for the retinopathy caused by those drugs.

Ageing and disease processes can alter the volume of distribution of drugs. For example, in uraemia the volume of distribution of digoxin is greatly reduced so that plasma levels may rise into the toxic range after only one dose. Where an active transport process is involved in tissue distribution, one drug may compete with another for that process. For example, tricyclic antidepressants prevent the uptake of adrenergic neurone blocking agents into the nerve terminal and therefore antagonise the hypotensive effect.

Renal Excretion

Only those drugs with poor lipid solubility can be excreted by the kidney. Two mechanisms are involved:

Glomerular filtration of drugs may be impaired in old age, hypovolaemic shock as well as intrinsic renal disease. Thus toxic accumulation of drugs such as digoxin and the aminoglycoside antibiotics may occur if appropriate dosage adjustment is not made.

Active tubular secretion of some drugs occurs. There may be competition between drugs for the excretory mechanisms. For example, probenecid inhibits the excretion of penicillin. Excretion of acidic or basic substances may be affected by pH changes. Alkalinisation of the urine causes increased ionisation of aspirin in the urine, rendering it less lipid-soluble and thus preventing reabsorption from the nephron tubule (*see* Table 13.2).

Hepatic Metabolism

The liver converts highly lipid-soluble drugs into water-soluble metabolites which may be excreted by the kidney. One or two phases of metabolism may be required. Phase I involves oxidation, reduction or hydrolysis and Phase II, glucuronidation, sulphation, methylation or acetylation. Many drugs undergo microsomal oxidation using a common system of enzymes. The activity of these enzymes is largely determined genetically, and it varies widely between individuals. For this reason, there is a tenfold range of steady state plasma levels of drugs such as phenytoin and nortriptyline in patients given the same dose. Acetylation is under the control of a single gene so that the population can be divided into slow or fast acetylators. In general, it is the slow acetylators who suffer the dose-related adverse effects, e.g. lupus erythematosus with hydrallazine and neuropathy with isoniazid, although the fast acetylators will suffer the adverse reaction if it is the acetylated derivative that is toxic, e.g. lupus erythematosus with procainamide.

In old age and hepatic disease, the drug metabolising capacity of the liver is reduced, increasing the possibility of toxic accumulation of drug. Some drugs have the power to increase the capacity of the microsomal oxidation system ('enzyme induction') and thus to increase the elimination of other drugs metabolised by that system. Thus, many hypnotics and anticonvulsants can alter the dosage requirement of warfarin (*see* Table 13.2). Over-anticoagulation can occur when they are withdrawn. Enzyme induction takes several days to develop as it involves protein synthesis. 'Enzyme inhibition' by drugs, however, is an immediate effect. Thus chloramphenicol can inhibit the metabolism and prolong the effect of chlorpropamide and isoniazid has a similar effect on phenytoin.

Commonly used drugs which induce hepatic enzymes

Anticonvulsants

Phenytoin
Phenobarbitone (all barbiturates)
Primidone
Carbamazepine

Sedatives/Hypnotics

Glutethimide
Dichloralphenazone
Chlorpromazine

Antimicrobials

Rifampicin
Griseofulvin

Diuretics

Spironolactone

PHARMACODYNAMIC MECHANISMS

Altered responsiveness to drugs in the body tissues can give rise to predictable drug reactions. Patient factors similiar to those which influence pharmacokinetic variability can influence drug sensitivity. Thus the aged are sensitive to the effect of hypnotics and sedatives such that they may cause hallucinations and mental confusion. They are particularly sensitive to the postural hypotensive effect of phenothiazines. Disease processes can alter drug sensitivity. Encephalopathy can be precipitated by sedatives in patients with hepatic failure, and respiratory depression can be profound if minor sedatives are given to patients with respiratory failure. Monoamine oxidase inhibiting drugs can interact with indirectly acting sympathomimetics, e.g. phenylpropanolamine, by increasing the amount of noradrenaline

which is released onto the receptor. There may also be genetic differences in receptor sensitivity. For example, occasional individuals are resistant to the actions of warfarin.

DRUG IDIOSYNCRASY

Many unpredictable drug reactions have a genetic or immunological mechanism. In most however the mechanism is ill-understood.

Glucose 6-Phosphate Dehydrogenase (G6PD) Deficiency

G6PD is responsible for the maintenance of reduced glutathione in the red cell. Reduced glutathione prevents the damaging effect of oxidising agents on the cell. Deficiency of G6PD is a sex-linked inherited defect common in Negroes and Mediterranean races. In such people drugs with oxidising properties can denature intracellular proteins including the globin part of the haemoglobin molecule and haemolysis may result. Such drugs include primaquine, sulphonamides, nitrofurantoin, aspirin, phenacetin, chloramphenicol, PAS, probenecid and quinine.

Hereditary Methaemoglobinaemia

People with congenital absence of the enzyme, methaemoglobin reductase, may become cyanosed if given oxidising drugs when large amounts of methaemoglobin will form.

Porphyria

The characteristic feature of the hepatic porphyrias is excessive production of the enzyme a-amino laevulinic acid synthetase. Hepatic enzyme inducing drugs may further increase the enzyme and precipitate an attack of porphyria.

Malignant Hyperpyrexia

This is a condition characterised by a rapid rise in body temperature during anaesthesia often in the presence of suxamethonium. Rigidity of skeletal muscle, acidosis, and hyperkalaemia accompany the pyrexia. The mortality is between 60 and 70 per cent. The genetic predisposition to the condition is inherited as an autosomal dominant trait with variable penetrance.

Drug Hypersensitivity

Immunological mechanisms are responsible for many unpredictable drug reactions. Such reactions include anaphylaxis, serum sickness, various skin rashes, blood disorders and lupus-like syndromes.

Table 13.2   Table of drug interactions

Site and mechanism of interaction	First drug	Second drug	Effect on first drug
1. *Formulation*			
Mixture in intravenous infusions	Penicillin	Hydrocortisone	Inactivates
	Heparin	Hydrocortisone	Inactivates
2. *Gut*			
Altered motility	Digoxin	Propantheline	Increased absorption
	Digoxin	Metaclopramide	Decreased absorption
Altered pH	Tetracycline	Sodium bicarbonate	Reduced absorption
Chelation	Tetracycline	Calcium, magnesium, aluminium + iron salts	Reduced absorption
	Warfarin	Cholestyramine	Reduced absorption
3. *Plasma protein binding*			
Displacement from sites	Warfarin	Aspirin	Potentiation
	Chlorpropamide	Phenylbutazone	Potentiation
	Phenytoin	Salicylates	Potentiation
4. *Hepatic enzyme induction*			
	Warfarin	Any enzyme inducer	Decreased levels
	Tolbutamide	Any enzyme inducer	Decreased levels
	Prednisone	Any enzyme inducer	Decreased levels
5. *Hepatic enzyme inhibition*			
	Warfarin	Phenylbutazone	Increased levels
	Warfarin	Clofibrate	Increased levels
	Phenytoin	Disulfiram	Increased levels
	Azathioprine	Allopurinol	Increased levels
6. *Renal excretion*			
Competition for tubular secretion	Penicillin	Probenecid	Increased levels (used therapeutically)
	Salicylates	Probenecid	Increased levels
	Acetohexamide	Phenylbutazone	Increased levels
Change in urine pH	Salicylates	Sodium bicarbonate	Decreased levels ⎱ used in severe
	Phenobarbitone	Sodium bicarbonate	Decreased levels ⎰ overdoses
	Fenfluramine	Acetazolamide	Decreased levels
7. *Receptor sites*			
Competition	Morphine	Nalorphine	Decreased effect
	Tubocurarine	Neostygmine	Decreased effect
Altered uptake	Guanethidine	Tricyclic antidepressants	Decreased effect
	Bethanidine	Tricyclic antidepressants	Decreased effect
	Debrisoquine	Chlorpromazine	Decreased effect
Altered metabolism of transmitter	Ephedrine	MAOIs	Potentiation (hypertensive)
	Phenylpropanolamine	MAOIs	Potentiation (hypertensive)
Additive effect at same receptor	Warfarin	Salicylates	Potentiation
	Tubocurarine	Gentamicin	Potentiation
	Nitrazepam	Alcohol	Potentiation

SUGGESTED FURTHER READING

Avery, G. S. (ed.) (1976) *Drug Treatment*. Adis Press.

British Journal of Hospital Medicine. December 1974.

Davies, D. M. (ed.) (1977) *Textbook of Adverse Drug Reaction*. Oxford.

Hansten, P. D. (1975) *Drug Interactions*. Philadelphia: Lea & Febiger.

Turner, P. and Richens, A. (1975) *Clinical Pharmacology*. Edinburgh & London: Churchill Livingstone.

Wade, O. L. and Beeley, L. (1976) *Adverse Reactions to Drugs*. Heinemann.

Nephrology

14

J. C. MACKENZIE

Nephrology is the practice of renal medicine. Though some renal diseases such as primary glomerulonephritis are uncommon, others such as uncomplicated lower urinary tract infections in women are not. In fact only 7,500 deaths directly attributed to renal disease are recorded in the Registrar General's Report each year and both in the UK and USA deaths from renal disease remain at about 10 to 15 per 100,000 per annum. Secondary involvement of the kidneys is, however, a common finding in many systemic diseases and conditions as diverse as diabetes mellitus, connective tissue disease, multiple myeloma or even congestive cardiac failure have renal components. The study of renal disorders is made difficult for the student for two reasons. Firstly, diseases of the kidney are often latent and lie dormant for many years with perhaps only minimal proteinuria, hypertension or an occasional attack of urinary tract infection to indicate their presence. The finding of proteinuria or hypertension at routine medical examinations is a common method of detection. Secondly, kidney diseases are capable of mimicking many different disorders. The 'uraemic syndrome', developing from covert chronic renal failure, may appear in many guises other than hypertension, producing conditions as dissimilar as anaemia, peripheral neuropathy or even gout.

The epidemiology of renal disease shows geographical variations; mismatched blood transfusions remain not an infrequent cause of acute renal failure in some areas and *Plasmodium malariae* is a common aetiological factor in the glomerulonephritis seen in Africa.

Diseases of the kidney may be acute, chronic, hereditary or congenital and the incidence of renal disorders is related to the age, sex, race, nationality, occupation, drug intake, and the family and past history of the patient. All of these factors must be considered in making a diagnosis or when predicting the likely outcome of the disease, i.e. the prognosis.

In the study of renal disorder it is helpful to think of the kidney as a structural and also a functional unit. Major symptoms and signs can be divided conveniently into two types. There are those relating to the anatomical fabric of the kidney, ureters, bladder and urethra, i.e. loin pain, renal swellings and the passage of blood or protein in the urine and those apparently unrelated clinical features of the 'uraemic syndrome' produced by the kidneys' failure to fulfil their main functions.

THE STRUCTURE AND MODE OF ACTION OF THE KIDNEY

Structure (Fig. 14.1)

The kidneys are paired retroperitoneal bean-shaped and encapsulated organs weighing 150 to 170 g and measuring 12.5 × 7.3 cm, but varying with the size of the individual.

As a rough guide, they correspond to three-and-a-half vertebral bodies as seen on an X-ray. Both kidneys are approximately the same length; a discrepancy of more than 1.5 cm is pathologically significant, e.g. unilateral pyelonephritis or rarely renal artery stenosis. They lie opposite T12, L1, L2 and L3 vertebrae with the hilum adjacent to the body of L2. The right kidney is about 1.5 cm lower than the left and both move about the length of a vertebra during respiration. The renal angles overlie the kidneys posteriorly and their surface markings comprise the lower edge of the 12th rib, the lateral border of the sacrospinalis muscle and the medial side of the attachment of the external abdominal oblique muscle to the 12th rib. Kidney tenderness may be elicited on palpation of this renal angle and it provides the best site for percutaneous biopsy. The capsule of the kidney and ureters receive their innervation from the 10th, 11th and 12th thoracic and 1st lumbar nerves and pain from the renal tract may be felt over the skin distribution of these nerves; the renal parenchyma does not contain pain fibres. The kidney receives its blood supply from the renal arteries which may be multiple. The main renal artery divides into segmental divisions with interlobar, arcuate and finally interlobular branches. The renal veins may also be multiple. The gross structure of the kidney and its collecting system is shown in Fig. 14.1. There are two or three major calyces in each kidney with up to fourteen minor calyces.

219

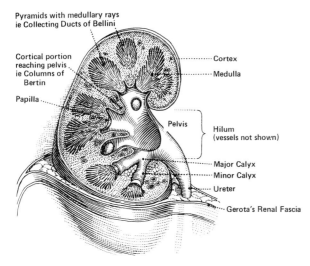

Fig. 14.1   The gross structure of the kidney.

Congenitally the kidneys may be abnormal in number, size, development, shape and position. A solitary normal kidney, a small under-developed hypoplastic kidney, horseshoe-shaped kidneys, formed by fusion of the lower poles across the midline, and ectopically placed kidneys in the bony pelvis all occur with an instance of about 1 in 500 to 1,500 of the population. The pelvis and ureter are sometimes duplicated on one or both sides producing a duplex kidney.

Each kidney contains one million functioning units or nephrons. A nephron consists of a tube about 35 μ wide and 50 mm long and the total length of the tubules of both kidneys is about 112 km (Fig. 14.2). The top end is

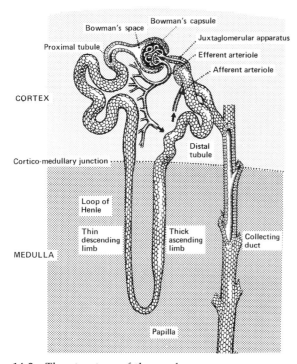

Fig. 14.2   The structure of the nephron.

invaginated around the cluster of the capillary network comprising four to six loops and forms the glomerulus, and the lower end enters the collecting duct. One important relationship often shown inaccurately in textbooks is that of the distal tubule. This lies adjacent to its own glomerulus and in close proximity to the afferent arteriole forming part of the renin-secreting juxtaglomerular apparatus. This allows a balance of function to be maintained between the arteriolar pressure and the sodium excretion into the tubules.

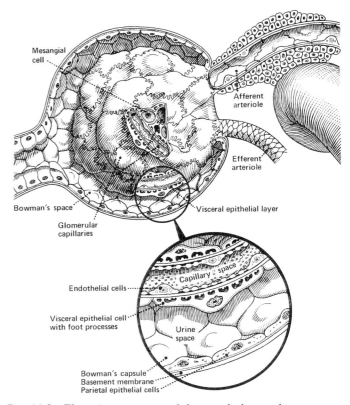

Fig. 14.3   The microanatomy of the renal glomerulus.

The glomerulus is 0.2 mm in diameter and histologically is made up of three types of cells, epithelial, endothelial and mesangial; the latter correspond to interstitial cells, have a mesangial matrix and are actively phagocytic. The invaginated top end of the tubule constitutes most of the basement membrane and the epithelial layer of cells (Fig. 14.3). The parietal epithelial cells line the inside of Bowman's capsule situated on the outer side of Bowman's space across which urine passes into the tubules. The visceral epithelial layer and basement membrane are closely applied to the capillaries, i.e. the endothelial cell layer. However, anatomically it is impossible for the epithelial layer to completely encompass the capillary circumferentially as it is reflected from one capillary loop to another. Therefore, in the stalk or core of the glomerulus the mesangium is in direct contact with the endothelial layer. This is important in the understanding of the histology of membrano-proliferative glomerulonephritis (*see* page 238). The visceral epithelial cells are unique as they stand on the basement membrane on foot processes or pedicles (Fig. 14.3). The endothelium of the capillary loops contain regularly spaced fenestrations with an average diameter of 70 nm and contribute to the inner layer of the basement membrane. The basement membrane itself is 300 nm thick. The epithelial cell layer has 'slits' or 'pores' which measure 30 nm across between the interdigitated foot processes. The total filtering surface of the two kidneys is equivalent to about 1.5 m². All the tubules are lined by cuboidal cells except for the thin segment of the loop of Henlé which is made up of flat epithelium. The proximal tubule cuboidal cells have a brush border and this corresponds to the segment of maximum reabsorption. The collecting duct is also lined with cuboidal epithelium.

Mode of Action

The two million nephrons receive 25 per cent of the cardiac output per minute giving a renal blood flow of 1,300 ml/min and allowing for a normal packed cell volume of 45 per cent, this corresponds to a renal plasma flow of 700 ml/min. From this the nephrons ultrafilter 120 ml/min or the equivalent of 180 l/24 hours. This varies with body size and is slightly less in women than men. The filtration pressure is the result of the glomerular capillary pressure of 8 kPa (60 mmHg), less the sum of the oncotic pressure of the plasma proteins 3.3 kPa (25 mmHg), plus the intracapsular hydrostatic pressure of 1.3 kPa (10 mmHg) and equals 3.4 kPa (26 mmHg). It is said that a kidney works on the principle of throwing out the baby with the bath-water and recovering the baby. Certainly the 180 l contains 25,000 mosmol or 580 g or sodium equivalent to $1\frac{1}{2}$ kg of salt and ultimately only about 1.5 l of urine containing about 4 g of sodium is excreted in 24 hours. Therefore, 576 g of sodium and 178.5 l of water are reabsorbed. This enormous filtration of sodium and water allows adequate amounts of the more slowly diffusing substances, such as urea, to be excreted and allows homeostasis or the 'milieu interieur' to be kept within narrow limits of ±2 per cent. The normal range of urine output is 0.5 to 20 ml/min representing a daily output of 720 to 2,880 ml. Assuming that the kidney is capable of concentrating urine to a level of 1,200 mosmol/l, then the compulsory 600 mosmol daily solute load to be excreted will require a minimum daily urinary volume of 500 ml. Some useful normal values are listed in Appendix II.

Sodium and Potassium Handling (Fig. 14.4)

The proximal tubule is responsible for the reabsorption of 80 per cent of the glomerular filtration, largely

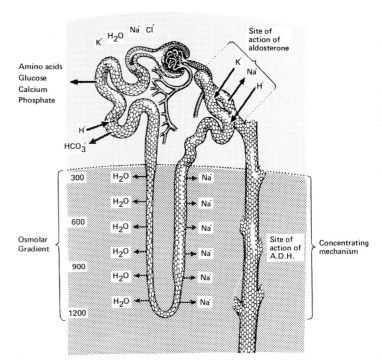

Fig. 14.4   Functions of the nephron.

sodium, potassium and water. As the *volume of the extracellular fluid is governed by sodium balance* an autoregulatory mechanism must operate within the kidney. The exact mechanisms are not known, but it is likely that the kidney makes the necessary adjustments to sodium excretion or reabsorption via the juxtaglomerular apparatus and through renin-aldosterone secretion. A decrease in pressure within the lumen of the afferent arteriole or an increase in the concentration of sodium in the distal tubule will initiate renin release and under the influence of aldosterone, sodium reabsorption, in exchange for hydrogen or potassium ions, will occur in the distal tubule. An increase in afferent arteriole pressure or a decrease in distal tubule sodium would switch off renin secretion.

The body has a great facility for regulating sodium balance and although reabsorption seems to be the most important mechanism there is probably in addition a natriuretic, or 'third' hormone, controlling excretion of sodium. Experimental evidence suggests that it may originate from the brain and it acts on both proximal and distal tubules to increase sodium excretion. This hormone is yet to be identified.

The kidney is less well able to control potassium balance in relation to serum levels or dietary intake. Potassium, like sodium, is almost all reabsorbed in the proximal tubule and then exchanged for sodium and hydrogen ions in the distal tubule under the influence of aldosterone. Diuretics increase sodium delivery to this distal site and the resulting exchange with potassium may produce hypokalaemia. It is suggested that serum potassium levels as well as renin-angiotensin mechanisms may control aldosterone secretion.

Just as the extracellular volume is controlled by sodium balance so *the osmotic concentration of the body fluid is dependent upon water balance*. The final adjustment following the enormous reabsorption of water in the proximal tubule is this time achieved by the concentrating mechanisms of the loop of Henlé and the collecting duct, under the action of the antidiuretic hormone (ADH). This is excreted by the posterior pituitary in response to changes in serum osmolarity (*see* page 165). As can be seen from the diagram (Fig. 14.4) the ascending limb of the loop of Henlé actively pumps sodium into the interstitium of the kidney and creates an osmotic gradient ranging from 300 mmol at the cortico-medullary junction to 1,200 mmol at the tip of the papilla. The descending loop loses water into the hyper-osmolar interstitium and gains sodium. This is the counter current multiplier principle and maintains the osmolar gradient within the medulla. Urea is freely diffusible and assists in maintaining the gradient. As the blood supply to the medulla, i.e. the vasa recta, is also a loop, this gradient down through the medulla is not dissipated. Incidentally, the very poor blood supply from the vasa recta has disadvantages as the papillae are very susceptible to ischaemia and toxic damage and may slough off. The concentration of the urine is adjusted as the collecting duct runs down through the pyramid. The effect of ADH regulates urine concentration between the range 300 to 1,200 by altering the permeability of the wall of the collecting tubules. The ratio of urinary osmolarity to plasma osmolarity ($U_{osm}:P_{osm}$) is usually 3 to 4:1, i.e. 900 to 1,200:300 mosmols, but urine may be as dilute as 40 mosmol/l.

Hydrogen Ion Excretion

Apart from their role in conserving glucose, amino acids, phosphate and calcium, largely in the enormous proximal reabsorption site, the tubules also maintain acid-base balance. The kidney's role in maintaining the body pH between 7.35 to 7.45 is secondary to that of the lungs. The lungs can only get rid of hydrogen ions in the form of carbonic acid as CO_2. The 60 mEq of 'fixed acid', i.e. phosphate, lactate, sulphate and hydroxybutyric acid produced daily from metabolites has to be buffered, mainly with bicarbonate. These 'fixed acids' are retained as the glomerular filtration rate falls, accounting for the acidosis of renal failure.

Hormones and Metabolic Function

In addition to renin the kidney produces erythropoetin (*see* page 372), probably from the region of the juxtaglomerular apparatus and also prostaglandins from the

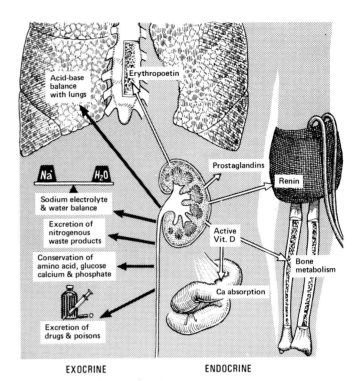

Fig. 14.5   The functions of the kidney.

medullary area. The other important function of the kidney is its ability to form the biologically active form of vitamin D, i.e. 1:25 dihydroxycholecalciferol (*see* page 192).

FUNCTION AND MALFUNCTION

The functions of the kidney are shown in Fig. 14.5. The exocrine functions comprise the excretory and regulatory roles and strictly the endocrine functions involve only secretion of the hormones renin, erythropoetin and prostaglandin, but the metabolism of vitamin D is included. Renin produces vasoconstriction and salt retention through the angiotensin-aldosterone axis. The intrarenal secretion of renin vasoconstricts the afferent arteriole and it is thought that prostaglandin, a potent vasodilator, is the balancing hormone. Prostaglandin also has a natriuretic action. Erythropoetin stimulates red blood cell formation. From knowledge of these functions it is possible to anticipate clinical manifestations that arise from acute or chronic failure of renal function. In addition to a general loss of nephron function the glomerular basement membrane may become permeable to protein from the damage produced by a glomerulonephritic lesion without any element of renal failure initially. Also selective tubular malabsorption of water, calcium, phosphate, glucose and amino acids produces a number of rare, usually hereditary tubular defects. Included in this group is renal tubular acidosis, where there is failure to excrete hydrogen ions.

Acute Renal Failure

When the kidney fails abruptly and there is sudden cessation of urine formation the following features develop:

1. Over-hydration from sodium and water retention.
2. Acidosis.
3. Hyperkalaemia.
4. Hyperphosphataemia causing hypocalcaemia.
5. Hypermagnesaemia.
6. Uraemia.
7. Toxic retention of drugs.

The acute onset and rapid course means that the long term toxic effects of a raised blood urea or serum phosphate do not have time to develop, and it is pulmonary oedema from overhydration or cardiac arrhythmias and asystole from hyperkalaemia that threaten life.

Chronic Renal Failure

The 'uraemic syndrome' proper refers to chronic renal failure and in contrast to acute renal failure, sodium, potassium and water retention is rarely found until the glomerular filtration rate is very low at levels of less than 5 ml/min. This explains the lack of oedema in patients with advanced yet not end-stage chronic renal failure.

During progressive destruction of the kidney, it is postulated that nephrons fail completely, i.e. glomeruli and tubules, and so glomerular-tubular imbalance does not occur. This 'intact nephron hypothesis' suggests that the residual intact nephrons hypertrophy and can cope with the normal daily solute load. This theory explains some of the findings in chronic renal insufficiency, such as the polyuria and excessive sodium and potassium loss in the urine. Polyuria, from the osmotic diuretic effect of urea, accounts for the nocturia in adults and enuresis in children with chronic renal failure. 'Salt-wasting' or more correctly a fixed sodium excretion may be a problem requiring active replacement with sodium chloride capsules or slow-Na tablets. Potassium may be lost excessively, but in end-stage renal failure hyperkalaemia is more of a problem, especially if potassium supplements or potassium-sparing diuretics are given.

Phosphate retention reduces the serum ionised calcium and this stimulates parathormone excretion causing secondary hyperparathyroid bone disease. This secondary phenomena of parathormone secretion as a result of a primary disturbance of phosphate and then calcium is an example of what is called the 'trade-off' hypothesis, i.e. one thing leading to another. In addition, as renal tissue is destroyed, less active vitamin D, i.e. 1:25 dihydroxycholecalciferol is produced, and calcium absorption from the gut is reduced. Thus renal osteomalacia, or rickets, indistinguishable from the nutritional type, will develop from both the low serum calcium and antagonistic effect of uraemic toxins on the action of vitamin D. Retained hydrogen ions are buffered by calcium carbonate, again from bone, causing further decalcification. Collectively these bone changes are known as uraemic bone disease or renal osteodystrophy. If the product of the serum calcium level × serum phosphate level exceeds 6 (e.g. 2.0×3.2), not an uncommon finding in chronic renal failure, spontaneous calcification develops in ectopic sites such as joints, blood vessels, muscles and eyes.

Terminal renal failure is characterised also by encephalopathy and neuropathy. The specific uraemic toxin has not been clearly identified, but in addition to rises in urea, creatinine and uric acid, phenols, indoles, guanides and parathormone are all found in increased quantities. Azotaemia is a term sometimes used instead of uraemia to include all nitrogen retention.

Uraemia has far reaching toxic effects in cell membranes and transfer mechanisms and on the peripheral action of hormones. For instance, insulin antagonism can lead to poor glucose utilisation, inhibition of growth hormone to dwarfism in children, and suppression of sex hormones to infertility in men and women.

The anaemia of chronic renal failure is of particular interest as it has many causes – the lack of erythropoetin and the suppression of its action on the bone marrow by uraemic toxins is one mechanism, but haemolysis, blood loss, iron, folate, pyridoxine and histidine deficiency also contribute.

As most endocrine glands are capable of producing excessive amounts of hormone as well as undersecreting, it is interesting that in some patients with renal carcinoma or polycystic kidneys secondary polycythaemia from excess erythropoetin secretion is seen.

Hypertension in chronic renal disease is thought to be due largely to hyperreninaemia. It is only in the end-stages of chronic renal failure that sodium and water retention causes a rise in blood pressure from hypervolaemia.

RENAL INVESTIGATIONS

1. Examination of urine.
2. Blood urea.
3. Serum creatinine.
4. Glomerular filtration rate.
5. Radiology.
6. Ultrasound.
7. Renal biopsy.

Early chronic renal failure cannot be detected clinically nor its progress monitored without the help of laboratory tests. Simpler, easier and cheaper investigations should be used initially. For example, the examination of a freshly voided urine specimen by the clinician is the most important test in clinical nephrology.

223

Examination of Urine

The lost art of simple urinalysis in favour of laboratory screening of stale urine is to be deplored.

Urinalysis. The 'Stix' tests, i.e. impregnated paper stick dipped into freshly voided urine have simplified urinalyses and have largely replaced all other urine tests. Albustix, Haemostix and Clinistix screen urine for the presence of albumin, blood and glucose respectively. Combistix, in addition to the above, tests for ketones and also estimates the pH of the urine.

Albustix are very sensitive to albumin and may pick up physiological amounts as a trace, i.e. 4 mg/dl; they do not detect the Bence-Jones protein of multiple myelomatosis. Boiling and salicylsulphonic acid tests are therefore still useful.

Haemostix are sensitive to free haemoglobin and less to intact red blood cells in the urine and the practice of placing the stick in the urine stream as it is passed is unreliable for detecting blood because the red cells have not haemolysed. Just as diabetic patients use Clinistix, so a nephrotic or proteinuric patient may also use Albustix to monitor protein loss in the urine.

Pathological amounts of protein (greater than 150 mg/24 hours) may be missed in aliquots of dilute urine and physiological amounts of less than 150 mg/24 hours detected as significant in aliquots of concentrated urine. Therefore, a 24-hour urine collection is the only accurate method.

The commonest cause of persistent proteinuria is glomerular disease and the commonest cause of transient proteinuria is a urinary tract infection.

24-Hour Urine Collections. An accurate timed collection usually over a period of 24 hours (occasionally 12 hours) is necessary to estimate the total daily excretion of a substance. Quantitative tests are applied mainly to urinary protein excretion in the investigation of persistent proteinuria and the nephrotic syndrome, but also to calcium, uric acid and cystine excretion in the investigation of renal stones (*see* page 249). Occasionally it is necessary to know the daily loss of sodium or potassium in patients with chronic renal failure with associated sodium and potassium losing states. The 24-hour urine collection is required to calculate clearances, i.e. creatinine clearance for measurement of glomerular filtration rate (*see below*).

Protein Selectivity. This refers to the ratio of the clearance of immunoglobulin, a large molecular protein, to the clearance of albumin, a small molecular protein. The selectivity of the urine protein contributes to the management of some patients with proteinuria. If albumin predominates in the urine, it suggests that the damage to the basement membrane is minimal and allows only the smaller protein through, i.e. minimal lesion nephritis. If concentrations of protein in the urine are roughly

---

Types of proteinuria
Pathological
Parenchymatous renal disease*
Glomerular damage
e.g. glomerulonephritis
Tubular lesions
e.g. congenital tubular disorders
Urinary tract infection
Physiological or functional
Fever
Exercise
Emotional stress
Extremes of temperature
Postural or orthostatic
Cardiac failure

*Some renal disease may not exhibit proteinuria, e.g. polycystic disease.

the same as those of the plasma, i.e. non-selective, then minimal lesion and/or steroid responsiveness are unlikely.

$$\text{Selectivity} = \frac{\text{C IgG}}{\text{C Albumin}}$$ (i.e. less than 0.16 'highly selective'; greater than 0.16 'non-selective').

Urine Microscopy. Before examining urine under the microscope the naked eye appearance and smell may assist diagnosis.

The urine is normally straw-coloured as a result of the presence of urochromes, but can become dark orange when concentrated. There are several causes of abnormal coloured urine.

Causes of coloured urine	
Cloudy	Bacteria, Pus, Urates, Phosphates
Smokey	Red blood cells
Red-brown	Haemoglobin, Urobilin, Myoglobin
Red	Drugs, e.g. phenindione, rifampicin Porphyria, Beeturia
Orange	Bile
Yellow	Drugs, e.g. mepacrine
Green-blue	Methylene blue, Fluorescein, Pseudomonas urinary infection.
Blue-black	Homogentisic acid (alkaptonuria), Melanin

Infected urine has a pungent 'fishy smell' and ketones as well as being detected on the breath impart a sweet 'pear-drop' aroma to urine.

Normal urine contains the odd red and white blood cell and a few hyaline casts, with squames from the lower urinary tract in the female.

To look at the urinary sediment or deposit microscopically, 10 ml of urine is spun for five minutes only at 2000 r/min so as not to break up casts – 9 ml is discarded. After resuspending the sediment in the remaining 1 ml a drop is examined under a cover-slip with the $\frac{1}{6}$ or high power objective. More than two red blood cells or five white blood cells per high powered field in the absence of vaginal contamination is considered abnormal. Several fields have to be examined to see any hyaline casts. Hyaline casts are impressions of the tubules made up of a normal tubular protein known as Tamm-Horsfall protein and about 400/hr are excreted as a normal finding. However, casts are also the most important abnormal constituents of urine and differentiate renal parenchymal lesions from other causes of haematuria and proteinuria. There are several kinds of pathological casts:

Cellular casts are hyaline casts filled with red cells or white cells, resulting from glomerulonephritis or inflammation of the renal parenchyma respectively.

Granular casts are degenerate cellular casts and sometimes break up and have a waxy appearance.

Broad casts are seen in renal failure, representing the larger hypertrophied structure of the remaining 'intact nephrons' in chronic renal failure.

Fatty casts are seen in the nephrotic syndrome.

Mid-stream Specimen or Urine (MSU). This is a method of obtaining a sample of urine for bacteriological studies without contamination and is sometimes known as a 'clean catch' specimen. It relies on scrupulous cleaning of the external genitalia and then, when a good flow of urine is established, catching a specimen in a sterile 'honey type' jar. The urine, i.e. mid-stream, is sent to the laboratory immediately for examination or stored in a refrigerator (4°C) until required as otherwise further growth will take place if the urine is infected. Quantitative bacterial counts define the presence of a urinary tract infection, i.e. 10^5 organisms/ml of urine indicates an infection. Urine containing 10^4 organisms/ml is considered doubtful and a repeat MSU is indicated. 10^3 organisms/ml is likely to be due to contamination.

An alternative to the MSU is the dip-slide incorporating a 'culture media' covered slide and container. The slide is dipped into a freshly voided urine specimen or passed through the urine stream during micturition. It can then be placed in the container and posted to the laboratory for bacterial counts, culture and sensitivity. It is very useful in general practice, and as a 'DIY' procedure for patients with recurrent infections allows early diagnosis and treatment.

Catheter Specimen of Urine (CSU). It is rarely necessary to obtain a catheter specimen of urine, but if a catheter is being passed for other reasons the opportunity of sending a sample should not be missed. The 10^5 organisms/ml rule does not apply to clean specimens of urine or to suprapubic aspiration specimens. Any bacteria found in these specimens are significant.

Suprapubic Aspiration. Using a small needle and syringe and having checked that either the suprapubic area is dull to percussion, or that the bladder is palpable, the needle is inserted in the mid-line immediately above the symphysis pubis and urine obtained by aspiration. This is a useful technique in young children and avoids the need for catheterisation and the difficulties of obtaining a mid-stream specimen for bacteriology.

Blood Urea

The blood urea is a common yet crude test of renal function. The level of urea in the blood does not rise until the glomerular filtration rate (GFR) has dropped to about 30 ml/min. Fig. 14.6 shows that renal function is severely compromised before the blood urea is elevated. Three stages of decline in GFR are recognised:
1. Diminished renal reserve before a rise in blood urea is obvious.
2. Chronic renal insufficiency as the blood urea rises,

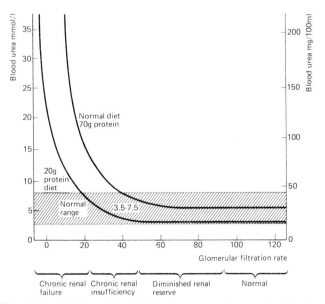

Fig. 14.6 Relationship of blood urea to glomerular filtration rate.

but no pathological changes of chronic uraemia have developed.

3. Chronic renal failure.

The concentration of blood urea is influenced not only by protein, i.e. nitrogen, intake, but also by its breakdown. Infection, starvation, steroids, tetracycline and other catabolic or anti-anabolic drugs will increase the blood urea without any alteration of the GFR. Similarly, high or low protein diets will alter the blood urea out of proportion to the GFR. Therefore, the blood urea is a useful measure of how well a patient is adhering to a low protein diet in chronic renal failure. In pregnancy because of the high renal blood flow and raised GFR (up to 200 ml/min) the blood urea should be below the normal lower limit. It may be falsely low in severe hepatic disease.

Serum Creatinine

The serum creatinine concentration is a much more reliable test of renal function than the blood urea. Although it still has a similar exponential relationship to the GFR, it is not so affected by the extrarenal factors influencing blood urea levels.

Glomerular Filtration Rate (GFR)

Endogenous creatinine clearance is used to measure the GFR; it is the most important test of renal function. It is used initially to assess the degree of renal impairment and thereafter to monitor changes in function. An accurately timed urine collection, to the nearest minute and millilitre over 24 hours, is required with a blood sample for the plasma creatinine concentration. The clearance concept can then be applied. Clearance of a substance is defined as the theoretical volume of plasma completely cleared of that substance in unit time. Provided the substance is completely filtered and not secreted or absorbed in the tubule, then the quantity of the substance recovered in the urine in a minute must be equal to the amount of plasma filtered to provide that quantity. The clearance is expressed in ml/min, as obtained from the formula:

$$Ccr = \frac{Ucr\ V}{Pcr\ T}$$

V   = volume of urine in 24 hours
Ucr = urinary creatinine concentration.
Pcr = plasma creatinine concentration.
T   = 24 hours = 24 × 60 = 1,440 min.

An example of the creatinine clearance worked out to give the GFR corrected to 1.73 m² is shown in Appendix II. It is important to allow for body size, otherwise a small person with a normally low clearance would be thought to have renal insufficiency. Ethylene-diamine-tetroacetate (EDTA) labelled with the gamma emitter ^{51}chromium (^{51}Cr) is another accurate method of measuring the GFR. The clearance principle may be used, but a simpler indirect method relates the plasma decay curve to the GFR after an IV injection of ^{51}Cr EDTA, thus avoiding the difficulties of accurate urine collection. This latter method is very useful in young children and in out-patients.

Radiology

Radiology is used extensively in the investigation of renal disease and its accompanying bone disease.

Plain or Straight X-rays of the Abdomen may be all that is required to assess renal size and position. Sometimes known as KUB (kidneys, ureters and bladder), it will show up renal calculi and other calcifications in the abdomen and pelvis and is always taken as a preliminary film to intravenous pyelogram.

An Intravenous Pyelogram (IVP) (also known as excretory urography) using contrast media opacifies the kidney and its collecting systems with progressive visualisation of the whole tract – calyces, pelvis, ureters and bladder on serial films. A post-micturition or void film is taken to assess the residual urine volume. Some of the more obvious renal pathologies diagnosed radiologically are shown in Fig. 14.7. Tomography is employed if the kidneys are poorly visualised. Tomograms are X-ray cuts taken at different depths or levels within the body at the same time as the IVP. They are known as nephrotomograms when used to examine kidneys.

Retrograde Pyelography. Sometimes a kidney does not show up on one side with an IVP, either because it is

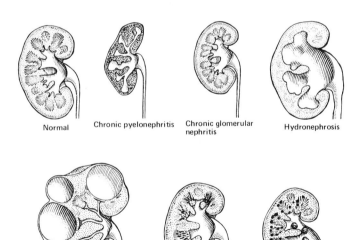

Fig. 14.7 Examples of renal pathology that may be diagnosed radiologically.

congenitally absent or non-functioning. After cytoscopy a catheter is passed up the ureter to the site of obstruction or into the renal pelvis and contrast media injected.

Antegrade Pyelography. This is sometimes used following insertion of a nephrostomy tube or cannula in an obstructed kidney.

Micturating Cystourethrography (MCUG). Retrograde flow of urine from the bladder up the ureters, i.e. vesico-ureteric reflux is diagnosed by filling the bladder *per urethrum* with contrast media and then taking a series of X-rays during the act of micturition. In the most severe forms contrast media will be seen flowing up the ureter and distending the pelvis giving the appearance of hydro-ureter or hydronephrosis, i.e. distension of ureters and pelvis respectively. Vesicoureteric reflux may be unilateral or bilateral.

Arteriography and Venography. The renal vasculature, both arterial and venous, can be outlined radiologically. Each renal artery or renal vein can be selectively cannulated via the femoral artery and vein respectively. Injection of contrast media shows up the vessels. The diagnosis of renal artery stenosis and the differentiation of renal masses, such as simple renal cysts from a renal tumour, requires renal arteriography. Renal vein or venous thrombosis is best diagnosed by renal venography.

Isotope Studies. The structure and function of the kidney can be examined using isotopic-labelled substances excreted by the kidney.

Isotope renography employs radioactive-I-labelled Hippuran (sodium-o-iodo hippurate). Following intravenous injection both renal angles are monitored using gamma counters and a curve is obtained for each kidney. The curve has a vascular, secretory and excretory component and unilateral differences in function are easily detected (Fig. 14.8). It is mainly used to screen

hypertensive patients for unilateral renal disease, e.g. renal artery stenosis or unilateral chronic pyelonephritis, but will also detect unilateral acute ureteric obstruction. Renography is only an adjunct to more conventional tests, e.g. IVP, but the radiation dose is less.

Renal scan or scintography. By using a gamma camera instead of a counter and several different isotopes, both structure and function of the kidneys can be examined.

Bone X-rays and isotope scans are used to detect renal bone disease, e.g. hyperparathyroidism.

Ultrasound. Ultrasonography is useful to detect accumulations of fluid, blood or pus around the normal or transplanted kidney. It will also differentiate a solid tumour from a cyst within the kidney.

Renal Biopsy

The main use of renal biopsy is in the investigation of proteinuria and occasionally in acute renal failure. A small sample of renal tissue is removed from one kidney under local anaesthetic using a cutting or aspiration biopsy needle. The needle is inserted percutaneously into the kidney through the renal angle. Rarely, an open biopsy through a surgical incision may be required. The sample must contain glomeruli and is examined by light, electron and immunofluorescent microscopy. Light microscopy is used up to 1,000 × magnification and electron microscopy up to 40,000×. Immunofluorescence is used to detect glomerular deposits of immunoglobulins, complement and fibrin. Human antisera to IgA, IgE, IgG, IgM plus anti-complement and anti-fibrin sera are run on to the biopsy section and exposed to a fluorescent light source. The depositions will fluoresce and classify the glomerulonephritis immunologically, for example IgA nephropathy. The pattern, either granular or linear, and the distribution around the capillary loops or in the mesangium are also demonstrated (Fig. 14.9). Apart from transient haematuria, complications such as severe haemorrhage, or loss of function, are rare. Relative contraindications to biopsy are a single functioning kidney, renal tumours or cysts, uncontrolled hypertension, a bleeding tendency or small contracted kidneys.

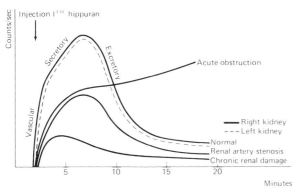

Fig. 14.8 Normal and abnormal renogram curves.

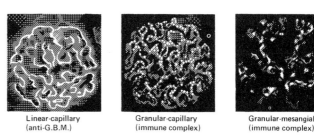

Linear-capillary (anti-G.B.M.)   Granular-capillary (immune complex)   Granular-mesangial (immune complex)

Fig. 14.9 Patterns of glomerular immunofluorescence.

MAJOR SYMPTOMS

Loin or Flank Pain

Pain from the capsule or pelvis is produced by distension of these structures, secondary to inflammation or obstruction. It is situated in one or other renal or costovertebral angle and is described as flank or loin pain. It is often difficult to differentiate from either vague low backache or, when radiating anteriorly, from abdominal pain of a variety of causes.

Renal Colic

This is a misnomer as it is caused by ureteric colic from obstruction with blood, stones, pus or papillae. It is not colicky but usually constant, varying only in intensity. It has a characteristic distribution from the loin around into the hypochondrium and descending into the groin and upper thigh, i.e. skin distribution of T12, L1, L2 and L3, and it may be accompanied by signs of shock, i.e. hypotension, rapid low volume pulse and sweating. If the pain is mainly anterior in distribution it may be mistaken for an acute abdomen, e.g. perforation, appendicitis or cholecystitis.

Bladder Pain

This is usually a dragging discomfort felt suprapubically, but in a more severe form, often as a result of cystitis, a painful and urgent desire to pass urine accompanied by a feeling of incomplete bladder emptying is known as strangury. 'Pis a deux' literally means to pass water twice and is also produced by a feeling of incomplete bladder emptying.

Pain may also be felt in the urethra or over the perineum in urethritis or prostatic inflammation.

Disturbances of Micturition

Frequency. The average man passes urine about four or five times a day, but women only twice or three times; anything in excess of this constitutes frequency. The desire to micturate is stimulated by about 300 ml urine in the normal sized bladder; therefore polyuria will produce frequency.

Dysuria. Burning, scalding or pain during the act of micturition felt in the urethra and commonly associated with frequency is known as dysuria. The symptoms of urgency and strangury can also accompany severe dysuria.

Polyuria. The persistent passage of 24-hour urine volumes in excess of 2.5 to 3 litres constitutes polyuria. It has many causes and, of course, produces frequency and nocturia (*see below*).

Nocturia. The necessity to get up at night to pass urine is singly the earliest and most consistent symptom of chronic renal insufficiency or failure. Enuresis, i.e. bed-wetting in children, may indicate underlying renal disease, just as nocturia may do in the adult.

Oliguria. Oliguria is defined as a volume of urine less than 400 ml in 24 hours.

Anuria. Anuria is defined as a volume of urine less than 100 ml in 24 hours. Total anuria means absolutely no urine, and raises the suspicion of obstruction to the ureters. It is important to emphasise that anuria does not mean retention of urine. Retention is an inability to pass urine although an adequate urine volume is present within the bladder.

Haematuria

Another classical sign of urinary tract disease is the passage of blood-stained urine and only 0.5 ml blood is required in a litre of urine to show up as frank or macroscopic haematuria.

Types of Polyuria

Type	Cause
Diabetes insipidus	Lack of antidiuretic hormone
Nephrogenic diabetes insipidus	Lack of response to antidiuretic hormone
Compulsive water drinker	Water diuresis
	Loss of concentrating ability
Diabetes mellitus	Glucose osmotic diuresis
Diuretic therapy	Sodium diuresis
Chronic renal failure	Urea osmotic diuresis
	±damage to medullary concentrating mechanism, e.g. chronic pyelonephritis

RENAL FAILURE

ACUTE RENAL FAILURE (ARF)

Definition

Acute renal failure is defined as a sudden decline in renal function over a period of hours or days when the inadequate quantity or poor quality of urine leads to a rise in plasma levels of nitrogenous waste products, i.e. acute uraemia.

Background

Although classically associated with oligo-anuria, acute renal failure may develop over a wide range of urine volumes and even in the presence of an apparently adequate output of 1 to 2 l/24 hours. However, the urine in these cases contains little urea and this high-output, non-oliguric or polyuric type of failure requires a high degree of clinical vigilance if it is not be missed.

The main causes are shown in Fig. 14.10.

Acute renal failure is divided into three categories: pre-renal, renal and post-renal.

Pre-renal or Incipient Renal Failure. This is simply physiological oliguria. Functional failure from a reduced renal blood flow and glomerular filtration rate produces acute uraemia without structural damage to the kidney. This stage is immediately reversible and return to normal function is possible with corrective therapy. The kidney is still capable of concentration and this ability is used as a differential diagnostic index (Table 14.1).

Shock or circulatory collapse is the commonest cause of under-perfusion of the kidney and three types are recognised.

1. *Hypovolaemic shock* follows loss of blood or plasma after major surgery, trauma, obstetric haemorrhage, acute pancreatitis or severe burns. Loss of water and electrolytes causing gross dehydration with circulatory collapse is seen in the polyuria of diabetes mellitus, in severe diarrhoea and vomiting and in paralytic ileus when fluid is sequestered within the gut.

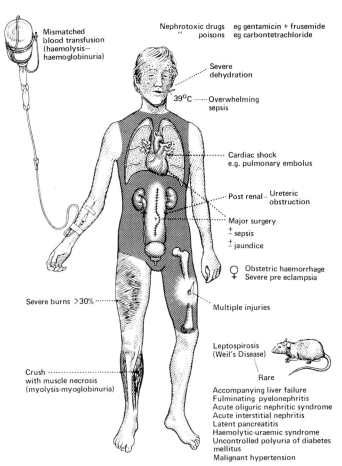

Fig. 14.10 The causes of acute renal failure.

2. *Septicaemic or endotoxaemic shock* follows overwhelming sepsis usually from a Gram-negative bacteraemia after intra-abdominal surgery but can occur with no apparent traumatic or surgical insult, for example following a viral pneumonia.

3. *Cardiogenic shock* is produced by the profound drop in blood pressure after a myocardial infarction, pulmonary emboli or cardiac tamponade. This rarely causes acute renal shut-down because in addition to simple under-perfusion, tissue damage is an important accompanying factor.

Table 14.1 Diagnostic indices in acute renal failure

	Insipient renal failure (pre-renal)	Established renal failure (renal)
Central venous pressure (CVP)	Low 2 cmH$_2$O or less	Normal or high 6 to 10 cmH$_2$O
Urine volume	Low	Low
Urine sediment	Usually absent	Often present
Response to: mannitol and/ frusemide	Diuresis	No effects or high output failure induced with frusemide
Urine osmolality	>500 mosmol/l	<350 mosmol/l
Urine urea	>250 mmol/l	<160 mmol/l
Urine sodium	<20mmol/l	>50 mmol/l
Urine: plasma (osmolal ratio)	>1.8:1	<1.1:1
Urine: plasma (urea ratio)	>15:1	<10:1
Urine: plasma (creatinine ratio)	>15:1	<10:1

Renal or Established Renal Failure. This results from structural damage to the kidney. The commonest cause is progression from an unrecognised or untreated pre-renal phase or from ingestion of nephrotoxic drugs and poisons. However, any severe parenchymatous lesion will interfere sufficiently with the renal blood flow to cause acute renal failure, i.e. acute glomerulonephritis, pyelonephritis or interstitial nephritis. Haemolysis is a potent cause of acute renal failure as seen in mis-matched blood transfusion, the haemolytic-uraemic syndrome and in leptospirosis and other severe infections. In fact the jaundiced patient is curiously susceptible to acute renal failure, for example hepato-renal syndrome and acute obstructive cholangitis.

'Post-renal' Renal Failure. This means acute obstruction to urine flow into the bladder and is also known as acute obstructive uropathy. The obstruction may be intrarenal with urates, sulphonamide crystals or myeloma protein blocking the collecting ducts. However, it is, more commonly, extrarenal with either bilateral ureteric obstruction or, more commonly, obstruction to the ureter of a solitary functioning kidney. The major causes of a blocked ureter are stones, blood, tumours, sloughed necrotic papillae or inadvertent ligation during surgery. Total anuria, i.e. no urine at all, is suggestive of post-renal failure. Rarely, a solitary kidney may be severely traumatised when either the ureter or the blood vessels of the ureter are avulsed causing acute anuria.

Pathology

Tubular necrosis is the commonest histological lesion in acute renal failure. The glomeruli are usually normal with destruction of the tubular epithelial cells and sometimes evidence of regeneration with intracellular mitotic figures. If shock is prolonged and profound, following obstetric haemorrhage or associated with disseminated intravascular coagulation, then acute cortical necrosis may develop. It is uncommon. The cortical area of the kidney including the glomeruli becomes ischaemic and infarcted and with acute cortical necrosis, recovery of normal renal architecture and function does not occur.

The pathophysiology of acute renal failure is not completely understood, but two mechanisms can produce tubular necrosis:
1. Impaired renal blood flow and perfusion causing an ischaemic or circulatory type of injury to the proximal and distal tubules.
2. Direct poisoning by nephrotoxic drugs or agents causing a nephrotoxic or toxic injury confined to the proximal tubule. There is no reduction in circulating blood volume, i.e. hypovolaemia in this latter type.

As a result of tubular damage and failure of reabsorption, the excess sodium chloride delivered to the distal tubule stimulates the secretion of intrarenal renin and angiotensin from the juxtaglomerular apparatus. Angiotensin produces vasoconstriction of the afferent arteriole and a drop in glomerular filtration and subsequent oliguria; prostaglandins may not reach the glomeruli from the medulla to counteract this action with vasodilation. Why, after the circulation is restored, no reflow of urine occurs remains conjectural. It is thought that there may be ischaemic swelling of the endothelial lining of the afferent arterioles with localised intravascular coagulation within its lumen reducing blood flow still further in an already constricted vessel. It is likely in conditions associated with haemolysis and myolysis that the subsequent filtration of free haemoglobin and myoglobin perpetuates oliguria by forming casts in the tubules. However, tubular obstruction with debris and back-diffusion of urine into the kidney substance through the damaged tubules may play a part, but are rarely the sole cause of acute renal failure. The other pathologies, including acute oliguric glomerulonephritis, acute fulminating pyelonephritis and acute interstitial nephritis, cause acute renal failure because of either the degree of damage to the glomerulus or from the direct interference to the flow of blood in the intralobular arteries, secondary to inflammatory swelling of the interstitium of the kidney. Rarely, direct occlusion either of both major renal arteries or veins will also cause acute anuria.

Symptoms and Signs

Pre-renal, renal and post-renal stages of acute renal failure have different clinical features. The two methods of presentation are either following some recognisable incident, for example surgery and trauma or unheralded 'out-of-the-blue', suggesting latent infection, nephrotoxins or post-renal obstruction. The onset of acute renal failure may be undetected, particularly in a seriously ill patient as a result of preoccupation with the primary pathology, for example major trauma. Sometimes it is obvious from the symptoms and signs that the patient has underlying chronic renal failure as well, i.e. acute-on-chronic renal failure.

Symptoms

Diminished urinary output – urine may be dark from concentration or presence of free haemoglobin.
Total anuria – no urine at all suggests post-renal obstruction.
Renal pain – makes post-renal obstruction a more likely cause.
Thirst and dry mouth – dehydration, i.e. pre-renal.
Hiccough and drowsiness from acute uraemia.
Dyspnoea due to pulmonary oedema from overhydration.

Signs

'Pre-renal' signs are those of dehydration, circulatory collapse or frank shock:
Low volume, rapid pulse.
Low blood pressure.
Constricted veins and cold cyanosed extremities.
Dry inelastic skin, dry tongue with occasional parotitis.
Low eyeball tension.
Oligo-anuria.

'Renal' signs are those of overhydration complicated by frank uraemia and hyperkalaemia.
Dyspnoea ⎫
Basal crepitations ⎬ from pulmonary oedema of over-⎭ hydration

Raised jugular venous pressure from increased circulatory blood volume of overhydration.
Cardiac arrhythmias from hyperkalaemia.
Uraemic bleeding from mucous membranes and anaemia.

'Post-renal' signs may be identical to those of established renal shut-down, but may include the signs of obstruction, i.e.
Tenderness in the loin or over the kidney anteriorly.
Palpable kidney from the acute ureteric obstruction.
Total anuria interpolated with periods of polyuria due to momentary relief of obstruction is considered pathognomonic, but rarely seen.

Investigations

1. Measurement of hourly urine volume via urethral catheter.
2. Haemoglobin, white blood cell and platelet counts – haemoglobin may be inappropriately high in dehydration; the white blood cell raised in bacterial sepsis and the plateletes low in continued haemorrhage. (Do other screening tests for disseminated intravascular coagulation (see page 420).)
3. Blood urea, serum creatinine and electrolytes to assess degree of uraemia, acidosis and serum potassium level.
4. ECG monitoring of serum potassium level.
5. Serum calcium, serum phosphate for hypocalcaemia and hypophosphataemia.
6. Renal indices (Table 14.1).
7. Radiological or isotopic examination to exclude acute obstructive uropathy (post-renal) and small contracted kidneys of chronic renal failure.
8. Mid-stream specimen of urine for sediment, culture and sensitivities.
9. Chest X-ray to demonstrate pulmonary oedema.
10. Blood gases to detect early respiratory failure and assess need for assisted ventilation.
11. Blood culture – high incidence of secondary septicaemia in acute renal failure.
12. Specific serological studies for bacterial and viral antibodies, e.g. leptospiral titres.
13. Renal biopsy. If no causative incident such as shock, sepsis, obstruction or exposure to nephrotoxins is obvious and the acute renal failure has come 'out-of-the-blue', then renal biopsy is justified to make a diagnosis. It is also performed if renal function does not return after two or three weeks and when the kidneys are of normal size.

As the treatment of acute renal failure is an exercise in intensive care, most of the investigations require to be repeated frequently, even six to twelve-hourly.

Basis of Treatment

Before treatment begins three questions have to be answered:

(a) Is there post-renal obstruction?
(b) Is there a pre-renal element or has established renal failure already supervened?
(c) Were the kidneys functioning normally before the present illness or could this be acute-on-chronic renal failure?

1. Exclude obstruction or relieve it by retrograde catheterisation or insertion of nephrostomy tube(s).
2. Replace all known losses with the correct quantity and quality of fluid, i.e. blood, plasma or electrolyte solutions depending on deficiency under central venous pressure monitoring.
3. Check serum potassium level and if high or rising give:
(a) 50 ml of 10 per cent calcium gluconate IV to protect myocardium from toxic effect of hyperkalaemia. This also corrects hypocalcaemia prior to giving 50 ml of 8.3 per cent of sodium bicarbonate IV to correct acidosis which lessens the risk of hypocalcaemic tetany.
(b) 100 ml of 40 per cent dextrose with 20 units soluble insulin to drive potassium back into the cells.
(c) Sodium or calcium resonium 50 g as retention enema or 30 g orally or via intragastric tube six-hourly. This ion exchange resin binds intestinal potassium and prevents absorption.
4. Trial of mannitol: 100 ml of 20 per cent mannitol as a rapid IV bolus.
5. Trial of frusemide: a slow IV infusion (4 mg/min) of 500 mg of frusemide. (Not if gentamicin or a cephalosporin have been given recently.) If renal failure is not established, urinary output will double to 40 to 50 ml/hour, otherwise there is no response.
6. In established renal failure overhydration should be avoided by restricting fluids to 400 ml each 24 hours plus all other losses until dialysis can be arranged.
7. Intubation and ventilation may be necessary to treat pulmonary oedema.
8. Hypercatabolism is common in acute renal failure, i.e. rise in blood urea of 10 mmol/day or more. It may be

suppressed by administering 50 per cent dextrose with insulin.

9. *All patients with established renal failure require dialysis whatever the level of blood urea.* The aim is to prevent uraemia rather than treat it. When uraemia is controlled, wounds heal better; the patient is fed properly and complications such as bleeding are less likely.

(i) Early, short and frequent dialysis – peritoneal or haemodialysis.

(ii) Maintain haematocrit at about 35 per cent.

(iii) Treat infection with appropriate narrow spectrum antibiotic.

(iv) Feed the patient with adequate calories as carbohydrates, fat and protein or give amino acids by infusion.

(v) Give water-soluble vitamins and folic acid.

(vi) Blood plasma supplies all the necessary trace elements or micro-nutrients.

The course and treatment of a hypothetical post-traumatic patient is shown in Fig. 14.11.

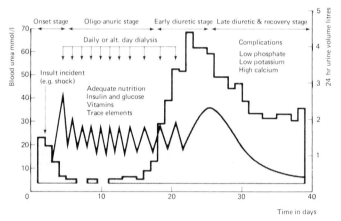

Fig. 14.11 Course of a hypothetical patient with post-traumatic shock and acute renal failure.

Complications

Hyperkalaemic cardiac asystole.

Pulmonary oedema and respiratory failure due to over-hydration or 'shock lung', i.e. multiple pulmonary emboli of leucocyte aggregates from unfiltered blood transfusion.

Secondary sepsis and septicaemia.

Hypophosphataemia and hypokalaemia during diuretic recovery phase.

Disseminated intravascular coagulation.

Malnutrition.

Mortality and morbidity of causative pathology.

Prevention

Recognise 'high risk' surgical patients: aged, dehydrated, diabetics, jaundiced, on nephrotoxic drugs, or with pre-existing renal impairment, and avoid a preoperative policy of 'nil by mouth'.

Recognise 'high risk' surgical procedures: cardiac and aortic

surgery, all gall bladder surgery with biliary obstruction, surgery with the presence of infection, particularly peritonitis and including that due to viruses.

In the above instances keep patient hydrated and give mannitol perioperatively. Avoid nephrotoxic drug combinations, particularly gentamicin, cephalosporins and frusemide.

Prognosis

The mortality rate in established acute renal failure is 40 to 90 per cent, despite early dialysis and feeding. Tragically, death may occur during the recovery phase, and is often the result of infection or from the primary incident.

If the patient with acute tubular necrosis survives, a return to normal renal function can be expected within six months to a year. In cortical necrosis only partial recovery may occur and the patient may be left with chronic-on-acute renal failure requiring long term dialysis support.

The outcome in the other causative pathologies, for example glomerulonephritis will depend on the effectiveness of specific treatment.

CHRONIC RENAL FAILURE (CRF)

Definition

A slow progressive decline in renal function over many months or years to an end-stage manifest by chronic uraemia or the 'uraemic syndrome'. It is irreversible.

Background

The expression 'diminished renal reserve' corresponds to a degree of impaired renal function when the blood urea may be normal, but the creatinine clearance shows that the glomerular filtration rate is below the expected level for age and body size (Fig. 14.6). 'Chronic renal insufficiency' is used to denote the next stage when the urea just begins to rise and the glomerular filtration rate has fallen to 30 to 40 ml/min. Chronic renal insufficiency or the state of diminished renal reserve may come to light if a patient is subjected to a further assault on renal function, for example surgery, dehydration or exposure to nephrotoxic drugs, and produces acute-on-chronic renal failure. Some of the commoner causes of chronic renal failure are listed on the following page. The chief primary diseases are glomerulonephritis and pyelonephritis. The onset is often so insidious that the disease may not be detected until the glomerular filtration rate has fallen to 5 to 10 ml/min and the kidneys are small and contracted.

The end-stage kidney defies histological classification and the need to establish a precise diagnosis is academic anyway. Renal biopsy in these cases is unhelpful and unwarranted, and the procedure may be difficult with

Causes of chronic renal failure

Chronic glomerulonephritis—Primary immune
                complex disease
Chronic glomerulonephritis—Secondary to
                systemic disease
Chronic pyelonephritis
Diabetic nephropathy
Chronic interstitial nephritis e.g. drugs
Chronic obstructive uropathy
Hypertensive nephrosclerosis
Gout
Polycystic disease
Amyloid
Myeloma

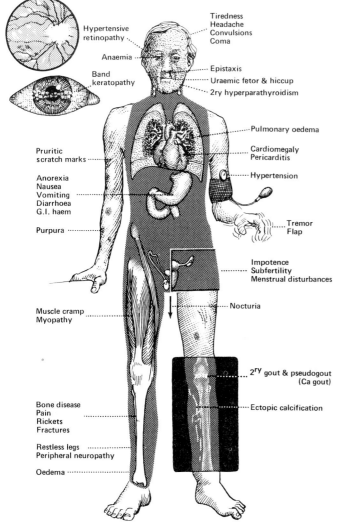

Fig. 14.12 Clinical features of chronic uraemia.

haemorrhage being more common. Most of the glomeruli are sclerosed, although the remaining functioning ones are often large and there are large areas of fibrosis and tubular atrophy. It would be possible to differentiate chronic pyelonephritis from glomerulonephritis, but not to identify the type of nephritis, i.e. proliferative or membranous.

It appears that as a destructive lesion decimates the nephron population it leaves the remaining nephrons intact and it is this so-called 'intact nephron hypothesis' that explains some of the pathophysiological events in chronic renal failure. Reduction in the number of functioning nephrons not only causes a retention of urea, phosphate, sulphate and other uraemic toxins, but places a heavy solute load on the remaining nephrons.

Table 14.2 Clinical features of chronic renal failure

Symptoms	Signs
Cutaneous	
Pruritus	Pigmentation
Dry skin	Scratch marks
Ocular	
Failing vision	Hypertensive retinopathy
Sore eyes	Corneal calcification
	Conjunctival calcification
	(red eye)
Cardiovascular	
Dyspnoea	Hypertension ± pulmonary oedema
	(uraemic lung)
Orthopnoea	Pericarditis ± effusion
Chest pain	Ischaemic heart disease (ECG)
Swollen legs	Cardiac failure
Gastrointestinal	
Anorexia	Fetor
Vomiting	Parotitis
Thirst	Oral ulceration
Diarrhoea	
Neuromuscular	
Drowsiness	Encephalopathy – tremor, flap
Fits	Peripheral neuropathy – sensory, motor
Coma	Myopathy – muscle wasting
Cramps	
Weakness	
Restless legs	
Skeletal	
Bone pain	Ectopic calcification – joints,
Joint pain	blood vessels and eyes
Gout	Uraemic bone disease (X-ray)
Endocrine	
Impotence	Growth failure
Infertility	Delayed puberty
Menstrual disturbance	Gynaecomastia
Haematological	
Fatigue	Anaemia
Dyspnoea	Bruises
Bruising	Purpura
Epistaxis	
Genito-urinary	
Thirst	Proteinuria
Nocturia	Abnormal urinary sediment
Enuresis	

This load subjects them to a continuous osmotic diuresis. The normal concentrating ability of the tubules cannot cope with the large urine flow and polyuria results. Retention of sodium and water does not usually develop until the GFR is under 10 ml/min. In diseases that damage mainly the medulla, such as chronic pyelonephritis and analgesic nephropathy and other chronic interstitial nephritides, selective damage to the concentrating ability may lead to chronic salt-wasting and a dehydrated state, i.e salt-losing nephropathy.

Symptoms and Signs (*see* Table 14.2, Fig. 14.12)

Investigations

Haemoglobin and a blood film to characterise anaemia.
Blood urea and creatinine clearance to estimate the renal function.
Serum uric acid.
Excretory urography with nephrotomography to assess renal size and to exclude obstruction.
Mid stream specimen of urine to examine the urinary sediment and detect any urinary infection.
Serum calcium, phosphate and alkaline phosphatase to detect the early biochemical changes of uraemic osteodystrophy, i.e. renal bone disease.
Skeletal survey or bone scan and bone biopsy to confirm renal bone disease.
Australia antigen screen (HBsAg) – outbreaks of

hepatitis B in renal units carries a high morbidity and mortality particularly amongst staff.
Tissue-typing if a transplant is contemplated.

Basis of Treatment

The three basic stages of treatment in the treatment of chronic renal failure are as shown in Fig. 14.13.

1. **Preservation of Remaining Nephron Function:**
(a) Control of hypertension and heart failure if present.
(b) Treatment of any superimposed urinary infection.
(c) Removal of other factors compromising renal function, in particular, urinary tract obstruction.
(d) Correction of salt and water depletion.
(e) Salt and water loading with covering diuretic therapy.
(f) Careful prescribing if drugs are potentially nephrotoxic.

2. **Conservative Management of Uraemic Syndrome:**
(a) Restriction of dietary protein intake, sometimes potassium restriction is also necessary.
(b) Administration of aluminium hydroxide to reduce intestinal phosphate absorption and the serum phosphate levels, thus delaying the onset of renal bone disease.
(c) Correction of low serum calcium levels with oral calcium supplements and vitamin D.
(d) Allopurinol to lower serum uric acid levels and control clinical gout.

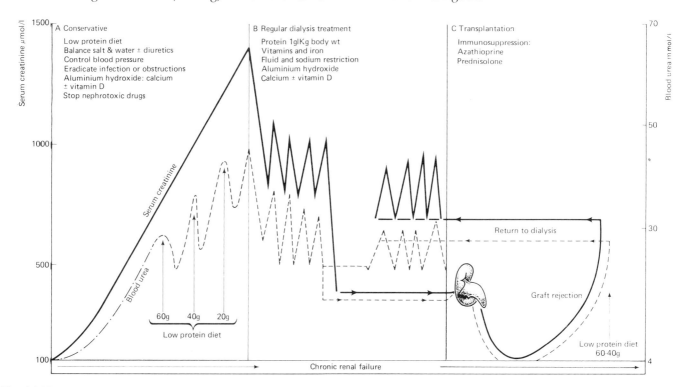

Fig. 14.13 Management of a hypothetical patient in a chronic renal failure programme.

(e) Acidosis is not usually treated but calcium can be given as carbonate.

A balance must be achieved therapeutically between controlling the blood pressure and keeping the patient oedema-free yet administering as much salt and water as possible and covering this with diuretic therapy to maintain a high urine flow. The rationale for this is that although the GFR cannot be improved it may well be reduced by sodium and water depletion. Urea is freely diffusable and is excreted by the tubules in a high urine flow state.

The sheet anchor in the treatment of chronic renal failure is the low protein diet. It does not improve function, but merely reduces the level of urea and other uraemic toxins. Decrements should be made initially when the blood urea levels reach about 25 to 30 mosmol/l and then again as the concentration returns to that level with further deterioration in function.

A 60 g diet is introduced when the GFR reaches 15 to 30 ml/min with further reductions to 40 g at 5 to 15 ml/min. The 20 g or Giovannetti diet is reserved for patients with GFRs of 5 ml/min or less. This last diet is given to patients unlikely to be accepted on to the chronic renal failure programme, i.e. dialysis and/or transplantation, as it barely maintains a positive nitrogen balance. The low protein diets rely on a high biological value content for their efficacy, i.e. high essential amino acid content. The body metabolises these diets more efficiently with less nitrogen waste production. Some urea may be recycled to provide a nitrogen source for non-essential amino acids.

3. Long Term Dialysis and Transplantation:

Indications for regular dialysis treatment:
Patients aged about 5 to 55 without systemic disease or neoplasia.
Clinical deterioration despite good conservative management.
Presence of uraemic pericarditis.
Onset of severe renal bone disease.
Development of peripheral neuropathy.
Serum creatinine greater than 1,200 μmol/l.
Glomerular filtration rate 3 to 5 ml/min.

Dialysis will replace all the exocrine but not the endocrine functions of the kidney. Anaemia will persist; hypertension is controlled in 90 per cent of patients without resorting to bilateral nephrectomy and bone disease can be arrested by adequate dialysis, control of serum phosphate levels, and vitamin D therapy in the form of 1:25 dihydroxycholecalciferol or occasionally by parathyroidectomy.

Transplantation: Most patients can be transplanted from regular dialysis programmes using living related or cadaver donor kidneys.

The two main contraindications to transplantation are the presence of chronic infection, and bladder outflow obstruction. Immunosuppressive drugs used to prevent rejection decrease response to infection.

Donor kidneys are matched with the recipient on dialysis for major blood groups and histocompatibility leucocyte antigens (HLA). Two-year graft survival is about 65 per cent for the living related donor and about 45 per cent for the cadaver kidney. Patient survival is 20 to 30 per cent better than this as a return to dialysis is possible. Five-year survivals with a cadaver kidney are about 35 per cent. About one-third of transplanted kidneys fail in the first six months and if the kidney lasts for two or three years then continued graft survival is likely. Recently, a recurrence of glomerulonephritis has been reported in transplanted kidneys after four to five years.

GLOMERULONEPHRITIS

Definition

Glomerulonephritis is a bilateral disease of the kidneys characterised by a variety of clinical syndromes and glomerular lesions. The term is used in two contexts: clinically, for example acute glomerulonephritis, and pathologically, for example proliferative glomerulonephritis describing the histological appearance of the glomeruli. Glomerulonephritis may be primary, for example acute post-streptococcal glomerulonephritis or secondary to a systemic disease, for example lupus nephritis in systemic lupus erythematosus (*see* page 119).

Background

Primary and secondary nephritis are initiated, in most cases, by immunological mechanisms, and two types of immune response are seen:
(a) Immune complex nephritis.
(b) Anti-glomerular basement membrane antibody nephritis (anti-GBM nephritis).

Immune Complex Nephritis. This is much the commoner of the two types.

The streptococcus is the best known nephritogenic antigen but many others have been recognised.

Large numbers of soluble immune complexes formed by the antigen-antibody reaction are conveyed to the kidney by the rich renal blood supply. They are trapped by the glomerular basement membrane and the ensuing damage and inflammatory nephritic lesions are caused by activation of the complement system and coagulation cascade. In fact, platelet aggregation and fibrin deposition are often seen within the glomerular capillary loops. The reason why some people exposed to one of the listed antigens develop nephritis and others do not is poorly understood. Susceptibility to nephritis is thought to be related to an individual's immunological competence, i.e. relatively immune deficient individuals

Antigens proved or suspected of causing immune-complex nephritis		
Exogenous		Antigens
Infections:	Bacterial:	Streptococcus, Staphylococcus
		Treponema pallidum, Pneumococcus, Salmonella
	Viral:	Coxsackie B, Hepatitis B, Epstein-Barr
	Parasitic:	*Plasmodium malariae*, Schistosomiasis, Toxoplasmosis
	Fungal:	*Candida albicans*
Drugs:		Penicillamine, Gold, Heroin
Endogenous		Desoxyribonucleic acid (DNA) i.e. lupus
		Tumour cell antigens, i.e. carcinoma
		Lymphoma
		Thyroglobulin, Cryoglobulin
		Glomerular basement membrane*

*Anti-glomerular basement membrane antibody nephritis.

may be prone to nephritis. Equally, it is difficult to explain why antigens produce different histological appearances. The streptococcus stimulates a proliferative glomerulonephritis response with immune complexes on the outside or epithelial surface of the basement membrane, and *Plasmodium malariae* produces a membranous nephropathy with immune complexes largely within the basement membrane. The simplest explanation is that it is related to the size of the formed soluble immune complexes or to the intensity of the antibody response.

Anti-glomerular Basement Membrane Antibody Nephritis (Anti-GBM Nephritis). This is a rare cause of glomerulonephritis. It is initiated by the formation of a direct antibody to the glomerular basement membrane and is accompanied by pulmonary haemorrhage, i.e. Goodpasture's disease (*see* page 241).

Pathology

The following main groups form a basic histological classification of glomerulonephritis:

1. Minimal lesion nephropathy.
2. Membranous nephropathy.
3. Diffuse proliferative glomerulonephritis.
   (a) without crescents
   (b) with crescents.
4. Focal proliferative glomerulonephritis.
5. Membrano-proliferative glomerulonephritis.
6. Focal glomerulosclerosis.
7. Chronic glomerulonephritis.

Several terms used in the classification require explanation. 'Diffuse' when applied to the whole kidney indicates that all the glomeruli are abnormal, but when referring to one individual glomerulus it means that all the loops are involved and 'global' would be a better

differentiating term. Similarly 'focal' means that only some glomeruli are affected within the kidney as a whole, but alternatively, that only part of the glomerulus is diseased – in this case 'segmental' is the better and more correct description (Fig. 14.14).

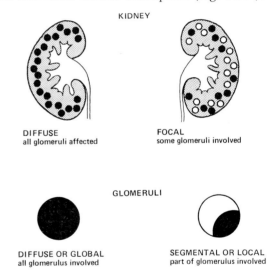

Fig. 14.14 Glomerulonephritis.

Minimal Lesion Nephropathy. The commonest cause of the nephrotic syndrome in children is minimal lesion nephropathy – it is also known as lipoid nephrosis, minimal change or nil disease. This glomerular lesion shows no abnormality on light microscopy, but on electron microscopy (10,000×) there is fusion or loss of the foot processes. Loss of foot processes is probably a non-specific finding related to the protein loss; it is seen in most of the other protein losing nephritides as well. The term 'nephropathy' is used in preference to 'nephritis' as there is no cellular proliferation; this applies also to the membranous lesion. Immunofluorescent studies are generally negative (Fig. 14.15).

236

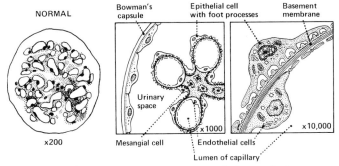

Fig. 14.15 Normal appearance: minimal change lesion. *Note:* Fusion and loss of foot process *not* shown.

Membranous Nephropathy. This is characterised by uniform thickening of the basement membrane without any cellular proliferation. It is also known as epi- or extra-membranous glomerulonephritis. Electron microscopy shows electron dense deposits representing immune complexes situated within the basement membrane just beneath the epithelial cell layer – subepithelial. This gives a classical 'spiky' appearance which is also seen with silver-staining of ultra-thin 1μ sections on light microscopy (Fig. 14.16). Immunofluorescence shows a granular picture with IgG mainly. In elderly patients this lesion may be the first indication of an underlying malignancy.

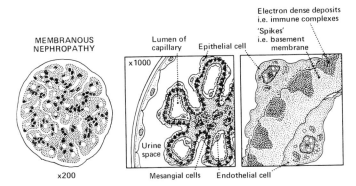

Fig. 14.16 Glomerulonephritis: membranous nephropathy.

Diffuse Proliferative Glomerulonephritis. One or all three of the cellular elements of the glomeruli, i.e. endothelial, mesangial and epithelial, show proliferation but the capillary loops are thin-walled showing no thickening of the basement membrane. Occasionally polymorphs may be seen in the glomeruli and then the term 'exudate' is applied. Epithelial cell proliferation causes capsular or tuft adhesions between the visceral and parietal layers and in extreme forms this is recognised as crescent formation (Fig. 14.17). Fibrin contributes to crescent formation. Glomerulonephritis with crescents carries a worse prognosis. Some classifications use the terms endo-capillary and extra-capillary to represent endothelial or epithelial proliferation. Both primary and secondary glomerulonephritis may show a

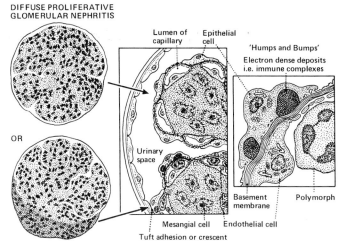

Fig. 14.17 Glomerulonephritis: diffuse proliferative.

similar diffuse proliferative picture, for example post-streptococcal and lupus nephritis. Immunofluorescence shows a granular appearance; IgG is the predominant immunoglobin. Electron microscopy shows electron dense deposits on the outside of the basement membrane. A number of cases of glomerulonephritis defy precise histological classification but are usually included as sub-groups within the proliferative category.

Many show some mild mesangial proliferation only, often with a focal segmental distribution and they often have IgA deposits within the mesangium. This latter group presents with recurrent haematuria in males particularly after exercise and is known as Berger's IgA nephropathy. Interestingly, in Henoch Schönlein nephropathy haematuria is a common feature and again IgA is the predominant immunoglobin to be seen on immunofluorescent microscopy.

Focal Segmental Proliferative Glomerulonephritis. Focal segmental proliferative glomerulonephritis is a more benign condition than the diffuse variety. It should not be confused with focal glomerulosclerosis (*see below*) which is progressive. Although the antigen is rarely recognised in the primary form, focal nephritis is

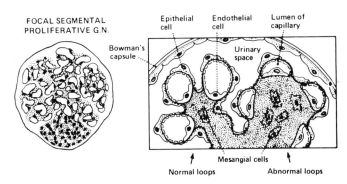

Fig. 14.18 Glomerulonephritis: focal segmental proliferative.

237

the commonest lesion in the nephritis of systemic lupus erythematosus, polyarteritis nodosa and Henoch Schönlein purpura. Proliferation is confined to a few loops. Immunofluorescent deposits are confined to the involved segment of the glomerulus (Fig. 14.18).

Membrano-proliferative Glomerulonephritis. Sometimes known as mesangio-capillary glomerulonephritis, this glomerular lesion was formerly thought to be a mixed type representing a combination of proliferative and membranous lesions. This was understandable as on light microscopy there was apparent thickening of the basement membrane plus cell proliferation. However, it is now known to be a truly proliferative lesion. It is associated with low levels of serum complement, i.e. hypocomplementaemia. The proliferation involves mainly the mesangial cells and matrix where it is contiguous with the endothelium and they grow around the capillary loops just underneath the endothelial cell layer, apparently thickening the basement membrane and giving it a split or tram-line appearance (Fig. 14.19). This is confirmed on electron microscopy or by silver-stained 1μ sections on light microscopy. Immunofluorescence shows a granular picture.

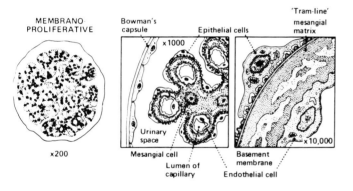

Fig. 14.19 Glomerulonephritis: membrano-proliferative.

Focal Glomerulosclerosis. The presence of sclerosis in a glomerulus irrespective of the type of histological appearance suggests a progressive lesion. In the specific lesion described as focal glomerulosclerosis, areas of

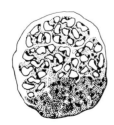

Fig. 14.20 Focal glomerulosclerosis.

segmental sclerosis ultimately obliterate the glomerular capillaries and the patient develops chronic renal failure, often within a few years. Many of the glomeruli look normal, and it is important that because of insufficient cortical tissue on renal biopsy that it is not mistaken for a minimal lesion nephropathy (Fig. 14.20). The juxtamedullary glomeruli are first to be affected. Therefore the biopsy sample may be unrepresentative if only a small piece of tissue is obtained.

Chronic Glomerulonephritis. Histologically, chronic glomerulonephritis exhibits the final common end-point of glomerular destruction and it is usually impossible to recognise the initial glomerular lesion, i.e. proliferative from membrano-proliferative, as many of the glomeruli are sclerosed. Renal biopsy does not contribute to diagnosis or management when chronic renal failure has already developed.

Clinical Syndromes

Glomerulonephritis, both primary and secondary, may present in the following quite distinct ways:

1. Acute nephritic syndrome – acute glomerulonephritis.
2. Rapidly progressive glomerulonephritis.
3. Persistent proteinuria.
4. Nephrotic syndrome.
5. Recurrent haematuria.
6. Acute renal failure.
7. Chronic renal failure – chronic glomerulonephritis.
8. Hypertension.

Until the glomerular lesion has been identified microscopically it is better to stick to these purely clinical descriptions. A particular mode of presentation cannot be definitely attributed to a specific histological appearance, although associations do occur between clinical features and the type of underlying glomerular lesion (Table 14.3).

Furthermore, transition from persistent proteinuria to the nephrotic syndrome may occur and a patient first presenting with an acute nephritic syndrome may pass on to a nephrotic stage. Many of the patients with glomerulonephritis, irrespective of the initial histological lesion, will inevitably progress to a stage of chronic renal failure (Table 14.3).

Acute Nephritic Syndrome. The acute nephritic syndrome or classical acute glomerulonephritis is an illness of rapid onset and comprises:
Haematuria.
Proteinuria.
Oliguria.
Hypertension.
Transient uraemia with a temporary decrease in renal function.

238

Table 14.3 Clinico-pathological correlation and outcome in the six basic types of glomerulonephritis

	Acute nephritic syndrome	Recurrent haematuria	Nephrotic syndrome	Persistent proteinuria	Chronic renal failure*
Diffuse proliferative GN	+++	−	±	±	?
Focal proliferative GN	+	+++	+	±	±
Focal glomerulosclerosis	−	++	+++	++	+++
Membrano-proliferative GN	+	+	++	±	+++
Membranous nephropathy	−	−	++	++	+++
Minimal change nephropathy	−	−	+++	++	−

GN = Glomerulonephritis.
*Sustained hypertension may precede a decrease in GFR.

It is now an uncommon disease in Britain, probably because of better living conditions and readily available antibiotics.

The other conditions sometimes presenting with an acute nephritic syndrome are Henoch-Schönlein purpura, disseminated lupus erythematosus and polyarteritis nodosa.

Rapidly Progressive Glomerulonephritis. These secondary nephritides, and others, including a minority of post-streptococcal glomerulonephritis and Goodpasture's disease, may follow the course of a rapidly progressive glomerulonephritis, with an accelerated deterioration in renal failure to end-stage chronic renal failure often within two years.

Persistent Proteinuria. The commonest presentation of glomerulonephritis is persistent proteinuria in excess of 0.2 g/day. The association was originally documented by Dr. Richard Bright in the nineteenth century. This finding, frequently uncovered at routine medical examinations – pre-employment, for insurance or mortgage purposes, at antenatal clinics, or on admission to hospital for other reasons such as elective surgery, may be the only indication of the disease. It is axiomatic that the difference between persistent proteinuria and proteinuria sufficient to cause the nephrotic syndrome is one only of degree and the same underlying histological changes in the glomeruli are capable of producing either. Furthermore, they should both be treated with equal seriousness.

Nephrotic Syndrome. In contrast to the rapid onset of the acute nephritic syndrome, producing a sick patient, the nephrotic syndrome develops insidiously and in the early stages the patient remains well and ambulatory apart from noticing slight oedema, particularly around the ankles or eyes. The main clinical features are:
Persistent proteinuria (0.05 g/kg body weight/day, or more).
Hypoalbuminaemia (less than 20 to 25 g/l).
Oedema.

Normal renal function (compare acute nephritic syndrome).
Normal or low blood pressure (compare acute nephritic syndrome).

Although the proteinuria of the nephrotic syndrome in the past has been described as 'massive', 'gross' or 'heavy', it is defined quantitatively as a sufficiently large urinary protein leak to produce a drop in serum albumin level to the critical levels of oedema formation, i.e. serum albumin levels less than 25 g/l. The sequence of events leading to oedema are shown in Fig. 14.21.

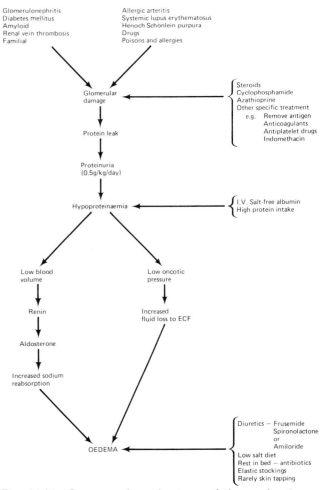

Fig. 14.21 Causes and mechanisms of the nephrotic syndrome and its treatment.

239

Glomerulonephritis is the commonest cause of the nephrotic syndrome, but several other diseases involving the kidney may cause protein-losing states and these are listed on page 239.

The patient first notices painless swelling of the ankles or develops facial or sacral oedema due to redistribution of fluid after lying flat. There may be dependent oedema of the genitalia, ascites, pleural effusions or effusions into knee joints. Some patients may notice large weight gains due to fluid accumulation. White nails or white bands across the nails is a specific sign of chronic hypoalbuminaemia and is seen in long-standing nephrotic patients. Hypercholesterolaemia, hypertriglyceridaemia and an increase in clotting factors are common accompaniments of the nephrotic syndrome. This explains the higher incidence of ischaemic heart disease in long standing nephrotic patients and also the occurrence of pulmonary emboli from thrombosis in peripheral or even major vessels. Renal vein thrombosis is more often a complication rather than a cause of the nephrotic syndrome. The low levels of plasma immunoglobulins make these patients susceptible to infection and was the commonest cause of death before the introduction of chemotherapy.

Recurrent Haematuria. Some types of glomerulonephritis may be heralded by the onset of recurrent episodes of painless haematuria. All investigations to exclude a surgical cause such as tumours, stones and infections are negative. The attacks may be precipitated by an intercurrent infection usually of the upper respiratory tract, or by exercise. Occasionally, the attacks are complicated by loin pain, and a small group of patients, mainly women, have recurrent loin pain only. The condition is commonly benign with no element of progressive glomerular destruction.

Acute and Chronic Renal Failure. Occasionally, a patient may present 'out-of-the-blue' with acute anuric renal failure and without obvious clinical features of acute glomerulonephritis. A renal biopsy may show the histological appearance of severe or proliferative glomerulonephritis often with crescents.

Similarly, a patient may be diagnosed as having chronic advanced end-stage renal failure without ever having had any obvious previous glomerulonephritic type of illness. Perhaps proteinuria has been present undetected for years and the disease has not come to light until hypertension or the stigma of chronic uraemia become obvious.

Chronic glomerulonephritis in a clinical sense is used to describe all the different nephritides which have not resolved completely but have progressed to a permanent stage of chronic renal insufficiency or failure.

Hypertension. An incidental finding of hypertension may be the first indication that glomerulonephritis is present and when proteinuria is minimal it is impossible to differentiate the clinical situation from essential hypertension without a renal biopsy. This hypertension may pre-date any deterioration in renal function.

Investigations

1. Urinalysis—glomerulonephritis shows proteinuria and/or microscopic or macroscopic haematuria, but also there are casts. This differentiates it from surgical lesions.
2. Blood urea.
3. Serum creatinine and creatinine clearance for glomerular filtration rate.
4. Serum albumin.
5. 24-hour protein output and selectivity.
6. Serum cholesterol and lipids.
7. X-rays of renal angles to assess size of kidneys prior to renal biopsy.
8. Serum complement – low in membrano-proliferative, lupus and sub-acute bacterial endocarditis glomerulonephritis.

Renal biopsy must be performed in all patients to differentiate primary and secondary glomerular lesions.

Complications

Hypertension and its complications.
Chronic renal failure.

Differential Diagnosis

1. Transient proteinuria – commonest cause of proteinuria in general practice is a urinary tract infection.
2. Haematuria may result from surgical lesions in the kidney – casts will not be present.
3. Other causes of dependent oedema – cardiac, hepatic, malabsorption, malnutrition or lymphatic obstruction of the legs.

Basis of Treatment

Therapy is divided into
1. General Treatment
2. Specific Treatment

General Treatment:

The acute nephritic syndrome:
1. Rest in bed and fluid restriction.
2. Control of hypertension.
3. Treatment of pulmonary oedema and congestive cardiac failure.
4. Control of acute uraemia by low protein diet or, if necessary, short term dialysis.
5. Penicillin, if aetiology is streptococcal, or by an appropriate chemotherapeutic agent.

The nephrotic syndrome:
1. Bed-rest to induce a diuresis.
2. Fluid and sodium restriction.

3. Diuretics for salt and water retention.
4. Aldosterone antagonist for secondary hyperaldosteronism.
5. Salt-free albumin infusion to mobilise extracellular fluid by increasing oncotic pressure.
6. Rarely, tapping of ascites and pleural effusions or skin incision for peripheral oedema.
7. Prompt treatment of infection.
8. Observation for venous thrombosis and anticoagulant therapy if necessary.
9. Occasionally, cholestyramine and clofibrate therapy is given for hypercholesterolaemia and hypertriglyceridaemia.

The treatment of acute and chronic renal failure are dealt with elsewhere. Symptomless proteinuria does not require treatment. Recurrent haematuria is seldom severe enough to cause anaemia and therefore does not warrant treatment.

Specific Treatment. Specific treatments for glomerulonephritis are singularly unsuccessful except in minimal lesion nephropathy. The following drugs are used:
1. Steroids.
2. Immunosuppressive drugs.
3. Anticoagulants.
4. Inhibitors of platelet aggregation.

Removal of the antigen is the first line of attack, for example penicillin for streptococcal infection or antimalarial drugs for malaria. Then attempts to reduce proliferation can be made with anti-inflammatory drugs, for example steroids and immunosuppressives. The non-immunological platelet deposition and fibrin formation may be arrested with anticoagulants and drugs reducing platelet adherence.

Very profound protein leaks have been improved in some cases using indomethacin. As many of the nephritides have a spontaneous remission rate of 25 to 75 per cent, it is difficult to assess the efficacy of treatment. Progress may be very slow and the more aggressive therapy with toxic drugs, for example steroids and immunosuppressives is confined to those patients with rapidly deteriorating renal function or with early evidence of sclerosis on serial renal biopsies. Even then, therapy should be confined to a short course of eight weeks. Long term steroid treatment is not used.

Prognosis (Fig. 14.22)

Minimal lesions and some proliferative glomerulonephritics, particularly those following streptococcal infections, have a high rate of total remission, but most of the other lesions are progressive. Recent work suggests that even acute post-streptococcal glomerulonephritis may be very slowly progressive.

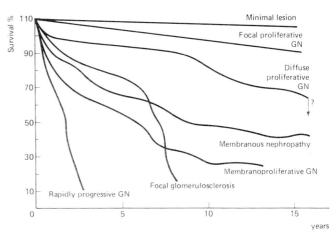

Fig. 14.22 An outline of survival or prognosis in the different types of glomerulonephritis (GN) in adults.

GOODPASTURE'S DISEASE

Definition

Rapidly progressive glomerulonephritis with lung purpura associated with the lineal appearance of anti-glomerular basement membrane antibody seen on immunofluorescent microscopy of renal biopsy material (*see* page 236).

Background

Young men are affected mainly. Haemoptysis precedes renal involvement and is often profuse enough to require multiple blood transfusions. The glomerular basement membrane itself becomes antigenic and antibodies are formed, i.e. anti-GBM antibody nephritis.

One theory suggests that inhalation of hydrocarbon causes injury to the pulmonary basement membrane, which is antigenically similar to GBM. Therefore, antibody formed against the fragments of the damaged lung basement membrane released into the circulation will cross-react with the GBM of the kidney. The clinical course is stormy and usually one of a very rapid deterioration in renal function similar to other rapidly progressive glomerulonephritides.

Pathology

The histological picture is of a proliferative glomerulonephritis often with crescents. The diagnosis is confirmed by a finding of a continuous electron dense deposit along the line of the basement membrane on electron microscopy supported by the classical linear appearance on immunofluorescence.

Symptoms and Signs

The symptoms and signs are those of the acute nephritic syndrome with haemoptysis.

241

Investigations

1. Similar to those for glomerulonephritis.
2. Renal biopsy – immunofluorescent or electron microscopy is diagnostic.
3. Anti-glomerular basement membrane antibody titres.
4. Chest X-ray – 'fluffy' areas throughout lung fields are indistinguishable from pulmonary oedema.

Basis of Treatment

Steroids and immunosuppressive drugs, e.g. azathioprine or cyclophosphamide.
Dialysis for acute renal failure.
Blood transfusion.
Plasmaphaeresis to eradicate antibody.
Long term dialysis for chronic-on-acute renal failure and transplantation later when antibody titre drops.
Bilateral nephrectomy is no longer performed as renal function may improve sufficiently to stop dialysis.

Prognosis

Without supportive dialysis mortality is 90 to 100 per cent. Death may occur as a result of lung haemorrhage even with dialysis and other supportive therapy.

URINARY TRACT INFECTIONS

Definition

Bacterial invasion of any part of the urinary tract including in ascending order, the bladder, ureters, pelvis, papillae and parenchyma of the kidney, producing a bacterial count in the urine of 10^5 organisms/ml or greater constitutes a urinary tract infection.

The term 'urethritis' is confined to venereal infections of the urethra, for example gonococcal urethritis (*see* page 150). Renal tuberculosis, renal carbuncles and perinephric abscesses arise from direct haematogenous invasion of the kidney rather than indirectly as an ascending infection from the bladder via the ureters.

Background

The shortness of the female urethra and its susceptibility to traumatic inflammation during sexual intercourse explains the higher incidence of urinary tract infections in females; the urethral orifice can become intravaginal during coitus. The attack rate is more than ten times that of males. Bacteria from faecal contamination of the perineum and vulva or from a vaginal discharge, infect the mechanically inflamed urethra and are able to pass easily into the bladder, multiply and ascend the ureters to the pelvis and kidney substance. More than 50 per cent of females have an attack of

dysuria at some stage in their life-time and with many of them it is a recurrent problem. Although infections occur largely in normal urinary tracts, the presence of an infection should raise the suspicion of an abnormality and therefore, infections should be considered as markers or indicators of underlying pathology, for example secondary to renal calculi, obstruction or rarely congenital anomalies causing stasis. This suspicion of an abnormality in the urinary tract is heightened if the invading organism is anything other than *Escherichia coli*, the causative bacteria in 70 per cent of urinary tract infections in the general population. This principle is particularly applicable to young males as urinary tract infections are uncommon until the fifth or sixth decade in men, when prostatic obstruction leads to infection and stasis. It is convenient to divide urinary tract infections into upper and lower, and this and some of the causes of precipitating factors are shown in Fig. 14.23.

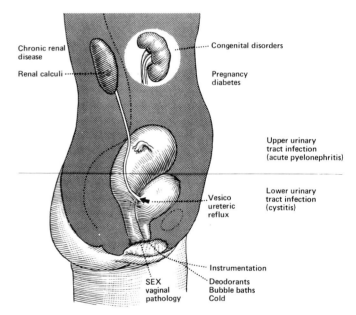

Fig. 14.23 Urinary tract infection: some causes and mechanisms.

Symptoms and Signs

Urinary tract infections present in the following ways:

Urethral syndrome.
Asymptomatic bacteriuria.
Cystitis.
Acute pyelonephritis.
Acute papillary necrosis.
Chronic pyelonephritis.

Urethral Syndrome. Dysuria, frequency, urgency, feeling of incomplete bladder emptying in the absence of significant bacteriuria constitutes the urethral syndrome. These findings suggest that this is the stage

242

when the urethra is merely inflamed but not infected. Sexual intercourse, allergy to nylon underwear, biological washing powders, bubble-baths and cold can all predispose to this condition.

Asymptomatic Bacteriuria. When significant bacteriuria (10^5/ml or greater) is found in the absence of symptoms it is known as asymptomatic bacteriuria. With asymptomatic bacteriuria, spontaneous eradication occurs in about 50 per cent.

Cystitis. This is the commonest presentation of urinary tract infections. In addition to the symptoms of the urethral syndrome, foul or fish-smelling, cloudy urine, suprapubic pain and tenderness and occasionally, haematuria are seen. 'Honeymoon' cystitis emphasises the relationship between cystitis and sexual activity. Although symptoms are confined to the lower urinary tract, infection may have spread upwards to involve the pelvis and kidney, without the specific symptoms of acute pyelonephritis.

Acute Pyelonephritis. Bacterial invasion of the renal substance is usually superseded by an attack of cystitis, but this is not always so. Symptoms include loin pain, rigors and malaise, plus the symptoms of cystitis. Signs are loin tenderness, fever, often very high, and an abnormal urinary sediment containing red blood cells, white blood cells and bacteria. Proteinuria of less than 3 g may be present and enlargement of the kidneys may be seen radiologically.

Acute Papillary Necrosis. Rarely, in an overwhelming infection of the kidney, particularly in patients with diabetes mellitus, the papillae of the kidney may become severely damaged. They become necrotic, slough off and pass into the ureter causing obstruction. Patients with diabetes mellitus are particularly susceptible to fulminating acute urinary tract infections of this type.

Pyelitis of Pregnancy. This term suggests infection confined to the pelvis of the kidney only, but as the renal parenchyma is invariably involved, the term should not be used.

Chronic Pyelonephritis. The relationship between acute urinary tract infections and chronic pyelonephritis is poorly understood.

Investigations

1. MSU for Gram-stain to detect bacteria; culture and antibiotic sensitivity; urinalysis and examination of sediment.
   Repeat MSU 48 hours and six weeks after cessation of treatment as a 'test of cure'.
2. Exclude vaginal pathology, e.g. *Trichomonas vaginalis* or infected cervical erosions.
3. Plain X-ray of the abdomen (KUB) or an IVP should be carried out after the first infection in males and the second in females.
4. Cystoscopy or urethroscopy may be necessary if symptoms are recurrent and confined to the bladder or urethra.

Basis of Treatment

General:
Bed rest and tepid sponging to lower very high temperatures. Convulsions are not uncommon in children with hyperpyrexia.
Analgesics for pain.

Specific:
High fluid intake (3 l/day) and regular bladder emptying, particularly last thing at night to avoid climax bacterial populations during the hours of sleep.

Chemotherapy. Before getting results of bacteriology give
(a) Cotrimoxazole (Septrin) 2 tabs. twice a day, or
(b) Sulphadimidine 1 g four times a day, or
(c) Ampicillin 500 mg four times per day; this is a good third choice and if the patient is vomiting can be given parenterally.
   As soon as the bacteriological culture and sensitivity are available the appropriate antibiotic can be substituted and continued for seven days.

Prevention

Women, prone to recurrent cystitis and urinary tract infection, should be retrained to take a high fluid intake and empty their bladder regularly, particularly after intercourse. They should also be encouraged to maintain a high standard of perineal toilet and have any vaginal discharge investigated and treated. Long term low-dose prophylaxis may be necessary: nitrofurantoin 50 mg, cotrimoxazole 1 tab., nalidixic acid 1 g or cephalexin 125 mg at night may prevent recurrent attacks. The first three drugs are preferred as they do not alter intestinal bacterial flora nor is the incidence of vaginal candidiasis increased, both of which occur with broad spectrum antibiotics.

CHRONIC PYELONEPHRITIS

Definition

Chronic unilateral or bilateral inflammatory disease of the kidney, diagnosed radiologically as a result of a scarred or shrunken appearance of the kidneys, and clubbed calyces on excretory urography constitute chronic pyelonephritis.

Background

Chronic pyelonephritis is an enigma. It does not seem to be the direct result of recurrent acute pyelonephritis or long-standing asymptomatic bacteriuria in adult women with normal urinary tracts. Urinary stasis seems to be a pre-requisite caused by a high pressure bladder from obstruction or neurological lesions. Vesico-ureteric reflux, pre-existing damage to the kidney from chronic interstitial nephritis, renal calculi or diabetic nephropathy all predispose to the development of chronic pyelonephritis.

Recent work suggests that chronic pyelonephritis without any obvious cause, for example non-obstructive, is initiated by vesico-ureteric reflux in childhood, with or without superimposed infection. It is suggested that infected or non-infected urine flowing back up the ureter and striking the delicate lining of the renal pelvis and even penetrating up the collecting ducts into the renal parenchyma itself, i.e. intrarenal reflux, causes the scarring and contraction seen later in adult life. Bilateral chronic pyelonephritis is a common cause of chronic renal failure and unilateral disease may produce hypertension in the presence of normal renal function.

By the time chronic pyelonephritis is picked up on X-ray during the investigation of, say, an acute intercurrent urinary tract infection or by the onset of hypertension or chronic renal failure the reflux will have disappeared and at this stage it is often a sterile disease. There may be no history of recurrent urinary tract infections in the past. The term 'chronic pyelonephritis' may well be replaced by 'chronic reflux nephropathy', for these latter cases. Bilateral chronic pyelonephritis is the most common cause of chronic end-stage renal failure, apart from chronic glomerulonephritis.

Pathology

Macroscopically one or both kidneys are small, misshapen with occasional polar areas of hypertrophy, in contrast to the bilateral small, regular and evenly contracted kidneys of chronic glomerulonephritis. The cut surface confirms the clubbed calyces seen on excretory pyelography with scars stretching in from the cortex opposite each dilated calyx causing reduction in the renal cortical thickness.

Microscopically the appearances are indistinguishable from any other chronic interstitial nephritis showing infiltration of the interstitium with lymphocytes and plasma cells. Areas of periglomerular fibrosis, tubular atrophy and fibrous scars are interspersed with normal parenchyma and arteriolar changes of hypertension may be superimposed. Sometimes tubules are dilated and filled with a homogenous eosin-stained material, giving the appearance of 'thyroid' areas. This histological appearance is said to be pathognomonic of chronic pyelonephritis.

Symptoms

Chronic pyelonephritis is often asymptomatic but may be uncovered by the finding of asymptomatic bacteriuria or proteinuria and on the subsequent excretory urogram. Other forms of presentation are non-specific:
Vague illness.
General malaise.
Tiredness and loss of appetite.
Low back pain.
Recurrent urinary symptoms with or without fever.
Symptoms of chronic renal failure.
Symptoms of hypertension.

Signs

Patient may have no abnormal signs.
Signs of chronic renal failure, e.g. anaemia.
Clinical finding of hypertension and its complications.

Investigations

1. Urinalysis – proteinuria, usually about 1 to 2 g/day.
2. MSU often sterile but with excess white blood cells, i.e. $10/mm^3$, greater than 400,000/hr, or significant bacteriuria 10^5 organisms/ml urine.
3. Creatinine clearance – to assess renal function and establish baseline for future follow-up.
4. Excretory urography shows chronic pyelonephritic changes.
5. Micturating cystogram – to exclude vesico-ureteric reflux.
6. Renography – to compare degree of impaired function on each side.

Basis of Treatment

1. High fluid intake.
2. Eradication of infection if present.
3. Removal of aggravating factors, e.g. obstruction and calculi.
4. Consider reimplantation of ureters if vesico-ureteric reflux is very gross in order to:
(a) Preserve renal function.
(b) Eradicate infection more readily.

Vesico-ureteric reflux will sometimes cure itself spontaneously around puberty, provided it is not gross and the child's urine is kept sterile in the intervening years. This requires regular follow-up with MSUs, and sometimes long term chemotherapy.

5. Consider nephrectomy for unilateral disease, if blood pressure is tending to rise, but only if the 'good' kidney is normal. The glomerular filtration rate of this remaining kidney should be equivalent to one-and-a-half functioning kidneys, i.e. hypertrophy has taken place and should be seen as enlargement on X-ray.

Other reasons for nephrectomy are non-functioning kidneys, pain and inability to eradicate infection.

6. Control of hypertension – drugs.
7. Control of uraemia – low protein diet.

Out-patient follow-up is important as these patients may be candidates for the dialysis and transplantation programme.

RENAL TUBERCULOSIS

Tuberculosis of the urinary tract develops first in the kidney, usually as a result of haematogenous spread from a primary pulmonary focus. Both kidneys are infected, but usually one more than the other and often many years after the initial infection has healed. Painless haematuria with or without loin pain and sterile pyuria, i.e. MSU sterile, is the commonest presentation. The diagnosis is confirmed by the excretory urographic appearance of chronic pyelonephritis, with overlying calcification in the diseased portion. The infection spreads downwards in contrast to other bacterial urinary infections involving first the pelvis, then the ureters and bladder, producing the appearance of a 'golf-hole' ureter on cystoscopy. Finally, the infection spreads to the genital tract, producing tuberculosis of the epididymis, prostate or seminal vesicles. The tubercle bacillus is best recovered from examination of six consecutive early morning mid-stream specimens of urine. Treatment follows the same lines as that for pulmonary tuberculosis with a regime including two or three drug combinations given for a period of two years (*see* page 339). Steroids are sometimes added to prevent fibrosis and subsequent obstruction in the ureter. Surgery is rarely undertaken nowadays.

SYSTEMIC DISEASES AND THE KIDNEY

The following diseases commonly involve the kidney and the renal manifestations may be the first and only sign of the disease:

Diabetes mellitis
Henoch-Schönlein
 purpura
Amyloidosis
Haemolytic-uraemic
 syndrome

Systemic lupus
 erythematosus
Polyarteritis nodosa
Scleroderma
Multiple myeloma
Gout

Other diseases include sarcoidosis, sickle cell anaemia, and infections where the causative agent produces a secondary glomerulonephritis, for example malaria, sub-acute bacterial endocarditis.

DIABETIC NEPHROPATHY

Chronic renal failure is the cause of death in 30 per cent of diabetics. Renal vascular damage in diabetes parallels that seen in the eye, i.e. the degree of diabetic retinopathy is a measure of the severity of diabetic nephropathy. In the follow-up of a diabetic patient the urine is tested routinely for protein as well as sugar. Proteinuria is the first sign of renal involvement in diabetes and this protein-losing nephropathy may progress to the nephrotic syndrome. Proteinuria does not appear for 15 to 20 years after the onset of diabetes mellitus, but it is an ominous sign and life prognosis is then about seven years. Once the blood urea rises with a glomerular filtration rate of 30 to 40 ml/min the prognosis is only two to three years. Several renal lesions are seen (*see below*).

Apart from controlling the diabetes and hypertension and treating urinary infections nothing can be done to slow the inexorable destruction of the kidney. As the glomerular filtration rate drops it is important not to rely on urine testing for the presence of sugar as these may be falsely low or negative and blood sugar levels are

Renal lesions in diabetes mellitus	
Type	*Description*
Diabetic glomerulosclerosis	Thick glomerular capillary walls
Kimmelsteil-Wilson lesions	Hyaline nodules replacing glomerular capillary loops
Acute pyelonephritis ± papillary necrosis	Acute interstitial inflammatory changes
Chronic pyelonephritis ± papillary necrosis	Chronic interstitial inflammation with scarring and periglomerular fibrosis ±nephrosclerosis

necessary for adequate control. Dialysis and renal transplantation is rarely successful in diabetes because of advanced arterial disease.

HENOCH-SCHÖNLEIN PURPURA (ANAPHYLACTOID OR NON-THROMBOCYTOPENIC PURPURA) (see page 414)

This condition is commoner in children and is characterised by:
Purpuric rash – commonly on the feet and skin.
Arthritis.
Abdominal pain with gastrointestinal haemorrhage.
Haematuria – 90 per cent.

A focal segmental proliferative glomerulonephritis is the commonest renal lesion presenting with mild haematuria, but more widespread proliferation with crescent formation can produce the acute nephritic syndrome.

Steroids appear to help the extrarenal manifestations, but have little effect on the glomerulonephritis. Immunosuppressive drugs are no more effective. Recovery rate is 90 per cent in children, but progression to chronic renal failure and/or hypertension within 5 to 10 years is a feature in 50 per cent of adults.

AMYLOIDOSIS

Amyloid is an eosinophil material of protein and chondroitin sulphate and is deposited in several sites including the kidney.

It is most commonly secondary to several chronic conditions. It appears to be an abnormal response to long-standing inflammation or suppuration such as chronic osteomyelitis, tuberculosis, multiple myelomatosis, rheumatoid arthritis, or ulcerative colitis, and the deposits are mainly in the kidney, liver and rectum. It may also be primary or familial. Familial amyloidosis occurs by itself or as a complication of a condition known as Familial Mediterranean Fever. The distribution in the familial and primary types is mainly in the tongue, heart, gastrointestinal tract and peripheral nerves. Paradoxically the secondary amyloidosis of multiple myelomatosis tends to have this primary distribution.

The kidneys are large and the glomerular loops are almost completely replaced by amyloid deposition giving them a structureless and bloodless appearance.

The condition should be suspected if persistent proteinuria or the nephrotic syndrome develops in a patient with one of the potential amyloid diseases, for example rheumatoid arthritis. Sudden acute renal failure may occur from bilateral renal vein thrombosis. Renal amyloid is best diagnosed indirectly by rectal biopsy as there is a 90 per cent correlation between the finding of amyloid in the rectum and the kidney.

Eradication of chronic sepsis may arrest amyloid deposition, but in the other diseases progression to death from chronic renal failure seems inevitable in a few years. Penicillamine and colchicine have been used with little success. Steroids worsen the condition.

HAEMOLYTIC-URAEMIC SYNDROME

This is a disease of early childhood usually heralded by fever, diarrhoea and vomiting and followed within a few days by severe haemolysis, thrombocytopenia, cerebral disturbances and acute oliguric renal failure. In adults, a related condition without a prodromal illness is known as thrombotic thrombocytopenic purpura (see page 420). Both conditions are closely related to a disseminated intravascular coagulation and are probably caused by hypersensitivity. Treatment has been successful using heparin, platelets, fresh frozen plasma and supportive dialysis, but mortality remains high, at 40 per cent in children and 75 per cent in adults.

SYSTEMIC LUPUS ERYTHEMATOSUS (see page 119)

A multisystem connective tissue disease, ten times more common in the female, involves the kidney in about 60 to 70 per cent of cases. It is a great masquerader of renal disease, both clinically and histologically. The sole manifestations may be renal with no rash or arthritis presenting with either the acute nephritic syndrome, nephrotic syndrome, persistent proteinuria or chronic renal failure. On examining biopsy material a wide spectrum of lesions are seen including minimal change, diffuse or focal proliferative glomerulonephritis and membranous nephropathy. The histological mimicry makes it essential that all glomerulonephritic patients are screened for antinuclear factor to exclude systemic lupus erythematosus.

Prognosis in lupus glomerulonephritis will, therefore, depend very much on the type of glomerular lesion.

The commonest lesion is a mild focal segmental proliferative glomerulonephritis, but if there is no sclerosis or hypertension the prognosis is fairly good.

High dose steroids, azathioprine and cyclophosphamide are all used to treat the more progressive proliferative lupus glomerulonephritics, and plasmaphaeresis to clear circulating immune complexes has been used empirically.

POLYARTERITIS NODOSA (see page 121)

The kidneys are affected in 80 per cent of cases and may produce the only abnormal findings. The condition is seen more often in males. When the arteritis affects the smaller vessels (microscopic polyarteritis) a focal proliferative glomerulonephritis is produced. This often presents initially as an acute nephritic syndrome, but advances to chronic end-stage renal failure in the manner of a rapidly progressive glomerulonephritis. A finding of hepatitis B virus antigenaemia is not uncommon in polyarteritis nodosa. The condition is steroid responsive. When the larger vessels are involved with the arteritic process, recurrent infarcts of the kidney and loin pain are major clinical features.

SCLERODERMA (*see* page 122)

This affects the kidneys in the late stages of progressive systemic sclerosis after the skin, joints, gut and lungs are obviously clinically involved. The scleroderma kidney shows histological changes of severe arteriosclerosis with fibrinoid necrosis indistinguishable from malignant hypertension. Terminally, proteinuria is followed in several years by chronic renal failure.

MULTIPLE MYELOMATOSIS (*see* page 402)

This shows a variety of renal lesions. The commonest lesion is distension of the renal tubules with laminated casts made up of Bence-Jones protein, with renal failure, but also pyelonephritis, neurogenic bladder from spinal compression by a myeloma tumour and direct infiltration of the kidney with myeloma cells are seen. Myelomatosis may be complicated by amyloidosis and even more rarely by renal vein thrombosis.

GOUT (*see* page 40)

In primary gouty arthritis two renal complications occur. Both are uncommon. Uric acid calculi form and tophaceous deposits similar to those in the pinnae of the ear and joints, are seen in the kidney. These deposits set up an inflammatory reaction, make the kidney susceptible to infection and in fact produce appearances of chronic pyelonephritis. This chronic gouty or urate nephropathy is an example of chronic interstitial nephritis. These patients develop chronic renal failure and hypertension.

Secondary gout complicates leukaemia and other myeloproliferative disorders and during drug therapy or irradiation an enormous urate load is presented to the kidney. Uric acid deposits can block the collecting ducts and cause acute renal failure, e.g. post-renal or acute obstructive uropathy.

Most of the renal complications of hyperuricaemia are prevented by a high fluid intake, allopurinol therapy or alkalinisation of the urine.

CONGENITAL AND HEREDITARY DISEASES

The presence of any obvious congenital defect, particularly of the pinna of the ear or the genitalia, should alert the clinician to the possibility of an underlying congenital renal anomaly.

CONGENITAL DISEASE

Congenital defects occur with an incidence of 1 in 500 to 1,500 of the population and include anomalies of number, size, shape and position of the kidneys, and also include reduplication of the ureters, obstruction of bladder outflow and urethral valves. Medullary sponge kidney is a rare benign congenital condition characterised by dilatation of the collecting tubules (pyelectasis) and is diagnosed on X-ray. Within the dilated collecting tubules calcification occurs giving the classical radiological appearance of 'rice-seed' opacities around each calyx. It is one of the causes of nephrocalcinosis. Single cysts are also congenital.

HEREDITARY DISEASE

Polycystic disease is the commonest hereditary condition of the kidney and is inherited as an autosomal dominant. It appears in the third to fourth decade and presents with haematuria, recurrent urinary infections, hypertension and in 10 per cent with secondary polycythaemia. Cysts in the liver and 'berry' aneurysms of the circle of Willis are common accompaniments – subarachnoid haemorrhage is not an uncommon cause of death. Infantile polycystic disease is a rarer and quite different disorder and results in death during the first month of life.

Medullary cystic disease, not to be confused with medullary sponge kidney, is a rare cause of chronic renal failure in childhood. Hereditary nephritis, described by Alport, is a glomerulonephritis with deafness in families and causes chronic renal failure in the second or third decade of life. The prognosis is worse in the males of the family. Hereditary tubular defects are discussed on page 628.

MISCELLANEOUS RENAL DISORDERS

INTERSTITIAL NEPHRITIS

Definition

Interstitial nephritis is characterised by inflammatory changes within the interstitium of the kidney with little or no involvement of the glomeruli initially. It can be acute or chronic and can cause acute or chronic renal failure respectively.

Background

The main causes are shown below.

Causes of interstitial nephritis

Pyelonephritis: acute and chronic
Allergic drug reactions
Analgesic and heavy metal nephropathy
Hyperuricaemic, hypokalaemic and hypercalcaemic nephropathy
Hereditary nephritis
Irradiation nephritis
Sickle cell anaemia
Balkan nephropathy

This essentially non-specific damage of the tubulo-interstitial region of the kidney may be produced by several different factors including infection, ischaemia, obstructive back pressure, hypersensitivity to drugs and exposure to toxic amounts of endogenous substances, for example calcium or uric acid, and also exogenous substances, for example analgesics or lead. Chronic hypokalaemia causes interstitial nephritis. The commonest cause is acute pyelonephritis or drug hypersensitivity and of chronic interstitial nephritis, chronic pyelonephritis or chronic analgesic nephropathy. This latter condition is seen in women mainly and is associated with many years of analgesic abuse. Anaemia, peptic ulceration, constipation and chronic laxative ingestion are common accompaniments.

Pathology

Oedema and infiltration of the interstitium with lymphocytes and plasma cells is seen in drug allergies and an arteritis may be present also. Hypokalaemia causes characteristic vacuolation of the tubular cells. Areas of fibrosis in the medulla and around the glomeruli, i.e. periglomerular fibrosis indicate chronicity. A kidney damaged in this way is more susceptible to pyelonephritis which in itself produces the histological appearance of interstitial nephritis.

Symptoms

Acute	Chronic
Fever	Polyuria
Itchy rash	Symptoms of chronic
Haematuria	uraemia
Oliguria	

Signs

Acute	Chronic
Generalised rash	Signs of chronic uraemia,
Joint swelling	e.g. anaemia
Signs of acute renal failure	Proteinuria (about
Occasionally jaundice	1 g/24 hours)

Investigations

1. Mid-stream specimen of urine. Examination of urinary sediment.
2. Haemoglobin and plasma viscosity.
3. Blood film for eosinophilia.
4. Blood urea and creatinine.
5. Skin and renal biopsy.
6. Plain X-ray abdomen – large kidneys.

Basis of Treatment

1. Treatment will depend on underlying pathology.
2. Acute interstitial nephropathy from drug allergies may respond to steroids.
3. Correction of hypokalaemia and hypercalcaemia.
4. Allopurinol for hyperuricaemia.
5. Antibiotics for infection.
6. Withdrawal of analgesics and other toxic agents.
7. Appropriate treatment for acute or chronic renal failure.

HEPATO-RENAL SYNDROME

In certain circumstances, simultaneous injury to the liver and kidney occurs, for instance with carbon tetrachloride poisoning and Weil's disease and generalised infection with haemolysis. However, acute renal failure is prevalent in patients with liver disease, particularly cirrhosis with fluid retention (ascites), but also following biliary tract surgery in the jaundiced patient. It seems that the jaundiced kidney is curiously susceptible to acute renal shut-down and it is more to these latter two conditions that the term 'hepato-renal syndrome' is applied.

RETROPERITONEAL FIBROSIS

Both ureters are encircled and obstructed by a spread of fibrotic tissue from the posterior abdominal wall. This peri-ureteric fibrosis usually arises from a retroperitoneal malignancy such as lymphoma or from the spread of a metastatic carcinoma in lymph nodes.

Idiopathic and drug induced forms (e.g. methysergide) are seen and usually present with chronic obstructive uropathy and uraemia. The intravenous pyelograms sometimes show a characteristic drawing of the ureters medially towards the vertebral column. Low backache and a high plasma viscosity are diagnostic features.

RENAL VEIN THROMBOSIS

There are five types of renal vein thrombosis:
1. Secondary to the severe hypovolaemia of the nephrotic syndrome, and commonly associated with a membranous nephropathy.
2. Secondary to leg vein thrombosis extending into the inferior vena cava and then to the renal veins.
3. Secondary to infiltration of the kidney with amyloid and from direct spread of renal carcinoma, for example hypernephroma, around the renal veins.
4. Following rejection of a renal transplant.
5. Following extreme dehydration from diarrhoea and vomiting in a neonate or infant.

The condition may be unilateral or bilateral.

Renal vein thrombosis is quoted as a cause of the nephrotic syndrome, but its association with the nephrotic syndrome accompanying membranous nephropathy suggests that it is likely to be a secondary phenomena to the hypercoagulable state and to hypoproteinaemic hypovolaemia. Specific clinical features are flank or abdominal pain and increasing gross proteinuria. It is diagnosed radiologically usually by selective venography or arteriography. Spontaneous recannulation may occur and anticoagulants are used to prevent extension of thrombosis. Direct installation of fibrinolytic agents into the renal veins via a cannula or surgical removal of the thrombus have been successful in a few cases, but prognosis in bilateral involvement is usually bad.

RENAL CALCULI

Definition

Renal or urinary calculi, renal calculous disease, nephrolithiasis are all terms used to describe stones within the kidney and other parts of the urinary tract.

Background

Renal calculi are commoner in men than women in contrast to the higher incidence of urinary tract infections in the female.

About 3 to 5 per cent of men suffer from renal stones and in 50 per cent they are recurrent. Table 14.4 shows the causes and frequency of renal stones. In 60 per cent of patients with stones no obvious cause can be found. Over 90 per cent of calculi contain calcium and even uric acid and cystine stones may become more radio-opaque to X-rays as a result of calcium accretion around them.

Aggravating factors in calcium stone formation include sedentary occupations, tropical and sub-tropical habitat, dehydration, geographical dietary and drinking

Table 14.4 Renal calculi

Type of stone	Urine pH	Frequency (%)
Calcium oxalate*	Alk.	70
Calcium phosphate*	Alk.	15
Calcium magnesium ammonium* phosphate (mixed stone)	Alk.	10
Uric acid†	Acid	2 to 5
Cystine†	Acid	1 to 3
Matrix†	Either	1 to 2

*Radio-opaque.
†Radio-translucent.

water differences, alkaline urine, urinary tract infection (urea-splitting organisms form an alkaline urine), analgesic abuse, obstruction and stasis in the urinary tract and the presence of foreign bodies, for example drainage tubes, suture material and bilharzia ova. Renal stones also tend to run in families. The commonest precipitating factor is hypercalcuria. Hypercalcuria is defined as an excretion of more than 8.5 mmol (350 mg) calcium in the urine per day in man or 7.5 mmol (300 mg) in women while on a normal calcium intake. In the USA the limits are 2.5 mmol (100 mg) less. The average urinary calcium excretion in idiopathic hypercalcuria is about 12.5 mmol/day (500 mg).

Hypercalcuria is classified into three types:
1. Absorption.
2. Resorption.
3. Excretory.

Absorption Hypercalcuria. This indicates excessive absorption of calcium from the gut, for example vitamin D intoxication in health fads, sarcoidosis, excessive intake of milk and alkalis for peptic ulceration (milk alkali syndrome), and of unknown cause.

Resorption Hypercalcuria. This follows excessive bone breakdown, for example hyperparathyroidism, multiple myeloma, secondary metastases, Cushing's syndrome, steroid therapy, immobilisation; these all cause hypercalcaemia initially and secondary hypercalcuria as a result. Renal tubular acidosis (see page 628) causes resorption of bone, hypercalcuria and an alkaline urine predisposing to stone formation without hypercalcaemia.

Excretory Hypercalcuria. This results from failure of renal tubular reabsorption of calcium and is idiopathic.

Uric acid stones form in an acid urine in gout, and in conditions causing secondary hyperuricosuria such as during treatment or radiotherapy for myeloproliferative disorders. Although secondary gout occurs in chronic renal failure the dilute urine prevents stone formation.

Cystine stones form in the hereditary tubular defect of amino acid reabsorption; cystine, ornithine, arginine and lysine are excreted, but cystine is the least soluble. The matrix is a mucoprotein and stones form around it.

Occasionally, soft pultaceous aggregations form in the urinary tract without sufficient calcium oxalate or phosphate to form hard stones, i.e. 'milk of calcium' stones.

Pathology

Calculi may form in any part of the urinary tract and can cause obstruction and/or infection. Sites of formation and obstruction are shown in Fig. 14.24.

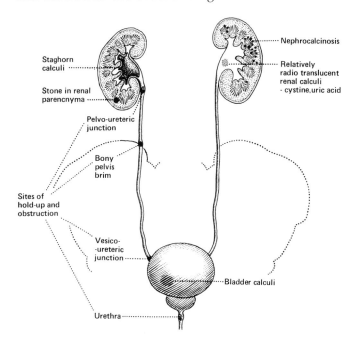

Fig. 14.24   Renal and bladder calculi and nephrocalcinosis.

Pyelonephritic changes in the kidney, hydronephrosis and pyonephrosis may be seen, but renal calculi are not an uncommon incidental finding at post mortem.

The mechanism of stone formation is related to supersaturation of the urine with crystalloid. Possibly, stone-forming patients have an excess of mucoprotein material supplying a nidus for calculus development or a deficiency of substances inhibiting stone formation, for example pyrophosphates.

Symptoms

May be none.
Vague central backache.
Loin pain without colic – unilateral.
Ureteric colic with occasionally signs of shock.
Haematuria.
Frequency if stone passes into bladder or urine becomes infected.
Anuria if a solitary functioning kidney becomes obstructed.
Passage of 'gravel', stone or milky-looking urine.

Signs

May be none.
On passage of stone there may be:
Tenderness and guarding over loin or course of ureter anteriorly.
Palpable kidney, due to hydronephrosis or if infected a pyonephrosis.
Sterile pyuria and trace of protein.
Haematuria – or microscopic blood cells in urinary sediment (sometimes painless).
Stigmata of chronic renal failure (rare).

Complications

Acute renal failure – post-renal, i.e. acute obstructive uropathy – calculus impacted in ureter of only functioning kidney.
Recurrent or persistent urinary tract infection – organisms are exotic, e.g. pyocyaneus or proteus often resistant to antibiotics and impossible to eradicate.
Chronic renal failure – chronic obstructive uropathy and/or chronic pyelonephritis.

Investigations

1. Plain X-ray abdomen—calcium containing stones visible.
2. Excretory urography—uric acid and cystine stones show up as filling defects. Distension of the ureter alone, (hydroureter) or hydronephrosis are seen.
3. Mid-stream specimen of urine to exclude infection and detect sterile pyuria or red blood cells.
5. Estimation of serum calcium, phosphorus and alkaline phosphatase. The serum calcium may be raised in hypercalcaemic states and the phosphate lowered in hyperparathyroidism, whilst a raised alkaline phosphatase may indicate metabolic bone disease.
4. Parathormone level—confirms hyperparathyroidism.
5. Serum uric acid—raised in gout.
6. 24-hour urinary calcium, uric acid and cystine screening test.
7. Blood urea and serum creatinine to monitor renal function.
8. Acid load test to measure ability of kidney to excrete an acid urine following ingestion of 0.1 g/kg body weight of ammonium chloride. Renal tubular acidosis is suspected if urine pH is not less than 5.6. A low serum bicarbonate and potassium with a high chloride are common findings.
9. Stone analysis—calculi passed or removed surgically are retained for analysis – urine should be strained to catch fragments or gravel.

Basis of Treatment

Renal colic. Analgesics and smooth muscle relaxants.
Urinary infection. Appropriate chemotherapy.
Ureteric obstruction. Stones of less than 6 mm often pass spontaneously with high fluid intake and exercise. Cystoscopy and dislodgement or trapping of stone by passing a wire snare basket up the ureter.
Indications for surgery:
(a) Unrelieved obstruction.
(b) Large staghorn calculus causing severe pain.
(c) Intractable infection causing deterioration in renal function.
(d) Recurrent haemorrhage.

Surgical procedures aim to preserve as much renal tissue as possible, i.e. nephrolithotomy rather than nephrectomy.

Prevention

High fluid intake as in the prevention of urinary tract infection for all stone formers.

Absorption Hypercalcuria. Stop vitamin D. Treat sarcoidosis with steroids. Reduce dietary calcium – soften drinking water if necessary. Cellulose phosphate treatment to bind intestinal calcium.

Resorption Hypercalcuria. Treat primary cause if possible, e.g. parathyroidectomy for hyperparathyroidism.

Excretory Hypercalcuria. Bendrofluazide increases calcium tubular reabsorption.

A combination of high fluid intake, bendrofluazide and cellulose phosphate will prevent recurrence in 60 to 70 per cent of renal stone formers.

Uric Acid Stones. Alkalinise urine. Allopurinol therapy – sometimes used in calcium stone formers, also to reduce total urine crystalloid.

Cystine Stones. Alkalinise urine. Penicillamine therapy.

Differential Diagnosis

1. Acute abdomen or musculo-skeletal backache.
2. Other causes of haematuria – tumours and tuberculosis.
3. Other causes of sterile pyuria – tuberculosis and analgesic nephropathy
4. Urinary tract infection.
5. Other causes of acute or chronic renal failure.

Prognosis

Chronic renal failure is extremely uncommon in renal calculus disease. Although morbidity is high from recurrences, urinary infection and ureteric obstruction, the prognosis in terms of longevity is excellent.

NEPHROCALCINOSIS

Definition

Nephrocalcinosis means calcification within the substance or parenchyma of the kidney.

Background

Nephrocalcinosis is diagnosed radiologically and often found as an incidental finding during X-ray of the gastrointestinal or genito-urinary tract.

Diffuse nephrocalcinosis represents miniature stones within the renal tubules. These micro-calculi rarely cause symptoms *per se*. Most of the aetiological factors in stone formation have the potential to produce nephrocalcinosis, i.e. hypercalcaemic states, sarcoidosis and renal tubular acidosis. It is also seen in the condition known as medullary sponge kidney. Nephrocalcinosis localised to one or other pole suggests calcification in an hypernephroma or tuberculous area. Papillary calcification occurs in analgesic nephropathy and tram-line calcification of the cortex develops in acute cortical necrosis if the patient survives for a year or more.

Symptoms and Signs

Usually symptomless.
Occasional haematuria or urinary tract infection.
Passage of micro-calculi.

Investigations

Similar to screening for renal stones.

Prognosis

The outlook as far as renal function is concerned is excellent.

PREVENTIVE NEPHROLOGY

Long term dialysis and transplantation are successful in supporting life and rehabilitating patients with chronic renal failure, but are at the wrong end of the therapeutic spectrum. These expensive and time-consuming treatments are necessary because of a failure to prevent or diagnose and treat renal disease at an early curable stage.

There are nine basic syndromes in nephrology, not including chronic renal failure:

Acute nephritic syndrome.
Nephrotic syndrome
Asymptomatic urinary abnormalities, e.g. proteinuria, or haematuria.
Acute renal failure.
Urinary tract infection.

Urinary tract obstruction.
Renal tubular defects.
Hypertension.
Renal calculi.

Not all of these syndromes progress to chronic renal failure, but many cause a loss of renal function. As only a few renal diseases can be actively prevented the aim must be accurate diagnosis and preservation of nephron function with appropriate treatment. There are several important areas of activity in preventive nephrology:

1. Early and sustained control of secondary renal hypertension.

2. Vigorous treatment of urinary tract infection, test of cure and prevention of recurrences.

3. Correction of gross vesico-ureteric reflux in children and control of infection with long term prophylactic antibiotics if necessary.

4. Removal of nephrotoxic drugs and industrial agents, e.g. analgesics and inorganic lead.

5. Correction of obstruction to the urinary tract.

6. Removal of renal calculi and prevention of recurrences.

7. Removal of potential antigens causing glomerulonephritis.

8. Further search for effective treatment in glomerulonephritis.

9. Genetic counselling for families with potentially hereditary renal disorders, e.g. polycystic kidney disease and hereditary nephritis (Alport's disease).

The inability to treat glomerulonephritis effectively remains the biggest challenge in renal medicine.

SUGGESTED FURTHER READING

General – Reference

Brenner, B. M. and Rector, F. C. (eds.) (1976) *The Kidney*. Philadelphia: W. B. Saunders Co., Ltd.
Black, D. A. K. and Jones, N. F. (1978) *Renal Disease*. 4th ed. Oxford: Blackwell Scientific Publications.
Jones, N. F. (ed.) (1975) *Recent Advances in Renal Disease*. No. 1. Edinburgh: Churchill Livingstone.

General – Short and Readable

De Wardener, H. (1973) *The Kidney*. 4th ed. Edinburgh: Churchill Livingstone.
Gabriel, R. (1977) *Renal Medicine*. London: Bailliere Tindall.
Newsam, J. E. and Petrie, J. B. B. (1975) *Urology and Renal Medicine*. 2nd ed. Livingstone Medical Text.

Renal Failure

Jones, N. F. and Ledingham, J. B. C. (1977) Chronic Renal Failure. *Medicine* 28: 1502–1517.
Evans, D. B. (1978) Acute Renal Failure. *Practitioner* 220: 893–900.
Bricker, N. S. (1972). On the Pathogenesis of the Uraemic State: 'Trade-off Hypothesis'. *New England Journal of Medicine* 286: 1093–1099.

Glomerulonephritis

Sharpstone, P. (1974) Renal Glomerular Disease. *Hospital Up Date* Pt. 1: 603–617; Pt. 2: 715–726; Pt. 3: 814–821.
Cameron, J. S. (1977) Treatment of Glomerulonephritis by Drugs. *British Medical Journal* 1, Pt. 1: 1457–1459; Pt. 2: 1520–1522.
Baldwin, D. S. (1977) Post-streptococcal Glomerulonephritis – A Progressive Disease? *American Journal of Medicine* 62: 1–11.

Urinary Tract Infections

Wing, A. J. (1977) Urinary Tract Infection in Adults. *Medicine* 29: 1571–1587.

Pathology

Heptinstall, R. H. (1974) *Pathology of the Kidney*. 2nd ed. Boston: Little, Brown & Co.
Dunhill, M. D. (1976) Pathological Basis of Renal Disease. Philadelphia: W. B. Saunders Co. Ltd.

Miscellaneous

Malek, R. S. (1977) Renal Lithiasis: A Practical Approach. *Journal of Urology* 118: 893–901.
Sharpstone, P. (1977). Prescribing for Patients with Renal Failure. *British Medical Journal* 3: 36–37.
Curtis, J. R. (1977). Drug-induced Renal Disorders. *British Medical Journal* 2, Pt. 1: 242–244; Pt. 2: 375–377.
Hosking, D. J. (1977) Renal Osteodystrophy. *British Medical Journal* 2: 110–112.
Neary, D. (1976) Neuro-psychiatric Sequelae of Renal Failure. *British Journal of Hospital Medicine* 15: 122–130.
Higgins, P. M. (1978) Haematuria. *British Journal of Hospital Medicine* 19: 325–334.

Disorders of Water and Electrolytes

15

G. WALTERS

On average, the total body water amounts to about 60 per cent of the body weight, approximately two-thirds of it (40 per cent of body weight) being intracellular and one-third (20 per cent of body weight) being extracellular. Plasma forms part of the extracellular fluid (ECF) and constitutes between one-quarter and one-fifth of it. Changes in the distribution of water between the intra- and extracellular compartments occur in accordance with changes in osmotic pressure across the cell membrane.

Much of our knowledge of intracellular electrolytes has been obtained from studies *in vivo* with radioactive isotopes. Such methods, however, take too long for them to be used routinely in clinical medicine, and in practice intracellular changes have to be inferred from observations made on the ECF, i.e. plasma. Measuring the plasma electrolyte concentrations does, of course, provide direct information only on the *composition* of the ECF whereas changes in the *volume* of ECF are often more important. It follows that measurements of plasma electrolyte concentrations are only useful if their interpretation is based upon a sound knowledge of physiological and pathological principles and a clinical assessment of the volume of the ECF.

SODIUM AND WATER

The amount of sodium in the body is of the order of 3,000 mmol (3,000 mEq), of which about two-thirds is located in the ECF and most of the remainder in the bone; the cells contain only very small amounts. The sodium in bones does not exchange readily with that in the ECF and so cannot be called upon to mitigate losses from the ECF. The normal intake of sodium is very variable, and the normal urinary loss of sodium is slightly less than the intake, by the small amount lost in the sweat and faeces.

The sodium concentration in the ECF is a major determinant of its osmotic pressure, and the total amount of sodium present governs the ECF volume. The relationship between osmotic pressure and volume is discussed in more detail below.

Osmotic Pressure, Osmolality and Osmolarity

Osmotic pressure is a function of the total number of particles in solution to which the membrane under consideration is impermeable. The concentration is expressed in terms of the milliosmole (mosmol). This takes account of dissociation, so that for substances like glucose which do not dissociate the milliosmole is the same as the millimole (mmol). But for ionisable substances, one millimole will give more than one milliosmole, e.g. one millimole of sodium chloride will, if completely dissociated, give two milliosmoles, namely one each of sodium ion and chloride ion. The osmotic concentration is expressed either as osmo*lality* or, less commonly, as osmo*larity*. The former refers to concentration in milliosmoles per kilogram of solvent, and the latter refers to concentration in milliosmoles per litre of solution. In aqueous solution there is very little difference between the two but in plasma the difference is about 7 per cent; this is because about 7 per cent of plasma volume is due to protein, and therefore the concentration of particles in the whole plasma is lower than it is in the plasma water.

The normal plasma osmolality is about 280 mosmol/kg of plasma water, and the electrolytes contribute about 95 per cent of this, with urea and glucose contributing the major part of the remainder. The plasma proteins contribute very little to the osmolality, their importance in relation to fluid shifts being that they do exert a significant osmotic pressure across the capillary wall which is freely permeable to electrolytes, urea and glucose. The plasma protein concentration therefore influences the movement of fluid through the capillary wall but not through the cell membrane. Urea and glucose both cross the cell membrane so that although a rapid change in their extracellular concentration will initially cause a shift of water, this will gradually be nullified as the intra- and extracellular concentrations attain equilibrium. The contribution made by the electrolytes to the total osmolality depends on the sodium concentration. This is because sodium is by far the most abundant cation, and any change in its concentration is always accompanied by an equivalent change in the total anion concentration in order to preserve cation-anion equivalence.

Regulation of the Body Sodium and Water Content

The body sodium content is regulated by renal tubular reabsorption. Some of this occurs in the distal tubule under the control of aldosterone, where sodium ions are reabsorbed in exchange for hydrogen ions and potassium ions, but most of it occurs in the proximal tubule under the influence of a postulated natriuretic hormone or 'third factor' (*see* Fig. 14.4, page 221).

The main stimulus to sodium reabsorption is a reduction of the ECF volume. This reduces renal blood flow which stimulates renin production and hence aldosterone secretion (*see* Fig. 10.5, page 166). In addition natriuretic hormone activity is reduced, possibly through an effect of the reduced blood volume on volume receptors, and this allows maximal sodium reabsorption in the proximal tubule. Conversely, expansion of the ECF volume promotes sodium excretion by reversal of the foregoing mechanisms. It must be emphasised that this volume effect occurs irrespective of the plasma sodium concentration.

The water content of the body is regulated by the antidiuretic hormone (ADH) which is formed in the hypothalamus and stored and secreted by the posterior pituitary gland. It increases the reabsorption of water by the renal collecting tubules and is secreted in response to a rise in plasma sodium concentration.

Loss of sodium from the ECF will initially produce a fall in osmolality. This will inhibit ADH secretion and water will be excreted in dilute urine until the sodium concentration is restored. This is clearly achieved at the expense of a fall in the volume of the extracellular fluid. When the resulting fall in blood volume exceeds about 10 per cent it becomes a stimulus to ADH secretion, strong enough to override the inhibiting effect of hyponatraemia which may then develop.

The addition of sodium chloride to the ECF without a corresponding volume of water increases the concentration of sodium so that antidiuretic hormone is secreted; hence the kidney initially secretes a small volume of concentrated urine and any water administered will be retained. However, the increased ECF sodium concentration causes a shift of water out of the cells and the resulting expansion of the ECF volume leads to inhibition of sodium reabsorption by the renal tubules; the excess sodium is therefore excreted. A combination of these mechanisms finally restores the ECF sodium content and concentration to normal and hence also the volume of ECF.

In summary, *if the regulatory organs are intact, sodium retention will lead to water retention and thus to ECF volume expansion. Conversely, sodium loss will result initially in water loss and hence in ECF volume depletion.*

WATER AND SODIUM DEPLETION

The term dehydration is used loosely to refer to depletion of the body fluids. In practice, it is important to distinguish between depletion of the body water without much loss of sodium, and depletion of water with depletion of sodium. There are important differences in their effects.

1. **Water Depletion**

The loss of water alone must lead to concentration of the remaining body fluid, so that the plasma sodium concentration must rise. This rise will be mitigated by a shift of water out of the cells because of the increased extracellular osmolality.

This shift of water also minimises the contraction of the ECF volume, and hence of the plasma volume, so that circulatory failure is not a common feature. Water depletion presents clinically as a cerebral disturbance due to dehydration of the brain cells. Secretion of the anti-diuretic hormone promotes the formation of a small volume of very concentrated urine; the sodium concentration of the urine will be low because such volume depletion as does occur will stimulate the sodium retaining mechanisms.

Thirst develops and ADH secretion ensures maximal retention of any water administered. However, if water loss continues without replacement there must be a progressive rise in the plasma sodium concentration; this is balanced by a corresponding rise in the concentration of anions, mainly chloride.

The causes of water depletion with resulting hypernatraemia are as follows (Fig. 15.1):

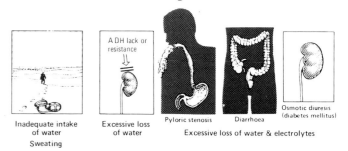

Fig. 15.1 Some causes of excessive losses of body water.

1. Low water intake. This may be due to non-availability, inability to swallow, or general weakness as in acutely ill elderly patients living alone.

2. Osmotic diuresis. This refers to the maintenance of a high urine volume by a large amount of solute passing through the tubules; diabetes mellitus and the excretion of a high urea load in hypercatabolic patients or when high protein feeds are given, are important causes. An increased volume of urine is necessary to excrete the solute load and may result in a negative water balance with a progressively rising plasma sodium.

3. Diabetes insipidus (see page 165). This only induces significant water depletion when there is restricted water intake or interference with the thirst mechanism; e.g. in traumatic diabetes insipidus, hypernatraemia may be the first indication of it in a comatose patient unless the urine output is measured.

4. Excessive loss of water from the skin, stomach or intestines.

Hypernatraemia due to water depletion must be distinguished from that due to excessive administration of concentrated sodium solutions. The latter has occurred due to over-zealous administration of hypertonic sodium bicarbonate solutions to correct acidosis, when isotonic solutions would have been more appropriate, and from the administration of some protein hydrolysates which contain large amounts of sodium. An unusual cause, but one which has proved fatal on occasions, is the administration of too much salt water to induce vomiting after swallowing a poison. The history, which may be in the form of the fluid balance charts, is the most important factor in making this distinction. There may be clinical evidence of a change in ECF volume, and the urine sodium concentration may also be helpful in difficult cases, as it is low in water depletion and high when the cause is excessive sodium intake.

2. Depletion of Water with Sodium

When loss of water is accompanied by loss of sodium the changes are somewhat different and vary with the sodium content of the fluid lost (see Table 15.1). When the total water loss exceeds the sodium loss, relative to their proportions in normal ECF, the plasma sodium concentration will tend to rise as before but to a lesser extent. Therefore, the shift of water from the intracellular fluid will also be less, so that the residual contraction of the ECF volume will be greater than with the loss of an equal volume of water alone, and circulatory failure

is a common feature of advanced cases. The greater the sodium content of the fluid lost the smaller the rise in ECF sodium concentration, and the greater the residual contraction of the ECF volume. Thus, the loss of bile which has a sodium content approximately the same as plasma will itself produce no change in the plasma sodium concentration and will induce no shift of water out of the cells. The whole of the biliary loss will therefore be borne by the extracellular fluid volume.

Any decline of the extracellular volume will be associated with a progressive rise in blood haemoglobin concentration due to reduction of the plasma volume, and a progressive rise in blood urea due to impaired renal blood flow. In a severe case the latter may be as high as 60 mmol/l (360 mg/100 ml).

In the early stages of sodium depletion, drinking water or the administration of inappropriately hypotonic solutions intravenously will lower the sodium concentration and switch off antidiuretic hormone secretion. The water will then be excreted in dilute urine and the ECF volume will continue to fall. A good urine output may be maintained in this way and may mislead an observer into thinking that the patient is being adequately treated.

When the circulating blood volume has fallen by about 10 to 15 per cent, antidiuretic hormone secretion is stimulated, water will be retained and if hypotonic solutions are given, hyponatraemia occurs. The inhibitory effect of hyponatraemia on ADH secretion is not strong enough to override the stimulus of volume depletion and the decline in volume will be slowed, but at the expense of the osmolality. The fall in extracellular osmolality now induces a shift of water *into* the cells and if this is large the syndrome of acute water intoxication will occur. There is apathy, confusion, nausea and vomiting in the early stages, progressing to convulsions, coma and death with increasing severity. Not all cases of hyponatraemia exhibit water intoxication.

With sodium depletion, sodium virtually disappears from the urine because contraction of the ECF volume stimulates renal sodium reabsorption, whether or not the plasma sodium concentration is low, provided of course that the regulatory mechanisms are normal.

The causes of sodium loss, which is always accompanied by water loss, are as follows:

1. The loss of body secretions: vomiting, diarrhoea (Table 15.1), drainage of peritoneal or pleural fluid, and even CSF if the volume is large.

2. Loss through the kidney:

(a) With deficiency of mineralocorticoids, as in Addison's disease (see page 169).

(b) Chronic renal disease in which an osmotic diuresis occurs (see page 232).

In (a) and (b) there will be significant amounts of sodium in the urine despite the presence of hyponatraemia.

(c) The use of diuretics.

Table 15.1 Some examples of the electrolyte concentration of body secretions (mmol/l)

	Na	K	Cl	HCO$_3$
Gastric juice (acid)	80	10	120	0
Pancreatic juice	130	4	60	60
Bile	130	4	110	25
Faeces in diarrhoea	30	30	50	
Colostomy:				
drainage fluid	60	20	50	

Basis of Treatment

The treatment of water depletion is to administer adequate amounts of water, either by mouth or intravenously as 5 per cent glucose.

In sodium depletion, appropriate amounts of sodium must also be given either as the chloride or as the bicarbonate, depending on the acid-base state.

When fluid losses are measured, replacement is straightforward. It requires only simple arithmetic based on the fluid balance charts, a table of the electrolyte composition of the secretions lost, and knowledge of the therapeutic fluids available.

When sodium and water loss have been severe before the patient comes under observation, assessing the therapeutic requirements is more difficult. It must be stressed again that measuring the plasma electrolyte concentrations gives information only on the composition of the ECF and does not indicate the extent of volume depletion. The latter has to be assessed crudely by clinical examination, although the plasma urea and blood haemoglobin concentration may be useful pointers.

The correction of volume deficit is usually more important than the restoration of normal composition. When this is to be achieved rapidly, as in shocked patients, solutions which are approximately isotonic with respect to sodium, such as 'normal saline' (150 mmol/l), should be used. Hypotonic solutions may resuscitate the patient if given rapidly enough, but will cause the plasma sodium concentration to fall precipitously with a risk of water intoxication.

It is impossible to give precise guidance about the amount of fluid required and the rate at which it should be given. In general, if there is acute hypotensive circulatory failure ('shock') fluid should initially be given rapidly at the rate of about one litre in 15 to 30 minutes until the blood pressure rises; the infusion rate may then be slowed. The blood pressure is then likely to fall again because the infused fluid now passes into the interstitial space faster than it is being infused, and the rate must be adjusted so that the blood pressure is maintained about 13.3 kPa (100 mmHg). After two or three litres in an adult it is possible to slow the rate of administration without a recurrence of hypotension. Thereafter, appropriate fluids may be administered at the rate of one litre in four to six hours. Given good kidney function the final adjustments will be made by the kidney. Once the circulation has been stabilised there is no longer any need for rapid infusion.

A rough guide to the volume of normal saline likely to be required is as follows. In an average adult male, if the history and examination indicate dehydration without circulatory impairment, up to two litres is probably required. An ECF deficit of three litres usually causes tachycardia, a small pulse volume and cutaneous vasoconstriction; a deficit of four litres is usually associated with hypotension.

The treatment of water intoxication consists of giving a hypertonic mixture of sodium chloride and sodium bicarbonate intravenously. This withdraws the excess water from the cells and expands the ECF volume. The possibility of an adverse effect on the circulation must be borne in mind in patients with renal failure or cardiac disease. The amount of sodium required is calculated as follows:

Sodium required (mmol or mEq) =
(Normal plasma Na – Observed plasma Na)
$$\times \text{ Total body water (litres)}$$

WATER AND SODIUM RETENTION

The retention of water alone in the presence of a normal extracellular sodium content occurs in oliguric renal failure, in the syndrome of inappropriate secretion of ADH (*see* page 164) and sometimes when oxytocin analogues, which have antidiuretic activity, are given intravenously in hypotonic solutions to induce labour. Excessive water retention may also occur during the first forty-eight hours after injury or surgical operation when ADH is secreted excessively.

In cases with good renal function, the plasma sodium and chloride concentrations are reduced in the same proportions, the bicarbonate level remaining normal. Characteristically, and unlike states of depletion, the plasma urea concentration is low or normal. The urine is inappropriately concentrated with a specific gravity exceeding 1.010 (corresponding to an osmolality of about 300 mosmol/kg of water). Despite the low plasma sodium the urine sodium concentration is relatively high (usually greater than about 15 mmol/l (mEq/l)) because the expanded ECF volume resulting from excessive water retention inhibits the renal tubular reabsorption of sodium.

Retention of both water and sodium in excessive amounts (Fig. 15.2) occurs in several important con-

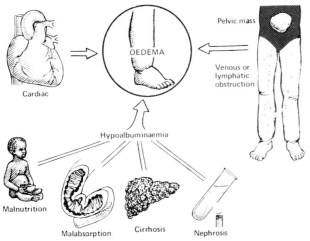

Fig. 15.2 The major causes of oedema.

ditions, for example, congestive heart failure, hepatic cirrhosis and the nephrotic syndrome. In all of these the amount of fluid retained may be sufficient to cause gross oedema, ascites and pleural effusions. When water and sodium are retained in normal proportions (i.e. in the proportions in which they are normally found in ECF), so that the plasma sodium and chloride concentrations are normal, the picture will be one of excess extracellular fluid. In severe cases of heart failure and cirrhosis treated with diuretics, the loss of sodium may not be accompanied by an equivalent loss of water so that hyponatraemia results. In these patients, despite the hyponatraemia, the total exchangeable sodium may still be greatly increased.

Sometimes, excessive use of diuretics reduces the total extracellular sodium below normal. The blood urea begins to rise and the patient feels unwell. The cautious administration of salt may then be beneficial.

POTASSIUM

Total body potassium is approximately 3,500 mmol (mEq). Almost the whole of this is in the cells, only about 60 mmol (mEq) being in the extracellular fluid. This disparity is important clinically, because shifts of comparatively small amounts into and out of the cellular mass will produce very large alterations in the extracellular concentration. The cell content of potassium is related to the water, protein, organic phosphate and carbohydrate content, so that when these substances are lost from the cell potassium is liberated. Potassium lost from the cells in this way is excreted in the urine. Such a loss is appropriate and does not constitute a true potassium depletion, but the latter may well occur when protein, carbohydrate or water are replenished without added potassium.

The normal dietary intake varies between 50 and 150 mmol (mEq) daily and practically all of this is excreted by the kidney, a small amount appearing in the faeces. In the kidney the filtered potassium is reabsorbed in the proximal tubule, and thereafter secreted in the distal tubule in exchange for sodium ions which are reabsorbed, under the influence of aldosterone.

POTASSIUM DEFICIENCY

This is usually, but not always, accompanied by hypokalaemia; there may be a normal or even a high plasma potassium concentration in patients with renal failure and dehydration, or acidosis. It arises from a number of causes and it is not unusual for some of them to coexist.

The important causes are:
1. Loss of gastrointestinal secretions (*see* Table 15.1). The excessive use of purgatives can produce very severe hypokalaemia, with plasma potassium levels as low as 1.0 mmol(mEq)/l. A history of such a cause is often difficult to obtain as the patient regards the frequency of bowel action as normal, or deliberately conceals the use of purgatives.
2. Excessive loss through the kidney.
(a) Primary hyperaldosteronism or Cushing's syndrome (*see* page 167).
(b) Secondary hyperaldosteronism (*see* page 166).
(c) Treatment with diuretics.
(d) Treatment with carbenoxolone for a peptic ulcer. This has an effect on renal tubules similar to aldosterone.
(e) Alkalosis. In this condition, as there is a deficiency of hydrogen ions, potassium ions are secreted in preference to hydrogen ions in exchange for sodium in the distal tubules (*see* page 221).
(f) Certain disorders of renal tubular function, e.g. congenital renal tubular acidosis in which hydrogen ion secretion by the distal renal tubules is deficient, so that sodium conservation depends largely on potassium secretion.

Starvation alone does not usually cause hypokalaemia, but it may occur in patients with anorexia nervosa if they vomit.

The clinical manifestations include weakness, depressed tendon jerks, and abdominal distension. On rare occasions the effect on skeletal muscle is such that a flaccid paralysis develops. However, even severe hypokalaemia may be attended by none of these. The ECG may be abnormal with prolongation of the Q-T interval, depression of the S-T segment and the appearance of U waves.

Prolonged depletion causes morphological changes in the kidney, notably vacuolation of the tubular cells. The concentrating power of the kidney is impaired, because it becomes resistant to the effect of ADH, and the patient may have polyuria and thirst. The potassium lost from the cells is replaced partly by hydrogen ions from the ECF so that there is an intracellular acidosis and an extracellular alkalosis. Hydrogen ion is secreted in preference to potassium ions by the renal distal tubule and, despite the extracellular alkalosis, the urine becomes slightly acid. In long-standing cases, glomerular damage may also occur.

The history is important in determining the cause of hypokalaemia. When there is doubt, measurement of the urinary excretion can be useful for distinguishing renal loss from other causes. If the potassium excretion is much greater than 30 mmol(mEq)/day when the plasma level is below 3.0 mmol(mEq)/l, the urinary level is inappropriately high and is presumably the route of the loss.

Basis of Treatment

Treatment consists of giving potassium supplements. It is not usually urgent unless there is severe muscle weakness, and supplements should be given by mouth whenever possible, provided the patient will take *enough*. If not, potassium should be given by intravenous infusion, as the chloride in cases of alkalosis or as the citrate in acidosis unless the acidosis is being corrected with sodium bicarbonate.

As a general rule intravenous infusions should be given slowly, the concentration of potassium not exceeding 50 mmol(mEq)/l. There is no way of calculating the total amount of potassium needed, which may be as high as 1,000 mmol(mEq). It is not usually necessary to give more than 150 mmol(mEq)/day, but as much as 300 mmol(mEq) daily can be given intravenously in cases where losses are high, and the plasma level should be measured daily until normal levels are restored. If the urine is alkaline, renal loss will be high. When large amounts are given over a short period the ECG should be monitored.

POTASSIUM INTOXICATION

This occurs when high plasma levels result from a failure to excrete potassium when intake or liberation from the cells is high. It is seen in renal failure especially in the presence of acidosis. In the latter, not only is potassium displaced from the cells by hydrogen ion but hydrogen ion secretion by the renal tubule is increased as part of the reaction to acidosis (*see* page 263), and therefore secretion of potassium ions is decreased for a given amount of sodium reabsorption.

Hyperkalaemia may give rise to sensory changes or skeletal muscle paralysis, but its most important effect is on the myocardium. The ECG first shows an increase in the height of the T waves, so-called 'peaking'. Then there are varying degrees of disturbance of intraventricular conduction and finally ventricular fibrillation or cardiac arrest. These may occur without prior warning, hence the need for great caution in any patient with hyperkalaemia. Levels of about 5 or 6 mmol(mEq)/l are not dangerous in themselves, but might be rising rapidly. Death occurs usually with levels greater than 10 mmol(mEq)/l.

When an arrhythmia develops, intravenous calcium chloride or gluconate will antagonise the effect of high levels of potassium and will quickly restore a normal rhythm. The hyperkalaemia, of course, persists and must be tackled simultaneously by other methods. Intravenous glucose and insulin will usually lower it to a safe level, but the effect may be short-lived. Haemo- or peritoneal dialysis are the definitive methods for treating persistently high levels.

In any patient with hyperkalaemia, dehydration and acidosis should be corrected and these measures themselves will often result in a shift of potassium into the cells and lower the plasma level to normal or even below normal. For persistently slightly raised levels an ion exchange resin taken by mouth or administered rectally may be an effective method of control.

SUGGESTED FURTHER READING

Taylor, W. H. (1970) *Disorders of Electrolyte Balance*, 2nd ed., reprinted 1974. Oxford: Blackwell Scientific Publications.

Acid-Base Regulation

16

G. WALTERS

The physiological approach to acid-base regulation is based on the Lowry-Brønsted theory, according to which an acid is a substance which donates a proton and a base is a substance which accepts a proton. Hence in the reaction:

$$HA \rightleftharpoons H^+ + A^-$$

HA is an acid and A^- is its conjugate base; it follows that all anions are bases, but all bases are not anions, e.g. nitrogen-containing compounds are able to accept protons, so that $R - NH_2$ becomes $R - NH_3^+$ and NH_3 becomes NH_4^+.

Some substances have both acidic and basic properties and are amphoteric. For example, water behaves as an acid in the reaction:

$$H_2O \rightleftharpoons H^+ + OH^-$$

and as a base in the reaction:

$$H_2O + H^+ \rightleftharpoons H_3O^+$$

Similarly, the dihydrogen phosphate ion $H_2PO_4^-$ can behave as an acid by dissociating into $H^+ + HPO_4^{2-}$, or as a base by accepting a proton to form H_3PO_4.

The extent to which acids dissociate in solution is variable. Those with a marked tendency to dissociate are called strong acids and those with little tendency to dissociate are called weak acids. Bases are similarly classified in terms of their affinity for hydrogen ions, so that the hydroxyl ion, which combines with hydrogen ion to form water, is a strong base, and the chloride ion, which has very little tendency to combine with hydrogen ion in aqueous solution, is a weak base.

The acidity of a solution is defined in terms of the concentration of hydrogen ion. This is traditionally expressed as pH where:

$$pH = \log \frac{1}{[H^+]} \text{ or } -\log[H^+] \qquad \textit{Square brackets denote concentration}$$

Some clinical laboratories now express hydrogen ion concentration directly in molar units, but this practice is not yet widespread and pH is used throughout this chapter. The following discussion is equally applicable when hydrogen ion concentration is expressed in nanomoles/l, except that a rise in pH corresponds to a fall in hydrogen ion concentration.

BUFFERS

Buffers are substances which in solution resist a change of pH upon the addition of acid or base. Optimal buffering requires components which will resist both the changes caused by added acid and by added base. A typical system would consist of a mixture of a weak acid and a salt of a weak acid, although other combinations, including organic compounds, may be used. The weak acid buffers the effect of added base and the salt buffers added hydrogen ions in the following manner.

The addition of a strong base is followed by its combination with protons in the solution, hence by a reduction in the acidity (i.e. an increase in the pH).

Example:
$$NaOH \rightleftharpoons Na^+ + OH^-$$
$$OH^- + H^+ \rightleftharpoons H_2O$$

If, however, there is a weak acid such as carbonic acid present, it provides a ready source of protons for the basic ions to combine with. As the acid is a weak acid its protons are initially held mainly in the undissociated molecule and are only released in significant amounts when there are basic ions to combine with.

$$NaOH \rightleftharpoons Na^+ + OH^-$$
$$H_2CO_3 \rightleftharpoons H^+ + HCO_3^-$$
$$H_2O$$

The addition of a strong acid contributes hydrogen ions to the solution, but they are largely prevented from changing the pH by the salt of a weak acid. This dissociates almost completely in dilute solution and thus makes available strongly basic ions which combine with added protons to form the largely undissociated weak acid.

Example:

$$HCl \rightleftharpoons H^+ + Cl^-$$
$$+$$
$$NaHCO_3 \rightleftharpoons Na^+ + HCO_3^-$$
$$\downarrow$$
$$H_2CO_3$$

Physiological Buffer Systems

The body contains a number of different buffer systems. In extracellular fluid it is the carbonic acid/sodium bicarbonate system which plays the major part. Proteins also have buffering properties by virtue of their carboxyl and amino groups, and haemoglobin makes a significant contribution to the buffering capacity of blood, a lesser contribution also coming from the plasma proteins.

Phosphate buffers make a relatively small contribution to buffering in blood, but are an important system in urine. Orthophosphoric acid, H_3PO_4, is able to release three hydrogen ions on dissociation, which it does in three successive stages thus:

$$(1)$$
$$H_3PO_4 \rightleftharpoons H^+ + H_2PO_4^-$$
$$\Big\downarrow (2)$$
$$H^+ + HPO_4^{2-}$$
$$\Big\downarrow (3)$$
$$H^+ + PO_4^{3-}$$

At physiological pHs, it is reaction (2) that is important (*see below*).

In a given solution all the buffers present are in equilibrium with each other and therefore the changes in the system as a whole can be evaluated by defining the changes in one of the buffer systems. In the case of blood it is the carbonic acid/bicarbonate system that is selected because it is possible to measure or derive all of its components.

The Henderson-Hasselbalch Equation

When an acid HA dissociates,

$$HA \rightleftharpoons H^+ + A^-$$

the equilibrium constant $K = \dfrac{[H^+][A^-]}{[HA]}$

and $\log K = \log H^+ + \log \dfrac{[A^-]}{[HA]}$

Transposing $\log K$ and $\log H^+$

$$-\log H^+ = -\log K + \log \dfrac{[A^-]}{[HA]}$$

or, $pH = pK + \log \dfrac{[A^-]}{[HA]}$

where $pH = -\log[H^+]$

and $pK = -\log K$

This is the Henderson-Hasselbalch equation.

For the first dissociation of carbonic acid,
$$H_2CO_3 \rightleftharpoons H^+ + HCO_3^-$$

$$pH = pK + \log \dfrac{[HCO_3^-]}{[H_2CO_3]}$$

And for the second dissociation of orthophosphoric acid

$$pH = pK + \log \dfrac{[HPO_4^{2-}]}{[H_2PO_4^-]}$$

The value of pK is, of course, different in each system since it is a characteristic of the acid concerned.

Blood pH

Although whole blood is used for pH measurements it is the pH of plasma that is measured, and this is represented by the equation:

$$pH = pK + \log \dfrac{[HCO_3^-]}{[H_2CO_3]}$$

Since K is a constant, pK is also a constant, so that pH depends on the ratio of $[HCO_3^-]/[H_2CO_3]$.

Carbonic acid is formed by the reaction $CO_2 + H_2O \rightleftharpoons H_2CO_3$, so that its concentration is proportional to the concentration of CO_2 in solution. Since the latter is proportional to the partial pressure of CO_2 (in the atmosphere in contact with the solution, i.e. alveolar air) we can say that pH depends on the ratio $[HCO_3^-]/P_{CO_2}$.

PHYSIOLOGICAL MECHANISMS IN ACID-BASE REGULATION (Fig. 16.1)

Normal metabolism produces hydrogen ions and these are dealt with first by buffers. Since the weak acids so formed do have some tendency to dissociate, buffers do not wholly prevent a change in pH, but minimise it. The effect of buffering by bicarbonate is to lower the bicarbonate concentration and to increase that of carbonic acid, and the slight alteration of pH which occurs will be reflected in the changed ratio $[HCO_3^-]/[H_2CO_3]$ consequent on these changes. Physiologically, however, this system is more effective than it would be *in vitro* because of the ability to excrete the product of buffering and to regenerate more buffer.

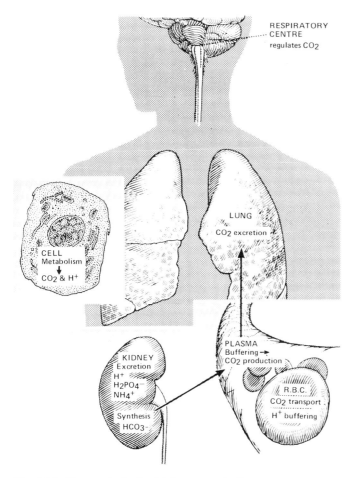

Fig. 16.1 The control of acid-base metabolism.

The carbonic acid dissociates into CO_2 and water, the CO_2 is expired and the hydrogen ion is excreted as water. The accumulation of even a small amount of hydrogen ion (or CO_2) stimulates the respiratory centre, and if the fall in HCO_3^- is large, hyperventilation will be sufficient to lower the P_{CO_2} to an abnormally low level which almost matches the low HCO_3^- and thus shifts the ratio $[HCO_3^-]/P_{CO_2}$, and hence the pH, back towards normal. Complete compensation by hyperventilation cannot occur as the maintenance of the compensatory low P_{CO_2} depends on the continuation of hyperventilation which requires continuation of its stimulus, the low pH.

Although this mechanism can shift the pH back towards normal it would ultimately become exhausted if the bicarbonate consumed was not replaced. A continuous supply of bicarbonate is ensured by the kidney, and this finally corrects the disturbance. Bicarbonate is filtered by the glomerulus, but in normal individuals on the usual acid-producing diet it is completely reabsorbed by the tubules. Moreover, when the bicarbonate in the extracellular fluid (ECF) is reduced through buffering, the renal tubular cells also synthesise bicarbonate which diffuses into the ECF to replenish the pool. The mechanism of these changes is as follows.

The renal tubular cells contain abundant carbonic anhydrase (CA) which catalyses the reaction:

$$CO_2 + H_2O \xrightleftharpoons{CA} H_2CO_3 \xrightleftharpoons{} H^+ + HCO_3^-$$

The H^+ is secreted into the lumen of the tubule, in exchange for sodium ions, and there some of it combines with the filtered bicarbonate to form carbonic acid. This dissociates into CO_2 and water and the CO_2 diffuses into the tubular cells where it is once more converted into carbonic acid and hence into H^+ and HCO_3^-. The bicarbonate ions thus produced diffuse into the ECF balanced by the reabsorbed sodium ions, and the hydrogen ion is secreted into the tubule and thus the process continues.

Hydrogen ions secreted into tubular fluid which contains little or no bicarbonate ions will be excreted either as free hydrogen ion, which lowers the pH, or combined with other buffers, notably the phosphate and the NH_3/NH_4^+ systems:

$$HPO_4^{2-}(+2Na^+) + H^+ \longrightarrow H_2PO_4^-(+Na^+) + Na^+$$

secreted by tubular cells   reabsorbed by tubular cells

The ammonia diffuses into the tubular urine from the tubular cells where it is formed from glutamine. It combines with secreted hydrogen ions to form NH_4^+ which is unable to diffuse through the tubular cell membrane. The total amount of hydrogen ion excreted in this way is therefore composed of three fractions:
1. Free hydrogen ion, the amount of which is very small and can be calculated from the pH.
2. Hydrogen ion incorporated in $H_2PO_4^-$ and, to a lesser extent, other buffers, e.g. creatinine; these can be estimated, together with the free hydrogen ions, as the titratable acidity.
3. Hydrogen ion as NH_4^+.

PATHOLOGICAL DISTURBANCES OF ACID-BASE BALANCE

Terminology

The terms acidosis and alkalosis are used respectively to indicate changes which in the absence of corrective mechanisms would cause the pH of the blood to become more acid or more alkaline than normal. In this respect the reference pH is the pH of arterial blood, about 7.40. The terms acidaemia and alkalaemia have been used to denote an actual change of blood pH beyond the limits of normal, but, nowadays, they are rarely used.

As the pH of blood varies with the ratio $[HCO_3^-]/P_{CO_2}$, alteration of either the bicarbonate concentration or the P_{CO_2} alone will cause a change of pH. The P_{CO_2} is regulated by pulmonary ventilation, and an acidosis or alkalosis due to alteration of the P_{CO_2} is said to be a respiratory disturbance. A change due to elevation or lowering of the bicarbonate concentration is said to be a non-respiratory or metabolic disturbance.

As seen above, mechanisms other than buffering have to be invoked to restore the pH to normal. A primary alteration of one component of the ratio provokes a compensatory change in the other component, aimed at restoring the ratio to normal. The compensatory change must, therefore, be in the same direction as the primary change. The P_{CO_2} is altered by adjustments to ventilation and the HCO_3^- concentration is altered by the kidney.

The partial pressure of CO_2 can be altered very rapidly. It takes very much longer, however, for the kidneys to produce a large change in the bicarbonate concentration; this is an important point when predicting the acid-base changes to be expected in given circumstances (see below). In practice, compensation is frequently incomplete, so that reference is made to a compensated, a partially compensated or an uncompensated disturbance.

The pH and P_{CO_2} can both be measured directly by electrodes, but various methods are used to determine bicarbonate concentration. In the discussion that follows, the term 'plasma bicarbonate' refers to the concentration of bicarbonate ion as it is used in the Henderson-Hasselbalch equation. This is referred to as the actual bicarbonate. It is usually calculated from the measured values of pH and P_{CO_2} and is often done automatically by the sophisticated instruments now used for these measurements.*

When the laboratory reports 'plasma bicarbonate' as part of the electrolyte profile, it has usually been estimated by a procedure which estimates all the CO_2 in the plasma after strong acid has been added to liberate the CO_2 present as bicarbonate ion; accordingly, some laboratories report this as plasma 'total CO_2' on 'T_{CO_2}'.†

The plasma bicarbonate or T_{CO_2} gives a close approximation to the actual bicarbonate as, under physiological conditions, the amount of CO_2 in physical solution and in the form of H_2CO_3 amounts to about 1.2 mmol/l (1.2 mEq/l) compared with about 24 mmol/l (24 mEq/l) for the actual HCO_3^-.

The 'standard bicarbonate' is the bicarbonate concentration when the P_{CO_2} is 5.33 kPa (40 mmHg). Its significance is explained later (see below 'Assessment of acid-base state').

Two other terms sometimes used are 'buffer base', used to denote the total buffering capacity of whole blood including haemoglobin, and 'base excess' which denotes the amount of acid or base necessary to bring the pH of whole blood back to 7.40. These two concepts are not universally accepted because they refer to changes in the blood only, rather than in the whole body, and they will not be discussed further.

METABOLIC, OR NON-RESPIRATORY, DISTURBANCES

Metabolic Acidosis

A metabolic acidosis results when hydrogen ions accumulate for reasons other than CO_2 retention. The bicarbonate level falls owing to buffering and there is increased formation of carbonic acid. The ratio $[HCO_3^-]/P_{CO_2}$ falls, and the acidosis stimulates the respiratory centre. It must be stressed that although the increased formation of carbonic acid tends to raise the P_{CO_2}, the rapidity of onset of hyperventilation and its efficacy are such that the P_{CO_2} does not rise but actually falls if the lungs are normal.

Increased production of hydrogen ion occurs in diabetic ketoacidosis and in lactic acidosis due to various causes including hypoxia and shock syndromes. A relative excess of hydrogen ion also occurs when bicarbonate ions are lost, for example, in pancreatic and small intestinal secretions, and in cases of transplantation of the ureters into the colon. The colonic mucosa is able to absorb chloride ions in exchange for bicarbonate ions, so that as the plasma bicarbonate falls the plasma chloride increases, i.e. there is a hyperchloraemic acidosis.

As the kidney is important for the elimination of hydrogen ions and regeneration of bicarbonate, renal failure is another cause of acidosis. With generalised renal failure, a fall in plasma bicarbonate is counterbalanced by increased levels of phosphate and other retained anions. The urine pH and titratable acidity may be normal but ammonia secretion is deficient and the total amount of hydrogen ion excreted, and hence of bicarbonate formed, is inadequate. In congenital renal

---

* The calculation assumes a pK of 6.10, but this value changes in some pathological states.

† Strictly speaking, to obtain the T_{CO_2} accurately the blood should be collected anaerobically and the plasma separated from the red cells and analysed under anaerobic conditions, as CO_2 will be lost from the plasma on exposure to air.

tubular acidosis, there is deficient tubular hydrogen ion secretion although ammonia formation is normal; as glomerular filtration is normal, phosphate and other anions are not retained and the low plasma bicarbonate level is counter-balanced by a high plasma chloride, i.e. acidosis is again hyperchloraemic.

Metabolic Alkalosis

This is due to the loss of hydrogen ion or to the administration of base. Loss of hydrogen ion in gastric juice is a common cause. The hydrogen ions in gastric juice are derived from the reactions:

$$H_2O + CO_2 \rightleftharpoons H_2CO_3 \rightleftharpoons H^+ + HCO_3^-$$

which take place in the parietal cells of the gastric mucosa. The hydrogen ions are secreted into the gastric lumen accompanied by chloride ions from the ECF, and the bicarbonate ions enter the ECF and replace the chloride ions. Since the chloride concentration of acid gastric juice is greater than that of the ECF, the plasma chloride concentration falls with vomiting and there is an equivalent rise in plasma bicarbonate.

Potassium depletion is another cause of metabolic alkalosis. The loss of potassium ions from body cells is replaced in part by hydrogen ions from the ECF, thus causing an extracellular alkalosis and an intracellular acidosis. In the distal renal tubule the secretion of hydrogen ions in exchange for sodium ions is linked to the secretion of potassium ions. In potassium deficiency, there is little potassium available for this exchange and proportionately more hydrogen ions are lost. The bicarbonate ions generated by this process increase the bicarbonate concentration in the ECF. The increased secretion of hydrogen ions by the renal tubules results in the unusual combination of a slightly acid urine associated with alkalosis in the blood (Fig. 16.2).

The ingestion of excessive amounts of bicarbonate for dyspepsia and the over-enthusiastic administration of bicarbonate intravenously, e.g. in cases of cardiac arrest, are other causes.

RESPIRATORY DISTURBANCES

Respiratory Acidosis

This is caused by any condition which results in CO_2 retention. A rise in the CO_2 tension will reduce the ratio of bicarbonate to P_{CO_2}, thus causing a fall in pH. The compensatory reaction will be a rise in plasma bicarbonate above normal levels so that the pH will return towards normal; the additional bicarbonate is formed in the renal tubules by the mechanisms outlined above, but it will take some time. Thus, in an acute respiratory acidosis the P_{CO_2} will be high with little change in the bicarbonate and therefore a low pH; in a well compensated chronic respiratory acidosis the bicarbonate will

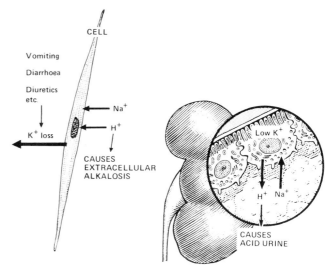

Fig. 16.2 The effects of potassium deficiency.

also be high and the pH normal or only slightly low. A large increase in plasma bicarbonate may take several days to develop maximally.

Respiratory Alkalosis

This is produced by hyperventilation. Increased excretion of carbon dioxide lowers the P_{CO_2} and, therefore, increases the ratio $[HCO_3^-]/P_{CO_2}$, and hence the pH. The compensatory reaction consists of excretion of bicarbonate by the kidney which ceases to secrete the hydrogen ion necessary for its reabsorption.

Causes of hyperventilation include hysterical overbreathing, drugs (e.g. salicylate), pulmonary embolism, cerebral lesions, septicaemia and hypoxia. The latter is a powerful stimulus of respiration. For example, when part of the lung is affected by oedema, oxygen is prevented from reaching the blood flowing through the inter-alveolar capillaries and desaturated blood returns to the left atrium. The resultant arterial hypoxia stimulates the respiratory centre so that the non-oedematous parts of the lung are hyperventilated, and this may be sufficient to produce a low P_{CO_2}.

MIXED DISTURBANCES

So far we have considered pure disturbances of the respiratory or non-respiratory types. Sometimes there is more than one process causing a primary disturbance. These may be such that their effects summate, or they may oppose each other. Such mixed disturbances must not be confused with the occurrence of a primary disturbance and a compensatory reaction to it.

One example of a mixed disturbance due to a single aetiological factor is aspirin poisoning. The salicylic acid released causes a metabolic acidosis. Although this stimulates hyperventilation, the salicylate ion itself is an even more powerful stimulant of respiration and causes a respiratory alkalosis. Whether or not the resultant state is an acidosis or an alkalosis depends on which of the two processes predominates; in adults it is usually the respiratory alkalosis.

In the respiratory distress syndrome of the newborn in which exchange of both oxygen and carbon dioxide in the lungs is severely impaired, hypoxia causes a metabolic acidosis which summates with the respiratory acidosis, causing a large fall in pH.

ASSESSMENT OF THE ACID-BASE STATE

The clinical information available, together with knowledge of the mechanisms described above, usually enables the type of acid-base disturbance to be predicted. Measurements can then be made to determine if these changes have occurred and, if so, their magnitude. For example, if the patient has chronic emphysema the changes are likely to be a respiratory acidosis, whereas a history of protracted vomiting would suggest a metabolic alkalosis. However, the prediction would be somewhat uncertain if the patient with emphysema had been treated with diuretics as a hypokalaemic alkalosis may have been superimposed on the respiratory acidosis.

The pH is usually extremely helpful when interpreting acid-base data because compensation is frequently incomplete, especially in metabolic disturbances, and overcompensation does not occur. Therefore, the pH usually indicates the nature of the primary change or, in a mixed disturbance, the dominant change. Thus, in a patient with a raised bicarbonate and a raised P_{CO_2}, a pH of 7.56 would indicate a metabolic alkalosis with a compensatory rise in P_{CO_2}, and a pH of 7.30 would indicate a respiratory acidosis with a compensatory rise in bicarbonate.

Consider a patient with the following values for arterial blood:

pH	7.62	Normal, about 7.40 ± 0.03
HCO_3^-	20 mmol/l (20 mEq/l)	Normal, about 27.0 ± 3
P_{CO_2}	2.66 kPa (20 mmHg)	Normal, about 5.33 (kPa) ± 0.65 (40 mmHg ± 5)

The pH is clearly alkaline, therefore the primary disturbance is one that causes an alkalosis. A fall in bicarbonate lowers the ratio of bicarbonate to P_{CO_2} and thus causes acidosis, hence the fall in bicarbonate cannot be the primary change; conversely, a fall in P_{CO_2} increases the ratio, thus causing an alkalosis. We conclude that the low P_{CO_2} is the primary change and that the low bicarbonate represents a compensatory change which is utterly inadequate.

However, it would still be possible for the low bicarbonate to represent (in part at least) another primary change due to a coexisting metabolic acidosis, as in the case of salicylate poisoning, or due to a hypoxic lactic acidosis. The final conclusion would depend on whether there was any evidence of such an additional primary disturbance.

The Standard Bicarbonate

The actual plasma bicarbonate does not depend solely on synthesis by the renal tubule. Its production by the gastric mucosa has been referred to (see page 263), and in addition it is formed in the erythrocytes. Carbon dioxide from the tissues is transported to the lungs in the red cells where carbonic anhydrase converts it to carbonic acid. The hydrogen ions produced by the dissociation of carbonic acid formed in the red cells are buffered by the haemoglobin, so that further dissociation occurs and the red cell bicarbonate level increases. Because there is much more protein available for buffering in red cells than in plasma, the red cells have the higher bicarbonate level and bicarbonate diffuses into the plasma, chloride ions moving into the red cell to replace them. The higher the P_{CO_2}, the greater the amount of carbonic acid formed in the red cells and the more bicarbonate ions diffuse into the plasma. This occurs both *in vivo* and *in vitro*.

It follows that with retention of carbon dioxide a rise in the actual plasma bicarbonate might not be due to increased production in the renal tubule, but to an increased shift of bicarbonate out of the red cells as a consequence of the high P_{CO_2}. This latter component is called the respiratory component of plasma bicarbonate. It is necessary to distinguish the respiratory component from the metabolic component in order to determine whether or not a compensatory change has occurred. For this reason Astrup introduced the concept of the 'standard bicarbonate'. This is the bicarbonate concentration of the sample of blood determined after equilibrating it with a P_{CO_2} of 5.33 kPa (40 mmHg) *in vitro*. Since this is the average normal P_{CO_2} it will result in restoring the respiratory component of the plasma bicarbonate to normal. Any remaining abnormality of the plasma bicarbonate will, therefore, be due to alteration in the metabolic component, thus indicating either a compensatory change or, perhaps, a separate metabolic factor.

The concept of standard bicarbonate is not universally accepted because the value obtained *in vitro* only approximates to that obtained by equilibrating the whole body, which is really what is required.

TREATMENT OF ACID-BASE DISORDERS

Effective treatment of an acid-base disturbance requires correction of the underlying cause. This is sometimes easy, but at other times may prove impossible. For example, if diabetic ketoacidosis is not severe, treatment with insulin will suffice to correct the acidosis. If required, a metabolic acidosis can be corrected by administering sodium bicarbonate.

In metabolic alkalosis, the bicarbonate can only return to normal if adequate chloride is provided. Isotonic sodium chloride solutions may be adequate, but if there is potassium deficiency it is necessary to give potassium chloride supplements at the same time.

In a respiratory acidosis, treatment must be aimed at increasing the elimination of CO_2. Tracheal intubation lowers the anatomical dead space sufficiently to achieve this in some cases but others need to be ventilated artificially. It must be remembered that although such measures may reduce the $P\mathrm{CO}_2$ rapidly, any compensatory elevation of the plasma bicarbonate will fall very much more slowly. Therefore, if the $P\mathrm{CO}_2$ is lowered rapidly the patient will swing from a state of partially compensated respiratory acidosis to what is in effect a state of uncompensated metabolic alkalosis, which will persist until renal excretion of bicarbonate catches up.

In a similar way, the rapid correction of a low plasma bicarbonate in renal failure may not immediately correct the intracellular acidosis, so that stimulation of the respiratory centre persists with the development of a respiratory alkalosis.

In respiratory alkalosis there is a need for hyperventilation to be reduced. This can be achieved easily if the patient is being artificially respired, but spontaneous hyperventilation is a more difficult problem. In this case the application of a rebreathing technique will gradually cause the $P\mathrm{CO}_2$ to rise.

SUGGESTED FURTHER READING
Zilva, J. F. and Pannall, P. R. (1975) *Clinical Chemistry in Diagnosis and Treatment*. 2nd ed. London: Lloyd-Luke.

Cardiology

17

D. W. BARRITT

MAJOR SYMPTOMS IN HEART DISEASE

Psychology

People fear heart disease because it is common knowledge that sudden death is often due to a disorder of the heart. Doctors must always be aware of this underlying fear when patients complain of symptoms they suspect may indicate any sort of heart disease. The situation is worsened by the expectation that any strain on the heart may be fatal. Thus, it is feared that any undue exertion or emotional upset is dangerous, and the pleasures of life may be squandered or destroyed by these considerations. When a diagnosis of heart disease is made the doctor should be sure that his advice as to levels of activity is clearly understood. Avoidance of unnecessary invalidism and anxiety largely rests on a clear understanding by the doctor of the nature of the disease, its severity, prognosis and management, and the instinctive appreciation by the patient that he is in competent hands.

Lack of Symptoms

It is not rare for serious heart disease to be unaccompanied by any symptoms. In particular, quite extensive occlusion of coronary arteries may develop unobtrusively and patients may then die perhaps without ever complaining of the first pain, or within minutes of experiencing it.

One needs also to be aware of the extent to which patients with severe heart disease may be protected from symptoms in modern surroundings. For example, patients with advanced rheumatic heart disease in congestive cardiac failure may insist that they are never breathless. The statement is true because they accustom themselves to a very low level of physical activity, never climbing stairs, never walking more than a few yards, and spending almost their entire day in a chair or bed. Ready availability of the motor car makes this situation possible. This is really an unrecognised symptom which could be called *contented invalidism* (Fig. 17.1).

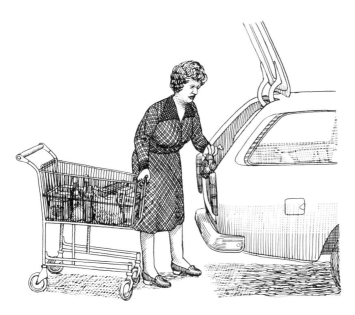

Fig. 17.1 Cardiac disease: the contented invalid.

SYMPTOMS

Breathlessness and pain are the two chief symptoms of heart disease.

Breathlessness

Nervous Breathlessness. This may be unassociated with heart disease. Unlike the action of the heart the mechanism of ventilation easily intrudes into consciousness. A manifestation of nervousness is that the breathing may feel restricted and that insufficient air is being taken in. This is accompanied by conscious efforts to control and increase ventilation. The anxiety causes tachycardia. Common language of this syndrome is that 'I can't get a big enough breath, the air seems to stick at the top of the chest'. Attacks of this type may occur at rest or on exercise. In patients with and without heart disease this symptom complex should be recognised as a nervous one. It does not indicate any functional impairment.

Pulmonary Venous Congestion. The common types of breathlessness in heart disease are related to disease of the left side of the heart and have the same basis. This is what will be called in this book pulmonary venous congestion. It is best exemplified in mitral stenosis when narrowing of the mitral valve orifice obstructs emptying of the left atrium and, thus, the pulmonary veins. The most easily measured consequence of this obstruction is that pressure rises in the left atrium and must therefore rise in the pulmonary veins, capillaries, arteries, and the right ventricle. This rise in pressure affects ventilation in a number of ways. In the first place the rise in pressure in these distensible structures inevitably causes increase in the vascular volume so that more blood is stuffed into the lung than normal. This must encroach on and diminish to a small extent the volume and compliance of the lung and slightly increase airway resistance so that there is some increase in the work of breathing. Also, if there is a considerable rise in pulmonary capillary pressure then the flow of lymph in the lung increases and there will be a risk of exudation into the alveoli. Pulmonary congestion may also cause changes in the reflex control of breathing.

Pulmonary venous congestion may be present at rest in severe cases but will always, of course, increase on exertion. More frequently, resting pressures are normal but as the flow of blood increases with muscular exertion, intrapulmonary pressures rise and the patient is aware of breathlessness on walking up hills or stairs, or hurrying.

Orthopnoea. In severe pulmonary venous congestion intrapulmonary pressures will be high at rest and patients may then be unable to lie flat in comfort. The symptom is called orthopnoea – inability to breathe comfortably when lying flat. Sitting up brings immediate relief, for venous return from the lower half of the body is diminished and cardiac output falls with a fall in work load for the left side of the heart. Perhaps more important, the weight of the liver and other abdominal structures falls away from the diaphragm, thus easing the work of breathing. Patients with severe orthopnoea may refuse to go to bed at night and prefer to sleep in an armchair.

Paroxysmal Nocturnal Dyspnoea. Such patients are also subject to attacks of paroxysmal nocturnal dyspnoea or cardiac asthma. This odd condition of threatened or actual pulmonary oedema comes on during sleep. It is a most important clue to the severity of left heart disease, but rarely witnessed by the doctor because the attack is over before he arrives. Skilful questioning is therefore the only technique available in this diagnosis. The characteristic features are as follows:

After going to bed at the usual time and falling asleep before midnight the patient is awakened in about an hour or longer by a feeling of suffocation or being unable to breathe. His first sensation on waking is

important. Waking in fright is *not* paroxysmal nocturnal dyspnoea. He is then very breathless and instinctively must sit up or sit on the edge of the bed or get out of bed, perhaps to go to the window. He continues to be severely breathless for perhaps ten minutes or more. There may be wheezing or rattling in the chest and a little sputum – frothy or blood-stained. After ten minutes or so the breathing begins to settle and in another few minutes all is well and the patient can go back to sleep without further trouble. Essential features of cardiac asthma are its timing in the early hours, the first sensation of suffocation, severe breathlessness for about ten minutes, and fairly rapid relief on sitting up. Examination during the attack reveals the presence of râles at the lung bases or all over the lung fields.

It is uncertain why the attack occurs during sleep. Cardiac asthma may occur during the day and is sometimes precipitated by effort. It may then be recognised as an attack of severe breathlessness lasting for several minutes at rest. There may be genuine and justifiable fear for life. The attacks will not always resolve so easily but develop into pulmonary oedema with the production of copious frothy sputum, a cold sweat, and central cyanosis.

Cough is not a prominent symptom in heart disease but it is an important clue to severe pulmonary venous congestion. The cough is usually not productive, but a little blood may appear. Usually, the complaint is of an irritating, troublesome dry cough, often when lying down. Beware the patient with left heart disease who begins an irritating cough. He is likely to produce full-blown pulmonary oedema, and die. Recurrent bronchitis with wheezing and sputum is a complication of pulmonary venous congestion (*see* mitral stenosis, page 295).

Pain in the Chest

After breathlessness pain in the chest is the most important symptom of heart disease. Its pathophysiology is of two types only.
1. Most frequently the cause is relative or actual impairment of blood flow to areas of left ventricular muscle, which are thus rendered hypoxic.
2. The second is inflammation of the pericardium in pericarditis.

Also common is pain around the left breast which is not due to heart disease at all, but is an expression of anxiety. This is conveniently called innocent left breast pain (*see* page 282).

Both types of pain are more fully discussed in the sections on angina pectoris and pericarditis.

Palpitations

This is the term used to describe undue consciousness of the heart beat. All normal people are aware of the

267

heart beat in moments of extreme stress or after violent exertion. The factors that seem to be responsible are the fast rate and forceful contraction. Introspective people may also be very conscious of the heart beat under less stressful conditions. By itself this condition is entirely innocent. Beware of thyrotoxicosis. The real importance of palpitations is in the recognition of cardiac arrhythmia. Most commonly, patients are aware of ectopic beats. The premature beat is felt and then the long pause and subsequent more powerful beat. Some people find the sensation very unpleasant. Paroxysmal tachycardia or paroxysmal atrial fibrillation declare themselves as attacks of palpitations.

Loss of Consciousness

A relatively uncommon, but important symptom of heart disease is attacks of loss of consciousness. Stokes-Adams attacks in heart block is one example. Less well recognised is *effort syncope*, which occurs in aortic stenosis. The attack occurs during effort. For example, a man may be hurrying in the rain or a woman pushing a pram up a slope. There may be a momentary dizziness and then abrupt unconsciousness lasting for a few moments only. The attacks are due to severe restriction of cardiac output. At rest, peripheral vasoconstriction protects central aortic pressure but during exercise, when muscle vessels dilate, the aortic pressure falls and perfusion of the brain ceases. Recovery comes with falling to the ground.

Fainting

This is an important phenomenon in those with and without heart disease. A faint can be defined as an attack of loss of consciousness in the upright position due to low central aortic pressure, which is immediately corrected by falling to the ground. The basic fault is the gravity pooling of blood in the veins and capillaries below the diaphragm. Medical students in the operating theatre and guardsmen stationary on a hot day are the classical victims. Fainting under these circumstances is not due to any sort of heart disease. On the other hand, low aortic pressure due to acute myocardial infarction or rapid blood loss may cause fainting of serious import.

Fatigue

This may be a symptom of serious heart disease or of none, and it is an even harder symptom to assess than breathlessness. Fatigue is one of the prominent symptoms of anxiety states and of malingering. Its diagnostic value in patients with heart disease is probably negligible. This is not to say that patients with heart failure do not experience it, or find relief with good treatment.

Cyanosis

This is important as a sign rather than a symptom. It is more likely to be remarked on by relatives than by the patients themselves. Patients with veno-arterial shunts may notice that their hands go blue when they exercise. Blueness of the lips in older people tells one nothing about the state of the heart.

Oedema

Swelling of the ankles and, occasionally, of the abdomen is the paramount symptom of congestive heart failure. Recurrent ankle swelling in middle-aged women and in the warmer months of the year is not a symptom of heart disease. Oedema is due to heart failure only if right atrial pressure is raised. *Gastrointestinal symptoms* may also accompany congestive heart failure. These include subcostal discomfort, which may be worse on exercise, loss of appetite and vomiting. Congestive swelling of the liver is the usual cause.

ARRHYTHMIAS

Definition

An arrhythmia is any condition in which the regular activation of the ventricles from the sino-atrial node is disturbed.

The term sinus arrhythmia (Fig. 17.2) raises a difficulty. At resting heart rates, the sino-atrial node quickens a little in inspiration and slows in expiration in all normal people. In children and fit young people this change in rate may be so abrupt and arresting that a more serious disorder may be suspected. The physiological nature of the phenomenon is always obvious if the

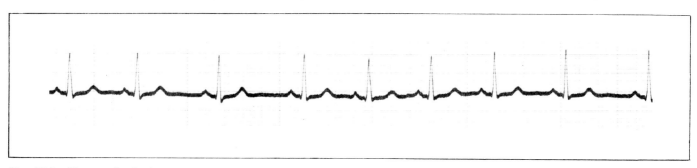

Fig. 17.2 Sinus arrhythmia.

pulse is observed through one or two slow, deep breaths.

Resting heart rates vary a good deal. In infants and small children rates of 100 or more are normal whereas in athletic youths it may be as slow as 50. Occasionally, sino-atrial activity seems to cease momentarily, leading perhaps to a halving of the heart rate. This condition is called sino-atrial block.

Background

Function. Forward propulsion of blood from the heart clearly calls for simultaneous activation and contraction of all the fibres of a chamber so that pressure is exerted on the blood within it. After contraction there must follow a period of rest to allow the chamber to refill. We can consider that the processes of activation and recovery within heart muscle are directed to this end.

The functional properties of myocardium concerned with this orderly sequence are rhythmicity, conductivity and refractoriness. Thus, an activating impulse must arise, be conducted rapidly to the whole heart, and no further activation occur for a short period. All parts of the heart chambers possess these three properties, but they are most highly developed in the specialised cells of the Purkinje system and the sinus and atrio-ventricular nodes. In particular, the rhythmicity of the sino-atrial node is more reliable, and normally at a higher rate than any other area, and it is this which makes it the pacemaker of the heart. Once an impulse originates in any part of the heart it will be conducted to neighbouring areas unless these areas are in a refractory phase. If an impulse begins to spread it is likely to activate the whole heart and give rise to a beat. The only processes that can halt it are a state of refractoriness, or pathological blockage in the central area of the conducting pathway – the bundle of His and its main branches.

The normal sequence of events therefore is impulse formation, conduction, and then refractoriness. When the impulse reaches myocardial cells they are depolarised and then contract. After contraction, repolarisation occurs and it is at this time that refactoriness is present.

Exercise, catecholamine activity, and drugs that have sympathomimetic activity increase rhythmicity and conductivity and diminish refractoriness, thus speeding the heart's action. Rest, with increased vagal tone, and drugs that block sympathetic activity diminish rhythmicity and conductivity and increase refractoriness. Digitalis acts directly on the myocardium to increase rhythmicity, but through its action in stimulating the vagus it increases refractoriness.

Structure. The anatomical pathways responsible for coordinating orderly activation of the myocardium consist of the sino-atrial node, atrio-ventricular node, and the bundle of His and its branches which penetrate the whole of the ventricular musculature (Fig. 17.3). In addition, there are specialised condensations of Pur-

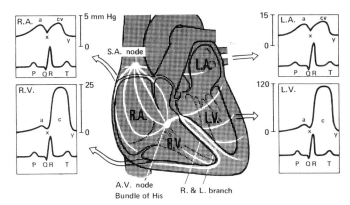

Fig. 17.3 Conducting pathways and intracardiac pressure pulses.

kinje cells carrying the impulse across the atria from the sino-atrial to the atrio-ventricular node.

Because of its high rate of rhymicity which makes it the pacemaker of the heart, the sino-atrial node in the right atrium is richly supplied with autonomic nerve fibres and thus the heart rate is under the constant influence of sympathetic and vagal factors. The atrio-ventricular node and Purkinje network are similarly influenced, particularly in respect of conductivity and refractoriness. The intactness and response of this system of neural control is readily tested by compressing the carotid sinus and observing immediate slowing of the heart.

Nature of Arrhythmias

Disturbances of rhythm can really only take three forms.

Depression of Rhythmicity. This is the least common. Sino-atrial block has been mentioned but loss of inherent rhythmicity usually indicates very profound sickness of the myocardium and is rarely of clinical importance except as a terminal event, when asystole may be the mode of death.

High Refractoriness, or Failure of Conductivity, or Block. This is also relatively uncommon. Major disturbance of the heart is only likely if the block is in the central conducting pathways such as the bundle or its main branches. The most frequent pathological causes are myocardial infarction, degenerative fibrosis in the elderly, and poisoning with digitalis or other cardiotoxic drugs.

Increased Rhythmicity from a Focus of Impulse Formation Outside the Sino-atrial Node. This is by far the commonest type of arrhythmia. Such a focus is called an ectopic focus and the arrhythmia an ectopic arrhythmia. All parts of the heart possess inherent rhythmicity. This, of course, confers the great advantage to the organism that, if the main pacemakers fail, or the normal impulse is blocked, then a lower pacemaker will emerge. Under these circumstances its rate of discharge is slow and the lower down the conducting tree the pacemaker is situated the slower is its inherent rate. Ventricular pacemakers are moreover little influenced by exercise and sympathetic activity so that there is little or no increase of rate with exercise.

Ectopic rhythms in the presence of a normally functioning pacemaker and conducting system can only be due to inappropriate impulse formation which captures the conducting system and activates the heart before the sino-atrial node is next due to do so. Any such ectopic impulse is therefore *premature.*

EXTRASYSTOLES (ECTOPIC BEATS = PREMATURE BEATS)

Atrial Ectopic Beats. These activate the atrium first (Fig. 17.4). Conduction through the atrio-ventricular node

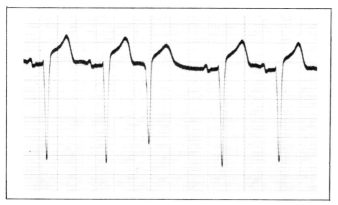

Fig. 17.4   Atrial ectopic beat.

and bundle of His may then be normal and the shape of the QRS in the electrocardiogram will be the same as normally conducted beats. However, as activation is premature it can be the case that the conducting path-

ways will not completely have recovered from the refractory phase of the preceding beat and the premature beat may then be conducted more slowly and in different directions than in the normal beat (aberrant conduction). This will mean that the premature beat will resemble a ventricular ectopic in the electrocardiogram.

Junctional Ectopics. These originate near the atrioventricular node and may spread backwards and forwards to activate atria and ventricles simultaneously. In the electrocardiogram the P wave is inscribed in the QRST complex and is difficult or impossible to recognise. Because the atrium contracts at the same time as the ventricle, when the tricuspid valve is closed, its energy is dissipated in the venae cavae and an unusually large venous wave is seen in the neck, synchronous with the carotid pulse (Cannon wave).

Ventricular Ectopics. These originate below the AV node and usually below the bundle of His. If the impulse arises in a division of the left branch it will spread backwards to the division of the bundles before passing normally down the fibres of the right branch.

The result will be a slow and aberrant activation of the ventricular system. Electrocardiographically, therefore, the ventricular complex will be widened and different in shape from the normal beats. Thus, the distinction between ectopic beats of ventricular and supraventricular origin is usually easy to see from the electrocardiogram (Fig. 17.5).

Symptoms

Awareness of the heart beat.
The heart stops for a moment.
Misses a beat.
Starts with a sudden bump.

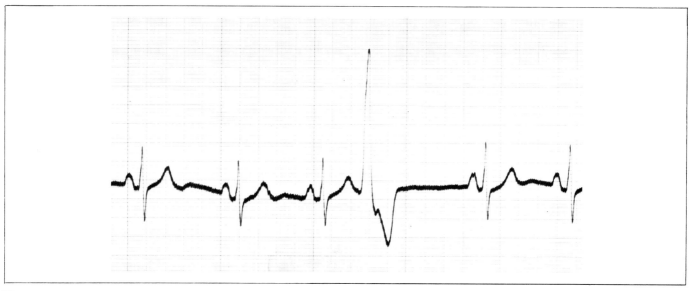

Fig. 17.5   Ventricular ectopic beat.

Signs

Irregularity of pulse; usually occasional breaks in regular sinus rhythm.

Pulse volume appropriately variable; big volume after pause.

Premature beat may be impalpable.

Very frequent ectopics resemble atrial fibrillation.

Significance

Occasional atrial ectopics are very common in normal people. Their occurrence calls for clinical examination of the heart. If nothing is found it is essential that the *patient understands* that the irregularity is unimportant and that there is no disease of the heart. Palpitation is to be ignored. No follow-up is indicated.

Frequent atrial ectopic beats are often the precursor of persistent atrial fibrillation. Thus, their presence in a patient with thyrotoxicosis, mitral stenosis or atrial septal defect may indicate that atrial fibrillation may subsequently occur.

Ventricular ectopics occur also in otherwise normal hearts and may be similarly benign. On the other hand, ventricular disease frequently manifests itself by giving rise to ventricular ectopics (e.g. myocardial infarction). Rather greater care should therefore be taken in deciding the prognosis of ventricular ectopic beats, for though persistent atrial arrhythmias are rarely fatal, persistent ventricular arrhythmias are always potentially so because they may presage ventricular fibrillation.

Basis of Treatment

In themselves, ectopic beats of ventricular or supraventricular origin call for explanation only. If the disturbance of rhythm is due to definable disease of the heart then appropriate treatment may diminish their frequency. Left ventricular failure, for instance, frequently gives rise to ventricular premature beats, and treatment with diuretics and if necessary digitalis will diminish their frequency.

Overdosage with digitalis compounds causes ventricular ectopic beats, but is no contraindication to full digitalisation where appropriate.

PAROXYSMAL TACHYCARDIA

Paroxysmal tachycardia is the term applied to a rapid arrhythmia lasting for minutes or hours. Rapid impulse formation from an ectopic focus may be responsible.

Normal and abnormal function of the atrio-ventricular (AV) node is clinically important. The normal function of the AV node is to delay transmission of the activating impulse on its way to the ventricles. This allows time for the atria to contract and fill the ventricle before systole. In addition, this delaying function and the degree of refractoriness of the node protect the ventricles from dangerously fast activation in conditions like atrial fibrillation or flutter when atrial impulses are evident at 300 to 500 per minute. Under certain conditions however, this protective function breaks down. One such circumstance is the presence of a conducting pathway from atria to ventricles by-passing the AV node. This is the anatomical basis of the Wolff–Parkinson–White syndrome (*see* page 272). Retrograde conduction through a portion of the AV node which has lost refractoriness is another. In both these circumstances the activating impulse may pass downwards to the ventricles but also be conducted backwards to the atrium and thence downwards again. A rapid circus movement is thus initiated giving rise to regular tachycardia.

PAROXYSMAL SUPRAVENTRICULAR TACHYCARDIA

This results from the rapid discharge of a focus in the atria or atrio-ventricular node, or the presence of a re-entrant circus. The features are a rate of 100 to 250 a minute and absolute regularity; P waves of abnormal shape may be seen in the electrocardiogram. The attack may occur in patients with otherwise normal hearts or in disease, for example myocardial infarction. It may complicate the passage of catheters or polythene tubes into the heart.

Symptoms

Sudden onset of rapid, regular beating.

Occasionally, dizziness or faintness or breathlessness.

The attack switches off abruptly after minutes, hours, or even days.

Diuresis may occur.

Signs

Rapid, regular pulse. May be a fall in blood pressure.

May be Cannon waves in jugular venous pulse if atria and ventricles contract simultaneously.

ECG—may show abnormal P waves; absolute regularity; QRS complexes usually of normal shape but bundle branch block may widen the complex.

Significance

The heart may be normal.

In the presence of heart disease a paroxysm of tachycardia may lead to temporary but dangerous deterioration. The rare condition of Wolff–Parkinson–White syndrome should be looked for (Fig. 17.6). The diagnosis is an electrocardiographic one with a short P–R interval and a pre-excitation wave with the appearance of right or left bundle branch block.

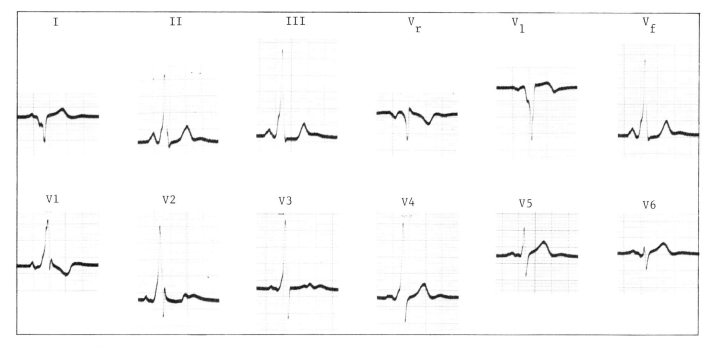

Fig. 17.6 Wolff-Parkinson-White conduction (pre-excitation).

Basis of Treatment

In patients without heart disease the attacks are not dangerous although they are sometimes highly unpleasant. Occasionally, and especially in atrioventricular nodal tachycardia, the patient may be able to stop the attack by making a forced expiration against a closed glottis (Valsalva manoeuvre), or by bending down the the head forcibly between the knees. The doctor may stop the attack by pressure on either carotid sinus or by eyeball pressure (vagal effect). Immersion of the face in ice cold water may also be effective.

If the attacks are frequent, consideration has to be given to long term treatment with drugs. The only really safe long term agents are digitalis and propranolol, and they may not be effective. Drugs such as quinidine or procainamide, which suppress the activation process in the myocardium are really too dangerous to use continuously in a prophylactic way.

Bed-rest and rapid digitalisation are the best treatment of a severe attack. If the situation becomes alarming, direct current countershock therapy can always be used with confidence. The newer anti-arrhythmia drugs, particularly disopyramide may terminate the arrhythmia and eliminate the need for anaesthesia. Long term treatment with oral disopyramide may prevent attacks.

PAROXYSMAL VENTRICULAR TACHYCARDIA

This results from rapid discharge of impulses from an ectopic focus below the bundle of His. The condition is much more serious than supraventricular tachycardia because it commonly occurs only in patients with myocardial disease and it can quickly progress to ventricular fibrillation, and is thus a potentially fatal arrhythmia.

Distinction from the supraventricular type is by the electrocardiogram. The QRS complex is wide and notched, usually there is slight irregularity, and rarely, a P wave may be seen followed by a normally conducted beat.

Significance

Ventricular tachycardia is a potentially fatal arrhythmia and always calls for management in hospital with electrocardiographic monitoring. The attack may upset the patient little and may stop without treatment but no risk should be taken as life is at stake.

Basis of Treatment

In The Attack. With continuous display of the electrocardiogram on an oscilloscope, lignocaine should be given intravenously in an initial dose of 100 mg injected slowly over three minutes. The injection is stopped if the arrhythmia reverts. If there is no response, a second 100 mg may be given without delay. In the seriously ill patient who responds to lignocaine an infusion should follow the intravenous bolus in a dosage of 1 to 2 mg a minute in order to keep the ectopic focus suppressed.

This type of therapy occupies at least thirty minutes and the defibrillator should be standing by, for the

272

arrhythmia may be terminated at once by DC shock if the patient's condition is seriously deteriorating. The only real disadvantage of electrical treatment is that it calls for a brief period of anaesthesia. Intravenous diazepam produces sufficient clouding of consciousness to be acceptable. Anti-arrhythmic drugs all depress myocardial contractility and in this medical emergency the risks of anaesthesia need to be weighed against the potential hazard of the continuing arrhythmia and increasing quantities of suppressant drugs.

Digitalis overdosage is a potent cause of ventricular tachycardia and needs to be considered in the initial diagnostic assessment. If over-digitalisation is responsible then treatment should begin with intravenous potassium and practolol and the serum K is rapidly measured. Electrical defibrillation is dangerous because when the heart restarts the rate may be very slow on account of depression of pacemaker activity and high degree atrio-ventricular block.

Prophylaxis. Myocardial damage is the most potent stimulus causing ventricular tachycardia. For this reason optimal treatment of left ventricular failure and the avoidance of hypokalaemia, hypoxaemia, acidosis or digitalis poisoning are the most important preventive measures. When the arrhythmia threatens to occur or recur in spite of good treatment it may be correct to use suppressive drugs prophylactically. In situations such as acute myocardial infarction, intravenous therapy with lignocaine is most effective. Treatment may be continued for days or weeks with procainamide by mouth (250 mg four times daily). Similarly, disopyramide or mexiletine may be given orally.

VENTRICULAR FIBRILLATION

Ventricular fibrillation (Fig. 17.7) is conveniently mentioned here. The essential physiological disturbance is rapid, disorderly activation of different portions of the ventricular myocardium so that contraction ceases, the pulse ceases, heart sounds are absent, and death ensues in minutes. As previously mentioned, ventricular fibrillation may follow ventricular tachycardia. It may also begin abruptly, particularly in the presence of repeated, very premature ventricular ectopic beats falling on the T

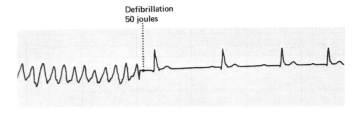

Fig. 17.7 Ventricular fibrillation converted to co-ordinated rhythm by DC shock.

wave of the preceding beat (vulnerable period, phase of super-normal conductivity).

Ventricular fibrillation may cease spontaneously or be arrested by improving oxygenation, correction of acidosis, or by external cardiac massage.

If the arrhythmia is recognised in a patient who has just collapsed, then the immediate use of the defibrillator is always indicated.

ATRIAL FIBRILLATION

Atrial fibrillation is the most important arrhythmia for the practitioner to study as it is the commonest persistent arrhythmia and its presence brings important modifications to haemodynamics and overall prognosis. The arrhythmia can be paroxysmal in just the same way as paroxysmal tachycardia already described, but it may persist for years or decades.

Mechanism. An ectopic atrial focus discharges at the rate of about 500 a minute. Because of differing degrees of conductivity and refractoriness or neighbouring myocardial fibres, the impulse spreads in a haphazard fashion and, thus, concerted contraction is lost. The first consequence therefore is functional paralysis of atrial contraction with different parts of the atrial muscle contracting inco-ordinately.

Impulses arrive at the atrio-ventricular node at very high speed. The node may be in a state of absolute refractoriness, or partial refractoriness or normally conductive. Its response is again unpredictable and therefore activation of the ventricle is quite irregular. The ventricular rate may be very rapid (200 to 300 a minute). The second major consequence of atrial fibrillation (Fig. 17.8) is therefore total irregularity of ventricular rhythm,

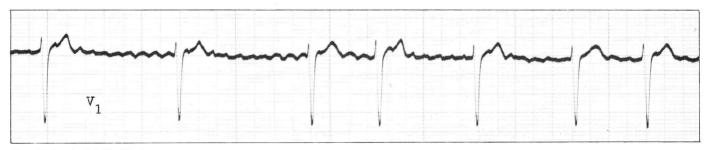

Fig. 17.8 Atrial fibrillation.

273

often with a rapid ventricular rate, especially at the onset of the disturbance and in the absence of digitalis.

These consequences will be more fully worked out in individual diseases, particularly mitral stenosis.

Background

Atrial fibrillation is due to disorder of the atrial myocardium. Potent pharmacological agents able to induce it are adrenaline, isoprenaline and thyroxine. Potent pathological causes are chronic rheumatic myocarditis, myocardial ischaemia and atrophy of the sino-atrial node.

Main Causes of Atrial Fibrillation

Mitral stenosis and reflux.
Thyrotoxicosis.
Old age (?ischaemia).
Myocardial infarction.
Long-standing coronary heart disease (relatively uncommon).
Hypertension (uncommon).
Acute and chronic respiratory disease.
Sino-atrial disease (see page 276).
Pharmacological agents: adrenaline, noradrenaline, isoprenaline.

Symptoms and Signs

Clinical Recognition. The onset of rapid ventricular rates may lead to breathlessness and heart failure, particularly in the presence of structural damage (e.g. mitral stenosis). It may equally be symptomless.

The patient may be aware of the irregularity (palpitations). The pulse is absolutely irregular (distinction from frequent ectopic beats and atrial flutter with varying block calls for electrocardiography). Note that it may not be easy to detect the irregularity, and at times careful palpation and auscultation for many seconds may be necessary.

The pulse volume varies according to the length of the previous cycle, hence systolic and diastolic blood pressure levels vary a little or a lot from beat to beat. Auscultation is the best bedside technique to recognise the irregularity. The pathognomonic feature that can be recognised is the occurrence of several long cycles (slow beats) in succession. This is unlike frequent ectopic beats where a long pause is always preceded by a premature beat.
Note: The presence of a fourth heart sound always excludes atrial fibrillation as it implies atrial contraction.

ECG Recognition. This is nearly always easy and it is inexcusable for the thoughtful student to fail to recognise atrial fibrillation unless the ventricular rate is exceptionally rapid.
1. Regular P waves do not precede each beat.

2. Absolute irregularity, that is to say the cycle lengths vary in unmathematical sequence.
3. Fibrillation waves can often or usually be recognised as irregular undulations of the baseline, especially in lead VI and limb lead II.
4. The QRS complex is normal in width in most instances.

Significance

The onset of atrial fibrillation always calls for an overall assessment of the state of the heart. Its continuance always carries a risk of thrombus formation in the atria and, thus, of systemic embolism. The latter risk is considerable only in mitral stenosis.

Ventricular function cannot be entirely normal, for the nature of the irregularity precludes normal physiological control of the heart rate. At low levels of physical activity and with normal ventricular diastolic pressures, blood will flow through the inert atrium entirely adequately. During exercise with fast heart rates, however, diastole is so short that inadequate filling of the ventricles in the absence of atrial contraction leads to inability to attain maximal cardiac output. Thus, it has been observed that race horses who develop atrial fibrillation *never win*.

In the same way, ventricular disease giving rise to high diastolic filling pressures calls for a powerful atrial contraction, and loss of this contraction as atrial fibrillation develops may cause further serious impairment.

Basis of Treatment

The following questions and their answers are helpful in deciding upon therapy.
1. Is there disease of the heart which can be corrected so that sinus rhythm will re-emerge? (e.g. thyrotoxicosis).
2. Is the arrhythmia likely to be transient and perhaps relatively devoid of danger? (e.gs. myocardial infarction, pneumonia, no detectable heart disease) or is it likely to persist? (e.g. advanced rheumatic heart disease).
3. Has atrial fibrillation been present for months or years or is it clearly of recent onset?

It is always correct to digitalise the patient first. This is easy to achieve within 24 hours. A frequent consequence is that the ventricular rate slows, myocardial metabolism thus improves, and sinus rhythm may be restored.

If the patient is not digitalised a decision should be made within a few days as to whether electrical defibrillation is sensible. The method is very safe with the proper apparatus, but there is a small risk of dislodging an embolism and it is not wise to intervene in this way unless there is a good chance that sinus rhythm will persist. Success is unlikely if the arrhythmia has been present for years. If there is a history of systemic embolism or in the presence of mitral stenosis the patient should be put on anticoagulants for four to six weeks prior to defibrillation.

In the majority of patients, atrial fibrillation will persist and it is a firm indication for the long-term administration of digitalis to control ventricular rate. Unduly rapid ventricular rates are uneconomical for three reasons:

(a) Much energy is used per unit time.

(b) Ventricular filling is inadequate and thus stroke volume will be small.

(c) The period of recovery is very brief and thus contractility of the myocardium is depressed.

In older patients whose resting ventricular rate is normal (70 or less), it may not be necessary to insist on continuous digitalisation, but with active patients an improved physical capacity can be expected with digitalis, because ventricular rates are bound to increase considerably during exercise.

ATRIAL FLUTTER

Atrial flutter will be dealt with briefly, for its background and management are essentially the same as for atrial fibrillation. It is less common, and rarely persists for very long periods of time.

Signs

Atrial rate is usually 300 per minute. This allows regular ventricular response with acceptance of every second or fourth atrial impulse and heart rates of 75 or 150 a minute, often perfectly regular.

The atrio-ventricular block may be variable with an irregular ventricular rhythm (Fig. 17.9).

ECG shows regular P waves at 300 a minute and 2 to 1 or 4 to 1 block.

There are pressure waves in the atria at 300 a minute.

Basis of Treatment

Digitalisation is always correct. It may stop the arrhythmia, slow the ventricular rate from 150 to 75, change flutter to fibrillation, or, quite often, fail to influence the situation.

Direct current conversion should be used under the same circumstance as for atrial fibrillation. It almost always responds to a low energy shock.

ATRIO-VENTRICULAR BLOCK

Heart block is caused by failure to conduct the atrial impulse across the atrio-ventricular node and bundle of His to the ventricular muscle. The condition may be congenital in association with abnormalities of the ventricular septum, especially ventricular inversion (corrected transposition). It can be induced by excessive doses of digitalis or produced by myocardial infarction, when it is usually transient (hours or days).

It is common in the elderly, when the usual pathological feature is unexplained degeneration of the Purkinje fibres in the bundle of His and its main branches.

In some patients the block is permanent, in others it alternates with periods of normal condition, and this intermittent block may continue to be troublesome for years (Fig. 17.10).

Symptoms

Brief attacks of loss of consciousness, usually due to ventricular arrest (Stokes-Adams attacks). The patient may feel giddy for a second or two and then 'dies'—that is, he falls unconscious, is pulseless, white, and respiration ceases; there may be convulsive movements. The heart then restarts (it may fail to) and the skin flushes. Consciousness then returns and in a moment or two recovery is complete. The attack may be very brief and consist only of transient giddiness and then recovery.

With slow ventricular rates (12 to 30/minute) cardiac output is low and the patient may be breathless, fatigued, in full congestive heart failure or with frequent angina pectoris.

ECG Diagnosis. This is not difficult, for the ventricular rate is slow and P-R interval unduly long and in complete heart block constantly variable (Fig. 17.10).

Differential Diagnosis

Differential diagnosis from epilepsy is very important but all too often not achieved, simply by failure to consider the possibility of heart block in the older age group. Anticonvulsant drugs are useless to control Stokes-Adams attacks.

A powerful new aid to diagnosis is the 24-hour tape record of an ECG carried out as an out-patient. Rapid analysis of the 100,000 complexes by an electronic

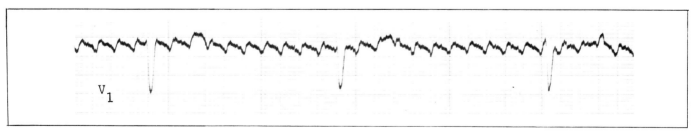

Fig. 17.9 Atrial flutter and complete heart block.

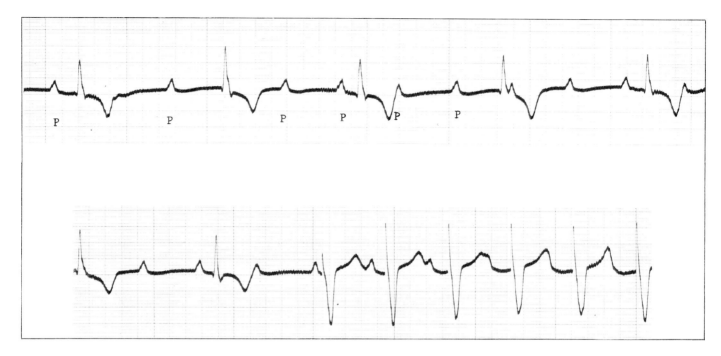

Fig. 17.10 Complete atrio-ventricular block. The last six beats are from an electrical pacemaker.

device soon identifies periods of atrio-ventricular block or tachycardia which may prove the diagnosis.

Prognosis

Sudden death may occur at any time. Some patients, however, survive for years. Frequent attacks of loss of consciousness is a very distressing condition and its correction with electrical pacemaking is accepted with gratitude by nearly all patients.

Basis of Treatment

If the ventricular rate is 40 or more (it rarely increases with exercise) and the patient has few complaints, it is reasonable not to prescribe treatment.

If Stokes-Adams attacks are not controlled or if heart failure is present then the ventricular rate should be increased and maintained by electrical pacing of the right ventricle. In an emergency, the ventricles will often respond to repeated sharp blows on the lower end of the sternum.

Method 1. Passage of a catheter electrode, usually through the subclavian vein to the right ventricle. The tip is positioned low in the apex of the right ventricle with the heart responding to low voltage current (<1 V). A reliable pacing unit discharging at 70 to 80 a minute is then attached distally and is implanted under the skin in the right axilla. With constantly slow ventricular rates a fixed rate unit is employed. With variable block it is essential to use a unit that will not fire into the

vulnerable period (T wave) of a spontaneous beat. This is usually achieved by an electronic device which records ventricular potentials from the catheter tip and inhibits the discharge for a second after each beat. Thus, the pacemaker will fire only if no spontaneous beat is sensed ('on demand' pacemaker).

Method 2. In the rare cases where the intravenous route fails, electrodes can be stitched on to the surface of the right ventricle at thoracotomy. Pacemaking should not be practised, except in emergencies, outside experienced cardiac units, for the passage of catheters into sick hearts is fraught with danger, and good positioning and expert electronic supervision is essential for the maintenance of trouble-free pacing, on which a happy life depends.

SINO-ATRIAL DISEASE

In some patients transient dizziness or Stokes-Adams attacks are due to profound slowing or standstill of the sino-atrial node. The usual pathological change is atrophy of the node. Heart rates of around 50 per minute with a poor response to exercise are the usual clues. Resting electrocardiograms, especially 24-hour tapes, may show loss of normal P waves with nodal beats keeping the ventricles activated. Not rarely, attacks of atrial fibrillation or flutter also occur and then rapid palpitations may be the cause of the patients' complaint. Anti-arrhythmic drugs are useless as they tend to make the heart rate still slower and troublesome symptoms are only effectively treated by electrical pacemaking.

HEART FAILURE

Heart disease of all types may kill the patient in minutes or hours, from serious disturbance of rhythm (e.g. ventricular tachycardia to ventricular fibrillation: heart block) or from pulmonary oedema or pulmonary embolism. These fatal conditions could all be classified as acute heart failure.

Alternatively, grave disturbances of ventricular function may exhibit themselves more slowly in the form of a series of symptoms, signs, and phenomena of altered physiology that we call heart failure.

It is convenient to discuss the entity of heart failure before describing individual types of disease.

Heart failure is difficult to define. The essence of the condition is a rise in diastolic pressure in the affected ventricle. In left ventricular failure due to high blood pressure, for instance, the resting ventricular diastolic pressure may be raised at rest from the normal 12 to 25 mmHg (1.6 to 3.3 kPa). The clinical evidence of this disturbance will be effort breathlessness and perhaps orthopnoea with the presence of a gallop rhythm and râles at the lung bases. One may, however, be able to recognise an earlier stage of ventricular breakdown when ventricular diastolic pressure is within normal limits at rest, but rises with effort or emotion or during sleep. Such a patient will also notice effort breathlessness and may be subject to dyspnoea; a gallop rhythm may be present, but basal râles are unlikely. The basis of the symptoms is, of course, pulmonary venous congestion, for it is clear that a raised left ventricular diastolic pressure causes an obligatory rise in pressure in the left atrium → pulmonary veins → pulmonary capillaries → pulmonary artery → right ventricle (Fig. 17.11, Table 17.1).

Right ventricular failure is rather easier to recognise because we do not need tubing and manometers to be certain of raised diastolic pressure in the right ventricle.

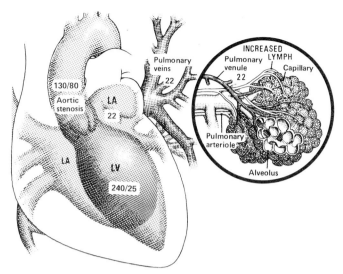

Fig. 17.11 Pulmonary congestion due to left ventricular failure.

With the uncommon exceptions of obstruction to the superior vena cava, tricuspid stenosis and large intrathoracic pressure swings with obstructive airways disease, right ventricular filling pressures can be read off at the neck by looking at venous pulsation.

The clinician who knows his business can always be distinguished from the unskilled by his technique in estimating right atrial pressure. The rules are:
1. Prop the patient up at an angle of less or more than 30° according to the height of pressure (Fig. 17.12).
2. Rest the head comfortably on a pillow so that the sternomastoid muscles are relaxed.
3. Lift the chin a little and turn the head slightly to the left to look at right-sided veins and to the right to study the left.
4. Look.

Table 17.1 Left ventricular failure

Abnormal physiology* (mmHg)			Symptoms	Signs	X-ray chest
A. *Incipient or early*	Rest	Exercise			
LV end diastolic pressure	15	25	Effort dyspnoea	±Forceful apex	Enlarged LV
LA mean	18	30	±paroxysmal nocturnal dyspnoea	±3rd sound gallop	
Pulmonary capillaries	18	30	Tendency to bronchitis	(Fig. 17.13)	±Prominent upper lobe pulm. veins
Cardiac output at rest. Fails to rise to normal exercising values					
B. *Established, frank LV failure*			Effort dyspnoea		
LV end diastolic pressure	18	30	±orthopnoea	Displaced apex	Enlarged LV
LA mean	20	40	±paroxysmal nocturnal dyspnoea	±3rd sound gallop	Distended upper lobe pulm. veins
Pulmonary capillaries	20	40	±bronchitis	±Basal râles	±Septal lines
Cardiac output may be low at rest. Restricted rise on exercise.					

*Normal physiology: LV end diastolic pressure: rest 12, exercise 12.

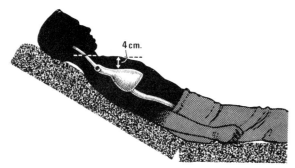

Fig. 17.12 The relationship of the neck veins to the right atrium (see text).

5. Look. Is there pulsation? Is it venous or arterial? How high above the angle of Louis (manubrium sterni) is it? Venous pulsation collapses abruptly in diastole as the tricuspid valve opens. This sharp downstroke should be the sign that the pulsation is venous.

6. To prove that it is venous pulsation, press the root of the neck with a finger to occlude the deep vein. If the pulsation ceases it is venous.

7. If pulsation cannot be seen it is usually possible to cause distension of the superficial jugular vein by pressure with a finger. If the vein empties immediately, the finger is removed, then right atrial pressure is normal (Fig. 17.13).

8. Beware the distended external jugular vein that is occluded in fascial planes at the root of the neck. It does not pulsate normally and will empty with movement of the neck or with inspiration. It is not a true manometer of right atrial pressure.

When there is difficulty in identifying neck veins, gentle, firm pressure over the liver will squeeze blood into the right atrium, temporarily raising pressure and filling the neck veins so that they are more easily recognised (hepato-jugular reflex).

RIGHT VENTRICULAR FAILURE = CONGESTIVE HEART FAILURE

Symptoms

Breathlessness.
Swollen ankles, legs, abdomen.
Upper abdominal discomfort, tenderness.
Nausea, vomiting, anorexia.
Fatigue.
Oliguria.

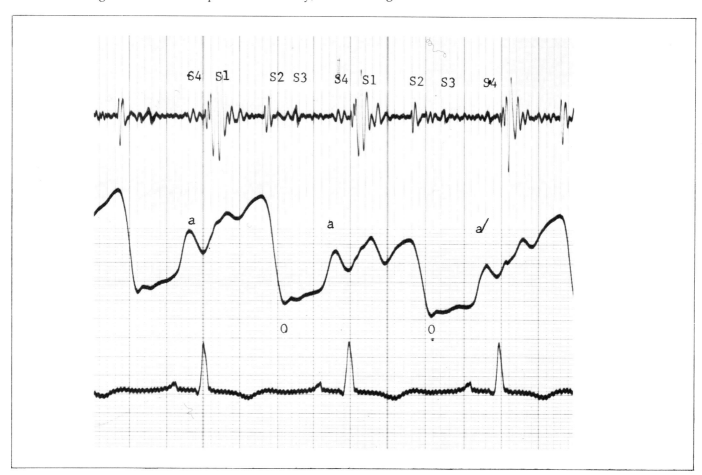

Fig. 17.13 Phonocardiogram (top) and apex cardiogram (middle) showing the relationship of third and fourth heart sounds to atrial contraction (a) and mitral valve opening (o).

Signs

Raised right atrial pressure (essential to diagnosis).
Enlarged liver (usually tender).
Pitting oedema of ankles, legs, sacrum, abdominal wall.
Ascites, pleural effusion.
Low urine output.
Weight gain.
Icteric tinge.
Albuminuria.

Congestive heart failure is one of the end-points of progressive heart disease. Death is then at hand at any moment as a result of fatal ventricular arrhythmia, pulmonary embolism, pulmonary oedema, or renal failure. On the other hand, if ventricular disease progresses very slowly, as is often the case in the elderly, patients may survive in heart failure for a number of years with continuous medication.

Basis of Treatment

Rest. The less the demands of the tissues the more chance the heart has to 'catch up'. Optimum position, well propped up.

Digitalisation

(a) In atrial fibrillation the ventricular rate is reduced thus increasing filling time and sparing energy requirements.
(b) In ventricular failure digitalisation improves contractility (positive inotropic effect). With improving stroke volume the heart rate tends to fall with further benefit.

Preparation of choice. Digoxin; become thoroughly conversant with the dose range. Disbelieve suggestions that digoxin may cause vomiting in some patients when other digitalis preparations do not.

Usual dosage by mouth: initial dose 0.5 mg, followed by 0.25 mg six-hourly for 24 hours and then 125 μg three tablets daily. Atrial fibrillation with rapid ventricular rate may call for a larger dose. Raised blood urea gives evidence of poor renal function with slow excretion of digoxin (maximum dosage 250 μg). In the elderly, 250 μg usually suffices.

Rapid digitalisation can be undertaken with absolute safety. Dosage is 0.5 mg given over five minutes intravenously, followed by 0.25 mg in three hours, followed by 0.25 mg six-hourly to a total of 1.5 mg. By this time the oral route will usually be appropriate. Intramuscular injections can be used for patients who are vomiting.

Digitalis overdosage. The margin between effectiveness and overdosage is very narrow. One constant problem is that heart failure causes vomiting, and so does excessive dosage. It may therefore call for sound judgement to decide if too much or too little digoxin is being given. In the same way, ventricular failure is often accompanied by ventricular ectopic beats which may also be caused by excessive dosage. Blood digoxin levels can now be measured and if this technique is available, the problem may be simplified.

Symptoms of digoxin poisoning:
Anorexia.
Nausea.
Vomiting.
Yellow vision.
Rarely mental confusion.

Signs:
ECG:
Frequent ectopic beats.
Severe bradycardia.
   Long P–R interval.
   Sagging S–T segments.
Paroxysmal atrial tachycardia with block.
Ventricular tachycardia.

If it is decided that overdosage has occurred, then the drug should be omitted for at least 24 hours. Low serum potassium levels potentiate the effect of digitalis on the heart. In the presence of an arrhythmia, therefore, the serum potassium level should always be determined urgently. An intravenous infusion of 25 mEq (mmol) of potassium chloride given over one hour can be started before the laboratory result is known.

Diuretic Therapy. Left ventricular failure must be accompanied by an increased intrathoracic blood volume, for pressures are raised in veins and capillaries. Circulating blood volume in the systemic circuit is also increased in heart failure because of diminished excretion of water and salt. The exact mechanism that leads to their retention is not entirely clear. When peripheral oedema is present there is also a very large increase in extracellular fluid volume.

Diuretic therapy helps to correct all these changes. The reduction of intrathoracic blood volume by diuretics in left ventricular failure does much to relieve breathlessness. In congestive heart failure diminishing blood volume not only removes oedema but improves ventricular failure as it reduces excessive venous filling pressure.

Thiazides. The first choice diuretic is a thiazide – tablets bendrofluazide 5 mg or hydrochlorothiazide 50 mg daily. The latter is best given combined with amiloride, to conserve potassium (Moduretic). Patients who also take digoxin will need potassium supplements, Slow-K 600 mg twice daily, if serum potassium falls.

Frusemide 40 mg by mouth has a more rapid and powerful action. Its disadvantages are: first, that it is several times as expensive as the thiazide diuretics; secondly, the very rapid diuresis may be a nuisance, especially for a man at work who will have to absent himself several times in the morning to pass urine. In older men, retention of urine can easily be precipitated by this rapid diuresis. In the crisis of acute left ventricular failure with pulmonary oedema, however, intravenous frusemide 20 mg is the drug of choice. An intense diuresis begins within minutes and breathlessness is relieved as quickly.

Aminophylline intravenously, 250 mg given over 5 to 10 minutes is also life-saving. The drug increases cardiac contractility and relieves any airways obstruction that may be present.

Morphine intravenously is also invaluable as it relieves the inevitable terror and dilates the venous system.

Aldosterone blocking agents are an additional potent weapon in severe heart failure. When added to thiazide diuretics they increase the diuresis and also conserve potassium so that potassium supplements are usually unnecessary. Dose: spironolactone 50 or 100 mg twice daily.

CORONARY HEART DISEASE

Definition

Obstruction to one or more branches of the coronary arteries that deprives an area of heart muscle of its blood supply, partially or completely. With rare exceptions such as coronary embolism, dissecting aneurysm, and periarteritis nodosa, the obstruction is due to the growth of plaques of atheroma within the intima. These encroach upon the lumen of the vessel impeding blood flow. Rupture of plaques into the lumen or thrombus formation upon them may rapidly cause infarction of the myocardium.

Partial obstruction of vessels causes no symptoms until the narrowing is severe enough to render the myocardium hypoxic during exercise – *angina pectoris.* Complete obstruction gives rise to acute *myocardial infarction.* Multiple major or minor infarcts give rise to extensive *fibrosis* with impairment of ventricular function.

Background

Coronary heart disease is a disease of the second half of life (80 years). With the increased effectiveness of medical care, which has largely eliminated pulmonary infection as a killing disease and improved life expectancy in many cancers, coronary heart disease has become the major cause of death in countries with a European culture. With the change in the clinical importance of these diseases, diagnostic standards have also been revolutionised so that coronary heart disease is now recognised with much greater certainty than even a generation ago. This last consideration does allow for some doubt as to whether the increased incidence of fatal coronary attacks can be attributed partly, or even wholly, to better diagnosis. The evidence for an increased incidence, however, seems overwhelming.

William Heberden wrote the classical description of angina pectoris in English, in 1772. Pathologists did not recognise the nature of myocardial infarction until it was described by Herrick in 1912 and 1918. Until that time cardiac aneurysms were being attributed to emotional or physical trauma, and fatty degeneration of the myocardium was given as a common cause of death. It will be impossible to prove how much of the increase in the proportion of deaths attributed to coronary heart disease is due to a change in the disease and how much to a change in reporting. There are strong reasons, however, for thinking that the disease is becoming commoner and affecting younger people as affluence, sophistication and physical sloth become more widespread. Contemporary necropsy studies by identical techniques carried out in different racial groups either in different parts of the world or in neighbouring, but culturally different, areas seem to show that an increasing incidence accompanies affluence.

No single cause has been identified to account for myocardial infarction. The search for the causative factors involves a study of population over a period of years and recording clinical, electrocardiographic and necropsy evidence in each person. A number of such studies have been completed and certain factors have been identifed which allow them to be regarded as 'risk factors'. The following appear to be established beyond all reasonable doubt.

1. **Age.** Rare before 30 years of age, coronary heart disease probably becomes increasingly common with every decade.

2. **Sex.** Men are affected about one decade earlier than women, and below the age of 60 years the proportion of men to women affected is of the order of 4:1.

3. **Hypertension.** Clinical disease and death from coronary obstruction is more common even with slight elevation of blood pressure, especially in men.

4. **Diabetes Mellitus.** Clinically apparent or in the pre-clinical phase is a causative factor.

5. **Hypercholesterolaemia (Hyperlipidaemia).** In many Americans or Britons, comparable in age and blood pressure, there will be a higher incidence of coronary disease in those with blood cholesterol levels in the upper third of the range than in those in the lower third. Moreoever, in families with hypercholesterolaemic xanthomatosis clinical cases may be seen even in childhood. In this respect it should be noted that in Britain the mean range of blood cholesterol levels in adults is

from 120 to 250 mg per cent (3.1 to 6.5 mmol/l), whereas in most African countries where the disease is considered rare the mean cholesterol level is of the order of 3.1 mg per cent. It may, therefore, be questioned whether 'normal' levels of cholesterol are ever found in Britain.

6. **Family Incidence.** There seems to be a weak family incidence of the disease. This must remain a weak statement when the disease is probably universal and affected by such factors as levels of blood pressure, blood cholesterol, and blood sugar.

Other possible risk factors have been postulated on what appears to be sound evidence.

7. **Cigarette Smoking.** The clinical incidence is roughly doubled in moderate cigarette smokers (15 a day) and trebled in heavy smokers (>30 a day). Carboxyhaemoglobin may have an injurious effect on the arterial intima, and initiate atheroma.

8. **Obesity.** Overeating is, of course, likely to affect body size, blood sugar levels, and blood lipid levels.

9. **Physical Sloth.** Lack of physical exercise – the hallmark of affluence – may be a factor.

10. **Social Class.** This, of course, will affect such other things as overeating, cigarette smoking and physical exercise.

11. **Mental Stress.** Those affected like to think that they have carried an unfair share of the world's troubles.

12. **'Soft'** domestic water supply may in some unknown way render a population more susceptible to arterial disease.

13. **The Contraceptive Pill** appears to increase the low incidence of myocardial infarction in young women, especially smokers.

Symptoms and Signs

With about equal frequency, coronary disease presents with repeated bouts of chest pain associated with effort – angina pectoris – or as the illness of myocardial infarction. A small number of patients are first aware of the symptoms of left ventricular failure due to infarcts which have not caused pain. Patients who already have one symptom may develop either of the other two. The disease progresses in an episodic way and the interval between new clinical incidents may be days or a considerable number of years. Recurrence is absolutely unpredictable. Death from arrhythmia is an ever-present threat.

ANGINA PECTORIS

Pathology

Coronary arteriography has shown that occasionally patients with angina pectoris have no obvious obstruction to the main vessels. In some, especially if pain

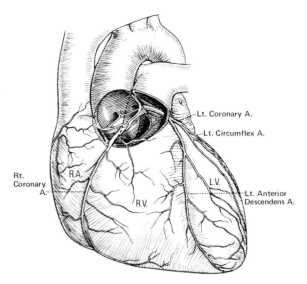

Fig. 17.14   The distribution of the main coronary arteries.

occurs at rest and there are accompanying ECG changes, coronary spasm can be demonstrated. That is to say that an obstructed vessel can be fully dilated by giving oral nitroglycerine.

The usual pathology, however, is atheromatous obstruction to the proximal segments of either the right coronary artery or the left anterior descending or circumflex branch of the left coronary artery or its main stem in the short segment before it divides (Fig. 17.14).

Symptoms and Signs

The characteristic symptom complex establishes the diagnosis. The art of medicine is in drawing out the story from one who may not be good at expressing his feelings. Time must be spent in listening and feeling with the patient. Key questions are:

1. Where do you feel the pain? (Fig. 17.15). The patient

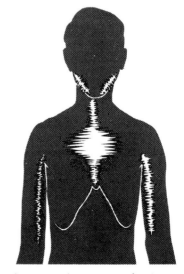

Fig. 17.15   Angina pectoris: pattern of pain.

places his hand on the centre of the sternum. Also felt in the left arm, throat, jaw and right arm.

2. What does it feel like? Pressure, tightness, heaviness, like a weight, a band across the chest.
3. Does it make you stop or slow up? Usually, yes.
4. If you walk quickly up a slope would you expect to get it? Yes.
5. Do you get it when you are sitting quietly in a chair? No?

There are really no signs. If there is evidence of left ventricular failure, this is due to an infarct or to hypertension. Predisposing conditions may be detected in a few cases. Thus, there may be glycosuria from diabetes or xanthelasma palpebrarum from hypercholesterolaemia.

Investigations

1. Electrocardiograms may be normal at rest or may show evidence of an infarct, either recent or long ago. If normal at rest, an exercise test mounting and dismounting a one-foot step for a number of minutes may induce the pain. At this time there will be a depression of the S–T segments in the electrocardiogram. The test takes 10 to 15 minutes to perform and an experienced electrocardiographic technician or doctor is needed. A doctor must always be present in case arrhythmia develops. An abnormal resting electrocardiogram renders the test unnecessary and dangerous.
2. Chest X-ray is indicated. The heart is normal in size.
3. Haemoglobin estimation is performed if anaemia is suspected. Low haemoglobin levels obviously accentuate myocardial hypoxia.
4. Coronary arteriography is being performed with increasing frequency because demonstration of the extent of obstruction determines, within limits, life prognosis and allows surgical treatment to be considered. It is essentially a preoperative investigation.

Differential Diagnosis

1. From oesophagitis. In oesophagitis the usual site of pain is below the xiphisternum, but it may be felt wherever angina is felt. The pain of oesophagitis is commonly burning or gnawing in character. It is not made worse by walking or hurrying. It is worse on lying or stooping and after food.
2. From innocent left mammary pain, the features of which are shown in Table 17.2.

Basis of Treatment

No treatment is known to stay the progress of atheroma formation. The patient soon learns that if he walks more slowly he will not get pain.

Trinitrin tablets sucked under the tongue, or chewed, cause widespread vasodilation with some fall in blood pressure and peripheral pooling of blood which temporarily reduces cardiac output and left ventricular work, with relief of pain. It is more effective if used before exercise. Occasionally, it causes throbbing headache.

Weight reduction relieves left ventricular work.

It is wise not to smoke cigarettes although the patient should not be led to believe that stopping smoking will abolish the risk of further attacks.

Beta-adrenergic blockade of the heart with propranolol or oxprenolol slows the heart rate and reduces cardiac output and left ventricular work. Most patients will be able to walk a little faster without getting pain if they take such tablets continuously. The alternative is to allow a little more time for walking, time that can be set against waiting in surgery for the prescription which also costs money. Dosage: propranolol and oxprenolol 80 to 640 mg a day.

Onset of angina pectoris or swift increase in its frequency or long attacks of pain, especially at night may mean that myocardial infarction has occurred or is threatened. This will be an urgent signal for a period of rest.

The nature of stable angina should be explained to the patient. Pain should be avoided as often as possible and should always be respected by resting. Normal work can continue unless frequent pain makes this impossible. The tone of advice should be cool and given without gloom.

Surgical treatment of coronary artery obstruction is now being very actively investigated. Many patients have successfully been relieved of troublesome angina by a vein by-pass graft being placed between the ascending aorta and a coronary artery distal to a major block. Coronary arteriography is essential to delineate patency of the vessel and a team of experienced cardiac surgeons needs to be available. There is an operative mortality of the order of three per cent in skilled hands. Long term results are not yet known, but the majority of grafts remain patent. Surgical treatment is indicated if pain seriously interferes with normal activity in spite of beta blockade or other measures. The prognosis of

Table 17.2 Features of innocent left mammary pain

Site	Vocabulary	Circumstances	Relief from
Around the left nipple	Aching	Any time	
(Tender to touch)	Stabbing	Worse *after* work	Time alone
Left shoulder to elbow	Sharp	Does not make me stop	
Left scapular area		May last hours	

obstruction of the left main stem is so unfavourable that its demonstration is an indication for surgery.

If angina pectoris has been present with little change in frequency for a period of weeks then it is unlikely that myocardial infarction has recently occurred or threatens. Under these circumstances the condition will stay without appreciable change for an indefinite time. This could be one day or possibly 20 years. Thus, the major problem of giving a prognosis is the unpredictability of the disease. From the time of diagnosis the majority of patients are alive seven years later. One may be dead next day.

MYOCARDIAL INFARCTION

Background

The risk factors have been enumerated. It is unusual for there to be any specific precipitating factors at the onset of an infarct. Occasionally, there may be such specific factors as a surgical operation, unaccustomed exercise (sweeping up snow), a moment of physical fear or intense grief. Outpouring of catecholamines and fast heart rates are common to these events.

Pathology

There is usually total loss of blood supply to an area of heart muscle as a result of thrombosis on a plaque of atheroma, or rupture of the soft contents of a plaque into the lumen of the vessel with additional thrombus formation. There is an area of necrosis of left ventricular muscle and this may extend to involve the endocardium or pericardium. There may be rupture of the ventricular wall into the pericardium or right ventricle. Papillary muscles may be affected and allow mitral reflux. The weakened wall may bulge to form an aneurysm.

Severity. It is not rare for myocardial infarction to occur without the patient being at all aware of it. Electrocardiography and laboratory evidence proves this. More commonly, the patient is dead within minutes or hours of the first symptom. Between these extremes is an obvious illness which calls for medical care but is soon resolved, or a severe illness perhaps lasting for weeks with permanent and severe damage to the left ventricle.

Symptoms

The commonest symptom is pain in the same sites and of the same nature as angina pectoris, but not usually precipitated by effort and not relieved by rest or by trinitrin tablets. The pain may be slight or severe, and last a half to twelve hours, or more. It may recur. Recent onset angina or recent worsening of angina is very common.
Sweating.
Nausea.
Fainting.
Breathlessness.
Fear.

Signs

Anxiety and cold sweat.
Fall in blood pressure.
Heart rate may be quick or slow.
Heart sounds may be diminished in intensity.
May be gallop rhythm.

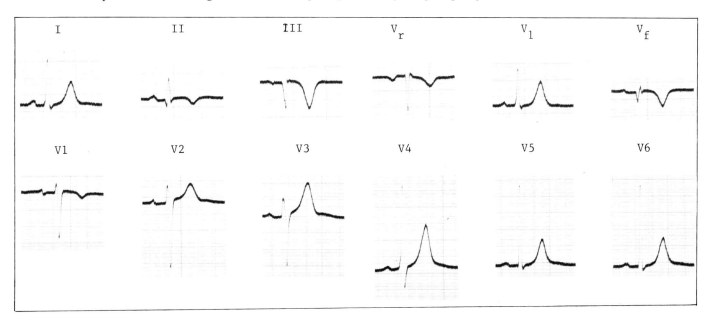

Fig. 17.16   Inferior myocardial infarction.

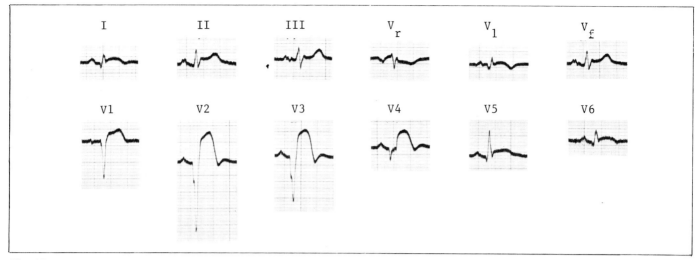

Fig. 17.17 Recent anterior myocardial infarction.

May be râles at lung bases.

Pericardial friction may occur on the second or subsequent days.

Investigations

1. Electrocardiogram at this stage is likely to be abnormal. Changes develop within 36 hours in nearly all patients.

A rise in level of S–T segments in leads II, III, AVF and perhaps V6 (inferior infarction, Fig. 17.16) or in I, II, AVL and V2-4 (anterior infarction, Fig. 17.17).

T wave inversion in appropriate leads as above.

Deep, wide Q waves in appropriate leads as above. T wave changes are the most constant feature. S–T segment elevation usually resolves within 2 to 4 weeks. Q wave and T wave changes begin to resolve more slowly but may remain permanently (Fig. 17.18).

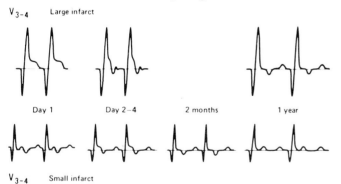

Fig. 17.18 Development of ECG changes in myocardial infarction.

2. A low-grade fever usually begins within 48 hours of the onset and lasts 2 to 4 days.

3. Leucocytosis and a raised ESR or plasma viscosity accompany it (Fig. 17.19).

4. More specifically there is a transient rise of enzymes

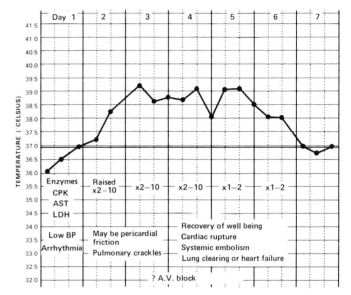

Fig. 17.19 Myocardial infarction: sequence of biochemical and clinical changes.

released from the infarcted myocardium which can be measured in the serum.

Complications (Fig. 17.20)

Any type of arrhythmia including ventricular fibrillation and ventricular standstill.

Left ventricular failure of all grades of severity.

Cardiogenic shock. That is a very low cardiac output with hypotension, cold sweating skin, and mental confusion.

Rupture of the left ventricle leading rapidly to tamponade and death.

Papillary muscle dysfunction or rupture giving rise to acute mitral regurgitation.

Systemic embolism, usually in the second week from intraventricular thrombus.

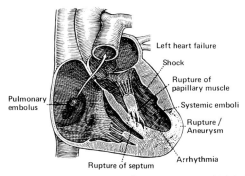

Fig. 17.20 Complications of acute myocardial infarction.

Aneurysm of the left ventricle.
Pulmonary embolism.

Basis of Treatment

An appropriate treatment regime needs to be instituted immediately, for more deaths occur within the first hour of the illness than at any other time and the risk of death diminishes progressively with every hour that passes. Early death will be due to arrhythmia, usually ventricular fibrillation. Both these eventualities may be prevented by inducing physical and mental rest. The first is easy and calls for a comfortable bed with the patient supported by pillows in a position he feels comfortable. Inducing mental tranquillity is more difficult, for almost all patients instinctively realise that this is a dangerous illness.

First, pain needs to be relieved. Heroin (5 to 10 mg intravenously) is the drug of choice in view of its effectiveness and lack of interference with the circulation. If it is not available morphine (15 mg intravenously) should be used. Its disadvantage is that it may induce vomiting. Both these drugs have also a strong narcotic effect and help to allay fear. In less severe circumstances pethidine (50 mg intramuscularly) or pentazocine may be preferred.

From family and nurses the patient needs to understand that his responsibilities are for the moment altogether shelved, that his physical needs will all be supplied by someone else, and that he needs quiet. From his doctor he needs sensible reassurance that this illness is commonplace in medical experience and that full recovery is the rule. He needs also to feel by instinct that there is competence, experience, and technical facility to cope with any complication.

If he is taken ill at home it may be sensible to leave him there, especially if the illness has been present for some hours before diagnosis, if it is mild, if he is elderly, and if the hospital is a good distance away.

The principal advantage of hospitalisation is that this will be most important in the *management of arrhythmias*. To this end all patients in hospital should have a monitoring oscilloscope with an alarm connected to them for the first two to three days. This allows disturbances of rhythm to be detected at once. Most major hospitals now have a specific ward area reserved for this type of medical care, the coronary care ward. Much sophistication of electronic monitoring machinery is possible.

1. Atrial fibrillation and other supraventricular tachycardias should be treated with full doses of digoxin. If the ventricular rate is very rapid and heart failure is feared, direct counter shock may be used to terminate the arrhythmia.

2. The occurrence of frequent ventricular ectopic beats, and especially ventricular ectopics which occur very early in the region of the T wave, may be followed by ventricular tachycardia or ventricular fibrillation. When ventricular tachycardia occurs during the course of myocardial infarction it progresses to ventricular fibrillation in a high proportion of cases. For these reasons ventricular arrhythmia should be treated with drugs that suppress the excitability of myocardial cells.

(a) *Intravenous lignocaine.* A bolus of 100 mg given over two minutes is appropriate first treatment for ventricular tachycardia. A continuous infusion will be needed, for the drug is rapidly metabolised. If a first bolus of 100 mg does not arrest ventricular tachycardia the dose can be repeated within a few minutes. If this fails, another drug may be used or intravenous diazepam given and the attack terminated with direct counter shock. After the attack, or in the presence of frequent ventricular ectopics, lignocaine should continue to be administered at the rate of 2 mg a minute, or less if the rhythm remains steady. This can be followed by procainamide by mouth (500 mg six-hourly).

(b) Two new anti-arrhythmic agents are currently being evaluated. *Disopyramide and mexiletine* given orally have a high success rate in restoring normal rhythm and as prophylactic agents. Propranolol and other beta blocking drugs seem also to be valuable agents in patients recovering from anterior myocardial infarction, but are of course contraindicated in severe left ventricular failure and in patients with airways obstruction.

3. Ventricular fibrillation may follow the warning arrhythmias mentioned above or it may occur without warning. It causes instant death, as the cardiac output falls at once to zero. If a direct counter shock of sufficient power is applied at once, the arrhythmia will almost always be corrected, and co-ordinated contractions return.

4. Monitoring the electrocardiogram is useless unless ventricular fibrillation can immediately be treated. If there is more than a few seconds' delay, external cardiac massage must be instituted and artificial respiration soon started. As the minutes pass, acidosis rapidly develops, and the chances of successful defibrillation fall off sharply.

5. Bradycardia may also call for treatment. At the onset, a slow sinus rate will depress cardiac output and increase the risk of ventricular fibrillation and a low output state. Atropine should be used to increase the

heart rate; dose 0.6 mg intravenously repeated in 10 minutes if the heart rate is below 50 a minute.

6. Atrio-ventricular block is a more serious matter. It is commonest with infarcts of the diaphragmatic wall of the left ventricle and may become progressive with a long P–R interval changing to higher degrees of partial block and then to complete block. Or it may develop suddenly without lengthening of the P–R interval. This is particularly likely with anterior infarcts affecting first one bundle branch and then the other. Stokes-Adams attacks may occur. If the patient is not seriously ill with an inferior infarct there is a good chance that normal conduction will be restored in a few days. With slow rates a dangerous fall in output is likely and ill patients need electrical pacing. An endocardial electrode is passed, as already described, and an on-demand unit attached and left in position for 10 to 14 days after normal rhythm returns. A decision about pacing and passage of the catheter calls for expert cardiological skill, for the ventricle is easily disturbed and repeated stimulation is dangerous.

7. Left ventricular failure and congestive heart failure should be treated in the ordinary way, with rest, effective diuretics and digitalisation.

In severe cardiogenic shock the head should be kept low and the foot of the bed raised to increase venous return and safeguard cerebral blood flow. It may be helpful to infuse up to a litre of dextrose saline to maintain good filling pressure for the left ventricle. New inotropic agents such as dopamine may be useful.

8. The use of oxygen needs to be considered. In all severe cases there is a fall in arterial Po_2, usually of modest proportion. Oxygen inhalation from a mask or nasal spectacles will correct this. It is unproven that this is helpful in preventing complications. No form of oxygen administration is available that does not disturb the patient to some extent and it is foolish to insist on oxygen therapy in a patient who is not obviously ill and who is upset by mask or spectacles.

9. Anticoagulant therapy. There is some evidence that when acute coronary incidents follow in rapid succession there may be benefit from a period of anticoagulation. Anticoagulant therapy, however, with heparin or oral prothrombin antagonists seems to be largely ineffective in preventing recurrence or extension of infarction. Such therapy does materially diminish the risks of pulmonary embolism and of intraventricular thrombus formation and systemic embolism. There is wisdom, therefore, in reserving anticoagulant therapy for those patients with severe infarction who are likely to be immobile for some weeks and are at greatest risk of developing leg vein thrombosis.

10. Period of bed rest. Initial bed rest is essential to allow monitoring and diminish the risk of arrhythmias. The patient feels ill and wishes to rest and this allows assessment of the severity. After a few days it is obvious whether or not there is any risk of heart failure or heart block. Those who have no complication and are feeling well can safely be allowed to move out of bed and begin to walk after a few days. Even those with a more severe illness and who may have a gallop sound calling for diuretic therapy can be allowed out of bed within two weeks if the situation is stable. Given normal home circumstances another week in hospital is as long as is required. There should then be a period of convalescence, first walking in the house, and then in the street.

The vital aspect of management in myocardial infarction is protection of the morale of the patient. It is safe to anticipate from the beginning that most men will return to their former employment and, probably, to their former level of activity within three months. It is crucial therefore not to allow patients and well-meaning relatives to slip into the misconception that the quality of life must change and that avoidance of risk must dominate all movements from then on. This means that after a short period of rest at home there should be active retraining in a low key, anticipating return to work. Gradually increasing exertion is to be encouraged and this can, with benefit, include physical training in a physiotherapy department, if accommodation is available.

It is safe to point out that in the majority of cases, life six months after infarction will have changed little from before the illness. Of course, a proportion of men will be troubled by angina pectoris or breathlessness, and this may limit their powers. The guide to activity should be that the time to rest and slow down is the development of central chest pain or breathlessness. Some men will be debarred from their usual occupation. Bus drivers and heavy truck drivers will lose their licences and be forced to find alternative employment. Men in business who work long hours under mental pressure may well lose their drive and lose their position with their firm unless they are actively encouraged not to weaken. Every man is entitled to decide how much over the minimum of effort he is going to make, but myocardial infarction should rarely be the excuse for opting-out altogether.

Long Term Prevention

There is little evidence that any known measure postpones the next attack but the following are sensible:
Stop smoking.
Avoid obesity.
Maintain a steady level of physical activity.
Treat hypertension.

Young men with repeated episodes may benefit from long term anticoagulant therapy if this can be adequately supervised.

The question of attempting to lower the level of blood lipids continues to pose a problem in management. Controlled trials of the effect of low fat diets in patients who have survived an attack of myocardial infarction failed to show any real benefit. More recent trials using clofibrate in survivors of myocardial infarction and in patients with angina pectoris appear to show a reduction in subsequent mortality, but it is now clear that clofibrate may cause gall bladder disease.

Prognosis

Of men of all ages who recover from an attack of myocardial infarction about 70 per cent are alive five years later. Naturally, the prognosis is worse for the elderly and for those with heart failure and is, therefore, very good for 5 to 10 years for the younger ones whose attack is not too severe. The next attack is unpredictable. Nothing is known of the factors that will precipitate it. These considerations underline the wisdom of making the most of life after recovery.

FIBROSIS OF THE LEFT VENTRICLE

Every major infarct destroys a portion of left ventricular muscle that cannot regenerate. In addition, minor scars add to the loss of contractile force. The end result may be left ventricular failure. There may be a clinical history of major infarcts or, occasionally, none. The electrocardiogram may give clear evidence of major infarcts or simply suggest diffuse fibrosis. When elderly people present with heart failure of this type it is uncertain how much of the loss of contractility is due to age alone.

Management is as for any type of heart failure.

In a few patients, severe heart failure may follow the first infarct. If the patient is not elderly it may be correct to study the ventricle by cardiac catheterisation and angiocardiography. Ventricular failure may be due to mitral regurgitation or to ballooning of one part of the cavity wall as a flap or an aneurysm which absorbs and dissipates contractile energy, detracting from forward flow. Surgical excision of such an aneurysm or flail segment now gives good results.

DISEASES OF OTHER ARTERIES

PERIPHERAL VASCULAR DISEASE

Definition

Ischaemia of the terminal portion of a limb due to atheromatous obstruction of major vessels by plaques or thrombosis. The disease is virtually confined to the legs.

Background

This is similar to that of coronary disease. Hypertension, diabetes, and hyperlipidaemia are important predisposing factors, and cigarette smoking plays a major role. The male sex predominates.

Pathology

Iliac, femoral, and popliteal vessels are affected by changes similar to those described in the coronary system. Severe obstruction at any level endangers the viability of peripheral tissues. Necrosis and gangrene of the toes and foot may therefore follow, often without a specific infection. In the presence of diabetes mellitus the addition of neuropathy and diminished resistance to infection more readily leads to infective gangrene.

Symptoms

Intermittent claudication (intermittent limp) is the usual presenting symptom in young patients. The features are:
Pain in the calf muscles, less often thigh or buttocks.
Pain usually described as 'like cramp'.
Comes on walking a certain distance, more quickly at higher speed and up inclines.
It makes the patient stop, relief comes with one to five minutes rest.
May be one leg or both.
Loss of sexual function may be a feature of aortic bifurcation occlusion in males.
Pain in the muscles or foot at rest, especially at night, is a feature of severe ischaemia.

Discolouration of the skin of the toes and dorsum of the foot, and pain are the symptoms of threatened or actual gangrene.

Signs

Patients with pain but without necrotic skin will virtually always have some diminution of peripheral pulses. Usually more than one and often all four foot pulses are impalpable or very much reduced. Popliteal or femoral pulses may also be lost with proximal obstruction. In doubtful cases oscillometry is useful.

Poor tissue perfusion can be demonstrated by the slow return of colour to the skin when finger pressure is released or on elevation of the leg.

Empty veins and dusky discolouration of the skin of the feet are signs of impaired blood flow.

Investigations

1. Diabetes needs to be excluded by examining the urine for sugar.
2. If surgical treatment is being considered *arteriography* will be required. The distal vessels are delineated by injecting the contrast material into the iliac or femoral arteries. More proximal obstruction calls for injection into the abdominal aorta by a translumbar needle.

Basis of Treatment

Little can be done to prevent progression of the arterial disease except to forbid cigarette smoking.

Intermittent Claudication. Drugs are probably all valueless. Peripheral vasodilator drugs do not produce any measurable increase in muscle blood flow. The patient should be encouraged to walk. Ischaemia is the most powerful vasodilator.

Surgical treatment is indicated if the symptom is so severe that the patient cannot work. Firstly, the major obstruction needs to be visualised by arteriography and patency of more peripheral vessels demonstrated; a vein by-pass graft may then be feasible. Subsequent thrombosis of the graft can occur. Alternatively, major blocks may sometimes be relieved by endarterectomy.

Threatened or Actual Gangrene. Protect the toes by taking care to wear shoes that do not chafe the skin. Forbid walking barefoot. Take care over cutting the toe nails. Avoid any injury. Institute frequent nursing care of any lesion of the skin, if necessary admit to hospital.

Explore the possibility of surgical relief of the obstruction.

Surgical sympathectomy or chemical sympathectomy by injecting the sympathetic pathways in the epidural space may sometimes be helpful by producing a degree of vasodilatation in the skin. The muscle vessels are probably unaffected.

Amputation will be necessary for extensive gangrene and, occasionally, for very severe pain.

BUERGER'S DISEASE (THROMBO-ANGIITIS OBLITERANS)

Doubt continues as to whether this is a real entity. The original description was of angiitis affecting peripheral arteries and veins, especially of young males. The diagnosis may nowadays be suggested in young men who are heavy cigarette smokers with severe obstructive disease of distal leg arteries. Cessation of cigarette smoking results in clinical improvement. The situation cannot be distinguished with certainty from atheromatous obstruction.

RAYNAUD'S DISEASE

Definition

Paroxysmal spasm of arteries supplying the digits of both hands causing coldness and blueness or pallor of the skin.

Background

The cause is obscure. Women are affected more often than men. The common age is 20 to 40 years. Cold is the essential causative agent and warmth invariably relieves. The reduction in blood flow may be so severe as to lead to gangrene of the digits. Severe attacks may be precipitated by the use of amine oxidase inhibiting drugs.

Symptoms

Attacks of deadness, pallor, coldness and blueness of the fingers with paraesthesiae. Immersing the hands in cold water or walking out into the cold may precipitate the attack.

Signs

There may be trophic changes in the fingers or nails. Major pulses are present and normal.

Differential Diagnosis

Attacks of paroxysmal spasm of digital arteries are known as *Raynaud's phenomenon*. They may occur as a complication of other conditions, notably in conditions like systemic lupus erythematosus and scleroderma (*see* page 119). The symptom complex is also found in workers with pneumatic or vibrating tools. Bilateral cervical rib may also be responsible.

The condition is common in patients treated with beta blocking agents.

Investigations

1. Examination of the blood to exclude systemic lupus.
2. X-ray of the chest to exclude cervical rib.

Basis of Treatment

The first line of treatment is to protect the hands from cold. Long-sleeved dresses and undergarments should be worn and gloves are essential out of doors. Smoking is harmful. Medication with Serpasil 0.25 mg twice a day, which depletes the peripheral tissues of vasoactive amines, may be helpful.

In very severe cases, surgical sympathectomy is necessary.

DISSECTING ANEURYSM

Definition

A disorder of the aorta and its main branches characterised by bleeding into the media or the vessels. There is usually rupture of the intima so that the haematoma is in continuity with the lumen. Rupture of the aorta usually follows.

Background

Dissecting aneurysm is not a complication of atheroma, although the two conditions almost always coexist, as only adults are commonly affected. It is a good deal commoner in hypertensives than normotensives.

Dissecting aneurysm is a specific feature of Marfan's syndrome (see page 627). Children and young adults may then be affected.

Pathology

The features are:
Haemorrhage into the vessel wall with the creation of a large haematoma.
Rupture into the lumen of the aorta especially in the ascending portion.
Dissection around the origin of the aorta's main branches with constriction or total obstruction of the lumen. Branches from the coronaries to the femorals may be affected.
Rupture of the outer wall of the aorta into the mediastinum, pleura, pericardium or abdomen.
Dissection in the first part of the aorta may cause disturbance or separation of an aortic valve cusp and lead to aortic reflux.
Histologically there is cystic necrosis of the media.

Symptoms

Pain. This is usually substernal and indistinguishable from myocardial infarction. There may, however, be severe radiation to the back, abdomen or any limb.
Neurological symptoms may occur including stroke or paraplegia.
Rapid death.

Signs

There may be none.
Loss of an arterial pulse in the neck or a limb.
Aortic reflux.
Signs of pleural effusion.
The blood pressure is not usually low.
Neurological signs, e.g. hemiplegia, paraplegia.
May be anuria – involvement of renal arteries.

Investigations

1. Chest X-ray most frequently gives the clue to diagnosis. The aortic knuckle is commonly deformed and subsequent radiographs show increasing size. There may be fluid in the left pleural sac.
2. Aortography confirms the diagnosis.
3. ECG may show evidence of left ventricular hypertrophy from pre-existing hypertension or it may be normal.
4. The urine may contain albumin or blood.

Differential Diagnosis

Usually from myocardial infarction. The distribution of pain and abnormal chest X-ray are points to look for.

Dissection can be complicated by myocardial infarction.
Limited dissection may be painless and is an occasional cause of aortic regurgitation.

Basis of Treatment

Medical. Rapid lowering of aortic systolic pressure reduces the risk of rupture. Relief of pain and anxiety with narcotics and medical expertise are important. Pressure lowering drugs should be given by injection to hold the systolic blood pressure at 100 mmHg (13.3 kPa).

Surgical. If an aortogram shows the dissection to begin below the left subclavian artery and to end above the renal artery, surgical replacement of the descending thoracic aorta is not too formidable a proposition. Severe aortic regurgitation is also amenable to surgical repair.

Prognosis

Untreated dissecting aneurysm has an extremely high mortality (of the order of 90 per cent within a week). Intensive pressure lowering therapy improves the outlook. A few patients survive for years.

HYPERTENSION

Definition

A hypertensive person has blood pressure levels which are constantly raised above the usually accepted range, except perhaps during sleep. Such a person is, of course, unaware of this circulatory statistic, but it renders him liable to heart failure and cerebral haemorrhage perhaps after many years. It is not possible to define normal levels of blood pressure. In populations where this book is likely to be read there are changes of levels with age so that during childhood the systolic blood pressure is of the order of 100 mmHg (13.3 kPa); during adult life 140/90 mmHg (18.6/12 kPa) is usually regarded as the upper limit of normal at rest, but in the elderly, systolic pressures as high as 160 to 170 mmHg (21.4 to 22.6 kPa) are not considered hypertensive. There are studies of primitive populations untainted by sophistication where it seems that the systolic pressure is rarely higher than 120 mmHg (15.9 kPa) and it seems probable therefore that, as with levels of blood cholesterol, our 'normal' values are suspect. Anxiety invariably causes some rise in blood pressure and allowance must be made for this before a diagnosis is made. Hypertension may be a complication of underlying renal or endocrine disease (Fig. 17.21).

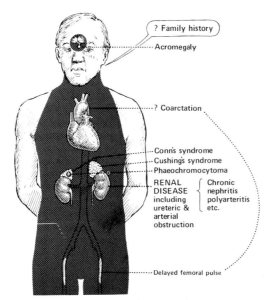

Fig. 17.21   Hypertension: some important causes.

Background

Idiopathic (Essential) Hypertension. In the great majority of patients with hypertension no single cause can be identified. In addition to race, genetic background may also be important for there is a strong tendency for hypertension to run in families. There is argument as to whether levels of blood pressure are determined by a single gene or are multifactorial. The latter seems probable and it is appropriate to compare the situation with that of height of the body which depends not only on genetic background, but also nutritional state and childhood disease.

Moments of anxiety cause a transient rise of blood pressure, but it is impossible to state whether sustained hypertension is related at all closely to psychological factors.

Dietary factors do not seem to be important when comparing one well-fed person with another. Obesity of the arm leads to falsely high readings from a blood pressure cuff.

One piece of abnormal physiology that excites interest is that if hypertensives are given an infusion of saline they excrete a bigger load of salt in the urine than do normotensives. It is clear that the sodium ion plays an important role in maintaining blood pressure levels but it seems more likely that this hypertensive natriuresis is the result of hypertension rather than a causative mechanism.

Height of blood pressure is, of course, determined by the cardiac output and the peripheral resistance. It is possible that in some patients with early hypertension, levels of cardiac output may be on the high side, but in the established disease it is the *peripheral resistance* that is always high. The state of the peripheral resistance is under the control of reflexes with receptors in the carotid sinus and aortic arch. Artificial increases in blood pressure due to increasing peripheral resistance lead to slowing of the heart with a fall in cardiac output. It is therefore the case in hypertension that those circulatory reflexes are set at too high a tone, and allow excessively high levels of pressure to exist at normal heart rates.

Renal Factors. Renal abnormalities cause hypertension.

Laboratory evidence. Goldblatt showed, and many subsequent investigators have confirmed, that hypertension can be produced by making the kidneys ischaemic. This is usually done by partially clamping renal arteries. Removal of the clamp relieves the hypertension. There are clinical parallels of this experiment, which will be discussed.

It has been postulated that the following reaction is responsible.

Renin produced by the kidney activates angiotensin I, which is present in the bloodstream to give rise to angiotensin II.

Angiotensin II can be prepared and it gives rise to sodium retention and a rise in blood pressure in normals when infused.

When patients with hypertension thought to be due to unilateral renal disease are studied it is not always possible to demonstrate any rise in angiotensin and renin levels.

Clinical evidence. Acute glomerulonephritis is almost always accompanied by some rise of blood pressure, and it may be severe. When healing occurs with accompanying diuresis, blood pressure promptly falls to normal again. In chronic glomerulonephritis with severe impairment of renal function, hypertension is almost invariable.

In other renal diseases, such as chronic pyelonephritis and polycystic kidney, severe hypertension occurs with much greater frequency than would be expected and may, therefore, be a result of the renal disease.

Renal artery stenosis may also cause hypertension. The clearest examples of this syndrome are young women with severe hypertension due to stenosis from fibromuscular hyperplasia of the renal artery. If the stenosis is unilateral, then relief of the obstruction or removal of the kidney may cure the hypertension.

Renal factors are also important in malignant hypertension.

Pregnancy. Blood pressure is almost always recorded in pregnancy. Many cases of hypertension are discovered in this way. Raised blood pressure in the first trimester usually indicates pre-existing hypertension.

Endocrine Causes of Hypertension. Pre-eclamptic toxaemia is now a much less important disease than formerly, but the contraceptive pill may cause hypertension.

Phaeochromocytoma. Excessive production of pressor amines from this tumour of the adrenal medulla causes severe hypertension, which is often markedly fluctuating.

Cushing's syndrome also causes excessive suprarenal activity and may be complicated by sustained hypertension.

Acromegaly by a different mechanism which is not fully understood.

Aldosterone secreting tumour of the adrenal (Conn's syndrome) leads to excessive retention of salt and water, which may lead to hypertension.

Coarctation of the Aorta. Mechanical obstruction beyond the left subclavian artery is alone responsible. Surgical excision of the stricture in childhood is curative.

Pathology

With the exception of hypertension due to renal or endocrine disease, the pathology of hypertension is that of its complications. Artery walls are thickened. Atheromatous degeneration is increased in amount.

Symptoms

The only symptom that may be attributed to the rise in blood pressure *per se* is headache. Thus, the great majority of patients even with severe hypertension are symptomless and the discovery is made at a routine examination or when complications occur. Malignant hypertension may cause a generalised headache, worse on waking and tending to improve after rising. Lowering the pressure relieves the headache. More frequently, hypertension is discovered when middle-aged patients consult their doctors for tension headache or transient dizziness. Then the symptoms are not directly attributable to the rise in pressure. Other members of the family may be hypertensive.

Investigations

The aims are to elucidate the background to the disease so that underlying renal or endocrine disease can be excluded, and to assess severity and the presence of complications such as incipient renal failure or left ventricular failure.

1. **Clinical Examination** detects the presence of retinal abnormalities. Retinal photography, if available, confirms the following grading or retinal changes which are of profound prognostic import.
   Grade I. Minor changes in the calibre of retinal arteries.

Grade II. Arterio-venous nipping with narrowing and irregularity of the lumen of arteries.
Grade III equals Grade II plus retinal haemorrhage. Exudates may also be present.
Grade IV equals Grade III plus papilloedema.
Femoral pulse. Coarctation is always diagnosed at the bedside from diminution and delay of the femoral pulse when compared with the wrist. Appropriate murmurs are also present over the heart and scapulae.
The apex beat is forceful from left ventricular hypertrophy. Audible 4th or 3rd sound gallops give evidence of hypertensive left ventricular disease.
Pulsus alternans may be present. This can rarely be felt with the finger, but the sphygmomanometer gives evidence of regular rhythm with alternate beats of differing strength; for example, systolic pressures of 220 to 190 and diastolics of 130 to 115. (This phenomenon may also be discovered in normotensive patients at fast ventricular rates.)
Repeated readings of blood pressure as the patient becomes familiar with the routine, help to establish how severe and continuous the hypertension is.

2. **Serum Electrolytes.** Raised blood urea signifies severe renal involvement. In patients not receiving diuretics diminished serum potassium level with a metabolic alkalosis raises suspicion of aldosterone secreting tumour (*see* page 168). Hyperaldosteronism may also be caused by severe hypertension.

3. **Urine Examination.** Absence of albuminuria largely excludes severe renal involvement and malignant hypertension.
Microscopy and culture of a freshly voided urine sample reveals the presence of pus cells and organisms in chronic pyelonephritis, and casts and perhaps red cells in malignant hypertension and chronic glomerulonephritis.
When renal involvement exists, urine concentrating power and creatinine clearance rates need to be measured.

4. **Intravenous Pyelography** is indicated in young hypertensives and when albuminuria, raised blood urea, low serum potassium, enlarged kidneys or abdominal bruit raise the possibility of primary renal disease. The following lesions may be obvious:
   Renal stones.
   Congenital polycystic kidneys.
   Grossly impaired function in one kidney.
   Careful exmination of frequent films may also reveal irregularities of the collecting systems as a result of scarring from chronic infection.
   Increased early concentration in one kidney compared with the other may be a result of diminished glomerular filtration in the presence of arterial stenosis.

5. When renal disease is suspected a **Radioactive Renogram** (page 227) gives further evidence of altered function.

6. **Renal Arteriography** confirms renal artery stenosis.

7. **Cystoscopy, Retrograde Pyelograms** and **Differential Urine Analysis** from both ureters may be called for.

8. **24-hour Catecholamine Estimation.** 24-hour urine collection allows phaeochromocytoma to be diagnosed. Antihypertensive drugs given in the previous three weeks vitiate the test.

9. **Electrocardiography** may show evidence of left ventricular hypertrophy in hypertensive heart disease.

Complications

Hypertensive Heart Disease:

Symptoms. Effort dyspnoea; paroxysmal nocturnal dyspnoea. Swollen ankles.

Signs. High blood pressure; gallop rhythm; basal râles; ECG changes; sometimes atrial fibrillation.

Prognosis. In the absence of advanced coronary disease effective pressure lowering treatment relieves heart failure for many years.

Cerebral Haemorrhage (*see also* page 526) Related to height of systolic pressure and to age, the haemorrhage may be intracerebral or subarachnoid.

Malignant Hypertension:

Definition. Severe hypertension manifested clinically by the presence of papilloedema (Grade IV retinopathy) and usually albuminuria, and pathologically by fibrinoid necrosis of renal arterioles. May complicate hypertension of any cause except aortic coarctation. (Kidney vessels are at low pressure.)

Background. Severe hypertension (usually with a diastolic pressure of 140 mmHg (18.6 kPa) or more) is accompanied by arteriolar necrosis in the kidney. There is, thus, an acute and worsening renal lesion and a vicious circle exists.

Signs. Papilloedema and retinal haemorrhage and exudates; albuminuria.

Complications. Headache; heart failure; renal failure; cerebral haemorrhage; visual deterioration.

Prognosis. Without treatment, the majority of patients are dead within one year of diagnosis and virtually 100 per cent within two years.

Coronary Thrombosis. Hypertension is an important risk factor in coronary disease as it increases the rate of development of atheroma, especially in men. Long term pressure lowering therapy does not offer much protection.

Cerebral Thrombosis. Similar situation to coronary thrombosis. Long term pressure lowering therapy, however, does diminish the risk of recurrent stroke in hypertension. This suggests that the majority of strokes in hypertension are due to bleeding and, perhaps, minor aneurysm formation.

Retinal Haemorrhage. This is an important complication as the visual disturbance it may produce leads to the discovery of hypertension. Also, as the hallmark of Grade III retinopathy it carries serious prognostic import.

Renal Failure. This is common with malignant hypertension and with primary renal disease complicated by hypertension.

Hypertensive Encephalopathy. This is a rare complication of severe hypertension characterised by status epilepticus or transient hemiplegia or monoplegia. Pressure lowering therapy relieves the neurological features. The pathological basis is not known (?Vascular spasm; ?Cerebral oedema.)

Basis of Treatment

If hypertension complicates renal or endocrine disease these primary conditions should be treated first. Phaeochromocytomas should be removed.

Renal artery stenosis and unilateral pyelonephritis may be cured surgically, but a kidney that is functioning reasonably well should not be removed without due consideration. In particular, renal artery stenosis is frequently a complication of long-standing hypertension and atheroma, and its relief will not affect blood pressure levels permanently. In many cases, therefore, treatment should be directed at lowering blood pressure with drugs. If this is successful, renal artery stenosis may best be left alone. In the presence of renal failure it is correct to lower the blood pressure intensively and observe the effect on renal function. If the blood urea then rises, it is probable that nothing but renal dialysis will save the patient's life. Renal dialysis by removing salt and water from the body may effectively lower the blood pressure without the use of other drugs.

The necessity to press continuous treatment is obvious in the case of malignant hypertension when the untreated prognosis is so serious. With effective treatment the prognosis becomes the same as for essential hypertension provided severe renal damage does not already exist. On the other hand, most patients with hypertension are entirely symptomless and may remain so for many years. It thus requires careful reasoning to persuade a busy and energetic man, who falls foul of his doctors when asked to undergo an insurance examination, that continuous medical management for years or for ever is wise. If the treatment also renders him impotent his cup is full with chagrin.

Clearly, the following situations carry such a serious prognosis as to demand long term treatment.
1. Malignant hypertension.
2. Hypertensive left ventricular failure.
3. Hypertension with stroke.
4. Hypertension with incipient renal failure (raised blood urea).
5. Hypertensive encephalopathy.
6. Hypertension with retinal haemorrhage (Grade III retinopathy), because the untreated prognosis approaches that of malignant hypertension.

With less severe grades of hypertension, it is necessary to decide whether to press medication on an unwilling patient, or how severe a degree of discomfort from therapy to accept. Certain clinical features worsen the prognosis and the presence of more than one leave little doubt that life expectancy will be quite seriously curtailed:

High levels of diastolic pressure (>110mmHg).
Grade II or greater retinopathy.
Male sex.
ECG evidence of left ventricular hypertrophy.
Family history of early death from vascular disease.
Hypertension before middle age.

Community studies now leave little doubt that even modest rises in blood pressure increase the risk of early vascular death, especially in men, and there is, therefore, clearly a case to be made for treating uncomplicated hypertension in early adult life. The treatment may be life-long and the burden on the patient and on the medical services may be intolerable.

Diuretic and Dietary Salt Restriction. All drugs that increase renal excretion of sodium and water have a slight hypotensive effect. They markedly potentiate all hypotensive drugs. Dietary salt restriction acts similarly. With current oral diuretics potassium supplements may be required, although a healthy person with a good appetite for potassium-containing foods may omit these additional tablets. In the presence of heart failure, digoxin will also be required, and then potassium supplements are essential.

Weight Loss. This will please the patient by improving the figure and reducing effort breathlessness. The doctor will find a fall in blood pressure with reduction in the thickness of the arm.

Intensity of Treatment (Table 17.3). Clearly, treatment should be aimed at reducing blood pressure to normal levels for as many hours of the day as possible. There is much to recommend beta blockade as first choice in those patients who never wheeze. Propranolol and oxprenolol have been used so extensively that they seem remarkably free from serious side effects. They may produce unpleasant or occasionally dangerous coldness of the hands and feet. One tablet (40 to 160 mg) once or twice daily suffices. Alone these drugs will rarely lower blood pressure by more than 40/15 mmHg (5.3/1.9 kPa).

Bendrofluazide 5 mg daily and other thiazide diuretics (not frusemide which is less effective and both inconvenient and expensive) lower pressure almost as much and some prefer to use them as first choice. Hypokalaemia is the most frequent unwanted effect, but gout may be precipitated. Beta blockade and thiazide diuresis are usually additive in effect and the two used together will suffice for most patients who are not in the severest category. Two or three tablets a day

Table 17.3 Hypotensive drugs

Name	Type of action	Effect on lying pressure	Postural hypotension	Disadvantages	Dose range	Daily cost
Propranolol, Oxprenolol, etc.	beta adrenergic blockade ?mechanism	Full	No	Cold extremities Contraindicated in asthma	80–320 mg	21 p 27 p
Thiazide diuretics	?On vessel wall as a result of sodium diuresis	Full	No	Hypokalaemia May induce gout and occasionally diabetes	5 mg	1 p
Methyldopa	Peripheral adrenergic blockade	Worthwhile	Yes	Lassitude Occasionally, impotence Rarely, haemolytic anaemia	0.5–1 g	16 p
Bethanidine, Guanethidine, Debrisoquine sulphate	Peripheral adrenergic blockade	Little	Yes++	Postural and exercise hypotension Sometimes impotence	30–120 mg	11 p 16 p 12 p
Reserpine	Central on vasomotor centre	Full	No	May evoke depression	0.1 mg thrice daily	1 p

are needed and the cost in money terms and unwanted effects is small.

Methyldopa has headed world sales for a few years. This is a tribute to its efficacy and safety. Lassitude is the most frequent side effect. There is less to be gained by increasing the dose above 500 mg twice daily than by adding a diuretic or other agent.

Methyldopa and adrenergic blocking agents like debrisoquine sulphate may induce symptomatic postural hypotension, especially in the elderly. Such a patient may not be hypotensive in the clinic or surgery, but on rising from bed or a chair in the morning, blood pressure can fall and the patient also, with the risk of injury.

Duration of Treatment. Probably indefinite unless myocardial infarction causes a permanent fall in pressure.

RHEUMATIC HEART DISEASE

Definition

The acute phase of the disease begins ten days after infection of the throat with haemolytic streptococci. Rheumatic fever presents as an acute polyarthritis which may be complicated by endocarditis, pericarditis and myocarditis. Sydenham's chorea is characterised by involuntary movements of the limbs, facial muscles and trunk. Both acute diseases resolve spontaneously within weeks unless heart failure causes early death. The chronic phase is due to scarring of valves and myocardium, which may advance insidiously over several decades.

Background

Haemolytic streptococcal infection of the throat is an essential pre-requisite to rheumatic fever and chorea, but these diseases that are the clinical manifestations of acute rheumatism follow the streptococcal infection only in about five per cent of cases; after an interval of at least ten days in the case of rheumatic fever, and four to ten weeks for chorea. In about 80 per cent of cases antibodies against streptolysin O (raised ASO titre) can be demonstrated in the blood. Anti-heart antibodies can also be demonstrated in the blood. These diseases are related to streptococcal infection in a similar way to acute glomerulonephritis, erythema nodosum and Henoch Schönlein purpura, when the two latter have a streptococcal origin. It is assumed that there is an immunological basis.

Successful treatment of the throat infection within the first few days eliminates the risk of the late complications.

In approximately one-third of patients with chronic rheumatic heart disease no acute illness has been recognised. Acute rheumatism may therefore be subclinical. In the majority of cases progressive scarring with deteriorating function continues without fresh manifestations of acute rheumatism.

Acute rheumatism has always been more common in the lower social class in Great Britain and with the increasing affluence of the last century the disease has been declining. Its virtual disappearance may have been abetted by the advent of penicillin, but it was dying before. Because of this relation to standards of living and nutrition, acute rheumatism has a changing geographical distribution. It is now much more prevalent and severe in Arab countries and in the Indian subcontinent than in Europe. Girls are affected nearly twice as often as boys.

Pathology of the Heart

In the acute phase, fibrinous pericarditis may occur. It heals with adhesions. Constrictive pericarditis never occurs.

Myocarditis can lead to early heart failure. The characteristic histological feature is the Aschoff nodule.

Endocarditis causes nodules to appear on the contact margins of the mitral and aortic cusps. They do not exceed 2 mm in size and do not cause emboli. The cusps are inflamed and oedematous.

Healing is by fibrous scars. At the mitral valve chordae tendinae are involved. Fusion occurs at the commissures, and the end result is the production of mitral stenosis with rigid cusps and a small orifice. Rigidity of the cusps and dilatation of the mitral ring may lead to predominant reflux. At the aortic valve similar changes produce aortic stenosis or reflux or a combination of the two.

With the passage of years either valve may calcify.

Involvement of the myocardium is more difficult to prove by histology.

Thrombus formation in the left atrium and appendage are common in mitral stenosis, especially after atrial fibrillation has begun.

The tricuspid valve is never affected in the absence of mitral involvement.

The pulmonary valve is virtually free from risk.

All the valve lesions may become the site of bacterial endocarditis.

RHEUMATIC FEVER

Symptoms

Ten days after a sore throat, pain and stiffness begin in one or more joints, which may be red and swollen. Malaise and fever.

Within about five days the joint symptoms improve but then a second crop of joints may be similarly affected.

The same cycle is repeated up to about three times. Fever then subsides.

Central chest pain accompanied by return of fever indicates pericarditis.

Symptoms of heart failure may accompany very severe cardiac damage.

Signs

Fever to 40°C for a week or two.
Signs of polyarthritis.
Sometimes erythematous rashes; erythema marginatum is characteristic.
Subcutaneous nodules occur in severe attacks. They are found on the backs of elbows and wrists, fronts of knees, ankles, occiput. They are hard and painless, 0.5 to 1 cm in diameter and persist for two weeks or more.

Heart:
Apex beat may be displaced.
Apical systolic murmur. Apical mid-diastolic murmur (Carey Coombs murmur).
Aortic diastolic murmur.
All can disappear. Persistence indicates valve damage.

Investigations

1. ESR – raised (100 mm/hr).
2. ASO titre – raised (>250 units).
3. ECG may show prolonged P–R interval.

Differential Diagnosis

1. Rheumatoid disease (persistent joint changes).
2. Henoch Schönlein purpura (purpuric rash diagnostic).
3. Disseminated lupus erythematosus (protracted course).

Basis of Treatment

Oral penicillin 500 mg three times daily for ten days.
Rest in bed to minimise heart work until fever and raised ESR abate.
Salicylates 600 mg four or six-hourly for fever and joint pains.
In very severe attacks corticosteroids are sometimes used.

Prognosis

Full recovery always, except for heart.

SYDENHAM'S CHOREA

Symptoms and Signs

One month after a sore throat involuntary, clumsy, unrhythmic, purposeless movements of a limb or limbs occur. Grimacing movements of the face may occur. Limb is clumsy. Handwriting spidery.
Movements cease during sleep. Hypotonia. Pendulum knee jerk.
Child appears highly nervous.
Subcutaneous nodules rare.
Heart affected as in rheumatic fever but often less severe.

Differential Diagnosis

From nervous tics.

Basis of Treatment

Exclude continuing streptococcal infection. Sedate with phenobarbitone or chloral hydrate.

Prognosis

Full recovery of central nervous system always; usually within two to four months. May recur during pregnancy or with the contraceptive pill for reasons not understood.

CHRONIC RHEUMATIC HEART DISEASE

Background

Mitral stenosis is always due to rheumatism and is its commonest manifestation. The lesion becomes established within weeks of an acute attack and symptoms may soon become apparent. Much more commonly, years or decades pass before the narrowing produces a sufficient rise in left atrial pressure to cause breathlessness.

Symptoms and Signs

Increasing effort breathlessness may be followed by orthopnoea and paroxysmal nocturnal dyspnoea.

Winter bronchitis is common, also cough and haemoptysis. At this stage resting pulmonary capillary pressure may be as high as 25 mmHg (3.3 kPa) and rise with little effort to 40 to 60 mm (5.3 to 8.0 kPa). Thus, pulmonary oedema readily occurs. This symptom complex is sometimes precipitated by the high output state of pregnancy and by the onset of atrial fibrillation with a rapid ventricular rate.

On the other hand, the build-up of symptoms may be very slow indeed so that a common pattern of events is:

20 to 30 years – pregnancies with little trouble.
40 to 50 years – increasing effort, breathlessness leading to frank heart failure. Onset of atrial fibrillation may bring obvious deterioration or pass unnoticed.

Perhaps as a result of the very long period over which pulmonary capillary pressure is rising, breathlessness can be very inconspicuous, or even absent, even with life-threatening pulmonary venous congestion. Changes in pulmonary arterioles can lead to very severe pulmonary hypertension with the pulmonary artery systolic pressure exceeding 100 mmHg (13.3 kPa). Right heart failure may follow, as with other causes of pulmonary congestion.

Other principal symptoms are systemic and pulmonary embolism.

In a few cases a full life span is achieved without symptoms.

Complications

1. Systemic embolism can occur with sinus rhythm but left atrial stagnation is clearly worsened when fibrillation supervenes. Emboli are often large, and obstruction of the aortic bifurcation or a common iliac artery threaten one or both legs with gangrene. Then pain, loss of sensation and coldness of the limb are at once obvious.
2. Cerebral embolism may be the worst disaster of the disease. A dense hemiplegia can recover in hours, as the neighbouring vessels are healthy and soon provide anastomotic circulation. In other cases no recovery occurs.
3. Renal embolism may lead to the production of hypertension.
4. Coeliac axis embolism may cause fatal gangrene of the gut.

Several emboli may occur in rapid succession or years may elapse between incidents.
5. Pulmonary embolism and infarction are common. The source is usually the leg veins where thrombosis is favoured by reduced peripheral blood flow and relative immobility.

Signs

Inspection:
High coloured cheeks (mitral facies).
Normal or raised right atrial pressure.

Palpation:
Pulse rather small volume. May be irregular due to atrial fibrillation. Apex beat may be displaced to the left. A loud first sound is palpable. At the left sternal edge a forceful right ventricle and pulmonary valve closure may be felt.

Auscultation:
Mitral area. Loud first sound, second sound, opening snap, diastolic rumble, loudest in very late diastole in those with sinus rhythm and contracting left atrium. The murmur is usually much louder with the patient turned on to the left side. Its duration is from the opening snap to the next first heart sound. The opening snap is usually loudest at the tricuspid or pulmonary area. Absence of a loud first sound or opening snap imply rigidity of the cusps.

Investigations

1. Chest X-ray to show size of heart, left atrium and severity of pulmonary congestion.
2. Cardiac catheterisation may be helpful if the severity of the stenosis is in doubt. Resting and exercising pulmonary wedge pressures establish severity.
3. Ultrasound scanning of the anterior cusp shows range and speed of movement, both limited in mitral stenosis.

Differential Diagnosis

Differential diagnosis from other causes of pulmonary congestion and systemic embolism. The auscultatory features are virtually always conclusive. However, echocardiography may be necessary to exclude left atrial myxoma. This is a soft mobile tumour growing from its base on the atrial septum. It may plug the mitral orifice in diastole and impede the cusps to cause mitral regurgitation. Major systemic embolism also occurs. The less common right atrial myxoma may similarly block the tricuspid orifice.

Basis of Treatment

Preventive. Once damage to cusps has begun, scarring and contraction will continue. As the acute stage may be subclinical and the infecting organism is ubiquitous, long term prophylaxis may be necessary.
(a) Treatment of sore throats. If acute rheumatism is to be prevented the steps should be: (i) Swab the throat. In 24 hours it should be known whether or not streptococci are responsible. (ii) If so, penicillin treatment should be given for ten days. Dose: oral penicillin 500 mg three times daily for ten days.
(b) In susceptible cases a continuous penicillin level can be achieved, thus covering the danger of subclinical episodes. Dose: oral penicillin 250 mg twice or thrice daily or a once monthly injection of benzyl penicillin (Penidural) 5 ml. This regime should be regarded as obligatory for all patients with rheumatic heart disease in the first half of life. There is no clear indication when prophylaxis can safely be withdrawn. The risk of further attacks diminishes with each decade.

Mitral Valvotomy. Severe mitral stenosis which threatens life by way of pulmonary oedema and congestive heart failure calls for surgical dilatation of the valve. In a proportion of patients severe breathlessness will cause such discomfort that surgical relief is requested. More often, valvotomy should be advised to prevent the more advanced manifestations of the disease. The indication for valvotomy is therefore the presence of severe mitral stenosis, not the severity of symptoms. Indeed, those with less severe obstruction may complain more if they seek attention. Naturally the age of the patient is important. In young women who may wish to bear children, valvotomy is indicated in the absence of symptoms if left atrial pressure is dangerously high. Over the age of 55 years valvotomy would not normally be advised in the absence of symptoms, for deterioration is likely to be slow. The onset of atrial fibrillation is a landmark that always calls for prognostic review. Symptoms are usually worse as a consequence of the faster ventricular rate and restricted diastolic filling time. It may be correct to dilate the valve and then attempt to restore sinus rhythm with direct counter shock. Long term maintenance of sinus rhythm is unlikely.

Dilation of the mitral orifice is now performed with a metal dilator introduced into the valve through the left ventricular cavity. Rupture of adherent commissures usually results, and the obstruction is relieved sufficiently to lower left atrial pressure without mitral reflux. Rigid calcified cusps split less well. There is always a risk (perhaps 5 per cent) that either cusp will tear and gross reflux be produced. In this case mitral valve function may be unimproved or made worse. An effective period of anticoagulant treatment is essential in all patients with atrial fibrillation before valvotomy, to minimise the risk of producing systemic embolism when the left atrium is disturbed.

Long term or permanent relief can be expected if the cusps are not excessively rigid and the commissures split well. There is some likelihood that the commissures may adhere again and cause re-stenosis but it is probable that most cases of so-called re-stenosis have been due to inability to relieve the stenosis adequately. Second operations are sometimes called for. Valve replacement may eventually be necessary.

Medical Treatment. Surgical success is not invariable, or may be inappropriate. Medical treatment is then, as for all cases of pulmonary venous congestion, with digoxin and diuretics. Digoxin is not helpful except in the presence of atrial fibrillation, as the left ventricle is not involved.

Long term anticoagulant treatment is to be considered for all patients who have had systemic embolism or who have atrial fibrillation. Cerebral embolism is the disaster to be feared. Well-controlled treatment does diminish the risk of emboli, but exceptions occur. Treatment is needed for life with the ever-present risk of spontaneous haemorrhage and the necessity for expert medical management with laboratory control. It is often the case, therefore, that life-long treatment is impracticable.

Prognosis

Prognosis has largely been covered in considering the basis of treatment. When mitral stenosis is discovered in the absence of symptoms it is impossible to forecast with confidence whether deterioration will occur. Severe stenosis with high left atrial pressure in younger patients will nearly always cause complications. Mild stenosis may never progress. At the stage of heart failure with obstruction that cannot be relieved, good medical treatment and restriction of activity may prolong life for as long as five or even ten years.

With the increasing safety of valve replacement, more cases are suitable for surgery.

MITRAL REGURGITATION

Symptoms

As in mitral stenosis, for these are due to pulmonary venous congestion: the rate of progress of symptoms is also similar.

Signs

Inspection:
Active precordium. Normal or raised venous pressure.

Palpation:
Displaced, hyperdynamic, left ventricular cardiac impulse.
May be systolic apical thrill.
Increased pulsation over the right ventricle and pulmonary area.

Auscultation
Diminished first sound.
Loud, long, high-pitched (blowing) systolic murmur at the apex and surrounding areas; accentuated by turning patient to the left.
Loud, clear third heart sound.
Short low-pitched diastolic murmur with and after the third sound. The presence of a short diastolic murmur at the apex in a patient with mitral reflux does not indicate concomitant stenosis, but is caused by much increased ventricular filling.
Loud and perhaps palpable pulmonary closure sound.

Investigations

1. Chest X-ray – large left ventricle and left atrium.
2. ECG? Atrial fibrillation. Clear evidence of left ventricular hypertrophy unusual.
3. Ultrasound shows rapid movement (rapid left ventricular filling).
4. Cardiac catheterisation essential if surgical treatment needs to be considered.
5. Left ventricular angiography demonstrates the volume of reflux, size of the chambers, degree of movement of the mitral cusps and contractility of the left ventricle. Severity of pulmonary changes measured simultaneously.

Complications

As for mitral stenosis, except that systemic embolism is less common.

On the other hand, subacute bacterial endocarditis is an important risk whereas it is almost unknown in advanced mitral stenosis.

Differential Diagnosis

Free reflux and pure stenosis are easy to distinguish. Mixed lesions are common, and the assessment is then one of deciding the dominant feature and the likelihood of successful valvotomy. Catheterisation is often essential.

If a systolic murmur is the only sign, aortic stenosis may wrongly be considered.

Non-rheumatic mitral regurgitation is common. Usual causes are prolapse of congenital abnormal cusp, papillary muscle dysfunction (coronary disease), ruptured chordae tendinae, cardiomyopathy. When there is no past history of rheumatism, sinus rhythm is the rule, and the left atrium may be of near normal size. The alternative aetiology may be obvious.

Basis of Treatment

The only effective surgical treatment is likely to be replacement of the valve. As this carries an appreciable operative mortality (5 to 10 per cent), and as present prostheses are not entirely satisfactory, surgical treatment is only considered as symptoms become severe and life clearly threatened. Mitral prostheses call for life-long anticoagulant treatment to diminish the considerable risk of thrombus formation and systemic embolism. Homograft and heterograph valves have an appreciable rate of breakdown.

Prognosis

There is often a long symptomatic course similar to mitral stenosis. Accurate prognosis is difficult, thus decision for valve replacement is also difficult. Sudden death is not uncommon from left ventricular arrhythmia.

AORTIC STENOSIS AND REGURGITATION

Severe rheumatic damage to the aortic valve with sparing of the mitral valve is relatively uncommon. Unlike mitral stenosis it is not commoner in girls.

Symptoms

A long period of freedom from symptoms.
Left ventricular failure leads to pulmonary venous congestion and its attendant symptoms. Deterioration is then usually rapid, especially with aortic stenosis.
Angina pectoris occurs with both but is commoner with stenosis than with reflux.
In aortic stenosis, effort syncope may occur.

Table 17.4 Signs of aortic stenosis and regurgitation

	Aortic stenosis	Aortic regurgitation
Pulse	Slow rising Notched upstroke	Rapid rise Large pulse pressure Hyperdynamic carotids

Palpation
  apex
  base
	Forceful
	Systolic thrill
		Hyperdynamic, displaced

Auscultation	Harsh aortic systolic
	  murmur
	Diminished aortic
	  closure sound
	May be slight reflux
		Very high-pitched
		  early diastolic murmur
		  in aortic and
		  tricuspid areas
		May be systolic
		  murmur also

Signs (see Table 17.4)

Complications

Subacute bacterial endocarditis.
Left ventricular failure.
Sudden death.
In patients with heavy calcification of the valve atrioventricular block may occur.

Prognosis

The onset of frank left ventricular failure carries a bad prognosis both with obstruction and reflux. Death is usual within two years.

In stenosis, both effort syncope and angina pectoris indicate that left ventricular hypertrophy is severe. There is a risk of unheralded ventricular arrhythmia and sudden death.

In severe reflux the left ventricle enlarges progressively and may become hugely dilated. It is very difficult to decide when left ventricular 'failure' can be said to have occurred.

Basis of Treatment

The only treatment that materially effects the long term outlook is surgical replacement of the valve.

Frank left ventricular failure is the clearest indication that life expectancy is seriously threatened.

NON-RHEUMATIC AORTIC VALVE DISEASE, INCLUDING SYPHILIS

CONGENITAL AORTIC STENOSIS AND CALCIFIC AORTIC STENOSIS IN THE SECOND HALF OF LIFE

Background and Pathology

Congenital fusion of the aortic valve commissures produces obstruction to the left ventricular outflow. The obstruction may be severe. The condition is dealt with on page 302, 'Congenital heart disease'. If the obstruction is less severe it is likely to escape attention in youth, but there is a strong tendency for calcium to accumulate on the cusps, probably as a result of platelet and fibrin aggregation. Heavy calcification may then produce severe obstruction in later life. Symptomatic deterioration is commonest in men after 45 years of age. Normal aortic valve cusps may possibly also calcify in later life.

Symptoms, Signs, Complications, Treatment and **Prognosis** are as set out under 'Rheumatic aortic stenosis' (page 298).

AORTIC REGURGITATION

This may complicate ankylosing spondylitis and Reiter's syndrome as a result of aortitis in the first few centimetres of the aortic root. The features are as set out on page 298.

SYPHILITIC AORTITIS OF THE AORTIC ROOT

Background

A complication of late syphilis usually becoming symptomatic 10 to 25 years after the primary infection (*see* page 153).

Pathology

Aneurysm of the aortic root. The intima is puckered and covered by bluish grey 'plaques' or elevations. There is considerable thickening which may result in a heaping up of intimal tissue around the coronary ostia causing severe narrowing of the inlet, the 'pinhole meatus'. The aortic cusps are shortened with rolling of cusp margins. Necrosis of muscle and elastic tissue in the aortic wall as a result of endarteritis of the vasa vasorum leads to weakening of the wall with dilatation of the valve ring and ascending aorta (aneurysm).

Symptoms

Breathlessness from left ventricular failure.
Angina pectoris from aortic reflux and obstruction of the coronary ostia.

Signs

Collapsing pulse.
Hyperdynamic displaced apex beat.
Aortic diastolic murmur.

Aortic systolic murmur and occasionally thrill due to the aneurysm.
The aortic closure sound may be loud.
May be undue pulsation in the aortic area.
May be obstruction of the superior vena cava.

Investigations

1. X-ray shows prominent ascending aorta and enlarged heart.
2. ECG – left ventricular hypertrophy.
3. Blood WR etc., positive in most cases.

Complications

Left ventricular failure.
Possible risk of subacute bacterial endocarditis.

Differential Diagnosis

From aortic reflux of other causation.

Basis of Treatment

Prevention by standard penicillin treatment of early syphilis.

In the established disease, penicillin treatment should also be given but its effect in improving prognosis is disputed. It is perhaps wise to give two or three weeks' treatment with oral iodides before beginning treatment.

Aortic valve replacement if left ventricular failure threatens life.

ANEURYSM OF THE AORTIC ARCH AND DESCENDING AORTA

Pathology

Weakening of the aortic wall as already described. Aneurysm of the arch is likely to compress the following structures:
Trachea and left bronchus.
Recurrent laryngeal nerve.
Oesophagus.
Thoracic sympathetic outflow.
Aneurysm of the descending aorta may also compress the oesophagus and the bodies of the thoracic vertebrae.

Symptoms

Breathlessness and unproductive cough (tracheal compression).
Hoarseness of the voice.
Dysphagia.
Back pain.

Signs

Stridor.
Increased cardiac dullness to percussion.
Horner's syndrome.
Diminished pulse in one arm.

Investigations

1. Chest X-ray will show the aneurysm.
2. Aortogram visualises the extent.
3. Positive blood WR.
4. Barium swallow confirms oesophageal obstruction.
5. Laryngoscopy shows paralysed left vocal cord.

Complications

Rupture of the aneurysm into the mediastinum or oesophagus or trachea.

Differential Diagnosis

From other mediastinal tumours. Aortography is the definitive investigation.

Basis of Treatment

Treatment with penicillin, as above.
Surgical resection of the aneurysm and its replacement with a prosthetic graft. This is clearly a less formidable procedure if the aneurysm begins beyond the left subclavian artery.

Prognosis

Rupture is the threat to life. In some patients the lesion advances very slowly and death is often due to other causes.

CONGENITAL HEART DISEASE

Congenital malformations of the heart may be single or multiple. Those with single defects are much more likely to survive infancy and are therefore much more commonly encountered outside baby units. Arterial oxygen saturation is not impaired in any of these defects unless severe pulmonary hypertension develops. Only the more common defects are described.

Lesions allowing a left to right (arteriovenous) shunt form a big group.

PATENT DUCTUS ARTERIOSUS

Mechanism

Failure of the ductus to thrombose and become obliterated in the first few hours or days after birth allows blood to flow from the high pressure aorta to the low

pressure pulmonary artery. Left ventricular work is therefore wasted as a proportion of its output flows uselessly back into the lungs. Left ventricular stroke volume is increased and aortic diastolic pressure falls unduly low, thus giving a high pulse pressure with an abrupt upstroke of brief duration (water-hammer pulse).

Symptoms

Usually none.

Signs

Left ventricular hypertrophy. Over the pulmonary area a long harsh murmur is audible which is loudest at the end of systole, at the time of the second sound, and persists throughout diastole. It waxes and wanes continuously (machinery murmur).
X-rays show a prominent aortic arch and pulmonary arteries.

Complications

Left ventricular failure.
Severe pulmonary hypertension.
Subacute bacterial endocarditis.

Basis of Treatment

Surgical closure in all cases, in childhood, unless pulmonary vascular resistance is excessive.

VENTRICULAR SEPTAL DEFECT

Mechanism

Failure of the upper portion of the ventricular septum to close completely.

Abnormal Physiology

Left to right shunt. In large defects the shunt flow is greater than forward flow through the aortic valve. This tends to raise right ventricular and pulmonary artery pressures. High pulmonary vascular resistance may develop with limitation or reversal of the shunt.

Symptoms

Usually none during childhood.

Signs

Enlarged left ventricle.
Systolic thrill and long systolic murmur maximal at the left sternal border at the third interspace. The pulmonary component of the second sound may be delayed

and increased. There may be an apical diastolic murmur due to increased flow through the mitral valve.
X-ray shows an enlarged heart and increased pulmonary arterial shadowing.

Complications

Left ventricular failure.
Severe pulmonary hypertension.
Subacute bacterial endocarditis.

Basis of Treatment

Surgical closure with cardiopulmonary by-pass if the left to right shunt is large enough to threaten life.

Severe pulmonary hypertension is a contra-indication. Spontaneous closure of defects is common in early childhood.

ATRIAL SEPTAL DEFECT

Mechanism

Failure of the atrial septum to close completely. The defect is usually large (2 cm or more).

Abnormal Physiology

Right ventricular muscle wall is thinner than the left and its filling pressure is lower. For this reason, blood flows from left to right through the defect. Right heart pressures are usually normal, left atrial pressure is reduced. Shunt flow usually exceeds systemic flow.

Symptoms

Usually none.

Signs

Unusually pulsatile right ventricle. Soft pulmonary systolic murmur. Delayed pulmonary component of the second sound in expiration. This is due to right ventricular overload and the fact that the phases of the respiratory cycle will not cause differential filling of the two ventricles.

The effect of the phases of the respiratory cycle on the second heart sound with *normally closed atrial septum* is shown in Table 17.5.

Investigations

X-ray shows increased heart size. There are unduly prominent pulmonary artery shadows.

Table 17.5 Normal splitting of the second sound

Inspiration	Expiration
Increased right ventricular filling	Diminished right ventricular filling
Right ventricular systole prolonged	Right ventricular systole shortened
P_2 delayed	P_2 not delayed
Diminished left ventricular filling	Increased left ventricular filling
Left ventricular systole slightly shortened	Left ventricular systole not shortened
A_2 slightly premature	A_2 not premature
Split S_2 0.05 sec	Split S_2 0.02 sec

Complications

Onset of atrial fibrillation or flutter in the second half of life is common. Congestive heart failure may then follow. Severe pulmonary hypertension rare.

Basis of Treatment

Surgical closure of the defect with cardiopulmonary by-pass in childhood if the heart is enlarged and the shunt considerable.

ISOLATED PULMONARY STENOSIS

Mechanism

Imperfect development of commissures of the valve leaflets so that the cusps do not flatten themselves against the wall of the pulmonary artery in systole but obstruct outflow. Less commonly, the obstruction is due to a fibrous stricture in the outlet of the right ventricle (infundibular stenosis).

Abnormal Physiology

Raised right ventricular systolic pressure 40 to 200 mmHg (5.3 to 26.6 kPa).

Symptoms

Usually none.
With severe obstruction breathlessness, fatigue, and effort syncope may occur.

Signs

Pulmonary systolic thrill and harsh murmur.
Widely split second sound due to prolonged right

ventricular systole and low pulmonary artery pressure. X-ray shows prominence of the main pulmonary artery (post-stenotic dilatation) and thin peripheral branches.

Complications

Subacute bacterial endocarditis.
Ventricular arrhythmias which endanger life.
Congestive heart failure may occur.

Basis of Treatment

Open pulmonary valvotomy with temporary arrest of the circulation except in mild cases (right ventricular systolic pressure <50 mmHg (6.7 kPa)).

AORTIC STENOSIS

Mechanism

Impaired development of the commissures.

Abnormal Physiology

Raised left ventricular systolic pressure.

Symptoms

None.
Effort breathlessness.
Angina pectoris.
Effort syncope.

Signs

Forceful left ventricle.
Systolic thrill and harsh murmur in the aortic area.
Ejection click at the mitral area.
Small pulse volume with slow rising upstroke (undetectable in children).

Complications

Left ventricular failure.
Subacute bacterial endocarditis.
Sudden death.

Basis of Treatment

Surgical treatment is unsatisfactory because free incision of the commissure allows the cusps to prolapse and, thus, severe reflux may develop. With severe stenosis, valvotomy is performed with partial incision of the commissure under cardiopulmonary by-pass to reduce obstruction. Heavy calcification of the valve is inevitable above the age of 30 years; left ventricular failure then necessitates valve replacement.

COARCTATION OF THE AORTA

Mechanism

Imperfect development of the aorta opposite the ductus arteriosus and below the left subclavian artery. There is usually a diaphragm across the vessel with a small central orifice.

Abnormal Physiology

High pressure in the proximal aorta and its branches. Low pressure below. Extensive collateral channels develop.

Signs

Absent, diminished or delayed femoral pulses.
Forceful left ventricle.
Palpable collateral channels.
Systolic murmur at the pulmonary area and continuous murmurs over collateral channels (internal mammaries, angle of scapula).

Complications

Rupture of aorta or aneurysm of the circle of Willis.
Left ventricular failure especially in infancy.
Subacute bacterial endocarditis.

Prognosis

Survival beyond middle life unusual.

Basis of Treatment

Surgical excision of the obstructed segment during childhood.

MULTIPLE CONGENITAL DEFECTS

All the defects already described may coexist in any possible combination. Combined defects that allow a right to left (venoarterial) shunt give rise to *cyanosis*. These are the complications of *cyanotic congenital heart disease*:
1. Effort breathlessness is inevitable for the blood reaching the respiratory centre contains an excess of CO_2 and deficiency of O_2.
2. Compensatory polycythaemia occurs and increases with time.
3. Thus, central cyanosis may be present at rest and becomes obvious with exercise. Finger clubbing is almost invariable.
4. Growth may be delayed.
5. The filtering of small clot particles by the lung is by-passed, and thus systemic abscess and embolism may occur.

6. Death in infancy is common in the absence of effective surgical treatment.

The commonest type of cyanotic congenital heart disease to be seen in older patients is Fallot's tetralogy.

Pathology

There is a large ventricular septal defect and severe pulmonary stenosis, which may be valvular or infundibular or both. Because a proportion of right ventricular output enters the left ventricle and aorta, the pulmonary artery is small and the aorta large. The aortic valve lies directly above the ventricular septal defect and outflow tract of the right ventricle.

Symptoms

Severe breathlessness, sometimes with squatting.
Cyanosis.
Fainting turns (cyanotic attacks).
Impaired growth.

Signs

Harsh systolic murmur and thrill at the pulmonary area.
Loud single second heart sound (pulmonary element inaudible).

Investigations

1. Chest X-ray shows normal-sized heart with small pulmonary arteries.
2. ECG – right ventricular hypertrophy.
3. Cardiac catheterisation and angiocardiography proves the diagnosis.

Basis of Treatment

Palliative. Anastomosis of the subclavian artery to a pulmonary artery (Blalock's operation) increases pulmonary blood flow and raises arterial oxygen saturation.

Corrective. The presence of marked cyanosis calls for surgical repair of the defect except in small infants. Under cardiopulmonary by-pass the ventricular septal defect is closed and pulmonary stenosis relieved by opening the pulmonary valve by incision, and any stricture in the right ventricle is also excised. A successful operation restores the heart virtually to normal.

The following are other common types of multiple lesions with cyanosis:
1. Transposition of the great arteries.
2. Total anomalous pulmonary venous drainage.
3. Tricuspid atresia (right heart hypoplasia).
4. Left heart hypoplasia.

5. Ebsteins' malformation of the tricuspid valve (plus patent foramen ovale).

Effective surgical operations are available to correct or ameliorate the majority of these defects, but their consideration is outside the scope of a general textbook.

INFECTIVE ENDOCARDITIS

Definition

Bacterial ulceration of heart valve cusps, especially those previously damaged by rheumatic endocarditis, or of congenital abnormalities of the heart such as persisting ductus arteriosus, ventricular septal defect, or aortic coarctation.

Background

The common causative organism is *Streptococcus viridans*. It enters the bloodstream from the root of an infected tooth, particularly after dental extraction. The organism is of low virulence and will not settle on healthy valve cusps. It may, however, become established on cusps previously affected by rheumatic endocarditis. *Staphylococcus aureus* and, occasionally, *Staph. albus* behave similarly. *Strep. faecalis* may gain entrance to the bloodstream as a result of urinary tract disease, especially during instrumentation (cystoscopy). It may attack previously healthy cusps. Other occasional invaders are *Rickettsia burneti* and *Candida albicans*.

Pathology

The affected cusp or congenital abnormality becomes ulcerated and fibrin and platelet debris aggregates upon it. These friable vegetations readily break off to cause systemic embolism in distant organs. Cusps may perforate and rupture. Heart failure results. Peripheral emboli cause infarction. The continuing infection gives rise to a constant bacteraemia and splenomegaly. Lesions of the right side of the heart give rise to pulmonary emboli and infarction. Renal infarcts may occur and there is a specific glomerulonephritis in some cases. Embolisation of distant arteries may give rise to mycotic aneurysm.

Symptoms

Of Infection:
Chills, rigors, fever.
Malaise and lassitude.
Weight loss.
Confusion.

Of Emboli:
Painful nodes in palm of hand and fingers or toes (Osler's nodes).
Pain in muscles.

Transient neurological symptoms (monoplegia, paraesthesiae).
Haematuria (usually microscopic).

Of Heart Failure:
Breathlessness.
Ankle swelling.

Signs

Fever.
Pallor.
Splenomegaly.
Microscopic haematuria.
Osler's nodes.
Finger clubbing.
Purpuric spots below finger nails, over trunk or limbs.
Heart murmur, especially aortic reflux.
Signs of heart failure.
Signs of cerebral infarction.
Loss of an arterial pulse in a limb.

Investigations

1. Blood cultures must always be taken in suspicious cases, before any antibiotic is given. The bacteraemia is constant and every culture can be expected to grow the infecting organism unless it is being suppressed by previous treatment. This does not, of course, apply to infections with rickettsia. In a few cases, for unknown reasons, positive blood cultures are not obtained.
2. Blood count – normocytic anaemia, leucocytosis, high ESR.

Complications (Fig. 17.22)

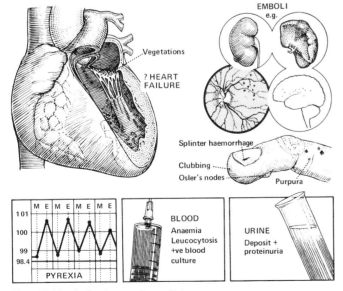

Fig. 17.22   Infective endocarditis.

Heart failure.
Systemic emboli with stroke or ischaemia of a limb.
Mycotic aneurysm, occasionally rupture.
Glomerulonephritis with renal failure.

Differential Diagnosis

From any cause of prolonged fever. The detection of a heart murmur is the vital clue.

Basis of Treatment

Prophylaxis. Patients known to have rheumatic damage to valves or congenital heart lesions should be advised to take particular care of their teeth and seek routine dental care for the whole of their lives. If teeth are to be extracted this must be performed under antibiotic prophylaxis. In patients not recently treated with penicillin, a mixture of 0.5 mega units of crystalline penicillin and 0.5 mega units of procaine penicillin by intramuscular injection one to two hours before extraction, followed by oral penicillin V 500 mg three times daily for two to three days. Patients already taking penicillin or with known penicillin sensitivity should be covered with cephaloridine or erythromycin.

Cure of the Established Disease. This depends on the eradication of the infection before there is severe damage to valve cusps. The following principles are important:
1. Early diagnosis. Suspicion is aroused whenever a patient known to have a heart lesion has a febrile illness.
2. Immediate and frequent blood cultures before any antibiotic is given.
3. The disease is only cured by bactericidal antibiotics.
4. Standard treatment of streptococcal or staphylococcal infection is with penicillin. Crystalline penicillin 1 to 3 mega units six hourly for four to six weeks. If the organism cultured is shown to be less penicillin-sensitive than usual, or the response of the temperature chart to treatment is not entirely satisfactory, larger doses of penicillin are given and streptomycin, 0.5 g twice daily, added. Probenecid may be used to delay renal secretion and increase blood levels of penicillin.
5. Penicillin-resistant organisms may call for treatment with cloxacillin, cephaloridine or gentamicin.

Heart Failure. This is treated in the usual way. Its presence denotes a poor prognosis and high risk of death from heart failure. Valve replacement under cardiopulmonary by-pass may then be indicated. The surgical prognosis is good.

Prognosis

In congenital heart disease, antibiotic cure is the rule. Severe damage to the heart is unlikely.

The greatest risk to life accompanies damage to the

aortic valve, when acute left ventricular failure may rapidly ensue.

Prompt treatment greatly reduces the risks.

VENOUS THROMBOSIS, PULMONARY EMBOLISM AND PULMONARY INFARCTION

Definition

Pulmonary Embolism. Embolism of the main pulmonary artery or its major branches from thrombus breaking free from veins in the leg or pelvis or, rarely, from the fibrillating right atrium.

Pulmonary Infarction. Infarction with partial collapse of a portion of lung as the result of complete or nearly complete occlusion of the branch of the pulmonary artery which supplies it.

Background

Leg vein thrombosis is almost unknown in childhood and adolescence.

An important predisposing factor is local disease of veins as a result of distension or varicosity. Varicose veins result from insufficiency or destruction of the valves in the thigh from previous thrombosis or obstruction due to high intra-abdominal pressure in pregnancy. Distension leads to relative stagnation and to changes in the intima.

The vast majority of cases occur when there is no pre-existing venous disease. Sluggish blood flow is then the principal factor. Bed rest is therefore the first risk factor and any adult lying in bed with any illness for a day or two is at risk. Naturally, the more severe the illness the more immobile the leg. Fractures of the leg and abdominal operations also produce a high degree of immobility.

Low cardiac output also contributes to sluggish blood flow as peripheral flow is severely reduced. Thus, the majority of patients hospitalised with myocardial infarction lay down thrombus in leg veins although there may be no clinical evidence.

Obstruction to the venous return in pregnancy has already been mentioned. Other abdominal masses act similarly.

Changes in coagulability of blood are also important. These changes defy precise measurement, but *in vitro* tests of platelet behaviour on glass surfaces and with certain chemicals and in electrical fields have shown abnormalities. These changes are present after surgical operations and injuries. Cancers may also lead to venous thrombosis by a similar mechanism as do the hormonal changes produced by contraceptive pills.

Any circumstances that lead to the formation of thrombus in leg veins may be followed by pulmonary embolism and infarction.

Pathology

Thrombosis of deep veins usually gives rise to little pain. Swelling of the lower leg may occur.

Thrombosis of superficial veins may be accompanied by signs of inflammation in the skin and subcutaneous tissues. It was customary to refer to the former as phlebothrombosis and the latter as thrombophlebitis. The distinction is out-dated.

Pulmonary embolism may occur without infarction. This is particularly important when embolism is massive. A large thrombus is then likely to embolise the bifurcation of the main pulmonary trunk or a main vessel to one lung. There is then severe obstruction to the circulation, but no single area of lung may be totally unperfused and if the patient survives, infarction may not occur.

Infarcts are usually haemorrhagic and an overlying fibrinous pleurisy is likely. The lower zones are affected with overwhelming frequency.

Symptoms and Signs

In the Legs:
Total absence. (Presence of the clot can now be detected by counting the concentration of injected labelled fibrinogen.)
Distended veins (sentinel veins).
Aching in the calf. Swelling of the lower leg or whole leg. Tenderness of the calf muscles to pressure.
Pain in the calf with forceful dorsiflexion of the foot (Homan's sign).
Redness, tenderness and swelling over the course of veins near the surface.

In the Cardiovascular System:
In a patient at risk (bed rest, thrombophlebitis) the following *symptoms* should arouse suspicion of pulmonary embolism:
Sudden feeling of faintness or loss of consciousness.
Breathlessness.
Central chest pain.

Signs:
Cold sweat, cyanosis.
Fall in blood pressure.
Tachycardia.
Tachypnoea.
Raised venous pressure.
Gallop rhythm.
Cardiac arrest.

In Pulmonary Infarction:
Symptoms:
Pleural pain.
Breathlessness.
Haemoptysis (may be tiny).

Signs:
Dyspnoea. Cyanosis.
Râles at affected base.
Loss of resonance to percussion.
Diminished breath sounds.
Fever.
Signs in the legs.

Investigations

1. ECG in major embolism is almost always abnormal, when there is a rise in venous pressure and hypotension. Axis shift to the right (S wave in I). Clockwise rotation (S > R V$_5$). T wave inversion leads III, II, V$_{2-4}$.
2. X-ray chest. May be normal. In major embolism it may show heavy central pulmonary artery shadows with relative translucency in peripheral lung fields.
In infarction: rise of diaphragm on affected side.
Loss of translucency at affected base and costophrenic angle.
Later: pleural effusion, linear streaks as infarct resolves.

Complications

Pleural effusion which may be blood-stained. Risk of further embolism.
In the legs there may be permanent swelling and late varicose ulceration of skin around internal malleolus.

Differential Diagnosis

Legs. Rupture of Baker's cyst of knee into calf muscles (sudden pain on bending). Cellulitis.
Cardiovascular System. Myocardial infarction. Gram-negative septicaemia.
Lungs. Pneumonia. Postoperative inhalation pulmonary collapse. Pleural effusion of other causation.

Prognosis

Legs. Full recovery with prompt treatment is the rule.
Cardiovascular System. Sudden death is not uncommon. Previous warning symptoms may have been ignored.

If the patient is still alive when the doctor arrives to make the diagnosis, death is unusual. Full clinical recovery is then almost certain. Repeated episodes can lead to permanent pulmonary hypertension and right heart failure, but this is excessively rare.

Similarly, with adequate treatment pulmonary infarction heals without detectable scars as constantly as does lobar pneumonia.

Recurrence is common in periods up to two months, but may also arise at any subsequent time with periods of immobility.

Basis of Treatment

Preventive:
Bed-rest should be discouraged except for sound reasons.
Regular leg exercises are advisable.
Raising the foot of the bed a few inches does much to speed the flow of blood in leg veins.
When bed rest is being relinquished, sitting still in a chair for more than a few minutes is forbidden.

In susceptible patients prophylactic anticoagulant therapy may be indicated.

Anticoagulant Therapy:
Heparin: route, intravenous.
Onset of action: immediate.
Half-life around two hours.
Dose: 30,000 to 60,000 units per 24 hours.
Method: continuous infusion or intermittent six-hourly.
Control: whole blood clotting time to two to three times control.
Danger of excessive dosage: spontaneous haemorrhage into all tissues – gut, retroperitoneal tissues, muscles, brain, skin.
Antidote: intravenous protamine.
Disadvantage: need for intravenous route.
Contraindications: peptic ulcer.

Oral Antithrombin Agents:
Warfarin sodium:
Route: tablets by mouth once or twice daily.
Onset of action: 48 hours.
Half-life: around 24 hours following peak.
Dose: variable, 1 to 20 mg daily.
Method and control: oral dose on day 1, prothrombin index day 3 and subsequent. One stage quick test (Manchester reagent) prolonged to three times control. During induction, prothrombin index three times weekly. Subsequent, weekly or at longer intervals according to stability.
Danger of excess dosage: as with heparin.
Antidote: Vitamin K intravenously. Whole blood transfusion (contains prothrombin).
Disadvantage: slow induction so that by day 3 there may be little or no demonstrable action. The dosage is increased and by day 5 it may still be the case that therapy continues to be inadequate. On a long term basis, control may be erratic and thus dangerous. Other drugs affect metabolism of warfarin in the liver and may thus interfere with control (barbiturates, alcohol, etc.).
Contraindications: impaired liver function as in heart failure may be accompanied by low blood levels of prothrombin or prothrombin synthesis. Dosage must therefore be small until control tests indicate the correct level of treatment. Peptic ulcer.

Routine Management of Venous Thrombosis and Pulmonary Infarction:

1. Immediate use of heparin and loading dose of warfarin sodium, day 1, up to 20 mg; day 2, 10 mg; day 3, 5 mg, then as indicated by prothrombin index. Heparin is discontinued after 48 hours.
2. Bed rest until fully anticoagulated. Foot of bed raised.
3. Pethidine for pleural pain.
4. No antibiotics unless indicated for other reasons.
5. When fully anticoagulated and recovering clinically, fairly rapid resumption of full mobilisation.
6. Anticoagulants to be continued at full dosage for three months if there is major evidence of pathology in the leg veins or any suggestion of recurrence of pulmonary embolism. Presumed pulmonary infarction with few signs in the legs and rapid clinical recovery may be treated for as short a period as two to three weeks if there is rapid recovery of full health (e.g. following herniorrhaphy).

Massive Pulmonary Embolism:

Monitor ECG and blood pressure.
Administer high concentration of oxygen by face mask.
Intravenous heparin 10,000 units.
Morphine if called for in presence of severe pain or panic.
Cardiac massage for cardiac arrest.
Pressor agents for severe, continuing hypotension.

If the clinical state of the patient deteriorates, two new methods of treatment may be available:

1. Thrombolytic therapy with streptokinase. This is relatively safe, but bleeding may occur. There is some evidence that it clears the pulmonary obstruction more rapidly than heparin and spontaneous fibrinolysis, but it is very costly.
2. Surgical embolectomy. Because recovery by medical management is the rule, this should *never* be attempted except in special centres by an experienced cardiac surgeon.

PERICARDITIS

Inflammation of the pericardium may be a manifestation of generalised disease or a primary affection. Pericarditis is, for example, a complication of systemic lupus erythematosus and malignant pericarditis may be found with bronchial or abdominal cancers. Pericardial friction accompanying myocardial infarction or rheumatic carditis merely gives auscultatory evidence of these diseases and is of no other importance. Nor is the fibrinous pericarditis that accompanies terminal renal failure of any great practical importance except as a prognostic sign.

Acute pericarditis due to pyogenic infection is very rare in Britain since lobar pneumonia has been treated with antibiotics. Similarly, acute tuberculous pericarditis has almost disappeared.

The two types of pericardial disease of great practical importance at present are acute idiopathic pericarditis and chronic constrictive pericarditis.

ACUTE IDIOPATHIC PERICARDITIS (BENIGN PERICARDITIS)

Definition

An acute inflammatory disease of the pericardium and underlying myocardium. The causative agent is not usually identified. Pleurisy and pneumonitis are sometimes present.

Background

This is a fairly common disorder of adults. Seasonal grouping of cases in spring and autumn and the tendency for the illness to follow upper respiratory infections suggest a virus aetiology. Sometimes rising antibody titres and/or isolation of viruses from the faeces appear to confirm this. The Coxsackie viruses have been implicated in some epidemics. On the other hand, some patients may have repeated attacks and it is suggested that autoimmune mechanisms are then important. An almost exactly similar disease may follow operations on the heart. There is strong evidence that this complication is related to blood in the pericardium, and it is usually known as the postcardiotomy syndrome.

Pathology

Little is known, for the condition is rarely fatal. Radiology and aspiration of the pericardium show that a sterile effusion may occur. It may be heavily blood-stained and, occasionally, is so great in quantity that the heart is compressed (cardiac tamponade).

Symptoms and Signs

Fever – malaise and chills.

Of Pericarditis:

Gripping central chest pain as in myocardial infarction; often worse with breathing or leaning forwards. Radiation to the jaw and arms is unusual.

Of Pneumonitis:

Pleural pain, dry cough, breathlessness.
Fever at the onset of illness (unlike myocardial infarction).
Pericardial friction – often transient and sometimes absent.
Occasionally raised venous pressure (tamponade or failure).
Basal râles (pneumonitis).
Pleural friction.

Investigations

1. ECG – characteristically raised S–T segments without pathological Q waves. Widespread T wave inversion may follow or be the dominant feature at the outset. Resolution of the changes in days or a couple of weeks is the important distinguishing point from myocardial infarction in cases of doubt.
2. May be leucocytosis and raised ESR.
3. Viral antibody titres may show diagnostic rise.
4. X-ray of chest may show patchy shadowing at the lung bases.

Complications

Recurrence (under 10 per cent).
Cardiac tamponade (very uncommon).
Congestive heart failure. This is very rare except as a result of tamponade. It implies that the myocardium is affected exceptionally severely.

Cardiac Tamponade.

This important complication requires elaboration. It is not only an occasional complication of idiopathic pericarditis, but may be due to malignant pericarditis or tubercle. Occasionally, it follows heart operations

Pathological physiology. High pressure in the pericardial sac hinders filling of both ventricles so that stroke output is very low. A fast heart rate at first compensates, but hypotension and gross diminution of peripheral perfusion follows.

Signs:
Very high venous pressure with liver enlargement.
A fast heart rate with gallop rhythm usually best heard at the tricuspid area.
Pulsus paradoxus – the pulse virtually disappears during a deep inspiration. This may be best felt at the femoral artery.
Low blood pressure.
Dyspnoea.

Emergency treatment of tamponade. Life is seriously threatened and relief of high intrapericardial pressure by aspiration an urgent necessity. An aspirating needle is introduced into the angle between the left costal margin and the xiphisternum and directed upwards, backwards, and slightly to the left until fluid is encountered. Heavily blood-stained fluid in the syringe may be indistinguishable from blood. In cases of doubt, blood from an arm vein should be taken in a second syringe and both placed by the bedside. Blood will clot but blood-stained effusion will not. If pure blood has been withdrawn the heart chambers have been entered. An oscilloscope should be monitoring the electrocardiogram. If the exploring needle touches the myocardium, ectopic beats are likely to be produced. Withdrawal of 200 ml of effusion gives dramatic relief. It may be wise to use a pericardial drain if tamponade recurs.

Differential Diagnosis

1. From myocardial infarction. A crucial distinction for coronary disease may easily be incorrectly suspected and needless serious anxiety produced (*see* Table 17.6).
2. Pericarditis with effusion. Malignancy and tubercle need to be considered. Tubercle bacilli may be isolated from the pericardial fluid.

Basis of Treatment

Idiopathic pericarditis is a self-limiting disease and usually remits spontaneously in seven to fourteen days. Only bed rest is called for or analgesics for chest pain. If tamponade occurs, aspiration will be needed.

Table 17.6 Differential diagnosis

		Myocardial infarction	Idiopathic pericarditis
Symptoms	Central chest pain	Rarely affected by breathing or posture Often arms and jaw	Quite commonly worse with breathing and posture. Rarely arms and jaw
	Pleural pain	Never at onset	May be present at onset
	Cough	Not a feature	May be a feature
Signs	Fever	Low temperature at onset Fever days 2–6	Fever usual at onset Declines over few days
	Pericardial friction	Transient 10%	Transient 50%, may be extensive and persist for days
	Pleural friction	Only with additional pulmonary infarction	Reasonably common
ECG		May be raised S–T segments in anterior or inferior leads May be pathological Q waves Extensive changes rarely remit within one month	May be widespread S–T segment elevation No pathological Q waves Extensive changes usually remit within one month

Occasionally, the symptoms persist for many days with a severe illness. Corticosteroids will then bring relief very rapidly, but care needs to be taken with withdrawal for relapse may follow. In the rare cases with numerous relapses, corticosteroids may need to be continued for weeks or months (prednisone 30 mg a day reducing to half this dose after two weeks).

CONSTRICTIVE PERICARDITIS

Definition

Gross fibrosis or calcific thickening of the pericardium encasing the heart and giving rise to congestive heart failure.

Background

This is a relatively rare disease but important as a cause of severe, protracted but curable heart failure. The disease may represent the late stage of healing of previous tuberculous pericarditis but it can follow other types of pericarditis, including that of rheumatoid arthritis, particularly if haemorrhagic effusion has occurred.

Pathology

The pericardium is dense, the cavity obliterated, and there is firm fibrous attachment to the myocardium. Calcification may be extensive. Occasionally there is histological evidence of tuberculous infection but this is now exceptional.

Symptoms

Swollen ankles, legs and abdomen.
Breathlessness.

Signs

Very high venous pressure invariable.
Enlarged liver, may be ascites.
Fast heart rate with 3rd sound gallop.
Small volume pulse (pulsus paradoxus unusual).
In older patients atrial fibrillation common.
May be pleural effusions.

Investigations

1. Chest X-ray. Heart size nearly normal (exceptional in other types of severe heart failure). Calcification of the pericardium may be seen.
2. ECG. Low voltage QRS complexes. Widespread flattening or inversion of T waves.
3. Liver function tests may show raised bilirubin, low serum albumin and prolonged prothrombin time.

Complications

Atrial fibrillation.
Impaired liver function.
Ascites and pleural effusions.

Basis of Treatment

Diuretics may hold the tide of oedema fluid at bay, but surgical excision of the constricting pericardium is usually indicated in all severe cases. Only skilled and experienced cardiac surgeons should attempt this surgical cure, for separation of the rigid and calcified pericardium from the atrophic myocardium is difficult, and perforation of the heart chambers with disastrous effects all too easy.

Prognosis

A successful operation lowers the heart filling pressures to normal and the long term prognosis is then good.

Differential Diagnosis

1. From other causes of heart failure. The near normal size of the heart in a patient with very high venous pressure is an important clue.
2. Low voltage ECG usually with no normal T waves is also important.
3. Calcification of the pericardium under these circumstances is pathognomonic.

CARDIOMYOPATHY

Definition

A usually fatal disease of the heart characterised by degenerative changes in the myocardium. The nature of the disease process is not usually identified.

Background

This is a group of primary disorders of the myocardium. In some types there is no identifiable cause of the myocardial failure. In others, a very strong family history leaves no doubt that genetic factors operate. Heavy alcohol consumption seems sometimes to be causative, although death from heart failure is uncommon in alcoholics. Moreoover, a considerable intake of alcohol is so widespread in affluent societies that it is impossible to tell what part it may play in cases of heart failure of uncertain origin. Occasionally, heart failure follows an influenza-like illness and virus myocarditis is considered to have occurred. There is rarely proof of the infection. Healing may occur or the damage progress. In some parts of the world, for example extensive areas of Africa, cardiomyopathy is the overwhelmingly common cause of heart failure. It is there often known as endomyocardial fibrosis.

In the majority of cases, heart failure is the presenting feature and the term congestive cardiomyopathy is used to categorise them. The following types can sometimes be recognised:

1. Idiopathic.
2. Familial.
3. Myocarditis.
4. Alcoholic.
5. Systemic lupus.
6. Amyloid.
7. Scleroderma.

In one group of cases, remarkable unexplained hypertrophy, particularly of the left ventricle, is the dominant feature. In some of these, hypertrophy of the septum and outflow tract obstructs the outlet of the left ventricle and produces severe sub-aortic stenosis. This disease has been very clearly delineated and is called, in Britain, hypertrophic obstructive cardiomyopathy (HOCM) and, in America, idiopathic hypertrophic sub-aortic stenosis (IHSS). Those cases with hypertrophy, but no demonstrable obstruction, can simply be described as hypertrophic cardiomyopathy.

These two main groups, congestive and hypertrophic, will be described separately.

CONGESTIVE CARDIOMYOPATHY

Pathology

Even with the aid of electron microscopy there is no clear pathological picture of the various types with the exception of florid endocardial fibrosis in East African cases. In general, there is loss of striation of the fibres with varying degrees of hypertrophy and fibrosis. Intracardiac thrombus formation and systemic embolism are not rare.

Symptoms

Effort breathlessness.
Paroxysmal nocturnal dyspnoea.
Swollen ankles.
May be family history of premature death.

Signs

Enlargement of the heart.
Third and fourth sound gallop rhythms.
High venous pressure when the disease is fully developed.
May be atrial fibrillation, ectopic beats or other arrhythmias.
The diastolic blood pressure is sometimes elevated.
Mitral reflux may be present and severe due to dilation of the mitral valve ring.

Investigations

1. Chest X-ray shows cardiac enlargement and pulmonary venous congestion.
2. ECG shows abnormal T waves over the left ventricle, ectopic beats, and sometimes low voltage QRS complexes.
3. Full blood count and antinuclear factor test to search for systemic lupus.
4. Cardiac catheterisation and angiography.

Complications

Heart failure.
Arrhythmia.
Systemic embolism.
Pulmonary embolism.

Differential Diagnosis

From all other causes of heart failure, especially rheumatic mitral reflux, coronary heart disease, and hypertensive heart disease. Coronary heart disease is usually excluded by the absence of angina pectoris or a history or ECG evidence of previous infarction. Coronary arteriography removes doubt.

Basis of Treatment

The destructive agent cannot usually be identifed and removed, but if alcohol is thought to be involved, abstinence must be insisted on. The myocarditis of systemic lupus erythmatosus responds to steroids.

Otherwise, heart failure is treated by appropriate physical rest, digitalisation, and a full diuretic regime. Systemic embolism and venous thromboembolism call for anticoagulant therapy.

Prognosis

Usually grave. Death from heart failure in months or a few years is common, in spite of well-directed treatment. Sudden death from presumed ventricular arrhythmia may also occur.

HYPERTROPHIC CARDIOMYOPATHY

Pathology

There is gross hypertrophy and some fibrosis of the myocardium, especially the intraventricular septum. The cavity of the ventricle tends to be small.

Symptoms

None.
Effort breathlessness.
Angina pectoris.
Effort syncope.
Sudden death.
May be family history of sudden or premature death.

Signs

Forceful left ventricle.
The upstroke of the pulse is rapid and not sustained.
Palpable and audible fourth heart sound at the apex.
Systolic murmur and sometimes thrill, maximal usually at the pulmonary and tricuspid areas.

Investigations

1. X-ray of the chest usually shows little cardiac enlargement.
2. ECG virtually always abnormal with gross evidence of left ventricular hypertrophy. The P–R interval is often rather short. Atrial fibrillation occurs.
3. Pulse and apex tracings show the rapid upstroke of the pulse (which may be followed by a deep notch before the diastolic notch) and exaggerated atrial pulsation.
4. Cardiac catheterisation may reveal the outflow tract obstruction.

Differential Diagnosis

1. From aortic valvular stenosis or congenital subaortic stenosis. Pulse tracings' echocardiograms and intracardiac pressure records and angiocardiograms are decisive.
2. From other causes of systolic murmurs. The specific features outlined usually allow a firm diagnosis.

Basis of Treatment

There is no specific treatment. Competitive sport should be forbidden for fear of precipitating a fatal arrhythmia.

Beta adrenergic blocking agents will slow the heart and reduce contractility and there are claims that prolonged treatment with propranolol 80 mg three times daily may diminish the risk to life and lessen symptoms. Surgical relief of outflow tract obstruction is practised, but the results are difficult to evaluate.

Prognosis

Variable. Many patients remain symptomless for years, but the disease is progressive and sudden death an ever-present risk.

SPECIAL PROCEDURES

The Electrocardiogram in Bedside Diagnosis

Direct writing electrocardiograms can be used to add accuracy to diagnosis with relative ease. The apparatus is portable, safe, painless and relatively inexpensive (about £300). Little knowledge is required to confirm such important diagnoses as atrial fibrillation or recent myocardial infarction in the majority of cases. The fact that long and intensive study is required to understand the electrocardiogram in difficult cardiological cases need not deter any doctor from using electrocardiography to prove his diagnosis. If he is not sure of the interpretation of any record he can ask for help through the post, or discard the investigation.

Many records taken by casual electrocardiographers are uninterpretable because of poor technique. Provided the machine is satisfactory there are really only three points to pay attention to:
1. The patient must be relaxed. He needs to be lying in comfort with his head resting on a pillow and all the limbs relaxed, as if he were alseep. The well-wishing by-stander who wishes to keep the patient chatting should be politely silenced.
2. Electrodes must be applied with care, and their screw connections should make faultless contact. A little electrode jelly is rubbed with vigour on to the skin and a light coating on to the electrode plate. The elastic strap holds the plate firmly without strangling the limb.
3. The limb leads are connected to the correct limb and the precordial leads applied exactly to the appropriate position.

A little time is allowed after selecting each new lead to allow electrical stability, otherwise the record slopes across the recording paper and is useless for analysis. Careless application of the electrodes leads to 50 cycle interference. Muscle tenseness also distorts the baseline and ruins the record.

Care over these few points will lead to the production of a steady record free of interference. Before any analysis, always write the name of the patient, the date, and identify each lead.

Analysis

The Rhythm. This is scanned for irregularities. P waves are identified, and their presence establishes that the heart is in sinus rhythm.

Heart Rate. This can be worked out by counting the number of squares between each R wave (Fig. 17.23).

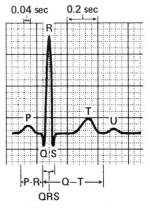

Fig. 17.23 Analysis of the electrocardiogram.

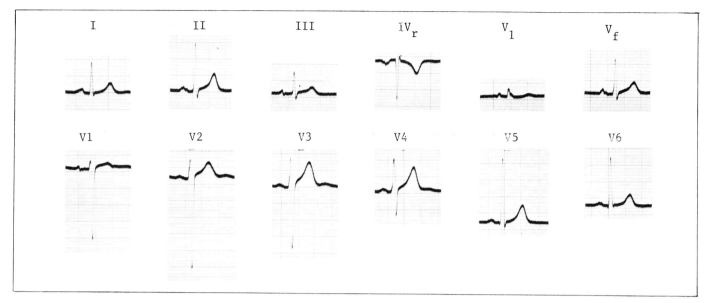

Fig. 17.24   Normal electrocardiogram.

Paper speed is 25 mm/second and if there are five large squares (25 small) between each R wave the heart rate is 60/minute. Four large squares equals 75/minute, and three equals 100/minute. Periodic changes in rate are likely to be due to sinus arrhythmia.

Large P Waves. These are due to atrial hypertrophy. Right atrial hypertrophy is characterised by a tall sharp P wave in V_1, and left atrial hypertrophy by a prolonged inverted P in V_1.

The P–R Interval. This is a measure of conduction time between atria and ventricles. It is measured by the time between the onset of the upstroke of P and the first deflection of the QRS complex. It should be assessed in more than one lead. At heart rates around 70/minute, the P–R interval should be less than 0.2 seconds (Fig. 17.24). Long P–R intervals are found in heart block, digitalis overdosage, and acute rheumatic fever.

Ectopic Beats. These are usually easy to identify because of the sudden change of R–R distance, with one short cycle followed by an unusually long one. If the ectopic arises in or above the atrio-ventricular node then the QRS is of usual shape and it may be preceded by an abnormal P wave. Ventricular ectopic beats are easier to pick out because their QRS pattern is totally different from the normal ones both in direction, duration, and voltage. The T wave is often inverted.

Other disturbances of rhythm have been dealt with in the appropriate section.

Voltage of the QRS Complex. This is relevant as measured by height of the R wave or depth of the S wave. All leads need to be inspected. There is no lower limit of normal, but low voltage throughout (less than 1 cm in nearly all leads) is characteristic of myxoedema and may also occur in severe heart failure, pericardial effusion, or constrictive pericarditis.

High voltage is a feature of ventricular hypertrophy, but separation between normal and abnormal is often not possible. Age is a factor. Right ventricular hypertrophy is best diagnosed in lead V_1. Except in children, an R wave greater than S in V_1 indicates right ventricular hypertrophy (except in some patients with inferior myocardial infarction). Left ventricular hypertrophy (Fig. 17.25) is best assessed by adding the depth of S in V_1 to the height of the taller R wave in V_5 or V_6. If the sum exceeds 35 mm, left ventricular hypertrophy is probable. Abnormal T waves in leads I, VL, V_{5-6} are, however, a commoner feature of left ventricular hypertrophy, especially in hypertension.

Width of the QRS Complex. This is a measure of the time taken for an excitatory impulse to activate the whole mass of ventricular muscle. Considerable hypertrophy of the ventricle leads therefore to slight widening of the QRS. More marked widening (greater than 0.1 sec, two and a half small squares) means abnormal delay in the activation process in one part of the conducting bundles and is characteristic of bundle branch block. Left bundle branch block gives a deep broad S wave in V_1 and a wide notched R wave in V_6. Right bundle branch block (Fig. 17.26) gives a notched R wave in V_1 and RS configuration in V_6. These abnormalities are seen most often in coronary heart disease and in heart block.

Abnormalities of the T Waves. These are very common, and frequently the experienced electrocardiographer is in doubt as to the cause. In most normal adults the T wave is upright in all the limb leads except AVR and in

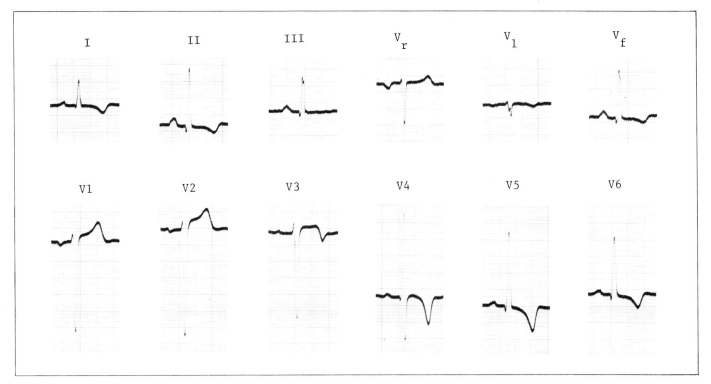

Fig. 17.25   Left ventricular hypertrophy.

all precordial leads except V_1. The T wave may, however, be inverted in lead III in normals, especially in obesity. Isolated inversion of the T wave in lead III can, therefore, be regarded as normal. Additional T wave inversion in leads II and AVF is abnormal. Abnormal T waves are flat or inverted. Common causes are digitalis therapy, old myocardial infarction, hypertension (leads I, AVL, V_{5-6}), myxoedema, hypokalaemia, pericarditis, etc. Very high T waves are sometimes a feature of hyperkalaemia.

Depressed S–T Segments. These can only usefully be analysed if the heart rate is below 90/minute. Digitalis therapy is one of the commonest causes. Others are ventricular hypertrophy and myocardial ischaemia. Depressed S–T segments during exercise or anxiety, which return to normal with rest or after TNT administration, are characteristic of angina pectoris.

Pathological Q Waves. Infarction or fibrosis of the wall of the left ventricle may give rise to an unduly deep or

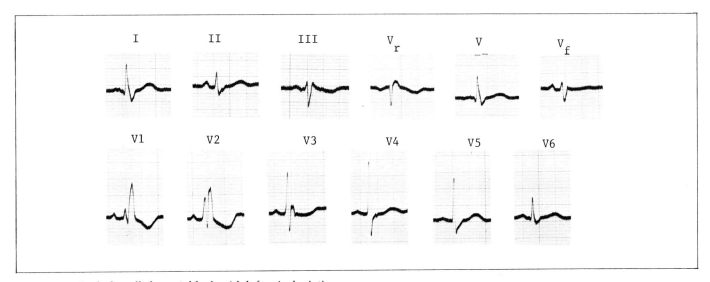

Fig. 17.26   Right bundle branch block with left axis deviation.

313

prolonged Q wave, that is, the potential recorded from the outer surface of the heart resembles a cavity lead. Pathological Q waves are seen in anterior myocardial infarction in leads V_{2-5} and in I and AVL. In posterior myocardial infarction they occur in leads II, III and AVF. A Q wave is considered pathological if its duration is 0.04 sec or its depth more than 25 per cent of the R wave in the lead in question (except in AVR).

CARDIAC CATHETERISATION

Measurement of pressures within the heart and great vessels, measurement of cardiac output, and visualisation of valves and intracardiac shunts have greatly increased the accuracy of diagnosis and paved the way to successful surgical treatment of heart disease. In experienced hands these procedures are relatively comfortable for the patient and carry little danger in the majority of cases. Passage of tubes along vessels is not felt, and once the skin is crossed and the lumen of the vessel entered only the discomfort of an X-ray table and the daunting sight of much apparatus and many medical attendants discomfort the patient. If, however, the total cost of such an investigation had to be borne by the patient, his discomforture would be extreme.

The right heart is normally entered by exposing an antecubital vein, and a radio-opaque catheter is then guided under X-ray control to the right atrium and ventricle and, thence, to the pulmonary artery. This allows all right heart pressures to be measured and a mixed venous blood sample to be withdrawn from the pulmonary artery. Cardiac output can then be estimated by measuring, simultaneously, oxygen uptake from a spirometer and oxygen content of mixed venous blood, and an arterial sample obtained by needle puncture.

$$\text{Cardiac output} = \frac{\text{Oxygen uptake}}{\text{Oxygen content of arterial blood} - \text{Oxygen content of venous blood}}$$

Other methods of measuring cardiac output include dye dilution and thermodilution techniques.

In congenital heart disease, right heart catheterisation has three other main uses apart from measuring pressures. Venous samples can be collected from the superior vena cava to the pulmonary artery. When left to right shunts are present, analysis of the samples will show a rise in oxygen saturation in and beyond the chamber the shunt enters. Thus, in ventricular septal defect, oxygen saturations will rise from 70 per cent in the right atrium to 80 per cent or more in the right ventricle and pulmonary artery. The bigger the shunt the greater the rise in oxygen saturation. Secondly, the catheter may pass to the left heart through the defect and thus prove its presence. Passage from the pulmonary artery to the thoracic aorta in patent ductus arteriosus is an example. Thirdly, contrast material can

be injected into the heart chambers, and rapid radiographs or cine film will outline the chambers, show the position of the pulmonary artery and aorta, and the existence of shunts.

Even in the absence of intracardiac defects that allow the venous catheter to enter left heart chambers, important information about left heart pressures can be obtained in the pulmonary artery. Under most circumstances, pulmonary artery and left ventricular pressure equalise at the end of diastole. The resistance of the pulmonary vasculature is so low that there is little gradient across it. Thus, at fairly slow heart rates and in the absence of mitral valve disease or raised pulmonary vascular resistance, the pulmonary diastolic pressure is an acceptable index of left ventricular diastolic pressure and, thus, of the presence or absence of left ventricular failure. Moreover, the catheter tip can be advanced far into the lung and wedged tightly in a terminal pulmonary artery. In this position the tip of the catheter, from which pressures are recorded, is now in contact only with pulmonary capillaries, veins, and the left atrium. Even if pulmonary vascular resistance is raised, pulmonary wedge pressure equals left atrial pressure.

Left heart chambers can be entered in three main ways:
1. From an open brachial arteriotomy the catheter is passed retrogradely across the aortic valve to the left ventricle.
2. The femoral artery is punctured and the ascending aorta entered by the Seldinger technique (through the needle a blunt-ended wire is inserted; over the wire a tight fitting and tapered end catheter is easily pushed into the artery; the wire is then withdrawn).
3. The femoral vein is punctured and a catheter containing a very long curved needle is passed to the inferior vena cava and right atrium. With the tip of the needle pointing towards the left scapula the inter-atrial septum is explored by feeling with the catheter containing the needle. Often, the foramen ovale is probe patent and the catheter enters the left atrium. If not, the septum is punctured by advancing the needle and the catheter passed over the top of the needle. Once the left atrium is gained the needle is withdrawn and the left ventricle can then be entered.

Left heart catheterisation is particularly helpful in chronic valvular disease and in the assessment of heart failure in adults. Cine angiography is valuable to give precise information about the state of both left heart valves and the behaviour of the left ventricle.

Right heart pressures can also be obtained more simply and without the need of X-ray facilities by introducing into an appropriate vein a very fine polythene tube which will be swept along by the blood flow as far as the pulmonary artery. A manometer and recorder displaying the shape of the pressure pulse allow one to recognise when the polythene enters the right ventricle and then the pulmonary artery. Care has to be taken not to introduce infection and to keep the tubing free of clot. The manometer and recorder are relatively costly, but the technique can be readily used at the bedside in very sick patients and may be a valuable guide to management.

Coronary arteriography is now also widely practised. Specially shaped catheters can be passed from a right brachial arteriotomy or Seldinger puncture of the femoral artery to the aortic sinuses. Small injections of contrast material show when the left or right coronary orifice has been entered. Cine films are then taken in several planes and the whole coronary tree can be well visualised. The information obtained is helpful in deciding the possible part played by coronary disease in older patients with valvular lesions, but its chief use is in selecting patients with symptomatic coronary disease who may be relieved of angina pectoris by surgical by-pass of coronary obstruction. The investigation carries a mortality of less than one per cent in expert hands.

ECHOCARDIOGRAPHY (Figs. 17.27, 17.28)

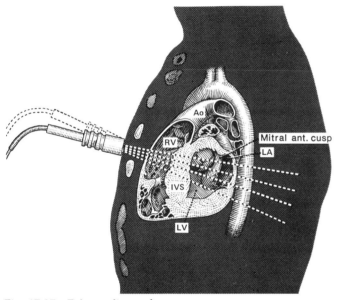

Fig. 17.27   Echocardiography.

A valuable non-invasive technique has been developed by using an ultrasound beam to detect intracardiac structures. The beam is emitted and sensed by the same small head which is held against the chest wall and directed between the ribs towards either heart chamber or any valve. Reflection from those surfaces within the heart on which the beam falls at right angles enables the valve cusps and ventricular walls to be mapped and their speed and range of movement measured. Thus both cusps of the mitral valve can be detected, any thickening appreciated, and failure of the valve to open adequately confirms mitral stenosis. Aortic and tricuspid valves can be similarly identified. In addition, the cross section of the left ventricle can be measured in systole and diastole and thus stroke volume and ejection fraction can be fairly accurately

deduced in most hearts. In congenital heart disease, abnormal placement of the aorta can be detected and abnormalities of heart chamber size and septal defects can be demonstrated. The technique is relatively inexpensive, without any hazard and is likely to be a standard procedure in most major hospitals.

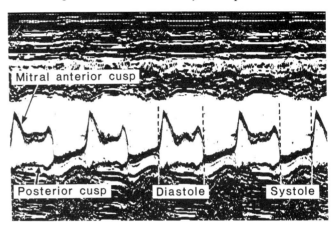

Fig. 17.28 (a)   Normal movement of mitral valve. In systole the anterior and posterior cusps are in apposition. In diastole the two cusps move in opposite directions but in mid-diastole the anterior cusp half as the ventricle fills; it then opens again with atrial systole.

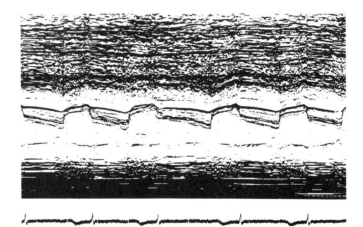

Fig. 17.28 (b)   Mitral stenosis. The range of movement of both cusps is limited. In diastole the posterior cusp moves in the same direction as the anterior. The downslope of the opening movement of the anterior cusp is blunted because the left ventricle fills very slowly. There are multiple echoes from the anterior cusp because it is thickened and calcified.

RADIO-ISOTOPE SCANNING

Another advance in technique which requires no more discomfort to the patient than an intravenous injection is radio-isotope scanning of the heart which is now being refined by the application of a computer. The shape and movement of the ventricles can be shown with considerable clarity and myocardial blood flow to left ventricular muscle can be quantitated in the assessment of coronary artery obstruction.

SUGGESTED FURTHER READING

General

Hamer, J. (ed.) (1977) *Recent Advances in Cardiology.* Edinburgh: Churchill Livingstone.

Anticoagulants in Heart Disease

Barritt, D. W. and Jordan, S. C. (1960) Anticoagulant drugs in pulmonary embolism. *Lancet* i, 1309.

M.R.C. Working Party (1959) An assessment of long term anticoagulant administration after cardiac infarction. *British Medical Journal* 1: 803–810.

Cardiac Arrhythmias

Stock, J. P. P. (1974) *Diagnosis and Treatment of Cardiac Arrhythmias.* London: Butterworth.

Cardiomyopathy

Goodwin, J. F. (1970) Congestive and hypertrophic cardiomyopathies: a decade of study. *Lancet* i, 731–739.

Coronary Artery Disease

Armstrong, A., Duncan, B., Oliver, M. F., Julian, D. G., Donald, K. W., Fulton, M., Lutz, W. and Morrison, S. L. (1972) Natural history of acute coronary heart attacks: a community study. *British Heart Journal* 34: 67–80.

Dewar, H. A. and Oliver, M. F. (1971) Secondary prevention trials (ischaemic heart disease) using clofibrate: a joint commentary on the Newcastle and Scottish trials. *British Medical Journal* 4: 784.

Hill, J. D., Hampton, J. R., Mitchell, J. R. A. (1978). A randomised trial of home versus hospital management for patients with suspected myocardial infarction. *Lancet* i: 837.

Royal College of Physicians of London and British Cardiac Society (1976) Prevention of coronary heart disease. *Journal of the Royal College of Physicians, London.* 10, 213; and Care of the patient with coronary heart disease, ibid. 10, 5.

Congenital Heart Disease

Jordan, S. C. and Scott, O. (1973) *Heart Disease in Paediatrics.* London: Butterworth.

Hypertension

Breckenridge, A., Dollery, C. T. and Parry, E. H. O. (1970) Prognosis of treated hypertension. *Quarterly Journal of Medicine* (new series) **39**: 411.

Marshall, A. J. and Barritt, D. W. (ed.) (1979) The hypertensive patient. London: Pitman Medical.

Subacute Bacterial Endocarditis

Cates, J. E. and Christie, R. V. (1951) Subacute bacterial endocarditis. A review of 442 patients treated in 14 centres appointed by the penicillin trials committee of the Medical Research Council. *Quarterly Journal of Medicine* **20**: 93–130.

Hayward, G. W. (1973) Infective endocarditis – a changing disease. *British Medical Journal* **2**: 706, 764.

Respiratory Medicine 18

G. LASZLO

This chapter describes the presentation and investigation of adults with disorders of the respiratory system. Diseases of the *upper* respiratory tract affect the nose, nasal sinuses, pharynx and larynx and the lymph nodes draining these. Common upper respiratory infections are mentioned, but not those surgical disorders, such as mastoiditis and nasopharyngeal tumours, usually treated by ear, nose and throat surgeons.

The mouth, pharynx and larynx are lined with squamous epithelium. At the level of the cricoid cartilage, the mucosa becomes columnar and ciliated like that of the nose. The *lower* respiratory tract is considered to start at this level; its mucosa normally is sterile.

The patient's symptoms, examination and investigations may lead to one or more anatomical diagnoses (Table 18.1), all of which may be caused by a number of diseases. Their classification in these pages follows as far as possible the standard pathological pattern: infection, trauma, new growth and secondary disturbances of metabolic, endocrine, immunological and circulatory origin. The important respiratory disorders of the newborn are omitted and those of children are described

superficially. Pulmonary thromboembolism and cardiogenic pulmonary oedema are discussed elsewhere (*see* Chapter 17). Several statements about the clinical presentation of disease apply mainly to the UK.

MAJOR SYMPTOMS OF LOWER RESPIRATORY DISEASE

The major symptoms of lower respiratory disease are cough, sputum, haemoptysis, shortness of breath, pain in the chest and fever.

Cough

A cough is a paroxysm of repeated forced expirations against a closed glottis. When involuntary, it is interspersed with sharp inspirations. It may be dry or productive. Coughing is provoked by stimulation of the irritant receptors of the mucosa of the respiratory tract which are most numerous between the larynx and the bifurcation of the trachea and for one or two divisions beyond.

Table 18.1   Presentation of important lower respiratory syndromes

Lower respiratory syndromes	Common clinical manifestations	X-ray
Mucosal irritation	Cough	
Haemorrhage	Haemoptysis	
Airway obstruction – localised	Dyspnoea, stridor, wheeze	*
diffuse	Dyspnoea, inspiratory effort,	*
	wheeze, abnormal lung function	*
Lung collapse	Diminished breath sounds, dullness, asymmetry	†
Lung consolidation	Dyspnoea, cough, bronchial breathing	†
Pulmonary oedema	Dyspnoea, cough, râles, sometimes characteristic sputum	*
Alveolar wall inflammation	Dyspnoea, cough, râles, abnormal lung function	*
Lung fibrosis – localised	Poor expansion, abnormal lung function	†
diffuse	Poor expansion, basal râles, abnormal lung function	*
Pleural inflammation	Pain, pleural rub	†
Pleural effusion	Pain, dyspnoea, diminished breath sounds	
	dull percussion note	†
Pneumothorax	Diminished breath sounds, hyper-resonance	†
Thoracic cage deformity	Poor expansion, deformity	*
Respiratory neuromuscular disease	Poor expansion	
Abnormal shadow on routine X-ray		†

*Characteristic X-ray findings may be present.
†Condition usually diagnosed by X-ray abnormality.

Inhalation of saliva, sputum and foreign bodies, inflammatory disease and neoplasms may stimulate coughing. A short dry cough is a feature of alveolar wall disease, thought to be mediated by receptors in the alveolar wall ('J' receptors).

Sputum

Sputum or phlegm is material secreted by the respiratory tract and expectorated; it may be mucoid, purulent or blood-stained. It may emanate from the nasal sinuses or nose as 'post-nasal drip', or from the bronchi. Most patients can tell whether it can be expectorated merely by clearing the throat or whether it has to be 'coughed up' from the chest. 'Catarrh' usually means 'tendency to form sputum'.

The production of mucoid sputum is a response to irritation, bronchial oedema or non-pyogenic infections such as those caused by viruses. The commonest cause of both nasal and bronchial hypersecretion is cigarette smoking, an intense form of atmospheric pollution. Non-smokers rarely expectorate regularly. 'Normal phlegm', as it is incorrectly described by smokers, emanates from hypertrophied bronchial mucus glands. These, however, react normally to changes of temperature, humidity and the presence of other irritants, such as dust, by increasing their secretion. Thus the first manifestation of a productive smokers' cough usually occurs in the winter months when a small amount of mucoid sputum is expectorated on rising. Ciliary activity is normally reduced at night. When there is more than about 100 ml of bronchial secretion in 24 hours there is enough pooling of secretions in the major airways at night to stimulate coughing.

Pus in sputum is recognised as yellow or green material. When it is associated with bronchial infection the pus is often mixed with mucus. Sputum from acute alveolar infections is usually more uniform in consistency. Pus indicates suppuration, a 'rusty' sputum from altered blood being characteristic of haemorrhagic pneumonias (Table 18.2).

Haemoptysis (Expectoration of Blood)

Frank blood in the sputum is frightening and usually leads to rapid investigation. No serious cause is found in about half such cases, with regular follow-up rarely producing an explanation not found initially. Haemoptysis occurs when a bronchial artery is eroded by neoplasia, infection or trauma. It is much more likely to occur when there are increased bronchopulmonary anastomoses or when the pressure in bronchial and systemic veins is elevated. The common serious causes of frank haemoptysis are tuberculosis and other cavitating lung infections, pulmonary infarction and bronchial carcinoma (Fig. 18.1). In the latter condition, the sputum is often mucoid and tinged with blood. Pulmo-

Table 18.2 Common causes of characteristic types of sputum

Types of sputum	Cause
Watery, scanty	Viral infections
Frothy, pink	Acute severe pulmonary oedema
Mucoid (M_1*)	Chronic bronchitis (simple) bronchial asthma
Mucopurulent	Infective bronchitis (usually *Haemophilus influenzae*)
(M_2* – mucus flecked with spirals of yellow pus) (P_1* – one-third pus) (P_2* – two-thirds pus)	
Rusty mucoid sputum	*Klebsiella pneumoniae* infections
Purulent (P_3*)	Suppurative broncho-pulmonary infections
Lurid green	*Pseudomonas aeruginosa* infections
Rusty	Pneumococcal or haemorrhagic viral pneumonia *Klebsiella pneumoniae* infections

*M_1, M_2, P_1, P_2 and P_3 defined above are useful phrases describing the naked eye appearance of sputum (MRC classification).
Occasionally, M_2 sputum contains mainly eosinophils and is allergic rather than infective in origin.

nary infarction causes clots, sometimes only over a period of a few days, while patients with tuberculosis tend to produce blood mixed with pus or blood clots over a longer period of time.

Certain conditions, notably mitral stenosis, bronchiectasis, and various forms of cystic lung disease including cystic fibrosis, are associated with increased bronchopulmonary anastomoses. It is usually these patients who suffer life-threatening haemoptysis complicated by secondarily infected lung consolidation and serious reduction of circulating blood volume. Tuberculosis is now a rare cause of such dramatic catastrophes

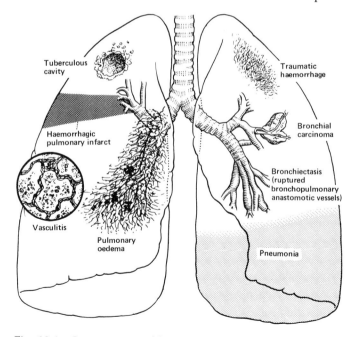

Fig. 18.1 Some causes of haemoptysis.

318

as those experienced by Chopin during his last piano recitals.

Shortness of Breath (Dyspnoea)

Some patients complain of awareness of the need for increased inspiratory effort because of alterations in respiratory mechanics which make breathing feel more difficult than normal. Others feel hunger for air which makes light exercise feel heavy. Breathless patients may complain of various unpleasant sensations about the chest (e.g. 'tightness') or a tendency to cough during severe exertion. Dyspnoea may occur:
1. During effort, consistently or variably.
2. At rest, continuously or in attacks.
3. In attacks during the night.

Effort dyspnoea is discussed further under 'respiratory function' (see page 320). When patients complain of it, they will often mention noticing it on stairs. When enquiring directly about effort tolerance, questions about ability to perform more prolonged exercise give a clearer idea of the severity of the disorder. For example:

Q1. Can you walk on the level at your own pace without stopping?
Q2a (if yes to Q1). Can you keep up with a normal person on the flat without being breathless?
Q2b (if yes to Q2a). Can you keep up with a healthy person on hills and stairs?
Q2c (if no to Q1). How far can you go without stopping?

According to the answers, effort tolerance can be graded numerically, but there is no general agreement about what to call these grades. Extremely fit people may complain of reduced effort tolerance, while still being normal in comparison with others.

The sensation of shortness of breath at rest is caused by acute changes of bronchopulmonary mechanics, such as an attack of pulmonary oedema or bronchial asthma, or by acute inflammatory disease of the lower respiratory tract, for example pneumonia or bronchitis. In these conditions, dyspnoea occurs at rest when pulmonary function is reduced only modestly to levels which would not cause similar discomfort to a patient with a chronic lung disease. The mechanism is not known; hypoxia and bronchial receptors responsive to local irritation are probably responsible for reflex hyperventilation and possibly altered awareness of breathing.

Nocturnal dyspnoea is described in Chapter 17. It may be a feature of bronchial asthma and is not pathognomonic of left ventricular failure as is sometimes thought. Shortage of breath when lying flat (orthopnoea) is a feature of heart failure, but patients with chronic bronchitis often choose to sleep with several pillows. This may be because lying flat provokes coughing which is relieved by sitting up.

Chest Pain

The majority of thoracic pains are not due to respiratory disease. A brief account of the differential diagnosis of this worrying symptom follows.

Angina pectoris, pericardial pain and the pain of acute pulmonary embolism are covered in Chapter 17, with their differentiation from oesophageal and other gastrointestinal pains. Apart from these, thoracic pain is most likely to originate from the parietal pleura, spine and chest wall.

Pleural pain caused by inflammation or malignant tumour is somatic, tends to be sharp, felt on one side and made worse by pressure on the chest, breathing and coughing. The patient sits still and takes shallow breaths. Simple analgesics usually provide relief, although of short duration in severe cases. Fractured ribs are similarly painful; accurate localisation may be possible. Pain from the diaphragmatic pleura may be referred to the shoulder tip or to the abdomen when it may be diagnosed as an acute surgical condition. Flitting pains similar to pleurisy may herald a recurrence of chest infection in patients with bronchiectasis, usually without an audible pleural friction rub. Spontaneous pneumothorax is the commonest cause of acute severe chest pain in the young adult. It may be pleuritic, but is often centrally placed or dull with little variation.

Mediastinal structures receive pain innervation, which is almost absent from the lung and visceral pleura. Acute conditions such as rupture of the oesophagus and aortic arch dissection are severely painful; inflammation of the oesophagus and trachea cause soreness. Pain may rarely arise from mediastinal tumours. Bronchial carcinomas situated within the lung may cause vague discomfort when situated near a major bronchus. More often, lateralised chest pain implies invasion of the intercostal nerves.

Irritation of dorsal nerve roots may be felt around the chest wall. Three or four days may elapse between the onset of pain from shingles (Herpes zoster) (see page 550) and the appearance of the rash. Root irritation from vertebral collapse is usually accompanied by central backache. Dorsal spondylosis may also cause pain in the chest wall. Examination reveals tenderness of vertebrae and limitation of thoracic rotation in such cases.

Many chest pains seen in general practice are of muscular origin. Repeated coughing causes flitting aches. Cough fractures occur. Interscapular pains occur in those who sit hunched over their work, the sewing machine being a frequent cause. Nervous tension causes sensations of stabbing or prolonged aching in the chest wall with local tenderness similar to 'tension headaches'; this may be where the patient thinks his heart is (less often under the left nipple than formerly).

Acute inflammation of one or more costal cartilages or its junction with rib or sternum causes pain with severe tenderness made worse by movement of the arms or trunk. This unpleasant acute condition usually lasts a few months (Tietze's disease). Simple analgesics or sedatives rarely affect chest wall pain.

Patients who have suffered any disease causing severe pain in the chest are thereafter liable to chest wall aches, and it is important when this occurs to persuade patients to ignore transient stabbing or prolonged dull aches as not heralding a recurrence of a serious disorder. After thoracotomy, pain may last for two years.

Almost one-quarter of all patients with ischaemic heart disease present with chronic atypical chest pains which are sometimes, but not invariably, related to prolonged or heavy exercise. These pains may be indistinguishable from muscular chest pain caused by tension or anxiety. When due to myocardial ischaemia, the pains usually change character over a few months and become more typical. The doctor must listen carefully to the description at each interview and be prepared to change his diagnosis. The intensity of the initial investigation will depend on the patient's health record, the presence of other classical manifestations of anxiety or pointers to a definite diagnosis and the likelihood that an electrocardiogram will draw attention to the heart (bearing in mind the fact that a normal trace may reassure the patient but not the doctor). It is important to find out before offering reassurance if the patient has any diagnosis in mind. (Heart disease or lung cancer may be feared if a relative or colleague has died recently of these.)

Reassurance that 'nothing serious' is present may relieve some, but not all of those troubled by this obstinate complaint, which patients learn to live with but rarely lose for ever.

TESTS OF RESPIRATORY FUNCTION USED IN CLINICAL PRACTICE

Three aspects of respiration which may be disturbed by disease and tested are pulmonary ventilation, pulmonary gas exchange and control of breathing. The common tests are those of:

1. Ventilation and lung volumes.
2. Blood gases.
3. Carbon monoxide (CO) transfer.

Pulmonary Ventilation

At the end of quiet expiration, when the muscles are at rest, the volume of air in the chest depends on the elasticity of the lungs, trying to empty, opposing the recoil of the chest wall tending to expand. Inspiratory muscles overcome first the lung recoil, then, if a deeper breath is taken, the combined recoil of the lungs and chest wall, and the thoracic cage is expanded beyond its resting position. Expiration is normally passive, the elasticity of the structures tending to expel air. Inspiratory work overcomes the *elastic recoil* and the *resistance of the bronchi to air flow*. To identify structural damage to the lungs by decreased alveolar or chest wall distensibility ('restriction') or by airway obstruction, one should in theory measure these, but the procedures are complex. Useful information emerges from simple static and dynamic lung volume measurements (Fig. 18.2). Vital capacity and its timed subdivisions may be measured on inexpensive portable apparatus.

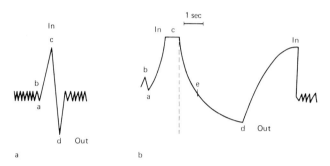

Fig. 18.2(a) Spirometric trace (diagrammatic) to show subdivisions of the static lung volumes.
18.2(b) Fast spirometric trace (diagrammatic) to illustrate timed ventilatory tests in a patient with airways obstruction. a = functional residual capacity; ab = tidal volume; ac = inspiratory capacity; c = total lung capacity; cd = vital capacity; d = residual volume; ce = forced expired volume in 1 sec (FEV$_1$).

Vital Capacity (VC). The maximum volume of air that can be expired after full inspiration. Normal values (3 to 6 litres) depend on sex, age and height, one standard deviation being about 10 per cent of the mean. VC may be reduced by:
(a) Loss of inspiratory reserve (lung fibrosis, obliteration of alveoli, rigidity of the chest wall, respiratory muscle weakness). Total lung capacity is reduced.
(b) Increased volume of residual air after full expiration (trapped by closure of obstructed airways). Total lung capacity is normal.

These may be distinguished by measuring total lung capacity. This may often be gauged from the clinical examination and X-ray. In restrictive disease, the total lung capacity is reduced. When the elastic recoil of the lungs is increased by fibrosis or consolidation, the lung volume (FRC) is reduced below normal and air flow is rapid during expiration.

Timed Forced Expiration and Expiratory Flow Rates. Simply, when airways are narrowed by obstruction of their lumen, air cannot be forced so rapidly through them. The rate at which air can be expelled during forced expiration can be expressed in various ways. FEV$_1$ (volume expired in the first second of forced expiration – Fig. 18.2) should be greater than 75 per cent of the vital capacity (80 per cent in young subjects and in women). A lower fraction indicates airways obstruction. When severely ill, patients with airways obstruction whose vital capacity is greatly reduced may be unable to expire for longer than one or two seconds. Under these conditions, a high ratio does not exclude airway obstruction. The absolute value of FEV_1 is a useful measurement which correlates well with the maximum breathing capacity. This is approximately FEV_1 (litres) × 30 litres per minute. When FEV_1 is less than 1.0 litre after a bronchodilator drug there is a considerable risk of respiratory failure.

Peak expiratory flow rate (PEFR) is flow rate at the beginning of a maximum forced expiration. Theoretically, it can be obtained from the traces of forced expired volume, but in practice it is measured with a flow meter (e.g. Wright's meter, Fig. 18.3). The normal range (380

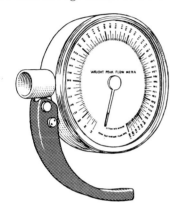

Fig. 18.3 Wright's peak flow meter.

to 700 litres per minute) is wide, but the test is useful for measuring changes in individual patients and for detecting fairly severe airways obstruction. Readings less than 100 litres per minute after bronchodilator drugs indicates a risk of respiratory failure.

Minor degrees of airways obstruction. The main sites of resistance to air flow are the larynx and trachea. Each of the 17 subsequent divisions of the 'bronchial tree' has a cumulative diameter greater (by a factor of about 1.3) than the parent branch.
Obstruction may occur:
(a) By narrowing of large airways.
(b) By obliteration of parallel small airways (Fig. 18.4). Obliteration of a few small airways, insufficient to reduce FEV_1 or peak flow measurably, may be detected by prolongation of forced expiration and reduction of air flow at low lung volumes (*see* Fig. 18.6).

Effects of variable airway calibre on tests. Airways become wider in inspiration and narrower on expiration in the same way as alveoli. Forcing expiration, although it ensures maximal rate of emptying of alveoli, compresses the airways. As a result, expiration cannot be hurried and may be *independent of effort* in diseases such as asthma and chronic bronchitis.

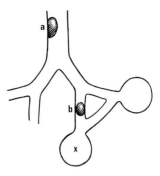

Fig. 18.4 Two ways (a) and (b), in which the flow of air to alveolus (x) can be impeded (obstructed).

The interpretation of measurements of air flow during forced expiration therefore depends on whether the airways are compressed to the point of closure (Fig. 18.5).

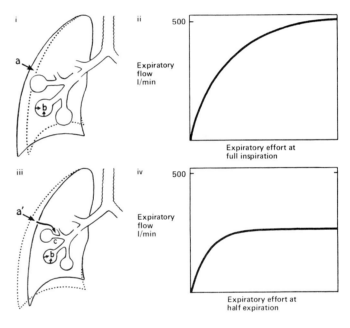

Fig. 18.5(i) and (ii) Normal lung at full inspiration. Expiratory flow is *aided* by expiratory force (a) and alveolar recoil (b); it is *resisted* by the resistance of the whole airway.
18.5(iii) and (iv) Expiratory muscle force applied around the lung (a') aids expiration by compressing the lung and hinders expiration by compressing the airways (c). These cancel, thus, the only force which empties the lung is the elastic recoil of the alveoli (b). Expiratory flow is almost independent of effort.

Maximum expiratory flow depends on:
(a) The elastic recoil pressure of the lungs.
(b) The conductivity of the airways between the alveoli and the collapsed segment of airway.
Radiographic studies suggest that closure normally occurs in the first few divisions of the major bronchi.

Patients with airways obstruction appear to have more tendency to airway closure and flow limitation occurs even at total lung capacity. Thus their measurements of peak flow and FEV_1 tend to be very reproducible, *if a full breath is drawn in*. Expiratory air flow is reduced when lung elasticity is lost (as in pulmonary emphysema, *see* page 344) or when there is narrowing of airways.

Obstruction of Larynx or Trachea. When this condition is sufficiently severe to cause dyspnoea, forced expiration is limited by it. A characteristic 'spirogram' is obtained:
(a) Peak flow is reduced proportionately more than FEV_1.
(b) Forced inspiration is affected more or less the same as expiration.

Variable airways obstruction. When airway obstruction is due to bronchial asthma (*see* page 345), the peak flow FEV_1 and other spirometric evidence all tend to vary together, for example after bronchodilators.

Early detection of bronchiolar disease. Early disease of peripheral airways may be detected by finding reduced flow rates at mid expiration, when FEV_1 and peak flow are normal (Fig. 18.6).

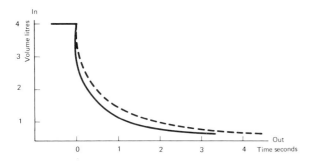

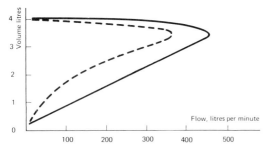

Fig. 18.6(a) Timed forced expiration recorded on a fast moving spirometer.
———: normal trace
----: from patient with early airways obstruction showing deceleration of expiratory flow at low lung volumes and prolongation of the time for forced expiration.
Fig. 18.6(b) The same subjects measured on a device which plots expiratory flow rate at different lung volumes.

Blood Gas Analysis

Interpretation of Arterial Pco_2. Ventilatory control mechanisms set arterial Pco_2 between 5.0 and 6.0 kPa (36 to 44 mmHg). This corresponds to an average alveolar concentration of around 5 to 6 per cent (at sea level). As

$$CO_2 \text{ excreted} = \text{ventilation} \times \text{alveolar concentration}$$

it follows that, to keep Pco_2 more or less constant, alveolar ventilation must remain proportional to metabolic rate: about 4 to 5 litres per minute at rest, about 40 to 50 litres per minute walking briskly uphill.

Low arterial Pco_2. Breathing which is excessive in proportion to metabolic rate and lowers arterial Pco_2 is called *hyperventilation*. This is not readily detected at rest unless quite severe. Increasing alveolar ventilation by a factor of one and a half reduces Pco_2 to 4 kPa (30 mmHg). At rest, increasing ventilation from 4 to 6 litres per minute is undetectable to subject or observer. The same proportional increase in exercise will reduce effort tolerance because patients tend to feel breathless when breathing at about 50 per cent of their maximum capacity.

The following mechanisms provoke overbreathing:

1. Anxiety.
2. Hypoxaemia (altitude, lung disease).
3. Metabolic acidosis (e.g. diabetes, excessive lactic acid production in exercise).
4. Conditions thought to irritate bronchial and lung nerve endings (asthma, bronchial irritation, pulmonary embolus, pulmonary oedema, pulmonary emphysema).

Overbreathing due to anxiety or acidosis causes a high Po_2 if arterial blood is sampled during a period of hyperventilation. When the lungs are abnormal Po_2 is low or not elevated.

High Pco_2. 'Alevolar hypoventilation' (*see also* ventilatory failure, page 367).

Normal subjects cannot hold their breath to allow Pco_2 to rise by more than a small amount. If made to breathe mixtures containing CO_2 they increase their ventilation. In some, CO_2 sensitivity is reduced or can be reduced by training (e.g. divers). Certain chronic lung diseases which cause increased inspiratory work are associated with a tendency for Pco_2 to rise, at first in exercise, later at rest, for example chronic bronchitis, chest restriction due to kyphoscoliosis and chronic paralytic diseases of respiratory muscles. Certain other lung diseases, for example heart failure, emphysema, bronchial asthma and pulmonary embolism, are accompanied by a tendency to hyperventilation. Therefore these disorders are accompanied by a high Pco_2 only if so severe that the lungs are unable to excrete all the CO_2

generated by metabolism. The patients feel strangled and are unable to exercise when they reach this condition.

Some patients have no intrinsic CO_2 drive, or lose it during sleep. Respiratory depressant drugs taken or given in excessive doses cause elevation of Pco_2 in normal subjects.

Interpretation of Arterial Po_2

Normal limits of arterial Po_2. Alveolar Po_2 may lie between 11 and 15 kPa (80 and 110 mmHg) when air is breathed. The exact result has little effect on arterial O_2 saturation (94 to 96 per cent).

The normal Po_2 may be predicted more accurately by the use of the alveolar air equation, which is obtained simply from the calculation of metabolic rate:

CO_2 output

$$= \text{Alveolar ventilation} \times \frac{\text{Alveolar } Pco_2}{\text{Bar press (dry)}}$$

and:

O_2 consumption

$$= \text{Alveolar ventilation} \times \frac{\text{Inspired } Po_2 - \text{alveolar } Po_2}{\text{Bar press (dry)}}$$

Combining these, and using the symbol R for the respiratory exchange ratio (CO_2 production/O_2 consumption) gives:

$$R = \frac{\text{Alveolar } Pco_2}{\text{Inspired } Po_2 - \text{Alveolar } Po_2}$$

and rearranging yields the *alveolar air equation*:

$$\text{Alveolar } Po_2 = \text{Inspired } Po_2 - \frac{\text{Alveolar } Pco_2}{R}$$

In the normal lung, the difference between alveolar and arterial Po_2 is less than 2 kPa (15 mmHg). R usually lies between 0.8 and 1.0. Thus arterial Po_2 and Pco_2 should add up to inspired Po_2 (20 kPa or 150 mmHg, breathing room air at sea level at a body temperature of 37°C saturated with water).

A useful approximation of this concept states that:

Arterial Po_2 should be more than 16 – arterial Pco_2 (kPa)
Arterial Po_2 should be more than 120 – arterial Pco_2 (mmHg)

If R is measured in the expired gas, the alveolar air equation provides an accurate assessment of the 'normal limit' of Po_2 under the conditions studied.

Low arterial Po_2 may be due to:

Underventilation (high arterial Pco_2).
Inefficient pulmonary gas exchange.
(a) Mismatching of pulmonary ventilation.
(b) (Rarely) reduced diffusing capacity.
Right-to-left cardiac shunt.

Mismatching of Ventilation and Perfusion. If unsaturated (venous) blood passes through areas of lung which do not receive their share of ventilation, abnormal amounts of reduced haemoglobin enter the arterial blood. If total ventilation increases, to try to compensate for this, the extra ventilation goes to the good areas where the blood is almost fully saturated anyway. Increasing ventilation can reduce Pco_2 in the blood leaving the well ventilated areas of lung to make up for the blood from which CO_2 is inadequately cleared. Therefore, when there is uneven distribution of ventilation and perfusion:

Pco_2 may be high, normal or low, according to the extent to which ventilation increases in response to the disease.
Po_2 is low for the amount of ventilation (judged by arterial Pco_2) and may be increased by breathing extra oxygen.

When there is patchy lung damage, the degree of hypoxaemia found when the patient is breathing air depends on whether the hypoxic pulmonary vasoconstrictor mechanism is intact. Po_2 may sometimes be surprisingly normal in such conditions as bronchial asthma, pneumothorax and pneumonia, because the blood goes where the ventilation is best. When this does not occur, the patient becomes hypoxaemic. This can be relieved only by increasing inspired Po_2 so that enough O_2 is supplied although ventilation remains low. When blood reaches totally unventilated alveoli, hypoxaemia persists even with O_2 enrichment. Cyanosis (visible capillary desaturation) is detectable if there is more than 30 g/l of reduced Hb (3 g/100 ml), i.e. less than 80 per cent saturation.

Respiratory failure is defined as inability to maintain normal blood gases at rest breathing air. Arterial Pco_2 does not normally rise above 6 kPa (45 mmHg), and a rise above 6.5 kPa (about 50 mmHg) defines ventilatory failure. Arterial Po_2 below 8 kPa (60 mmHg) when breathing air at sea level is abnormal under all circumstances.

Carbon Monoxide (CO) Transfer ('Diffusing Capacity')

CO is useful to test the capacity of the lung to transfer gas because it has a high affinity for haemoglobin and can be analysed in air in minute quantities. The ability of the lungs to extract CO from inspired air is usually measured after 10 seconds of breath-holding at full inspiration.

A breath of air with helium and 0.3 per cent CO is taken, held for 10 seconds and exhaled. Helium is insoluble; its dilution indicates the volume of accessible lung. Because of uptake, more CO is apparently extracted.

$$\frac{\text{CO inspired/CO expired}}{\text{Helium inspired/Helium expired}} \text{ is greater than 1.}$$

This ratio rises exponentially with time in normal subjects so its logarithm, divided by breath-holding time, forms the basis for a reproducible index of CO uptake.

The results are expressed in mmol uptake per min per kPa (or ml. min^{-1}. $mmHg^{-1}$).

Predicted mean ('normal') values vary with age and height and lie between 7 and 15 mmol. min^{-1}. $kPa^{-1} \pm 20$ per cent.

Clinically, the test is most useful when vital capacity and FEV_1/VC are normal. Then, if Hb is normal, reduction of CO transfer to 80 per cent or less indicates probable disease at the alveolar level, for example diffuse lung fibrosis. The test is simple and relatively sensitive, but a normal result does not exclude disease.

Interpretation of CO transfer

Reduction	*Increase*
Anaemia	Pulmonary
Reduced pulmonary	plethora
capillary bed	Polycythaemia
Reduced alveolar	
surface area	
Maldistribution of	
inspired gas	
Thickened alveolar walls	

CHEST RADIOLOGY

Only an introduction to the postero-anterior film is possible here. A systematic search of each plate can proceed as follows:

Name, Date, Technique ('portable' anterior posterior (AP) or the usual PA film).

Posture, Rotation, Penetration (Fig. 18.7).

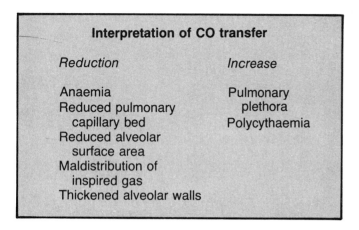

Fig. 18.7   Chest radiology: posture, rotation, penetration.

Shoulders, Neck, Abdomen, Breast and Nipple Shadows.

324

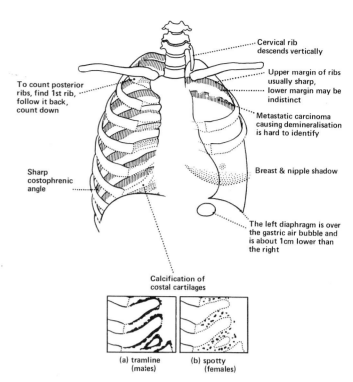

Fig. 18.8   Chest radiology: ribs, diaphragm.

Ribs, Diaphragm (Thoracic Cage) (Fig. 18.8). The diaphragm is normally at the 6th rib anteriorly, 11th rib posteriorly; 7 and 12 respectively suggest over-inflation, 5 and 10 suggest poor inspiration or reduced lung volume. If a dome is high, it may be paralysed. Pleural effusion obscures the diaphragm as does consolidated lung along its surface.

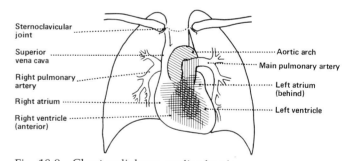

Fig. 18.9   Chest radiology: cardiac borders.

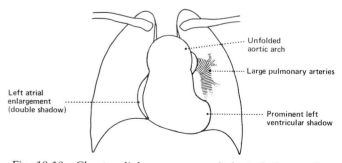

Fig. 18.10   Chest radiology: some cardiological abnormalities (diagrammatic).

Cardiac Borders (Fig. 18.9). Abnormal enlargement of various chambers (Fig. 18.10) and mediastinal shadows (Fig. 18.11) alter the normal appearance of the heart in the mediastinum.

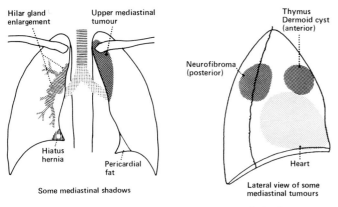

Fig. 18.11 Chest radiology: some mediastinal shadows.

Lung Fields. The lungs consist of air with a branching system of vessels (Figs. 18.12 and 18.13). The normal distribution is subjective. Excessive filling of vessels

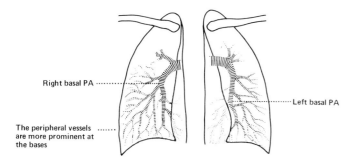

Fig. 18.12 Chest radiology: pulmonary arteries – branching fanwise.

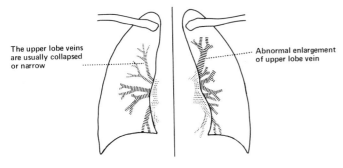

Fig. 18.13 Chest radiology: pulmonary veins – 'Staghorn' configuration.

(plethora) occurs when left atrial pressure is elevated or when there is left-to-right cardiac shunt. Poor filling of blood vessels locally indicates pulmonary vascular destruction or occlusion. Generalised loss of peripheral

vessels is usually accompanied by enlargement of the main pulmonary artery (pulmonary hypertension).

Abnormal Densities (Opacities) in the Lung Fields (Fig. 18.14)
(a) Look for obvious shadows.
(b) Search in apparently normal areas for small shadows (side to side, space by space).

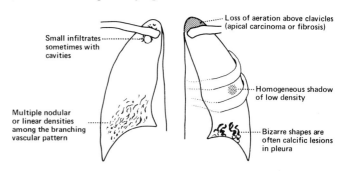

Fig. 18.14 Chest radiology: some shadows in the lung fields that often are not immediately visible.

SPECIALISED TECHNIQUES

Examination of Sputum and Bronchial Secretions

Sputum may contain mucus, pus or blood. Naked eye examination has been described (*see* page 318). Microscopic examination, using appropriate staining techniques, may show:

Neutrophilia or eosinophilia.
Malignant cells.
Rarely, employing Gram's stain, the presence of pathogenic organisms in typical form (but not acid-fast bacilli).
Mycobacterium tuberculosis (by special techniques).

Culture of Sputum. This may demonstrate respiratory pathogens. Unfortunately, the common pyogenic organisms which cause bacterial pneumonia are occasionally commensal organisms in the throat. Thus normal people may carry *Haemophilus influenzae, Streptococcus pneumoniae, Staphylococcus pyogenes* and *Streptococcus pyogenes*, as well as the common commensal organisms *Brahmanella catarrhalis* (formerly Neisseria), and diphtheroid bacilli.

Any course of antibiotics changes the normal throat flora, showing colonisation for several weeks by intestinal organisms and the saprophytic yeast *Candida albicans*. Their isolation from sputum very rarely indicates serious lower respiratory infection with these organisms. These may interfere with the isolation of more delicate species: more commonly, they mislead the clinician into treating a viral infection with antibiotics directed against a saprophyte. When there is clear evidence of pulmonary suppuration, isolation of a heavy growth of a single pathogenic organism from purulent sputum is reliable evidence of its pathogenicity.

Tracheal aspiration (through a bronchoscope, or, with some risk, by crico-thyroid puncture) has not been adopted outside certain specialised units because, surprisingly, misleading isolates are sometimes obtained.

Percutaneous, fine needle aspiration of the lung provides material for cytology and culture. Its value in severe cases of pneumonia is being investigated.

Virology

Viruses may be isolated from the throat during the first 24 to 48 hours of an infection: usually they have disappeared before the patient reports.

Only a few specific virus infections with a considerable systemic effect may be diagnosed retrospectively by the discovery of changing titres of antibodies during convalescence.

Virological studies have been most valuable in demonstrating that a high proportion of respiratory diseases are not bacterial, thus helping to define rational antibiotic policies (*see* 'Pneumonia', page 329).

Bronchoscopy

The larynx and major bronchi may be examined directly through a bronchoscope. The *rigid bronchoscope* is a tube through which the patient can breathe or be ventilated. The segmental bronchi can be examined, and foreign bodies removed. Most operators employ general anaesthesia. *Flexible fibre-optic bronchoscopes* are narrower and allow examination and sampling from more distal subsegmental bronchi. Ventilation takes place around the tube: closure of the airway around the instrument is very rare. Local anaesthesia may be used. The instrument allows diagnosis and localisation of about 70 per cent of bronchial tumours, by direct vision or cytological examination of bronchial brushings.

Percutaneous or Per-bronchial Biopsy

This is used in obscure and difficult cases of diffuse alveolar disease and for solid tumours. Experts are cautious in the application of these techniques, which may cause pneumothorax, occasionally haemorrhage, and, rarely, air embolism. The hazards are common to all methods. The safest instrument is the high speed trephine, but the technique is difficult to learn and the initial failure rate high. Though rarely dangerous, pneumothorax requiring aspiration occurs quite often. The acquisition of histological information should be important enough to management to justify the inconvenience of the procedure. The procedure is safer in consolidated lung or solid tumour.

Thoracotomy

Excision biopsy may be the only way of excluding malignancy when X-ray shows a peripherally placed lesion. It is preferred to percutaneous needle biopsy if one lesion is resectable, to avoid the risk of spread. Thoracotomy and biopsy may be employed to diagnose pleural lesions. Occasionally, open biopsy is used to diagnose diffuse lung diseases.

Technique of Chest Aspiration and Pleural Biopsy (*see* section on pleural effusions)

Fluid in the pleural cavity may be aspirated through a needle and subjected to chemical analysis, microscopy and culture. The first choice of site is indicated in Fig. 18.24. If this area is not dull to percussion, one space lower may be attempted (after checking the X-ray to make sure that the lesion is not anterior), but the effusion is likely to be thin and small. Failure is usually because of going too low, thus entering the diaphragm and subphrenic structures and failing to obtain fluid.

Pleural Biopsy. Pleural biopsy employing Abrams' needle is simple when an effusion is present.

Biopsy of a Scalene Lymph Node. This may yield histological diagnosis of sarcoidosis, lymphoma or neoplasm.

FATE OF INHALED PARTICLES

Deposition

Particles greater than 20 μ are nearly all deposited by sedimentation on the upper airway (e.g. visible dust).
Particles of 5 to 20 μ are deposited on nasal and bronchial airway (e.g. many pollutants).
Particles less than 0.1 μ diffuse towards the bronchial walls.
Particles 0.1 to 5 μ penetrate the alveoli. Most are exhaled because they sediment slowly (many aerosols, fibrogenic mineral dusts).

Clearance of Non-toxic Particles

Dust and non-pathogenic organisms are cleared from healthy bronchi by mucociliary action in two hours.

Clearance from alveoli is by the alveolar macrophage system in about five hours. Secretory IgA in bronchial mucus may inactivate organisms.

Damage by Inhaled Particles

This depends on the immunological response and the toxicity of the agent to phagocytes and macrophages. Phagocytosis may kill a non-pathogenic organism, or remove an inert particle. If the ingested material is toxic to leucocytes (e.g. pyogenic bacteria) or macrophages (e.g. silica) the cells are killed with liberation of mediators of inflammation and fibrosis.

ACUTE INFECTIONS OF THE AIR PASSAGES

MINOR RESPIRATORY INFECTIONS IN HEALTHY ADULTS

Background

Viruses cause a number of very common syndromes of upper respiratory tract infection, which are separated for convenience but which overlap. The viruses listed below have in common:

1. Spread by droplet infection.
2. Isolation of virus for 48 to 96 hours after onset.
3. Short incubation period.
4. High infectivity in the early stages.
5. Occasional serious complications in susceptible victims.

Viral syndromes affecting the upper respiratory tract

Common cold:

Rhinoviruses
Respiratory syncytial viruses (RSV)
Parainfluenza
Occasional enteroviruses (Coxsackie, Echo)

Pharyngo-conjunctivitis:

Adenovirus
Influenza, parainfluenza
Enteroviruses

Croup:

Parainfluenza
RSV
Adenovirus
Influenza

Viruses may be isolated from the whole respiratory mucosa and upper respiratory syndromes are associated with demonstrable but often asymptomatic bronchial disease.

Pathological changes in the respiratory tract persist for four to six weeks.

Similar symptoms may occur during systemic illnesses such as influenza, typhoid, and bubonic plague.

(Ring a ring of roses, a pocket full of posies,
Atishoo, atishoo, we all fall down.)

COMMON COLD

Symptoms and Signs

Increased nasal discharge, first watery, then mucous
Nasal obstruction with mucosal swelling, watery eyes, conjunctival inflammation
Sore throat, felt in the soft palate and nasopharynx
Systemic upset (fever, aching muscles, headache) is usually mild and often absent.

Complications

Middle ear pain caused by Eustachian tube obstruction with retention of serous fluid.
Bacterial otitis media. Pharyngeal commensal organisms such as *Strep. pneumoniae*, *H. influenzae* and *Strep. pyogenes* may be responsible: many are susceptible to benzyl penicillin or to ampicillin.
Osteomyelitis of the mastoid bones (mastoiditis), formerly a dreaded complication of otitis media, is now very rare and more cases are caused by *Pseudomonas aeruginosa* than formerly.
Recurrent otitis media is common among children, notably those with large adenoids. Even minor deafness may cause learning difficulties and under-achievement at school.

Sinusitis. The maxillary antra are most commonly affected. Nasal mucosal oedema prevents drainage with retention of secretions. Secondary bacterial infection, usually by *Strep. pneumoniae* and *H. influenzae* results in pus which fills the sinuses. Facial pain, which may radiate widely, is accompanied by local tenderness. Tetracyclines are transported well into infected sinuses and bring rapid relief in most acute cases. They are indicated when the nasal secretions do not drain spontaneously after the nasal swelling subsides.

Local or systemic alpha-adrenergic agents such as pseudoephedrine cause reduction of nasal congestion for short periods of time. They may aid discharge of serous secretions from the middle ear and nasal sinuses and are prescribed for patients with recurrent colds to prevent nasal congestion and possibly abort sinusitis.

PHARYNGITIS AND TONSILLITIS

'Sore throat' occurs when there is infection of the tonsils, the lymph nodes draining them and pharangeal lymphoid tissue. Pain and discomfort in swallowing are greatest after lying down and relieved by salicylates. Fever and neck stiffness occur. The tonsils and throat appear swollen; initially pale, they become 'injected' with visible blood vessels and then red. Conjunctivitis occurs frequently. *Mycoplasma penumoniae* presents in the same way: epidemics caused by this organism probably account for those cases which appear to respond dramatically to tetracyclines or erythromycin.

Streptococcal Tonsillitis (*Strep. pyogenes*). This is less common than it was. Fever and malaise are dramatic, pain may be intense. The tonsillar surface is pustular and there may be a yellow membrane over the whole tonsil.

Bacteriological examination of a *tonsillar swab* yields the diagnosis.

Complications

Streptococcal infections, if not treated with bactericidal drugs such as benzylpenicillin in adequate doses, may be complicated by acute glomerulonephritis, rheumatic fever, or chorea (*see* page 294). These are now rare, as is peritonsillar abscess (quinsy). The incidence started to fall before the advent of chemotherapy. A few strains cause scarlet fever.

Basis of Treatment of Streptococcal Tonsillitis

Treatment is with penicillin. Severe cases should receive intramuscular benzylpenicillin; most will respond to oral penicillin (erythromycin for patients allergic to penicillin).

Oropharyngeal Thrush

Infection of the mouth by the saprophytic yeast *C. albicans* is characterised by white plaques of fungus on the pharynx and palate which peel easily ('thrush'). Rare in healthy individuals, this may complicate treatment with broad spectrum antibiotics (which kill the resident saprophytic bacteria) and with oral or inhaled corticosteroid drugs. It is often found when immunity is defective. The infection may spread to the oesophagus or, rarely, the lungs (although candida is found often in sputum). The infection may be eradicated by sucking lozenges, or inhaling sprays of nystatin, amphotericin B or other antifungal antibiotics which are not absorbed when swallowed. Infection recurs in susceptible individuals. False teeth should be treated.

LARYNGOTRACHEITIS

Laryngeal infection causes cough, loss of voice, loss of vocalisation during cough, pain in the throat. Tracheitis causes cough and a sore sensation or pain behind the sternum. The symptoms are aggravated by cold and dryness and eased by steam. Laryngeal obstruction is rare in adults except when there is laryngeal paralysis. In children under four the laryngeal airway is small enough to close if the mucosa swells, a process aided by adherence of mucus and by reflex adduction of the vocal cords. This causes a characteristic noisy inspiration (stridor, 'croup') and a distressing sensation of inspiratory obstruction in the throat. Hyperventilation precedes respiratory failure. Most cases are viral.

Basis of Treatment of Croup

If the child is active, the mother should fill a small room, for example the bathroom, with steam and support the child by sitting him upright on her knee. This reduces hyperventilation and laryngeal adduction, aids expectoration of mucus, and may cause apparent relief. The development or persistence of cyanosis, tachycardia of 140 or more or persistence of obvious inspiratory difficulty, necessitates admission to hospital. This is discussed further (*see* page 367, ventilatory failure).

ACUTE BRONCHITIS

The symptoms are fever, cough and shortness of breath. At first sputum is absent, frothy or mucous. Secondary bacterial infection causes purulent sputum. If the bronchial tree is previously healthy, this usually remits spontaneously with regression to mucoid sputum and resolution of the cough in two to six weeks. Recurrent acute bronchitis of childhood is a manifestation of allergic disorders, more rarely cystic fibrosis and very rarely immune deficiency, especially IgG deficiency.

POTENTIALLY SERIOUS RESPIRATORY INFECTIONS

DIPHTHERIA (*see* page 24, infectious diseases)

EPIGLOTTITIS

A rare epidemic infection of children and adults with capsulated Type B *H. influenzae* may cause swelling of the epiglottis and aryepiglottic folds. After a few hours of minor respiratory symptoms the patient develops sore throat, dysphagia for saliva (dribbling is the alerting sign in children) muffling of the voice as opposed to hoarsening, progressing to restlessness and prostration. The uvula is oedematous. In adults, laryngoscopy shows the red swollen redundant epiglottis which may also be demonstrated by lateral X-rays of the neck. The lesion may be visible with depression of a child's tongue (*dangerous*). Throat swabs and blood culture are often positive for *H. influenzae*. Microabscesses are present in the epiglottis; the glottis is rarely infected.

Basis of Treatment

Treatment, as for meningitis caused by capsulated *H. influenzae*, is parenteral chloramphenicol, or parenteral ampicillin in high doses (15 to 20 g/day in adults: strains resistant to ampicillin are emerging. Hydrocortisone may reduce swelling. Tracheostomy may be needed. There is a significant mortality, reduced by early treatment.

BRONCHIOLITIS

An acute infection of the respiratory tract with serious obstructive swelling of bronchioles, usually affecting infants under two years. Most cases are caused by the respiratory syncytial virus. The manifestations are cough, signs of airways obstruction with hyperinflation of the chest and limpness. Treatment consists of hydration, oxygenation and artificial ventilation if P_{CO_2} rises. Corticosteroids, bronchodilators and antibiotics are ineffective.

WHOOPING COUGH (Pertussis see page 22)

Chronic respiratory illness (bronchiectasis) commonly follows unmodified pertussis.

INFLUENZA

An endemic, epidemic and occasionally world-wide (pandemic) illness, causing fever, rigors and muscle pains with upper and lower respiratory symptoms of varying severity. Complications include myocarditis, polyneuritis, myelopathy, encephalitis. Pneumonia is discussed later.

Epidemiology

There are three major strains (A, B, C), epidemics of the first two occurring every two or three years. Pandemics occurred in 1969, 1957, 1918 and 1889. The disease kills a higher proportion of those with chronic heart and lung disease. The attack rate is highest in pandemics, which follow antigenic mutation to forms against which there is no naturally occurring antibody. Cross-immunity between strains is slight. Vaccination confers partial immunity for one to two years at the cost of a significant short febrile illness which may cause serious disability in those most susceptible. Preparation of vaccines against new strains is not usually sufficiently rapid to avoid pandemics. The prophylactic administration of antiviral drugs is being studied. There are no drugs which alter the course of the established infection, apart from those which attack established bacterial pathogens.

Incubation period: 24 to 48 hours.
Excretion of virus: 2 days to 1 week.

PNEUMONIA

Definition

Pneumonia generally means any inflammation of the alveoli and their walls. The pneumonias have in common inflammatory cells and exudate in the alveolar walls and the alveolar spaces. When the latter are filled there are signs of consolidation.

The unnecessary and additional term 'pneumonitis' is occasionally used to indicate that the inflammation is minor ('subsegmental pneumonitis') or not infective ('chemical pneumonitis'). A new word 'alveolitis' is employed in the UK to describe inflammations of the alveolar wall not caused by infection or neoplasia ('fibrosing alveolitis', known in the USA as interstitial pneumonia).

Background

Classification of the pneumonias is best done on the basis of anatomical distribution of the detectable lesions and supposed cause, for example lobar pneumonia caused by Strep. pneumoniae.

Classification of pneumonias

Anatomical:
Lobar
Segmental
Lobular (bronchopneumonia)

Aetiological:
Viral, primary or complicated
Bacterial, primary or secondary
Fungal
Mycobacterial
Protozoal
Chemical
Physical, e.g. radiation
Allergic and 'autoimmune'

Classical descriptions of the condition distinguished lobar and bronchopneumonia. Lobar pneumonia was an acute illness of healthy adults caused by pneumococci, preceded by a 'cold' or exposure to cold and wet conditions. It lasted ten days, and resolved by crisis with a rapid subsidence of the fever and return of well-being thanks to the development of antibody. Most cases recovered: occasionally fever subsided gradually or recurred, thus indicating healing with excessive fibrosis and residual infection in the lungs or pleura. The mortality was between 20 per cent and 50 per cent: devoted physicians and nurses used to wait up all of the tenth night for the 'crisis'. This practice did a lot for the image of the family doctor who shared the family's relief or sorrow at the outcome in fact and in fiction.

Hippocrates recognised that fever and cough in an ill young man had a good prognosis (lobar pneumonia). If the patient appeared well, the outcome was likely to be fatal (pulmonary tuberculosis).

Bronchopneumonia was a killing disease of the young, the very old and the debilitated, as well as taking its toll as a complication of influenza (the 'old man's friend'). The role of viruses was not known until after chemotherapy had altered the course of bacterial pneumonia, but most bacterial cases were caused by staphylococci and streptococci with permanent damage to the most affected lobules in those who recovered.

An account now follows of the manifestations and principles of diagnosis and treatment common to all infectious pneumonias. Some important types are then discussed insofar as they have features which are additional or different.

Symptoms

Upper respiratory symptoms.
Fever, rigors.
Cough.
Sputum – absent, mucoid, watery, blood-tinged in viral illness. Purulent when a pyogenic organism is present.
Pleuritic chest pain in bacterial cases, rare in others.
Dyspnoea at rest.
Confusion (usually with hypoxaemia; common in the elderly).

Signs and X-rays

1. The presence of lower respiratory infection is diagnosed by rapid breathing, cyanosis or arterial blood gas disturbance, usually hypoxaemia with low $P{CO_2}$.
2. Clinical and radiological signs of consolidation do not always overlap. When present, they aid diagnosis:

Bronchiolo-alveolar inflammation: patches of inspiratory râles.

Consolidation: (dense) bronchial breathing, increased vocal resonance and whispering pectoriloquy (resolving) râles.

Pleural inflammation: pleural rub or effusion (*see* page 365).

Investigations and Differential Diagnosis

Pointers to the cause are:
1. Virus washing of throat (in first 48 hours of illness).
2. Acute and convalescent serum for viral antibodies (useful in epidemics and for retrospective diagnosis).
3. Culture and microscopy of sputum.
4. Rarely, aspiration of bronchi or lung.
5. Blood culture (positive in 50 per cent of fulminating bacterial pneumonias).
6. Differential blood count, for polymorphonuclear

leucocytosis (bacterial origin), eosinophilic leucocytosis (allergic conditions).

Complications

Pleurisy and pleural effusion are much more common after bacterial than viral pneumonia. Empyema (pus in the pleural cavity) is now rare.
Poor resolution, leading to abscess formation or fibrosis.

Basis of Treatment

Specific chemotherapy: the general principles of initial treatment are described below:

All Forms of Life-threatening Pneumonia. Rapid deterioration is most likely to be due to staphylococci, streptococci, pneumococci, haemophilus or klebsiella. Combinations of benzylpenicillin, flucloxacillin, and aminoglycoside drugs or certain cephalosporins have a suitable spectrum.

Lobar pneumonia. This is usually due to *Strep. pneumoniae:* use benzylpencillin.

Mild Pneumonia of Non-lobar Distribution. The use of tetracycline or erythromycin will eradicate *Mycoplasma pneumoniae* and *Strep. pneumoniae* in most cases and is recommended when mycoplasma is epidemic. Penicillin or ampicillin are more effective when *Strep. pneumoniae* is the pathogen.

Pneumonia Complicating Debilitation or Alcoholism. Gram-negative organisms and anaerobes are common (especially in the USA). Gentamicin with clindamycin, sometimes with penicillin, sometimes with metronidazole are drugs of first choice.

In all cases, material obtained for bacterial examination before treatment improves management of those patients who fail to respond in 24 to 48 hours.

Other treatments include oxygen for hypoxaemia and analgesics for pleuritic pain (aspirin and paracetamol or a mild opiate if necessary). If sputum becomes copious or abscess formation occurs, physiotherapy with postural drainage is prescribed. Little physiotherapy can be tolerated during the acute phase.

BACTERIAL PNEUMONIAS OF LOBAR DISTRIBUTION

PNEUMOCOCCAL PNEUMONIA

Definition

Pneumonia, usually of lobar distribution caused by *Strep. pneumoniae.*

Background

Classical lobar pneumonia (*see also* page 332) is caused by the pneumococcus (*Strep. pneumoniae*). The organism is inhaled. There is usually a predisposition to the retention of aspirated material or some factor which affects mucociliary clearance, for example, upper respiratory infection in the preceding 14 days, an alcoholic bout, possibly prolonged exposure to cold. The illness is of abrupt onset with chest pain, chills and the expectoration of rusty sputum. Estimates of the mortality of the untreated disorder were from 20 per cent to 50 per cent. Healing was accompanied by 'crisis' (sudden resolution of the fever and symptoms after five to eleven days) or by 'lysis' – a more gradual resolution. The incidence was beginning to fall before the introduction of sulphonamides (1935) and penicillin (1943) which have reduced the mortality to a small fraction.

Pathology

The characteristic naked eye changes are seen in the affected lobes – initially there is exudation of serous fluid into the alveolar spaces where bacteria can be found. Haemorrhage follows (red hepatisation), then the arrival of polymorphs (grey hepatisation) and macrophages which engulf them about this time that the alveolar fluid becomes sterile. Pneumococcal pneumonia is remarkable for the complete restoration of the lung architecture in most cases without fibrosis. Fibrosis and scarring occurred more commonly when there was resolution by 'lysis'.

Symptoms

Minor respiratory infection for a few days.
Abrupt onset of fever, chills, malaise; *later*, reddish-brown sputum, cough and dyspnoea.
Chest pain is pleuritic, may affect shoulder tip (diaphragmatic pleurisy).
Abdominal pain is a common diagnostic trap.

Signs

Labial herpes is common.
Mild cyanosis, tachypnoea.
Initially lobar consolidation, with bronchial breathing, whispering pectoriloquy, increased fremitus, later coarse râles. Signs are anterior and in the axilla in upper and middle lobe disease.
Confusion, occasionally related to fever and blood gas disturbance.

Investigations

1. Chest X-ray shows lobar or segmental consolidation, usually confirming the clinical signs.
2. Blood culture (positive in 50 per cent).
3. Sputum culture – pneumococci readily isolated in untreated cases.
4. Polymorphonuclear leuococytosis, often greater than 20 per fl.

Complications

Septicaemia.
Pleural effusion – serous or purulent, may precede empyema in inadequately treated cases.
Pericarditis.
Meningitis.
Peritonitis.
Arthritis.
Dehydration.
Circulatory collapse.
Slow resolution with pulmonary fibrosis.

Differential Diagnosis

1. Other pneumonias.
2. Pneumonia distal to malignant bronchial obstruction.
3. Pulmonary infarction. (Haemoptysis is usually bright red, fever and systemic upset slight or absent, leucocytosis rare.)

Basis of Treatment (specific)

Benzylpenicillin, 1 to 2 g six-hourly IM or possibly IV. May need to be combined with other antibiotics for severely ill patients who may have staphylococcal, klebsiella or other bacterial pneumonia until diagnosis confirmed. Other penicillins are less effective: bacteriostatic therapy may not prevent empyema if effusion develops.
Larger doses of benzylpenicillin needed for severely septicaemic patients with peritonitis or meningitis.

Prognosis

Response to penicillin is accompanied by a brisk fall of temperature to subnormal levels, like a crisis, sometimes followed by a low-grade fever for a few days. Serous pleural effusions occupying less than one-quarter of the hemithorax clear spontaneously, but increasing purulence increases the likelihood of residual pleural fibrosis: purulent effusions should be aspirated. Diagnostic aspiration is necessary in all instances.
The mortality with penicillin (or cephalosporins in allergic subjects) is less than five per cent.

Strep. pyogenes rarely causes a pneumonia which may behave in the same ways as pneumococcal pneumonia. The condition responds to benzylpenicillin in adequate doses: empyemas and post-streptococcal complications occur more commonly if inadequate doses of oral penicillins or tetracyclines are used.

Klebsiella pneumoniae and *Staph. pyogenes* may affect mainly one lobe. These cause pulmonary suppuration and invariably heal with fibrosis: residual cysts are common (Fig. 18.15).

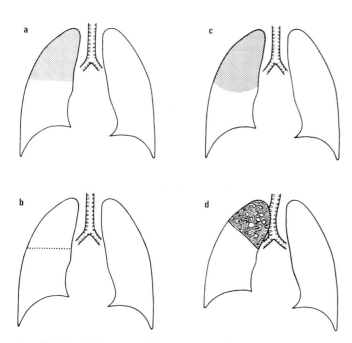

Fig. 18.15   Right upper lobe pneumonia.
(a) and (b) Pneumococcal: resolution with pleural thickening, restoration of lung architecture.
(c) and (d) Suppurative (e.g. Klebsiella): (c) bulging shadow; (d) resolution with fibrosis and cavitation.

Kleb. pneumoniae (Friedlander's bacillus) causes a specific pneumonia, most commonly seen above the age of 45 and associated with alcoholism and poor hygiene. The illness starts abruptly and may lead rapidly to prostration or may cause a prolonged illness, especially when treated with antibiotics such as ampicillin to which the organism is not adequately sensitive. The characteristic features which distinguish it are the expectoration of brownish, gelatinous sputum and the intense inflammatory alveolar oedema which often makes the lobe appear to bulge beyond its anatomical confines. Treatment is by the aminoglycoside drugs, tetracycline 2 g/day orally, chloramphenicol or cotrimoxazole. Penicillins and cephalosporins are inactive. Mortality remains high in fulminating cases. Affected lobes are destroyed.

PYOGENIC LUNG ABSCESS

Definition

A suppurative focus in the lung, associated with necrosis of tissue.

Background

Abscess formation is part of suppurative pneumonias and bronchiectasis: the term is reserved for lesions which are primary. These follow the inhalation of infected material: periodontal infection is a common source.

Inhalation occurs in sleep: distribution of abscesses depends on sleeping position.

Bacteriology

Mixtures of aerobic pyogenic organisms and anaerobes are found.

Symptoms

Fever, chills.
Pleurisy. Sudden expectoration of large volumes of pus.
Signs may be absent apart from occasional pleural rubs.

Investigations

1. Characteristic chest X-ray. Wall may be thin and regular (Fig. 18.16).

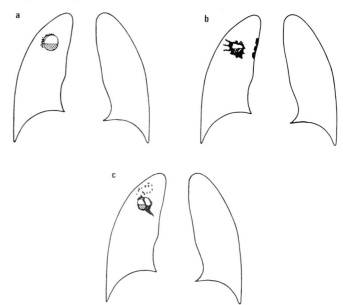

Fig. 18.16   Cavitating lung lesions.
(a) Lung abscess: wall regular, thin.
(b) Necrotising carcinoma of the bronchus: wall irregular, thick; peripheral spread; sometimes hilar node enlargement.
(c) TB: multiple variegate lesion; (sometimes) appearance of radiation from hilum.

2. Polymorphonuclear leucocytosis, rarely positive blood cultures.
3. Sputum culture for aerobes and anaerobes.

Basis of Treatment

Mobilisation if possible.
Antibiotics. *If ambulant*, flucloxacillin, ampicillin, metronidazole: *if ill*, aminoglycoside with clindamycin or metronidazole.
Bronchoscopy, if resolution does not occur within two weeks, to exclude endobronchial obstruction.
Bronchoscopy immediately if there is a history of inhalation of a foreign body.
Rarely, surgical excision of chronic benign lesion.

Differential Diagnosis

1. Carcinoma of the bronchus.
2. Pulmonary tuberculosis.
3. Amoebiasis.

NON-LOBAR PNEUMONIAS

NON-LOBAR PNEUMONIA CAUSED BY PYOGENIC BACTERIA (BRONCHOPNEUMONIA)

Definition

Patchy suppuration of the alveoli spreading from bronchioles.

Background

Aspiration of infected material in the presence of impaired immunity or bronchial clearance mechanisms. Predisposing causes include viral infection, malignancy, heart failure, chronic bronchitis, prolonged immobility, chest injury, surgical operation and coma. The disease is often bilateral and usually involves the lung bases.

Bacteriology

After virus infections, especially influenza, *Strep. pneumoniae*, *Staph. pyogenes* and *Strep. pyogenes* are the most commonly found pathogens; *H. influenzae* and *Strep. pneumoniae* in chronic bronchitis and in postoperative cases. Gram-negative enterobacilli frequently cause pneumonia and septicaemia especially in alcoholics and those with liver disease.

Symptoms and Signs

Cough.
Purulent sputum.
Fever, which may be moderate.
Rapid respirations.
Signs of consolidation.

Investigations

1. Sputum culture, blood culture.
2. Arterial blood gases.

Basis of Treatment

Specific antibacterial chemotherapy.
Assisted coughing and deep breathing.
Oxygen therapy.

ACUTE PNEUMONIA CAUSED BY VIRUSES AND SIMILAR ORGANISMS (Table 18.3)

Pneumonia of varying severity may be caused by a number of organisms which are not cultured easily, some of which respond to antibacterial agents. Formerly considered as large viruses, they are now classified separately.

The onset of the respiratory illness may be insidious or acute. Fever is often out of proportion to pulse rate or clinical condition. The presence of alveolar disease is detected by tachypnoea, hypoxaemia, reduction of vital capacity, râles and radiological shadowing. Chest X-ray changes may not match clinical signs or fit into segmental anatomy. Sputum is absent or mucoid, leucocytosis unusual. The organisms are not isolated in routine laboratories, the diagnosis usually being serological and confirmed during convalescence by a fourfold rise in circulating humoral antibody two to six weeks after the onset of the illness. Lung suppuration and pleural effusions are unusual, though they may occur. Pulmonary function tends to remain impaired for several months after clinical recovery, suggesting that the process is often widespread.

1. *MYCOPLASMA PNEUMONIAE* PNEUMONIA (PREVIOUS SYNONYMS: PRIMARY ATYPICAL PNEUMONIA, EATON AGENT PNEUMONIA)

This organism is epidemic in England, about every three years. Usually causing pharyngitis, myringitis and otitis, it is occasionally responsible for acute pneumonia. Incubation takes one to three weeks. The disease may be prolonged, treatment being relatively ineffective if started after a few days of fever. Complications (rare) are polyarthritis, haemolytic anaemia, erythema multiforme, renal failure. Cold agglutinins are found in the blood in about 50 per cent of cases after two days. Prompt treatment of upper and lower respiratory infections with erythromycin or tetracycline is worthwhile when this organism is epidemic.

2. PSITTACOSIS (ORNITHOSIS)

Parrots, budgerigars, pigeons, ducks and turkeys and humans may be infected by this organism, which may

Table 18.3 Pneumonias caused by specific non-bacterial organisms

Organism	Characteristic features	Specific treatment	Pathology
Varicella	Commoner now in adults, mortality 20% Multiple small shadows which calcify		Multiple small haemorrhages.
Measles	Often secondary bacterial infection, primary commoner in children with chronic illnesses	–	Giant cell and round cell infiltration of alveolar walls
Adenovirus	May cause very destructive bronchiectasis if complicating measles	–	
Influenza	Primary less common than secondary bacterial infection: often fatal, with bronchial mucosal necrosis and lung haemorrhage	–	Round cell infiltrate in alveolar walls with intra-alveolar haemorrhage and exudate
Mycoplasma pneumoniae	Epidemic and endemic Lobar, single or multiple; segmental or multiple nodular shadows	T E	Pathology may be similar to lobar pneumonia with considerable alveolar wall inflammation in areas which are less affected
Coxiella (Q fever)	Caught from farm animals, manure Segmental or nodular shadows	T C?	
Psittacosis	Bird or human vectors Segmental or nodular shadows	T C?	
Legionnaires' bacillus	Newly described, may be very severe Epidemic and a few sporadic cases Lobar or segmental changes often.	E	

T = tetracycline 2 g/day oral adult dose.
E = erythromycin 2 g/day oral adult dose.
C = chloramphenicol 1 g/day oral adult dose.

be caught from convalescent or well birds. The incubation period is seven to fourteen days or longer. Particular features include relative bradycardia, late development of X-ray changes, occasional hepatosplenomegaly, erythema nodosum and rose spots.

3. Q FEVER (*COXIELLA BURNETI*) (*see* page 29)

4. LEGIONNAIRES' DISEASE

A newly described epidemic febrile illness (1976 American Legion Convention at Philadelphia) causing pneumonia, often lobar, frequently severe and usually without pleural effusion. The organism is a coccobacillus, still unclassified (1977), grown with difficulty on eggs and identified by silver staining lungs and by a rise of fluorescent antibody titre. Several previous epidemics are known to have been caused by this. Erythromycin is probably the drug of choice.

LOWER RESPIRATORY INFECTIONS SECONDARY TO OTHER CONDITIONS

PNEUMONIA DISTAL TO BRONCHIAL OBSTRUCTION

Benign tumours, malignant tumours and inhaled foreign bodies are occasionally causes of pneumonia and of delayed resolution. In the absence of specific virological diagnosis, diagnostic bronchoscopy is usually advised if pneumonia fails to resolve after six weeks. *Peanuts* are often inhaled, especially if tossed into the mouth. The irritant peanut oil causes swelling of the bronchial mucosa; partial collapse becomes complete over one to two days. This condition should be suspected in children with cough and segmental lung shadowing. Bronchoscopic removal is necessary, as the peanut becomes wedged.

ASPIRATION PNEUMONIA

The aspiration of food may cause recurrent 'bronchopneumonia', diffuse lung fibrosis and attacks of nocturnal choking or wheezing.
   Causes include:
   Neurogenic dysphagia.
   Oesophageal reflux.
   Strictures of the oesophagus, especially benign lesions, achalasia, pharyngeal pouch.
Inhalation of gastric acid may cause severe respiratory failure, with inflammatory oedema and secondary infection. When occurring during childbirth this is called Mendelson's syndrome.

POSTOPERATIVE CHEST INFECTIONS

Collapse and consolidation of the lower lung lobes is common after surgery, occurring in 80 per cent of smokers with upper abdominal wounds (but only 10 per cent of non-smokers with lower abdominal incisions). The vital capacity is decreased by about one-half after major operation. Coughing and deep breathing are painful and may be suppressed. These predispose to mucus retention. Pathogenic organisms are almost always found in the sputum (usually *Strep. pneumoniae* and *H. influenzae*). These are the cause of lung infection. Prophylactic bactericidal antibiotics reduce the incidence of postoperative pneumonia but this practice has disadvantages and is not generally recommended. The lesions are usually well established by 24 hours. Chest infections are the major cause of pyrexia in the first two days after an operation. Prophylactic physiotherapy, given early, is under trial. Treatment is with physiotherapy, mobilisation in mild cases, and antibiotics in severe or persistent cases. The mortality is under one per cent and the long term effect on lung function unknown.

INFECTED PULMONARY INFARCT

Less than one in ten of pulmonary infarcts become infected, but when they do, anaerobic organisms are often present.

PNEUMONIA IN THE PRESENCE OF ABNORMAL IMMUNE RESPONSE

Patients receiving immunosuppressive therapy are subject to overwhelming infections with pathogenic bacteria and to symptomatic, often terminal, infections caused by ubiquitous saprophytic organisms. Steroid drugs given in daily doses equivalent to 30 mg prednisolone given for several weeks provoke the same hazard.

Treatment, which may prolong life, depends on accurate diagnosis. Open lung biopsy is most reliable. Alternatively the diagnosis may often be made by sputum cytology and culture, fine needle aspiration of the lung, bronchoscopic lung biopsy and percutaneous lung biopsy. Notable are the following:

Cytomegalovirus Pneumonia

Systemic Candidiasis. Invasive pulmonary candidiasis is very rare; culture of aspirated lung material is required to establish the diagnosis because *C. albicans* is often isolated from sputum.

Pneumocystis carinii Pneumonia.

Epidemic 50 years ago in European orphanages, this disease affects marasmic babies and patients being treated for leukaemia and by renal transplantation. The organism,
a protozoon, causes interstitial and alveolar pneumonia. Presentation is with cough, dyspnoea and fever. The X-ray appearances resemble bilateral pulmonary oedema, without any obscuring of the hila. Treatment is with pentamidine isethionate 2 to 4 mg/kg daily or trimethoprim 20 mg/kg with sulphafurazole 80 mg/kg/day. The mortality is 30 per cent with treatment, 100 per cent in immunosuppressed patients and 50 per cent in untreated infants. There is considerable residual pulmonary fibrosis after recovery.

Diffuse Pulmonary Cryptococcosis. *Cryptococcus neoformans* may produce a similar interstitial pneumonia. There may be a response to systemic antifungal agents such as amphotericin or miconazole.

NON-INFECTIVE PNEUMONIAS

EXOGENOUS LIPOID PNEUMONIA

This is consolidation caused by the inhalation of oily material (commoner in the days of oily nose drops and liquid paraffin treatment).

CHEMICAL PNEUMONIA

Acute respiratory illnesses may be caused by the inhalation of agents such as petroleum, burning plastics, and a wide variety of irritant gases, for example ammonia, nitrogen dioxide. Cough with mucoid frothy sputum and dyspnoea are the main presenting features. Radiological shadowing may be patchy or absent. Bronchial and pulmonary oedema may dominate the findings. Bronchiolar fibrosis with permanent bronchiolar stenosis may ensue. Corticosteroids are often given in the acute phase: their value has not been subjected to trial or experiment.

RADIATION PNEUMONIA

Radiotherapy to wide areas of lung or mediastinum may cause alveolar wall inflammation with intimal proliferation leading to occlusion of arterioles. This causes dry cough and dyspnoea starting one to twenty weeks, usually three to six weeks, after treatment. The symptoms subside in four to six months, usually with good symptomatic recovery but permanent reduction of vital capacity. On X-ray the hila are usually obscured with lung opacification and septal thickening. Irradiated lungs are susceptible to infection.

EOSINOPHILIC PNEUMONIA (pulmonary eosinophilia, Löffler's syndrome)

Widespread or localised consolidation, with dense infiltration by eosinophilic granulocytes and blood

eosinphilia (>1.0 cells/fl). Caused most commonly by:
Aspergillus fumigatus (*see* page 340) – about half of English cases.
Migrating ascarial and filarial larvae (tropical eosinophilia, *see* pages 350 and 595).
Polyarteritis nodosa.
Drug allergy.

Non-productive cough and dyspnoea, usually of insidious onset are the main features. Sputum, when present, looks purulent, but grows no bacterial pathogens and contains more than 25 per cent eosinophils.

Corticosteroids relieve the symptoms and signs. Maintenance may be required when the cause cannot be eradicated. Diethylcarbamazine kills microfilariae and is used in tropical cases, but some require corticosteroids for relief.

TUBERCULOSIS

Definition

An infection by the tubercle bacillus (*Mycobacterium tuberculosis*) in the lungs and elsewhere characterised by granulomatous lesions which tend to become necrotic and heal by fibrosis.

This section deals mainly with pulmonary tuberculosis.

Background

The discovery, between 1948 and 1952, of effective antituberculous chemotherapy, has hastened the end of a pandemic of tuberculosis of 400 years' duration, which reached its height in the UK 100 years ago. Where overcrowding and poor nutrition persist, the incidence remains higher (India, South East Asia). New cases are now notified in England at a rate of 10 to 20 per 100,000 per year: the mortality is very low, deaths occurring mainly in the elderly and in occasional undiagnosed cases. About half of the cases notified in the UK are in patients born in Asia.

Two strains have caused disease, *human* and *bovine*, easily differentiated in culture. Infection with the bovine strain is by ingestion in milk. The bovine strain is virtually extinct in N. America, the UK and Scandinavia. It is still found in Europe. Unboiled cow's milk is not drunk much in Asia and Africa.

Spread of the human strain is by inhalation of heavily infected droplets. Resistance to infection is lowered by:
Malnutrition and alcoholism.
Diabetes mellitus.
Smoking.
Corticosteroid drugs (given long term) and immunosuppression.
Silicosis.
Pregnancy.

Health care workers have always had a higher risk than others. Other examples of occupational incidence probably reflect economic status and the fact that it is possible to continue working when ill for longer in jobs not requiring extremes of physical activity.

Bacteriology

Koch discovered the acid alcohol-fast bacillus (AAFB) which can be stained by the Ziehl-Nielsen technique in smears of sputum, concentrated urine and cerebrospinal fluid. The organism grows in six weeks on special media. The guinea pig is highly susceptible, but inoculation is now used rarely as laboratory culture gives almost as good results.

Primary and Post-primary Infection: The Tuberculin Test

The changes caused by *M. tuberculosis* depend on the number of infecting organisms and on the immune state of the patient. The initial exposure is the *primary* infection, which normally provokes hypersensitivity in six weeks ('Type IV', cell-mediated hypersensitivity appears to correlate with clinical response). Subsequently, reinfection or recrudescence of dormant organisms causes 'post-primary' disease.

Hypersensitivity is identified by means of the *tuberculin test*. Standardised preparations of capsular protein injected into the skin cause local inflammation, with induration, erythema and perhaps blistering 48 to 72 hours after injection. The *Mantoux* test consists of the sequential *intradermal* injection of 1, 10 and occasionally 100 tuberculin units (TU) in 0.1 ml of saline (0.1 ml of 1/10,000, 1/1,000 and 1/100 tuberculin respectively). A wheal of more than 1 cm diameter is unequivocally positive and when obtained with 10 TU indicates infection at some time with *M. tuberculosis* antigens. Very large eruptions indicate current disease. The reaction usually remains positive, but becomes progressively weaker over 20 to 40 years. Weak reactions may occur as a result of exposure to atypical mycobacteria. The international standard for research is the response to 5 TU.

The Heaf multiple puncture test, employing a concentrated purified antigenic protein is a convenient substitute.

Positive tuberculin tests correlate with *in vitro* evidence of sensitisation of lymphocytes.

PRIMARY TUBERCULOUS INFECTION

Where the disease is common, this occurs in childhood. The organisms set up a minor inflammatory reaction at the site of entry and spread rapidly to regional lymph nodes where inflammation is brisk. Some degree of blood borne dissemination may occur at this stage. The commonest manifestation is a small area of consolidation near the periphery of the middle and lower lobes of the lungs, with hilar adenopathy; the adenopathy is predominant in children and is often bilateral in Asian patients. Tonsillar infection with cervical adenopathy and intestinal entry with mesenteric node tuberculosis were more common formerly. Clinical manifestations may go unnoticed:

Malaise.
Loss of well-being.
Weight loss or failure to grow.
Brief febrile illness.
Cough.
Occasionally, erythema nodosum or phlyctenular conjunctivitis.

Symptoms usually accompany conversion to a positive tuberculin test.

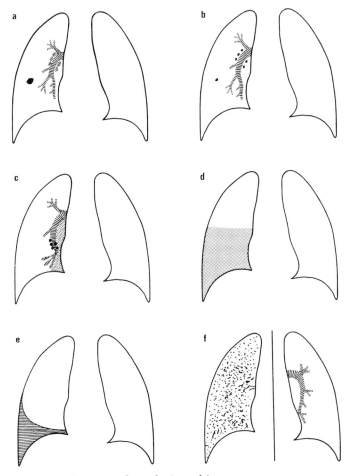

Fig. 18.17 Primary tuberculosis and its consequences:
(a) Primary complex; (b) calcified (healed primary) complex; (c) bronchiectasis; (d) pneumonia; (e) pleural effusion; (f) miliary TB (2 mm nodules obscure the pulmonary blood vessels).

Progression of the Primary Infection (Fig. 18.17)

1. Healing and calcification, without further consequences in the great majority.

Occasionally:
2. Obstruction of lobar bronchi by enlarged node (causing collapse, bronchiectasis).
3. Bronchial seeding with confluent pneumonia.
4. Erythema nodosum.
5. Phlyctenular conjunctivitis.
6. Pleural effusion (see page 365) at the time of tuberculin test conversion (a common cause of unexplained pleural effusion in patients under 30 years old).
7. Pericardial effusion.
8. Blood borne spread – miliary, renal, bone, meningeal, adrenal (causing Addison's disease) (usually 12 weeks to 1 year).

POST-PRIMARY PULMONARY TUBERCULOSIS

Background

Post-primary pulmonary tuberculosis arises by:

Direct progression of a primary lesion (rarely before puberty in Europeans).
Reactivation of a dormant lesion.
Haematogenous spread back to the lungs.
Reinfection.

The illness has a slowly progressive course.

Pathology

There is a healed primary focus.

Usually the posterior segment of upper lobe or apical segment of lower lobe are affected (contrast primary TB). In most animals, TB affects regions of low pulmonary blood flow.

The histological hallmark of the infection is the tubercle or caseating granuloma. (Granulomata occur when macrophages accumulate around insoluble foreign material.)

The centre of the more developed tubercle consists of necrotic broken down macrophages and contains acid-fast bacilli which are toxic to these cells. They are surrounded by sheets of 'epithelioid' cells (macrophages) which coalesce to form multinucleate giant cells. Around this is a cuff of lymphocytes and fibroblasts. These lesions, in which the bacilli reproduce, may coalesce, causing extensive areas of 'caseation' (necrosis with formation of white cheesey material). Healing is by fibrosis, without regeneration.

Blood borne spread may cause miliary tuberculosis. The pleura may be affected. The disease may seed on to the larynx, tongue and intestines.

Symptoms

Inconspicuous, or
Loss of well being.
Loss of weight.
Fever, 37°C to 39°C.

Anorexia.
Cough – dry, or with purulent sputum.
Haemoptysis.
Amenorrhoea.

Signs

Patient often looks well, with high colour.
Post-tussive râles occasionally.
Amphoric breathing, signs of cavitation, consolidation collapse and fibrosis in advanced cases.

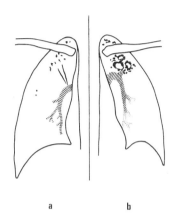

a   b

Fig. 18.18   Pulmonary tuberculosis
(a) Early infiltration = 'consolidation'.
(b) Extensive consolidation, lobar contraction, cavity formation. There is peribronchial thickening and fibrosis extending to the hilum.

Investigations

1. **Chest X-rays** (Fig. 18.18). The X-ray is of overriding importance. The appearances that may be present include:
    Patchy, irregular opacities, centred usually on one upper lobe.
    Cavities within such lesions.
    Streaks of fibrosis radiating from the hilum.
    Calcification.
    Solitary round shadows.
2. **Sputum.** For microscopy (immediate) and culture (six weeks) (or gastric washings or bronchoscopic aspirate).
3. **Granulocyte Count.** Usually not elevated. Occasional eosinophilia, lymphocytosis.

Complications

Tuberculous empyema.
Tuberculous pneumonia.
Tuberculous pericarditis.
Miliary tuberculosis.
Massive haemoptysis.
Amyloidosis

Differential Diagnosis

1. Bronchial neoplasm (age, cytology of sputum).
2. Pyogenic lung abscess and pneumonia (leucocytosis, sputum).
3. Fungal infections of the lung (specific serological and skin tests, sputum culture).
4. Drug-induced infiltrates.
5. Wegener's granuloma.
6. Resolving pulmonary oedema and chest infections can resemble pulmonary TB, but the rapid progress will prevent confusion.

The conditions mentioned are often diagnosed when failure to grow AAFB after six weeks *and* failure to respond to chemotherapy call for re-evaluation, with appropriate serological tests and perhaps lung biopsy. Most of these clinical conditions do not deteriorate rapidly over six weeks. While accurate diagnosis is desirable before treatment, it is often sensible to treat a patient in whom the suspicion of TB is very strong, pending the results of culture.

Basis of Treatment

Hospital admission, bed rest, etc., are now unnecessary, except in advanced cases, those unlikely to co-operate in treatment at home and those who are systemically ill. Chemotherapy has reduced the mortality to very low figures (Table 18.4).

Table 18.4   Drugs used in the treatment of infection with *Mycobacterium tuberculosis*

Drug	Dose (adults above 50 kg)	Side effects
Rifampicin	600 mg daily	Urine and sweat coloured orange Enzyme induction (oral contraceptive doses must be doubled) Abnormal liver function With isoniazid, hepatocellular jaundice Allergic reactions (fever, rash, rare)
Isoniazid	300 mg daily	Rarely peripheral neuropathy (pyridoxine 50 mg daily – given in high dose regimes and to malnourished patients) Jaundice (less than 1%) Fever, rashes, lymphadenopathy rare
Ethambutol	15 mg/kg/day	Optic neuritis (heralded by colour blindness, scotoma) with doses of 20 to 25 mg/kg
PAS	12 g/day	Gastrointestinal symptoms Allergy in 15% (fever, rashes, lymphadenopathy)
Streptomycin	0.5 to 1 g/day according to renal function	Vestibular damage (heralded by dizziness, may be irreversible) Allergy in 10%

Optimal chemotherapy of adults since 1972 has been with individual doses of:

Isoniazid 300 mg daily,
Rifampicin 600 mg daily (450 mg daily in patients under 50 kg),
Ethambutol 15 mg/kg daily.

The first two drugs are bactericidal for the organism. Three drugs are given for three months; one is then discontinued when it is shown that the organism is not resistant. Rifampicin and isoniazid are given for a total of nine months if serial X-rays show closure of cavities and sputum cultures become sterile by six months (this is usual). Other combinations of two drugs require eighteen to twenty-four months treatment to achieve similar cure rates (over 95 per cent free from relapse at five years).

The efficiency of 9-month courses of treatment of extrapulmonary (bone, kidney) TB have not been tested. Caseating lymph node tuberculosis appears to require eighteen months of treatment.

The very great expense of rifampicin, not yet overcome by mass production because it is semisynthetic, prevents its use as a universal drug. Other combinations of drugs have a cure rate of over 90 per cent if given for eighteen to twenty-four months. The cheapest are isoniazid and thiacetazone. The traditional treatment everywhere until 1972 consisted of:

Streptomycin, 0.75 to 1 g daily.
Isoniazid 300 mg daily, divided, in combination with Para-aminosalicylic acid (PAS) 12 g daily.
Other 'second line' drugs are available.

Drug combinations are used to prevent the selection of resistant strains, which occur wild in low numbers (about 1 in 10^6).

In very advanced cases when the patient is feeble, exhausted or moribund, corticosteroids are life-saving, given with appropriate chemotherapy.

Prognosis

Residual ventilatory defect is common. Death is now rare, and almost invariably due to neglect.

Prevention

BCG (Bacilli Calmette-Guerin) is an attenuated tubercle bacillus used as a vaccine to induce a positive tuberculin test. In Birmingham, England, the infection rate in a group of unvaccinated children in 1955 to 1960 was 5 per cent in five years, reduced to 1/10 of that figure by BCG inoculation at the age of 13. The protective value of the natural primary infection was intermediate. Life-threatening TB (miliary, meningeal) was virtually abolished. The programme is now being discontinued, because it has been calculated that in 1977 one case is prevented by the inoculation of about 40,000 children. Medical laboratory and 'health care' workers are still vaccinated in England, as are the newborn infants of mothers with the disease. The procedure has never been shown to be effective in the USA, where the practice has been to assume that a strongly positive tuberculin test indicates infection requiring chemotherapy for eradication. This policy of Mantoux surveillance may well be adopted in the UK.

Retreatment and Insurance Chemotherapy. These are often advised for older patients found to have extensive fibrotic pulmonary tuberculosis, which, although inactive, was not treated or treated by a regime now known to carry a high risk of reactivation perhaps with drug resistance. These are essential if steroids are prescribed or conditions such as lymphoma or diabetes require treatment. All forms of active tuberculosis should be treated with chemotherapy, even when a lesion has apparently been removed entirely at surgical operation (e.g. nephrectomy, excision of cervical nodes). Recurrence rates in these circumstances are very high unless chemotherapy is given.

MILIARY TUBERCULOSIS

Blood borne dissemination of TB organisms, with widespread granulomatous disease, may present as pyrexia and weight loss with no localising features. Diagnosis, when suspected, is by:

Chest X-ray. Discrete 2 mm shadows throughout both lung fields, usually without bilateral hilar adenopathy. Diagnostic changes not invariable.
Fundi. Visible miliary granulomata.
Bacteriological Diagnosis. Positive cultures obtained in 60 to 70 per cent of cases from large samples of concentrated urine, sputum, gastric washings or bronchial aspirate and culture of bone marrow.
Histology. Bone marrow sections, liver.
Tuberculin Test. Negative test common.
Lumbar Puncture. When meningeal signs present.
Therapeutic Test. Justified in cases where diagnosis cannot be established.

Basis of Treatment

Standard antituberculous chemotherapy; response of fever usually rapid (one to two weeks). Corticosteroids (predisolone 15 mg/day for two to three weeks) may be given to hasten clearing of pulmonary lesions: best reserved until response of fever to therapy has excluded other simultaneous causes of fever (e.g. lymphoma).

Prognosis

A significant mortality remains especially when the diagnosis is delayed.

SOME PULMONARY MYCOSES

ACTINOMYCETES

These may cause chronic segmental pneumonias, occasionally distal to carcinomas, sometimes discharging through the chest wall. They are often diagnosed at thoracotomy. Actinomyces responds to penicillin, Nocardia to sulphonamides.

HISTOPLASMOSIS

Endemic in Central and Northern USA *Histoplasma capsulatum* is a dimorphic fungus causing acute and chronic granulomatous disease, similar to primary TB, chronic pulmonary TB, miliary TB and chronic sarcoidosis. The condition responds to intravenous amphotericin B given for fourteen days; rifampicin is under trial. Adrenal failure is common in the disseminated form of the disease. Serological tests are available (preferable to the skin test).

CRYPTOCOCCOSIS

Cryptococcus neoformans, a ubiquitous yeast, causes chronic pulmonary disease and infects skin and bones. Acute or subacute meningitis is the commonest syndrome, often presenting as obscure pyrexia. Amphotericin B is given for several weeks.

ASPERGILLOSIS

The fungus *Aspergillus fumigatus* occurs as hyphae. It spores throughout the year, but mainly around October. Disease is due to hypersensitivity to the spores, with an immunological reaction. In some situations the inflammatory reaction creates a favourable environment for growth of the organism, in its filamentous form. Diagnosis is by one (possible) or two (probable) of:

Isolation of a heavy culture of the organism in sputum, using special media.

Immediate hypersensitivity (Type 1 reaction) on skin test, or specific IgE.

Late (8 to 24 hours) hypersensitivity on skin test, or, better, IgG (precipitating) antibody.

Clinical Syndromes (Table 18.5) are:

(a) Asthma.
(b) Pulmonary eosinophilia (hypersensitivity pneumonia with eosinophilia): May develop upper lobe fibrosis.
(c) Mucoid impaction with lobar collapse, simulating carcinoma: may resolve leaving proximal bronchiectasis.
   (b) and (c) may occur with or without asthma.
(d) 'Aspergilloma' fungus ball in old lung cavity. Asymptomatic, or haemoptysis, weight loss.

Asthma is treated according to severity (*see* page 349).
(b) and (c) respond to oral corticosteroids without antimicrobial drugs. Relapsing cases may require steroid maintenance: prednisolone 7.5 mg is the average daily requirement. Aspergillomas are removed surgically if possible (about 50 per cent). Antifungal agents (e.g. clotrimazole) may be instilled through the chest wall into infected cavities. The role of corticosteroids in reducing symptoms is under study.

AIRWAYS OBSTRUCTION

Definition and Background

Conditions characterised partly by reduction of the expiratory airflow rate are described in the next sections. Some definitions are needed at the outset.

Table 18.5 Clinical syndromes caused by hypersensitivity to *Aspergillus fumigatus*

Syndrome	Skin test	Precipitins	Treatment
Asthma	+	+ or −	As for asthma. Maintenance steroids often needed
Fleeting lung shadows* with blood eosinophilia	+	+(more than 70%)	Corticosteroids by mouth
Leading to:			
Bronchiectasis of proximal airways Bilateral upper lobe fibrosis Recurrent lobar collapse with aspergillus growing in bronchi as plugs	+	±	Corticosteroids, postural drainage
Mycetoma – fungus ball in old cavity	+	+ +	Excision sometimes practicable Corticosteroids?

*See 'pulmonary eosinophilia'.

Localised Obstruction of Large Airways. This occurs when the lumen of the larynx, trachea or major bronchi are narrowed from within the lumen, by distortion of the wall or by extrinsic pressure or distortion. Stridor and slow inspiration, with a catching of the breath in exercise or sleep, are the most obvious features. There may be a fixed wheeze when the obstruction is intrathoracic.

Diffuse Airways Obstruction. This occurs in chronic conditions such as bronchial asthma and chronic bronchitis where there is widespread narrowing of airways.

Chronic Bronchitis. By the MRC epidemiological definition, *simple chronic bronchitis is chronic cough with the expectoration of sputum from the chest for most days in the winter months (for at least three months of the year for at least two years).*

Localised causes of chronic cough are excluded. The only symptom of simple chronic bronchitis is the cough. The condition may be accompanied by:

Chronic airways obstruction.

Recurrent infections with increase of sputum volume and purulence.

Airways Obstruction. This term refers to the narrowing of airways with reduction of the maximum airflow rates that can be achieved in expiration (and, for differing reasons, in inspiration).

Bronchial Asthma. Episodic wheezing and dyspnoea accompanied by airways obstruction caused by variations of bronchial calibre. At least in the early stages the severity varies spontaneously and with treatment. Bronchial oedema secondary to heart failure and acute pulmonary infections are excluded from this definition.

Emphysema. Increase in the size of the alveoli (the air spaces distal to the terminal bronchiole) with destruction of their walls.

This definition, increasingly accepted, implies a pathological change in the structure of the lung, with loss of surface area for alveolar gas exchange. Previously, the term was used to mean any condition in which alveolar size was increased, including hyperinflation of the lungs. Compensatory hyperinflation (still known as compensatory emphysema) occurs when lung dilates to fill the space left by shrinkage or excision of a lobe. Such lobes function normally.

There are three main types of emphysema.

Centriacinar (syn. centrilobular) – changes are near the respiratory bronchiole. The lesion predominates at the lung apex and is associated with smoking and chronic bronchitis. It is discussed with chronic bronchitis and respiratory failure.

Panacinar emphysema occurs through the affected acini and can occur as a primary condition, without chronic bronchitis. This is the subject of a separate section.

Emphysematous cysts or bullae are over-expanded air spaces which compress surrounding lung. They may rupture, or cause dyspnoea.

Atopy. *The tendency to develop specific IgE antibody to common foreign proteins.*

Atopic individuals may manifest eczema, asthma, rhinitis, urticaria, angioneurotic oedema and anaphylactic shock.

The majority of patients with bronchial asthma and perennial rhinitis and almost all with seasonal rhinitis and with eczema are among the 10 per cent of the population who are atopic. Not all attacks of bronchial asthma or eczema are due to agents to which 'allergy' can be identified.

CHRONIC BRONCHITIS

Definition

Chronic bronchitis is characterised by the regular expectoration of sputum in the winter and an increased liability to develop recurrent bronchial infection and chronic airways obstruction. The rigorous epidemiological definition used in the British Medical Research Council surveys is given above.

Background

Ninety per cent of those with chronic bronchitis smoke, or have smoked, cigarettes. Many of the remainder have bronchial asthma or are atropic individuals. The pathological changes to be described are caused mainly by cigarette smoking.

Pathology

The trachea normally produces about 100 ml secretion per day. This is cleared by the cilia and swallowed. If this volume doubles, there is expectoration of sputum after nocturnal reduction of ciliary activity. The sputum is secreted in hypertrophied bronchial mucus glands and increased bronchiolar goblet cells. In early cases these may be the only histological changes that are readily detectable. Recently, it has been claimed that careful examination of the respiratory bronchioles of a few smokers coming accidentally to post-mortem reveals inflammatory changes not found in non-smokers. Breathing tests suggest that smokers, and those with asymptomatic simple chronic bronchitis, have narrowing of small airways, especially at the lung bases.

In more advanced cases there is obstruction of small bronchi by mucus, and obliteration by fibrosis. Centrilobular emphysema may accompany the changes, though they do not have the same distribution in the lungs. The tracheal and bronchial epithelium are no longer intact, the ciliated columnar epithelium being broken in places and replaced by *squamous metaplasia*. This impairs mucociliary clearance. The submucosa is infiltrated with polymorphonuclear leucocytes when infection is a major feature.

Changes secondary to alveolar hypoxia occur in the muscular pulmonary arteries. These hypertrophy, with intimal thickening, and result in right ventricular hypertrophy – 'cor pulmonale'. The pulmonary hypertension is only partially reversible by oxygen therapy. The polycythaemia that occurs secondary to arterial hypoxaemia is not usually severe (some 30 per cent increase in circulating red cell mass) but causes further pulmonary hypertension, especially in exercise. These factors predispose to pulmonary artery thrombosis.

Fluid retention may affect the lungs as well as the periphery. The mechanism is unknown, but it further worsens pulmonary gas exchange.

Epidemiology

Studies on a large scale between 1955 and 1965 have employed four techniques:
1. Questionnaires on respiratory symptoms, especially morning sputum.
2. Simple ventilatory tests (FEV, peak flow).
3. Statistics on hospital admission and working days lost because of chronic bronchitis.
4. Mortality statistics.

These have shown:
(a) A major effect of cigarette smoking, varying with number smoked.
(b) A marked interaction between cigarette smoking and living in London (but non-smoking Londoners and countrymen were similar).
(c) A marked rise in mortality during episodes of 'smog'.
(d) Manual workers have six times the mortality from chronic bronchitis of professional workers.
(e) Occupational dust exposure interacts with cigarette smoking and may be responsible for a small incidence in non-smokers (these figures have been hard to obtain).
(f) Childhood respiratory infections may be significant (uncertain).

The effects of the 1957 Clean Air Act have yet to be seen, as has the increasing cigarette consumption among women.

In Britain at present, between age 40 and 65:

About 40 per cent of the adult male population admits to morning cough and sputum from the chest.

About 17 per cent of men and 8 per cent of women aged 40 to 65 are seen by their general practitioners with symptoms of chronic bronchitis.

About 8 per cent of men and 3 per cent of women have chronic bronchitis with infective exacerbations most winters and breathlessness on the level.

The annual death rate registered as due to chronic bronchitis is about 80/100,000 for men and 25/100,000 for women, about one-sixth of that for ischaemic heart disease. The mortality increases with age. The average age of presentation with symptomatic chronic bronchitis is about 55 and the average age at death about 65.

The population of serious symptomatic chronic bronchitics is drawn from smokers with simple bronchitis. Many do not contract serious disease. The causes of the rapid progression of the changes in one-fifth of the individuals are unknown.

Chronic bronchitis has been an important cause of death in industrial Britain (the 'English disease'). Mortality statistics are unreliable because of variations in terminology. Where cigarettes are smoked bronchitis tends to be found if sought. There are pockets of the disease around the world, for example New Guinea.

SIMPLE CHRONIC BRONCHITIS

This has been regarded by smokers as 'the normal man's cough' or 'smokers' cough'. It usually improves on cessation or reduction of cigarette consumption, as may some of the subtle changes of pulmonary function that are detectable and, often, physical fitness. As long as simple ventilatory tests remain within normal limits, the condition does not cause major disability.

Simple bronchitis has one symptom and no signs. The next section describes progressive chronic bronchitis. Many of these patients will also have centriacinar emphysema, the severity of which is difficult to diagnose in life, but this does not affect management. The term 'chronic obstructive lung disease' and others like it have emerged to indicate those patients with chronic airways obstruction who may have emphysema and who may have had bronchial asthma.

EPISODES OF ACUTE BRONCHIAL INFECTION

These are characterised by increased cough, sputum volume, sputum purulence and dyspnoea, often with fever. In the early stages, these exacerbations are clearly related to cold affecting other members of the family and contacts. Episodes of atmospheric pollution may also precipitate infection, but are much less frequent in cities since the adoption of smokeless fuels.

Purulence of sputum is usually associated with *H. influenzae*, occasionally *Strep. pneumoniae*. Chemotherapy (tetracyclines, ampicillins or cotrimoxazole) against these shortens the episode. This standard practice has not been shown to affect the long term course of the disease.

Later, exacerbations may became more frequent and Haemophilus is never eradicated. The relative importance, in individual and in general, of viral and bacterial infection, of fluid retention and of true bronchial asthma in causing exacerbations is difficult to determine.

CHRONIC AIRWAYS OBSTRUCTION

Reduction of FEV_1 to 1.8 litres or less is associated with reduction of normal walking speed on the flat. Symptoms vary with weather and change of humidity. Reduction to below 1.0 litre is associated with an increasing likelihood of arterial hypoxaemia and elevation of arterial Pco_2, which may deteriorate sharply during exacerbations (see section on respiratory failure).

Effort dyspnoea correlates with ventilatory impairment, but is also affected by individual variations of ventilatory drive and tolerance to hypoxaemia. The average chronic bronchitic is dyspnoeic on effort, but not at rest, except during acute respiratory illnesses. A few patients behave differently. *Hypoventilation and polycythaemia* are caused by loss of chemoreceptor sensitivity to CO_2 and perhaps to hypoxaemia. These patients may complain of very little dyspnoea, but they underventilate, develop cor pulmonale and congestive heart failure (often described as 'blue and bloated'). Pco_2 and Po_2 falls abnormally in sleep. This syndrome can occur without chronic lung disease. Arousal, exercise or voluntary hyperventilation may actively improve blood gases when FEV_1 is above 1.5 litres. As lung damage advances, effort tends to be limited by syncope due to cerebral anoxia.

Panacinar emphysema (see page 344) is associated with the opposite response. Arterial Pco_2 is low or normal when airways obstruction is severe. Po_2 is relatively well preserved. Exercise causes intense dyspnoea and ceases before the blood gases change. Right heart failure occurs only terminally (sometimes called 'pink and puffing').

Symptoms

Cough with sputum from the chest, mucoid or purulent, usually present before other symptoms.
Effort dyspnoea, progressive over the years, punctuated by episodes of bronchial infection. Often dated to a particular illness or injury. Usually recognised as the need for increased work of breathing.
Ankle oedema.
Fatigue after day's work.

Signs

Cyanosis or polycythaemia may be detectable.
Signs of increased respiratory work: laryngeal tug on inspiration, use of scalenus anterior during quiet breathing, respiratory oscillation of venous pressure and of soft tissues of the neck.
Signs of hyperinflation: lack of lateral expansion, poor basal movement, liver dullness low, cardiac dullness absent. The trachea may be hidden behind the manubrium sterni.
Signs of airways obstruction: quiet breath sounds, wheeze or both.
Occasionally patches of râles.
Right heart failure is present if JVP elevated in inspiration with oedema and hepatomegaly.
Ventilatory failure (see page 367).

Complications

Cough fracture.
Cough syncope.
Depression.
Inguinal hernia.

Investigations

1. Haemoglobin, haematocrit for secondary polycythaemia.
2. Platelets normal.
3. Lung function, especially peak flow, FEV_1 and VC, serially.
4. Arterial blood gases if acutely ill.
5. Estimate arterial Pco_2 if FEV_1 below 1.0.
6. Chest X-ray: only specific feature is low position of diaphragm – excludes concurrent disease such as TB, neoplasm, confirms heart size.

Differential Diagnosis

Important sources of confusion are:
1. Primary polycythaemia (very high RBC mass; WBC, platelets or leucocyte alkaline phosphatase may be elevated).
2. Bronchial asthma, which may respond dramatically to treatment (see appropriate section for distinguishing features).
3. Cough and dyspnoea due to pulmonary fibrosis, allergic alveolitis.
4. Chronic left heart failure – ischaemia, mitral valve disease.
5. Pulmonary tuberculosis, lung cancer.

Basis of Treatment

Cessation of smoking.
Chemotherapy against *H. influenzae* or *Strep. pneumoniae* in sputum. Tetracycline 1.5 g/day, cotrimoxazole or ampicillin 1 g/day are bacteriostatic. Ampicillin 4 g/day or amoxycillin 2 g/day may be needed; they are bactericidal and effective in obstinate infections. Therapy is usually advised at the onset of infective exacerbations.

A few individuals who relapse, relapse rapidly and frequently may profit from regular bacteriostatic chemoprophylaxis (tetracycline 0.75 g/day, cotrimoxazole one twice daily or long-acting sulphonamides one weekly).

Advice about change of home is often sought. While Mediterranean climates are helpful in general, individuals vary and should be encouraged to try a short stay in the area of their choice without a permanent move until they are sure it suits them. The benefits of moving away from industrial British towns are much less obvious than they were 20 years ago. Even humidity at home, lifts or lack of stairs and areas where the patient can walk without encountering steep hills are helpful.

Troublesome paroxysmal cough with viscid secretions is sometimes treated with expectorants and 'mucolytics' which alter sputum viscosity. These are liked by some patients but are of no value other than for symptomatic relief.

Inhaled bronchodilators, for example salbutamol, ipratropium bromide, may relieve dyspnoea at rest and effort even when their effect on FEV_1 is only marginal.

Diuretics are given for peripheral oedema.

Respiratory failure and oxygen therapy are discussed elsewhere. Assisted expectoration is emphasised.

Surprisingly useful short term improvement can be achieved in patients on the brink of respiratory failure by admission to hospital, physiotherapy, oxygen, antibiotics and diuretics if indicated and nebulised salbutamol. Retraining can improve mobility, as can weight reduction where appropriate. In some instances the improvement is due to removal from undeclared tobacco or unsuspected allergies.

Exchange venesection to normal red cell volume (35 ml/kg) may relieve symptoms of secondary polycythaemia (check red cell mass). An exchange technique, replacing an equal volume of low molecular weight dextran, is essential.

EMPHYSEMA

Definition

Emphysema is a pathological term indicating that alveolar walls have broken down and are reduced in number (discussed fully above).

Background

Centriacinar emphysema accompanies many cases of chronic bronchitis. Panacinar emphysema causes a characteristic disorder presenting with progressive shortness of breath on exertion. Hereditary deficiency of the a_1 globulin, a_1-antitrypsin, causes progressive emphysema, starting in middle life, but earlier and more severely in smokers. The disease starts at the lung bases, becoming generalised. The damage may occur as a result of unopposed tryptic enzymes being liberated from leucocytes. (Trypsin injected into the trachea of experimental animals causes a similar lesion.) About one-third of cases are of this type. The cause of the remainder is unknown. A proportion are asthmatic, but the hyperinflated lungs of severe asthmatics do not in general have broken alveolar walls. Some have had respiratory infection in childhood.

About one-third of patients with emphysema have expanding air-containing cysts or bullae which expand by a check valve mechanism to achieve high positive pressures. These may cause symptoms by compression of normal lung. They may be excised or drained with at least temporary benefit in some cases, depending on overall lung function and the degree of compression that is relieved.

The abnormal mechanics of breathing are explained by the loss of elasticity. The unsupported bronchioles collapse in expiration and cause obstruction to air flow. The rate of inspiratory flow is less abnormal, but the work of inspiration is also increased because the thorax is hyperinflated and is harder to expand further than normal. The capacity to transfer gas is reduced because of the loss of alveolar and capillary surface area, but arterial O_2 saturation is usually not reduced at rest, and the disease causes intense hyperventilation. For this reason, the heart remains normal in size and appears small on X-ray, because of its vertical position in the chest. Hypoxaemia, ventilatory failure and heart failure follow prolonged severe dyspnoea and are terminal. Prolonged immobility predisposes to pulmonary embolism which is a frequent cause of increasing disability and death.

Symptoms

Dyspnoea of effort, inexorably progressive over several years.
Sputum scanty or absent except during respiratory infections.
Loss of weight.

Signs

Thin. Often rather desperate.
Pursed lips breathing often seen. Appearance of silent respiratory effort after brief exercise.
No cyanosis until very severe.
Large chest, horizontal ribs, low diaphragm, absent cardiac dullness.
In spite of hyperinflation, trachea often palpable, laryngeal tug absent.
Accessory muscles used in inspiration. Breath sounds quiet. In severe cases occasional râles at bases.

Investigations

1. Reduced FEV_1, well preserved VC, very low FEV_1/VC.
2. Reduced peak flow.
3. High total lung capacity, reduced CO transfer.
4. Pco_2 low or normal.
5. Hb, PCV normal.

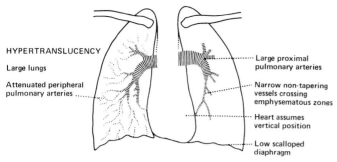

HYPERTRANSLUCENCY

Large lungs

Attenuated peripheral pulmonary arteries

Large proximal pulmonary arteries

Narrow non-tapering vessels crossing emphysematous zones

Heart assumes vertical position

Low scalloped diaphragm

Fig. 18.19 Radiological changes associated with advanced emphysema.

6. a_1-antitrypsin (or globulin electrophoresis) to detect hereditary cases.
7 Chest X-ray (Fig. 18.19).

Basis of Treatment

Cessation of smoking and advice to relatives in hereditary cases.
Treat reversible airways obstruction if present (increases comfort usually without improving effort tolerance).
Treat respiratory infections.
Investigate for possible benefit by resection of bullae.
In some cases: walking frame; oxygen at home if hypoxaemic at rest or on exercise (minority of cases).
(Radiotherapy to shrink affected areas has fortuitously helped a few patients and is under trial. Lung transplantation so far has not proved practicable.)

BRONCHIAL ASTHMA

Definition

A condition characterised by episodic wheezing and dyspnoea, accompanied by diffuse airways obstruction caused by variations of bronchial calibre. At least during the early stages, the severity varies spontaneously or with treatment over short periods of time. The definition excludes bronchial oedema caused by heart failure and acute pulmonary infection.

'Asthma' is used here synonymously with bronchial asthma. The term 'cardiac asthma', which denotes pulmonary oedema (sometimes with wheezing) is better avoided.

Background

The asthmatic has abnormal variability of bronchial calibre. Variations occur as a result of:

1. Bronchial smooth muscle constriction.
2. Bronchial mucosal cell swelling.
3. Submucosal inflammation and oedema.
4. Plugging of small airways with mucus and shed epithelium.

(1) and (2) may vary over very short times, while (3) and (4) take some days to resolve.

A variety of factors trigger the bronchial constriction. Some of these cause bronchoconstriction in all subjects but require less stimulus in asthmatics. Others cause bronchoconstriction only in susceptible subjects (Table 18.6).

Table 18.6 Factors precipitating bronchoconstriction

Factors causing bronchoconstriction in all subjects, to which asthmatics are highly susceptible	Trigger factors causing asthma in susceptible subjects
Acetylcholine*	Diurnal variations of bronchial calibre
Histamine*	Episodes of respiratory infection
Burning plastics	Inhaled or ingested allergens
Cigarette smoke	(a) *proteins*, e.g. house dust mite,
Formaldehyde	pollen, animal fur, moulds,
	egg, shell fish, horse serum
Foggy atmospheres	(b) *sensitisers*, e.g. aspirin, isocyanates
Inert dusts	Exercise (worse in cold air)
	Cold air (worse with exercise)
	Change of humidity
	Hyperventilation, respiratory alkalosis,
	repeated forced expirations
	Psychological stress

* May be used in laboratory tests.
Note: All above factors interact. Thus exercise induced bronchoconstriction or marked diurnal variation may occur only when the airways are sensitised, e.g. during the pollen season.

Even in the absence of disabling symptoms, the majority of untreated asthmatics show considerable variability of bronchial calibre, and of ventilatory function (e.g. peak expiratory flow rate, PEFR).

There are different *patterns of variability* and each patient has variable severity, which accounts for some of the difficulty in describing the condition. These patterns will be described in some detail as they determine treatment. We consider first the *triggers of individual attacks* and then the natural history of different manifestations of the disorder.

Pathology

The changes in fatal severe asthma are:
1. Hyperinflation of the lungs, not necessarily with destructive emphysema.
2. Mucus plugging of small airways – the material contains protein as well as mucus and may contain eosinophils.
3. Histological evidence of smooth muscle hypertrophy.
4. Eosinophilic infiltrate, submucosal oedema and hyperaemia.
5. Widespread shedding of ciliated epithelium.
6. There may be evidence of bronchial infection, with pus cells.

A few post-mortem examinations of lungs of asthmatics who died accidentally while in remission have shown patchy distribution of these changes to a varying degree in most cases. It is a generally held hypothesis that all types of asthmatic reaction provoke muscular bronchoconstriction and bronchial inflammation as described above, but that instantaneous reversibility is mainly due to the former, perhaps with mucosal oedema, while a preponderance of inflammatory change provokes a chest illness with incomplete reversibility lasting at least a few days after cessation of exposure to the trigger.

Immunopathology of Allergic Reactions Causing Bronchoconstriction. The majority of agents which cause allergic asthma do so mainly by immediate hypersensitivity (Type 1 reaction). Experimental work suggests that the sequence may be as follows:

Specific IgE is bound to mast cells in the bronchial walls. The reaction between antigen and IgE on the mast cell surface causes liberation of kinins from the cell – histamine, SRS, bradykinin, eosinophil-attracting factor. These substances are bronchoconstrictors and cause increase of vascular permeability. The reaction to a single experimental challenge lasts ten minutes to two hours. A minority of patients then experience a second (late) reaction, eight to twenty-four hours after challenge. This is often accompanied by a febrile reaction, with neutrophil leucocytosis. In some instances (e.g. allergic reactions to the mould aspergillus) the delayed reaction has been shown to be due to precipitating – IgG antibodies combining with the allergen and fixing complement (Type III reaction). The increased vascular permeability induced by the Type I reaction may cause deposition of IgG in the bronchi. The late bronchoconstriction is thought to be due partly to the liberation of kinins from leucocytes.

In each case there may be bronchial wall inflammation as well as the reversible effects of bronchoconstrictor agents, making the effects of the challenge more severe and long-lasting. The effects of repeated, prolonged or heavy exposure are more difficult to study experimentally. There may be a refractory period in which second exposures do not provoke constriction or the effects may be additive.

It is possible to block the liberation of kinins from mast cells pharmacologically by giving β_2 adrenergic agents and theophylline. These increase the intracellular concentration of 3' 5' cyclic adenosine phosphate (cyclic AMP). Premedication with these agents, and with cromoglycate may inhibit the bronchoconstrictor response to an allergen. Corticosteroids are more effective at blocking the delayed reaction than the immediate reaction. Immediate reactions are relieved by bronchodilator agents; late reactions respond only partially and for short periods to bronchodilators.

Mode of Action of Bronchodilator Drugs

Bronchial smooth muscle contraction is controlled by vagal fibres (numerous) via acetylcholine, circulating adrenaline and noradrenaline and affected by kinins released in the inflammatory process.

There is considerable evidence that the state of bronchodilatation is related to cyclic AMP in bronchial smooth muscle cells; if the concentration falls, there is bronchoconstriction. (There may be a modulating effect of constrictor cyclic guanidine monophosphate.)

Bronchodilators increase the intracellular cyclic AMP concentration:

β_2 sympathetic action (by adenyl cyclase activation).
Theophyllines (by inhibition of phosphodiesterase).
Prostaglandin E_1.

Some physiological substances causing bronchoconstriction can be blocked, notably:

Acetylcholine (vagal mediator blocked by atropine and analogues).
a-sympathetic agents (blockers exist, of little therapeutic value).

There are no therapeutically useful antagonists to released kinins.

Corticosteroid action is poorly understood. They increase depleted levels of cyclic AMP, and they rapidly reverse acquired resistance to β_2 sympathetic agents. They appear to block the Type III, but not the Type I inflammatory process. Reduction of vascular permeability may hypothetically be important in severe asthma.

EXTRINSIC, INTRINSIC AND ATOPIC ASTHMA

These terms are prevalent. *Atopy* is now generally defined as on page 341, and means a tendency to develop unusually high concentrations of specific IgE with consequent Type I hypersensitivity reaction demonstrable on skin tests to common environmental allergens. Most frequently positive in the UK are house dust mites, pollens, animal furs, feathers, foods and moulds. Atopic subjects are liable to develop eczema, asthma, hay fever or urticaria. It is not clear why an individual should suffer some but not all of these at different times. A large number of positive skin tests indicates a 'highly atopic' patient more likely to develop the classical syndrome of eczema in infancy, asthma in childhood, and hay fever in adolescence (the original meaning of 'atopic').

'Intrinsic asthma' is generally applied to cases where skin tests are negative, where there is no evidence of allergy to common inhaled antigens and asthma is most commonly precipitated in the first instance by infection. The syndrome of *anosmia, nasal polyposis, intrinsic asthma and aspirin sensitivity* is distinctive. The natural history of the intrinsic type of asthma is in some respects different from the extrinsic type, but there is considerable overlap. Both types may be associated with nasal polyposis and sensitivity to aspirin (1 to 10 per cent). Both may have eosinophilia, and both may have a personal or family history of allergic disorders. Excess IgE is not found in skin or blood of intrinsic asthmatics, but a role for IgE at the cellular level in the lungs and nose is not excluded.

A few atopic children develop chronic respiratory infection and bronchiectasis. In most, the tendency is to improve or remain well between attacks, with good response to cromoglycate. Intrinsic asthmatics tend not to respond to cromoglycate and a high proportion deteriorate progressively to chronic airway obstruction.

ALLERGIC ASTHMA AND RHINITIS

Air borne allergens may cause itching and watering of the eyes, sneezing, rhinorrhoea or blockage of the nose, itching throat or bronchial asthma. Pure allergic asthma occurs in under half of patients with seasonal rhinitis. The symptoms may go together, or the asthma may develop as rhinitis improves spontaneously or with treatment. Allergic factors identified from the history and knowledge of local ecology. Examples of seasons in the UK are:

Tree pollen	March to May
Grass pollen	May to July
Mould spores	July to December
Aspergillus fumigatus	All year, maximal September to January
House dust mite	All year, maximal September to December

Local variability, for example:

Ragweed pollen sensitivity in USA.
Earlier and longer pollen seasons in Mediterranean and tropical climates.
House dust mite scanty above 4,000 feet altitude.

Identification may be easy when reactions are immediate or when exposure is episodic (e.g. horse-riding, haymaking, bedmaking, consuming yeast in alcoholic drinks) or when symptoms are strictly seasonal.

The short and long term effects of perennial exposure, for example to a pet, are more difficult to evaluate. The role of the house dust mite *Dermatophagoides pteronyssimus* is still argued. It is $\frac{1}{3}$ mm long, digests moist keratin and cotton. Mite faeces is the major allergen of house dust: not highly antigenic, it is ubiquitous and thus causes the most commonly positive skin test (60 to 80 per cent of all atopics) which correlates with inhalational challenge. Avoidance is advised (washable synthetic bedding, dry vacuum cleaning of bedrooms and bed bases). A significant number of children and a few adults will improve symptomatically.

Skin sensitivity to common foods, for example eggs, cow's milk, justify investigation in obstinate cases. At present this is cumbersome and requires observation over a substantial period of dietary exclusion, followed by re-challenge if improvement occurs. The true inci-

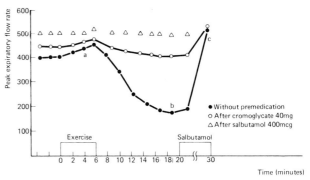

Fig. 18.20 Measurements of PEFR before, during and after exercise induced asthma.
(a) Transient rise of PEFR at start of exercise.
(b) Fall after exercise. This fall takes place more rapidly in children than in adults and is shown here beginning to resolve spontaneously after 20 minutes.
(c) The attack is terminated rapidly by the administration of a bronchodilator aerosol.

dence of symptomatic food allergy is unknown. Breast fed babies have a lower incidence of eczema than those fed with cow's milk.

EXERCISE INDUCED ASTHMA

Most children and about 50 per cent of adult asthmatics have this (Fig. 18.20). Wheeze and ventilatory changes occur *after* short periods of exercise but *during* longer periods. The symptom remits spontaneously with rest and is rarely prolonged (contrast allergen challenge). It is prevented by premedication with β-sympathetic bronchodilators in most patients and by cromoglycate in most children and some adults. After it has worn off exercise can often be resumed up to two hours later without recurrence ('running off'). Running is the most powerful trigger (100 per cent), cycling less so (60 per cent) and swimming even less (40 per cent). Cold air aggravates exercise induced asthma. Rather similar is the bronchoconstriction caused by repeated forced expirations (e.g. breathing tests), coughing, sneezing and laughing and by voluntary hyperventilation and alkalosis.

'PSYCHOLOGICAL ASTHMA'

This is still a contentious subject on which expert opinion has changed radically.

Asthma is a constitutional disturbance usually associated with a demonstrable immunological disorder. Psychological upsets in patients and their families are secondary to the fear of recurrence or of dying in an attack. Childhood neurotic traits and maternal anxiety are hardly commoner among children with intermittent asthma than among controls, but occur to excess with severe chronic asthma. Unrelieved asthma causes anxiety and a manipulative child or parent may appear to use this. If the asthma is treated successfully (90 per cent of children respond), the anxiety will usually go away.

Many asthmatics experience occasional attacks provoked by frustration, annoyance or occasionally anxiety or its relief. These may be involuntary, associated with overbreathing, laughing or running about or, rarely, self-induced for manipulative reasons. The mechanism is unknown (?vagal). Such attacks are usually relieved by most bronchodilators and prevented in some by cromoglycate.

Conditioning may cause bronchoconstriction (e.g. a picture of pollinating grass, or an attack on discovering that the inhaler has been left at home).

A very few adult patients give a history of onset of chronic asthma after some severe psychological stress (e.g. death of a relative, air raid) with no other accountable factors.

The treatment of severe asthma with sedation, hypnosis, etc., is dangerous and at best unhelpful.

The concept of 'nervous asthma' and the belief that it would go away if ignored are half-truths. They have resulted in occasional maltreatment and in considerable friction between many asthmatics and their doctors, teachers and friends. Appropriate reassurance, careful explanation of the treatment, supervision of withdrawal of medication and education about sensible self-medication over a period of time are highly rewarding. Asthmatics, like diabetics, should be well-informed about their condition and its treatment.

ASTHMA PRECIPITATED BY INFECTION

Wheezing complicates coryza, tracheitis and bronchitis in asthmatics at all ages. Infection is a predominant trigger in infancy (0 to 8 years) and in asthma of late onset. The immunopathology is unknown. There is poor, but not absent, response to bronchodilators. Corticosteroids are beneficial except in children under three. Cromoglycate may abort some attacks, but cannot be used if cough and wheeze are severe.

CHRONIC ASTHMA

As well as episodes of wheezing triggered by the factors in Table 18.7, lung function and symptoms depend on:
1. Diurnal variation of ventilatory capacity (a common pattern is shown in Fig. 18.21).

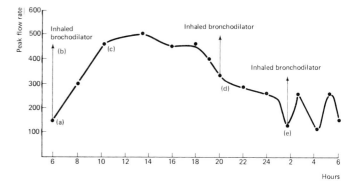

Fig. 18.21 Diurnal variation of PEFR in an asthmatic. Exercise induced asthma may be superimposed upon this variability which occurs spontaneously:
(a) morning dip; (b) relief by bronchodilator; (c) near normality during the day; (d) fall during the evening; (e) nocturnal awakening.

2. The effects of prophylactic treatment which may reduce the short term variability.
3. In a few patients, gradual or sudden progression to a form of irreversible chronic airways obstruction.
4. Individual variation in the perception of bronchoconstriction (from 20 per cent to 70 per cent reduction of ventilatory tests at rest).

Natural History of Asthma

Prognosis is related to age at onset and initial trigger factors shown in Table 18.7.

Table 18.7 Onset of bronchial asthma

Age	Major precipitating causes	Prognosis
0 to 7	(a) Wheezy bronchitis in respiratory infections	50% have no further attacks 50% become asthmatic with positive skin tests
	(b) Eczema, asthma	Majority are chronic, multifactorial 5% become dependent on corticosteroids
7 to 15	Allergic, exercise	80% remit age 15 to 19 Half of these relapse at some time
15 to 25	Pure seasonal asthma	Half gradually improve Half become perennial (especially those of late onset)
25 to 70	(a) Perennial rhinitis, nasal polyposis asthma (b) Precipitation by infection or, rarely, emotional shock	Most become steroid-dependent for life Majority become chronic steroid-dependent A small proportion develop polyarteritis

Patients may have:

Intermittent wheezing, mild or severe.

Chronic wheezing, with intermittent exacerbations.

While asthma is intermittent, trigger factors may be identified in many cases. All types of asthma may become chronic.

Asthma Mortality

Most asthmatics survive to old age. Unexpected deaths still occur, now mostly in those patients allowed to deteriorate. In hospital, almost all unexpected deaths occur in the early morning, or in patients given aminophylline without oxygen. The death rate fell with the introduction of steroids and rose in the 1960s in those countries where high dose isoprenaline was available. Recognition of unresponsiveness to bronchodilators as an indication for steroid therapy has overcome this problem. There are now about 1,000 deaths per year in the UK.

Symptoms

Variable dyspnoea, induced by trigger factors described. Airways obstruction is sensed in inspiration and in expiration.
Wheeze.
Cough is common, sputum – thick jelly, with spirals of eosinophilic pus, occasionally purulent.
Nocturnal dyspnoea and cough. Dyspnoea.
Intolerance of cigarette smoke.
Well-described variants include presentation with cough or dyspnoea alone.

Signs

Abnormally red or oedematous nasal mucosa.
Prolongation of expiration.
Hyperinflation of the lungs during attacks.
Wheeze.
When severe, absent breath sounds and use of accessory muscles.
Normal cardiac findings, except tachycardia.

Danger signals of severe asthma:
Progressive reduction of bronchodilator response.
Progressive reduction of effort tolerance.
Inability to talk.
Distress without audible wheeze.
Pulsus paradoxus. Pulse rate >130 beats/min.
Mental confusion.
Cyanosis.
Peak flow below 100 l/min after bronchodilator.

Investigations

1. **Chest X-ray.** May show hyperinflation with normal vascular pattern or concomitant emphysema, exclude pneumothorax.

2. **Blood Eosinophilia.** (>0.3 cells/fl) not invariable, suppressed by steroids.
3. **Skin Tests.** Help to identify atopic individuals and occasionally point to specific allergens. Nasal, bronchial and food challenge may help the expert in difficult cases.
4. **Lung Function.** Demonstration of variability of airway obstruction during the day or *after* 6 min exercise – measure PEFR, alternatively FEV_1 and FEV_1/VC. Response to bronchodilators or steroid treatment. Large FRC and T_LC. Normal T_Lco except in severe exacerbations or chronic severe airways obstruction (cf emphysema). Exercise tests or challenge tests in *asymptomatic* patients.

Risk of ventilatory failure if PEFR cannot be elevated above 100 l/min with treatment. Blood gases near normal except during acute attacks. Pco_2 reduced except in very severe asthma.

Differential Diagnosis (only common pitfalls leading to inappropriate treatment are given)

1. Between infective asthma of late onset and chronic bronchitis.
2. Between exercise induced asthma and other causes of dyspnoea.
3. Between nocturnal asthma and attacks of acute ventricular failure or, rarely, inhalation of gastric juice.
4. Between severe asthma and spontaneous pneumothorax.
5. Wheeze due to proximal airways obstruction (laryngeal, bronchial tumour, inhalation of food).

Complications

Ventilatory failure.
Spontaneous pneumothorax.
Antibiotic and other drug sensitivity.

Basis of Treatment

In all cases look for danger signs and immediately institute treatment for severe asthma.

Treatment of Acute Chest Illnesses (usually infective):
Rest, preferably out of bed.
Oral bronchodilators, for example salbutamol 2 mg six to eight-hourly.
Broad spectrum antibiotics if sputum purulent.
Course of corticosteroids (except in infants) if unacceptable dyspnoea at rest or progression towards danger signs; five to six days (prednisolone 30 mg decreasing) are sufficient. These courses cause no serious adrenal suppression.
Steam inhalations may aid expectoration of viscid sputum.

Treatment of Episodic Wheezing. Occasional reversible wheeze, asthma induced by exceptional exercise may be treated by salbutamol inhalations 100 to 400 μg four-hourly as required.

Regular wheeze (requiring frequent inhalations) and nocturnal wheeze merit prophylaxis in addition.
(a) Sodium cromoglycate, 20 mg by inhalation one to four times daily; if this provokes wheezing use after salbutamol inhalation or, rarely, in compound form with isoprenaline, or
(b) Theophylline, for example aminophylline. As effective as cromoglycate in high doses giving blood levels of 10 μg/ml (gastrointestinal and central nervous side effects may be troublesome), or
(c) Oral β-sympathetic drugs, for example salbutamol 2 to 4 mg six-hourly, or
(d) Ephedrine (α and β-sympathomimetic) is cheap and acceptable to some. If trials of the above are ineffective in reducing the daily use of the inhalers, corticosteroids by inhalation or mouth may restore reversibility.

Continuous Unresponsive Wheeze and Cough. Long term corticosteroids. Oral steroids, if severe obstruction, given to restore optimal pulmonary function. Several weeks prednisolone (10 to 15 mg) after a few days at a higher dose may sometimes be needed. Change to inhaled steroids, for example beclomethasone 200 μg four times daily and reduce with PEFR readings. May be more effectively distributed in lungs after salbutamol inhalation. Some patients require continuous oral steroids.

Acute Severe Unresponsive Asthma (Status Asthmaticus):
Intravenous hydrocortisone 200 mg. Until response, 1,200 mg/24 hours.
Oxygen.
Aminophylline, 250 to 375 mg then 1 mg/kg/hour by IV infusion.
No sedation.
Artifical ventilation usually needed when Pco$_2$ elevated for more than a few hours or patient unconscious.
Antibiotics if evidence of infection (include anti-staphylococcal treatment during influenza epidemics).
After initial improvement:
Continue steroid therapy with prednisone 30 to 40 mg decreasing rapidly as peak flow rises.
Salbutamol 5 mg six-hourly by nebulised inhaler or by tablets and pressurised inhaler.
Theophylline orally, occasionally aminophylline per rectum at night.
Broad spectrum antibiotics if sputum purulent or infection suspected.
On discharge:
Maintenance therapy with corticosteroids one to six weeks until airways obstruction, cough, dyspnoea and hyperinflation have resolved. Then withdraw observing

PEFR, with cromoglycate or inhaled steroids. Enquire retrospectively for possible precipitating causes (shell fish, etc.).

Treatment of Seasonal Rhinitis

Antihistamines if tolerated: nocturnal may be sufficient (alcohol intolerance).
Sodium cromoglycate spray, three-hourly.
Desensitisation during the winter to pollen where this is sole allergen (other desensitising injections are usually ineffective).
Local or systemic steroids may be needed.

ALLERGIC PULMONARY INFLAMMATION

Background

A number of organic agents may cause an acute inflammatory response mediated by a hypersensitivity reaction. Some are micro-organisms (e.g. the spore of actinomycetes from mouldy hay), but the illnesses are classified as allergic rather than infective because the organisms do not reproduce in the lungs and the inflammation is mediated by the defence mechanism. Bronchopulmonary aspergillosis is intermediate in this respect (*see* page 340).

PULMONARY EOSINOPHILIA (EOSINOPHILIC PNEUMONIA)

Definition

Segmental lung consolidation or diffuse nodular shadowing, with high blood eosinophilia, responding to corticosteroids, occurring with or without asthma.

Background

Aspergillosis. Over half of UK cases of pulmonary eosinophilia are caused by this. Other common causes of asthma may precipitate it.

Drugs. Sulphonamides, nitrofurantoin (which cause a distinctive type with pleural effusions).

Intestinal Parasites. Larva migrans from human ascaris or from toxocara (dog and cat worms requiring antibody titres for diagnosis since adult forms are not harboured by humans).

Tropical Eosinophilia. Filarial infestation. Many cases are associated with nocturnal larval migration. Diethylcarbamazine eradicates these. Steroids may be required to restore pulmonary function.

Polyarteritis Nodosa. May present with this syndrome in a form which often does not affect the kidneys and responds to corticosteroids (*see* page 121).

Course

A six-week illness with cough, sputum, dyspnoea and pleurisy. Some residual pulmonary dysfunction is the rule.

Basis of Treatment

Prednisolone 30 mg aborts rapidly, with gradual reduction of the dose over six weeks. Some cases relapse.

EXTRINSIC ALLERGIC ALVEOLITIS (HYPERSENSITIVITY PNEUMONIA)

Definition

Pulmonary alveolar inflammation in response to inhaled organic dusts, mediated principally by circulating antibody.

Background

Farmers' lung, pigeon and budgerigar fanciers' lung, are the best known examples, with demonstrable specific circulating antibody (*see* Table 18.8). There is a systemic and pulmonary reaction to exposure to the antigens. The time course of the febrile reaction (4 to 48 hours) and presence of 'precipitins' – IgG antibodies – in many cases suggests that this is an example of Type III hypersensitivity, but the histology is variable. The condition affects a small minority of those exposed.

Pathology

Infiltration of alveolar walls and respiratory bronchioles with lymphocytes and plasma cells. Severe cases may show granuloma formation superficially resembling sarcoidosis. Vasculitis is not a major feature, unlike experimental Type III hypersensitivity. Healing takes place with diffuse pulmonary fibrosis. Bronchiectasis occurs in progressive cases, with recurrent infection. Right ventricular enlargement and failure are secondary to hypoxaemia.

Symptoms and Signs

On acute exposure, there may be an immediate asthmatic reaction in some cases.
Chest tightness, dyspnoea, and cough with fever, muscle pains and malaise.
Fine râles are characteristics: these may persist.
The attacks subside after 2 to 4 days. Progression to chronic fibrosis produces a condition indistinguishable from bronchiectasis or fibrosing alveolitis.
Budgerigar fanciers are exposed continuously to small doses of the bird's serum (excreted in droppings). Cough and dyspnoea progress insidiously, with lung granulomata and fibrosis.

Investigations

1. **Chest X-ray.** No abnormality in early cases. Minor nodular shadows in heavy exposure. Later: upper zone fibrosis and honeycomb lung.
2. **Precipitins.** To budgerigar in all cases of budgerigar lung, to thermophilic actinomycetes in most patients with acute farmers' lung. Twenty per cent of exposed farm workers and pigeon fanciers have precipitins without symptoms. Circulating antibody not yet identified from many other types.
3. **Blood.** Usually leucocytosis, no eosinophilia.
4. **Lung Function.** Typical reaction shows hypoxaemia, low vital capacity and lung volumes, reduced CO transfer. There may be airways obstruction in patients with associated asthma or when there is chronic respiratory failure.

Table 18.8   Examples of extrinsic allergic alveolitis

Disease	Cause	Precipitin test
Farmers' lung Mushroom workers' lung	Spores of thermophilic actinomyctes	10% false −ve +20% false +ve among farmers
Pigeon fanciers' lung	Pigeon serum in excreta	+20% false +ve among breeders
Budgerigar fanciers' lung	Budgerigar droppings	+ in symptomatic patients
Malt workers	*Aspergillus clavatus* spores	+
Grain handlers	Grain weevil	−
Pituitary snuff	Animal antigens	−
Humidifier fever	Thermophilic actinomyctes Saprophytic amoebae	± ±

Basis of Treatment

Corticosteroids, 30 mg prednisolone or more per day, until maximal improvement, then withdrawal, watching pulmonary function. Chronic fibrosis does not improve. Treat bronchial infection.

Removal from exposure is essential to prevent respiratory failure (farmers' lung is a registered industrial disease). Masks must be used properly.

Preservation of hay in a dry state will reduce the incidence of farmers' lung.

BRONCHIECTASIS

Definition

Localised or generalised dilatation of bronchi, with susceptibility to sputum production and recurrent bronchopulmonary infection.

Background

The incidence is falling. Most cases result from chest infection in childhood, notably measles, whooping cough and perhaps adenovirus infections. Some have allergic bronchopulmonary aspergillosis. Local obstruction, for example tuberculous adenopathy, may cause localised resectable disease.

Pathology

There may be traction on bronchial walls by local fibrosis. The dilated bronchi have a squamous lining, lacking the normal ciliary clearance. Pooling of secretions leads to chronic bronchial infection, which is not localised to the most affected segments. *H. influenzae*, staphylococcus and *Pseudomonas aeruginosa* are common pathogens. The bronchi are crowded together, due to alveolar fibrosis, and there may be no functioning lung distal to the most affected areas. The lingula is commonly affected. Bronchopulmonary vascular anastomoses may bleed.

Symptoms and Signs

Classical:
Daily sputum > 30 ml/day, purulent during exacerbations, with offensive taste.
Cough on lying down, exercise.
Haemoptysis of fresh blood.
Dyspnoea in advanced cases.
Episodes of pneumonia with fever and pleuritic pain, with vomiting during expectoration.
Clubbing. Splenomegaly.
Coarse râles over affected lobes.
Cyanosis and respiratory failure are late.

Mild: In mild cases the patient may be normal in between chest colds, or may have a tendency to expectorate chronically. There may be a few peristent râles, but there is no clubbing or gross pulmonary dysfunction.

Investigations

1. **Sputum Culture.**
2. **Chest X-ray.** *Mild* cases normal. Bronchography (justified only when localised disease or complications are suspected) shows lesions.
   Moderate cases – reticular changes over affected lobes.
   Severe cases – cystic changes visible on plain films, with surrounding consolidation during exacerbations.
3. **Vital Capacity and FEV$_1$** with Po$_2$ and Pco$_2$ in severe exacerbations are guides to the effectiveness of treatment. Sometimes there is airway obstruction.

Complications

Cerebral abscess.
Amyloidosis.
Life-threatening haemoptysis.

Basis of Treatment

Postural drainage at home (may be intolerable on first day of febrile exacerbation): ten minutes three times daily until no sputum is produced by the procedure.

Antibiotics. When the disease is mild, the patient may experiment by delaying a day or two to see if exacerbations are cut short by antibiotics. Usually these are beneficial. Tetracycline or cotrimoxazole may be adequate against *H. influenzae*. If not, ampicillin 2 to 4 g/day or amoxycillin 1.5 to 3 g/day continued for ten days, followed by doxycycline 100 mg or erythromycin 1 to 2 g/day until purulence is eradicated. Maintenance chemotherapy is justified when there is immediate relapse followed by a second successful treatment.

Overgrowth with *Ps. aeruginosa:* this may be pathogenic or may conceal *H. influenzae* infection. In pneumonic illnesses, aminoglycosides and carbenicillin are infused. These are not given to try to eradicate the organism from the sputum.

Prognosis

Severe cases progress to respiratory failure and chronic airways obstruction in the fifth or sixth decade, regardless of remission as a result of removal of most affected lobes. Mild and moderate cases have a normal life span.

CYSTIC FIBROSIS (FIBROCYSTIC DISEASE, MUCOVISCIDOSIS)

Definition

A hereditary disease of exocrine secretory organs with abnormal mucus production, the main manifestations of which are pancreatic steatorrhoea recurrent or chronic bronchopulmonary suppuration and high concentrations of sodium in sweat.

Background

The disease is caused by a recessive gene of high incidence (1/25). There is an association with allergic disorders. Many of the symptoms are explicable by obstruction of tubules by mucus (thought formerly to be abnormally viscid): ciliary function is hypothetically impaired. Pancreas, lung, sinuses, bile ducts and seminiferous tubules are affected. Severe cases present in infancy with intestinal obstruction, failure to thrive, steatorrhoea and associated vitamin deficiency, or with recurrent respiratory infection leading to bronchiectasis, progressive respiratory impairment. Milder cases are surviving to adulthood in increasing numbers, especially boys. Hepatic cirrhosis, sinusitis and pneumothorax are frequent problems. Diabetes mellitus is rare. Most males have azoospermia, but girls are fertile.

Pancreatic deficiency is treated with oral enzymes taken before meals with enzyme supplements (see page 93).

Respiratory Symptoms and Signs

Recurrent or chronic bronchial infection with purulent sputum.
Progressive shortness of breath.
Haemoptysis, which may be life-threatening.
Clubbing of fingers and toes, at least to a minor degree, is usual.
Minor chest deformity.
Râles, often over upper lobes, during exacerbation, continually as condition advances.
Respiratory failure.

Diagnosis and Assessment

1. **Sweat Sodium.** In children sweat sodium greater than 50 mM (adults, 70 mM doubtful; 90 mM likely).
2. **Chest X-ray.** Bronchiectasis, cysts, nodular changes in upper and middle zones, fibrosis and recurrent consolidation, occasionally abscess formation.
3. **Sputum.** *H. influenzae*, *Staph. aureus* or *Ps. aeruginosa* are the common pathogens, occurring usually in that order during the patient's life-time. When the latter is the only isolate during acute infections, it may be regarded as the pathogen.

4. **Lung Function.** Reduction of vital capacity, especially during exacerbations. Evidence of some airways obstruction. Reduced Po_2 during exacerbations. Elevated Pco_2 is a late finding.

Complications

Heat stroke (loss of sodium in sweat).
Pneumothorax.
Haemoptysis.

Basis of Treatment

Postural drainage, as for bronchiectasis.
Antibiotics according to bacteriology, until sputum mucoid or absent. *Ps. aeruginosa* requires high doses of gentamicin or tobramycin to achieve peak levels of 10 to 12 $\mu g/ml$ in serum with carbenicillin 20 to 40 g/day. Up to three weeks' treatment may be required; eradication is virtually impossible.

Long term antibiotics are given for frequent recurrences caused by a persistent sensitive organism.

In the chronic stage antibiotic treatment is indicated for fever, acute pneumonic illnesses, and when vital capacity falls.

Prognosis

Ps. aeruginosa infection with recurrent infection occurring at more than three-monthly intervals is at present likely to cause death in five years.

THORACIC CAGE DISEASE

Background

Ventilatory impairment may be caused by impaired expansion of the thoracic cage. The consequences depend on the degree of lung involvement.

PARESIS OF RESPIRATORY MUSCLES

Poliomyelitis is now rare; acute polyneuritis, injury to the spinal cord and relatively rare neuronal and muscular diseases are now the major causes of this problem. Paralysis of the diaphragm, with intact intercostal muscles, causes 50 per cent reduction of vital capacity. Loss of respiratory muscles below C2, with preservation of sternomastoids, yields a vital capacity of under 1 litre with a loss of automatic breathing during sleep. In general, reduction of VC below 1 litre is associated with the risk of ventilatory failure, especially if Po_2 is reduced by lung damage.

Muscular weakness causes impairment of cough, which increases the hazard of lung damage during respiratory infections.

The management is discussed under 'respiratory failure' (see page 368).

RESPIRATORY COMPLICATIONS OF SEVERE KYPHOSCOLIOSIS

Maldistribution of pulmonary ventilation and perfusion with low arterial Po_2 occurs in proportion to the reduction of lung size. Ventilatory failure, with cor pulmonale and congestive heart failure usually occurs between the ages of 30 and 50, but some patients survive into old age. The prognosis correlates with the vital capacity. Children with severe deformity may remain remarkably active, but some limitation is common.

ANKYLOSING SPONDYLITIS

The costovertebral joints may fuse in this condition to yield a fixed chest, ventilation being achieved by the diaphragm. The inspiratory capacity is reduced by up to 30 per cent, but this is not a cause of blood gas disturbance or of dyspnoea. Respiratory infection is not a major problem. The patients are in danger when diaphragmatic function is impaired, for example after abdominal infection or surgery. Bilateral upper zone fibrosis may occur.

SARCOIDOSIS

Definition

A systemic disease of unknown cause with non-caseating granulomata in lymph nodes and other characteristic sites. The course is benign in the majority of patients.

Background

Sarcoidosis was recognised as a skin condition in the nineteenth century. A chronic pulmonary form was clearly identified as being distinct from tuberculosis by 1940. The prevalence of an early acute stage was recognised and distinguished from rheumatic fever in 1946. In London, the prevalence rate in those born in the UK is 27/100,000, rising to 97 and 213 for Irish immigrant men and women. There is no evidence that the prevalence rate has changed over the past decade. The cause of most cases of sarcoidosis is unknown. Clinically indistinguishable disorders may be caused by chronic exposure to industrial beryllium (berylliosis) and by large areas of tattoo. Crohn's disease (see page 79) is historically similar, but clinically distinct.

Pathology and Aetiology

The characteristic feature of sarcoidosis is a granulomatous lesion (Fig. 18.22), with multinucleate giant cells, epithelioid cells and lymphoid cell infiltration of the surrounding tissues. Unlike the granulomata of TB, central necrosis is absent, minimally present in very severe cases. These may heal, leaving no residue, or

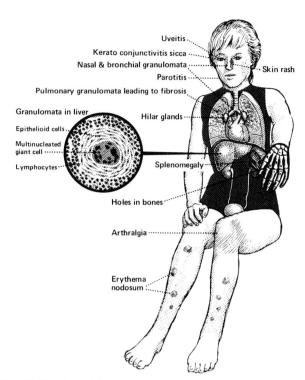

Fig. 18.22 Sarcoidosis.

there may be residual fibrosis after about two years, starting with sclerosis of the follicles. No pathogens are detected. Foreign body granulomata are similar. The epithelioid cells are derived from macrophages. Experimentally, granulomata may be induced by a wide variety of insoluble agents, for example insoluble antigen-antibody complexes, schistosoma eggs and finely particulate foreign bodies.

The *Kveim* test is positive in about 80 per cent of active cases. Kveim antigen is extracted from large spleens excised from patients with the active disease. The injection of 0.1 ml of extract into the skin causes a nodular granuloma with typical histology on punch biopsy in positive cases. Batches vary in specificity: some have produced positive reactions in patients with Crohn's disease.

Immune complexes circulate in patients with acute erythema nodosum. Delayed hypersensitivity tests (such as the tuberculin test) often become negative in the course of the disease. There is evidence that this is a consequence, and not a cause of sarcoidosis. Antibody synthesis appears to be normal.

Symptoms and Signs

Acute sarcoidosis frequently presents in young people with erythema nodosum and bilateral enlargement of the hilar lymph nodes in the chest (HAEN). This form of the disease has an excellent prognosis, and some 95 per cent of cases recover spontaneously in a few months. A few develop pulmonary infiltrations and may go on to become breathless. The lung changes may progress to a chronic, destructive, fibrotic disease, which may, occasionally, be fatal.

CHRONIC SARCOIDOSIS

This may present in a variety of ways (Table 18.9, Fig. 18.22). Pulmonary sarcoidosis may present with rapid

Table 18.9 Systemic manifestations of chronic sarcoidosis

Eye	Anterior uveitis: glaucoma Posterior uveitis Kerato-conjunctivitis (occasionally dryness) Lachrymal gland enlargement
Skin	Recurrent erythema nodosum (rare) Papules and nodules: 'lupus pernio' Hypertrophic scars are common
Joints	Polyarthralgia: polyarthritis Bone cysts (accompanied by skin changes)
CNS	Neuropathy Meningomyelitis Posterior pituitary lesions, diabetes insipidus
GI	Hepatomegaly, splenomegaly
ENT	Nasal granuloma
Lung	Bronchial inflammation Lung granuloma and fibrosis, rarely pleural Hilar adenopathy
General	Hypercalcaemia and renal complications Painless parotitis Enlarged lymph nodes Fever (rare) Cardiomyopathy (congestive)

or slow progression of cough, dyspnoea or chest pain or may be detected at routine chest X-ray. Cardiac sarcoidosis (rare) causes arrhythmias, sudden death and congestive cardiomyopathy.

Examination reveals the manifestations listed. Râles are usually scanty or absent. Cor pulmonale may result from progression to severe fibrosis.

Investigations

1. **Diagnostic.** Kveim test. Histology of affected node or site. Liver granulomata in 80 per cent.
2. **Chest X-ray.** Hilar adenopathy. Diffuse nodular shadows, especially in upper and middle zones. *Later:* upper zone or generalised pulmonary fibrosis. Honeycomb lung. 'Egg shell' calcification of hilar nodes.
3. **Hand X-ray.** Punched out cysts.
4. **Blood.** Raised serum calcium (about one in ten) falls with steroid treatment. Abnormal liver function. Variably raised ESR, plasma viscosity.

5. **Tuberculin Test.** Negative (important if positive previously).
6. **Lung Function.** Reduction of vital capacity and CO transfer occurs with chronic alveolar wall infiltration and fibrosis and does not mirror exactly the severity of radiological granulomatosis. Good correlation with degree of dyspnoea. Fibrotic disease or bronchial disease cause chronic irreversible airways obstruction combined with small lung volumes and considerable hypoxaemia.

Differential Diagnosis

HAEN is characteristic. The chronic glandular form occasionally resembles Hodgkin's disease.

Prognosis

Ninety per cent of acute cases with HAEN recover. Ten per cent develop pulmonary infiltrates. About half of these, and of those who present without an acute flare-up, remit in a few years. A few progress rapidly. The disease is more aggressive in patients of African descent.

Basis of Treatment

The condition responds to corticosteroids which, given early, appear to suppress granuloma formation and prevent progression to fibrosis, but do not alter the prognosis for eventual remission or relapse. Since moderate doses of prednisolone (5 to 17.5 mg daily) are usually sufficient to maintain remission, powerful immune suppressants have no advantage. Higher doses are needed to induce initial remission (prednisolone 30 mg daily for one to four weeks, followed by 20 mg daily until manifestations improve). There is no known 'radical' cure.

Absolute indications for corticosteroid control include:
Anterior uveitis (drops are effective).
Posterior uveitis.
Hypercalcaemia.
CNS involvement.
Dyspnoea.
The efficacy of prednisolone in cardiac sarcoidosis is not known.

Judgement may be exercised:
When there is asymptomatic chest X-ray change. If this does not remit in one to two years, fibrosis will ensue. When duration is unknown, intermittent treatment is indicated.

Skin lesions and nasal disease may be treated if they are disfiguring or unpleasant.

In cases of symptomatic lymphatic or glandular swelling.

DIFFUSE PULMONARY INFILTRATION AND FIBROSIS

Background

A number of conditions cause diffuse infiltration of the alveolar walls with inflammatory cells, with or without alveolar exudate and eventually diffuse lung fibrosis (Table 18.10). Bronchiolar fibrosis may occur. Many of these conditions may present acutely either as an acute pneumonic illness or insidiously. In general, the manifestations of these disorders are clubbing, fine basal râles, reduction of vital capacity, lung volumes and CO transfer, variable hypoxaemia and hyperventilation. Progression may occur to 'honeycomb lung': large areas of the lung may be replaced by cysts formed of dilated bronchioles pulled open by fibrosed and obliterated alveoli.

Radiological change is most obvious in diffuse granulomatous disease, and may not be proportional to the functional abnormality.

Some characteristic causes are listed in Table 18.10 which is not complete. Most of the conditions mentioned are *not common*. Their distinction is of importance to the specialist in advising treatment. The table is given for interest to show how clinical judgement is used to start differentiation, but students will not wish to memorise it.

CRYPTOGENIC FIBROSING ALVEOLITIS
(US synonym: interstitial pneumonia)

Definition

A progressive condition of unknown cause character-

Table 18.10   Some of the disorders leading to diffuse pulmonary fibrosis

Disorder	X-ray lung fields	Rales	Clubbing	Histology
Cryptogenic fibrosing alveolitis – acute	(a) Widespread (b) Nodular shadows	+	0	Inflammation
Cryptogenic fibrosing alveolitis – chronic	(c) Basal fibrosis (d) None	Early	80%	Inflammation and fibrosis
Asbestosis	Basal fibrosis plus pleural disease	Early		Inflammation and fibrosis
Silicosis	Nodular, confluent shadows	Late	Late	Typical nodules near bronchioles, massive fibrosis
Coal pneumoconiosis	Nodular shadows	Absent	Absent	Carbon nodules
Sarcoidosis	Nodular shadows Hilar adenopathy	Few, late	Rare	Granuloma, fibrosis
Eosinophilic granuloma	Nodular shadows Adenopathy sometimes. A few progress to reticulation	Late	Sometimes	Eosinophilic granuloma, 'honeycomb lung'
Extrinsic alveolitis	Variable nodulation	Acute	Late	Inflammation, variable granuloma, bronchiectasis
Systemic sclerosis	Basal reticulation	Variable	Rare	Dense fibrosis
Disseminated secondary carcinoma	Nodulation or lymphatic obstruction	Variable	Rare	Malignant cells
Lymphoma	Large or fine nodules	Late	Rare	Round cells in alveolar walls
Leukaemias	Nodular or linear infiltrates	Usual	Rare	Fibrosis after therapy
Radiation fibrosis	Variable	Variable	Rare	Vasculitis, fibrosis
Paraquat poisoning	Progressive basal reticulation	Usual	0	Fibroblast proliferation within alveoli
Recurrent pulmonary oedema	Sequence of films showing incomplete resolution	During acute attacks	Sometimes	Diffuse fibrosis

ised by acute or insidious inflammation of the alveolar walls leading to fibrosis.

Background and Pathology

Nomenclature and classification have made this difficult to study. In 1933, Hamman and Rich described the terminal stage of the condition in four patients with dyspnoea, râles, cyanosis and signs of cor pulmonale who were thought to have primary heart disease. Later, an acute pneumonic illness was described with round cell infiltration of alveolar walls and in some cases with considerable desquamation of Type II alveolar cells and macrophages into the alveolar spaces, often responding to corticosteroids. In the UK most cases between 1950 and 1965 were referred to the Brompton Hospital whose large biopsy specimens showed that desquamation, interstitial round cell infiltration and apparently irreversible fibrosis could coexist. A single descriptive name was therefore proposed to indicate that there was inflammation of the alveoli which could fibrose and was of unknown aetiology – cryptogenic fibrosing alveolitis. In America, the acute form is known as 'desquamative interstitial pneumonia' and distinguished from 'usual interstitial pneumonia'. Other detailed pathological findings are sometimes included in the classification.

There is overlap with the systemic 'autoimmune' diseases. At least five per cent of patients with rheumatoid arthritis have an identical condition. Forty per cent with cryptogenic fibrosing alveolitis without rheumatoid disease have antinuclear antibodies in their serum. The same is true of patients with asbestosis, which is often indistinguishable. There is an association with chronic active hepatitis, Sjogrens' syndrome and renal tubular acidosis. Recently circulating and pulmonary immune complexes have been demonstrated in the acute forms of the disease. These disappear in the fibrotic stage.

Most patients present between the age of 40 and 70.

Symptoms and Signs

The *acute* form presents with rapid onset of dry cough and dyspnoea at rest or slight exertion. Fine râles are heard at the bases. Cyanosis or clubbing are present in a minority.

The *chronic* form presents with insidious onset of exertional dyspnoea and variable cough. The hallmark is fine râles, easy to miss, heard at the end of inspiration, often only at the bases or in the axilla. Clubbing occurs in 80 per cent.

Complications

Bronchial infection.
Respiratory failure.
Cor pulmonale.

Investigations

1. **Chest X-ray.** Progressively: fine nodulation, basal fibrosis, generalised honeycombing.
2. **Blood.** Elevated plasma viscosity and ESR, 40 per cent have positive antinuclear factor.
3. **Lung Function.** Low vital capacity and subdivisions of lung volumes. Usually high expiratory flow rates. CO transfer reduced (this is earliest abnormality in insidious cases). If changes are considerable (50 per cent of normal or less) reversibility is unlikely. PO_2 varies with clinical state, but may be only slightly reduced in early cases. PCO_2 low except terminally.

Differential Diagnosis

The numerous causes of diffuse lung fibrosis and diffuse X-ray changes have been discussed. Conditions clinically very like the spectrum of cryptogenic fibrosing alveolitis are:
1. Some drug-induced pulmonary fibroses (hexamethonium, busulphan, occasionally other cytotoxic drugs).
2. 'Rheumatoid lung' and associated diseases such as chronic active hepatitis.
3. Asbestosis.
4. A few cases of viral pneumonia.
5. A few cases of recurrent left heart failure.
6. All diffuse fibroses in the end stage of 'honeycomb lung'.

Basis of Treatment

Unsatisfactory.
For Dyspnoea: corticosteroids in high doses (prednisolone 40 to 60 mg/day), tailing to maintenance doses as clinical improvement occurs. A few acute cases can tail steroids completely. There are instances described of irreversible relapse after withdrawal. Controlled trials to determine the value of suppression in mild asymptomatic cases are not available (e.g. using ESR as criterion) and there is no standard therapy. When symptoms or functional deficit progress in spite of tolerable steroid therapy, azathioprine or penicillamine may appear to arrest the disease. About 50 per cent are rapidly progressive.

DISEASES CAUSED BY INHALED MINERAL DUSTS

Background

Inhalation of different dusts provokes varying degrees of functional disturbance. Some, of high molecular weight (iron oxide, barium sulphate, tin oxide), are impressively radio-opaque but are relatively inert. Talc and beryllium provoke granulomatous disease and fibrosis. Silica, asbestos and coal are discussed fully.

Most dust inhaled is transported out of the lungs. The bronchial tree is cleared directly by the mucociliary escalator. Inert particles deposited in the alveoli are carried, engulfed in macrophages, either to the bronchi or to the lymph nodes. With heavy exposure, the lymphatics become blocked, which accounts possibly for the worsening of the dose/response relationship for highly fibrogenic dusts when they are mixed with inert dusts.

Pneumoconioses occur as a result of a fibrous reaction to dusts retained in the lung; severity of the lung condition depends on:

Dose inhaled.
Particle size (*see* page 326)
Toxicity to macrophages.
Asbestos and silica are notably toxic to macrophages.

Chronic bronchitis and emphysema are additional hazards, although their industrial incidence has been hard to evaluate because of the small numbers of non-smoking men working in the industries concerned.

COAL WORKERS' PNEUMOCONIOSIS

Definition

Simple pneumoconiosis refers to the nodular lesions affecting the lungs of coal miners caused by carbon deposition. They are associated with focal emphysema, but may not necessarily cause symptoms. *Complicated pneumoconiosis* describes the progressive massive fibroses which cause respiratory disability and failure.

Background

Some 40,000 workers are at risk in the UK. An estimated incidence of 20 per cent of coalminers of more than 20 years' service with simple pneumoconiosis is falling, because of improved dust extraction.

Pathology

The deposition of coal in the lungs leads to nodular fibrosis, mainly reticulin, near the respiratory bronchioles. When the lymphatics are blocked, the deposition of pigment and fibrosis affect the septa and lymphatics in them. Progressive fibrosis results in sheets of collagen being deposited. An immunological reaction is the likely cause. A higher proportion than normal have IgM rheumatoid factor. The condition is no longer thought to be due to tuberculosis.

Miners with rheumatoid arthritis are especially prone to develop crops of necrobiotic nodules in the lungs (Caplan's syndrome). These are typical rheumatoid nodules surrounded by sheets of fibrous tissue, 1 to 5 cm diameter.

Symptoms and Signs

Simple pneumoconiosis is identified on X-ray by widespread nodular lesions, mainly in the middle zones. If symptoms are present, they are caused by associated asthma, chronic bronchitis, emphysema or other disorders.

Progressive massive fibrosis (PMF) causes dyspnoea, low vital capacity and lung volumes, progressive arterial hypoxaemia and death from respiratory failure.

Compensation

The International Labour Organisation has published standard films for comparison. Lesions are graded according to size and extent into categories.

Compensation may be given to those in the higher categories 2 and 3. Disability is judged on clinical, radiological and functional grounds, and is classified as 0, 10 per cent to 100 per cent. Associated emphysema is compensated if disability is 50 per cent or more. This rule may be changed as studies of non-smoking miners becomes available. 'Safe' work is not excluded for those receiving pensions. The deaths of those receiving benefit for pneumoconiosis or suspected of dying of its complications must be reported to the coroner.

Basis of Treatment

This is directed against infection, airways obstruction and heart failure, if present.

SILICOSIS

Definition

A pneumoconiosis caused by the inhalation of finely particulate silica.

Background

Risk of Silicosis:
1. Mining of precious metals, tin, copper, graphite, mica, anthracite.
2. Quarrying and dressing of slate, granite, sandstone, road drilling.
3. Sand blasting.
4. Pottery and ceramics.
5. Boiler scaling.
6. Grinding (new techniques avoid silica).

Silica is more fibrogenic than coal and function relates more closely to radiographic category. There is a predisposition to tuberculosis not seen in other pneumoconioses. PMF may occur.

Pathology

The fibrotic patches are grey. Sclerotic nodules, which may be confluent, are concentric rings of collagen. Lymph nodes may calcify. The pleura is often involved.

Symptoms and Signs

Early disease may show little change.
Slowly progressive dyspnoea with respiratory infections.
Exertional cough.
Acute silicosis (mill stone fever) with a generalised bronchiolitis, fever and very high mortality, is now extremely rare.

Investigation

1. **Chest X-ray.** Miliary and nodular lesions on the upper and middle zones. Egg shell calcification. Pleural thickening. Massive fibrosis, sometimes cavitating. Signs of cor pulmonale.
2. **Sputum.** For tubercle bacilli (X-rays may be indistinguishable).
3. **Vital Capacity.** This is reduced, with preservation of FEV/VC ratio.

Differential Diagnosis (of X-ray appearances)

1. Sarcoidosis.
2. Miliary tuberculosis.
3. Other causes of diffuse pulmonary mottling.

DISEASES RELATED TO ASBESTOS EXPOSURE

Background

Asbestos (Greek for 'indestructible') has been used for 100 years, known since prehistory. It is a natural fibre consisting of aluminium, calcium, iron, nickel and magnesium silicates. Its consumption is increasing. Very fine fibreglass can be used instead, but this is very expensive and may prove no less harmful (inhalation of coarse fibreglass is not harmful to lungs). Several forms exist, the main ones being:

Chrysotile (white asbestos) – USA and Canada, Russia, Central Africa.
Crocidolite (blue asbestos) – South Africa, particularly dangerous.

Fibres may be $20 \mu \times 3 \mu$. They are heavy, so are distributed axially in the air stream to lower lobes, but are deposited according to their narrow diameter and penetrate to the pleura.

Chrysotile is soluble and curved, so deposited more in bronchi and more readily removed.

Asbestos bodies (dissolving fibres covered with protein) found in sputum or in the lungs are proof of exposure.

Conditions Caused by Asbestos

1. Asbestosis: diffuse, mainly basal, pulmonary fibrosis, clinically similar to fibrosing alveolitis. Râles, clubbing, reduced vital capacity and CO transfer appear early, with progressive dyspnoea. Raised plasma viscosity, blood antinuclear factors and rheumatoid factors occur in one-third. The chest X-ray usually shows basal fibrosis, often with pleural thickening, plaques or calcification. Cessation of smoking is urged (see (4) below). Corticosteroids are usually tried and found to be unhelpful.
2. Hyaline pleural plaques are found pathologically and radiologically. They calcify. They do not cause symptoms.
3. Mesothelioma of the pleura. A rare malignant pleural tumour presenting with pain or unexplained pleural effusion, fatal in two years. No treatment known at present is effective. The tumour spreads by invasion locally. Occasional cases start in the peritoneum. Nine-tenths of cases have been exposed to asbestos. Crocidolite, with its straight fibres, is particularly implicated.
4. Carcinoma of the bronchus (see page 360). Up to 50 per cent of known patients with asbestosis die of this condition. There is a marked interaction with smoking.

Incidence

Asbestosis presents 10 to 25 years after first exposure. About 8 per cent of naval dockyard workers with 25 years of exposure were found to have the disease. Mesothelioma has occurred 15 to 25 years after slight exposure. Groups at risk included:

Dockers.
Naval dockyard workers.
Boiler attendants (lagging).
Gas mask manufacturers.
Building workers, especially pipe-laggers
Demolition men.
Brake lining workers.
Those washing contaminated overalls.

The risk to populations 'down wind' from concentrated sites is unknown; it has probably been exaggerated but may increase as more asbestos is mined and dumped.

Compensation

The pulmonary hazard was described in the first decade of this century. Legal measures to control exposure were introduced in 1931 and yet the hazard of asbestos was only general medical knowledge by about 1950 and public knowledge in about 1965. Gas masks, issued to civilians in 1940 but never used except in drill, contained asbestos filters. In 1965, over half of the 30,000 to 40,000 people estimated to be at risk worked for firms employing three men or less and were unaware of the hazard.

Wages were high, and safety gear generally not worn.

Stringent regulations now in force have reduced dust exposure, and failure to wear suitable gear leads to dismissal. When exposure is proved, pneumoconiosis panels are generous in their acceptance of the diagnosis of asbestos related disability and death. Retirement is not now enforced from work in safe areas.

The former lack of publicity about the hazards of asbestos, for which there was no industrial substitute, appears like a 'cover-up' motivated by economy. This has led to accusations of negligence and claims for substantial damages are currently (1978) being filed against firms, some of whom may in fact have complied with the inadequate regulations of the day.

TUMOURS OF THE LUNG

BRONCHIAL CARCINOMA

Definition

A malignant growth of the bronchial mucosa.

Background

Bronchial carcinoma is almost entirely a disease of affluent populations in which cigarettes have been freely available for 20 years or more. In England and Wales, male mortality from the disease has risen ten times from 1930 to 1966. Mortality for females is much lower, but rises each year as more women smoke more cigarettes. Doll and Hill's studies of British doctors, which followed their original observation of the very low incidence of non-smokers among patients with bronchial carcinoma show a thirty-fold increase in the disease in men smoking 25 or more cigarettes a day compared with non-smokers. Doctors who gave up smoking became safer as the years passed and reduced their risk of developing lung cancer several fold. Cigars and pipe tobacco were much less dangerous. Exposure to asbestos dust carries a high risk of bronchial carcinoma.

Pathology

Cell Types. Squamous cell carcinoma is the most frequent, accounting for about 60 per cent of all growths. The lesion is virtually confined to cigarette smokers. Anaplastic (mainly small cell or oat cell) carcinoma, very poorly differentiated and highly malignant, constitutes about 30 per cent. Adenocarcinoma causes about 10 per cent. These are mostly peripheral growths and are probably not related to cigarette smoking. Alveolar cell (bronchiolar) carcinoma constitutes about 1 per cent. These are related to other lung diseases, for example fibrosing alveolitis.

With the exception of adenocarcinoma, most growths occur in the large bronchi close to the hilum. The mass is mostly outside the lumen of the bronchus but intrudes into it, thus causing partial obstruction and interference with drainage of the segment of lung beyond. Pulmonary collapse and infection are common complications. Metastasis is to local lymph nodes and directly into the pulmonary veins, hence to the brain, liver, bones, etc.

Symptoms (Fig. 18.23)

May be none. The diagnosis may be made by routine X-ray, or the patient die of cerebral or disseminated metastases without there being any suspicion of intrathoracic disease until after death.
Cough. Most heavy smokers have a cough, and may produce small amounts of sputum, especially in the morning. A change in frequency of cough or in the nature of the sputum is suspicious.
Haemoptysis, small or large, often mixed with mucus.
Breathlessness on effort.
Anorexia, dyspepsia, and weight loss.
Symptoms from pulmonary collapse, pulmonary infection or pleural effusion:
Breathlessness.
Pleural pain.
Purulent sputum.
Chills and rigors.
Hoarseness of the voice (recurrent laryngeal nerve compression at left hilum).
Pain in the arm, occasionally dull chest or shoulder pain.
Symptoms from metastases (see 'complications').
Note: patients with Cushing's syndrome and hypercalcaemia may present with mental confusion, stupor, or coma. This may be wrongly thought to indicate metastases.

Signs

None, or

Signs of Large Airways Obstruction:
Stridor.
Fixed wheeze.

Signs of Pulmonary Collapse:
Loss of resonance.
Loss of breath sounds and voice sounds.
Mediastinal shift towards the affected side.

Signs of Pleural Effusion:
Friction.
Loss of resonance at the affected base.
Loss of breath sounds.
Loss of voice sounds.
May be bronchial breathing at upper level.
Finger clubbing.
Superior vena caval obstruction with distended veins in the neck and over the upper chest wall.

Palpable hard lymph nodes in the supraclavicular fossa and axillae.
Irregular, nodular hepatomegaly.
CNS manifestations.

Investigations

1. Chest X-ray is the commonest clue to diagnosis. Radiological appearances include:
   (a) No detectable change.
   (b) Slight enlargement or distortion of a hilar shadow or an obvious hilar mass.
   (c) An area of pulmonary collapse with or without a hilar shadow.
   (d) Pleural effusion.
   (e) Lung abscess.
   (f) A peripheral mass.
   (g) Occasionally lymphatic carcinomatosis.
Emphysematous change may be present with any of these as a result of smoking.
2. Cytological examination of the sputum is a reliable method of diagnosing bronchial carcinoma in experienced hands. A negative result does not exclude the diagnosis.
3. Bronchoscopy may allow the lesion to be seen and biopsied.
4. Pleural biopsy and cytology of the fluid can be carried out if there is an effusion: these will diagnose most malignant effusions.
5. FEV_1, vital capacity and Pco_2 should be measured as well as effort tolerance. Respiratory failure will probably ensue if, after resection of a tumour, FEV_1 is less than 1.0 litre.
6. Thoracotomy and lobectomy may be necessary for peripheral masses whose identity may not be established in any other way.

Complications (Fig. 18.23)

Pneumonia, lobar collapse, lung abscess.

Metastatic:
Pleural effusion.
Invasion of chest wall and brachial plexus (apical tumours) (Pancoast's syndrome).
Metastases in local lymph nodes.
Superior vena caval obstruction.
Metastases to brain, liver, bones, pericardium.
Atrial fibrillation.

Non-metastatic:
Pulmonary hypertrophic osteoarthropathy with painful wrists or ankles.
Endocrine syndromes: Cushing's syndrome, dilutional hyponatraemia, hypercalcaemia, gynaecomastia from abnormal secretion by tumour cells of ACTH, ADH, parathormone and oestrogens respectively.
Neuromuscular syndromes, particularly peripheral

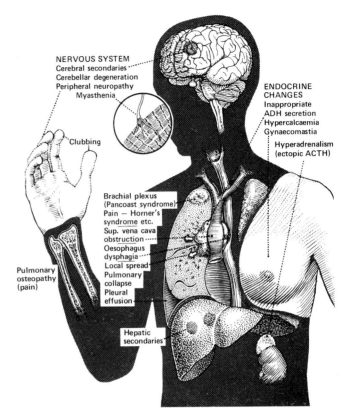

Fig. 18.23 Carcinoma of the bronchus.

neuropathy, cerebellar dysfunction, dermatomyositis and a form of myasthenia (Eaton-Lambert syndrome).

Differential Diagnosis

This covers a very wide field of medicine.

Suspicion of malignancy must be high in any case of lung abscess and in any unexplained pneumonia, especially if slow to resolve. Similarly, pleural effusion needs careful investigation. Tuberculosis and neoplasm may be hard to distinguish or may coexist. Bronchoscopy is indicated if there is doubt. Bronchial neoplasm is also to be excluded in obscure cases of neuropathy, endocrinopathy, liver metastases and brain tumour, even if a plain chest X-ray is normal.

Basis of Treatment

Prevention. Every doctor should show uncompromising hostility to all forms of tobacco smoking. Major changes of social habits are relatively commonplace in history and social disapproval or disgust of cigarette stench is to be fostered. Those already addicted need sympathetic help to give up the habit. It should not be forgotten that the medical profession's conversion to regarding cigarette smoking as harmful is barely two decades old.

Cure:
(a) *Surgery*. Removal of the affected lobe or lung is

the treatment of choice. Extensive spread of the growth often makes resection impossible or unwise. Persisting pleural effusion usually precludes success. Old age and poor respiratory function are other relative contraindications. In all, about one-quarter of patients are suitable for surgical resection at the time of diagnosis. The five-year survival of operated cases is around 25 per cent so that of all patients first diagnosed as having bronchial carcinoma only 5 to 10 per cent are alive at the end of five years. These figures have shown no improvement in recent years.

(b) *Radical radiotherapy*. Randomised trials of resection or irradiation in patients considered to have operable lesions have been carried out. For squamous cell growths surgery was obviously preferable. For anaplastic types the results were very poor with both methods, but five-year survival was as good with radiotherapy as with resection. Intensive cytotoxic chemotherapy is under trial; the role of stimulation of immunity is being investigated.

Palliation. This is sometimes useful with irradiation or cytotoxic chemotherapy. Obstruction of the superior vena cava or trachea may be very distressing and may respond to either form of treatment. Local treatment of pain in the chest wall may be helpful and intrapleural chemotherapy slows the rate of re-accumulation of malignant effusion. Haemoptyses may be arrested.

Counselling. Relief of physical and mental stress in the patient and family often calls for time and trouble from the physician. The diagnosis is often suspected by the patient. The issues of what to tell have to be faced conscientiously and discussed with the family and all those involved. It is not necessary to mention withdrawal of tobacco at this stage.

BENIGN TUMOURS

Tumours of the bronchial mucosa other than carcinoma are uncommon. Carcinoid tumours and, more rarely, cylindromas may arise. Their presence in the bronchial lumen give rise to troublesome cough, wheeze and sometimes repeated haemoptyses. Collapse of a lobe with added infection may also occur. In a small proportion of cases the carcinoid syndrome may be produced (*see* page 89).

Bronchoscopy reveals the lesion, and surgical removal is then indicated.

The patients are usually young (men aged around 30). *Haemartomas* are fetal rests which grow in middle life. They may calcify. The resemble peripheral carcinoma and are usually removed by segmental resection.

LYMPHOMAS (*see* page 405)

Lymphomas, leukaemia and proliferative disorders of the reticuloendothelial system may develop hilar lymphatic gland enlargement, diffuse pulmonary infiltrates, or, rarely, present as localised tumours. Clinically, they produce dry cough, effort dyspnoea and the characteristic functional disturbances of alveolar wall disease.

SECONDARY CARCINOMA OR SARCOMA

Some are diagnosed at X-ray as a single or a few round lesions. Haemoptysis, cavitation and disturbance of lung function are late manifestations. Surgical resection is sometimes advised for the lesions secondary to renal cell carcinoma, laryngeal carcinoma and osteogenic sarcoma (under trial). Malignant melanoma and most other secondary tumours are not resected. Other cases present with multiple smaller irregular lesions more likely to cause cough and dyspnoea. Prostatic lesions may rarely regress with hormone therapy. Choriocarcinoma is treated with cytotoxic agents in special centres; cures are known. Secondaries from thyroid tumours rarely take up ^{131}I, but may respond if they do. Breast tumours may arrest for a while with hormone therapy: trials of cytotoxic agents are in progress. The outlook for secondary malignancy of the lungs is poor.

CARCINOMATOUS LYMPHANGITIS

Retrograde obstruction of pulmonary lymphatics from hilar nodes, usually from breast or bronchial tumours. The classical presentation is with dyspnoea, cough, reduced vital capacity and hypoxaemia, but this is not invariable. Some patients present with wheezing and airways obstruction, which occasionally responds to corticosteroids and bronchodilators.

PULMONARY OEDEMA

Most cases are due to left ventricular failure (*see* page 277). Cough may be dry, or associated with mucoid or frothy sputum. Dyspnoea of effort, orthopnoea and paroxysmal nocturnal dyspnoea are the classical presentations. Wheeze occurs in asthmatic and bronchitic subjects. In the early stages the oedema is peribronchiolar and in the alveolar walls. Fine râles are heard. Later, there are pleural effusions and silent zones in the lungs as the alveoli fill with fluid and collapse. Later still, frothy, sometimes pink, sputum, wells up into the bronchi, with coarse bubbling râles. Vital capacity is reduced, airways obstruction variable, hypoxaemia is a late development.

NON-CARDIOGENIC OEDEMA

Increased pulmonary vascular permeability may lead to exudation of serum into the alveolar walls and alveoli.

Chronic pulmonary oedema occurs in uraemia (>35 mmol/l).

Acute non-cardiogenic pulmonary oedema occurs in intensive care units as:
'Shock lung'.
Oxygen toxicity.
Part of the syndrome of fat embolism (with vascular occlusion).
Part of the response to lung contusion (with lung haemorrhage).
In viral pneumonias.
Perhaps, some types of haemoperfusion and in response to toxic chemotherapeutic agents.

PULMONARY MANIFESTATIONS OF SOME SYSTEMIC DISORDERS

RHEUMATOID ARTHRITIS (*see also* page 32)

Pulmonary complications are commoner in men, although the disease predominates in women. They are commoner in severe nodular disease with positive rheumatoid factor. If these manifestations precede arthritis, rheumatoid factor may only appear with joint disease.
(a) Cryptogenic fibrosing alveolitis in 5 to 10 per cent: asymptomatic râles and gas transfer defect in 30 per cent.
(b) Necrobiotic nodules: single or multiple. Caplan's necrobiotic nodules with scar tissue in coalminers with rheumatoid factor.
(c) Pleural effusions, responding to corticosteroids.
(d) Recurrent bronchopulmonary infection.
(e) Acute pleuro-pericarditis.

POLYARTERITIS NODOSA (*see also* page 121)

This may present with intrinsic asthma, eosinophilic pneumonia or both. Pleuro-pericarditis occurs.

SYSTEMIC LUPUS ERYTHEMATOSUS (SLE)

(a) Recurrent pleural effusions.
(b) Syndrome like acute pulmonary oedema.
(c) Small volume lungs.
(d) Dyspnoea with reduced vital capacity and gas transfer, hypothetically due to pulmonary vasculitis.
(e) Diffuse pulmonary fibrosis (rarely, typical fibrosing alveolitis).

SCLERODERMA (*see also* page 122)

Progressive basal alveolar and pulmonary vascular fibrosis. Dyspnoea and gas transfer defect precede X-ray changes.

CRANIAL ARTERITIS (*see also* page 522)

Non-atopic asthma and chronic airways obstruction occur in association with this disease.

WEGENER'S GRANULOMA

Acute systemic and pulmonary disease may occasionally mimic tuberculosis clinically, radiologically and histologically.

DRUG-INDUCED LUNG DISEASE

Various syndromes are produced by drugs. This list is incomplete. Some regimes are obsolete (indicated with*).

Drug-induced SLE. This has the features of non-renal SLE – the antinuclear antibody found reacts with single-stranded DNA. Steroids and withdrawal result in cure.
Hydrallazine in high doses.*
Phenytoin.
Procainamide.

Pulmonary Eosinophilia. Reversible.
Nitrofurantoin (with small pleural effusions).
Sulphonamides (usually without pleural effusions).

Diffuse Pulmonary Fibrosis, Acute and Chronic. Partially reversible.
Nitrofurantoin.
Hexamethonium.*
Gold.
Busulphan, other cytotoxic agents.
High dose intravenous bleomycin.* Invariably fatal.

Pulmonary Oedema. Pathology unknown.
Amitriptyline overdose.

Pleuro-pulmonary Fibrosis. Irreversible.
Long term oral practolol.*
Methysergide.

Asthma – Anaphylaxis.
Aspirin and non-steroidal anti-inflammatory agents.
Penicillin.
Sera (e.g. antitetanus):* rarely pollen and other desensitising 'vaccines'.

PARAQUAT POISONING (*see also* page 211)

Acute changes include renal failure and painful oral, pharyngeal and oesophageal ulceration. Progressive bronchiolo-pulmonary fibrosis develops secondarily, in some cases, usually with renal failure and delayed excretion. O_2 enhances toxicity and should be used only if hypoxaemia is severe and symptomatic. The disease is invariably fatal. Treatment of poisoning is discussed elsewhere.

PLEURAL DISEASE

SPONTANEOUS PNEUMOTHORAX

Definition

The entry of air into the pleural cavity through a spontaneous rupture of the pleural surface of a lung.

Background

The entry of air into the pleural cavity allows partial or complete retraction of the lung with opening of the chest wall and of the mediastinum towards the full expanded side. This occurs suddenly, usually by rupture of a subpleural emphysematous bleb. Rapid decompression in aircraft or after diving may provoke pneumothorax. Forceful movements of the chest or arms are sometimes blamed.

The condition presents as acute chest pain, often severe, usually pleuritic and lateralising, occasionally central. It is the commonest cause of severe organic non-traumatic chest pain in the young.

Most cases occur in young men 18 to 35 (male: female ratio 5:1). Many have asthma which may be mild or in remission. Some have arachnodactyly. More than half will experience two or three episodes. Most older patients have emphysema or previous tuberculosis. Rare predisposing causes include cystic fibrosis, 'honeycomb lung', lung abscesses and infarcts and ectopic endometriosis.

Haemorrhage, when it occurs, may be profuse. One hemithorax (3.5 l) may contain one half the blood volume. The mortality of massive spontaneous haemopneumothorax is significant (up to 1 in 4).

Pathology

As air enters the pleural space there is partial or complete collapse of the lung on the affected side. As the lung shrinks, the hole becomes sealed and air will slowly be reabsorbed from the pleura. Resorption occurs because Po_2 is higher in the pleural air than in the capillaries. Breathing 24 to 28 per cent oxygen speeds resorption by increasing the gradient for nitrogen. This normally allows healing of the torn pleura with spontaneous cure. Occasionally, the tear acts as a valve allowing air to enter the pleural space during inspiration. More and more air enters the pleura, especially as respiratory movements become more forceful. Tension pneumothorax is then present. There is pressure over the opposite lung and obstruction to venous return to the right side of the heart. Death may result.

Symptoms

Sudden chest pain of pleural type, occasionally central. Effort breathlessness in some cases.

Signs

May be hard to detect.
May be increased respiratory rate.
Diminished breath sounds on the affected side.
Diminished movement and increased resonance to percussion on the affected side, which may be larger than the other.

In Tension Pneumothorax:

Severe breathlessness and fright.
Cyanosis.
Distended neck veins.
Hypotension.

Investigations

Chest X-ray shows the pneumothorax. The pleural edge is seen separated from the rib cage. Lung markings are absent outside it.

Complications

Tension pneumothorax.
Bilateral pneumothorax.
Haemorrhage, usually slight, occasionally profuse.
Mediastinal 'emphysema'.
Persistent bronchopleural fistula, chronic pneumothorax.

Basis of Treatment

If there is no dyspnoea, and the pneumothorax is not greater than one-third of the hemithorax, it may be left to resorb spontaneously in seven to fourteen days. Oxygen, 24 to 28 per cent for two to three days, speeds resorption.

Larger pneumothoraces, or those causing dyspnoea are aspirated. Usually an intercostal catheter is inserted to an underwater seal. If the air is not coughed out, and the lung expanded fully in a few hours, suction is applied to expand the lung using a special pump which cannot generate more than 30 to 40 cmH_2O pressure within the pleural cavity (not suction apparatus). Rapid expansion may cause transient pulmonary oedema and may unseal a pleural tear, so the treatment is not hurried unnecessarily, but the catheter should not be left dangling for too many hours in the pleural cavity nor should the lung be left collapsed for long.

For the procedure, premedication with diazepam or an opiate is advisable to prevent shock. Good pleural analgesia is necessary.

Catheters should be at least 10 English (16 French), i.e. 5 mm internal diameter. Fine tube block and air may be forced through the tissues of the chest wall (surgical emphysema). This complication is treated with adequate drainage of the pneumothorax, and oxygen to speed resorption of the tissues. The second anterior space is convenient. Some prefer the axilla, which should be used if there is fluid present. A larger catheter is then needed. Substantial haemothorax should be drained to prevent fibrosis and calcification. Anti-staphylococcal chemotherapy is given if this occurs.

After resolution, the tube is clamped, and removed if there is no recurrence in a few hours. Large broncho-pleural fistulae require more suction than is possible with one tube. Patients with ruptured emphysematous bullae may require up to six weeks suction with two tubes.

Tension pneumothorax is a medical emergency. A wide bore needle is inserted into the pleural space to allow the escape of gas, relieving compression of the great veins. The needle is then replaced as soon as possible by a valve or underwater seal.

Recurrent pneumothorax is treated by pleurectomy, a painful but successful surgical operation which cures the condition. Various forms of chemical 'pleurodesis' – induction of adhesions with iodised talc, camphor in olive oil, etc., have incomplete success, but the agents used are fibrogenic and may be carcinogenic so the procedures are under review.

TRAUMATIC PNEUMOTHORAX

Background

The usual causes are:
1. Penetrating stab wounds.
2. Fracture of ribs with penetration of the lung by a spicule of bone.
3. Chest operations.
4. Artificial ventilation at high pressures.

Complications

Haemothorax is very common.

Basis of Treatment

Aspiration by catheter or open operation.

PLEURAL EFFUSION AND PLEURISY

Definition

Pleurisy is the name given to painful inflammation of the pleural surfaces.
Pleural Effusion denotes the presence of fluid in a pleural cavity.

Background

Pleural effusions complicate a number of conditions and may be the principal manifestation. They usually consist of serum, but blood, pus and, rarely, lymph may also be found.

Serous effusions may be *transudates* caused by altera-tions in the balance of colloid osmotic pressure and lymphatic and vascular pressures. These barely favour resorption under normal conditions. The protein con-tent is low (typically less than 20 g/l). Inflammatory or neoplastic effusion are *exudates*, in which capillary per-meability is high and protein content approaches that of serum (typically more than 40 g/l).
Transudates are caused by:
1. Congestive heart failure or left ventricular failure of any cause.
2. Hypoproteinaemia, especially nephrotic syndrome.
3. Rarely, myxoedema and ovarian fibroma (Meigs' syndrome).
Exudates may be:
1. Acute infection – bacterial pneumonia.
2. Chronic infection – tuberculosis, toxoplasmosis.
3. Subphrenic infection.
4. Pulmonary infarction.
5. Malignant disease: bronchial, metastatic (especially breast, ovary), (rarely) pleural mesothelioma (*see* 'asbes-tos related disorders').
6. Autoimmune disease: rheumatoid arthritis, SLE and other types of vasculitis.

In the UK, 80 per cent of pleural effusions occupying more than half the thorax are caused by malignancy or tuberculosis.

Symptoms

Dyspnoea.
Pleural pain, usually relieved by separation of the pleural surfaces when effusion enlarges.

Signs

Increased respiratory rate, pleural rub.
Decreased movement of the affected side of the chest.
Stony dullness to percussion at the base.
Diminished or absent breath sounds.
(Sometimes) bronchial breathing and whispering pec-toriloquy above the effusions.
(When large) displacement of the trachea and apex towards the opposite side.

Investigations

1. Chest X-ray shows the characteristic concave upwards shadow when fluid is present.
2. Needle aspiration shows the presence and nature of fluid.
3. Pleural biopsy is valuable in cases of suspected malignancy and tuberculosis – it is best performed at the time of the first aspiration.

Differential Diagnosis

1. Large effusions – 80 per cent are malignant or tuberculous.
2. Blood-stained effusions are usually malignant or thromboembolic.
3. Cytology or culture may reveal aetiology. Lymphocytes may occur in malignant as well as tuberculous effusions. Numerous non-malignant mesothelial cells suggest pulmonary infarction.

Basis of Treatment

The underlying cause is treated.

Large effusions are drained (Fig. 18.24) if they are a

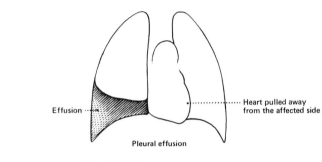

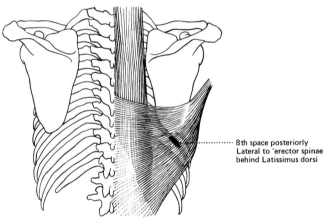

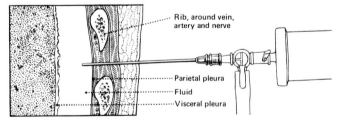

Fig. 18.24 Pleural effusion:
(a) radiological appearance; (b) best site for aspiration of fluid; (c) aspiration.

major cause of discomfort. Infected effusions heal with considerable fibrosis and should be aspirated as far as possible. Purulent pleural effusions are drained surgically if they loculate and become inaccessible to

repeated aspiration. When fibrosis causes restriction, surgical decortication of the pleura may improve function.

Malignant effusions may be arrested by instillation of cytotoxic agents or sclerosants.

LUNG COLLAPSE

Background

Pulmonary collapse is not a disease, but a complication of a number of intrathoracic abnormalities. The presence of air or fluid in the pleura leads to a reduction in volume of the lung that could be considered as collapse.

More intensive shrinkage of lung volume results from complete obstruction of a lobar bronchus. Absorption collapse then occurs as oxygen from the alveoli is quickly taken up by the circulation and nitrogen follows more slowly.

The main causes are:
1. Bronchial carcinoma when the obstruction is due to the growth, surrounding inflammatory changes and retained excretions.
2. Inhaled foreign body.
3. Compression of a bronchus by enlarged hilar nodes (e.g. Hodgkin's disease, primary tuberculosis).
4. Viscid, inspissated mucus which is not coughed up. This is especially likely after operation when coughing is painful, in whooping cough, and asthma.
5. Aspergillosis (see page 340).

Shrinkage of lung volume leads to a rise in the diaphragm on the affected side, over-distension of the rest of the lung, shift of the mediastinum towards the affected side, and flattening and diminished movement of the affected side.

Symptoms

Breathlessness.
Sometimes, pleural pain.

Signs

Increased respiratory rate.
Diminished chest wall movement.
Partial loss of resonance to percussion.
Diminished breath sounds on the affected side.
Diminished voice sounds.
Diminished vocal fremitus.
Trachea and apex beat shifted towards the affected side.
Rarely, cyanosis.

Investigations

1. Chest X-ray. Occasionally, the lesion is difficult to detect as the rest of the lung hyperinflates to fill the

hemithorax. A linear shadow of the collapsed portion can usually be detected. The rise in the diaphragm is often conspicuous.

2. Bronchoscopy will reveal the nature of the bronchial obstruction.

Complications

Bronchiectasis.
Lung abscess.

Differential Diagnosis

From pneumonic consolidation, pulmonary infarction and pleural effusion.

1. In pneumonic consolidation there is characteristically bronchial breathing and increased voice sounds.

2. Pulmonary infarction is accompanied by reduction of volume of the affected segment of the lung. Râles are much commoner with infarction, and the presence of haemoptysis and evidence of venous thrombosis weight the scales in favour of infarction.

3. Pleural effusion is likely if the loss of resonance to percussion is absolute. X-ray changes of effusion may be decisive. Both conditions may be present together.

Basis of Treatment

Obstruction to the bronchus needs to be relieved if possible. Foreign bodies can be removed at bronchoscopy.

Physiotherapy is important to aid the coughing up of mucous plugs in postoperative patients. Methods include positioning the patient to get maximum help from gravity, percussion of the chest wall to help dislodge the tenacious material, and encouragement to cough forcefully. Corticosteroids are given in asthma and allergic aspergillosis.

VENTILATORY FAILURE

Definition

Failure to oxygenate the blood in the lungs and to keep arterial carbon dioxide pressure at or below normal level when breathing fresh air at normal Po_2.

Background

Ventilatory failure will be discussed under three headings:

1. Acute ventilatory failure. Previously healthy patient (e.g. drowning, laryngeal obstruction, bronchial asthma).

2. Neurogenic respiratory failure.

3. Acute-on-chronic ventilatory failure (e.g. acute exacerbations of chronic bronchitis).

This subject can only be touched on, but a few points are worthy of note.

ACUTE VENTILATORY FAILURE

A 'Brook airway' facilitates mouth-to-mouth respiration.

In all cases, false teeth should be removed, and a finger used to hook out material from the back of the tongue (seaweed, regurgitated food) before mouth-to-mouth ventilation begins. Cardiac massage is given for the usual indication (absent carotid pulse).

DROWNING

Salt water drowning may be complicated by fluid overload with hypernatraemia: fresh water drowning by haemolysis, water intoxication and pulmonary vascular haemorrhage. A child may be held upside down for a second to pour water out of the mouth and airways: a heavy adult should be resuscitated in the most convenient position.

LARYNGEAL OBSTRUCTION

Causes include angio-oedema, epiglottitis, diphtheria (rare), inhaled foreign body (e.g. dummy). (See also croup, page 328.)

In the casualty department, laryngoscopy and intubation is usually possible. Tracheostomy may be done with a needle, through which enough oxygen can be given or air blown to save amateur surgery. This is ideal for the emergency treatment of infants.

Cricothyroid Puncture is easily performed in adults, but is dangerous in children.

INHALATION OF FOOD

Sudden death in restaurants is nearly always caused by the inhalation of large pieces of food, usually meat. This is provoked by talking while eating, coupled with impaired co-ordination of the swallowing mechanism caused by alcohol. Supraglottic obstruction may be relieved by hooking out the food with a finger. Inhalation into the trachea is the least reversible catastrophe, because air cannot be inspired to generate cough. Emergency treatment consists of a vigorous upward push on the upper abdomen, in the hope of displacing the diaphragm upwards and dislodging the wedged food (artificial cough).

ACUTE SEVERE BRONCHIAL ASTHMA OR BRONCHIOLITIS

In a previously healthy patient when consciousness is impaired or Pco_2 elevated above 8 kPa, 60 mmHg, artificial ventilation is required unless it is seen that the patient is improving rapidly.

The dangers of increasing hypercapnia are:
1. Arrhythmia due to respiratory acidosis.
2. Respiratory depression due to CO_2 narcosis.

Pco_2 rises more slowly than Po_2 falls (because of blood and body tissue buffers). Therefore give oxygen at once (by a mask giving generous concentrations, or by anaesthetic equipment if there is respiratory arrest) and assess adequacy of ventilation later. Healthy children tolerate a low pH better than adults: not all children with bronchiolitis and Pco_2 of 8 kPa will be given artificial ventilation, though careful monitoring is required to ensure stable rhythm, steady Pco_2 and adequate Po_2.

NEUROGENIC RESPIRATORY FAILURE

LOSS OF RESPIRATORY DRIVE (SLEEP APNOEA)

Several rare syndromes of unknown cause have in common *periodic apnoea during sleep* causing transient hypoxaemia and its consequences: polycythaemia, pulmonary hypertension, heart failure, sudden infant death, daytime hypersomnolence, morning headache, intellectual deterioration and eventually chronic respiratory failure. Snoring and upper airway obstruction may coexist (*obstructive apnoea*) as may obesity ('*Pickwickian*' *syndrome*) and complete loss of metabolic control of breathing ('*Ondine's curse*'). Treatment is individual and may include weight reduction, diuretics, adenoidectomy, tracheostomy, phrenic nerve pacing, nocturnal oxygen or artificial ventilation. Chronic CO_2 retention with papilloedema may mimic cerebral tumour.

NEUROMUSCULAR WEAKNESS

Acute paralytic disorders such as myasthenia, polyneuritis and poliomyelitis may cause respiratory insufficiency. There is progressive reduction of vital capacity. In the early stages Pco_2 is low, but when vital capacity falls below 1.0 litre there is an increasing risk of hypoventilation. When the disorder is curable or self-limiting, artificial ventilation is then given.

Involvement of the respiratory muscles in chronic paralytic diseases does not cause symptoms if the patient is immobile. Occasionally, there is preservation of the muscles in the neck with loss of diaphragmatic and intercostal power. When this occurs, ventilation may be adequate during the day but cease or fall in sleep. Cor pulmonale may then ensue.

Basis of Treatment

Artificial ventilation may be given at night to those with sufficient muscle power to breathe during the day. Various devices are used (specially moulded cuirasses applying intermittent negative pressure to the thoracic cage; rocking beds which apply upward pressure to the diaphragm by the action of gravity on the abdominal contents). Continuous artificial ventilation by negative or positive pressure ventilation may continue for many years when a patient has survived a paralytic illness without recovery of the respiratory muscles.

PULMONARY INSUFFICIENCY: CHRONIC AND ACUTE-ON-CHRONIC RESPIRATORY FAILURE

Severe chronic bronchitis is accompanied by increased work of breathing and disturbances of the pulmonary gas exchanging mechanism. Characteristically, these are accompanied by adaptation to moderately severe hypoxaemia, with mild CO_2 retention. Results such as:

Pco_2: 50 mmHg (6.7 kPa)
Po_2: 50 mmHg (6.7 kPa)
pH: 7.38

are not uncommon in ambulant patients who appear quite well. When such patients develop acute bronchial infections or fluid retention, they usually suffer severe rises of Pco_2 and deterioration of Po_2. Relief of hypoxaemia or sedation further reduce respiratory drive without improving the underlying condition and cause progressive underventilation with acute respiratory acidosis.

There are no consistent physical signs of CO_2 retention and hypoxaemia. The following may occur:
Mood disturbance.
Confusion or aggression.
Coma.
Flapping tremor.
and with severe CO_2 retention:
Almost absent respiratory movement.
Warm hands, dilated veins.
Papilloedema and raised intracranial pressure.

Example:
Pco_2: 70 mmHg (9.5 kPa)
Po_2: 30 mmHg (4.0 kPa), breathing air
pH: 7.20

If such a patient were given unlimited oxygen therapy, perhaps with a sedative, a typical result would be:

Pco_2: 100 mmHg (13.5 kPa)
Po_2: 150 mmHg (20 kPa), breathing O_2
pH: 6.90

Artificial ventilation is now required for CO_2 narcosis. The use of controlled oxygen therapy, usually with 24 per cent, elevates arterial Po_2 somewhat, usually with only a minor effect on arterial Pco_2:

Pco_2: 75 mmHg (10 kPa)
Po_2: 45 mmHg (6 kPa), on 24 per cent O_2
pH: 7.15

Less than 1 in 4 of such patients will develop progressive hypoventilation. This improvement in oxygenation relieves some distress.

Other forms of treatment are aimed at maintaining ventilation and inspiring the lungs:
Regular arousal (half to two-hourly, according to condition, day and night).
Assisted coughing (at each arousal).
Antibiotics.
Bronchodilators (aminophylline has a mild stimulant effect).
Diuretics.
Avoidance of sedation.
Intravenous fluids, usually dextrose with 120 mEq (mmol) daily of KCl.
Artificial ventilation is used if the patient becomes:
Unconscious.
Unco-operative.
Unable to cough.
Exhausted.
The family of a severe chronic respiratory cripple may request palliation rather than artificial ventilation under these circumstances.

When arterial Pco_2 rises after oxygen therapy the oxygen should not be withdrawn – this results in severe hypoxaemia.

OXYGEN THERAPY

1. For acute severe dyspnoea with hyperventilation (e.g. LVF, bronchial asthma, pulmonary embolism) use generous oxygen therapy. Use a firm plastic mask with holes capable of taking 10 litres/min of O_2 flow (e.g. Hudson). O_2 concentration depends on O_2 flow, rate and depth of breathing.

2. **Ventimasks.** For controlled oxygen therapy. Ventimask delivery of 24 per cent regardless of O_2 flow. These masks use the high flow O_2 enrichment principle. DRY O_2 running at 4 litres/min *or more* entrains 20 times its own volume of air, delivering a draught of 24 per cent at 80 litres/min *or more* at the face. There is no CO_2 retention. Do not use humidified O_2 (spoils performance of mask, no benefit because only one-twentieth of mixture is humidified).

Twenty-eight per cent Ventimasks are available. The thirty-five per cent/forty per cent design affects entrainment ratio. An adequate draught requires higher O_2 flow above twenty-eight per cent.

3. **Nasal Cannulae.** For continuous O_2 therapy when exact O_2 concentration is uncritical. Humidified O_2 is run in through cannulae at the nostrils, half to one-and-a-half litres/min.

Indications. Continuous O_2, convenient for eating, talking. Well tolerated by convalescent patients and those with chronic lung disease.

Oxygen at Home

This may be prescribed for occasional relief of distressing attacks in the severely disabled patient with chronic bronchitis and emphysema.

The value of continuous O_2 at night for the treatment of chronic hypoxic pulmonary hypertension is under trial.

ARTIFICIAL VENTILATION

The doctor should be able to perform mouth-to-mouth breathing and airway toilet, to use a hand operated resuscitator with airway and face mask and to intubate the trachea.

A few pointers may help those who have to care for patients admitted to intensive care wards. This section is not a comprehensive guide.

Indications

Hypoxaemia unrelieved by tolerable O_2 therapy.
Raised arterial Pco_2 when there are embarrassing vital functions, progressive or likely to deteriorate acutely.
Exhaustion.

Principles

Intermittent positive pressure breathing (IPPB) is usually employed. Mechanical ventilators deliver breaths through a cuffed endotracheal tube and a valve to prevent rebreathing. Sedatives (e.g. diazepam IV), relaxants (e.g. pancuronium) or both are given.

Tracheostomy is performed after ten to fourteen days to prevent permanent damage to the larynx.

The apparent sophistication of modern equipment conceals the simplicity of the principles. The operator controls ventilation (l/min) by setting:

1. Tidal volume.
2. Frequency of breathing.

Settings are approximate, so the ventilation achieved is checked. Oxygen is added at a known rate.

Ventilatory Requirement

The artificially ventilated patient is sedated, and has to do no respiratory work. Metabolic rate is therefore basal and depends on temperature (approximately 200 to 250 ml/min of O_2 consumption and CO_2 output, doubling for each degree C of temperature).

$$\text{Alveolar ventilation l/min} = \frac{CO_2 \text{ output (ml/min)} \times .11}{Pco_2 \text{ (kPa)}}$$

$$= \frac{CO_2 \text{ output} \times .86}{Pco_2 \text{ (mmHg)}}$$

i.e. 4 l/min if CO_2 output is 200 ml/min.

To this must be added the ventilation of the 'dead space', which includes the trachea, endotracheal tube and piping between them and the valve *plus* any areas of poorly perfused lung. On average, the ventilatory requirement if the lungs are normal is 5 l/min, while the 'dead space' effect of disease adds another 3 to 5 l/min when bronchopulmonary disease is present.

Control of Tidal Volume and Frequency

The machine generates pressure in the bellows and delivers volumes of air according to the dynamic compliance of the lungs (a function of resistance of the airways and stiffness of the alveoli).
1. Normal lungs require a low rate and tidal volume.
2. Obstructed airways admit air and empty *slowly*; a low respiratory rate (11 to 12 breaths/min) is used, with long expiratory pauses.
3. Stiff lungs (e.g. lung contusion) are most efficiently ventilated at lower pressures requiring higher frequencies (16 to 20 breaths/min).
4. High inspiratory pressure obstructs venous return, which occurs during expiratory pauses.
5. Some ventilators deliver set volumes, pressure being recorded (a useful check on progress in airways obstruction). Some drive at set pressures, volume being checked; 10 to 15 cmH$_2$O is average for normal lungs, 20 to 30 for stiff lungs, 30 to 40 for chronic bronchitics, up to 70 cmH$_2$O in severe status asthmaticus.

Added Oxygen

Sufficient O$_2$ is added to achieve arterial O$_2$ saturation of 90 to 95 per cent when possible. Sustained ventilation with concentrations greater than 40 per cent causes pulmonary O$_2$ toxicity (pulmonary oedema and fibrosis). Pco$_2$ is measured on a meter, but may be guessed from ventilated minute volume and O$_2$ flow into a ventilator.

End Expired Pressure

Stiff lungs collapse in expiration. Alveoli may be kept open during expiratory pause with *positive end expired pressure* (PEEP), usually a valve set at 5 to 10 cmH$_2$O. Disadvantage: embarrasses venous return; increases cardiac pressures.
Advantage: usually improves Po$_2$ without increasing inspired O$_2$.

Incorrect Ventilation

Hyperventilation causes alkalosis and hypotension. Arterial blood gases are checked early. If Pco$_2$ is low, reduce ventilation (or add external 'dead space').

Inadequate ventilation (high Pco$_2$) almost invariably means faulty technique or inadequate sedation except in severe bronchial asthma.

Rapid correction to Pco$_2$ 5.5 kPa (40 mmHg) of compensated respiratory acidosis yields profound metabolic alkalosis, hypokalaemia and hypotension. Large quantities of KCl are needed (up to 200 mEq/day) to replete lost chloride store.

Initial Management

1. Intubate: check position of tube by X-ray.
2. Ventilate: check blood gases.
3. Drip.
4. Naso-gastric tube (gastric stasis almost invariable for 24 hours).
5. Endotracheal toilet (suction with disposable catheter through endotracheal tube).
6. Observe: Blood pressure, ECG monitor, ventilator volumes and pressures.
7. Central venous pressure only if fluid balance problems.

Maintenance

Restlessness means increased ventilatory requirement. Remember that the paralysed sedated patient may be awake. Avoid paralysis after 24 hours if possible. Always assume patient is awake; talk to him, explain actions.
Daily X-ray; blood gas assessment for improvement.

Weaning

Attempt when condition is *improving*. Be prepared to wait 48 hours after any setback. Most chronic bronchitics require 5 days.
Withhold sedation.
See if patient breathes adequately given humidified O$_2$ enriched air around the tracheostomy tube. Be prepared to restore mechanical ventilation (with patient's agreement) for fatigue. On the second day, the tube can almost always be removed.

Complications of Artificial Ventilation

Pneumothorax and pneumomediastinum (high pressures).
Laryngeal damage (bronchotomy after seven to fourteen days, average ten).
Tracheal stenosis (25 per cent have some) and necrosis.

ADULT RESPIRATORY DISTRESS SYNDROME

This is high-protein pulmonary oedema which complicates almost all seriously ill patients requiring ventilation. The pulmonary vessels are abnormally leaky. Known causes include:

1. Pulmonary contusion.
2. Endotoxic shock.
3. Fat embolism
4. Oxygen toxicity.

SUGGESTED FURTHER READING

General Reference Books

Crofton, J. W. and Douglas, A. C. (1975) *Respiratory Diseases*. Oxford: Blackwell.

Fraser, R. G. and Paré, J. A. P. (1970 and 1977) *Diagnosis of Diseases of the Chest: An Integrated Study Based on the Abnormal Roentgenogram*. Philadelphia: Saunders.

Asthma

Clark, T. J. H. and Godfrey, S. (1977) *Asthma*. London: Chapman and Hall.

Chronic Bronchitis and Emphysema

Fletcher, C. M., Peto, R., Tinker, C. and Speizer, F. (1976) *Natural History of Chronic Bronchitis and Emphysema: An Eight Year Study*. Oxford: Oxford University Press.

Thurlbeck, W. M. (1976) in *Respiratory Disease* (ed. Lane, D. J.). London: Heinemann.

Cigarette Smoking

Smoking or Health (1977) Royal College of Physicians, 3rd Report. London: Pitman Medical.

Clinical Signs

Brewis, R. A. L. (1975) Chapters in *Lecture Notes on Respiratory Disease*. Oxford: Blackwell.

Forgacs, P. (1978) *Lung Sounds*. London: Baillière Tindall.

Immunology

Turner-Warwick, M. (1978) *Immunology of the Lung*. London: Arnold.

Occupational Disease

Morgan, W. K. C. and Seaton, A. (1975) *Occupational Lung Diseases*. Philadelphia: Saunders.

Parkes, W. R. (1974). *Occupational Lung Disorders*. London: Butterworths.

Pathology

Spencer, H. (1977) *Pathology of the Lung* (excluding pulmonary tuberculosis), 3rd ed. Vols. i and ii. Oxford: Pergamon Press.

Respiratory Failure

Cumming, G. and Semple, S. J. G. (1973) In *Disorders of the Respiratory System*. Oxford: Blackwell.

Respiratory Physiology: Introduction

Cherniack, R. M. (1977) *Pulmonary Function Testing*. Philadelphia: Saunders.

Saunders, K. B. (1977) *Clinical Physiology of the Lung*. Oxford: Blackwell.

West, J. B. (1974) *Respiratory Physiology*. Oxford: Blackwell.

West, J. B. (1977) *Pulmonary Pathophysiology: The Essentials*. Oxford: Blackwell.

Haematology: Including Disorders of Lymphoid Tissue

19

G. L. SCOTT and A. E. READ

HAEMOPOIESIS

In the adult, haemopoiesis occurs exclusively in the bone marrow, in the ribs, sternum, pelvis, vertebral bodies and the ends of the long bones. In certain pathological states, for example myelofibrosis, the liver and spleen may be involved (extra-medullary haemopoiesis). Although there are toti-potential stem cells, capable of differentiation along any of the major cell lines – erythrocytes, granulocytes and platelets (and probably lymphocytes), blood cells are normally produced from committed stem cells, which give rise to one cell line only.

THE RED CELL

Red cell production requires an adequate number of stem cells (normoblasts), essential nutritional requirements (iron, B_{12}, folic acid) and hormones (thyroxine, androgens). The major stimulus to erythropoiesis is arterial oxygen desaturation. This causes the release of a glycoprotein, erythropoietin, from the renal cortex (?juxtaglomerular apparatus). This probably acts as an enzyme converting a protein, produced by the liver, into the active substance. The major function of red cells is the transport of oxygen by means of haemoglobin. The mature red cell is non-nucleated and has limited synthetic capacity. Its life span is 100 to 120 days (each day over 200×10^6 RBCs are produced by the normal bone marrow). Marrow output can increase up to six-fold by extension of haemopoietic tissue into fatty marrow in the skeleton. It is, therefore, possible to compensate for blood loss and haemolysis provided that there is no lack of factors needed for erythropoiesis. Destruction of red blood cells occurs in the reticuloendothelial system where cleavage of the four-ring haem molecule results in the production of bilirubin and biliverdin, which are handled by the liver (see page 61), the iron and globin being reutilised.

ANAEMIA

Definition

Anaemia is usually said to be present when the haemoglobin concentration falls below the accepted lower limit of the normal range, depending on age and sex (see Table 19.1). This is an over-simplification. A more precise definition would be in terms of the delivery of oxygen to the tissues. In pregnancy and splenomegaly, where there is expansion of the plasma volume, apparent anaemia exists without any alteration of the red cell mass. In some congenital disorders of the red cell, oxygen transport to the tissues may be facilitated so that normal tissue oxygenation occurs despite a low haemoglobin level.

Pathophysiology

The delivery of oxygen to the tissues by haemoglobin depends on the shape and position of the oxygen dissociation curve (Fig. 19.1). These are determined by the structure of the haemoglobin molecule, the pH of

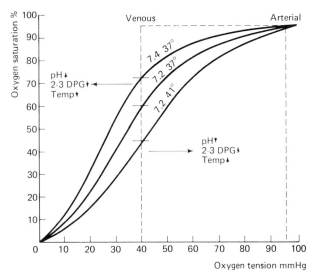

Fig. 19.1   Oxygen dissociation curve of haemoglobin showing influence of pH, 2–3 DPG concentration and temperature.

Table 19.1 Normal red cell values

Measurement	SI Units	Normal range (adults) Males	Females
Haemoglobin	g/dl (decilitre)	13.0–18.0	11.5–16.5
Red cell count	×10^{12}/l	4.5– 6.5	3.9– 5.8
Packed cell volume (PCV)	decimal fraction*	0.40– 0.54	0.37– 0.47
Mean cell volume (MCV)	fl (femtolitre)*	75–95	
Mean cell haemoglobin (MCH)	pg (picogram)	27–32	
Mean cell haemoglobin concentration (MCHC)	g/dl*	31–35	
Reticulocytes	%	0.2–2.0	

Note: Some automated cell counters (e.g. Coulter S) may give different ranges because of the method of calculating the PCV. In particular the range for the MCV is higher (84 to 99) and MCHC is less useful in identifying hypochromic anaemias.

the blood and the concentration of the intracellular metabolite, 2–3 diphosphoglycerate (2–3 DPG).

Alkalosis or a fall in 2–3 DPG shifts the curve to the left and reduces delivery of oxygen. Acidosis and a rise in 2–3 DPG shifts the curve to the right and increases delivery of oxygen.

The principal mechanisms of adaptation to anaemia are increased synthesis of 2–3 DPG and an increase in cardiac ouput. In adults, with a normal cardiovascular system, symptoms of anaemia are unusual, except on exertion, until the haemoglobin level falls below 9.0 g/dl (g/100 ml). Prolonged, uncompensated anaemia causes a hyperdynamic circulation and anoxic changes in the tissues.

Diagnosis

The use of automated electronic cell counters (e.g. Coulter 'S', Haemalog D) has simplified the diagnosis of anaemia and has revived interest in the value of the red cell indices. Mild abnormalities may be detected before they are readily visible on the blood film and iron deficiency and megaloblastic anaemia may be recognised at an earlier stage. It has also been necessary to revise the previously established range of normal values (*see* Table 19.1).

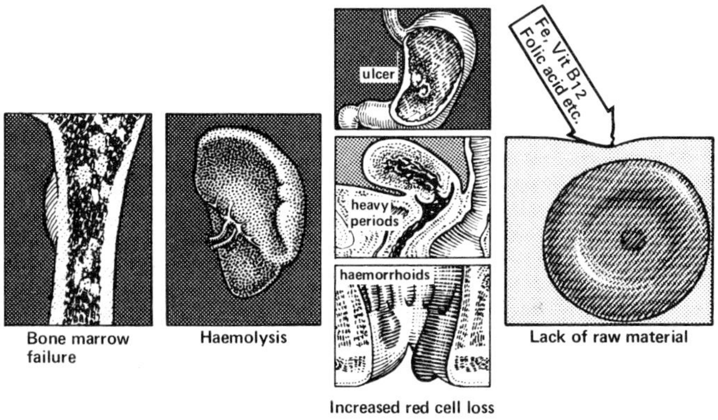

A morphological classification of anaemia, based on the red cell indices is useful because it gives a lead to the underlying cause for the anaemia. On a morphological basis, anaemias can be divided into the following types:

Types of anaemia

Normochromic/Normocytic:
Normal MCV, Normal MCH
e.g. anaemia of chronic disease, malignancy, renal failure, aplastic anaemia.

Hypochromic/Microcytic:
Low MCV, Low MCH
Iron deficiency (*most important*) but also thalassaemia, sideroblastic anaemia, anaemia of chronic disease (severe).

Macrocytic:
MCV raised
Megaloblastic anaemia (*most important*) but remember other causes of macrocytosis:
i.e. reticulocytosis (haemolysis or haemorrhage), liver disease, alcoholism, sideroblastic anaemia, cytotoxic therapy, aplastic anaemia (sometimes), hypothyroidism.

Fig. 19.2 The main causes of anaemia.

Causes (*see* Fig. 19.2)

A Decreased Red Cell Production:
I *Failure of haemoglobin synthesis:*
Iron deficiency.
Thalassaemia.
Sideroblastic anaemia.
Anaemia of chronic disease.

II *Failure of DNA synthesis:*
Megaloblastic anaemia due to:
(a) B$_{12}$ deficiency.
(b) Folate deficiency.
(c) Other rare causes.

III *Bone marrow failure or replacement:*
Aplastic anaemia.
Infiltration due to leukaemia, myeloma, lymphoma, carcinoma or myelofibrosis.

IV *Miscellaneous:*
Hormone deficiency – hypothyroidism.
Erythropoietin lack – chronic renal failure.

B **Increased Red Cell Destruction:**
I. Haemolysis.
II. Chronic blood loss (usually causes iron deficiency anaemia).

Symptoms (of any type of anaemia)

May be none or due to increased cardiac output and tissue anoxia.
Fatigue.
Lassitude.
Dyspnoea.
Palpitations.
Angina.
Intermittent claudication.
Fainting.
Ankle oedema (occasionally due to cardiac failure).

Signs

Pallor.
Tachycardia (hyperdynamic circulation).
Signs of cardiac failure.

A. ANAEMIA DUE TO DECREASED RED CELL PRODUCTION

I ANAEMIA DUE TO FAILURE OF HAEMOGLOBIN SYNTHESIS

CHRONIC IRON DEFICIENCY (Fig. 19.3)

Background

Iron deficiency is the commonest cause of anaemia in the world. It usually results from a combination of inadequate intake and excessive loss. Pre-menopausal women and children are particularly susceptible and in some underdeveloped countries it is almost universal, due to a combination of poor diet and chronic blood loss from parasitic infestation, principally hookworm.

The normal iron requirements are approximately 1 mg/day for men and 2 mg/day for pre-menopausal women. Pregnancy and lactation cause an average net loss of 750 mg. The average Western diet contains 15 to 20 mg of iron/day and only about 10 per cent of this can be absorbed. The principal food sources are shown in Table 19.2.

Table 19.2 Food sources of the major haematinics

	Food sources of haematinics (all uncooked mean values)		
	Fe mg/100 g	Folate µg/100 g	Vit B$_{12}$ mg/100 g
Meat	3	10	6
Liver	10	300	100
Flour	1.5–7	14–20	0.4
Green vegetables	10	50	0
Milk and	0.2	0.2	0.2–0.6
eggs	2	8	1 (per egg)

Factors promoting iron absorption from food include:

(a) Ascorbic acid.
(b) Hydrochloric acid.
These reduce ferric to ferrous iron in which form it is more easily absorbed.
(c) Iron deficiency.
(d) Active erythropoiesis.

Factors diminishing iron absorption include:

(a) Partial gastrectomy – which limits intake and causes malabsorption by increasing the rapidity of intestinal movement past the upper small bowel site of iron absorption (duodenum and upper jejunum).
(b) Combination of iron with dietary phosphates and phytates.

Iron absorption takes place in the upper small bowel by an uncertain mechanism. A storage form, in the epithelial cell, and a disposable form compete for retention. In conditions of iron saturation, iron is shunted to a disposable pool and exfoliated with the intestinal cells into the gut lumen. In iron deficiency and active erythropoiesis iron enters the storage pool and is freely absorbed. In the plasma, iron is transported, bound to a specific β-globulin (transferrin), to the marrow and reticuloendothelial system, where it is either used for erythropoiesis or is stored as ferritin or haemosiderin. There is normally about 1 g of storage iron in the body and this can be mobilised if needed for erythropoiesis. In iron deficiency, the iron stores become depleted before there is any change in the red cells. Anaemia is a late feature of iron deficiency. In iron overload, for example haemachromatosis, or transfusional haemosiderosis, the total iron stores are increased and may be as much as 50 g compared with the normal.

Factors that help to cause iron deficiency (*see* Fig. 19.3) include:

In Women: Menstruation, menorrhagia, pregnancy (particularly multiple).
Poor intake (common in the average housewife).
Malabsorption and chronic intestinal bleeding (e.g. analgesic use, haemorrhoids).

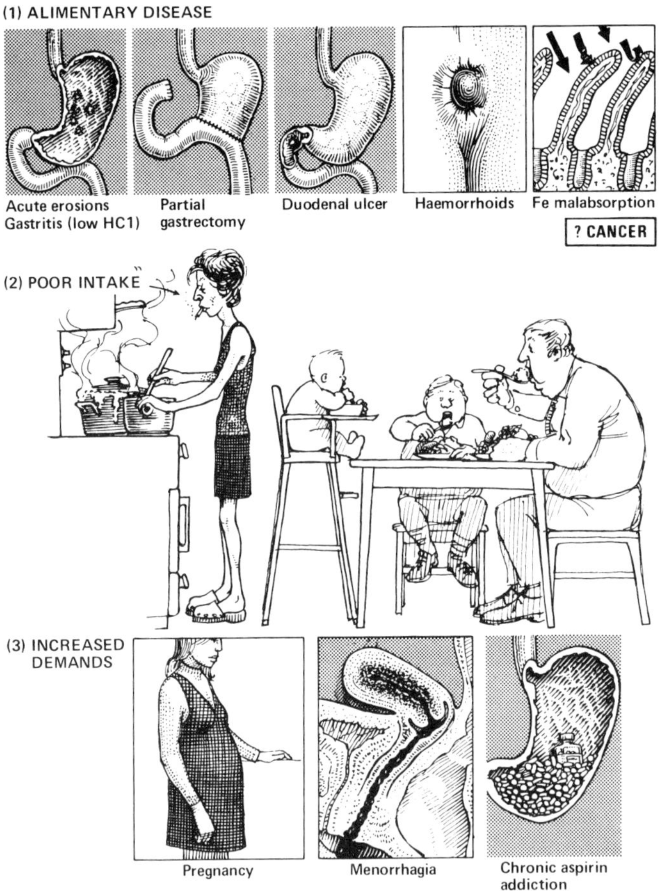

(1) ALIMENTARY DISEASE

Acute erosions Gastritis (low HC1) | Partial gastrectomy | Duodenal ulcer | Haemorrhoids | Fe malabsorption | ? CANCER

(2) POOR INTAKE

(3) INCREASED DEMANDS

Pregnancy | Menorrhagia | Chronic aspirin addiction

Fig. 19.3 The causes of chronic iron deficiency.

In Men: Poor intake (rare).
Chronic intestinal bleeding.

In the Tropics: Hookworm, geophagia, etc.

Pathology

Severe iron depletion causes tissue changes. There may be atrophy of the mucosa of the tongue and gastric mucosa. In some cases this latter feature is reversible and gastric secretion, which is often diminished, may return to normal. Atrophic changes in the mucosa of the upper oesophagus may result in the formation of a web (Paterson–Kelly–Brown syndrome). This causes dysphagia and may be pre-malignant.

Symptoms

May be none or may be due to anaemia (*see above*) or due to tissue iron deficiency.
Lassitude.
Dyspnoea.
Brittle nails.
Sore tongue – rarely.

Indolent cracking at corners of mouth.
Dysphagia.
Pica.

Signs

Pallor.
Spoon-shaped brittle nails (koilonychia).
Smooth, usually pale, tongue.
Angular stomatitis (cheilosis).
Rarely splenomegaly.

Investigations

Note: In latent iron deficiency there may be no changes apart from diminished stainable iron and a lower serum iron level. At a later stage, red cell changes may be present, although the haemoglobin may be normal. In clinical iron deficiency the following are found:
1. The haemoglobin is reduced.
2. The red cells are small (microcytic, MCV less than 75 fl), poorly haemoglobinised (hypochromic, MCH less than 27 pg) and of varying shapes (poikilocytosis) and sizes (anisocytosis).
3. The serum iron is low and the serum transferrin is raised giving a high total iron binding capacity (TIBC). The percentage saturation is less than 15.
4. The bone marrow shows reduced or absent stainable iron and normoblastic hyperplasia.
5. The serum ferritin level is reduced.

Differential Diagnosis

The main types of anaemia likely to be confused with iron deficiency are other hypochromic anaemias, namely:
Thalassaemia, especially thalassaemia minor.
Sideroblastic anaemia.
The anaemia of chronic disease.
The serum iron/TIBC is helpful in distinguishing these conditions.

Basis of Treatment

Treatment should be along two lines – to erradicate the cause for iron deficiency and to correct the anaemia and replenish the iron stores. For the former, dietary advice, a gynaecological opinion in females, and the treatment of gastrointestinal lesions may all be required. The basis of the treatment of the anaemia is the administration of iron, preferably by mouth, but occasionally parenterally. Very rarely, blood transfusion (packed cells) may be needed.

Oral Therapy (Table 19.3). A multitude of oral preparations exists, but there is no evidence that any preparation is more effective than simple Ferrous Sulphate BP 200 mg three times daily taken after meals. In the occasional patient who cannot tolerate this preparation, because of anorexia, constipation, abdominal pain, etc., Ferrous Gluconate BP 300 mg three times daily may be used. These preparations contain 60 and 36 mg of iron in each tablet respectively. Provided there is no malabsorption or other limiting factors the haemoglobin should start to rise 5 to 10 days after starting treatment, and continue to rise at a rate of around 1 g each week. Iron therapy should be continued for at least three months after the haemoglobin has returned to normal in order to replenish the iron stores. Continuous therapy may be needed if the underlying lesion cannot be corrected. Vitamin C can be given with oral iron preparations to increase absorption. Slow release capsules are not only expensive but also ineffective in many cases, because the iron is released in the lower part of the small intestine where absorption is minimal. The commonest reason for not responding to oral iron is failure to take the tablets regularly. Other reasons include malabsorption (rarely), use of the wrong preparation, continuing blood loss and misdiagnosis.

Parenteral Therapy. Parenteral iron should not be used without adequate reason. The main reasons are genuine intolerance of iron (rare, except in patients with inflammatory bowel disease), failure to take oral iron, severe malabsorption, uncontrollable bleeding and severe anaemia in the late stages of pregnancy. Intramuscular iron is preferable because severe side effects are more common with IV iron. These include fever, severe back pain, headache, vomiting, joint pains and occasionally anaphylactic reactions. IV iron also frequently causes severe painful phlebitis at the site of infusion. There is little evidence that IM or IV rather than oral iron causes a faster rise in haemoglobin.

The preparations available are:

Ferrivenin – saccharrated iron oxide for IV use (multiple weekly doses of 100 mg).

Imferon ⎤ ⎧ (Iron dextran and iron sorbitol citrate acid)
Jectofer ⎦ ⎨ Preparations, for IM use and in the case of
      ⎩ Imferon for total dose IV infusion.

Total dose. IV infusion of iron by which 1 g or more of iron, as Imferon, is given slowly by IV infusion diluted in 1 litre of 5 per cent dextrose and normal saline, has become popular in the past few years, particularly for severe anaemia in pregnancy. There is evidence that this technique does produce a more rapid rise in haemoglobin, but it may be accompanied by alarming side effects, especially in pregnancy.

There is always a danger that iron deficiency anaemia will be incompletely investigated, particularly as the anaemia can be so readily cured. A most careful watch

Table 19.3 Treatment of iron deficiency anaemia

Route	Preparation	Advantages	Disadvantages
Oral	Ferrous sulphate 200 mg tds (180 mg Fe)	Cheap (1 month's treatment 2.5p)	Occasional intolerance Nausea, constipation, abdominal pain, etc.
	Ferrous gluconate 300 mg tds (108 mg Fe)	Cheap, but costs three times that of ferrous sulphate	
	Feospan 2 capsules daily (90 mg Fe)	Once daily treatment	Costs 22 times that of ferrous sulphate (Slow and expensive)
	Slow Fe 2 tablets daily (100 mg Fe)	Once daily treatment	Costs 18 times that of ferrous sulphate
Intramuscular	e.g. Jectofer (iron sorbital) 2 ml → 100 mg Fe	?Slightly more rapid effect	Painful. Contraindicated in renal or hepatic disease
	Imferon (iron dextran) 2 ml → 100 mg Fe		Painful – occasionally fever, arthralgia. Skin staining. Avoid? risk of neoplasia (based on animal experiments). Contraindicated in hepatic and renal disease
Intravenous	Ferrivenin (saccharated iron) 2 ml → 100 mg Fe	Given as calculated series of injections of 2–5 ml (100–250 mg Fe)	Injections must *not* be given outside veins. Contraindicated in hepatic and renal disease
	Imferon (iron dextran) 2 ml → 100 mg Fe	May be used as total Fe infusion, i.e. 1–2 g Fe diluted in 5% dextrose drip	Occasional alarming side effects, e.g. collapse, generalised muscle pain, thrombophlebitis

Note: To form 1 g of haemoglobin requires 250 mg of iron.

for causes, such as intestinal (particularly colonic) cancer, must be kept in patients in whom a diagnosis of idiopathic iron deficiency has been made. A solitary barium meal should not be the reason for assuming that no intestinal lesion is present. Investigations should be thorough and hospital directed.

THALASSAEMIA (see under Disorders of haemoglobin page 388)

SIDEROBLASTIC ANAEMIA

This term describes a heterogenous group of anaemias in which there is failure to incorporate iron into haem, possibly due to a congenital or acquired defect in the enzymes concerned with haem synthesis. Pyridoxine is a co-factor in haem synthesis and relative deficiency of this vitamin may be a factor. There is usually a moderately severe anaemia (Hb around 8 g/dl) and the blood film shows a characteristic picture of dimorphic red cells, i.e. a mixture of hypochromic and normochromic cells and there may be macrocytosis. A high serum iron level and increased saturation of transferrin distinguish these anaemias from iron deficiency. The diagnostic feature is the presence of normoblasts containing a perinuclear ring of iron-laden granules (ring sideroblasts) in the marrow.

This disorder occurs in two main forms, a rare primary sex-linked form found in males and a secondary acquired form. The acquired form may be idiopathic, mainly found in the elderly, or secondary. Secondary causes include drugs (e.g. antituberculous drugs, INAH is a pyridoxine antagonist), alcoholism, lead poisoning, malabsorption and malnutrition. It may also complicate myeloproliferative disorders, haemolysis, megaloblastic anaemia and leukaemia. Some idiopathic forms may be pre-leukaemic.

Treatment is unsatisfactory. Most patients with the congenital form and a smaller number with the idiopathic form will respond to pyridoxine. Large doses (up to 300 mg daily) may be needed and treatment may be required for several months before a response occurs. Some patients will respond to folic acid or crude liver extract. Transfusion should be avoided if possible because iron overload usually makes the condition worse.

ANAEMIA OF CHRONIC DISEASE

Anaemia is a common complication of chronic infections (e.g. SBE, tuberculosis) chronic inflammatory conditions (e.g. rheumatoid arthritis) and malignancy. In these conditions there may be multiple causes for anaemia, for example chronic blood loss in rheumatoid arthritis due to ingestion of analgesics and folate deficiency in malignancy. Nevertheless, there is also a common, and incompletely understood, refractory anaemia due to a disturbance in iron transport. Iron accumulates in the reticuloendothelial system and is not available for erythropoiesis. The haemoglobin level falls slowly to around 8 g/dl, and the red cells are normochromic, although they may become hypochromic if the disease is prolonged. The serum iron level is low and so is the TIBC, so that the percentage saturation of transferrin is either normal or only slightly reduced. In the marrow there is abundant storage iron in the reticuloendothelial cells, but little in the normoblasts. This form of anaemia must be distinguished from iron deficiency because iron therapy is not indicated. There is no treatment apart from treatment of the primary condition and, in severe cases, blood transfusion.

II ANAEMIA DUE TO DEFECTIVE DNA SYNTHESIS

MEGALOBLASTIC ANAEMIA

Definition

Megaloblastic anaemia is caused by defective DNA synthesis, most commonly due to B_{12} or folate deficiency, although other rarer causes exist. It is characterised by the appearance of the red cell precursors in the marrow which have large nuclei with an open chromatin pattern.

Background

Both B_{12} and folate are needed for purine and pyrimidine synthesis which are essential constituents of DNA. Deficiency of B_{12} and folate interfere with DNA synthesis and the effects are seen in all rapidly proliferating tissue, particularly the bone marrow, epithelial cells and the gonads. In addition, B_{12} deficiency may affect the tissue of the CNS, although the biochemical basis of this is unknown.

Folate. Folic acid is pteroylglutamic acid. In food, folate is present in a variety of forms including larger molecules – polyglutamates. Folates are found in many foods, particularly fresh green vegetables, yeast and liver (Table 19.2). The folate content of food may be destroyed by cooking and the polyglutamates are inactive until split by intestinal enzymes—conjugases. Folic acid is absorbed in the small bowel, there being no specific absorption site. The average daily intake is around 400 μg, the average daily need being 100 μg. The body stores, mainly in the liver, are about 10 to 15 mg. Folate needs are increased where there is rapid cell proliferation, for example haemolysis, malignancy and pregnancy.

Folic acid may be measured in serum and in red cells. The former is not a reliable guide to body folate stores as it is very labile; the latter is more useful. Folate is usually assayed by a microbiological technique using *Lactobacillus casei*. Normal values are:

Serum 6 to 20 μg/l.
Red cell 150 to 650 μg/l.

Interpretation of folate levels may depend on the B_{12} level (Table 19.4).

Vitamin B_{12}. Vitamin B_{12} is a group of compounds, the cobalamins. Various forms exist in the body; the most important being methylcobalamin. Hydroxycobalamin is usually used in treatment. Cyanocobalamin, formerly used, is contraindicated because it is partially inactive, at least as far as the neurological effect, and it may even promote changes in the CNS. Absorption involves combination with a glycoprotein, intrinsic factor (IF), secreted by the gastric fundal cells. The combined B_{12}:IF complex is absorbed in the terminal ileum where absorption takes place at a specific receptor site with splitting of the complex. In the plasma, B_{12}, in the form of methyl B_{12}, is transported on specific transport proteins – the transcobalamins.

B_{12} is found only in animal produce. The average daily intake is about 100 μg and the average daily need is 2 μg. Body stores, mainly in the liver, amount to between 2 to 4 mg.

B_{12} can be measured in serum. There are two principal methods of assay – a microbiological one using *Lactobacillus leichmanii* and a radioassay. These two techniques give different normal ranges:

L. *leichmanii* assay   160– 900 ng/l.
Radioassay   300–1000 ng/l.

Very high B_{12} levels may occur in liver disease and in myeloproliferative disorders (*see* Table 19.4).

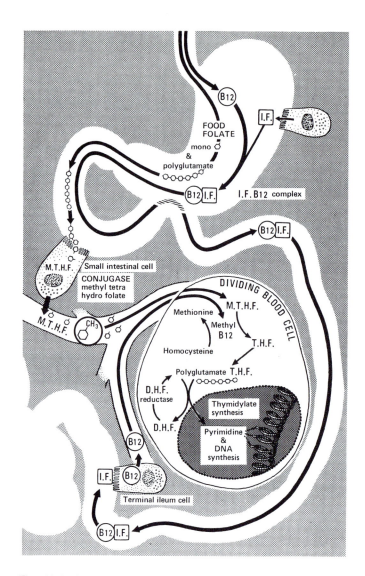

Fig. 19.4 B_{12} and folate metabolism.

Table 19.4   Interpretation of B_{12}/folate levels

	Serum B_{12}	Serum folate	Red cell folate
B_{12} deficiency	↓	N or ↑	N or ↓
Folate deficiency	N or ↓	↓	↓
Combined deficiency	↓	↓	↓
Doubtful significance*	N	↓	N

Note:
1.* Low serum folate levels are common in ill patients and do not necessarily denote folate deficiency.
2. Antibiotics may interfere with microbiological assays.
3. High levels of B_{12} and folate will be found in treated patients.
4. High levels of B_{12} are also found in liver damage and some myeloproliferative disorders.

B_{12} and Folate Metabolism (Figure 19.4). B_{12} and folate metabolism are interrelated. Folates are converted in the small intestinal cells to methyltetrahydrofolate (methyl THF) which is the principal form in the plasma. Methyl THF enters cells where it is demethylated to give THF and this is used to form THF polyglutamates, the active folate co-enzymes. These take part in many reactions involving the transfer of one-carbon fragments. An important folate-dependent reaction is thymidylate synthesis, required for the formation of pyrimidine. In this reaction, THF is oxidised to dihydrofolate (DHF), which is inactive, and which is re-converted to THF by the enzyme DHF reductase. Inhibition of this enzyme by some drugs – for example methotrexate, is an important cause of folate deficiency.

The most important known reaction of methyl B_{12} is the methylation of homocysteine to methionine, because this is needed to convert methyl THF to THF, an essential step in folate metabolism. Thus B_{12} deficiency causes a block in folate metabolism as a result of which the serum folate level rises because it is no longer metabolised and intracellular folates become depleted.

Causes of B₁₂ deficiency

Inadequate intake:
    Strict vegetarianism, vegans
    Extreme malnutrition

Malabsorption – gastric:
    Pernicious anaemia
    Congenital intrinsic factor deficiency
    Partial or total gastrectomy

Malabsorption – intestinal:
    Blind loop syndrome
    Coeliac disease
    Tropical sprue
    Crohn's disease
    Ileal resection
    Fish tapeworm – rare, except in Scandinavia
    Congenital B₁₂ malabsorption

1. PERNICIOUS ANAEMIA (Figure 19.5)

Definition

Megaloblastic anaemia due to B_{12} deficiency caused by intrinsic factor deficiency, resulting from immunological damage to the gastric mucosa.

Background

This is a disease of the elderly, being rare under the age of 40, although a rare juvenile form is known. The patients often have grey hair and blue eyes, or give a family history of premature hair greying and/or vitiligo. Pernicious anaemia has a known familial tendency and is not uncommonly associated with diseases of immunological significance, such as idiopathic hypothyroidism, rheumatoid arthritis or diabetes. The finding of antithyroid antibodies in many patients with pernicious anaemia and the existence of both gastric and IF antibodies supports an immune aetiology.

Pathology

There is marrow hyperplasia in the long bones. Epithelial surfaces show degenerative changes, particularly marked in the stomach which is thin-walled and shows marked atrophy of the body and fundus.

Symptoms

Those of anaemia.
Painful glossitis.

CNS symptoms:
    Numbness and tingling in hands and feet.
    Weakness of limbs.
    Unsteadiness of gait.
    Occasionally dimness of vision and symptoms of psychiatric disorder, depression, confusion, hallucinations, etc.

Signs

Pallor.
Pyrexia.
Jaundice, usually slight (related to haemolysis and ineffective erythropoiesis).
Vitiligo.
Splenomegaly.
Occasionally haemorrhagic retinopathy.
Neurological:
    Peripheral neuritis.
    Spastic paraplegia.
    Posterior column signs, e.g. loss of proprioception and vibration sense.
    Confusion.
    Dementia.
    Optic atrophy.
Note: Look for other evidence of immune diseases and enquire carefully of the family history.

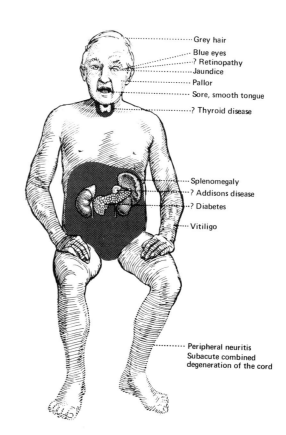

Fig. 19.5 Pernicious anaemia.

Investigations

Haematological:

1. There is anaemia of varying degree. In severe cases the haemoglobin level may be as low as 3 g/dl, but in early cases the haemoglobin level may be normal.

2. There is macrocytosis, MCV greater than 100 fl and in severe cases it may exceed 130 fl, but if iron deficiency also exists the MCV may be normal.

3. The blood film shows macrocytic red cells, usually oval in shape, and anisocytosis and poikilocytosis. The red cells are fully haemoglobinised and the MCH is normal. In combined iron and B_{12} deficiency, there may be a dimorphic picture with macrocytes and hypochromic cells.

4. The white cell and platelet count are often low.

5. The bone marrow shows megaloblastic erythropoiesis and also white cell changes with giant metamyelocytes.

6. The serum B_{12} level is low, but occasionally may be at the lower limit of normal and in patients with neurological complications it is often very low. Serum folate levels are variable (see Table 19.4).

7. The diagnosis is confirmed by radioactive B_{12} absorption tests. The most usual technique employed is the Schilling test which depends on the estimation of urinary labelled B_{12} excretion over 24 hours following a small dose (1 μg) of oral labelled vitamin B_{12} and a large (1 mg) dose of cold vitamin B_{12} by intramuscular injection to produce urinary excretion. Characteristically, in pernicious anaemia the 24-hour labelled urinary excretion is less than 5 per cent, but there is full correction (greater than 10 per cent excretion) if the test is repeated with an effective source of IF.

(Note: patients with high gastric IF antibody levels may show incomplete correction with IF). A modern technique, with both free and IF bound forms of vitamin B_{12} differentially labelled, allows simultaneous absorption of both varieties of B_{12} to be measured. This is provided in a pre-formed pack as Dicopac. However, false results may be obtained by this technique and it is more expensive than the standard Schilling test.

8. Immunological. Gastric parietal cell antibodies are found in around 90 per cent of patients with pernicious anaemia; these may also be found in patients with gastric atrophy and in normal subjects. Antibodies to IF are diagnostic of pernicious anaemia but they are found in only 60 per cent of patients with pernicious anaemia. Other auto-antibodies particularly anti-thyroid antibodies are commonly found.

9. Miscellaneous. The production of gastric basal and maximal acid is impaired. The latter is best shown after effective stimulation of the stomach with Pentagastrin 6 μg/kg. The volume and acid response is reduced and pH does not fall below 6.

10. Radiology is important in the exclusion of other causes of vitamin B_{12} deficiency and often the stomach shows evidence of mucosal atrophy (tubular or 'bald' stomach).

11. Serum bilirubin is mildly raised. The serum iron is also raised unless there is coexistent iron deficiency.

Complications

Sub-acute combined degeneration of the cord, and other neurological symptoms.
Gastric cancer.
Other autoimmune diseases, particularly myxoedema.

Differential Diagnosis

Other forms of megaloblastic anaemia.

Basis of Treatment

This is with vitamin B_{12} in the form of hydroxycobalamin. It is usual to give an initial high dosage – i.e. 1 mg by injection for six doses on alternate days, particularly if there is neurological involvement. Following this, 250 μg is given by intramuscular injection at monthly intervals for the rest of the patient's life. After treatment, signs of response include a reduction in pyrexia, increased well-being and, on the sixth day, a maximal reticulocytosis depending on the initial haemoglobin level, followed by a steady rise in haemoglobin. If iron deficiency also exists, this may reduce the rate of response.

Severe cases, often accompanied by toxic confusion and neurological disorders, are worrying problems. Transfusion with packed cells may be required, although this must be done with great caution and with a simultaneous administration of a diuretic. The patient's cerebration may deteriorate after vitamin B_{12} treatment and before improvement eventually begins. Recent work has stressed the importance of potassium depletion in the cause of this syndrome, but there is no need to give potassium supplements except in the most severe cases.

Treatment with folic acid alone is highly dangerous and on no account should it be given because of the risk of lowering the serum vitamin B_{12} and precipitating neurological damage.

Patients on regular vitamin B_{12} injections often complain, at follow-up, of feeling weak and tired prior to the monthly injection. There is little to support the validity of such claims and generally pernicious anaemia remains a most satisfactory disorder to treat. Two provisos have to be made about this last statement. First, as the stomach remains atrophic (though it has been shown that structure and function can be improved with steroid therapy) there is a ten-fold risk, compared with normal controls, of gastric cancer. Second, other autoimmune disorders may develop and myxoedema in particular needs prompt recognition. These two reasons are the major ones for regular follow-up.

Rarely, patients with sub-acute combined degeneration of the cord sustain permanent neurological damage. There is no place nowadays for the use of other forms of vitamin B_{12} and/or IF therapy.

The treatment of patients with severe megaloblastic anaemia of unknown aetiology is a difficult problem. The best course is to take blood for B_{12} and folate assays and then to start treatment with high dose B_{12} and then to follow this 24 hours later with folate.

2. ANAEMIA DUE TO OTHER CAUSES OF B_{12} DEFICIENCY

Inadequate Intake. This is a rare cause in developed countries, except in vegans.

Gastrectomy. Due to loss of IF by surgical resection and subsequent atrophy in the gastric remnant. To this must be added the effects of afferent loop stasis and poor intake. Anaemia takes two years or more to develop because of hepatic vitamin B_{12} stores, occasionally it may not become apparent until after 10 to 15 years.

Malabsorption. Vitamin B_{12} deficiency is found in 10 per cent of coeliac patients, but is more common in tropical sprue, particularly when it is chronic.

Childhood Forms:
(i) Congenital intrinsic factor deficiency. (*Note:* gastric acid and pepsin normal, which differentiates it from juvenile pernicious anaemia.)
(ii) Congenital B_{12} malabsorption.
(Due to failure of ileal absorption. Gastric function and IF normal. Proteinuria found.)
(iii) Juvenile pernicious anaemia identical with the adult disease and often found with other endocrine diseases, e.g. hypoparathyroidism, Addison's disease.
(iv) Coeliac disease, etc. (*see above*).

Note: The importance of these conditions lies in their ability to produce both anaemia and neurological disease.

3. FOLATE DEFICIENCY (Fig. 19.6)

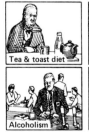 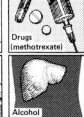 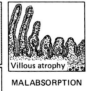 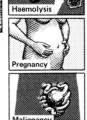 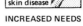

Fig. 19.6 The major causes of folate deficiency.

Causes of folate deficiency

Inadequate intake:
  Malnutrition
    old age
    poverty
    psychiatric disturbance
    alcoholism

Malabsorption:
  Coeliac disease
  Tropical sprue
  Dermatitis herpetiformis enteropathy

Excess demands:
  Pregnancy
  Prematurity
  Chronic haemolysis
  Malignancy
    leukaemia
    lymphoma
    myeloproliferative disorders
    (e.g. myelosclerosis, polycythaemia)
  Exfoliative skin disorders

Drugs:
  Anticonvulsants
  Alcohol
  Oral contraceptives
  Folate antagonists
    e.g. methotrexate
    pyrimethamine (Daraprim)
    cotrimoxazole (Septrin)

Deficiency of folic acid produces an exactly similar type of anaemia. The diagnosis is made by the finding of low folate levels and a response to oral folic acid, provided malabsorption is not present. Diagnosis of folate deficiency secondary to malabsorption may be confirmed by proving malabsorption of nutrients such as fat and carbohydrates and by using a folate absorption test.

Pregnancy

Megaloblastic anaemia of pregnancy is found in 0.5 to 5 per cent of pregnant women and is commonest in Asia and Africa. It is more likely with multiple pregnancies and is related to dietary intake. Its cause is the increased demands for folate by the growing fetus. These outstrip the nutritional intake. It is important because of the increased risk of accidental haemorrhage. Prophylaxis is

381

with folate and iron supplements (folate 100 μg daily, in addition to a normal diet).

Malabsorption

This is most often seen in coeliac disease where folic acid deficiency is almost universal and determinations of serum and red cell folate are good screening tests for this disease. In mild cases, folate deficiency may occur without any other symptoms of malabsorption. Deficiency may be due to architectural abnormality in the small bowel mucosa or, perhaps, intestinal conjugase deficiency.

Drugs

Drugs may produce folate deficiency in a variety of ways. Methotrexate inhibits dihydrofolate reductase. The mode of action of anticonvulsants is not certain, although it is thought that they interfere with the action of intestinal conjugases. There is also often a diminished folate intake. It is certainly common, and about one-third of epileptics on long term treatment have biochemical or haematological evidence of deficiency. The detection of folate deficiency is important as its correction may lead to a lessening of fits. Alcohol has a direct anti-folate action, although diminished intake is an important additional factor in alcoholics. Low folate levels are not uncommon in women on oral contraceptives but megaloblastic anaemia is rare.

Malignancy and Myeloproliferative Syndromes

With the exception of leukaemia, which may be exacerbated, beneficial clinical and haematological effect may follow the use of folic acid supplements when secondary folate deficiency develops.

Therapy

The usual dose of folic acid is 5 to 15 mg daily. A rise in the reticulocyte count and in the haemoglobin follows treatment. In patients with malabsorption the dose used is such that enough of the drug crosses the intestinal barrier to cause a marrow response. Where B$_{12}$ deficiency is present therapy with folic acid alone may precipitate neurological complications.

III ANAEMIA DUE TO BONE MARROW FAILURE OR INFILTRATION

1. APLASTIC ANAEMIA

Definition

Aplastic anaemia is caused by reduction in the number of, or the disorderly function of, the haemopoietic stem cells, in the absence of marrow infiltration and in the presence of all of the essential factors required for normal haemopoiesis. Usually all haemopoietic cell lines are involved so that there is neutropenia and thrombocytopenia as well as anaemia, although the degree of each is variable.

Background

Most cases of aplastic anaemia result from damage to the marrow due to drugs, chemicals or viruses. Some cases appear to be 'idiopathic' in that no obvious cause can be identified, although many of these may be due to unusual susceptibility to some unrecognised toxic agent. The known cause of aplastic anaemia can be classified as follows:

(a) Marrow Suppressant Drugs. These will produce marrow aplasia in all patients if given in sufficient dosage. These are the cytotoxic drugs, especially the alkylating agents, used in the treatment of malignant disease. Busulphan (Myleran) is particularly hazardous as its effects may be delayed and some patients may be susceptible to relatively small doses. Excessive radiation is another cause.

(b) Other Drugs. The action of these drugs is unpredictable. Only a small percentage of patients receiving them will react adversely. Usually several courses, rather than continuous treatment, are needed although the total dose received may be small. At present there is no known way in which susceptible subjects may be identified by laboratory tests. A large number of drugs have been suspected of causing aplastic anaemia although there is considerable difficulty in establishing a causal relationship.

Known high risk drugs include:

*Chloramphenicol	Gold
Sulphonamides	Penicillamine
*Phenylbutazone and	Anticonvulsants – phenytoin
derivates	Oral hypoglycaemic agents
*Amidopyrine (now no longer used)	

*indicates particularly high risk.

Chloramphenicol is now rarely used for antibacterial therapy in the United Kingdom although it is still widely used in some parts of the world, including Europe.

Phenylbutazone is probably the commonest cause of aplastic anaemia in the UK and in many cases it is prescribed unnecessarily, when another simple analgesic would suffice.

Note: possibly most drugs may cause aplastic anaemia in the rare susceptible subject and therefore *indiscriminate prescribing without definite indication* should be avoided. Regular blood counts should be carried out on patients receiving courses of gold and penicillamine, as aplasia may be preceded by a gradual reduction in white cells and platelets and if this occurs the drug should be stopped immediately.

(c) Chemicals. The high risk ones include:

Benzene
Toluene
DDT
Gammabenzene hexachloride

Hair dyes and modelling glue have also been implicated. *All chemicals*, particularly solvents, insecticides and weed-killers should be handled with *extreme caution*.

(d) Viruses. Aplasia following infectious hepatitis is well recognised. The hepatitis is often mild and aplastic anaemia develops several months after recovering from hepatitis. The fatality rate is high. Temporary marrow aplasia (usually with a cellular marrow) may complicate other viral infections.

(e) Other Recognised Types. These include
(i) Congenital aplastic anaemia. Several rare varieties exist, e.g. Diamond–Blackfan syndrome – red cell aplasia, possibly a metabolic defect.
(ii) Pure red cell aplasia. Red cell series alone are affected. May have an immunological basis as it is often associated with autoimmune disease and a thymoma.

Symptoms

These are due to:
Anaemia.
Neutropenia – infections, especially of throat and tonsils.
Thrombocytopenia – bruising, bleeding from mucous membranes, cerebral haemorrhage.

Signs

Pallor.
Purpura and ecchymoses on skin, mucous membranes and sometimes haemorrhagic retinopathy.
Tonsillitis, pharyngitis, skin infections, septicaemia.

Investigations

1. Blood count. Anaemia is invariable and may be severe. The red cells are usually normocytic, although they may be macrocytic. Reticulocytes are usually low or absent.
2. Granulocytes and thrombocytes are variable in number.
3. Bad prognostic features are:
   Platelets $<20 \times 10^9/l$.
   Neutrophils $<0.4 \times 10^9/l$.
   Reticulocytes $<10 \times 10^9/l$ or 0.1 per cent.
4. Bone marrow aspiration usually yields a 'bloody tap' without fragments.
Bone marrow trephine biopsy is *mandatory* in all cases of suspected aplastic anaemia to exclude other causes of pancytopenia.
5. Ferrokinetic studies using ^{59}Fe. Useful in assessing erythropoiesis.
6. HLA typing – The patient and all siblings should be HLA typed in case bone marrow transplantation is indicated.
7. Ham's Test – To exclude paroxysmal nocturnal haemoglobinuria (PNH).

Differential Diagnosis

Other causes of pancytopenia:
   'Aleukaemic leukaemia'.
   Marrow infiltration due to carcinoma, lymphoma.
   Severe megaloblastic anaemia.
   Miscellaneous, including hypersplenism, miliary tuberculosis.

Basis of Treatment

Aplastic anaemia is a serious disease. Fifty per cent of patients die within six months, and of those with the bad prognostic features listed above 90 per cent are dead at the end of one year.

An exhaustive search should be made for a toxic cause and if a drug is suspected this should be withdrawn immediately. Chelating agents are of use in gold or heavy metal poisoning.

The basis of treatment is supportive therapy to prevent death due to anaemia, haemorrhage and infection until spontaneous recovery occurs. Patients in whom anaemia is the major problem may be maintained for many years by regular blood transfusions, although difficulty may arise from lack of veins, antibody production and haemosiderosis. Haemorrhage may be prevented by platelet transfusions, but patients invariably become resistant to random platelet transfusion because of antibody formation. Infections should be treated vigorously with wide spectrum antibiotics if the cause cannot be identified.

Corticosteroids help to reduce bleeding although they have no long term effect. The role of androgenic steroids is still debatable although it is probable that they do have a beneficial effect in some cases. Oxymethalone is the most widely used due to its low androgenic effect. It must be used at a high dose (2 to 5 mg/kg/day) and treatment may be needed for several months before any effect is seen. Regular liver function tests are needed to detect impending liver damage.

For poor risk patients the only hope for cure lies in bone marrow transplantation, provided that a suitable donor, usually a sibling, is available. Bone marrow transplantation is a hazardous procedure and an unpleasant experience for the recipient. Nevertheless the results so far suggest that the prognosis is better for transplanted patients than for those treated conservatively. There is a good case for referring poor risk patients to a centre experienced in bone marrow transplantation as soon as possible after the diagnosis is made, before they become sensitised to foreign antigens by repeated transfusion or die from overwhelming infection.

2. ANAEMIA DUE TO BONE MARROW INFILTRATION

Carcinoma and other malignant diseases may infiltrate the bone marrow and cause anaemia. The blood picture is usually leuco-erythroblastic, i.e. both immature white cells and red cells (normoblasts) are seen. Although lymphomatous infiltration may respond to cytotoxic therapy, the prognosis in carcinoma is usually very poor.

IV ANAEMIA DUE TO MISCELLANEOUS CAUSES

Anaemia is found in a number of medical diseases and often multiple factors are involved.

In *uraemia*, bone marrow function is depressed possibly due to a direct toxic effect. Erythropoietin lack is an important additional cause and persists despite removal of toxic factors by regular dialysis.

The anaemia of *liver disease* is complicated and includes marrow depression as well as haemolysis (q.v.), hypersplenism, iron and folate deficiency.

In *hypothyroidism*, marrow depression is perhaps related to diminished tissue needs for oxygen (and there is also a dilutional factor associated with fluid retention). The anaemia in hypothyroidism is often macrocytic and responds directly to thyroxine therapy.

The anaemia of *scurvy* similarly responds to vitamin C, but there is also a haemolytic element. Iron deficiency due to bleeding and poor oral intake as well as folate deficiency may also occur.

B. ANAEMIA DUE TO INCREASED RED CELL DESTRUCTION

HAEMOLYTIC ANAEMIA

Definition

Haemolytic anaemia occurs when the red cell life span (normally 100 to 120 days) is shortened by premature destruction and the capacity of the bone marrow to compensate for it is exceeded.

Background (Fig. 19.7)

Premature destruction of red cells (haemolysis) may be due to intrinsic abnormalities of the red cells or extracorpuscular factors, for example antibodies. In all types of haemolytic anaemia there is evidence of increased red cell production shown by a reticulocytosis and erythroid

hyperplasia in the marrow. The blood film shows polychromatic red cells (reticulocytes), which may be macrocytic, and in severe cases nucleated red cells may be present. Red cell abnormalities, for example spherocytes and fragmented red cells, may occur in some types of haemolytic anaemia.

There are also changes in bilirubin metabolism due to increased haemoglobin breakdown. The characteristic changes are an increase in serum bilirubin and an increased urinary and faecal uro- and stercobilinogen. Bilirubin is not found in the urine in uncomplicated haemolysis.

Red cell destruction may occur either in the reticuloendothelial system (extravascular haemolysis) or, more rarely, in the bloodstream (intravascular haemolysis). In the latter, free haemoglobin is liberated into the plasma where it combines with a transport protein haptoglobin and is transported to the reticuloendothelial system. When the haptoglobins are fully saturated, haemoglobin may combine with albumin, forming methaemalbumin, and it also appears in the urine, haemoglobinuria. Some haemoglobin in the urine is resorbed by the renal tubular cells, where it is broken down and excreted in desquamated cells as haemosiderin. Evidence of intravascular haemolysis is found, therefore, in haemoglobinaemia, methaemalbuminaemia, lowered or absent haptoglobins (note: this may occur in other conditions – especially liver disease), haemoglobinuria and haemosiderinuria. Finally, conclusive evidence of haemolysis may be obtained by measuring the rate of destruction of red cells labelled with the radioactive compound ^{51}Cr (sodium chromate). Surface counting over the liver and spleen may show the major site of red cell destruction and is useful in deciding whether splenectomy should be undertaken.

Pathology

Increased haemolysis leads to expansion of the marrow into the shafts of the long bones. In children with severe congenital haemolytic anaemia expansion of the marrow cavity may lead to changes in the cortical bone, producing clinical and radiological evidence of bone expansion. Pigment gall stones are commonly found in chronic haemolysis and splenomegaly occurs in many types of haemolytic anaemia.

Symptoms

Symptoms of anaemia (q.v.), and increased haemoglobin breakdown.
Jaundice, usually mild.
Haemoglobinuria.
Upper abdominal pain due to gall stones.
Leg ulceration in chronic haemolytic anaemia.
Specific symptoms of the causative lesion, e.g. bone pain in sickle cell disease.

Signs

Pallor.
Jaundice.
Splenomegaly.
Leg ulceration.
Bone changes (in chronic cases).
In congenital haemolytic anaemia—infantilism.

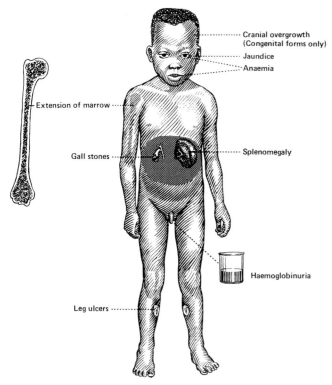

Fig. 19.7 Features of haemolysis.

1. HAEMOLYSIS DUE TO CONGENITAL ABNORMALITIES OF RED CELLS

Hereditary Spherocytosis

This is the commonest form of congenital haemolytic anaemia in Caucasians. It is inherited as an autosomal dominant character with incomplete penetrance, which means that the family history is not always obtained, although symptomless affected relatives may be discovered by laboratory tests. The nature of the lesion is not known for certain, but it is most likely an abnormality of the membrane protein. This causes the formation of spheroidal red cells which are abnormally sequestered in the spleen. The commonest clinical picture is recurrent episodes of anaemia and jaundice in childhood due to a temporarily increased rate of haemolysis and/or bone marrow suppression, usually caused by infection. Severe cases may present at birth as haemolytic disease of the newborn. Other modes of presentation include gall stones and intractable leg ulcers. Some

Causes of haemolytic anaemia

1. Congenital red cell defects

Membrane defects:
  Hereditary spherocytosis
  Hereditary elliptocytosis
Enzyme defects:
  Pyruvate kinase (PK) deficiency
  Glucose-6-phosphate dehydrogenase
    deficiency
Haemoglobin defects:
  Structural abnormalities e.g. Hb S. C. D
  Abnormal chain synthesis – Thalassaemia

2. Acquired haemolytic anaemia

Immune:
  Autoimmune haemolytic anaemia (AIHA)
  Isoimmune – incompatible blood tranfusion
  Haemolytic disease of the newborn
Infections:
  Malaria
  Septicaemias
Drugs and chemicals
Membrane disorders:
  Paroxysmal nocturnal haemoglobinuria
    (PNH)
  Liver disease
  Uraemia
Mechanical:
  Microangiopathic haemolytic anaemia
  Cardiac value prothesis
  March haemoglobinuria
Hypersplenism
Miscellaneous:
  Liver disease
  malignancy, etc.

patients may be completely asymptomatic and diagnosed as a chance finding when a blood count is done for some other reason. The spleen is usually palpable. As with all chronic haemolytic anaemias, folate deficiency may occur, especially in women when they become pregnant. The diagnosis is readily made from the clinical picture, family studies and the finding of a haemolytic anaemia with spherocytic red cells, and increased red cell fragility. The only condition which may cause confusion is autoimmune haemolytic anaemia (*see* page 389). Here the direct antiglobulin (Coombs') test is positive.

Treatment is splenectomy, which does not affect the basic red cell abnormality, but removes the major source of red cell destruction. Splenectomy also improves the leg ulcers and development when there is infantilism. Splenectomy should be recommended, in all but the mildest cases, to prevent complications due to gall stones, aplastic crisis and congestive cardiac failure.

Congenital Non-spherocytic Haemolytic Anaemia

These rare diseases may be caused by red cell enzyme or haemoglobin defects. The commonest is pyruvate-kinase deficiency, an abnormality of glucose metabolism. The clinical picture mimics spherocytosis, but the red cells are not spherocytic. The diagnosis depends on enzyme assays. Splenectomy is less successful but may be indicated if there is symptomatic anaemia.

Hereditary Elliptocytosis

This condition resembles HS, but the red cells are elliptical rather than spherocytic. Haemolysis does not usually occur; when it does, splenectomy may be helpful.

Glucose-6-Phosphate Dehydrogenase (G6PD) Deficiency

This is one of the most widespread genetic abnormalities in the world occurring commonly in negroes, and in certain Mediterranean and Oriental groups. It is a sex-linked character and only becomes manifest in males or homozygous females. G6PD is a key enzyme on the pentose phosphate pathway, which is the chief protective mechanism in red cells to oxidant stress. Haemolysis in G6PD deficiency is caused by oxidation of red cell constituents, including haemoglobin, which forms methaemoglobin and Heinz bodies – precipitated oxidised globin. Removal of Heinz bodies in the spleen damages the red cell membrane and eventually leads to haemolysis. Most subjects are asymptomatic except when exposed to oxidant drugs or chemicals, when severe self-limiting haemolysis may occur. Commonly used oxidant drugs include the anti-malarials (primaquine), phenacetin, sulphonamides, dapsone, nitro-

furantoin and vitamin K, in the newborn. Patients with the Mediterranean variety of G6PD deficiency may also be susceptible to the broad bean (*Vicia faba*). The disorder, known as Favism, is seen mainly in children and adolescence. Some varieties of G6PD deficiency found in Caucasians and in the Mediterranean can cause a chronic non-spherocytic haemolytic anaemia.

There are screening tests available for the recognition of G6PD deficiency, but the diagnosis is most readily made by enzyme assay.

Congenital Abnormalities of Haemoglobin

The haemoglobin molecule is made up of four polypeptide chains arranged in pairs. The structure of the principal forms of haemoglobin is shown in Table 19.5. Haemoglobin F is found in the fetus and its formation ceases in early neonatal life when synthesis of haemoglobin A begins. In certain pathological states, synthesis of haemoglobin F may continue. The disorders of haemoglobin are of two types – the structural variants in which an abnormal form of haemoglobin is produced and the thalassaemias in which there is failure to produce one or more of the normal haemoglobin chains at the required rate.

The structural variants are congenital abnormalities and most are due to a change in one of the amino acids making up the polypeptide chains. Each chain contains over 140 amino acids, and the theoretical number of abnormal haemoglobins is very large, but the majority of these are of no clinical significance – in fact many cannot be identified unless very advanced techniques are employed. A haemoglobin variant is only important clinically if it alters the function of haemoglobin in such a way that it causes anaemia or other symptoms. Structural variants were originally designated by letters,

Table 19.5 Some disorders of haemoglobin

Clinical state	Haemoglobins present	Globin chains	Amino acid changes
Normal Fetus	F	$\alpha_2\gamma_2$	
Adult	A (c.97%)	$\alpha_2\beta_2$	
	A$_2$(c.3%)	$\alpha_2\delta_2$	
beta-Thalassaemia			
Heterozygous (thal. minor)	A / A$_2$(3.5–7.5%) / F (Variable)		
Homozygous (thal. major)	F (up to 100%) / A / A$_2$ (Variable)		
alpha-Thalassaemia (Hb H disease)			
Fetus	Barts (small amounts) γ_4		
Adult	H (up to 30%) β_4		
Sickle cell disease trait	S (up to 100%)	$\alpha_2\beta^S_2$	β_6 Glutamic acid→valine
	A / S (up to 50%)		
Hb C disease	C	$\alpha_2\beta^C_2$	β_6 Glutamic acid→lysine

e.g. Hb S, C, D. Now they tend to be named after the place in which they were first discovered, for example Hb Hammersmith, Bristol or Köln, or more correctly, by indicating the correct nature of the amino acid substitution. The most important of the structural abnormalities is Hb S, sickle haemoglobin in which the sixth amino acid of the beta chain, normally glutamic acid, is replaced by valine. The importance of this change lies in the fact that deoxygenated molecules of Hb S can link to one another and form insoluble chains which distort red cells forming the characteristic sickle cells. These cells are rigid and become impacted in the small blood vessels causing micro infarcts.

The Sickling Disorders (see Fig. 19.8)

These are a group of conditions in which Hb S is present either alone or with other haemoglobins, and in which sickling can occur under appropriate circumstances. The most important one is sickle cell disease, the homozygous form (SS), in which the major haemoglobin present is Hb S. This disease occurs principally in negroes of whom one per cent have homozygous SS disease, there are also smaller racial groups in the Middle East and India. The conditions inducing sickling include hypoxia (especially during anaesthesia) acidosis, infection, dehydration and cold. The symptoms result from a combination of infarction and haemolysis. Infarcts may occur in most tissues but particularly bone, the spleen, the kidneys, the gut, the lungs and central nervous system. The disease is characterised by a series of crises due to sickling episodes produced by one of the above mentioned factors. In children, infarcts in phalanges cause painful swelling of the hands and feet (the hand and foot syndrome). Repeated splenic infarcts result in splenic atrophy and therefore the spleen is rarely palpable in adults. Gut infarcts may mimic an acute abdomen and sickle cell disease must be excluded in all negroes presenting with this symptom. Bone infarcts may cause confusion with acute arthritis or osteomyelitis. Infection is common in patients with sickle cell disease and salmonella osteomyelitis is a frequent complication. Severe haemolysis may accompany a sickling crisis. In children, massive sequestration of sickle cells in the spleen may cause severe anaemia. Pregnancy is a particular hazard and the maternal and fetal mortality is high, unless the patients receive close medical attention. Intractable leg ulcers are a common complication. It should be noted that the severity of sickle cell disease is influenced very much by the degree of medical attention which the patient receives. Sicklers in the immigrant population in England are far less affected than those in the West Indies and these less so than the native population in Africa.

The most important aspect in management is *prevention*. The nature of the sickling process should be explained to patients with this disease and they should be encouraged to avoid any situation likely to provoke

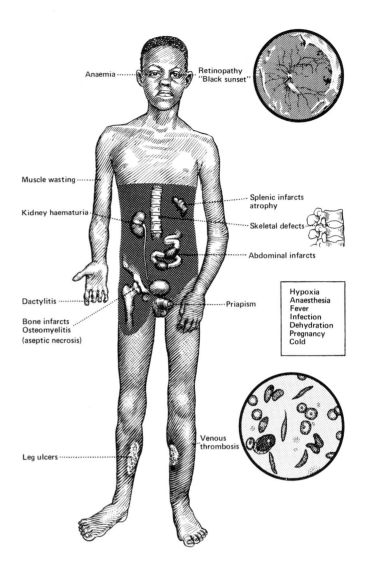

Fig. 19.8 Features of sickle cell disease.

sickling episodes. Anaesthesia should only be induced under the best possible circumstances and all infections should be treated promptly. The management of a sickling crisis depends on ensuring adequate oxygenation, rehydration, the correction of acidosis and vigorous treatment of infection. Blood transfusion should be avoided unless absolutely necessary, because the increase in blood viscosity may precipitate further sickling episodes. In severe cases exchange transfusion may be needed. In pregnancy, it is essential to ensure that folate deficiency does not develop. Newer forms of treatment with urea and cyanate have not been proven to be of value. Genetic counselling is an important part of the management of patients with sickling disorders.

Sickle cell trait (SA) is not a serious disease although it is widespread – 10 per cent of negroes carry the gene for Hb S. Sickling only occurs under conditions of extreme hypoxia, namely bad anaesthesia or air travel in unpressurised aircraft. Haematuria may occur in these patients.

The geographical distribution of Hb S coincides with that of other abnormal haemoglobins, particularly C, and these may occur in combinations. The combination of Hb S and Hb C (SC disease) is a particularly dangerous one because, although the patients are usually asymptomatic, certain conditions, for example anaesthesia and pregnancy, may induce severe and often fatal sickling crises.

The diagnosis of sickling disorders is not difficult. There are simple screening tests, normally depending on the differential solubility of Hb S and A which will readily identify patients with Hb S. A blood count and examination of a blood film will usually indicate whether this is sickle cell disease or sickle cell trait. The exact diagnosis can only be made by haemoglobin electrophoresis. Tests for Hb S should be carried out as routine on all patients of negro origin.

Other Haemoglobinopathies

Mention has already been made of haemoglobin C which occurs in negroes of West African origin. The homozygous form (CC) may cause anaemia and splenomegaly, but is relatively innocuous. Other abnormal haemoglobins, such as D and E do not give rise to disease. Other types such as haemoglobin M interfere with haemoglobin function, but they are very rare. The rare, unstable haemoglobins such as haemoglobin Köln cause a congenital, non-spherocytic haemolytic anaemia.

Thalassaemia (Fig. 19.9)

The thalassaemias are a group of congenital disorders of haemoglobin synthesis in which there is defective synthesis of one or more of the globin chains which make up normal adult haemoglobin (see Table 19.5). In the common form, beta thalassaemia, there is a deficiency of beta chains causing a reduction in the amount of haemoglobin A. To some extent this is compensated for by continuing production of haemoglobin F which normally ceases at birth, and of Hb A_2. The inheritance is complicated but, simply, two forms of the disease can be recognised – the homozygous form – thalassaemia major and the heterozygous form – thalassaemia minor, or thalassaemia trait.

Thalassaemia Major. This is also known as 'Mediterranean or Cooley's anaemia' and is a serious disease. There is severe anaemia and the red cells show gross hypochromia, microcytosis, anisocytosis and poikilocytosis, with target cells. There is destruction of newly formed red cells in the bone marrow (ineffective erythropoiesis) and this leads to expansion of the marrow cavity with resulting skeletal deformities, particularly noticeable in the skull ('hair on end' appearance in skull X-ray) and in overgrowth of the facial bones.

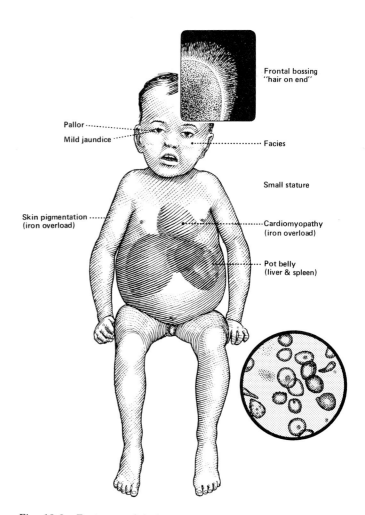

Fig. 19.9 Features of thalassaemia.

Growth is stunted and there is also marked hepatosplenomegaly. The only form of treatment is blood transfusion, and without this death usually occurs in early infancy or childhood. With regular blood transfusions, survival is possible into adolescence. Prolonged survival is limited by the effect of transfusional haemosiderosis, particularly cardiomyopathy. Splenectomy may be of value in reducing transfusion requirements, and the value of iron chelation and a hypertransfusion regime have yet to be evaluated.

Thalassaemia Minor. This is not a serious condition. The haemoglobin level is seldom less than 10 g/dl and is often normal. The red cells, however, are hypochromic and microcytic and the blood picture may be confused with iron deficiency. The condition is distinguished by the finding of a normal serum iron and TIBC. In most cases the Hb A_2 level is raised (above 3.5 per cent), and the Hb F level is usually normal or slightly raised, but occasionally family studies may be needed to establish the diagnosis. The main importance of this condition is that it should be recognised so that patients are not continually investigated and treated for non-existent iron deficiency.

β thalassaemia is common around the Mediterranean, the Middle East, India and the Far East. It should be remembered that thalassaemia minor has been found quite frequently in patients of Northern European origin.

In α thalassaemia there is defective synthesis of α chains. The genetics are complicated and depend on several pairs of genes. The homozygous condition is incompatible with life and results in stillbirth. One heterozygous form, Hb H disease, causes a clinical picture resembling β thalassaemia minor, although usually more severe. The haemoglobin level is often lower, and there is often splenomegaly. The blood picture resembles β thalassaemia and the diagnosis is made by finding Hb H (β4) in the red cells. There is no treatment apart from splenectomy in severe cases. This disease occurs in the Eastern Mediterranean and in the Far East.

2. ACQUIRED HAEMOLYTIC ANAEMIA

There are many causes of acquired haemolytic anaemia. Details of some of the more important forms are given below.

Autoimmune Haemolytic Anaemia (AIHA)

AIHA is due to the destruction of red cells by auto-antibodies. There are two main types depending on the nature of the antibody. These are IgG (warm) and IgM (cold) antibodies.

Autoimmune haemolytic anaemia

'Warm antibody'

Primary: Idiopathic
Secondary: Lymphomas, especially Hodgkin's
                  disease, CLL
                  Autoimmune disease, especially
                  SLE
                  Infections, particularly viral
                  Drugs, especially methyldopa

'Cold antibody'

Primary: The cold haemagglutination dis-
                  ease (CHAD)
Secondary: Lymphoma
                  Infections, especially mycoplasma
                  Paroxysmal cold haemoglobinuria
                  (PCH)

Warm Antibody AIHA. IgG antibodies cause mainly extravascular haemolysis and the clinical picture is typical of an haemolytic anaemia. The idiopathic variety may occur at any age. The onset is usually acute and anaemia may be severe. The blood film usually shows spherocytosis and the diagnosis is confirmed by finding a positive direct antiglobulin (Coombs' test). An exhaustive search should be made for a secondary cause, such as SLE. Treatment is initially by steroids, depending on the severity of anaemia a high dose, i.e. prednisolone 80 mg daily may be needed. This should be rapidly reduced as soon as the haemolysis comes under control. Some cases remit completely, but many become chronic requiring continuous therapy. If the haemolysis cannot be controlled by a low dose of prednisolone, splenectomy may be indicated. Red cell survival studies with surface scanning should be carried out first. Immunosuppressive drugs, for example azathioprine, have a small part to play in treatment and may allow reduction of steroid dosage. Blood transfusion should be avoided if possible because it may accentuate the haemolytic process.

Of particular importance is AIHA due to methyldopa. About 20 per cent of patients treated with this drug will develop a positive anti-globulin test, although less than one per cent have significant haemolysis. The drug need not be withdrawn unless haemolytic anaemia occurs. Most cases respond rapidly once the drug is stopped although the direct AHG test may persist for many months. The only other drug which regularly causes AIHA is mefenamic acid (Ponstan).

Cold Antibody AIHA. IgM antibodies cause agglutination and intravascular haemolysis of red cells when the temperature falls. Agglutination occurs mainly in the small vessels in the periphery, where the temperature is lower, and causes peripheral ischaemia, resembling Raynaud's phenomenon. Haemoglobinuria is common. The cold haemagglutination syndrome is found in elderly people. It is a form of dysproteinaemia and some cases terminate as a lymphoma. Usually no treatment is needed apart from advice about avoidance of cold, and the necessity to wear warm clothing. If haemolysis persists despite these measures then treatment with a cytotoxic agent, for example chlorambucil, may be needed. Steroids and splenectomy are less effective than with the warm antibody type.

Cold antibody AIHA complicating infections such as mycoplasma pneumonia is transitory and responds to treatment of the infection. Paroxysmal cold haemoglobinuria is an extremely rare form of AIHA and usually complicates viral infections. It used to be commoner when it was a complication of congenital syphilis.

Haemolytic Anaemia and Infection

These include malaria, including the dramatic type of intravascular haemolysis seen following an anti-malaria therapy, usually quinine, when massive haemoglobinuria gives its name to the condition 'blackwater fever' *see* page 588). Haemolytic anaemia may complicate gas gangrene infection (*Clostridium welchii*) and staphylococcal septicaemia, due to liberation of haemolysins. Mycoplasma pneumonia and some viral infections may cause AIHA.

Haemolytic Anaemia due to Drugs and Chemicals

Drugs and chemicals may induce haemolytic anaemia by three mechanisms:

1. *Direct toxicity*, due to membrane damage, e.g. phenylhydrazine.
2. *Oxidant damage*, mainly in subjects with an enzyme deficiency. Although certain drugs, for example dapsone, will cause haemolytic anaemia in normal subjects.
3. *Immunological haemolysis*. Methyldopa, already mentioned causes an AIHA. Some other drugs, for example penicillin and phenacetin, act as haptens and may cause an immune haemolytic anaemia which responds as soon as the drug is withdrawn.

Acquired Membrane Disorders

Abnormalities of the red cell membrane leading to haemolysis may be found in a wide variety of conditions, including liver disease and uraemia. One condition is of special importance.

Paroxysmal Nocturnal Haemoglobinuria (PNH) (Marchiafava-Michaeli Syndrome).

This is a rare acquired disorder of the red cell membrane. The nature of the defect is uncertain, but it makes the cells particularly sensitive to lysis by complement. Usually two populations of red cells can be demonstrated, one normal and the other with the PNH defect and as the disease progresses the percentage of abnormal cells increases. It is supposed that the PNH cells develop from a mutant clone which eventually suppresses the normal cells. There is a relationship between aplastic anaemia and PNH, and red cells with a PNH defect have been found in patients with myeloproliferative syndromes. The white cells and platelets are also involved and the disease may present as a pancytopenia. The usual presentation is as a chronic haemolytic anaemia. The classic symptom of nocturnal haemoglobinuria is often absent. The diagnosis is made by finding evidence of intravascular haemolysis and by a specific test, the acid serum lysis test, or Ham's test. Venous thromboses are common and often give rise to episodes of abdominal pain. The Budd-Chiari syndrome may develop as a result of hepatic vein thrombosis.

The only treatment is blood transfusion and as transfused plasma may cause increased lysis and severe reactions, washed red cell suspensions should be used. Iron deficiency may result from continuing haemosiderinuria, and parenteral iron should not be used because it may precipitate haemolysis. Anticoagulants may be required for treatment of venous thrombosis.

Mechanical Haemolytic Anaemia

Mechanical haemolytic anaemias arise from the destruction of red cells within the bloodstream. There are three main types.

Cardiac Valve Protheses. Leaks from valve protheses cause turbulence which breaks up red cells. These most commonly occur from incompetence of the aortic valve, but the mitral valve may also be involved. The blood film is characteristic showing many fragmented cells. Blood transfusion to maintain a normal haemoglobin level is helpful because it reduces cardiac output due to anaemia and thereby reduces turbulence. Severe cardiac haemolysis may necessitate replacement of the valve prothesis. Cardiac haemolytic anaemia has also been noted in patients with severe valve disease in the absence of a prothesis.

March Haemoglobinuria. This disorder was originally noted by the Greeks. It occurs in young men after prolonged running or soldiers after route marches. Haemoglobinuria is the presenting symptom. The red cells are basically normal and haemolysis is the result of destruction of the red cells by trauma in the small vessels in the soles of the feet. The condition is curable by the insertion of sorbo-rubber insoles into the shoes of affected patients.

Microangiopathic Haemolytic Anaemia. The basis of this type of anaemia is the formation of fibrin meshwork in the small blood vessels. The red cells passing through this are damaged and subsequently haemolyse. The blood film is characteristic with fragmented red cells of bizarre shapes, such as burr cells and helmet cells. Fibrin deposition in small vessels may occur in a wide variety of conditions as a result of either disease of the vessels themselves or as a part of the disseminated intravascular coagulation (DIC) syndrome (*see* page 420). Examples of the former are malignant hypertension, glomerular nephritis and malignant invasion of small vessels, especially by mucin-secreting carcinomas. Intravascular haemolysis resulting from microangiopathy may itself induce intravascular coagulation. A bleeding tendency resulting from consumption of platelets and clotting factors is therefore not uncommon.

Two syndromes deserve special mention. The haemolytic-uraemic syndrome occurs in children, usually after infection. There is a combination of renal failure and microangiopathic haemolytic anaemia, often with thrombocytopenia and evidence of DIC. A similar condition occurring in young adults is known as thrombotic thrombocytopenic purpura (TTP). The features of this disease are anaemia, thrombocytopenic purpura and bizarre disseminated neurological signs, due to multiple small thrombotic lesions. Both of these diseases are now thought to have an immunological basis, possibly due to immune complex formation. Treatment is unsatisfactory. The use of heparin to block the coagulation process is still debatable.

WHITE BLOOD CELLS

The white blood cells are of two main types – myeloid and lymphoid. The myeloid cells arise in the bone marrow and are either granulocytes or monocytes (macrophages) – these two types probably arising from a common stem cell. These cells are principally concerned with protection against infection by phagocytosis. Lymphoid cells are concerned with the immune defence mechanisms, both humoral and cell mediated (see page 116). They are heterogenous – some arising in the bone marrow and others in the lymphoid organs.

The normal distribution of white cells in the peripheral blood is shown in Table 19.6.

Table 19.6 Normal distribution of white cells (Total white count 4.0 to 11.0 × 10⁹/l)

Cell	Absolute number ($\times 10^9$/l)	Per cent
Neutrophils	2.5 to 7.5	40 to 75
Lymphocytes	1.5 to 3.5	20 to 45
Monocytes	0.2 to 0.8	2 to 10
Eosinophils	0.04 to 0.44	1 to 6
Basophils	0 to 0.10	0 to 1

Note:
1. Above ranges are for adults only.
2. White cell counts should be expressed in absolute numbers, percentage values can be very misleading depending on the total white count.
3. Racial variation exists. In particular negroes often have low total and neutrophil counts.

The major variations in white cells are as follows:

Neutrophil Leucocytosis ($>7.5 \times 10^9$/l)

Note: Considerable variation occurs in an individual during the day, influencing factors being exercise, food and stress.
Physiological, e.g. late pregnancy.
Infection, especially pyogenic infections.
Tissue necrosis.
Haemorrhage.
Malignant neoplasms.
Metabolic disorders, e.g. diabetic ketosis.
Myeloproliferative disorders (see page 392).

Eosinophilia ($>0.4 \times 10^9$/l)

Allergy, asthma, drug sensitivity.
Parasitic infestation – usually tissue invasion required, e.g. filaria, toxocara.
Pulmonary eosinophilia (Löeffler's syndrome) probably parasitic in origin.
Skin diseases, e.g. pemphigus, exfoliative dermatitis.

Infections – usually in the convalescent period.
Polyarteritis nodosa.
Malignant disease (particularly Hodgkin's disease).
Rarities – e.g. eosinophilic granuloma, eosinophilic leukaemia (a doubtful syndrome).

Lymphocytosis ($>3.5 \times 10^9$/l)

Viral infections – especially in children:
    Infectious hepatitis.
    Infectious mononucleosis.
Leukaemia – acute and, especially, chronic lymphatic leukaemia.
Note: 'Atypical lymphocytosis' may occur in many viral diseases, especially infectious mononucleosis.

Monocytosis ($>0.8 \times 10^9$/l)

Infections, especially chronic – e.g. TB, SBE:
    Protozoal infections.
    Infectious mononucleosis.
Malignant disease – monocytic leukaemia, carcinoma.
Chronic inflammatory intestinal disease – e.g. Crohn's disease.

Neutropenia ($<2.5 \times 10^9$/l)

Aplastic anaemia (see page 382).
Bone marrow infiltration, e.g. leukaemia, carcinoma, etc.
Infections, especially viral, or, if bacterial due to overwhelming infection.
Hypersplenism (enlarged spleen), particularly Felty's syndrome (rheumatoid arthritis with a big spleen – depression of neutrophil production may be a factor in this condition).
Immune, e.g. SLE.
Chronic idiopathic neutropenia and 'cyclic neutropenia' (a rare condition with a cyclic change in the neutrophil count).

Drug Induced Agranulocytosis

A number of drugs are known to cause agranulocytosis, either as part of the aplastic anaemia syndrome or else selective. Amongst the principal drugs involved are:
Chloramphenicol
Phenylbutazone
Gold
Anti-thyroid drugs – thiouracil
Isoniazid
Sulphonamides
Great care should be taken over the prescription of all drugs known to cause agranulocytosis and their use should be restricted to those in whom there is a genuine need for the drug which cannot be met by use of a less dangerous treatment.
Regular blood counts should be done on all patients receiving high risk drugs on a long term basis.

Agranulocytosis (neutrophils $<0.5 \times 10^9/l$)

This is a serious condition and often fatal. The clinical features include fever and infective lesions of the skin and mucous membranes, for example ulcerative stomatitis, and entirely due to facilitated invasion of tissue by bacteria, fungi, etc. Immediate withdrawal of the drug is mandatory. Otherwise treatment is supportive with antibiotic therapy. The value of corticosteroids and granulocyte transfusions is debatable.

MALIGNANT AND PROLIFERATIVE DISEASES OF HAEMOPOIETIC TISSUE

These diseases cause confusion because they are difficult to classify satisfactorily. By custom they have been grouped together according to their clinical picture. Recent developments in investigation and treatment have emphasised the difference between these diseases. A more logical classification would depend on the type of cell involved and the nature of the malignant transformation. Further confusion arises because some of these diseases show common features and may evolve into another form – thus they should be regarded as part of a spectrum rather than as isolated entities. A simple division may be made between diseases of the myeloid cells, i.e. those giving rise to blood cells – red cells, granulocytes and platelets – and diseases of the lymphoreticular cells. Clinically, it is convenient to consider these diseases under the following headings even though it should be realised that the diseases grouped together may have different origins and overlap between them may exist.

1. Myeloproliferative disease.
2. Acute leukaemia.
3. Immunoproliferative disease.
4. Lymphoma.

I. THE MYELOPROLIFERATIVE DISORDERS (Fig. 19.10)

Definition

This term was introduced by Dameshek to describe a group of diseases thought to arise from a primitive totipotential stem cell and showing common features and transition from one form to another. There may be

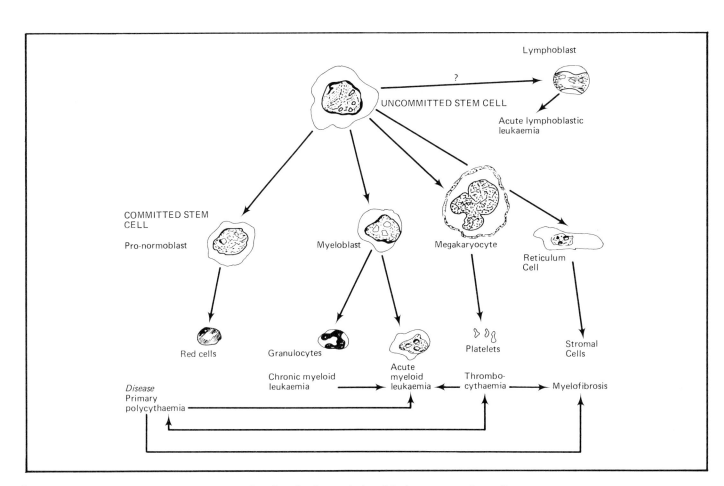

Fig. 19.10   Myeloproliferative syndromes showing the interrelationship between various diseases.

either uncontrolled, but relatively orderly, cell proliferation giving rise to normally functioning cells or proliferation of more primitive blast cells without further differentiation.

Pathology

The principal diseases concerned are:

Primary polycythaemia. Overproduction of red cells and usually granulocytes and platelets as well.

Essential thrombocythaemia. Excessive production of platelets.

Chronic myeloid leukaemia. Excessive production of granulocytes.

Myelofibrosis. Replacement of bone marrow with fibrous tissue.

Acute myeloid leukaemia (see under acute leukaemia). This may be a terminal event in all types of myeloproliferative disease.

1. POLYCYTHAEMIA

Background

Polycythaemia may be either *true* or *relative* (Fig. 19.11). In *true* polycythaemia there is an increase in the total body red cell mass. In *relative* polycythaemia there is an apparent increase in the circulating red cell mass due to a reduction in plasma volume.

True polycythaemia may be either primary or secondary.

PRIMARY POLYCYTHAEMIA (P. rubra vera)

This occurs mainly in middle-aged and elderly patients.

Symptoms (*see* Fig. 19.12)

Due to increased blood viscosity (raised packed cell volume):
Headache.
Dizziness.
Recurrent arterial and venous thromboses (e.g. retinal coronary and peripheral vascular disease).
Congestive cardiac failure.

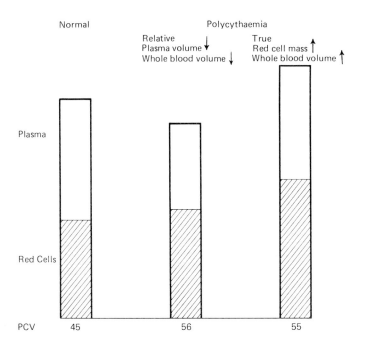

Fig. 19.11   True and relative polycythaemia.

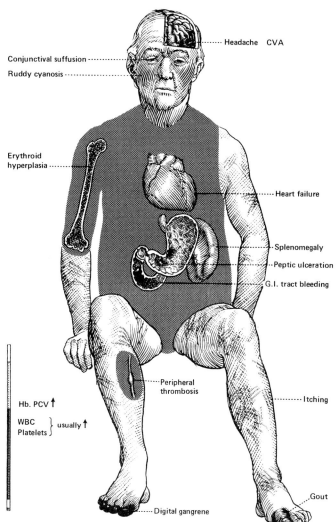

Fig. 19.12   Features of primary polycythaemia.

Due to a bleeding tendency:
Abnormal platelet function and vascular engorgement.
Cerebral, intestinal bleeding, etc.
Note: Patients may present with *iron deficiency anaemia.*

Due to histamine overproduction (probable):
Dyspepsia due to peptic ulcer.
Pruritus (especially after hot baths).

Due to increased cell turnover:
Hyperuricaemia and gout.

Signs

Ruddy cyanosis.
Moderate splenomegaly (70 per cent of cases only).
Signs of haemorrhage (e.g. skin, retina) and venous thrombosis.
Cardiac enlargment and heart failure.
Gout.

Investigations

1. The haemoglobin level and PCV are above the upper limit of normal
(*Men:* Hb>18.0; PCV>0.54 *Women:* Hb>16.5; PCV>0.47).
In approximately 70 per cent of cases the total white count is >10×10⁹/l and the platelet count >500×10⁹/l.
Note: Iron deficiency changes may be present especially if bleeding has occurred or the patient has been venesected.
2. The red cell mass (measured by ⁵¹Cr dilution) is increased. The plasma volume may be slightly raised.
3. The bone marrow shows myeloid hyperplasia and the reticulin content is usually increased.
4. The blood uric acid is usually elevated.
5. The neutrophil alkaline phosphatase (NAP) is usually raised.

Differential Diagnosis

The principal differential diagnoses are:
Secondary polycythaemia.
Relative polycythaemia (*see below*).

SECONDARY POLYCYTHAEMIA

This is caused by increased erythropoietin production due to:
1. Hypoxia (low arterial oxygen tension).
(a) High altitudes.
(b) Congenital heart disease with right to left shunt.
(c) Chronic pulmonary disease, e.g. severe chronic bronchitis or in extremely obese subjects with normal lungs due to diminished ventilatory effort.
2. Erythropoietin-secreting lesions.
(a) Renal – adenocarcinoma, renal cysts, hydronephrosis.
(b) Miscellaneous tumours – uterine fibroids, hepatoma, cerebellar haemangioblastoma.
(c) Abnormal haemoglobin structure – congenital methaemoglobinaemia, high affinity haemoglobins.

Differential Diagnosis

The differential diagnosis is shown in Table 19.7.

Complications

The main complications of untreated polycythaemia are vascular thrombosis, haemorrhage and cardiac failure. Gout may often be precipitated by cytotoxic therapy. Thrombosis of the portal vein (portal hypertension) hepatic veins – Budd-Chiari syndrome (ascites, hepatomegaly, and liver failure) may occur as well as cirrhosis, the latter for no known reason.

Myelosclerosis is a frequent end-stage of this disease and acute myeloid leukaemia may also occur (*see below*).

Table 19.7 Differential diagnosis of polycythaemia

Type of polycythaemia	PCV	WBC	Platelets	Red cell mass	Plasma volume	Po₂	Neutrophil alkaline phosphatase	IVP	Erythropoietin level
Primary	↑	N or ↑	N or ↑	↑	N or ↑	N	N or ↑	N	N
Anoxic	↑	N	N	↑	N	↓	N	N	↑
Renal	↑	N	N	↑	N	N	N	Abnormal	↑
Other secondary causes	↑	N	N	↑	N	N	N	N	↑
'Pseudopolycythaemia'	↑	N	N	N	↓	N	N	N	N

Basis of Treatment

All patients with primary polycythaemia require treatment. The objects of treatment are:
1. To maintain a PCV of less than 0.50. The increase of thrombotic complications rises sharply as the PCV exceeds this level.
2. To maintain a normal platelet count.
3. To prevent other complications for example gout and pruritus.

The mainstay of treatment is venesection and many patients can be managed by this only. Venesection should be carried out two or three times weekly until the PCV is below 0.50 and at varying intervals thereafter depending on the rate of rise of the PCV. Iron deficiency may develop after repeated venesections and iron therapy may be needed to avoid severe iron deficiency, which stimulates erythropoiesis by the hypoxic drive.

If venesection alone cannot maintain a normal PCV or if the platelet count is raised, additional therapy is necessary. This may be by either ^{32}P or cytotoxic drugs. The former is easier for the patient. The usual dose is 5 millicuries and more than one dose may be needed. The maximum effect on the PCV is not seen for two or three months. There is evidence that ^{32}P may be leukaemogenic, increasing the incidence of acute leukaemia and therefore it should, perhaps, be avoided in younger patients. The total dose should not exceed 30 millicuries. Cytotoxic drugs useful in the treatment of polycythaemia include, busulphan (Myleran) chlorambucil (Leukaeran) and cytarabine. Much more careful supervision of the patient, with repeated blood counts, is necessary.

Gout may be prevented, especially if cytotoxic therapy is given, by allopurinol. Pruritus may be a very troublesome symptom and difficult to relieve. It often responds to treatment of the primary condition, if it does not, some antihistamine, e.g. diphenylpyraline (Lergoban) and cyproheptadine (Periactin) may be helpful.

The treatment of secondary polycythaemia depends on the treatment of the cause, if possible. Polycythaemia may reverse after removal of renal or other tumours. Severe polycythaemia in non-reversible cardiac lesions may need treatment by venesection to prevent thrombosis. This should be carried out with caution and preferably with simultaneous replacement with low molecular weight dextran.

Relative polycythaemia occurs after dehydration, burns, etc. There is also a syndrome known unsatisfactorily as 'stress polycythaemia', 'pseudopolycythaemia' or Gaisböck's syndrome. It usually affects middle-aged males, who are overweight, cigarette smokers, hypertensive and under nervous strain. There is reduction in the plasma volume of unknown mechanism. There is increased mortality due to cardiovascular complications.

Treatment is directed towards weight reduction, control of hypertension and avoidance of stress.

2. ESSENTIAL THROMBOCYTHAEMIA

A rare form of myeloproliferative disease in which there is excessive production of platelets so that the platelet count is raised above the normal $500 \times 10^9/l$ and may be as high as $2,500 \times 10^9/l$. There is overlap with primary polycythaemia and transition to myelofibrosis is common. The platelets are morphologically and functionally abnormal. Symptoms are due to thrombosis and/or abnormal bleeding. Peripheral ischaemic lesions may cause confusion with degenerative arterial disease but the peripheral pulses are normal. Distinction must be made from other causes of thrombocytosis, for example postoperative, post-splenectomy, infection and malignant disease. This can usually be made from finding other evidence of myeloproliferation, abnormal platelet morphology and platelet function studies. Treatment should be aimed at reducing the platelet count to normal levels. This is by either busulphan or ^{32}P. Treatment is very rewarding; long survival is not unusual.

3. CHRONIC MYELOID LEUKAEMIA (CML)

Background

This is a disease with a peak incidence in middle age although a juvenile form exists. Characteristically it progresses through three stages –
1. A benign phase in which there is excessive production of granulocytes although the condition is responsive to treatment.
2. A malignant phase unresponsive to treatment.
3. A terminal phase resembling acute leukaemia.
    Not all three stages inevitably occur.

Symptoms

The onset is usually insidious, some cases are discovered as a chance finding.
Non-specific: weakness, lethargy, etc.
Due to anaemia (q.v.).
Due to increased metabolic rate: weight loss, sweating, etc.
Abdominal discomfort due to splenomegaly or splenic infarct.
Bone pain.
Abnormal bleeding due to abnormal platelet function or thrombocytopenia.
Gout.

Signs

Anaemia.
Splenomegaly.

Hepatomegaly.
Abnormal bleeding.
Gout.
Tissue infiltration, e.g. skin (late stages only).

Investigations

1. By the time symptoms occur there is usually anaemia (normochromic/normocytic). The white count is increased, usually >50 and occasionally as high as $500 \times 10^9/l$. The differential white count shows a neutrophilia with more immature forms, i.e. bands, metamyelocytes, myelocytes and a small number of blasts. There may be an increase in basophils.

The platelet count is usually normal or raised with abnormal forms. It falls as the disease progresses.
2. The bone marrow shows marked granulocytic hyperplasia, usually with an increase in megakaryocytes.
3. Cytogenic studies show an abnormal chromosome, the Philadelphia chromosome (deletion of long arm of 22), in about 80 per cent of cases.
4. The neutrophil alkaline phosphate (NAP) is low.
5. The serum B_{12} level is high, >1,000 ng/l, due to increased production of transcobalamins by the granulocytes.

Differential Diagnosis

Advanced cases present little difficulty. Those presenting with a WBC of around $50 \times 10^9/l$, may need to be distinguished from other cases of a myeloid leukaemoid reaction, for example severe infection, malignancy, and from granulocyte hyperplasia in other forms of myeloproliferative disease, for example primary polycythaemia.

Basis of Treatment

Treatment of CML remains unsatisfactory and there has been relatively little progress in the past 20 years. The mean survival remains under four years although a few patients survive for ten years or more. In the benign phase no treatment has been shown to be superior to busulphan (Myleran). This is given at a daily dose of 2 to 6 mg, until the WBC falls to around $20 \times 10^9/l$. Further courses are given when the WBC has risen to a level at which anaemia develops, usually around $100 \times 10^9/l$. Continuous treatment with busulphan is not recommended. Frequent blood counts are required to prevent marrow aplasia, often fatal. Other complications of busulphan include pulmonary fibrosis (often irreversible) and an Addison-like syndrome with pigmentation. Other cytotoxic drugs which may be used in the resistant phase include mitobronitol (Myelobromol), hydroxyurea (Hydrea), mercaptopurine and thioguanine. Allopurinol (300 mg daily) should be given

routinely with these drugs. As with all forms of malignant haematological disease, treatment should be supervised by a physician with experience in the use of oncolytic drugs.

The value of splenectomy in the benign stage of CML is still debatable. It certainly prevents the distressing complications arising from a rapidly enlarging spleen in the malignant phase and for this reason alone it is probably justified in fit patients. There is no evidence, as yet, that it prolongs overall survival.

Most cases eventually terminate as acute leukaemia, commonly myeloid, although sometimes lymphoblastic. Treatment is as for these conditions (*see* page 399), but the prognosis is very poor and seldom exceeds a few months.

4. MYELOFIBROSIS

In this disease there is replacement of the bone marrow by fibrous tissue and new bone formation. There is usually a leuco-erythroblastic anaemia with extramedullary haemopoiesis in the spleen and liver and occasionally other organs, for example the lymph nodes. Myelofibrosis is often the terminal stage of primary polycythaemia or thrombocythaemia, although these diseases may be clinically silent.

Symptoms

Of anaemia (q.v.) – weakness and dyspnoea are often out of proportion to the haemoglobin level.
Abdominal discomfort due to splenomegaly and acute pain due to splenic infarction.
Due to a raised metabolic rate – sweating, loss of weight.
Bleeding due to abnormal platelet function and/or thrombocytopenia.
Joint pain due to secondary gout.

Signs

Anaemia.
Massive splenomegaly.
Abnormal bleeding.
Gout.

Investigations

1. The blood picture is that of a leuco-erythroblastic anaemia, i.e. an anaemia with immature red and white cells in the peripheral blood. Anaemia may be severe and typically the blood film shows 'tear-drop' poikilocytes. The white count is variable but usually raised, with immature granulocytes. The platelet count is also variable, it is usually normal or low although in cases evolving from thrombocythaemia it may be high.
2. Bone marrow aspiration is usually unsuccessful, yielding a 'dry tap'. The diagnosis is made by bone

marrow trephine which shows increased fibrosis, new bone formation and often increased granulocytic precursors and megakaryocytes.

3. Liver or splenic biopsy shows extra-medullary haemopoiesis, but this is rarely required and may be hazardous due to the haemorrhagic tendency.

4. The Philadelphia chromosome is absent and the NAP is raised.

5. Radio-isotope studies show an increased plasma volume giving rise to a 'dilutional anaemia'. Ferrokinetic studies identify the spleen and liver as being the major sites of erythropoiesis, although this is largely ineffective.

Differential Diagnosis

Marrow fibrosis, with accompanying leuco-erythroblastic anaemia may be secondary to a number of other conditions including infiltration by carcinoma or other malignant disease, chronic infection particularly TB, irradiation, chemicals, fluoride, benzene, marble bone disease. Splenomegaly is not usual in these conditions and differentiation can usually be made by bone marrow trephine.

Complications

Termination as acute myeloid leukaemia may occur. Gross splenomegaly causes dilutional anaemia, haemolysis through hypersplenism and sequestration of red cells. Splenomegaly may also cause portal hypertension and bleeding from oesophageal varices due to increased splenic blood flow and increased hepatic resistance to blood flow. This is associated with portal infiltration by the myeloproliferative process.

Basis of Treatment

There is no effective treatment for this disease. Blood transfusion is usually required. If transfusion requirements are excessive, splenectomy may be indicated. The argument against splenectomy, that this organ is the major site of erythropoiesis, is probably not justified. Early splenectomy, when the operation is technically simple and before the complications of hypersplenism and repeated infarction arise, is probably to be recommended. Splenic irradiation may produce some of the benefits of splenectomy without the chances of a surgical operation.

Folic acid may produce a small increase in haemoglobin. The role of androgens is still not proven, but they are worth a trial in refractory cases.

II. ACUTE LEUKAEMIA (AL)

Definition

The acute leukaemias are diseases in which there is uncontrolled proliferation of primitive haemopoietic cells (blasts) in the bone marrow with replacement of the normal marrow cells. Blast cells usually appear in the peripheral blood but not invariably so.

Background

The cause of all types of leukaemia is unknown. Possible causes include:

(a) Viruses. A viral aetiology has been established in animals, but no conclusive evidence exists for man. The high incidence in young children and the occasional familial or locality clustering of the disease suggests that a viral or other environmental cause may be implicated.

(b) Genetic Abnormalities. There is a marked increase in leukaemia in patients with chromosomal abnormalities, for example Down's syndrome and Fanconi's syndrome.

(c) Ionising Radiation. The association between excessive irradiation and leukaemia is well established. The main points of evidence being, the use of X-ray therapy in the treatment of ankylosing spondylitis, inadequately protected radiologists and the survivors of the atomic bomb explosions. Radiation induced leukaemia is usually of the myeloid variety.

(d) Drugs. Certain drugs and chemicals, for example the alkylating agents, phenylbutazone and benzene may be leukaemogenic.

Two main types of acute leukaemia are recognised – acute lymphoblastic leukaemia (ALL) and acute myeloid leukaemia (AML). Correct identification is critically important because the treatment and prognosis in each type is very different. Both types of acute leukaemia can be subdivided on morphological, cytochemical and immunological criteria. In ALL, such studies have enabled the identification of poor risk cases, particularly those with 'T' cell leukaemia, who need more intensive therapy. AML exists in a variety of forms – in particular a monocytic component is often present. So far subdivision of AML into myeloblastic, monoblastic, myelomonoblastic, etc. has not proved to be important in patient management, and therefore it is reasonable to consider all forms of AML together.

Acute leukaemia is, fortunately, a rare disease. There are two peaks in incidence – one in early childhood, mainly ALL and the other in the elderly, mainly AML. The incidence of AL in children is approximately 4/100,000 children/year and in adults approximately 5/100,000 adults/year. All types are more common in males and there seems to be a real increase in frequency in recent years.

Pathology

There is extensive replacement of normal bone marrow causing suppression of normal haemopoiesis with resulting anaemia, thrombocytopenia and neutropenia. Other tissues notably the lymph nodes (in ALL), the spleen, the skin and the CNS may be involved.

Symptoms (Fig. 19.13)

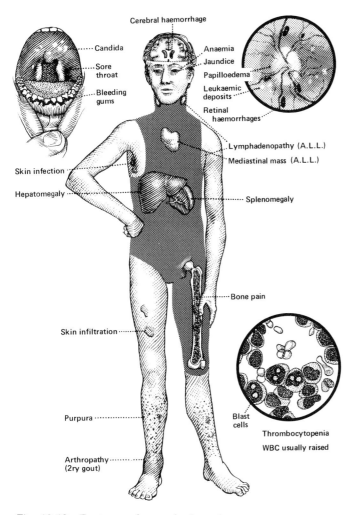

Fig. 19.13 Features of acute leukaemia.

The onset of acute leukaemia is usually acute or subacute. The symptoms are mainly *due to bone marrow replacement*, namely:
Anaemia
Bleeding (due to thrombocytopenia) – purpura, bleeding from mucous membranes, visual disturbance from retinal haemorrhages.
Infection (due to neutropenia) – fever, prostration (septicaemia), mouth ulceration, skin lesions.

Others:
Non-specific – weakness, anorexia, weight loss.
Bone pain.
Joint pain due to hyperuricaemia.
Headache – CNS symptoms, due to raised intracranial pressure from meningeal deposits.

Signs

Anaemia.
Bleeding – skin, mucous membranes, retina, gastrointestinal tract.
Fever – mouth ulceration (often with candida).
Skin lesions – infective or infiltrative.
Jaundice.
Retinal deposits and sometimes papilloedema.
Lymph node and tonsillar enlargement (especially ALL).
Splenomegaly.
Gingival overgrowth (especially monocytic leukaemia).

Investigations

1. **Blood Count.** Most patients are anaemic (normochromic). The white cell count is very variable and may be low, normal or high (occasionally $>100 \times 10^9/l$). *There is no typical blood picture of acute leukaemia.* Morphological distinction of peripheral blast cells may be very difficult. Thrombocytopenia (often severe $<20 \times 10^9/l$) is very common.

2. **Bone Marrow Examination** is essential. In aleukaemic cases it is the only way to make a diagnosis. The true cytological nature of the cells can only be established by this procedure. The percentage of blast cells may approach 100 per cent. Appropriate cytochemical staining should be performed.

Differential Diagnosis

The diagnosis is not usually difficult, if the combination of clinical and laboratory findings is taken together. Occasional confusion may arise with glandular fever and aplastic anaemia.

Basis of Treatment

Untreated, the prognosis in AL is usually less than a few months. Recent advances in the treatment of ALL have radically altered the prognosis in this disease and can rightly be claimed as one of the greatest successes in modern therapeutics. At least 50 per cent of children are alive and well after five years, and there is reason to believe that a high percentage of these are cured. The outlook in AML is less optimistic and the majority of patients still do not survive for much longer than one year. The improvement in treatment has depended upon:
1. The more successful use of oncolytic drugs to reduce or eradicate the leukaemic cell population.
2. The better use of supportive facilities, for example blood and platelet transfusions and antibiotics to enable the patient to survive the period before normal bone marrow function is re-established.

This type of treatment is expensive of time and

hospital resources and has been shown to be more effective when special units are established, accustomed to dealing with the effects of cytotoxic drugs and the problems of infection related to chronic marrow depression. The quality for the life of the patient is usually good and overnight admission for therapy can be arranged so that there is as little interference with schooling or employment as possible.

No child with AL should be treated without supervision from a specialised centre. The same principle applies to young adults.

In the elderly, the prognosis is much less good and it is doubtful whether removal to a specialised centre many miles away, with the inevitable separation from family and friends that this entails, is justified for the small prolongation of life that can be offered.

Oncolytic Therapy. The mainstay of treatment of AL is the effective use of oncolytic drugs. The mode of action and special side effects of the principal drugs used in the treatment of leukaemia and other haematological malignancies are shown in Fig. 19.14 and Table 19.8. Animal studies have shown that these drugs are best used in combinations administered at intervals – pulsed therapy. It is to be hoped that further success will be obtained by applying cytokinetic principles to the timing of the administration of drug combinations. The aims of treatment are:

(a) *Remission induction.* Intensive treatment is given with the object of reducing the leukaemic cell population to the point where normal bone marrow function is re-established. At this stage the patient is clinically and haematologically normal and is said to be in *remission*. Even so, a substantial leukaemic cell population probably still exists at this point.

(b) *Consolidation and maintenance therapy.* The object of this is to try and eradicate completely the remaining leukaemic cell population. Either the same drugs are used at less frequent intervals or else different drugs to try and prevent the development of resistance. The length of time that maintenance therapy should be continued is debatable, but it should probably be continued for at least one year and probably longer. If relapse occurs, remission induction is re-attempted with more intensive therapy.

(c) *Prophylactic therapy.* The fact that in ALL, CNS relapses were common, led to the concept that leukaemic cells might persist in protected sites, such as the CNS, which are not exposed to the effects of cytotoxic therapy. Prophylactic CNS irradiation and intrathecal methotrexate administration have helped to reduce the incidence of this complication dramatically.

The treatment of AL should not be undertaken by physicians without adequate experience in the use of the drugs concerned or of the natural history of the disease. Also no ideal drug regime has yet been devised and constant modifications are being introduced. For this reason detailed drug protocols are not given but only the broad outlines. For more detail, reference is best made to the current *MRC Leukaemia Trial protocols*.

ALL. The most useful drugs for achieving remission are vincristine and prednisolone. Colaspase (asparaginase) and daunorubicin or doxorubicin (Adriamycin) may also be useful. Approximately 95 per cent of patients should achieve a complete remission within a few weeks. CNS prophylaxis is essential. Maintenance therapy with mercaptopurine and methotrexate is necessary for at least two years.

AML. The most useful drugs are cytarabine, daunorubicin and thioguanine. Remission is more difficult to achieve than in ALL and may take up to ten weeks. Severe marrow aplasia is the rule before remission occurs. In the best centres remission rates of up to 70 per cent have been obtained, although many of these do not last more than a few months. Maintenance therapy is usually given at monthly intervals using combinations of the above drugs in rotation. Because the long term prognosis is relatively poor, CNS prophylaxis is not usually given.

There is no doubt that the present treatment of AML is unsatisfactory and that new approaches are needed. Immunotherapy has not proved to be a significant improvement. At the moment bone marrow transplantation appears to offer the best chance of a long survival for a small number of selected patients.

Supportive Therapy. Cytotoxic therapy alone has not been responsible for the improved survival in acute leukaemia. The transfusion of blood and blood products, especially platelets, has been particularly valuable. Prompt treatment of infections is also an important part of management. In pyrexial patients every effort should be made to find a source of infection, including repeated blood cultures. Treatment with a broad spectrum antibiotic combination should be started as soon as the necessary samples have been taken. The combination of gentamicin and carbenicillin is a very effective one in 'blind treatment' of infections. Oral and oesophageal moniliasis should be treated with oral amphotericin or miconazole. The value of granulocyte transfusions, gut sterilisation and the use of sterile isolation facilities is still not proven.

The overall management of the patient and relatives is of vital importance if morale is to be maintained. Successful treatment of AML is likely to be an unpleasant experience for the patient, perhaps requiring many weeks of hospitalisation. Such intensive therapy is not indicated in the elderly, and may actually worsen the prognosis, nor should it be persisted with in younger patients, when it is clear that treatment is having little effect.

Table 19.8 Oncolytic drugs used in treatment of haematological malignancy

Drug	Action	Mode of use	Clinical use	Side effects and special precautions
1. Alkylating agents (I)	Alkylation of DNA bases Interference with formation of DNA strands			*All* – myelosuppression, nausea vomiting
Mustine		IV	Hodgkin's disease Non-Hodgkin's lymphoma	Tissue necrosis. Brain damage, convulsions, vertigo *Note:* Give into fast running drip
Cyclophosphamide (Endoxana)		Oral or IV	NHL, Myeloma, ALL, AML	Less thrombocytopenia than mustine, alopecia Haemorrhagic cystitis – ensure high urine output
Melphalan (Alkeran)		Oral	Myeloma	
Busulphan (Myleran)		Oral	CML and other myeloproliferative syndromes	Amenorrhoea, sterility Skin pigmentation, pulmonary and liver fibrosis, hypotension May cause severe and irreversible marrow aplasia
Chlorambucil (Leukeran)		Oral	CLL, NHL	Dermatitis, hepatotoxicity
2. Antimetabolites	Interference with DNA synthesis			*All*—myelosuppression
Methotrexate (II) (Amethopterin)	Folate antagonist Inhibits dihydrofolate reductase	Oral, IV Intrathecal	ALL, AML, (NHL)	Mucosal ulceration, especially stomatitis, pharyngitis, and intestinal. Diarrhoea Liver damage Use with care in renal failure Can be antagonised with folinic acid (Leucovorin)
Mercaptopurine (III) (Puri-nethol) Thioguanine	Purine antagonists	Oral	ALL, AML, CML	Anorexia, nausea, vomiting Jaundice, hyperuricaemia Dose should be reduced if used with allopurinol (MP only)
Cytarabine (IV) (Cytosine arabinoside-cytosar)	Pyrimidine antagonist	IV SC Intrathecal	AML, ALL, (NHL)	Megaloblastic change. G–I disturbances, hepatic damage, dermatitis Usually used in combination Safe in renal failure
3. Antibiotics Daunorubicin (V) (Cerubidin)	Complexes with DNA binding both strands and preventing coiling	IV	AML, ALL, NHL	Myelosuppression – often prolonged. Nausea, vomiting, alopecia, skin rashes, fever
Doxorubicin (Adriamycin)				Thrombophlebitis *Myocardial toxicity* seen especially with daunorubicin. Cumulative dose should not exceed 600 mg Tachycardia, ectopics, arrhythmias, severe irreversible failure. Do not use in patients with cardiac conditions

Note:
1. Dosages are not given as they vary widely according to the treatment protocol.
2. Roman numerals refer to Fig. 19.14.

Table 19.8 continued

Drug	Action	Mode of use	Clinical use	Side effects and special precautions
4. Miscellaneous action Vinca alkaloids' (VI) Vincristine (Oncovin) Vinblastine (Velbe)	Uncertain Causes metaphase arrest by inhibiting spindle formation	IV	HD, NHL, ALL, (AML)	Myelosuppression, especially vinblastine Peripheral neuropathy, including autonomic, leading to ileus Hepatic necrosis, especially vincristine Alopecia Tissue necrosis – give into fast running drip
Procarbazine (Natulan)	Uncertain. Prolongs interphase and arrests mitosis	Oral	HD, NHL, (Myeloma)	Nausea and vomiting Neurological changes Sedative action Marrow depression May be oncogenic
Colaspase (Asparaginase) (VII)	Reduces level of L-asparaginase – an essential amino acid for some malignant cells	IV	ALL, AML	Anaphylatic reactions, fever nausea, vomiting, liver damage, neurological damage, mental changes, hypoglycaemia
Corticosteroids (Prednisolone)	Uncertain Lymphocytolytic inhibits mitotic activity. Reduces protein synthesis	Oral or IV	ALL, HD, NHL	Moon facies. Hypertension. Suppression of normal cortical activity. Psychosis, G–I bleeding Osteoporosis, immunosuppression Usually used in combination therapy

Note:
1. Dosages are not given as they vary widely according to the treatment protocol.
2. Roman numerals refer to Fig. 19.14.

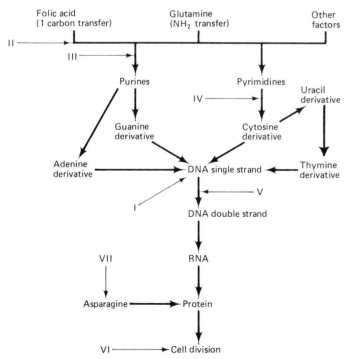

Fig. 19.14 Site of action of oncolytic drugs. (*See also* Table 19.8)

III. THE IMMUNOPROLIFERATIVE DISEASES

Definition

This term describes a group of diseases arising from malignant proliferation of immunocytes – cells concerned with the immune response. They are not interrelated, but are grouped together because they are characterised by a failure of the immune response.

CHRONIC LYMPHATIC LEUKAEMIA

This is a common form of leukaemia occurring in middle-aged and elderly subjects.

Pathology

There is a progressive proliferation of lymphocytes (usually B cells) with infiltration of the bone marrow and a lymphocytosis in the peripheral blood. Usually there is enlargement of the lymph nodes and splenomegaly.

Normal lymphocyte function is impaired and immune paresis develops.

401

Symptoms

Often none – the disease is discovered by chance.
Anaemia.
General non-specific – malaise, weight loss, etc.
Lymph node enlargement.
Recurrent infections, particularly chest infections.

Signs

May be none.
Lymphadenopathy.
Splenomegaly.
Signs of infection – pulmonary, skin – herpes zoster is a common complication.
Skin infiltration.
Salivary gland enlargement.
Pleural effusions due to pleural deposits.

Investigations

1. Blood count. The essential finding is a lymphocytosis ($>5 \times 10^9$/l). Occasionally, the lymphocyte count may reach $>500 \times 10^9$/l. 'Smear' cells (disintegrated lymphocytes) are usually seen in the blood film. Anaemia may develop in the later stages, so may thrombocytopenia, although in many cases these are normal at presentation.
2. The bone marrow is infiltrated by lymphocytes and normal haemopoietic tissue is reduced to a variable degree.
3. Lymph node biopsy (rarely needed) shows replacement of normal lymph node structure by small lymphocytes without invasion of the capsule or surrounding structures.
4. Immunoglobulin levels are usually reduced, IgM often being the first affected.

Complications

Autoimmune haemolytic anaemia occurs in some cases. Recurrent infection, especially chest infection sometimes with opportunistic organisms, is a common cause of death. Massive lymph node enlargement may lead to pressure symptoms, for example superior vena caval obstruction. Hypersplenism is a complication with marked splenomegaly. There is an increased incidence of other malignancies, especially of the skin.

Basis of Treatment

Many cases of CLL require no treatment. A raised white count alone is not an indication for treatment. Treatment should be directed towards preventing progressive marrow failure (anaemia and thrombocytopenia) reversing lymph node enlargement or treating complications, for example AIHA. Localised lymph node masses respond well to radiotherapy so do skin or pleural deposits. The drug of choice is chlorambucil and prednisolone should be added if there is bone marrow failure. The response may be slow, and careful haematological supervision is required to prevent overdose. Infections require prompt treatment. A few patients with recurrent infections may benefit by regular gammaglobulin replacement.

Prognosis

Some forms of CLL, especially in the elderly, are very benign and may persist for 10 to 15 years. Others are more malignant – the overall survival being about 50 per cent at five years.

MYELOMATOSIS

Definition

A disease due to malignant proliferation of plasma cells.

Background

Myeloma arises from the malignant transformation of a single line or *clone* of plasma cells. These cells are antibody-producing and according to the theory that each clone of plasma cells produces a single antibody, the malignant clone secretes identical immunoglobulin molecules. These molecules move together on serum electrophoresis and can be identified as a *monoclonal* or *paraprotein band*. The normal immunoglobulin molecule consists of two paired heavy and light chains (*see* page 116). In malignant plasma cells the synthesis of these chains may be asynchronous, so that an excess of light chains is produced, or the synthesis of heavy chains may be suppressed completely. Excess light chains appear in the plasma and are excreted in the urine as *Bence-Jones* protein.

The clinical features of myeloma are the result of the proliferation of plasma cells in the bone marrow causing bone lesions, and of the effects of the overproduction of immunoglobulin molecules or fragments of these. High levels of paraprotein make the plasma hyperviscous giving rise to the hyperviscosity syndrome. Bence-Jones protein can damage renal tubular cells and cause renal failure. Hypercalcaemia, from bone destruction, is an important additional cause of renal failure. Accumulation of light chains in the tissues can lead to amyloidosis. Normal immunoglobulin production is suppressed so that immune paresis and susceptibility to infection results. Occasionally, plasma cell tumours may be localised and may involve soft tissue forming *plasmacytomas*.

Pathology

Osteolytic lesions in the skull, long bones and axial skeleton are characteristic. Pathological fractures may result. Collapse of vertebrae, together with extramedullary extension may cause compression of the spinal cord. The kidneys are often damaged by hypercalcaemia, the toxic effect of excess light chains on the tubular cells, direct infiltration or amyloid (myeloma kidneys). Amyloid may be found in the skin, mucous membranes, nerves, kidneys, spleen and liver.

Symptoms (Fig. 19.15)

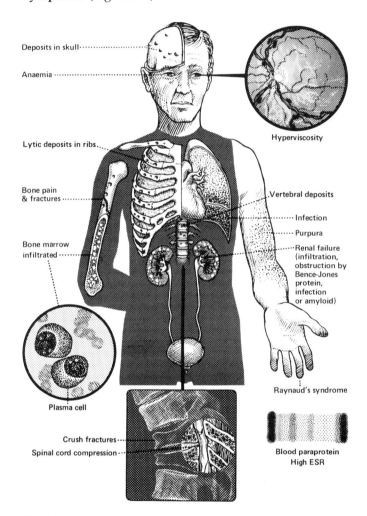

Deposits in skull

Anaemia

Hyperviscosity

Lytic deposits in ribs

Bone pain & fractures

Vertebral deposits

Infection

Purpura

Renal failure (infiltration, obstruction by Bence-Jones protein, infection or amyloid)

Bone marrow infiltrated

Plasma cell

Raynaud's syndrome

Crush fractures

Spinal cord compression

Blood paraprotein High ESR

Fig. 19.15   Clinical features of multiple myeloma.

Of bone lesions – bone pain, especially the spine, pathological fractures.
Of neurological complications – parasthesiae, weakness due to spinal cord compression.
Of anaemia.
Of renal failure (*see* page 231).
Of hypercalcaemia (*see* page 194).
Of hyperviscosity – weakness, visual disturbance, abnormal bleeding.

Signs

Bony tenderness.
Of spinal cord compression (*see* page 507).
Retinopathy – due to hyperviscosity.
Infiltration of skin, joints, mucous membranes, due to amyloid.

Investigations

1. **Haematological.** In early cases the peripheral blood may be normal. In more advanced disease a normochromic anaemia is usual, together with leucopenia and thrombocytopenia. A leuco-erythroblastic anaemia occurs in extensive disease.
Plasma cells are not usually seen in the peripheral blood but sometimes occur in large numbers in plasma cell leukaemia.
There is usually marked rouleaux formation due to the hyperglobulinaemia. This also causes a raised ESR and plasma viscosity.
Note: In cases where light chains only are produced the ESR may be *normal*.
The bone marrow shows plasmacytosis of varying degree, the distribution may be patchy and several aspirations at different sites may be needed to establish the diagnosis. The plasma cells are often of abnormal morphology.

2. **Biochemical.** A monoclonal protein (IgG, A,M,D) can be detected in the serum in approximately 80 per cent of cases. In about 70 per cent of these, excess light chains can be found in the urine (Bence-Jones protein). In most of the remaining 20 per cent of cases Bence-Jones protein only may be found. In a small percentage of cases no paraprotein can be demonstrated (*non-secretory myeloma*). Light chains may be either Kappa (K) or Lambda (L) but not both.
Note: To detect B-J protein, urine concentration and electrophoresis is necessary. Tests depending on the differential solubility of B-J protein by warming urine will detect only gross B-J proteinuria.
Normal immunoglobulin levels are reduced often severely. The serum albumin level may be reduced. Hypercalcaemia is common – correction of the serum calcium level for the albumin level must be made.
Hyperuricaemia is a common finding especially after cytotoxic treatment.
Assessment of renal function is essential.

3. **Radiological.** Osteolytic lesions, especially in the skull, long bones and vertebrae are characteristic. They have a sharply defined edge which helps to distinguish them from secondary deposits. A skeletal survey is essential, because lesions may be isolated. In some cases, osteoporosis alone is found and in others no bone lesions may be demonstrated.

Differential Diagnosis

Diagnosis depends on demonstrating:
(a) Plasmacytosis.
(b) Monoclonal immunoglobulin or light chain production with associated reduction in normal immunoglobulin levels.
(c) Bone lesions.

Advanced cases present no problem but if not all the three criteria listed above are present distinction has to be made from:
(a) Other causes of plasmacytosis, e.g. chronic infection, or inflammatory disease, e.g. rheumatoid arthritis.
(b) Other causes of paraprotein, e.g. benign, macroglobulinaemia lymphomas with an associated paraprotein.
(c) Other causes of osteolytic lesions – mainly secondary carcinoma.

Complications

The main ones have already been mentioned above – multiple fractures, renal failure and recurrent infections.

Basis of Treatment

There are two aspects of treatment:
1. Supportive treatment and management of complications.
2. Treatment directed to reducing the myelomatous tumour mass.

1. An early assessment should be made to establish the degree of hypercalcaemia and renal failure. Hypercalcaemia requires urgent treatment with rehydration, low calcium diet, corticosteroids and possible phosphate infusion. It usually responds to these measures and in the long term, to treatment of the myeloma. Renal failure may need to be treated with haemodialysis. Hyperviscosity should be treated by plasmaphoresis. Anaemia requires blood transfusion.

Orthopaedic procedures, for example pinning pathological fractures may reduce pain and increase mobility. Mobility should be encouraged and spinal corsets, walking frames, etc. may be very helpful. Bone pain can be severe, especially in the terminal stages and adequate and regular analgesics must be given.

2. There are two methods of attacking the myeloma tumour mass. Radiotherapy is invaluable in treating local bone lesions. The role of more extensive radiotherapy, for example hemi-corporeal irradiation is still to be evaluated. No treatment has yet been shown to be superior to the combination of an alkylating agent – phenylalanine mustard (Melphalan) and prednisolone given in seven-day courses at four to six-weekly intervals depending on the blood count. The addition of other cytotoxic agents, procarbazine and vincristine

may improve survival in advanced cases, but as yet their role is not proven. As with other malignant haematological disease routine allopurinol must be given.

The response to treatment should be monitored by serial measurements of paraprotein or Bence-Jones protein levels. In most cases there is a reduction in the paraprotein level, and presumably the tumour mass, until a plateau level is reached. The value of maintenance therapy at this point is still not confirmed.

Local plasmacytomas are often treated successfully by local irradiation.

Some patients who present with evidence of myeloma as judged by plasmacytosis and a paraprotein, but without bone lesions or other complications may require no treatment. These patients should be reviewed at three to six-monthly intervals and treatment started only when there is evidence that symptomatic disease is developing.

Prognosis

The prognosis is most influenced by the plasma cell tumour mass at presentation. Indications of a high tumour mass, and a bad prognosis, include anaemia, hypercalcaemia, renal failure, a high level of paraprotein and extensive bone lesions. A smaller number of poor prognosis patients show a response to treatment. Of patients responding to treatment, the medium survival is between three and four years. There is no doubt that the effective use of supportive and cytotoxic therapy has considerably influenced survival in myeloma. An increasing number of successfully treated patients are reported as developing acute leukaemia – whether this is due to the use of alkylating agents or the natural history of the disease seen in the longer survival is debatable. However, the longer survival and better quality of life offered by treatment with alkylating agents offsets the relatively small risk of acute leukaemia.

Patients with indolent myeloma may survive many years without treatment.

WALDENSTRÖMS MACROGLOBULINAEMIA

This is a rare disorder, affecting elderly patients, resembling myeloma in that there is overproduction of a monoclonal immunoglobulin – invariably IgM. There is proliferation of lymphoid cells with plasmacytoid features. Lymphadenopathy and hepatosplenomegaly are common features. Bone lesions are rare. The clinical features are due principally to hyperviscosity caused by high levels of IgM and bone marrow failure due to marrow infiltration. Hyperviscosity symptoms include weakness, abnormal bleeding (due to platelet malfunction) visual disturbance and in several cases, neurological symptoms including coma. Renal failure and immune paresis is less common than in myeloma.

Treatment is directed initially towards reducing the plasma viscosity which is most easily accomplished by plasmaphoresis. Long term treatment, aimed at reducing the number of malignant cells is best achieved with alkylating agents, especially chlorambucil, usually combined with prednisolone. The prognosis is very variable. Some patients run a benign course for many years requiring minimal treatment. In other patients, the disease is more aggressive and pancytopenia may be a limiting factor in continuing cytotoxic therapy.

BENIGN MONOCLONAL GAMMOPATHY

Monoclonal (M) bands may be found in up to 5 per cent of patients aged 70 and over. Many of these are of no significance. In the absence of any other signs of malignancy no treatment is required. Regular follow up at six to twelve-month intervals is probably advisable to assess the progression of the disease, if any. Benign M bands show little or no increase in amount over long periods. M bands are also found in a variety of other conditions, e.g. carcinoma, lymphoma, liver disease, infections, etc. They are of no significance and often transitory. Treatment is directed towards the primary condition.

IV. THE LYMPHOMAS

Definition

The lymphomas are a group of disorders caused by proliferation, presumably malignant, of lymphoreticular tissue.

Background

The major sites of lymphoreticular tissue are the lymph nodes, the liver, spleen, bone marrow, thymus and that which develops in relation to the alimentary tract, namely the tonsils and Peyer's patches. The lymphomas may involve any or all of these sites and, further, they may invade other organs where lymphoid tissue is not normally found, for example the central nervous system and skin. The clinical picture of the disorders is very variable and, so far, no entirely satisfactory classification exists.

Lymphoreticular tissue contains two main types of cell – lymphocytes and histiocytes (macrophages). Lymphomas may originate from either, or both, of these cell lines. Furthermore, there are several forms of lymphocytic cells (B, T and Null, see page 116) and these are capable of undergoing transformation in the presence of antigen. Lymphomatous change may affect any of these cell types and at any stage in the transformation process. Hence the histological picture may be very varied and in the past, confusion has arisen because transformed lymphocytes have been mistaken for histiocytes or 'reticulum' cells.

Modern techniques, involving the use of ultra-thin section, electron microscopy, cytochemistry and immunological detection of surface markers, have clarified the situation to some extent and the latest classification of the lymphomas subdivides them according to the nature of the cell involved. Other histological features which are of diagnostic value are the degree of differentiation of the cells and whether or not they are arranged in a diffuse or follicular pattern. On clinical and histological grounds one type of lymphoma – Hodgkin's disease – can be separated from the rest – the non-Hodgkin's lymphomas. A simplified attempt at classification of the lymphomas is given in Table 19.9.

The aetiology of the lymphomas is unknown. There is still speculation as to whether they are truly malignant diseases or an aberrant immunological response to some

Table 19.9 Classification of the lymphomas: A simplified attempt to compare the older classification with a more recent histological classification (Rappaport) and one based on immunological criteria (Lukes and Collins)

Old classification	Histological classification	Immunological classification
Hodgkin's disease	**Hodgkin's disease**	B Cell lymphomas
	Non-Hodgkin's lymphoma	CLL – small lymphocytes
		Waldenströms – plasmacytoid lymphocytes
	Lymphocytic (May be well or poorly differentiated and nodular or diffuse)	Most lymphocytic lymphomas
Giant follicular lymphoma		Some mixed (L and H) lymphomas
Lymphosarcoma		Some histiocytic and stem cell lymphomas ⎫ Follicular lymphocytes
	Mixed lymphocytic and histiocytic (The 'histiocytic component' probably represents transformed lymphocytes)	Burkitt's lymphoma
Reticulosarcoma		
		T Cell lymphomas
	Histiocytic (Many of these are probably transformed lymphocytes)	Some poorly differentiated lymphocytic lymphomas
Malignant histiocytosis		Some histiocytic lymphomas
		Some forms of ALL (with mediastinal tumours)
	Undifferentiated stem cell (Probably mainly lymphocytic)	Skin lymphomas – mycosis fungoides and Sezary's syndrome
		?Hodgkin's disease
		Histiocytic lymphomas
		Malignant histiocytosis

foreign agent, for example a virus. Another suggestion, possibly more likely, is that they start as the latter and then undergo malignant transformation. Evidence for a viral aetiology comes from studies of animal lymphomas and in man from Burkitt's lymphoma which is known to be associated with Epstein Barr (EB virus) infection. The possibilities of a viral aetiology have been strengthened by the finding of clustering of cases within communities and a tendency for an increased incidence in those who have had operations, such as tonsillectomy and appendicectomy, to remove lymphoid tissue. There is an increased incidence of lymphomas in patients with immune deficiency disorders, for example ataxia telangiectasia, certain autoimmune disorders, for example Sjögren's syndrome, in coeliac disease and as a result of immunosuppressive therapy.

HODGKIN'S DISEASE

This form of lymphoma may be separated from the others because of its unique histology and clinical features, and because it is the most amenable to treatment. It occurs in all age groups with two peaks, one in early adult life and the other in the elderly. There is a male predominance. A characteristic feature of the disease is the early loss of cellular immunity (delayed hypersensitivity reactions) leading to infections with opportunist organisms, for example fungi. In the early stages, the disease is usually confined to a localised group of lymph nodes and it spreads by orderly progression to involve other groups of lymph nodes and later extra-nodal structures.

Pathology

The hallmark of the disease is the Reed-Sternberg cell. This is a large cell with abundant cytoplasm and two (or more) large nuclei, often arranged as a mirror image, each with a prominent nucleolus. The nature of this cell is unknown, previously thought to be a 'reticulum' cell it is now thought that it might be a transformed 'T' cell. The lymph node architecture is destroyed and replaced with a variable cellular infiltration consisting of lymphocytes, fibrous tissue, eosinophils and plasma cells. The relative preponderance of lymphocytes and fibrous tissue is important in predicting prognosis. The greater the lymphocyte proliferation, the better the prognosis. Four histological varieties of the disease are recognised:

1. Lymphocyte predominance (least malignant).
2. Nodular sclerosis.
3. Mixed cellularity.
4. Lymphocyte depletion (most malignant).

The histologica picture is reminiscent of a graft–versus–host reaction and, possibly, represents the beneficial effects of the host immunological reaction. A plentiful lymphocyte production would represent an effective immune defence, in accord with the more benign course.

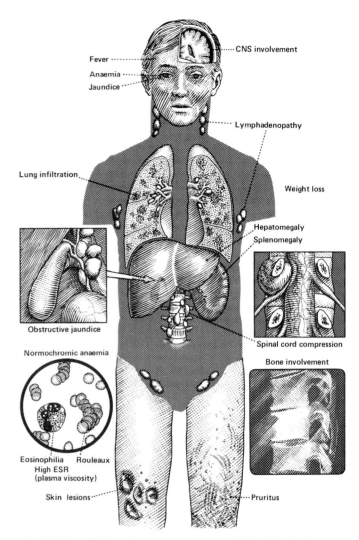

Fig. 19.16   Clinical features of advanced Hodgkin's disease.

Symptoms

Lymph node enlargement. The commonest presentation is painless enlargement of cervical and, less commonly, axillary or inguinal lymph nodes.

Systemic symptoms (of uncertain aetiology):
Fever (sometimes undulant and known as 'Pel Ebstein fever') – occasionally, pyrexia may be the only finding (PUO – pyrexia of unknown origin).
Malaise, weakness, weight loss, night sweats.
Anaemia (only in late stages).
Pruritus.
Alcohol–induced pain. An interesting, though rare, symptom is the occurrence of pain, and sometimes systemic symptoms of malaise, etc. following the ingestion of alcohol. Though not confined to Hodgkin's disease, pain is often related to the site of disease, particularly in bones. It occurs particularly where there is histological evidence of fibrosis.

Symptoms due to infection:
Fever. (An intective cause for fever should be excluded before ascribing it to the disease. *Note:* TB and opportunist infections, e.g. cryptococcal meningitis may occur because of the immune defect.)
Root pain and skin lesions due to *Herpes zoster.*

Signs (Fig. 19.16)

Lymphadenopathy – the nodes are 'rubbery', painless and often matted.
Splenomegaly.
Hepatomegaly.
Weight loss, jaundice and anaemia.
The following signs are less common:
Pulmonary collapse or pleural effusion (due to bronchial obstruction or pleural involvement). Rarely there may be vena caval obstruction.
Ascites, due to peritoneal or cysterna chyli involvement.
CNS involvement, e.g. paraplegia.

Differential Diagnosis

The causes of lymph node enlargement are shown below:

Causes of lymph gland enlargement

Generalised: Infectious mononucleosis
Chronic lymphatic leukaemia
Lymphoma
Rheumatoid arthritis (and Stills' disease)
Sarcoidosis
Syphilis (secondary)
Tuberculosis
Toxoplasmosis
Drug therapy, e.g. Epanutin, PAS, etc.

Localised: Local infection (pyogenic, TB, pediculosis)
Cat scratch fever
Rubella (occipital)
Lymphoma, Hodgkin's disease or NHL
Secondary carcinoma

Investigations

1. The diagnosis can only be made by histological examination of affected tissue, most usually a lymph node, but occasionally splenic or liver tissue, bone marrow or skin. *Any enlarged lymph node persisting for six weeks for which no cause can be found should be biopsied.* Prior consultation with the surgeon concerned helps to ensure a successful outcome histologically. Needle aspiration of lymph nodes is not recommended because it does not allow inspection of the nodal architecture. If infiltration of other organs, for example skin, liver or bone marrow, is suspected, biopsy of one of these may be an easier and alternative approach to lymph node biopsy. Scalene node biopsy may be of value when hilar nodes only are involved.

2. The blood picture may be normal in localised disease. Changes which may occur include a normochromic anaemia, eosinophilia and a raised ESR or plasma viscosity. Haemolytic anaemia may occur and is sometimes autoimmune (positive antiglobulin (Coombs') test). If there is marrow involvement a leuco-erythroblastic anaemia may be present. In the absence of marrow involvement a marrow biopsy is not helpful. *Note:* Hodgkin's tissue is rarely seen in aspiration biopsies – a trephine biopsy is always needed.

3. The serum copper level is raised (this test is helpful in following the course of the disease and in detecting early relapse).

4. Liver function tests may be abnormal if there is hepatic involvement.

5. Radiology is invaluable. A chest film may show bilateral hilar nodes or infiltration of the lung parenchyma. Bone involvement may be shown by osteolytic or occasionally, sclerotic lesions (ivory vertebrae). Lymphangiography is useful in some cases in demonstrating involvement of the para-aortic nodes (*see below* – Staging).

Staging

For the successful treatment of Hodgkin's disease, it is essential to know the extent of the disease so that all affected areas can be treated. Four stages of the disease are recognised:

Stage I. Involvement of a single lymph node region.

Stage II. Involvement of two or more lymph node regions on the same side of the diaphragm.

Stage III. Involvement of lymph node regions on both sides of the diaphragm or the spleen.

Stage IV. Involvement of extra lymphatic organs (excluding the spleen) with or without lymph node involvement.

Each stage is subdivided into either A or B depending on the presence of the systemic symptoms – weight loss, fever and night sweats. The prognosis in subgroup B is less good.

Staging based on clinical signs alone is unreliable and much of the recent success in treating Hodgkin's disease can be attributed to the improvement in the methods of

407

revealing subclinical disease, so that these areas can be treated. The most difficult diagnostic area is the abdomen. Lymphangiography is not entirely reliable as it does not demonstrate involved nodes in the upper abdomen, splenic pedicle or mesentery. Splenic involvement is also difficult to assess. Splenic enlargement does not necessarily indicate infiltration with Hodgkin's tissue, nor does absence of splenomegaly exclude it. The staging procedure includes the investigations listed above together with laparotomy in Stages I to III. The object of laparotomy is to biopsy the intra-abdominal lymph nodes and the liver and to perform splenectomy. Apart from revealing splenic involvement, splenectomy facilitates subsequent radiotherapy. There is no necessity for laparotomy in Stage IV disease.

Basis of Treatment

The object of treatment of Hodgkin's disease should now be cure not palliation. For Stages I, II and III the treatment of choice is irradiation, preferably using supervoltage techniques. For localised disease, wide field irradiation is given to cover all the lymph node groups above or below the diaphragm – the so-called 'mantle' and 'inverted Y' techniques. For Stage III disease, with involvement on both sides of the diaphragm, both fields are irradiated. The treatment fields are so planned as to exclude sensitive organs such as the lungs and kidneys.

Stage IV (and possibly Stage IIIB) is treated by oncolytic drugs. Single drug therapy has no place and considerably worsens the prognosis. Oncolytic drugs should be given in combination and in cycles, with gaps between each cycle to allow marrow recovery. The two most successful combinations in use at present are MOPP and MVPP (see Table 19.10).

Remission is usually achieved by six courses. The value of continuing maintenance therapy once remission has been obtained is still uncertain. Further treatment increases the chance of complications of drug therapy without apparently offering any real improvement in survival. The management of patients who relapse is also an unsolved problem. A number of other drug regimes are under trial, using nitrosoureas, doxorubicin (Adriamycin) imidazole and bleomycin.

All the drug regimes used in the treatment of Hodgkin's disease are very toxic and can cause severe marrow depression. Infectious complications, often with opportunist infections, are common. Important factors are the drug-induced neutropenia, the immune deficiency associated with the disease and the effects of high dose corticosteroids.

Prognosis

The use of wide field irradiation and energetic cytotoxic therapy has dramatically altered the prognosis in Hodgkin's disease, once almost invariably fatal. Over 80 per

Table 19.10 Oncolytic drug regimes used in the treatment of lymphoma

Drug regime	Dosage
MOPP (HD)	
Mustine hydrochloride	6 mg/m^2 IV on days 1 and 8
Vincristine (Oncovin)	1.4 mg/m^2 IV on days 1 and 8
Procarbazine (Natulan)	100 mg/m^2 orally on days 1 to 10
Prednisolone	40 mg/m^2 orally on days 1 to 10
	(given in cycles 1 and 4 only)
10-day course. Cycle frequency 28 days.	
MVPP (HD)	
As for MOPP except substituting	
vinblastine (Velbe) for vincristine	6 mg/m^2 IV on days 1 and 8
and prednisolone and procarbazine	Continue for 14 days
14-day course. Cycle frequency 42 days.	
COP (NHL – less well differentiated lymphocytic lymphoma)	
Cyclophosphamide (Endoxana)	800 mg/m^2 IV on day 1
	(Reduce to 400 mg/m^2 at bone marrow failure)
Vincristine	2 mg IV on day 1
Prednisolone	60 mg/m^2 orally days 1 to 5 then
	40, 20, 10 mg/m^2 for three days
8-day course. Cycle frequency 14 days.	
CHOP (poorly differentiated lymphocytic and histiocytic lymphomas)	
Cyclophosphamide	750 mg/m^2 IV on day 1
Doxorubicin (Adriamycin)	50 mg/m^2 IV on day 1
Vincristine	1.4 mg/m^2 (maximum 2 mg) IV on day 1
Prednisolone	100 mg on days 1 to 5
5-day course. Cycle frequency 14 to 21 days depending on degree of myelosuppression.	

HD = Hodgkin's disease; NHL = Non-Hodgkin lymphoma.

cent of patients with Stage I and II disease are alive and well at five years, and many of these are probably cured. The prognosis in Stage III and IV disease is less good but even so, the five-year survival is still in the order of 75 per cent. There is no cause for pessimism even in advanced Hodgkin's disease.

THE NON-HODGKIN'S LYMPHOMAS (NHL)

This is an unsatisfactory term as it embraces a group of diseases of widely different origin and natural history. These diseases are often much more widely spread than Hodgkin's disease, and they tend to progress in a much less orderly fashion. The lymphoid tissue of the alimentary canal is a common site of origin. Involvement of non-lymphoreticular tissue, for example skin, CNS and marrow, is more common than in Hodgkin's disease.

Background

These malignancies are thought to arise from either lymphocytes or histiocytes (monocytes). Histiocytic lymphomas are much less common than previously thought. Formerly these were classified as *reticulosarcomas*, but this term also included some lymphomas now thought to be lymphocytic. Most of the lymphocytic lymphomas were included in the classification of *lymphosarcomas*. The lymphocytic lymphomas should be regarded as a spectrum of disease, with overlap between them.

The variable clinical picture and cell morphology may be explained on the basis that each disease represents a malignant deviation at some stage in the normal differentiation of lymphoid cells. Modern studies have shown that most of the lymphocytic lymphomas are derived from B cells. The spectrum of B cell malignancies is wide ranging from CLL through the mainly solid-tumour lymphocytic lymphomas, to myeloma, representing the end-stage of B cell differentiation into antibody producing, or plasma cells. T cells are more difficult to identify, but some examples of T cell lymphoma have been recognised. These include some cases of CLL and ALL and two lymphomas, characterised by skin involvement – Sézary's syndrome and mycosis fungoides. Initially there are skin lesions only, which may simulate eczema, or they may form plaques or frank tumours (tomato tumours). Eventually, involvement of lymph nodes and other tissues causes a generalised lymphoma.

Of particular importance in determining treatment and prognosis is the presence of a nodular pattern in the lymph node architecture. This, presumably, represents an attempt on the part of the malignant cells to form follicles and, if so, these cells would be expected to be of B cell origin. Nodular lymphomas have a distinctly better prognosis than diffuse ones. A particularly benign form of nodular lymphoma used to be called *giant follicular lymphoma* or *Brill Symmer's disease*. Usually

only a single lymph node group or the spleen is involved. The disease progresses slowly over a long period of time, up to twenty years, and is very responsive to local DXR. Eventually most cases transform into a much more malignant lymphoma, which spreads rapidly.

Another form of lymphoma deserving special mention is Burkitt's lymphoma, a B cell malignancy. It is common in Equatorial Africa and tends to occur in children and to involve the facial bones (maxilla and mandible) with retroperitoneal and abdominal involvement, while sparing the peripheral lymph nodes and spleen. Because of its geographical limitation, a search for possible infective causes has led to the finding of a herpes group virus (Epstein-Barr (EB) virus) in a large percentage of tumour cells and corresponding antibodies in the serum. The precise part played by this virus is not known. The disease may show natural remissions and a dramatic response to cytotoxic drugs. Recently a similar cell line has been demonstrated in some cases of ALL.

The clinical picture in NHL is very variable, depending on the extent of the disease and the organs involved. Gut lesions may cause haemorrhage, perforation and obstruction. Ascites may occur from obstruction of intestinal lymphatics or the cysterna chyli. Retroperitoneal involvement may be difficult to diagnose as physical signs are few and the symptoms are non-specific, for example fever, loss of weight, malaise, etc. CNS lesions may be due to tumour deposits or to a demyelinating process 'multifocal leuko-encephalpathy'. Anaemia and thrombocytopenia may result from invasion of the bone marrow. Secondary immune deficiency may result and therefore infections are common, particularly with viruses, for example herpes, or opportunist organisms.

Basis of Treatment

There is no general agreement on the treatment of NHL. Precise histological diagnosis is essential and every effort should be made to define the extent of the disease, using a staging procedure similar to that described for Hodgkin's disease. The two alternatives for treatment are radiotherapy and cytotoxic drugs. Localised disease is probably best treated by DXR. Generalised disease requires oncolytic drugs. The more well differentiated B cell lymphomas are possibly best treated with chlorambucil alone or in combination with steroids. More malignant varieties require combination therapy – the two most widely used regimes being COP and CHOP (*see* Table 19.10). At present, there is considerable interest in whole body irradiation as a method of treatment, and a trial is in progress to try and assess the relative benefits of this compared with combination chemotherapy. It is not meaningful to give an overall prognosis for such a diverse group of diseases. The more benign nodular lymphomas have a long term survival, but the prognosis in the generalised diffuse lymphocytic or histiocytic form remains poor, with a mean survival of under two years.

THE BLEEDING DISORDERS

Background

The arrest of haemorrhage is a complicated process (Fig. 19.17). It depends on the interaction between:

1. The vessel wall.
2. The platelets.
3. The coagulation system.
4. The fibrinolytic system.

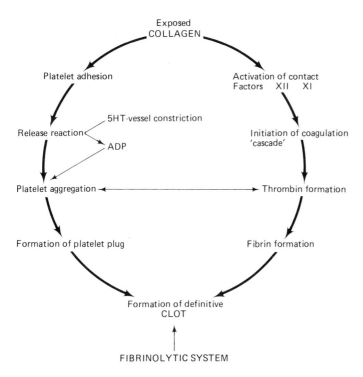

Fig. 19.17 Mechanism of haemostasis.
Note: There is an interaction between platelets and the coagulation system.

The initiating event in the formation of a clot, or thrombus, is damage to vascular endothelium with the exposure of collagen. Circulating platelets adhere to exposed collagen and, in doing so, release a number of intracellular constituents. These include 5-hydroxy-tryptamine (5HT), which causes constriction of small blood vessels, and ADP, which promotes platelet aggregation. Aggregated platelets form a platelet plug which provides a primary mechanism for the arrest of haemorrhage. This plug retracts and breaks down unless it is reinforced by the formation of a fibrin clot.

Fibrin formation is the product of the coagulation system (Fig. 19.18). This involves the activities of a number of factors, normally circulating as inactive pre-cursors. The active factors are usually enzymes which activate the next factor in the chain. The coagulation system is a cascade phenomenon, each step leading to the activation of a greater number of molecules, so that the activation of a small number of molecules of contact factor can give rise to the formation of large amounts of fibrin. The coagulation system can be activated by two pathways – the *intrinsic pathway*, depending on the activation of the contact factors XII and XI, and the *extrinsic pathway* activated by tissue thromboplastin released from damaged tissues. These two pathways interact and both are probably needed for normal haemostasis *in vivo*.

There is an interaction between platelets and the coagulation system. Activation of the coagulation factors occurs on the surface of aggregated platelets and thrombin formation promotes further platelet aggregation. Inappropriate fibrin formation *in vivo*, i.e. thrombus formation, is prevented by the presence of naturally occurring inhibitors.

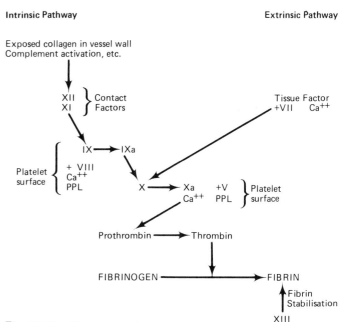

Fig. 19.18 The coagulation system.

Fibrin formation *in vivo* activates the fibrinolytic system which maintains the patency of the blood vessels. Rarely, overaction of the fibrinolytic system may cause abnormal bleeding. It is possible that defects in this system may lead to thrombosis.

Bleeding disorders may arise from defects in any of the steps needed for normal haemostasis as follows:

1. Vascular disorders (Table 19.11).
2. Thrombocytopenia (Table 19.12).
3. Platelet function disorders (thrombocytopathy).
4. Coagulation disorders.
5. Excessive fibrinolysis.

THE INVESTIGATION OF BLEEDING DISORDERS

The investigation of a patient with an actual or suspected bleeding disorder depends on a combination of clinical history and examination and laboratory investigations. The former should indicate the probable nature of the disorder and appropriate investigations should be used to confirm this. The investigations should follow an orderly scheme.

Clinical History

The patient should be questioned carefully about the following points:

Type and Extent of Bleeding. Bleeding into the skin, bruising and purpura, and into mucous membranes suggests a platelet or vessel defect. Bleeding into joints, and soft tissues is characteristic of a coagulation defect. Bleeding from multiple sites occurs in a generalised bleeding disorder, for example DIC. Bleeding from a single site, for example nose, gastrointestinal tract or uterus, may be due to a localised cause.

Onset of Bleeding and Past History. The sudden onset of bleeding in adult life usually indicates an acquired disorder, although it should be noted that some patients with mild congenital bleeding disorders may present for the first time with severe postoperative bleeding.

Surgical Operations. Of particular importance are dental extractions and tonsillectomy. These are major haemostatic challenges and any patient who has undergone these procedures without excessive bleeding is unlikely to have a severe congenital bleeding disorder.

Type of Bleeding. This should be established. Platelet and vessel disorders cause bleeding from the onset of trauma. Oozing continues for a variable period, but once stopped it does not usually recur. In coagulation defects, bleeding may not start for several hours after trauma. It is difficult to stop and does not usually respond to pressure. Recurrence of bleeding after stopping is usual.

Family History. This is of importance in congenital bleeding disorders. As many members of the family as possible should be seen and investigated, because in some mild congenital disorders affected relatives may be asymptomatic until faced with a major haemostatic challenge.

Systemic Disease. Liver disease, renal disease, malignancy and autoimmune disease may cause an acquired bleeding disorder.

Drugs. These may cause thrombocytopenia or affect platelet function, especially important are aspirin, other anti-inflammatory drugs, including steroids and drugs known to cause thrombocytopenia, for example thiazides.

Examination

The skin and mucous membranes should be inspected for bruises, purpura, petechial haemorrhages and localised vascular malformations. Joint deformities may indicate previous haemarthroses. Hepato- or splenomegaly may be present in systemic disease.

Hess Test. This simple test is abnormal in most small vessel and quantitative and qualitative platelet defects. A sphygmomanometer cuff should be inflated to 80 to 100 mmHg for five minutes. More than a few purpura over the forearm is abnormal (Fig. 19.19).

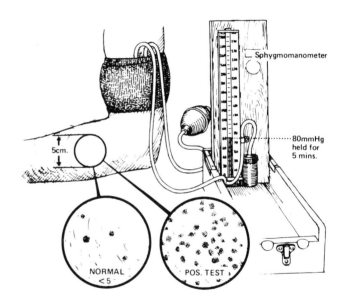

Fig. 19.19 The Hess test.

Laboratory Investigations

The laboratory investigation of a suspected bleeding disorder should include the following screening tests.

1. **Blood Examination** (including platelet count and film examination). This will detect thrombocytopenia. In some myeloproliferative disorders, for example thrombocythaemia, bleeding may occur from platelet dysfunction – the platelets are increased in number and are of abnormal morphology. The cause of thrombocytopenia may be revealed, for example in leukaemia.

2. **Bleeding Time.** This test is abnormal in thrombocytopenia and platelet function defects. It is usually normal in small vessel disease and in coagulation defects. It is particularly useful in the diagnosis of von

411

Willebrand's disease. It is important that it is performed under standardised conditions. The *Ivy* technique, in which three incisions are made in the forearm, is the best method. Normally, bleeding stops within ten minutes.

3. **Screening Tests of Blood Coagulation** (Fig. 19.20). These tests are carried out on citrated plasma. The citrate chelates the calcium required for coagulation to occur. Various substances are added to the plasma which is then recalcified and the time taken for fibrin clot formation is noted. The normal range for these tests varies according to the technique used in different laboratories. Note that the method of collection of blood is of critical importance. A clean venepuncture is essential. An exact amount of blood must be added to the measured amount of citrate contained in the collecting tube, and the sample should be analysed within a few hours of collection.

(*Note:* Whole blood clotting time. This test is very insensitive and if abnormal indicates gross pathology. It is never used now, having been superseded by the screening tests described below.)

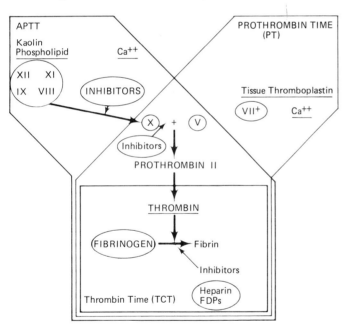

Fig. 19.20 Screening tests for coagulation system showing interrelationship between TCT, APTT and PT. Factors tested in each assay are enclosed in circles; substances added to citrated plasma in each test are underlined.

(a) *Thrombin clotting time.* Thrombin is added to citrated plasma. This tests the conversion of fibrinogen to fibrin. It is abnormal in *fibrinogen* deficiency, and in the presence of *inhibitors*, particularly *heparin* and *fibrinogen degradation products* (FDPs). It is useful in the diagnosis of DIC and can be used to monitor heparin therapy.

(b) *Prothrombin time (PT).* A test of the extrinsic system. Tissue thromboplastin (usually derived from brain) is added to citrated plasma together with calcium. It is particularly sensitive to deficiency in Factors VII, II, X and V and may be abnormal in severe hypofibrinogenaemia. It is useful in the diagnosis of coagulation defects secondary to liver disease or vitamin K deficiency. It is used to monitor oral anticoagulation therapy.

(c) *Activated partial thromboplastin time* (APTT). A test of the intrinsic system. The contact factors (XII and XI) are activated by kaolin. Added phospholipid takes the place of platelets. It is particularly useful in the diagnosis of deficiency of the contact factors and Factors VIII and IX. In these conditions the PT is normal. The APTT is also prolonged in deficiency of Factors X, V, II and fibrinogen. In these conditions the PT is also abnormal. The APTT is also sensitive to the presence of inhibitors of the coagulation system.

(d) *Fibrin degradation products* (FDPs). These are raised in the defibrination syndrome and disseminated intravascular coagulation.

4. **Special Tests**

(a) *Factor assays.* Abnormalities in the screening tests need to be confirmed by individual factor assays.

(b) *Platelet function tests.* Platelet adhesiveness and aggregation can be measured in suspected functional platelet defects.

(c) *Tests of fibrinolytic activity.* These are technically difficult and rarely requested clinically.

A. ABNORMAL BLEEDING DUE TO VASCULAR DEFECTS

Bleeding disorders due to vascular defects may be congenital or acquired. They are characterised by bleeding into the skin, easy bruising, purpura, and bleeding from mucous membranes. They are caused by either inflammation or damage to small vessels or changes in the supporting matrix.

1. HEREDITARY HAEMORRHAGIC TELANGIECTASIA (RENDU–OSLER–WEBER DISEASE)

This disorder is inherited as an autosomal dominant trait. It is characterised by multiple telangiectasia – dilatation of capillaries and arterioles – in the skin and mucous membranes. Involvement of nasal, respiratory, gastrointestinal and renal tracts is common where the lesions are submucosal. Large arteriovenous shunts and aneurysms may occasionally develop in the lungs, central nervous system and alimentary tract, including the liver, where cirrhosis may occur.

Symptoms

Patients commonly present with anaemia and a history of repeated epistaxes and haemoptyses. Recurrent gastrointestinal bleeding frequently occurs. The lesions tend to become larger with age and therefore symptoms may not be manifest until middle age. There is usually a family history of similar bleeding.

Signs

Lesions are found in the mouth (including under the tongue), the lips and finger tips (Fig. 19.21). They are bright red, raised and fade on pressure.

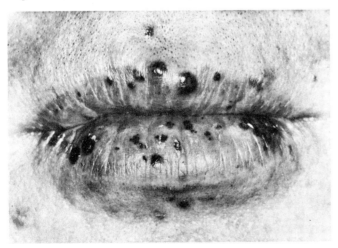

Fig. 19.21 Hereditary haemorrhagic telangiectasia.

Occasionally, an arterial bruit over the head, lung fields or abdomen suggests the presence of an arteriovenous anastomosis.

Investigations

1. The diagnosis is essentially a clinical one and must be thought of (and evidence looked for) in all patients with chronic iron deficiency anaemia, particularly where there is a suggestive family history and recurrent gastrointestinal bleeds.
2. Tests of haemostatic function are normal.
3. There may be iron deficiency anaemia and the occult blood tests may be intermittently positive.
4. Gastrointestinal endoscopy or examination of the nose may show classical submucosal lesions.

Complications

These are of haemorrhage and arteriovenous aneurysm formation. Serum hepatitis from multiple transfusions may partially explain the increased incidence of cirrhosis.

Differential Diagnosis

Distinction must be made from cherry angiomata (Campbell De Morgan spots) spider naevi and purpura.

Basis of Treatment

Nose bleeds should be treated initially with packing and cauterisation. Repeated nose bleeds may be helped by oestrogen therapy (ethinyloestradiol 0.5 to 1 mg daily) which produces squamous metaplasia of nasal mucosa and alteration of connective tissue ground substance with protection of lesions from trauma and subsequent bleeding. Anaemia requires iron therapy and, in severe cases, transfusion. Severe gastrointestinal haemorrhage may be an indication for laparotomy, but lesions are scattered throughout the alimentary tract and localisation of the site of bleeding may not be possible. Localised angiomata may, however, be removed.

2. SIMPLE EASY BRUISING

This is a common condition, occurring almost exclusively in young women, and thought to be due to abnormally fragile capillaries. It is characterised by the occurrence of crops of bruises on the limbs and trunk in the absence of trauma. There is often periodicity associated with the menstrual cycle and the condition is usually self-limiting. All tests of the coagulation system are normal. Apart from the cosmetic aspect, the condition is harmless. There is no treatment apart from the avoidance of aspirin, which may accentuate the bruising.

A somewhat similar condition, also mainly restricted to women, is *auto-erythrocyte sensitisation*. Crops of raised, often tender, bruises appear on the limbs. It has been suggested that this is caused by an abnormal immune response to extravasated red cells. There is a strong psychological component and the condition is usually precipitated by emotional stress.

3. ATROPHIC BRUISING: SENILE PURPURA

Areas of subcutaneous bleeding on the extensor surfaces of the hands and forearms are commonly seen in elderly people. They are caused by easy tearing of the subcutaneous vessels because of degeneration of the supporting elastic tissue. Similar lesions may be found in patients with Cushing's disease or on long term corticosteroid therapy.

In *scurvy* skin haemorrhages occur due to defective formation of the small vessel walls (*see* page 103).

4. BLEEDING DUE TO VASCULITIS

HENOCH-SCHÖNLEIN PURPURA

Definition

A disease of presumed immunological origin, characterised by widespread vasculitis and manifesting with a combination of purpura, arthritis, renal and intestinal involvement.

Background

This disease occurs most commonly in children and young adults. It is often preceded by streptococcal infection or drug ingestion particularly sulphonamides, aspirin, tetracycline and the thiazide diuretics. The combination of vasculitis, arthritis, gut and renal involvement is suggestive of immune complex formation and deposition. Some cases have been recorded in patients with positive hepatitis B antigen (HBsAg).

Pathology

Widespread inflammation of small vessels is seen leading to increased permeability and extravasation into the tissues. This may cause glomerular damage usually in the form of focal glomerular nephritis and oedema and haemorrhagic infiltration of the gut. Renal disease may progress to destruction of glomeruli and renal failure.

Symptoms and Signs

There may be a preceding history of drug ingestion or streptococcal infection. The disease manifests with:

1. *A skin rash* usually maximal over the buttocks and lower limbs. Lesions are red, about 5 mm in diameter, macular, sometimes raised and occasionally, with central ulceration. Recurrent crops may occur and itching may be severe.

2. *Arthritis.* Usually of knees and ankles, but also affecting hands and feet (this lasts for two to three days). Affected joints are swollen and painful.

3. *Abdominal pain*, colicky, may occur in attacks over several weeks. There may be vomiting, diarrhoea and blood in the stools. Laparotomy may reveal red, thickened oedematous areas of ʰowel and even intussusception.

4. *Haematuria* and other evidence of acute or subacute renal failure may be found (*see* page 246). Hypertension may develop. Occasionally oedema, often localised and recurrent, is present, and haemoptysis may occur.

Investigations

1. The blood count shows non-specific features, including a leucocytosis and raised ESR. The platelet count is normal and tests of coagulation normal.
2. The urine may show microscopic or macroscopic haematuria and casts.
3. Biopsy of skin lesions shows acute perivascular inflammation and an arteriolitis.
4. The blood urea may be raised and creatinine clearance reduced.
5. Barium studies of the gastrointestinal tract may reveal submucosal oedema in the small bowel.
6. Occasionally, considerable hypoproteinaemia, presumably due to intestinal protein loss, may occur.

Differential Diagnosis

Other causes of non-thrombocytopenic purpura, especially those caused by vasculitis due to drugs and infections.

Basis of Treatment

In most patients, the disease settles with bed rest and analgesics. The major worries are recurrent relapses of the symptoms, which may occur over several weeks or months, and the problem of renal involvement. Some degree of renal involvement is common, but progressive renal disease, even in adults, is rare, though it can be fatal. In patients with renal failure, there is considerable disagreement concerning the value of corticosteroids. Azathioprine is probably more helpful in those with progressive proliferative glomerular disease.

Prognosis

In a recent review it was shown that three of seventy-seven adult patients had chronic renal disease and in one this was fatal.

5. DYSGLOBULINAEMIC PURPURA

Bleeding disorders are common in hyperglobulinaemic states due to interference with platelet function, and the coagulation mechanism. This is particularly so in macroglobulinaemia where purpura and retinal haemorrhages are common. *Benign hyperglobulinaemic purpura* is a condition occurring in middle-aged women and characterised by crops of purpura on the legs. The IgG is greatly increased and the platelets are normal in number. Some cases develop an autoimmune disease, for example Sjögren's syndrome, in due course. Very careful investigation is required to exclude other causes of hyperglobulinaemia, for example DLE.

B. PLATELET DISORDERS

Platelets are produced in the bone marrow from megakaryocytes, derived from the toti-potential stem cell. Megakaryocytes are multinuclear cells – nuclear division continues until there are between 8 and 32 nuclei per cell when cytoplasmic budding occurs with the formation of platelets. Circulating platelets have a life span of eight to ten days. The normal platelet count is 150 to 450×10^9/l.

Platelet disorders may be due to:
1. Deficiency of platelets – thrombocytopenia.
2. Abnormal platelet function– thrombocytopathy.

1. THROMBOCYTOPENIA

Thrombocytopenia causes bleeding into the skin (petechiae, purpura and ecchymoses), mucous membranes (respiratory, gastrointestinal and urogenital tracts) and, most seriously, the CNS. Spontaneous bleeding does not occur, in the absence of infection, unless the platelet count falls below 20×10^9/l.

IDIOPATHIC THROMBOCYTOPENIC PURPURA (ITP)

Background

In this disorder, thrombocytopenia is caused by the production of anti-platelet antibodies. The cause is unknown although in some forms, especially in children, a viral aetiology is suspected.

The onset is usually acute with bleeding into the skin and mucous membranes. The most serious complication is intracerebral bleeding. Apart from bleeding manifestations, physical signs are absent. The presence of lymphadenopathy or splenomegaly should suggest an alternative cause.

In children, spontaneous recovery usually occurs within a few weeks. In adults, the disease usually pursues a chronic course.

Causes of Thrombocytopenia

1. Failure of platelet production

  (a) Congenital
  (b) B_{12}/folate deficiency
  (c) Marrow replacement, carcinoma, leukaemia, lymphoma, myeloma, myelofibrosis
  (d) Aplastic anaemia:
      Drugs, chemicals, irradiation

2. Excessive platelet destruction

  (a) Immune:
      Idiopathic thrombocytopenic purpura (ITP)
      Drug-induced
      AIHA (Evan's syndrome)
  (b) Consumption:
      Disseminated intravascular coagulation (DIC)
      Haemangioma
      Hypersplenism

Investigations

1. The platelet count is low but the blood count is otherwise normal.
2. The bone marrow shows an increased number of megakaryocytes with reduced ploidy and little evidence of cytoplasmic budding.
3. Anti-platelet antibodies may be demonstrated in most cases, but the technique is difficult and is not available routinely.
4. Screening tests for SLE should always be carried out because some cases of SLE present with immune thrombocytopenia.

Differential Diagnosis

The diagnosis of ITP is usually made by excluding other causes of immune thrombocytopenia. The conditions which have to be excluded are:
1. Drug-induced thrombocytopenia.
2. SLE.
3. Immune thrombocytopenia complicating lymphoma and CLL.

Basis of Treatment

Acute thrombocytopenia in children is usually self-limiting and unless bleeding is severe, with retinal haemorrhages, no treatment is required. The most effective treatment is corticosteroids. In immune thrombocytopenia, steroids increase the platelet count by depressing antibody formation. They also decrease capillary fragility and are, therefore, useful in the treatment of all forms of thrombocytopenia. These should be given in a high dose initially, i.e. prednisolone 60 mg daily, and should be reduced rapidly as soon as the platelet count rises. In chronic thrombocytopenia the dose of steroids should be titrated to maintain a platelet count above $30 \times 10^9/l$. At this level, serious bleeding is unlikely and if the platelet count can be maintained above this with 10 mg prednisolone daily, or less, no further treatment is necessary.

The second line of treatment is splenectomy but this should not be undertaken lightly because at least 20 per cent of the patients fail to respond. There is no easy way of predicting which patients will benefit by splenectomy, although failure to respond to steroids is an adverse feature.

Immunosuppressive drugs, for example azathioprine, have a small part to play in the treatment of ITP. In particular, they may enable a reduction in steroids, if an unacceptably high dose is needed to maintain the platelet count. Platelet transfusions are not very effective because the transfused platelets are rapidly destroyed by the same immune mechanism. Nevertheless, they should be given if there is severe bleeding or if splenectomy is contemplated. In fulminant cases, plasmaphoresis may be indicated.

DRUG INDUCED THROMBOCYTOPENIA

Drugs are an important cause of thrombocytopenia. There are two mechanisms of action:

(a) **Immune.** The drug usually acts as a hapten and is absorbed onto the platelet surface. Antibodies are formed against the drug and platelet complex. Examples of drugs acting in this way are the thiazide diuretics, methyldopa, quinine and quinadine.

(b) **Megakaryocyte Depression.** The action is on the stem cells in the bone marrow, with reduction in the number of megakaryocytes. Examples of such drugs are cytotoxic drugs, for example busulphan and methotrexate, chloramphenicol, chlorpropamide, the thiazides, gold and phenylbutazone.

Recovery is usually rapid in the former following discontinuation of the drug, but it may be prolonged or not occur at all in the latter.

2. THROMBOCYTOPATHY

These disorders present with similar clinical features to thrombocytopenia, but the platelet count is normal. They may be either *congenital* or *acquired*. The congenital disorders are rare, the commonest being *Glanzmann's disease (thrombasthaenia)*. In this condition the platelets fail to aggregate normally with ADP. Acquired causes include drugs (aspirin and the other non-steroid anti-inflammatory drugs), uraemia, macroglobulinaemia and

the myeloproliferative syndromes. Hess test and the bleeding time are usually abnormal and the diagnosis can be made by platelet function tests.

C. BLEEDING DUE TO COAGULATION DEFECTS

These are due to a deficiency in one or more of the factors needed for fibrin formation, or, more rarely, to the presence of inhibitors. They may be congenital or acquired.

Coagulation disorders

1. *Inherited factor deficiencies*

   VIII Haemophilia
   IX   Christmas disease
   VIII Related protein, von Willebrand's disease
   Other rare deficiencies
      I, II, V, VII, X, XI, XII, XIII

2. *Acquired factor deficiences*

   Prothrombin complex deficiency
      (II, VII, IX, X) vitamin K dependent factors
   Liver disease – prothrombin
      complex, +V and fibrinogen
   Intravascular coagulation syndrome
      (consumption coagulopathy; disseminated
      intravascular coagulation) – fibrinogen,
      II, V, VIII (+platelets)

3. *Inhibitors of blood coagulation*

   Factor VIII inhibitors –
      Haemophiliacs
      Pregnancy
      Collagen diseases
      Multiple factors – SLE

---

1. THE HAEMOPHILIAC SYNDROMES

HAEMOPHILIA

Definition

A genetically determined bleeding disorder manifest in males and caused by a deficiency of Factor VIII (AHG).

Background

The gene controlling the synthesis of the Factor VIII molecule is carried on the X chromosome. The haemophiliac gene causes the formation of a functionally abnormal molecule, although immunologically it is identical with normal Factor VIII. The abnormal Factor VIII molecule causes defective coagulation and therefore a bleeding tendency. The severity of this depends upon the level of Factor VIII (*see* Table 19.11).

Females with one abnormal X chromosome do not normally exhibit features of the disease (although they may have low Factor VIII and may bleed abnormally postoperatively), but they are carriers. The principles of the inheritance of haemophilia are shown in Fig. 19.22. The essential points to remember are:

1. *No child of a haemophiliac male, married to a normal*

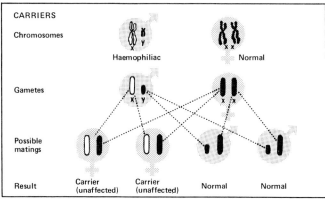

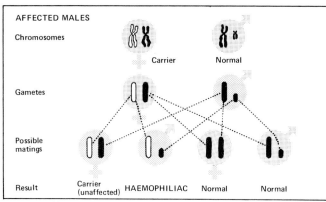

female will manifest the disease, but all his daughters will be carriers.

2. *If a female carrier marries a normal male, there is a 1:2 chance that her sons will be affected and that her daughters will be carriers.*

It is theoretically possible for a female to have haemophilia, if a female carrier marries a haemophiliac, but such a mating is exceedingly rare.

Haemophilia is a rare disease, the frequency being in the order of 1 per 10,000 of the male population.

Pathology

Haemophilia is characterised by bleeding into joints, muscles and soft tissues. Less often there is bleeding from the mucous membranes of the respiratory, renal and gastrointestinal tracts. Purpura *does not* occur. Bleeding into joints and tissues leads to destruction and deformity of the surrounding structures.

Symptoms and Signs (Fig. 19.23)

The principal manifestation of severe haemophilia is *spontaneous* bleeding into joints – usually the large weight-bearing joints – causing tender, painful swollen joints.

Bleeding may also occur into soft tissues, e.g. muscles. *Retroperitoneal haemorrhage* may mimic an acute abdomen.

Haematuria, gastrointestinal and occasionally intracerebral haemorrhage may occur.

Repeated haemarthroses can lead to *severe osteoarthritis.*

Haemorrhage into soft tissues may lead to compression of vital structures such as nerves (femoral nerve paralysis in ileo-psoas haemorrhage), arteries (ischaemia) and airways (asphyxia).

Mucous membrane haemorrhage may cause iron deficiency anaemia.

Severe bleeding may result from surgical operation or dental extraction.

All daughters of haemophiliacs are carriers. All sons are normal.

Haemophiliacs are the sons of a normal father & carrier mother. Female sibs. are normal or carriers.

Fig. 19.22   The inheritance of haemophilia.

Table 19.11   Relationship between Factor VIII level and bleeding

Condition	Factor VIII level	Bleeding tendency
Normal	50 to 200% (0.5–2.0 u/ml)	None
Carriers	25 to 100% (0.25–1.0 u/ml)	Usually none (may bleed postoperatively)
Haemophilia:		
Very mild	25 to 50% (0.25–0.5 u/ml)	Bleeding after major surgery
Mild	10 to 25% (0.1–0.25 u/ml)	Bleeding after minor surgery
Moderate	2 to 10% (0.02–0.1 u/ml)	Severe bleeding after minor injury Spontaneous haemarthroses
Severe	0 to 2% (0–0.2 u/ml)	Severe and frequent spontaneous bleeding and haemarthroses

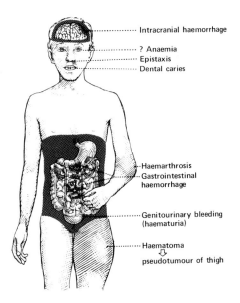

Fig. 19.23 Haemophilia and its complications.

Investigations

1. Of the coagulation screening tests (Fig. 19.20) only the APTT is abnormally prolonged.
2. The diagnosis is established by assaying the Factor VIII level. Factor VIII can be measured in two ways:
(a) *Coagulant activity.* This is invariably low in haemophilia.
(b) *Immunological activity* (Factor VIII related antigen). This is normal or high in haemophilia. This assay is useful in the diagnosis of von Willebrand's disease (*see below*) and in the detection of female carriers of haemophilia, who have low coagulant with high immunological activity.

Differential Diagnosis

Other congenital bleeding disorders, for example Christmas disease, resemble haemophilia but they may be distinguished by appropriate factor assays. The condition most likely to be confused with haemophilia is von Willebrand's disease (*see below*). Occasionally, in some conditions, for example SLE, pregnancy, malignancy, antibodies to Factor VIII may be produced causing a form of 'acquired haemophilia'.

Basis of Treatment

The essential principle of treatment is to arrest haemorrhage as quickly as possible by raising the Factor VIII to an appropriate level. Spontaneous haemarthroses are usually cured by raising the Factor VIII level to above 20 per cent (0.2 u/ml); for surgery it is necessary to maintain a level above 50 per cent (0.5 u/ml) until healing has occurred. Ileo-psoas and retroperitoneal haemorrhage may require treatment for several days. The amount of

Factor VIII concentrate to be given may be calculated from the formula.

Dose in units =

$$\frac{\text{Patient's weight (in kg)} \times \text{Required rise in Factor VIII}}{1.5}$$

Factor VIII has to be given intravenously. Sources are shown in Table 19.12. The half-life of Factor VIII is under twelve hours and therefore treatment twice daily is required.

For dental extractions the Factor VIII level should be raised preoperatively to 50 per cent and an antifibrinolytic drug, for example tranexamic acid 0.15 mg/kg should be given for up to seven days.

Table 19.12 Sources of Factor VIII for therapeutic use

Material	Average Factor VIII content (u/ml)	Comments
Fresh plasma	0.5 to 0.9	Factor VIII content varies. Large volume needed. Frequent reactions. Rarely used now. Must be stored at −20°C
Cryoprecipitate	3 to 5	Factor VIII content varies. Frequent reactions. Fairly large volume. Difficult to make up. Must be stored at −30°C
Freeze-dried human AHG	25 to 30	Factor VIII content known accurately. Small volume. Easily made up. Stored at 4°C. Reactions rare. Expensive. Hepatitis risk
Freeze-dried animal AHG	25 to 50	Very high potency. Allergic reactions frequent. Antibodies usually develop. May cause thrombocytopenia

The availability of Factor VIII concentrate has radically altered the management of haemophilia and many patients can now be treated at home, either by a relative or by themselves.

The management of the haemophiliac patient as a whole is of great importance. Attention should be paid to such matters as conservative dentistry, physiotherapy following joint bleeds, and the control of analgesics to prevent drug-dependence. Haemophiliacs should be encouraged to live as normal a life as possible, but they should avoid body-contact sport and other pursuits likely to lead to physical injury.

The family with a haemophiliac child require constant support and guidance and advice should be readily available on schooling, training for a job and also genetic counselling. For these reasons all haemophiliacs should be seen regularly and have their treatment supervised by a recognised Haemophilia Centre.

CHRISTMAS DISEASE

This is another sex-linked congenital disorder resembling haemophilia, but with deficiency of Factor IX. The clinical picture resembles haemophilia, although usually less severe. Its frequency is approximately one-seventh of that of haemophilia. There is a freeze-dried Factor IX concentrate available for replacement therapy and the principles of treatment are as for haemophilia.

VON WILLEBRAND'S DISEASE

Unlike haemophilia and Christmas disease this disorder is inherited as an autosomal dominant character and therefore affects both sexes. There is defective synthesis of the part of the Factor VIII molecule which carries the immunological determinants. This factor is needed for normal platelet function. As a consequence there is a low Factor VIII level and abnormal platelet function. The characteristic findings in this disease are low Factor VIII, clotting and immunological activity, a prolonged bleeding time, diminished platelet aggregation with the antibiotic ristocetin and defective platelet adhesiveness. It is now realised that this disease represents a spectrum and that not all patients demonstrate all the features. Furthermore, in an individual the abnormal findings may fluctuate and therefore repeated testing may be necessary to establish the diagnosis. The clinical picture is a mixture of a coagulation and platelet defect. The commonest mode of presentation is with epistaxis, menorrhagia, gastrointestinal bleeding or abnormal bleeding following surgery or dental extraction; haemarthrosis is uncommon.

Treatment is with cryoprecipitate or Factor VIII concentrate as for haemophilia, although usually a smaller dose is required.

2. DEFICIENCY OF VITAMIN K-DEPENDENT FACTORS (PROTHROMBIN COMPLEX DEFICIENCY)

Vitamin K is required for the intrahepatic synthesis of prothrombin (Factor II) as well as Factors VII, IX and X. Vitamin K being fat-soluble, requires bile salts for its absorption and, thus, when there is obstructive jaundice present, or in severe cases of liver cell disease, a deficiency of prothrombin complex may result. This possibility must always be borne in mind in the jaundiced patient when surgery is planned, and it is prevented by the administration of intramuscular vitamin K 10 mg daily. If a particularly rapid response is required it is achieved by giving water-soluble vitamin K by intravenous injection.

In an emergency, a more rapid response may be achieved with fresh frozen plasma or freeze-dried Factor IX concentrate, which contains Factors II, IX and X. The causes of vitamin K deficiency are shown in Fig. 19.24.

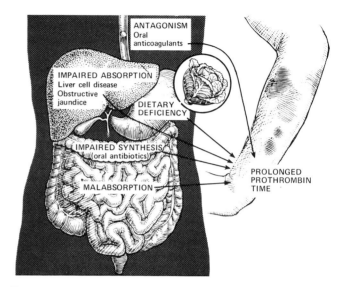

Fig. 19.24 Vitamin K and prothrombin metabolism and antagonism.

Oral anticoagulants, for example Warfarin, compete with vitamin K and depress the synthesis of Factors II, VII, IX and X. Attention is also drawn to the interactions between various drugs and oral anticoagulants which may render them more or less effective (*see also* page 217):

Chloral, phenylbutazone, clofibrate and Septrin increase the level of free anticoagulant drug by competing for plasma protein binding and thereby increase the sensitivity to the drug.
Aspirin has a complicated action; it increases the sensitivity to anticoagulants by reducing the synthesis of other coagulation factors and altering platelet function. Barbiturates cause increased metabolism of anticoagulants by induction of hepatic microsomal enzymes and thereby decrease sensitivity.

In prothrombin complex deficiency both the prothrombin time and the APTT are prolonged. The prothrombin time is particularly sensitive to deficiency of Factors II, VII and X and is used to monitor anticoagulant therapy. The introduction of a British Standard Thromboplastin has lead to standardisation of this test and the results are usually expressed as a ratio (the British Corrected Ratio or BCR). This is the ratio of the prothrombin time of the patient's plasma in seconds compared with a standard normal control plasma. *Example:*

$$\frac{\text{Patient's time} - 26 \text{ seconds}}{\text{Control} - 13 \text{ seconds}} \quad \text{BCR} = 2.00$$

For therapeutic purposes the BCR should be kept around 3.0. Serious bleeding does not usually occur until it rises above 5.0.

3. BLEEDING DUE TO LIVER DISEASE

Abnormal bleeding is common in patients with liver disease and the cause is often complex. As well as deficiency of vitamin K dependent factors, synthesis of Factor V and fibrinogen may also be impaired in severe liver disease. In addition, there is often thrombocytopenia and in some cases a degree of disseminated intravascular coagulation (DIC) may be present. Abnormalities of the fibrinolytic system may also contribute to abnormal bleeding.

4. THE INTRAVASCULAR COAGULATION SYNDROME

Background

Intravascular coagulation occurs in many conditions. The clinical picture and laboratory findings vary widely depending upon the cause, the extent and the speed of onset, and, as a consequence, a number of seemingly different syndromes exist. These have been described by a number of terms, for example disseminated intravascular coagulation (DIC), consumption coagulopathy and the defibrination syndrome. They all have in common the formation of fibrin within the vascular tree, the consumption of clotting factors (including platelets) to a variable degree, and the stimulation of fibrinolysis.

Factors which may trigger intravascular coagulation include:
(a) *The release of thromboplastin into the bloodstream*, e.g. obstetric accidents, carcinoma and leukaemia.
(b) *The activation of factor XII*, e.g. by contact with foreign surfaces, adrenaline, and complement components.
(c) *Platelet aggregation*. This can be induced by bacterial endotoxin, immune complexes, and contact with a foreign surface.
(d) *Endothelial damage*, as in malignant hypertension, renal disease, and acute hepatic necrosis, activates Factor XII and stimulates platelet aggregation. Exposure to foreign surfaces as in extra-corporeal circulation has a similar effect.

As a result of activation of the clotting mechanism fibrin formation occurs with consumption of some of the clotting factors, the principal ones involved being platelets, fibrinogen, prothrombin and Factors V and VIII. In chronic cases, increased synthesis of these factors may balance excessive consumption and their level may be normal or even raised. Intravascular coagulation activates the fibrinolytic system which causes dissolution of formed fibrin with the production of fibrin degradation products (FDPs). FDPs have an anticoagulant effect by inhibiting fibrin formation and this may potentiate the bleeding tendency. Fibrin formation in small vessels may lead to micro-thrombi and micro-infarcts and these may be responsible for the clinical picture. They may also be the cause of microangiopathic haemolytic anaemia (*see* page 390).

The causes of the intravascular coagulation syndrome are shown below:

The intravascular coagulation syndromes

Acute

1. Obstetric complications:
   Abruptio placentae
   Amniotic fluid embolism
   Eclampsia
   Retained products of dead fetus
   Septic abortion
2. Infections:
   Septicaemia – especially Gram-negative, meningococcal
   Malaria
3. Operations:
   Especially on the lungs and prostate
   Extra-corporeal circulation
4. Trauma and burns
5. Shock
6. Snake bites – e.g. vipers
7. Incompatible blood transfusion

Chronic

1. Neoplasms, e.g. carcinoma of lung, stomach, colon
2. Leukaemia, especially acute promyelocytic
3. Thrombotic thrombocytopenic purpura (TTP)
4. Haemolytic-uraemic syndrome
5. Giant haemangioma
6. Miscellaneous causes – e.g. collagen disease, amyloid, allergic vasculitis

---

The acute causes usually result in depletion of the clotting factors with, consequently, a severe bleeding tendency. In the *obstetric complications*, coagulation is due to the release of thromboplastin into the circulation. In *septicaemia*, endotoxin activates Factor XII and platelet aggregation. *Shock* is an important cause of DIC and it may potentiate other causes such as the obstetric complications and incompatible blood transfusion. The factors responsible are acidosis and adrenaline release.

In the chronic syndrome, consumption of clotting factors is often compensated by increased synthesis. Bleeding manifestations are not always present; the commonest being due to thrombocytopenia. The clinical picture is often due to micro infarcts and microangiopathic haemolytic anaemia (*see* page 420). In *carcinoma* intravascular coagulation results from the release of thromboplastin from the malignant cells and also from vascular change in the tumour circulation. In *promyelocytic leukaemia*, severe bleeding may occur shortly after treatment is started due to the liberation of thromboplastins from destroyed promyelocytes. Chronic DIC may persist for years in patients with *giant haemangiomas*. Vascular change in the abnormal circulation is the cause.

Investigations

1. **Clotting Tests.** The laboratory findings depend on the cause. In the acute syndromes the blood may fail to clot in the test tube. Depletion of fibrinogen, prothrombin and Factor V and VIII leads to prolongation of the TCT, PT and APTT (see Fig. 19.20). If a clot is formed it is usually wispy and may dissolve on standing due to excessive fibrinolysis. A fibrinogen assay is useful in assessing the degree of hypofibrinogenaemia. Fibrin degradation products (FDPs) are raised.

In chronic cases the clotting tests may be normal or even shortened due to circulating activated clotting factors. FDPs are usually raised and radioactive fibrinogen studies show increased fibrinogen turnover.

2. **Blood Count.** In most cases the platelet count is reduced. Anaemia may be due to bleeding or microangiopathic haemolytic anaemia. In the latter case, fragmented cells and other evidence of haemolysis will be present.

Basis of Treatment

Treatment of intravascular coagulation is unsatisfactory. The main object should be to remove or treat the cause if possible. Thus, in septicaemia treatment of the infection and reversal of shock is of prime importance. If bleeding is severe, replacement therapy is needed. Thrombocytopenia requires platelet transfusion. Multiple factor deficiency is treated with fresh frozen plasma. Fibrinogen may be needed in severe hypofibrinogenaemia.

The role of heparin to block the coagulation system and prevent fibrin formation is still debatable. It probably has no part to play in the acute syndromes, particularly if severe thrombocytopenia is present. It may be useful in some of the chronic syndromes. Likewise, the value of anti-platelet drugs such as dipyridamole or aspirin is unproved. The use of these drugs is worth considering, because they may be of some value and they are considerably less dangerous than heparin.

There is no place for antifibrinolytic drugs, for example EACA (*see below*). These may encourage generalised fibrin deposition giving rise to the Schwarzmann type reaction.

Prognosis

This is variable depending on the primary cause and whether it can be removed. Thrombotic thrombocytopenic purpura has a high mortality.

D. BLEEDING DISORDERS DUE TO EXCESSIVE FIBRINOLYSIS

Primary fibrinolytic disorders are very rare. Usually excessive fibrinolysis is secondary to intravascular coagulation. Primary fibrinolysis may occur in some neoplasms, especially prostatic carcinoma, during some operations, for example on the prostate and lung and in severe hepatic necrosis.

Excessive fibrinolysis may be blocked by antifibrinolytic drugs, for example epsilon-amino-caproic acid (EACA) or tranexamic acid. These should be used with care because of the danger of precipitating extensive intravascular thrombosis, but they do have a part to play in the management of postoperative bleeding following prostatectomy and in dental extractions in haemophilia.

DISORDERS OF PIGMENT METABOLISM

A. METHAEMOGLOBINAEMIA

Methaemoglobin is derived from haemoglobin by oxidation of the ferrous atom in haem to the ferric form. Methaemoglobin does not transport oxygen normally and as a consequence cyanosis occurs when it is present in amounts exceeding 1.5 g/dl. Large amounts of methaemoglobin cause symptoms of tissue hypoxia, i.e. those of anaemia, and may result in secondary polycythaemia. Small amounts of methaemoglobin are formed continuously in the normal red cell and its accumulation is prevented by enzymatic reducing systems including methaemoglobin reductase and the glutathione system. Methaemoglobin can be identified spectroscopically by the presence of an absorption band in the red part of the spectrum at 632 nm.

Causes of methaemoglobinaemia are:

1. **Drugs and Chemicals.** Oxidant compounds may overcome the normal reduction mechanisms and form methaemoglobin. This is especially so in enzyme deficiencies affecting the pentose-phosphate pathway (e.g. G6PD deficiency *see* page 386) in which there is failure to detoxicate oxidants. Drugs particularly likely to cause methaemoglobinaemia include nitrites, phenacetin, sulphonamides and the sulphones (Dapsone). The aromatic amines, for example nitrobenzene and nitrotoluene, are important industrial hazards causing methaemoglobinaemia.

2. **Haemoglobin Abnormalities.** Congenital abnormalities of haemoglobin involving amino acid substitution around the haem pocket can lead to excessive methaemoglobin formation. Examples are the haemoglobins M and the unstable haemoglobins, for example Hb Köln.

3. **Congenital Enzyme Deficiencies.** Congenital deficiency of methaemoglobin reductase is a rare cause of methaemoglobinaemia. Methaemoglobin levels may reach 50 per cent. Symptoms are rare below 25 per cent. Above this exertional dyspnoea and headaches occur. Treatment is required if the condition is symptomatic. Oxidant drugs should be avoided. Reduction of methaemoglobin can be achieved by ascorbic acid 500 mg daily. Methylene blue, which acts by stimulating the PPP, can also be used (1 mg/kg).

SULPHAEMOGLOBINAEMIA

Sulphaemoglobin is a further oxidation product of haemoglobin and its formation is irreversible. It frequently coexists with methaemoglobin and with denatured globin, i.e. Heinz bodies. The usual cause is oxidant compounds and it does not occur in the congenital forms of methaemoglobinaemia. It is probable that gut bacteria provide the source of sulphur from the breakdown of sulphur-containing compounds and the release of H_2S. It is identifiable spectroscopically. Small amounts, i.e. more than 0.5 g/dl cause cyanosis. There is no treatment apart from the removal of the cause.

B. PORPHYRIA

Porphyrin Metabolism

Porphyrins are tetrapyrolles, i.e. compounds containing 4 pyrolle rings. The pyrolle ring is, in turn, formed by the condensation of 2 molecules of delta aminolaevulinic acid (δ ALA). δ ALA is, in turn, formed from glycine and succinate, the latter in the form of succinyl CoA. An important enzyme δ ALA synthetase regulates the speed of this reaction. The monopyrolle, which is the structural unit, is porphobilinogen, and condensation of four of these units forms a porphyrin. Porphyrins are either Type I (symmetrical structure) or Type III (asymmetrical structure) while they can also be divided into copro- and uroporphyrins depending on the side chains, i.e. uroporphyrin (side chains, proprionyl and acetyl) or coproporphyrins (side chains proprionyl and vinyl). Protoporphyrin has a structure intermediate between uro- and coproporphyrin with side chains containing methyl, vinyl and proprionyl groups. It should be noted that uro- and coproporphyrins are found, despite their names, in both urine and faeces.

Types of porphyria are as follows:

ERYTHROPOIETIC PORPHYRIA

Congenital

This rare inborn error of metabolism is associated with increased production of Type I (symmetrical) uro- and coproporphyrins. There is severe photosensitivity with vesiculation and scarring of exposed areas – pink discolouration and fluorescence of teeth and bones and episodes of haemolytic anaemia. Red cells also fluoresce.

Erythropoietic Protoporphyria

This is probably the commonest type of porphyria. There is mild photosensitivity, hepatic cirrhosis, a tendency for early gall stone formation and a tendency also to death from liver failure. Though the defect is in bone marrow haem production, the protoporphyrin accumulates in the liver where it seems to be hepatotoxic. Urinary porphyrin excretion is normal.

HEPATIC PORPHYRIAS

Acute Intermittent Porphyria

This inherited disorder seems to be due to excessive activity of δ ALA synthetase with resultant increased hepatic production of porphyrins mainly of Type III. There is no photosensitivity, but the other clinical features include acute attacks of *abdominal pain* due to intestinal spasm, *paralysis* due to muscle denervation or peripheral neuritis, *psychiatric episodes and epilepsy*, which together with *tachycardia and hypertension*, produce a bizarre and often confusing clinical picture. A variety of drugs may precipitate acute bouts, the reason for this being the induction by them of more δ ALA synthetase in the liver (enzyme induction). Dangerous drugs therefore include alcohol, barbiturates and sulphonamides, while safe sedatives for this painful and distressing condition include morphine and chlorpromazine. Recent studies have confirmed that the basic abnormality in acute intermittent porphyria seems to be one of profound neurological dysfunction, while certain evidence, for example hyponatraemia, suggests central, i.e. hypothalamic dysfunction too.

There is no effective therapy, but avoidance of dangerous drugs is important, and skilled nursing, including treatment of respiratory failure may be needed. Corticosteroids have been used and because of evidence to suggest overactivity of the sympathetic nervous system, propranolol or other beta adrenergic blockers may help.

Porphyria Cutanea Tarda

This occurs in middle-aged and elderly patients with liver disease, often alcoholic in origin. Patients present with a picture of mild light sensitivity with a blistering eruption on exposed surfaces, and pigmentation. Porphyrins of Type I and III are excreted.

Care must be taken to avoid precipitant drugs of which oestrogens (given for carcinoma of prostate, etc.)

are important. Some degree of hepatic iron overload exists in those patients with alcoholic liver disease. Following venesection therapy there may be a worthwhile improvement in symptoms due to the porphyria.

Varigate Porphyria

This type of porphyria is recorded mainly from South Africa and its origins can be traced to the early Boer settlers. As its name implies, the clinical features are mixed, both acute type symptoms (abdominal pain, etc.) and skin photosensitivity are seen.

Investigations. Patients with *acute intermittent porphyria* and *porphyria cutanea tarda* excrete porphobilinogen in the urine. This is detected by mixing Erhlich's aldehyde reagent 1.0 ml with a similar volume of urine. A pink or red colour can be due to excess porphobilinogen or urobilinogen. Differentiation is made by adding a little chloroform. Urobilinogen (but not porphobilinogen) enters and gives a pink colour to the chloroform (lower) layer, while porphobilinogen remains in the aqueous phase. Patients with congenital porphyria do not excrete porphobilinogen in their urine and formal examination of the urine for porphyrins is required in this condition. It is, of course, helpful also in categorising those forms where there is porphobilinogen.

SUGGESTED FURTHER READING

Three comprehensive textbooks on haematology which cover all the subjects dealt with in this chapter and contain abundant references are:

de Gruchy (Penington *et al.*, eds.) (1978) *Clinical Haematology in Medical Practice*, 4th ed. Oxford: Blackwell Scientific Publications.

Hardisty, R. M. and Weatherall, D. J. (eds.) (1974) *Blood and Its Disorders*. Oxford: Blackwell Scientific Publications.

Williams, W. J. *et al.* (eds.) (1977) *Hematology*, 2nd ed. New York: McGraw-Hill Inc.

An important work providing up-to-date reviews of almost all aspects of clinical haematology, especially the oncological ones, is:

Hoffbrand, A. V. *et al.* (eds.) (1977) *Recent Advances in Haematology*. 2. London: Churchill Livingstone.

An invaluable series, which over the past few years has reviewed all the major topics in haematology is:

Clinics in Haematology. W. B. Saunders Co. Ltd.

This series is published three times each year and reference should be made to the complete list for relevant subjects.

The following books deal with special topics and are useful for references.

Biggs, R. (ed.) (1978) *The Treatment of Haemophilia A and B and von Willebrand's Disease*. Oxford: Blackwell Scientific Publications.

Girdwood, R. H. (ed.) (1974) *Blood Disorders Due to Drugs and Other Agents*. Excepta Medica.

Lehmann, H. and Huntsman, R. G. (1974) *Man's Haemoglobins*. North-Holland Publishing Company.

Mental Health

H. G. MORGAN

20

A. THE NATURE, HISTORY AND SCOPE OF PSYCHIATRY

Psychiatry is that branch of medicine concerned with abnormal states of mind and the resulting disorders of individual and group behaviour. Throughout the ages, society's attitude towards mental illness has been characterised by cruel repression and segregation, due to underlying fear and ignorance. In the Middle Ages, mentally ill persons were often burnt at the stake and their disturbed behaviour attributed to demoniacal possession. Even as late as the eighteenth century the mentally ill were chained, beaten, publicly exhibited, and unashamedly ridiculed by the public. Little distinction was made between paupers, criminals and so-called lunatics. The social ferment at the time of the French Revolution was accompanied by a humane and liberalising attitude towards mental illness, and men such as Esquirol, Pinel and Tuke unlocked doors of mental institutions and removed the inmates' chains. In the nineteenth century there was a return to an attitude of segregation, and large mental institutions were built throughout the country, each often at considerable distance from the homes of its patients. Today, the emphasis is on treatment of the mentally ill in the community, wherever possible, since it has become recognised that prolonged hospital stay, particularly when the institution is large, impersonal, and authoritarian, can in itself have many harmful effects on any individual, especially one who is mentally ill.

Like every rapidly developing field, psychiatry tends to have ill-defined boundaries. For example, it is often difficult to determine the demarcation between normal variation in behaviour and that due to mental illness, or to assess the precise role of psychological causes in the realm of somatic illnesses: in the field of antisocial behaviour and criminality, the distinction between 'badness' and 'madness' is often ambiguous and arbitrary. It is particularly important that in these areas the psychiatrist should not overstate his case by expounding unproved psychological explanations with deceptive facility. He should resolve the present ambiguities regarding his role and responsibilities in society by stating in simple and clear language the extent and limits of his skills.

B. APPROACHES TO CLINICAL PSYCHIATRY

Psychiatry is still to a considerable extent at the descriptive stage. Relatively little is known about the aetiology of mental illness, except to be sure that it is usually complex and multifactorial. The subject abounds with a plethora of theoretical approaches: it is important that the student should not regard them as mutually exclusive and so automatically side with one to the exclusion of all others. Although the basic clinical phenomena of mental illness can be elicited and described reliably, it must be recognised that the clinical syndromes in psychiatry are crude and ill-defined, not to be regarded in the same light as the more specific disease entities of general medicine. The student must satisfy himself from the outset that he can define all new concepts and terms before using them. Only in this way will he avoid ill-understood jargon, which merely confuses both himself and those with whom he tries to communicate. He must learn to depend on reliable descriptive clinical terms, and eschew those that imply mechanisms or value judgements; terms such as 'immature' or 'inadequate' are dangerous, and certainly have no place in first stage clinical assessment. The student's training may have led him to mistrust diagnoses made in the absence of physical signs and pathological correlates, and he may prematurely reject the study of human behaviour based on psychological and sociological norms. He may also find it difficult to move away to some extent from the traditional directive medical approach, but it is important that he does so if he is to be effective in treating mental illness. Further, he will find that to discuss emotional difficulties can be upsetting and embarrassing to any untrained individual, who tends to identify with his patients' problem and finds it hard to remain objective about them: as a result he may avoid discussing these topics altogether, or he may make the common mistake of adopting unrealistic and overambitious therapeutic aims.

Proper assessment and treatment of mental illness must be based on a thorough knowledge of normal and morbid anatomy and physiology, psychology, and sociology. Without understanding structure and function, it is impossible to distinguish organic from psychologically determined symptoms or to evaluate and utilise somatic treatment with safety. Knowledge of normal psychological processes, especially their variability from person to person, provides a baseline against which development of mental disturbance in an individual must be compared before its full significance can be assessed.

The student must also learn to see mental illness in a wider context than that of intra-individual disturbance, and he must evaluate each case in terms of the patient's relation to others. Disorders of interpersonal relationships may not only be the main cause of certain mental illnesses but frequently follow them closely as secondary complications. Some treatments in psychiatry are carried out in a group setting, and arise out of recognition of the fact that the powerful interpersonal forces existing in such situations can, for certain types of mental illness, be more therapeutic than the conventional one-to-one doctor–patient interview. Psychiatry, therefore, concerns itself with abnormality both within an individual and outside him in terms of his relationship with others, and his reaction to life events and social conditions.

C. CLINICAL ASSESSMENT IN PSYCHIATRY

THE CLINICAL HISTORY

The interview is of crucial importance in psychiatry, and its techniques must be fully understood if it is to yield accurate and reliable information. Common sources of error, apart from a hurried, careless approach on the part of the doctor or bias in his assessment arising from his own prejudices, include distortions or resistance in provision of information by the patient, particularly concerning embarrassing or painful topics. The doctor must learn to put the patient at ease and it may take several interviews before the patient can talk freely. For example, many persons feel guilty at discussing their marriage because they feel they are letting the other partner down by doing so. Reassurance on this point may pave the way to open discussion. One of the most important yet difficult topics is suicidal intent, about which the doctor must always satisfy himself. To do so, he must take care to introduce the subject at an appropriate time in the interview, and not by a blunt confrontation such as, 'Do you want to kill yourself?', which may well produce a denial. A more appropriate sequence would be: 'You have obviously felt very unwell, have you ever had desperate thoughts during this time?' 'Have you ever wondered about the future and

whether you could face it?' 'Have you ever felt so desperate that you have seriously thought of ending your life?'

The following sequence of enquiry is recommended as the most convenient to follow in history taking. More important than the precise sequence is a systematic method. Errors in clinical medicine may accrue from haphazard method as well as through ignorance on the part of the doctor.

Presenting Complaints

It is important to record these in the patient's own words, and to find out what he means by them. It is well known throughout the whole of medicine that words used to describe symptoms may convey entirely different meaning to the patient on the one hand, and the doctor on the other. This is particularly important in psychiatry. Terms such as 'tension', 'anxiety', 'depression' can be so non-specific that unless the doctor takes care to clarify what the patient means, they may in fact be talking completely at cross purposes.

At the outset, it is wise to find out why the person has come for help. In this way, the motivation of the patient may be assessed: he who is pushed or coerced by others may be a poor prospect for successful therapy.

History of the Present Illness

First of all the illness itself is assessed, including the type of symptoms, their duration, mode of onset (sudden or gradual) and their progression with time (deteriorating, static, or improved). Attention is then turned to the life situation leading up to and during the present illness. While interaction between life events and mental upset is usually close, it is important to remember that a temporal association between events and illness does not necessarily mean that a causal relationship exists between them. The fallacy of the post hoc ergo propter hoc argument (i.e. arguing that because B followed A, then A must have caused B) must always be kept in mind in assessing causes of mental disturbance. Many hypotheses regarding the aetiology of mental illness invoke mechanisms in which there is considerable lapse of time, sometimes many years, between supposed precipitant and onset of illness. Such theories should always be subjected to the most critical assessment before being accepted. In formulating causal connections between life events and mental illness it must be remembered that the illness may itself condition the way in which the patient sees the situation, and his explanations should not be accepted uncritically. Thus, a depressed patient with excessive self-blame may regard his inadequacies at work as the cause of his illness; he may even want to resign his job, only to regret this when he recovers.

Family History

Families of patients with mental illness frequently show a greater incidence of psychiatric disorder than does the general population. This may reflect genetic aetiological factors, but could also be due to the pathogenic effects of early family environment or, possibly, a combination of these mechanisms. When genetic factors predominate, it may be possible to detect Mendelian patterns of disease incidence in the family. For example, Huntington's chorea is transmitted via a Mendelian dominant hereditary mechanism, and it is possible to predict morbid expectancy rates in sibs and children of an affected person. In most mental illnesses, however, the relative importance of genetic versus environmental causes is still far from clear, and it is not easy to distinguish the two. The following information is required in a full family history: the family structure, the incidence and type of psychiatric disturbance in its members, deaths and separation from the patient, especially in childhood, the general home atmosphere, economic status, and the patient's relationship with relatives.

Personal History

Under this heading are recorded facts pertaining to early experience and development, marital, and socio-economic situation.

Illnesses. The development of mental illness or handicap later in life may stem from early life events, for example:

In utero: infection (rubella in first three months, syphilis), rhesus incompatibility.

At birth: brain injury, severe prematurity.

During infancy: infection (meningitis) trauma (head injury).

It is probable that relatively minor traumatic or anoxic brain injury at birth, for example due to toxaemia or antepartum haemorrhage, may play a role in the later development of a variety of neuropsychiatric complications such as behaviour disorders, as well as obvious organic mental impairment in severe cases.

Pattern of Development:

Intellectual. The earliest evidence of mental handicap is delay in reaching milestones in development (age at walking, talking). Less severe impairment may not become obvious until there is consistently poor academic performance at school.

Emotional. It is now increasingly recognised that many items of deviant childhood behaviour such as thumb-sucking and nail-biting are not necessarily indicators of emotional disturbance, and in the past their pathological significance has been over-emphasised. In assessing deviant behaviour it is important to take into account the age of the child (age appropriateness) and the effects on the child's development. Even at ten to twelve years, thumb-sucking has little association with psychiatric pathology. Persistent antisocial behaviour in childhood does tend to herald poor adult adjustment, but otherwise, almost any kind of behaviour can occur at some time in normal childhood development and care should be exercised before pathological significance is assumed.

Social. The normal child usually builds up friendships easily, although a certain degree of shyness or unwillingness to separate from the mother is common at certain stages in development. Severe impairment in relating to others is seen in extreme form as autistic withdrawal in childhood psychosis. Social difficulties may not fully declare themselves until the child leaves school and begins work, when he has to embark on a more independent life.

Psychosexual. Sexual maturation tends to need more adjustment in girls than boys. Menarche usually begins between 13 to 15 years and in most instances it is not accompanied by any emotional disturbance, especially when the child has been well prepared by discussion with parents or teachers. Puberty in the male is probably less often accompanied by emotional upset. Once puberty is passed the future sexual orientation is established. A transient phase of homosexual interest is common in adolescence and is not of any pathological significance, but persistence of deviant sexual interests beyond 18 years suggests that they may represent more enduring traits of personality.

Marital History. Enormous variation in normal marital behaviour occurs even within single cultural or social groups. For example, a certain degree of aggressive behaviour in the marriage, particularly on the part of the husband, may be regarded as compatible with a viable relationship in some groups, yet would be taken as immediate grounds for divorce in others. An objective assessment of a marital situation can be obtained only by interviewing both man and wife. Sexual drive and interest may differ in the two partners, and this may be a major source of disharmony. A marriage undergoes a series of stresses as it progresses. For example, birth of children (leading to loss of mother's working role outside the home), departure of children to school at five years, or later to college, or on marriage (leaving mother alone at home) are examples of events that may precipitate emotional upset in the vulnerable parent.

Work Record. Apart from indicating the socio-economic status of himself and his family, a patient's occupational history may provide a useful empirical index of his personal attributes: for example intellectual potential (type of work and success in it), persistence and drive (employment record, spells off work and changes of jobs), ability to get on with others (type of work, ability to work with or command others).

A progressive fall off in potential and academic promise, for example in a student who has a brilliant school record yet fails to continue his studies or to find satisfactory employment, may signify incipient mental illness.

Previous Illnesses. These, both physical and psychiatric, must be fully documented: the interrelation between the two is often close. A psychosomatic illness such as asthma presents in a somatic form, but may largely be psychologically determined. Psychiatric syndromes, when repetitive, tend to follow the same stereotype in any individual: thus, an illness is likely to be depressive in nature if the patient has suffered several depressions before. The precise character of previous mental illness in the patient helps both to clarify the diagnosis in later illnesses, and may even help in making prognostic predictions. For example a succession of schizophrenic illnesses is less compatible with eventual complete recovery than if there has been a similar pattern of depressive breakdowns.

Previous Personality

Figure 20.1 shows the ways in which knowledge of premorbid personality can assist in the assessment of a mental illness. The degree to which the patient has become different from his normal self can be determined, and provided the time of onset of symptoms is known, the rate of development of the illness then becomes clear. This may be relatively sudden, out of a good premorbid personality (A) or gradual in the context of long-standing psychological difficulties (B, C) when the illness may not be very different from his 'normal self'. This distinction is of practical importance, because prognosis in general tends to be better in those cases with good premorbid personality, especially when the illness is of sudden onset and an adequate environmental precipitant can be found. Knowledge of premorbid personality may also help us to understand why any individual has become ill in the circumstances prevailing at the time, especially when his symptoms constitute an accentuation of life-long psychological difficulties. Finally, knowledge of personality helps in the formulation of realistic aims in treatment.

The final outcome is to a considerable extent a function of previous personality. Patient A, it is hoped, will recover with outcome 1. Patients B and C are more likely to have outcomes 2, 3 or even 4, with varying residual difficulties, although the amount of personal support available and the degree to which life difficulties are resolved are also important in deciding the exact outcome. Care should be observed in applying these principles in younger patients (those less than 20 or even 25 years of age) because here psychological development is probably still taking place and an enduring personality pattern has still to be established.

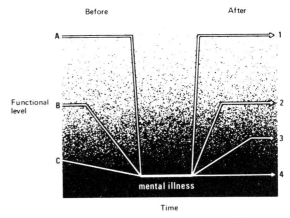

Fig. 20.1 Premorbid personality and mental illness.

Knowledge of the patient's previous (premorbid) personality, that is the sum total of his life-long psychological adjustment in life, provides the baseline without which adequate assessment of any mental illness is impossible. Previous personality is the equivalent of the physical norms of general medicine. It differs from them in that it is entirely a psychological assessment, and is subject to enormous variation even in the normal. In evaluating previous personality, it is crucial to obtain information not only from the patient but also from his friends and relatives, having first, of course, obtained his permission to do so. Certain personality types can be distinguished in the normal population, each having a characteristic constellation of traits, although in detail every individual is unique. The following headings are used in personality assessment:

Conation (drive, initiative, ambition, energy). At one extreme, rigidity of habit is most developed in the obsessional personality who gets anxious and irritable unless his life is conducted according to a fixed meticulously tidy routine. At the other is the happy-go-lucky individual who is the epitome of disorganisation yet still seems to get through life without any significant loss of efficiency.

Emotional. In a well-adjusted individual, the mood is stable, and in spite of life difficulties it does not show gross persistent deviations. The cyclothymic individual shows regular mood swings from one to the other. Some persons lack emotional warmth in relating to others: this is most obvious in the *schizoid personality*, who appears cold and lacks *rapport*. This contrasts with the *histrionic personality*, who is quick to express enthusiasm and displeasure, enjoys attention or being the centre of attraction, and in general tends to overreact emotionally. Anxiety is a universal experience, and there is considerable individual variation in the extent to which it is manifest in day-to-day behaviour. It is characterised by subjective apprehension, a sense of foreboding, with somatic equivalents of tension, restlessness, and, in extreme cases, tremor and tachycardia. Anxiety may in any individual be situationally specific or may be generalised over a wide variety of circumstances.

Social. The ability to make and keep friends is an important attribute of personality. Social isolation is a well-known predisposing factor in mental illness and suicidal behaviour. It is necessary to enquire about the number of social contacts both with family and friends, and whether the relationships are close or superficial. Recreational habits also provide useful insight into personality. Enquiry is also made about both alcohol and drug intake, remembering that the account given may be grossly distorted when the patient is abnormally dependent on them. An individual may be socially isolated either because he is too shy and anxious in company, or he may feel little need for social contact. He may then present the picture of a schizoid personality, seclusive, isolated, often with eccentric habits. This contrasts with the gregarious individual who seems most happy when he is actively involved in organising and attending social functions.

Cognitive. In assessing intellectual capacity, care should be taken in interpreting educational record. Poor reading or vocabulary may merely reflect inadequate schooling (poor quality or attendance) or lack of stimulus in the home. Type of work may provide a crude index of intellect potential, assuming of course that opportunity for advancement was adequate in the first place. On the other hand, high intelligence in itself is no guarantee to success in life, which depends also on sound personality structure, especially the attributes of persistence and ease of social communication.

THE MENTAL STATE

Assessment of the mental state should be carried out systematically under well-defined headings. Unless done in this way, mental processes will be incompletely elicited and a biased assessment will result. The following headings are the most convenient:

General Behaviour

Disturbances in mental state are closely mirrored in general behaviour, which should be noted in detail.

Activity may be increased. For example, the anxious patient is restless and tense, or the hypomanic patient may show extreme physical overactivity, be unable to rest, consistently embarking on fresh errands and activities. At the other extreme the general level of activity may be diminished: the retardation of depression is manifest as apathy, loss of interest, and slowness of movement. Apparent absence of responsiveness to the environment without loss of consciousness constitutes a state of stupor: it may complicate depression or catatonic schizophrenia.

The Patient's Attitude to Those Around Him may vary from genial helpful co-operation, to hostility, suspiciousness, and reticence. This last is seen in certain paranoid illnesses, and during clinical assessment it is then necessary to anticipate guarded replies and concealment of information. Hostility may occasionally erupt into aggression and violence, perhaps unexpectedly. The mute, catatonic schizophrenic patient may sometimes assault a by-stander, especially he who talks indiscreetly in front of the patient whom he thinks is inaccessible. Assessment of general behaviour should not be based entirely on the doctor–patient interview. Evidence from others, for example nursing staff or relatives, enables discrepancies to be detected in behaviour from one situation to another. For example, a patient may appear sad and apathetic when seeing the doctor, yet at other times he may be reported to be the life and soul of all social activity. Such inconsistency in behaviour would make it necessary to hesitate before diagnosing a depressive illness.

Abnormal Movements may vary from fine tremor, fidgeting, restlessness in anxiety, to the more bizarre features to be found in chronic schizophrenic patients: *mannerisms* are odd, stilted but otherwise normal movements, *stereotypies* are repetitive, pointless movements, e.g. grimacing for no apparent reason. *Catatonic disorders of movement* are most commonly associated with catatonic schizophrenia. The patient may appear completely mute or show violent aggressive overactivity. Negativism is shown when he does the opposite to what is requested, and ambivalence is said to occur when there is gross hesitancy and indecision. Flexibilitas cerea (waxy flexibility) may also be seen as a tendency to remain spontaneously in one statue-like posture for long periods, or to maintain a fixed posture into which he is placed by the examiner.

Speech

Here it is useful to distinguish between form and content. The content refers to topics about which the patient talks: thus, a depressed patient tends to be preoccupied with self-blame and a pessimistic outlook, the anxious patient is apprehensive about day-to-day events, or the paranoid patient is concerned with the imagined hostile attitude of others towards him. The form of speech refers to its structure, i.e. its quality, rate and cohesion. In hypomania there may be pressure of talk, in which rate of speech and change of topic are both increased. Mutism, or complete absence of speech may complicate any psychotic illness, particularly catatonic schizophrenia or depressive psychosis, and it may be accompanied by stupor, a state of marked reduction in general activity, without loss of consciousness. Mutism is also sometimes seen as a hysterical reaction to stress: this is hard to distinguish from malingering, which is a deliberate conscious pretence on the part of the patient. Between these extremes, slowing of speech with reduction in its quantity may be seen in the depressed patient, who is then said to show retardation with poverty of ideation.

Normal speech follows a logical, understandable sequence of ideas. This may be disturbed in a variety of ways. Flight of ideas, seen in hypomania, consists of pressure of talk which tends to flit in content rapidly from one topic to another because of the patient's distractibility by the environment. Although disjointed, it is usually possible to understand the sequence in terms of distractibility. For example, as a patient is discussing his illness, an aeroplane flies overhead and he switches to discussion of his last air trip to America, and how he enjoys cowboy films: a nurse comes into the room and he then talks about how pretty she is, perhaps flirting with her, and he goes on to describe his own daughter's nursing ambitions. In the hypomanic patient this sequence would occur at a rapid rate accompanied by marked jocularity. The disturbance of schizophrenic thought disorder is more subtle. It also takes the patient off the point but it is difficult to pin-point the logical discontinuities. The observer reacts by redoubling his own concentration but still fails to understand how the topic changes. This phenomenon has been called the 'knight's move', and reflects a disturbance in associative thinking in schizophrenia. In extreme form, utterances are reduced to gibberish, often containing new words (neologisms) manufactured by the patient. This is to be distinguished from dysphasia (in which the patient has difficulty in remembering words), to be found only in organic brain disorders. Routine assessment of speech should include writing down samples of the patient's talk verbatim: this is the most accurate way of illustrating the abnormalities involved.

Mood

Under this heading is included the emotional status of the individual as opposed to his thinking processes, although, of course, a close inter-relationship exists between the two. Although it is conventional to describe emotional (affective) status under certain headings, it must be emphasised that these are artificial entities which do little more than highlight the most obvious mood characteristics. They fall far short of describing the many subtle variations in mood state that may occur, these often changing rapidly, one merging into another.

Anxiety has been experienced by most persons: it may become severe in a wide variety of psychiatric disorders. It has both subjective and objective manifestations. The former comprise feelings of tension, foreboding, and worry. Apprehension may be related to certain life events, or it may bear little obvious relationship to environmental factors. Objectively, there is restlessness with inability to relax and sit quitely, and there may be signs of sympathetic overactivity with sweaty palms and palpitations. When severe anxiety becomes centred around specific situations, it is called phobic anxiety. This may be related to highly specific situations such as handling insects, or may be less circumscribed, for example related to being in open spaces or crowds (agoraphobia) or closed spaces (claustrophobia). Anxiety may also cause loss of appetite leading to significant weight loss.

Overt Depression of Mood is an important clinical feature to be found in a wide variety of mental illnesses. The patient looks miserable and unhappy. While in some cases he can brighten up from time to time, in severe depression there is no break in his gloom. Tearfulness may be obvious, although (particularly in males) this may not be mentioned by the patient unless he is directly asked about it. Diurnal variation of mood, where depression is worse in the mornings, is also a common feature in depressive illness, which may also be accompanied·by either reduced physical activity, as in depressive psychomotor retardation, or agitation when anxiety accompanies the depressed state.

Elation (elevation of mood above the normal) is, of course, the opposite to depression. Typically, it occurs in hypomania or following abuse of stimulants such as amphetamines or methedrine, when it is seen as a state of sustained abnormal good humour and hilarity which soon becomes tiresome to all except the patient, and generally accompanied by marked physical overactivity.

The degree of frankness in the patient is closely related to his mood. The suspicious patient will say very little, the paranoid patient may even question the doctor's credentials. The psychotic patient who is receiving treatment grudgingly, perhaps even under compulsion or under pressure from others, will impart as little information as possible and will tend to show resentment and hostility towards the doctor and the treatment regime. It is conventional to note the degree of emotional *rapport* that a patient can establish with others, although this is probably a highly unreliable clinical exercise. Lack of *rapport* is seen typically in certain schizophrenic states, when the patient presents a cold, distant front, with little apparent warmth of feeling. In schizophrenia there may also be incongruity of affect, when the patient giggles or smiles to himself while discussing serious issues; sometimes he may spontaneously complain of this symptom himself.

Disorders of Perception

A clear distinction should be made between hallucinations and illusions. A hallucination is a false perception in the absence of any adequate stimulus, whereas an illusion, in the strict medical sense, is a misinterpretation of actual sensory stimuli. Thus, a person who hears voices when clearly no voices are present is experiencing auditory hallucinations, while he who misinterprets a pattern on a curtain (e.g. believes that it contains frightening animals) is suffering from visual illusions. Hallucinations may affect any sensory modality: they may be auditory, visual, tactile, olfactory, or gustatory in form. They may complicate any kind of major psychiatric disorder: while there is much overlap, it is a useful clinical rule that organic mental disturbance tends to lead to visual hallucinations and the functional psychoses are more often characterised by the auditory type.

The content of hallucinatory experiences varies from the ill-defined (e.g. indistinct mumbling voices) to highly complex and organised experiences, e.g. recognisable voices talking to the patient, or visions of complex scenery. Hallucinations are often accompanied by emotional disturbance: in organic delirium there is severe anxiety as well as visual hallucinations. In derealisation, the perception of the surrounding environment is altered and strange. Depersonalisation is a sense of estrangement from the self, with a feeling of loss of identity or loss of one's own reality; the physical body may even appear to belong to someone else. Although transient episodes of depersonalisation may occur in the absence of mental illness, the more persistent severe disturbances of this kind can be disabling, and tend, in particular, to complicate depressive or schizophrenic illnesses.

Obsessional Compulsive Phenomena

These are recurrent thoughts or motor activity the patient feels compelled to repeat time and time again. He tries to resist them, only to become anxious in doing so. He is able to recognise, on quiet reflection, that his symptoms have no rational basis and that they are part of his own thinking processes rather than attributable to outside influences acting upon him. Obsessional compulsive symptoms are therefore accompanied by insight, because the patient recognises their abnormal nature. In this way obsessional compulsive symptoms are distinguished from delusions of passivity to be found in the schizophrenias: here, the individual may also feel compelled to act or think in a certain way but he attributes his experience to the action of outside forces, and does not believe that he himself is ill.

Obsessional compulsive phenomena are almost universal experiences. They are very common in childhood, and in adults they are to be found most frequently in the obsessional personality, when they are accompanied by rigidity of habits, meticulousness, and a need for orderliness and strict routine in daily life. Such an individual from time to time may develop accentuation of his obsessional symptoms to the extent that they interfere with his normal daily activities, and he is then said to have developed an obsessional neurosis. Obsessional thoughts may take the form of repetitive counting of numbers, recurrent musical tunes or phrases, sometimes accompanied by an impulse to shout them out loudly. Obsessional motor activity commonly takes the form of recurrent checking (e.g. gas and water taps, doors, locks) dressing rituals or handwashing. Repetition is, of course, greatest in the most severe obsessional neuroses, when the patient's whole day may be devoted to his obsessional behaviour to the exclusion of normal work and social activities.

Disorders of Thinking

Attention and Concentration. In some conditions the patient may be so preoccupied with his own psychic experiences that he does not attend to ordinary conversation. This is often seen in organic confusional states, for example in incipient and florid delirium tremens. In any severe psychiatric illness there may be severe difficulty in concentration, for example as a presenting symptom in a depressive illness, or in a schizophrenic patient preoccupied with his own fantasies. It is important to ensure that attention is adequate before proceeding to assess a patient's cognitive and intellectual status. Some idea of the patient's level of attention may be gained by noting his general reaction to the interview and by asking him to recite the months of the year, the days of the week in reverse, or to subtract seven serially beginning at an arbitrary number. It is wise to explain to the patient that these are tests of concentration and not intelligence.

Delusional Thinking. This constitutes a break with reality and is one of the hallmarks of the psychotic type of mental illness. A delusion is a false belief held against all evidence to the contrary and out of context with the cultural background of the patient. A delusion is therefore a disorder of thinking. It is incorrigible because all reasoned argument and evidence against it has no effect upon it. Nowadays, the man who maintains that the earth is flat might be considered to entertain a delusional idea. Some centuries ago, however, this was a universally held belief and not delusional because there was no evidence to the contrary. It is also necessary to take into account the cultural background of any patient suspected to have delusional ideas; for example an individual who believes that he experiences bodily pain due to magical interference by others is more likely to be deluded if he comes from a European cultural background than if he originates from a country where such ideas occur commonly as part of traditional folklore, for example the West Indies.

Having established the presence of delusional ideas, it is also important to note their content. Delusional *ideas of reference* are false beliefs that people talk about and deliberately centre their attention on the patient. *Paranoid delusions* are characterised by false ideas of persecution and injustice, resented by the patient who feels that he does not deserve such treatment. They may complicate any major mental illness, occurring most commonly in the older age groups and in schizophrenic illnesses. *Depressive delusions* are understandable in the light of the patient's mood disturbance. He may show morbid guilt over trival imaginary trespasses in the past (pecadilloes). The spinster who believed that she had contracted venereal disease through being kissed at a Christmas party many years before may be said to entertain morbid depressive guilt. The depressed patient may feel that others are hostile to him, but he accepts that their attitude is justified because of his own misdeeds. The patient with a hypomanic illness may show grandiose delusions which are understandable in terms of his expansive, euphoric mood, perhaps believing himself to be a millionaire or otherwise exalted in identity. The crucial clinical feature of delusions which complicate mood disturbance (affective psychoses) is that their content is understandable as a result of the mood change. In schizophrenic illnesses no such correlation is seen between disorder of mood and thought content. Delusions of *passivity* and *influence* are said to be confined to the schizophrenic illnesses, and consist of beliefs that thoughts or bodily functions are influenced and controlled in some strange way by outside influences, for example radar, electricity or radio waves.

Intellectual Functions

Organic brain disturbances produce characteristic disorders of cognitive function which are clearly delineated from the phenomena so far described. The organic disturbance of mental state consists of impairment of orientation, memory (amnesia), and intellectual capacity. Before these can be examined adequately it is necessary to ensure that the patient is able to attend to questions put to him; otherwise, assessment becomes highly unreliable. Orientation is examined in the dimensions of time, place and person: the patient is asked the day of the week and full date, where he is, and who he is. Organic disorders cause impairment of recent memory while distant recollections remain relatively intact. Old persons suffering from dementia may thus appear to live in the past because more recent memories have been lost. Occasionally, gross memory loss is seen, affecting both recent and distant memory: for example, as found in a person who walks into hospital apparently unable to remember any facts about himself, not even his name. Such global amnesia is in itself unlikely to be due to organic causes and may be due to hysterical reaction or malingering. Physical examination should never be omitted in such cases, however, because physical disorder such as head injury or epilepsy may have precipitated the hysterical reaction.

Routine assessment of any psychiatric problem must always include testing for recent memory loss, otherwise gross disturbances may easily be missed. The simplest way to test recent memory is to give the patient a full postal address, asking him to learn it. The number of times it has to be administered before it is learnt to perfection is noted, and the patient after being forewarned is asked to repeat it after five minutes, when his response is recorded.

Intellectual function can be difficult to assess clinically without special psychological tests. Grasp of general information (e.g. names of capital cities, basic geographical knowledge, recent events in the news) is dependent on educational experience and interests as well as intelligence. It can be useful, however, when unexpectedly poor performance is found in someone whose occupation and educational background is good. Reasoning and grasp of arguments are both impaired in chronic organic mental disorders (the dementias), and social indiscretion or disinhibition may be presenting features in these conditions. Formal tests of intellectual function are the most reliable of all psychological instruments, and they should be used to supplement routine clinical examination whenever intellectual impairment is suspected.

Insight

It is useful at the end of formal examination of the mental state to assess the patient's insight (the way he sees himself, his illness and his life situation). A few carefully worded questions serve this purpose, for example, 'Do you think all this has been due to illness?', or 'Do you believe yourself to be ill in any way?' If so, 'Do you think your illness is nervous or physical in nature?' In the psychoses, there is, by definition, a break with reality, and the patient may not accept that he is ill, or he distorts reality in a delusional way. Such a patient poses many problems in treatment. He may see no reason to take medication offered to him and he tends to be unreliable in taking it. The doctor, in recognising these attitudes in the patient can make appropriate adjustment in his treatment programme and he is able to understand the patient's mistrust or hostility towards him. In contrast, the neurotic patient has full insight into the fact that he is ill (though not necessarily into the cause of his illness) and he sees reality in a relatively undistorted way. As a result he is more likely to trust and confide in his doctor and he is usually prepared to accept regular medication. Assessment of insight thus provides a correct perspective in which a treatment regime may be planned for the individual patient.

PHYSICAL ASSESSMENT

It is important to remember that systemic organic disease may often present in the guise of mental disturbance. The anxiety of thyrotoxicosis, the depression or paranoid reaction of myxoedema are classic examples. In reverse, mental illness may present with physical complaints, and such patients tend to be exhaustively investigated in medical clinics before the true nature of the illness becomes recognised. The relation between physical and mental illness is, therefore, very close. Grave errors of diagnosis and management will ensue unless physical examination is included routinely in psychiatric assessment. It should be carried out in all cases presenting with mental illness, and not restricted to those in which somatic or organic mental symptoms clearly suggest the presence of organic disease.

D. CAUSES

The causes of mental illness are still in the main poorly understood. A variety of theoretical approaches exist. It is likely that each orientation contains some element of truth and the diversity between the various theories merely reflects the complexity of factors involved in leading to mental disorder. It is important not to adopt a partisan approach by patronising one orientation to the exclusion of others. It is necessary to assess each case from all theoretical viewpoints and to select the approach that is most likely to lead to successful treatment. Not infrequently, the patient himself has sympathies of his own, and it is wise to take these into consideration in choosing the type of treatment. It is not only a question of which approach is valid, but also which seems most likely to be successful in any particular patient.

In understanding the causes of mental illness, we must be prepared to consider both distant (predisposing) and recent (precipitating) factors as well as adverse sequelae which may perpetuate the disorder. We must try to understand why the individual has previously been rendered vulnerable by predisposing factors in such a way that he develops an illness at the time he does, possibly as a reaction to adverse precipitating events.

THE SOMATIC APPROACH

When mental illness is directly related to structural or physiological brain disorder, it takes a distinct form: in the acute stage it presents with delirium, confusion and disorientation, and in the chronic form as disorder of memory and intellect. This type of mental disorder forms only a small proportion of all mental illnesses. The search for physical causes in the remainder (the major psychoses, the neuroses and personality disorders) has, in spite of much enthusiastic work, produced few positive results. No structural or physiological disorders have been found consistently in association with these conditions, either in the central nervous system or elsewhere. Theories have been put forward attempting to explain certain mental illnesses in terms of biochemical disorder. A whole range of inborn errors of metabolism may lead to mental subnormality, although such cases form only a small proportion of the total subnormality problem. A great deal of work has been done in the search for a possible biochemical cause of the schizophrenias. The original stimulus in this field came from Gjessing's demonstration that a rare type of catatonia is associated with changes in thyroid function. Further leads in this field have come from the study of side effects of certain drugs: the paranoid hallucinatory symptoms that may complicate excessive and habitual intake of amphetamine are identical with those seen in certain types of schizophrenia; the hallucinogenic effects of mescaline bear some resemblance to schizophrenia, although in a very atypical way. Both amphetamine and mescaline, in terms of chemical structure, could conceivably be derived from disordered adrenaline breakdown, which has, therefore, been suggested as a possible cause of the schizophrenias. So far, however, attempts to detect abnormal metabolites in schizophrenic patients have not led to consistent results. The most recent claims for 3–4 dimethoxyphenylethylamine (DMPE), a theoretically possible breakdown product of adrenaline by methylation, and itself resembling mescaline, have not proved reproducible, and could be due to failure by investigators to control dietary factors. In the affective psychoses, biochemical research has demonstrated certain abnormality in the distribution of electrolytes between the inter- and extracellular fluids, but here again the exact significance of these findings is not yet clear: they could precede the illness or be secondary to it.

THE GENETIC APPROACH

This seeks to explain mental illness in terms of personal predisposition due to heredity. For example, the major psychoses tend to occur more often in the families of patients than in the general population. Twin studies have figured prominently in this approach. It is argued that monozygotic twins, having identical genetic endowment, should show a high concordance rate (i.e. both twins in a pair having the same illness) in those illnesses that are mainly genetically determined. Very high concordance rates have been demonstrated in monozygotic twins with schizophrenia or depressive psychosis, but the exact significance of these findings remains uncertain as there is at present no unequivocal way of distinguishing the effects of genetic endowment from those due to shared early pathological environment.

THE PSYCHOLOGICAL APPROACH

1. Causes in the Individual

Freud pioneered this kind of approach, dispensing with the traditional medical search for physical causes. In his theory of neurosis, he postulated that traumatic psychological experiences in childhood may lead to impaired emotional development, characterised by unresolved conflicts between incompatible drives and rendering the individual vulnerable to neurotic breakdown at a later date. Three hypothetical compartments of mental activity were suggested:

(a) The ego denotes the conscious thinking processes.
(b) The id represents the unconscious psychic processes containing basic drives and instincts.
(c) The superego is equivalent to conscience or the sum total of the individual's moral values.

It is postulated that neurotic breakdown occurs when unconscious conflicts break into the ego, and these have to be resolved by discussion aimed at gaining insight before complete recovery is possible. Although the concept of the unconscious has stimulated a fuller understanding of mental processes, it is perhaps one of the most widely abused in psychiatry. Too easily it becomes a readily invoked explanation for symptoms of obscure origin.

Understandable psychological interconnections in a person's mind are called psychodynamics. Freud formulated processes which he called defence mechanisms of the ego, whereby a person copes with the psychological stresses of living. They may be found both in what he called the psychopathology of everyday life as well as in mental illness itself.

Repression results in not being able to remember material which for some reason is unpleasant, and so is relegated to the unconscious.

Displacement refers to the shifting of feelings from one idea or object to another which is similar but for some reason more acceptable to the ego.

Reaction Formation involves transforming an unacceptable impulse into its opposite: hostile feelings towards an important figure are replaced by overt expressions of affection.

Rationalisation is a process of explaining away by the ego to make its irrational attitudes appear logical.

Denial is used widely in normal as well as pathological states. It may involve denial of the memory of an experience, or apparent lack of consideration of all implications of the reality situation.

In Projection the individual attributes to others his own feelings and motives that he finds difficult to tolerate in himself.

Regression is an attempt to return to an earlier (less mature) stage of function in order to avoid the difficulties evoked by the current situation.

Sublimation involves renunciation of direct gratification in a certain direction (usually sexual) in favour of pursuit of another that is more socially acceptable.

Defence mechanisms are incomplete solutions of psychological difficulties and, at best, can be efficient only for short periods. They relegate conflict to the unconscious level and do not permit their complete resolution. Neurotic breakdown is, therefore, always liable to occur.

The psychological explanation of mental illness emphasises the use of discussion (psychotherapy) of various kinds in treatment. When disturbance within the individual is regarded as paramount, attempts are made to resolve this in discussions between patient and therapist.

Learning theory has also made contributions to the understanding of mental illness in terms of abnormal psychological processes in the individual. Pavlov, in his work on conditioning in animals, pioneered the development of a theoretical approach which emphasises the process whereby adverse psychological reactions may be learnt. A stressful situation may lead to a fear or phobia which recurs in the individual whenever he is re-exposed to it, or even when he anticipates it. It is possible that a variety of morbid symptoms arise as learnt patterns of behaviour. For example, certain sexual deviations may result from exposure to an abnormal relationship with parents in childhood or adolescence. Somce cases of alcoholism may arise as a learnt response by habitual use of alcohol to reduce anxiety in a stressful situation. Behaviour therapy, which utilises learning theory principles, aims at getting the patient to unlearn certain morbid psychological responses.

Experiments with animals exposed to chronic frustrations in learning situations can produce disordered behaviour which suggests an analogy to certain emotional disorders in man. In terms of learning theory, inability to choose between two alternative actions either because of ambiguities between them or inconsistent reward or punishment, may be important factors whereby emotional disturbances become learnt. Experiments in man suggest that states akin to depression may be developed as protective devices in the face of intolerable psychological conflicts.

2. Disorders of Interpersonal Relationships

This approach emphasises the part played by disordered relationships between the patient and others in leading to mental illness. Man is a social animal and to remain mentally well he needs healthy relationships with others. Disturbed interpersonal relationships not only follow closely on mental illness but may themselves precede and directly precipitate breakdown. One of the clearest examples of this is the close correlation between suicidal behaviour and social isolation and estrangement from others in the community. Disturbed interpersonal relationships may act as precipitating causes of illness, for example arising out of marital disharmony, or they may have predisposed the individual to breakdown by their action years before. It is suggested, for example, that certain schizophrenias in adults may stem from exposure to pathogenic interpersonal influences in early family life.

The interpersonal approach to mental illness encourages attempts to understand the symptoms as a means of communicating with others, and in terms of their effects on other individuals: this approach has no analogy in other fields of medicine, treatment based on utilising group situations and the principles of the therapeutic community.

3. Environmental and Social Causes

Sociologists tend to look at mental illness in yet a wider sense, and see its causes in terms of social disturbance. For example, the preponderance of schizophrenia in social class V leads to the theory that the illness is caused by stress peculiar to this section of the community. It is, of course, difficult to disentangle social factors from other possible explanations such as vulnerable individuals sliding down the social scale as a result of incipient psychosis.

Many kinds of traumatic events, apart from disturbed relationships with others or social class factors, play a part in precipitating mental illness. It has, in the past, been customary to regard the functional psychoses (schizophrenias and affective psychoses) as entirely endogenous illnesses and not related to environmental upset in any way; the neuroses were thought to be mainly exogenous and reactive to life upsets. It is probably much more profitable to avoid such a rigid dichotomy and to regard mental illness of any kind as due to varying combinations of both long-standing personal predisposition and more recent precipitating factors. In all cases the possible reciprocal relationship between symptoms and the 'here and now' life situation must be assessed in detail. By dealing with the immediate life situation in therapy it is often possible to achieve results when treatment aimed at distant predisposing factors fails.

E. TREATMENTS

NON-PHYSICAL

Psychotherapy

This consists of a discussion between therapist and patient or a group of patients. Its general aim is to enable the patient to learn about himself and to establish ways of dealing with his personal problems.

Supportive Psychotherapy. Too little recognition is accorded to the value of constructive listening. Though apparently passive it may be an inestimable source of help to persons with psychological difficulties even when the therapist's time is very limited. Certain rules should be observed very carefully:

1. Concentrate on listening and say little. Avoid glib reassurance, which so often merely makes the patient feel that the true extent of his distress is not appreciated.
2. Do not interrogate. Ask questions if they really are appropriate, but try to encourage the patient to be at ease and to do the talking himself. Remember the immense therapeutic value of letting a patient talk about the problems which distress him even when you may produce no answers to them.
3. Make it clear that you accept the patient's intrinsic worth as an individual in need of help and without prejudice on your part. Therapy is most likely to succeed when it starts in a setting of genuine acceptance.
4. Do not pronounce on general matters and avoid directing the patient with regard to which course of action he should take. A harmful state of over-dependence on the therapist is easily produced, and when it does occur it is often the therapist's fault. Facile interpretations of behaviour should be avoided.
5. Keep your personal feelings out of it. They contribute nothing to therapy and are often an embarrassment to the patient who may find them a hindrance when he tries to communicate his own feelings.
6. Identify with the patient up to a point. This helps you to tune in to the problem, but do not take this too far. A therapist may so easily lose objectivity and by identifying too much with the patient becomes anxious and unable to set realistic goals.
7. Define aims clearly and explain fully to the patient the nature of the help which you are offering. Some kind of contractual arrangement, for example with agreement on the number of sessions and the problems to be looked at, is far better than open-ended interminable unstructured discussions.
8. Respect the confidentiality of what your patient says to you and make it clear that it will not be discussed with anyone else without his permission. Encourage the patient to discuss the behaviour of other persons when this is relevant to his treatment, but discourage gossip.

Interpretive Psychotherapy. This is a radical, planned form of discussion which may extend over months or even years, attempting to give the patient insight into his psychological problems to enable him to come to terms with them. This kind of treatment is based on the principle that promotion of a patient's insight into the nature and origins of his symptoms will lead to improvement. Such an approach is not appropriate in florid psychotic illness, which may be made worse by attempts to get the patient to understand the origin of his symptoms. Formal psychotherapy involves the use of interpretation by the therapist whereby psychological explanations for symptoms are offered in terms of their unconscious symbolic significance and other psychodynamic mechanisms. The therapist never dictates explanations to the patient. The emphasis is on encouraging the patient to reach the correct conclusion himself. The novice therapist usually makes the mistake of being authoritarian and allowing himself to pronounce to the patient. Much skill is required both in choosing which patients are likely to benefit from interpretive psychotherapy and in dealing with the emotional upsets that may arise during treatment. Not the least of these is the transference situation, an intense emotional relationship (either dependent or hostile) on the part of the patient towards the therapist. Psychoanalysis is a specialised form of psychotherapy in which early life events are scrutinised in detail and interpretations are offered in terms of Freudian theory.

Group Psychotherapy. This involves discussion between small groups of patients, all determined to talk openly about their problems. It is used in those non-psychotic illnesses where interpersonal difficulties play an important part, but it can also be useful in conditions where group identification is marked, e.g. chronic alcoholism and other addictions, or adolescent behavioural disturbances. Again, the therapist plays a non-directive role, and encourages the patient to follow constructive lines of discussion. The use of joint discussions with man and wife who have marital problems is a variant of group psychotherapy.

Hypnosis

Suggestion has been an important element in the healing art throughout the ages in all cultures. The eighteenth century Swiss physician, Mesmer, was the first to subject it to systematic study, but he ran into difficulties when he overemphasised the theatricals involved. He believed that hypnosis was due to animal magnetism, which could be transmitted from one person to another. For this purpose his subjects were asked to grasp tubs filled with iron filings. Hypnosis has to this day a mystique which dates not only from Mesmer's approach, but also that of Charcot, who utilised strong elements of suggestion in his clinical demonstrations of hysteria. The truth is that hypnosis is merely a state of heightened suggestibility, induced by relaxation and monotonous repetitive stimuli. It is neither sleep nor a state of unconsciousness: attention and awareness are restricted in range, and focussed intensely on to the therapist's conversation. Susceptibility to hypnosis varies considerably from one person to another, a small proportion of individuals being quite resistant. Post-hypnotic automatism is said to occur when a person subsequently carries out apparently blindly and automatically an act suggested to him under hypnosis. Such claims are difficult to validate because it is not possible to measure objectively the full extent of the subject's recall. Hypnosis cannot in this way induce behaviour that is contrary to the subject's normal moral and ethical code.

Hypnosis is used:
1. In the treatment of anxiety symptoms of neurotic origin.
2. In the treatment of hysterical symptoms: it is said that hysterical patients are extremely suggestible.
3. As an aid to anaesthesia by suggesting analgesia: in this way the total amount of anaesthetic drugs required may be reduced considerably in appropriate subjects. Hypnotic suggestion has a wide application in obstetrics by helping to prepare the anxious individual for childbirth.
4. In psychotherapy: by suggestion it may be possible to overcome resistances and thereby aid recollection of early traumatic experiences. This method should be used with great caution and only by the expert.

Hypnosis has limitations as a radical form of treatment because although it may erase symptoms by suggestion, it does not remove their underlying cause. A hysterical paraplegia may indeed disappear dramatically with the help of hypnosis, only to be replaced very rapidly by another hysterical symptom unless the underlying cause of the reaction is also treated.

Behaviour Therapy

This helps the patient to unlearn certain morbid psychological reactions, most commonly:
1. Neurotic anxiety, especially when it is restricted to certain situations, for example insect phobias.
2. Certain sexual deviations.
3. A very limited number of cases of chronic alcoholism.

Two main techniques are involved. Anxiety is treated by desensitisation, whereby the patient is taught to relax and then encouraged in fantasy to proceed along a previously constructed hierarchy of situations provoking increasing degrees of anxiety, while at the same time the therapist encourages full relaxation. Aversion therapy gets the patient to unlearn a morbid attitude by presenting it to him at the same time as an unpleasant stimulus, usually a mild but painful electric shock. Certain types of sexual deviation may respond to this approach. Behaviour therapy may fail for the same reasons as hypnosis does when it merely treats symptoms and ignores underlying causes. It is more successful when combined with psychotherapeutic discussion.

PHYSICAL TREATMENTS

Drugs

This section highlights important aspects of drug therapy in psychiatry. It is not intended to be a substitute for a full discussion of their pharmacology and therapeutics, which must be obtained elsewhere.

1. **Sedatives.** These are in general overprescribed. They are given to many patients who do not really need

them, and often the more potent and dangerous kinds are used when milder safer alternatives could be equally effective.

Non-barbiturates should be given as the drugs of first choice: chloral, dichloralphenazone, nitrazepam and glutethimide are safe and effective.

Barbiturates are very effective sedatives, but they are also highly dangerous because overdose may so easily prove lethal, and dependence due to habituation may develop quickly in certain individuals. Their use is acceptable in short courses for treatment of acute disturbances where sleep is impossible to procure by other means. They should be avoided:
(a) As long term medication, especially when the patient requests increasing doses.
(b) As a day-time sedative.
(c) In young adults except in acute illness as above.
(d) In any person with evidence of addictive propensities such as a history of alcoholism.
(e) In patients who are likely to injure themselves by drug overdose or otherwise.

2. **Minor Tranquillisers** (chloradiazepoxide, diazepam). These constitute a popular form of treatment of anxiety, mainly that complicating neurotic and affective disorders. They are of little value in the treatment of psychotic symptoms. They are relatively free from side effects at therapeutic doses, but minor dependence with marked accentuation of anxiety on sudden withdrawal is sometimes seen, especially if a prolonged course of the drug has been prescribed. It is wise to use these drugs in short, planned courses, and prolonged medication is rarely justified.

3. **Major Tranquillisers** (phenothiazines, haloperidol). These are used primarily in the treatment of the major psychoses (schizophrenia, hypomania). Their efficacy in controlling very disturbed behaviour and psychotic symptoms is said to have played a major part in facilitating the change to an open-door policy which took place in mental hospitals in the 1950s. This is probably only part of the story, because liberalising attitudes in hospital staff were also important and, in fact, these preceded the introduction of these drugs.

Phenothiazines. Addiction does not develop with the phenothiazines, but in routine psychiatric practice side effects are often seen, particularly when high doses are employed. The most common of these are tremor and muscle spasm due to extrapyramidal stimulation, and it is wise to prescribe an atropine-like drug (benzhexol or orphenadrine) especially when high doses are used. Photosensitivity may also cause problems, and patients receiving phenothiazines should be warned against sunbathing. Intrahepatic obstructive jaundice is a rare but relatively benign complication of chlorpromazine medication.

When a schizophrenic psychosis relapses because the patient does not take oral medication regularly, it is sometimes useful to use long-acting intramuscular phenothiazine preparations, usually injected every three weeks. A test dose must always be given under surveillance in hospital before a full dose regime is started. Extrapyramidal side effects may appear at any time during this form of treatment and can be severe. It is necessary for the family doctor in particular to be aware of this complication, and to prescribe anti-Parkinsonian drugs, if necessary intravenously, when muscle spasm is marked. Long-acting phenothiazines are useful only in those schizophrenic psychoses which respond well to full medication and where relapse seems attributable to inadequate oral intake by the patient.

Haloperidol (gamma aminobutyric acid antagonist). This may sometimes succeed in controlling psychotic symptoms when phenothiazines have failed. Extrapyramidal side effects may be particularly troublesome.

4. **Antidepressants.** Assessment of the antidepressant effect of drugs presents many difficulties in trying to disentangle placebo action from true therapeutic response. The self-limiting nature of most depressive illnesses also means that any drug given for long enough might appear to have antidepressant effects. The *tricyclic drugs* (imipramine hydrochloride, amitriptyline hydrochloride) have been shown in several double-blind trials to facilitate recovery of depression. Their side effects are mainly extrapyramidal in type (fine tremor, blurred vision, accentuation of prostatic obstruction or glaucoma) and in themselves are relatively mild. These drugs are worth using when significant depressive features are present. When these are severe and accompanied by suicidal risk it is not safe to depend on antidepressant drugs without also seeking specialist advice urgently.

Monoamine oxidase inhibitor (MAOI) antidepressants have not been shown effective by clinical trials. Their possible side effects can be dangerous. Severe hypertensive crises may be precipitated by concomitant intake of tricyclic antidepressants or sympathomimetic drugs, or a variety of foodstuffs including broad beans, cheese (especially the well-ripened varieties such as cheddar and camembert), Marmite, Bovril, Yoghurt, yeast extracts, game, chicken livers, beers, wines and creams. Severe liver damage may also sometimes occur. Monoamine oxidase inhibitors are probably too dangerous to be used as routine antidepressants, and they are unlikely to achieve more than can a judicious use of other less toxic drugs and electroconvulsive therapy. Patients who present with surgical emergencies need very careful management if they happen already to be receiving monoamine oxidase inhibitors, because of possible adverse reaction to drugs that may be used during anaesthesia. Adrenaline, noradrenaline, amphetamine, phenylephrine and ephedrine should not be administered to patients on MAOI therapy. Dangerous potentiation of alcohol, barbiturates, ether, pethidine, morphine, cocaine, procaine and insulin may occur. Excitation may develop with reserpine or methyldopa. Care must always be observed in changing from MAOI to tricyclic antidepressants: at least 1 week should be allowed after stopping the MAOI before beginning a tricyclic drug.

5. **Lithium.** Administered in the form of lithium carbonate, this may be helpful in the treatment of acute manic episodes. There is usually a delay of some days before clinical benefit occurs, and when urgent control of symptoms is required, lithium carbonate is usually combined initially with a major tranquilliser. It is also used as a prophylactic against relapse of manic illness, and long term maintenance therapy is then required.

It is important to monitor blood levels, especially in the early months of treatment in order to ensure that they remain within the range 0.6 to 1.5 mEq/l. Toxic effects can be extremely dangerous and they readily occur if the blood level remains above 2 mEq/l for long. The drug is accumulative and in severe poisoning haemodialysis may be necessary. It is, therefore, important to be vigilant for early signs of toxicity; these include fine tremor, nausea and abdominal discomfort, leading later to diarrhoea and vomiting. Drowsiness is a particularly important symptom because it may herald coma which can be fatal. Lithium is contraindicated in persons with serious renal or cardiac disease, and it may interfere with thyroid metabolism to produce frank myxoedema in some cases.

6. **Electroconvulsive Therapy (ECT).** The precise mechanism whereby this effective and widely used form of treatment exerts its action is unknown. Its discovery originated from the observation that mental hospital patients tended to lose psychotic symptoms if they developed spontaneous convulsions. Statistical figures also showed that epilepsy and schizophrenia rarely occurred in the same patient. Von Meduna, in 1935, argued that artificial induction of epileptic fits may help in the treatment of psychosis. He first used intravenous camphor in oil, but this has been superseded by electrical stimulation, which is safer and more easily controlled. The technique involves adequate premedication with atropine, followed by a short-acting intravenous anaesthetic (usually a barbiturate) with a short-acting muscle relaxant (e.g. scoline). The electrical stimulus is then applied by electrodes to the temples, either in the form of a static discharge from a condenser or as alternating current. The patient then has a modified (mild) convulsion, which may vary from fluttering of the eyelids to non-violent clonic body movements, lasting for about half a minute, the patient regaining consciousness several minutes later. Treatment consists of a course of such applications, usually five or six, but

sometimes up to twelve times in number. Recurrent courses are undesirable, but sometimes necessary in cases that are resistant to therapy or, where relapse occurs. Periods of several months should be allowed to lapse between each course of treatment. Not least in the technique of ECT is the adequate psychological preparation of the patient. The nature of the treatment must be explained in commonsense terms to each individual, emphasising that it is painless and, as far as the patient is aware, involves no more than an anaesthetic injection in his arm.

ECT is indicated:

(a) In severe depression of any kind when suicide risk is real.

(b) In depression of disabling degree in which environmental difficulties are not the limiting factor and where there has been inadequate response to other treatment.

(c) In mania or hypomania which is not adequately controlled by medication.

(d) In acute schizophrenic or other functional paranoid psychoses which have not responded to a few weeks of adequate drug therapy. ECT is especially useful in treating catatonic motor symptoms.

Complications of ECT although infrequent are not negligible.

They include:

The complications of any anaesthetic.

Cardiac arrythmias. Muscle relaxants increase this risk by their strong cholinergic action. Atropine premedication is thus necessary to counteract this as well as to dry secretions.

Physical injury (now infrequent since muscle relaxants were introduced).

Memory disturbance. This occurs in a small number of patients as a transient difficulty in recent recall lasting for minutes or hours after treatment, but it may take the form of florid confusion, particularly if ECT is inadvertently given to a patient with organic brain disorder.

All candidates for ECT should be thoroughly assessed physically beforehand. Senility in itself is no contraindication, but ECT should, as a general rule, be avoided where there has been severe recent physical illness such as cardiac infarction, cerebrovascular accident, severe hypertension, or organic brain disorder.

7. **Frontal Leucotomy.** In 1935 it was shown that frontal lobe extirpation in monkeys led to increased tolerance of frustration without obvious intellectual defect. Following this finding, Freeman and Watt, in 1942, introduced a procedure for treating certain mental illnesses in man by cutting fibre tracts in the frontal lobes. Early techniques were carried out blindly either via temporal burr holes or through the roof of the orbit. Various modifications of this operation were widely used in psychiatric practice up to the introduction of phenothiazines, which have to a considerable extent superseded it. Leucotomy today usually takes the form of an open neurosurgical

procedure involving very localised frontal section or ablation, and it is now not often used. The operation is considered in cases of severe tension due to mental illness when all other methods have failed. It must always remain a last resort in therapy because, of necessity, it inflicts brain damage. Recent onset schizophrenia that has defied intensive therapy over several years, yet seems destined to lead to chronic institutionalisation, is the most common indication. Less frequently, intractable depression with much tension in older patients, or intractable obsessional neurosis may warrant the operation. Complications may be neurological (haemorrhage at the operation, or fits) or psychological (social disinhibition or loss of initiative). Intellectual deterioration does not occur after an uncomplicated leucotomy. The operation should not be done on patients in which antisocial, particularly aggressive features or apathy are marked, and it cannot be expected to achieve much in patients lacking satisfactory premorbid personality.

8. **Insulin Therapy.** Modified insulin therapy involves administration of insulin to chronically debilitated patients with weight loss in doses sufficient to stimulate appetite without causing disturbance of consciousness. It must be distinguished from deep insulin therapy (once very popular as a treatment of chronic schizophrenia) in which, by a gradual increase in the dose of insulin, deep coma was induced for short periods and then terminated by administration of glucose. Deep insulin therapy is no longer in general use. Its apparent beneficial effects were probably more related to the extra care and attention the patient obtained in undergoing it and the more hopeful approach it stimulated in the staff, rather than due to any specific effects of insulin itself.

I. PSYCHOPHYSICAL RELATIONSHIPS

Physical and mental illnesses are closely interrelated in four ways:
1. The organic brain disorders, either structural or physiological in origin are associated with characteristic disturbances of cognitive mental functions (orientation, memory, intellect).
2. Systemic physical disease may be accompanied by a wide variety of psychological reactions, in the absence of organic brain pathology, and which are understandable in terms of the person's previous personality and experience.
3. In the psychosomatic illnesses, chronic psychological disturbance may play an important part in both initiating and maintaining systemic physical disease.
4. Mental illness may closely mimic physical disease by producing or even presenting with somatic symptoms. Exhaustive physical investigations may be performed

with negative results before the primary psychological basis for the illness is recognised.

A. MENTAL SYNDROMES DUE TO ORGANIC BRAIN DISORDER

Mental disturbance due to organic brain disease consists of characteristic clinical features which are usually quite distinct from those found in the functional (non-organic) mental illnesses. The full organic mental syndrome includes:
1. Memory loss (most severe for recent events).
2. Impairment of consciousness (particularly in acute illnesses).
3. Disorientation (in time, place, person).
4. Intellectual impairment (defects of grasp, reasoning, learning ability).
5. There may also be a variety of non-specific mental symptoms such as hallucinations (especially visual), mood disturbance, delusional ideas.

The organic mental syndrome is characteristically variable in its manifestation both from day to day or even hour to hour: typically, it is worse at night. The memory loss (amnesia) is mainly for recent events, in contrast to distant recollections which tend to remain relatively intact. Thus, the patient with senile dementia seems to live in the past, and day-to-day events do not appear to be recollected or even registered in his mind. This contrasts with functional (usually hysterical) amnesia, which tends to be global, extending over the whole of the patient's past, perhaps rendering it impossible for him to remember his identity. Such gross amnesia complicates only the most severe and obvious organic brain disease. Impairment of consciousness in the organic brain syndrome affects both the level (intensity) and extent of awareness (*see* Fig. 20.2).

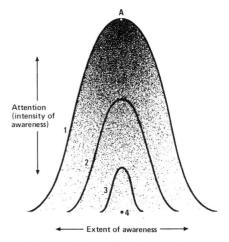

Fig. 20.2 Organic brain disorder and attention.

Normally (1), attention is focussed clearly on a small part of the environment (A), total awareness extending more widely although with much less degree of attention. Severe organic impairment of consciousness

438

may lead to unconsciousness (4), in which there is, of course, no awareness; less severe impairment leads to clouding of consciousness (2) and (3), when the intensity and extent of awareness are both reduced. Typically, a patient may fluctuate from one to the other. He finds it difficult to persist with a conversation, or to grasp what is said to him because he cannot concentrate fully, and he requires constant exhortation to prevent him from losing interest in what is said to him.

Disorientation follows if memory and conscious awareness are impaired to a sufficient degree. The patient may be unable to state where he is, who he is, or give the correct time, day and date (disorientation in place, person and time). Confusion is present when severe disorientation is combined with a sense of bewilderment.

Intellectual Impairment affects the ability to reason, especially in abstract form, to act with caution and in a socially acceptable way, or to anticipate and plan future events. Intellectual deficit may be difficult to detect in its early stages. It may present as loss of normal social inhibitions; for example, there may be deterioration in personal hygiene and care with dress, or indecent sexual exposure may occur for the first time. In progressive disorders, there is increasing impairment of ability to follow conversation or to calculate money. Conscious mental activity may ultimately become grossly restricted, and verbal responses fleeting and stereotyped, such as 'nice day' and 'nice drop of rain', without real involvement in day-to-day events.

Other Psychiatric Disturbance. A variety of non-specific mental symptoms may be found in organic brain disturbance. Hallucinations, when they occur, are more often visual than auditory in type and this may sometimes be useful as a diagnostic point. Mood may be labile, shallow, with rapidly fluctuating depression and tearfulness. The acute organic disturbance is often accompanied by bewilderment, with intense anxiety or fear and resulting agitation or aggressive behaviour. Paranoid delusions may develop, especially when there has been clouding of consciousness such as may occur following a severe overdose of sedatives. The physical examination is of paramount importance in clinical assessment of organic mental disturbance. Both neurological and systemic disease may constitute the underlying cause of the mental disturbance. Unless sought carefully, organic disease may remain undetected, particularly in the elderly.

1. Mental Syndromes Due to Acute Organic Brain Disorder

The acute organic mental syndrome is characterised by disorientation and clouding of consciousness. If severe, then the full picture of delirium is seen, when there is also bewilderment in association with anxiety, fear, illusions and hallucinations, most frequently visual in type. The condition is characteristically variable in severity from hour to hour, often worse at night and accompanied by restlessness. There are many possible causes (Table 20.1) and it is most important to carry out a complete physical examination in all cases.

Table 20.1   Causes of the acute organic mental syndrome

Organ system	Disease process
Neurological disorders	
Traumatic	Head injury. Epilepsy (post-traumatic)
Infective	Meningitis/encephalitis: bacterial, viral, spirochaetal (neurosyphilis)
Neoplastic	Primary tumour or secondary deposits
Nutritional	Cerebral beri beri
Vascular	Cerebral arteriosclerosis, cerebral haemorrhage or thrombosis
Degenerative	Chronic dementias with acute exacerbation
Idiopathic	Epilepsy
Systemic disorders	
Infections	Sepsis, e.g. tonsillitis, abscesses
Respiratory	Respiratory failure from any cause, e.g. chronic bronchitis, emphysema, bronchopneumonia
Circulatory: Cardiac	Cardiac infarction
Vascular	Shock from any cause
Drug intoxication	Overdose of drugs (alcohol, sedatives, hallucinogens). Bromide accumulation. Withdrawal syndromes including delirium tremens (alcohol, barbiturates)
Hepatic	Liver failure from any cause
Renal	Renal failure from any cause, e.g. nephritis, chronic obstruction due to prostatism
Metabolic disorders	
Nutritional deficiency	Malabsorption states, surgical complications (fistulae, ileus) unbalanced diet
Vitamin deficiency; electrolyte imbalance	Neglect of diet in chronic alcoholism or senility
Endocrine disorders	Addison's disease, Cushing's disease, thyrotoxicosis, myxoedema, diabetes mellitus, insulin overdose
Hyperpyrexia	Heat stroke, status epilepticus
Blood dyscrasias	Addisonian anaemia, leukaemia

The natural history of an acute organic mental disturbance depends on the cause and the effect of treatment on it. In some cases the condition is self-limiting. For example, delirium from drug withdrawal (alcohol, sedatives) in habituated individuals usually ends in a few days, provided complications are avoided by adequate care. Drug withdrawal delirium must always be suspected when such mental disturbance occurs unexpectedly and without obvious cause a few days after admission to hospital for any reason. It is likely that such a patient had not declared his habituation to sedatives or alcohol and then reacted to their sudden cessation at the time of hospital admission.

2. Mental Syndromes Due to Chronic Organic Brain Disorders: The Dementias

Chronic degenerative brain damage if extensive may lead to dementia, which is an acquired impairment of intellectual function. The main characteristics of this chronic organic mental state centre around deficiencies of memory and intellect, with secondary effect on general behaviour. It may be complicated from time to time by episodes of confusion and delirium. The term dementia implies that there has been an actual deterioration in intellectual capacity from the previous personality level.

The dementias are for clinical purposes divided arbitrarily into those in which onset occurs at 65 years or more (the senile dementias), and those which develop earlier (the presenile dementias).

SENILE DEMENTIA

Some progressive deterioration in intellectual ability always occurs after the fourth decade, but in healthy individuals this remains negligible in effect throughout life, and is more than compensated for by accumulated life experience. When disabling intellectual impairment develops after 65 years of age, it is termed senile dementia. The affected individual shows progressively less interest in day-to-day happenings, becomes preoccupied with events of the distant past and increasingly restricted in his activities. Acute confusional episodes with wandering may occur, especially at night, and persecutory delusions may be present. The general physical health is often good initially, but is progressively endangered by self-neglect and physical injury: the latter often occurs during night wandering, especially when ataxia is present.

Senile dementia is usually due to accentuation of normal ageing processes in the brain, although cerebral arteriosclerosis may be a superadded factor. While it is ill-judged to subject a senile individual to needless investigations, it should be remembered that occasionally senile dementia has a treatable cause (e.g. metabolic, neoplastic, vascular, or toxic disorders).

Management of senile dementia is in its early stages possible at home, although this can place a considerable burden on the family. Sedatives should be used sparingly because of the risk of precipitating acute confusion and delirium. Tranquillisers (chlordiazepoxide 5 mg three times daily; promazine 25 to 50 mg three times daily) may help to control agitated and wandering behaviour and hence reduce the likelihood of self-injury. The development of acute confusion may signify coincidental systemic physical complications (infections, cardio-respiratory complications, or metabolic disorders) which should be sought and treated. Advanced dementia leads to a bed-ridden existence, often with double incontinence, and at this stage hospitalisation may well become necessary.

THE PRESENILE DEMENTIAS

Dementia that appears before the age of 65 years is called presenile dementia. It may be due to a variety of causes (Table 20.2).

Table 20.2 Causes of dementia

	Aetiology	Examples
Senile (onset after 65 years)	Usually idiopathic (Accentuation of ageing process ±cerebral arteriosclerosis)	
Presenile (onset usually 40–65 years)	Idiopathic	Altzheimer's disease
	Traumatic	Head (brain) injury Post-traumatic encephalopathy
	Infective	Post-meningitis (acute bacterial or tuberculous) Encephalitis (GPI, viral)
	Vascular	Cerebral arteriosclerosis Cerebrovascular accident (haemorrhage, thrombosis)
	Metabolic	Hypothyroidism Severe hypoglycaemia Pernicious anaemia
	Toxic	Carbon monoxide poisoning Lead poisoning Chronic alcoholism
	Genetic	Huntington's chorea Pick's disease
	Neurological diseases	Cerebellar degeneration Multiple sclerosis Cerebral tumours (primary or secondary) Non-metastatic carcinomatous encephalomyelopathy

Idiopathic

In the majority of cases of presenile dementia, the exact aetiology is unknown. This diagnosis is permissible only after all known causes have been eliminated by full investigation. Prominent in the idiopathic group is the syndrome of Altzheimer's disease, which constitutes about four per cent of all autopsies for presenile dementia. Apart from dementia, this syndrome is often accompanied by lability of mood and tearfulness, with disorientation in place, which leads to a recurrent tendency to get lost. This correlates with marked parietal lobe involvement in the atrophic degenerative brain process which consists of an exaggeration of normal senile changes (neuronal loss, argentophil plaques and neurofibrillary cellular changes).

Traumatic

Severe head injury may cause subsequent dementia if brain damage is sufficiently extensive and diffuse. The severity of this damage, in terms of functional recovery, correlates well with the duration of post-traumatic amnesia, which is defined as that period of time after the injury before continuous memory recall is established.

Prolonged symptoms occasionally develop after relatively trivial head injury, for example when no loss of consciousness or neurological damage has occurred. Such a reaction is likely to be psychological in origin and is called the *post-traumatic syndrome*. It is usually understandable in terms of the person's previous personality and current life situation. Commonly, an element of gain may be detectable, whether it is related to a compensation claim or aimed at influencing the family or job situation. The distinction between unconscious hysterical mechanisms and deliberate malingering is very difficult to make, and neither should be considered before organic factors have been eliminated by thorough physical assessment. Once this has been done, the policy should be to hasten resolution of life situation difficulties. The patient's symptoms will tend to last as long as litigation and compensation claims continue.

Recurrent minor brain injury due to boxing may lead in a small proportion of cases to a picture of chronic post-traumatic encephalopathy. This can develop many years after cessation of the sport and is most usually seen in men aged 50 to 55 years. It consists of neurological symptoms (intention tremor of hands and head, dysarthria, with pyramidal and extrapyramidal signs) as well as psychiatric disturbance (dementia with memory loss, morbid jealousy, rage reactions, impotence).

Infective

Any infection of the central nervous system, whether bacterial, viral or spirochaetal may lead to dementia if the resulting brain damage is diffuse and severe. In the preantibiotic era, dementia was a common complication of those cases of meningitis that survived, particularly in tuberculous meningitis, presumably because here the arteritic process is especially severe. When neurosyphilis is complicated by dementia it is called general paralysis of the insane (GPI), or, if tabetic signs are also present, taboparesis. In the days before the cause was known or adequate therapy available, this disease was a terrible scourge. Esquirol wrote in 1874: 'When paralysis is a complication of dementia, all the paralytic symptoms appear one after the other. First of all articulation of sounds is laboured, soon after locomotion is difficult, finally there is loss of control of excretions.'

In all cases of neurosyphilis it is important to search carefully for evidence of dementia, which usually presents with disordered (usually disinhibited) social behaviour which is out of context with the individual's previous personality, and memory impairment for recent events. GPI presents most commonly with depression, or in ten per cent of cases with a grandiose paranoid psychosis.

Vascular

Severe cerebral arteriosclerosis may lead to dementia in the presenium or later, presumably by impairing cerebral blood supply. It is said that this form of dementia may present in its early stages with severe depression because the patient retains insight into his progressive impairment of memory and intellect. Care should be taken before a dementia is attributed to arteriosclerosis, which in itself is a common finding and may be merely coincidental with a dementia due to a different and possibly treatable cause. A useful clinical rule is to regard arteriosclerosis as a possible cause of dementia only if episodes of vascular accidents have occurred in the past (either cerebral or cardiac) and there is current clinical evidence of severe vascular disease (e.g. as seen in the retinal and peripheral vessels and by measurement of blood pressure).

Metabolic

Hypothyroidism. Severe thyroid deficiency in childhood (cretinism) may, if untreated, lead to permanent retardation of intellectual development. In adults, thyroid deficiency (myxoedema) at first causes impairment of concentration, and memory. If prolonged and severe it may leave a state of irreversible dementia. Early diagnosis and treatment of thyroid deficiency is important if irreversible intellectual impairment is to be prevented.

Hypoglycaemia of mild degree can lead to confusion: when severe it leads to loss of consciousness, and if prolonged it may cause irreversible coma or dementia. These symptoms may be seen in overdose of insulin or in spontaneous hypoglycaemia due to an insulinoma. The effects of hypoglycaemia can be reversed rapidly by glucose, provided this is administered without delay.

Toxic

Prolonged severe hypoxia may lead to irreversible dementia. It is seen most commonly in carbon monoxide poisoning, usually from coal gas. Unconsciousness may, in some cases, be succeeded by full recovery, but occasionally dementia may follow. Late complications may occur, when sudden deterioration with extrapyramidal signs and dementia leading to coma and death can occur about ten days after an initial, apparently full recovery. In order to prevent relapse of this kind, it is wise to treat cases of carbon monoxide with bed rest for one week after recovery of consciousness, taking care, of course, to prevent any complication of bed rest itself (particularly venous thrombosis or chest infection).

Genetic

Huntington's Chorea is inherited in the pattern of a Mendelian dominant gene. The condition is not sex-linked. Its clinical manifestations usually begin between 30 and 50 years of age, and consist of progressive dementia with choreiform involuntary movements. A variety of other psychiatric abnormalities may also occur, for example depression or paranoid states, and affected families have a high incidence of suicide or psychopathic behaviour.

Management of a patient with Huntington's chorea not only involves provision of adequate care of a relentlessly progressive disability for which no specific treatment is yet available, but in addition the family as a whole must be given assistance. Eugenic advice poses problems because by the time the illness declares itself in the patient he or she usually already has children, each of whom has a 50 per cent chance of developing the disease. The only certain way to prevent the disease from being transmitted further is to advise the patient not to have more children, and the existing family members not to plan children of their own. Rigorous directive advice of this kind can be tolerated only by the most robust of families, and it is then usually sought by them directly from the doctor. More frequently, when the family uses denial as a defence mechanism and cannot face up to the possibility that its members may become affected, more harm than good may accrue from such a direct approach unless it is requested. Family members who intend to marry should be encouraged to insure that their prospective partners have been fully informed about the disease.

Pick's Disease is also said to be inherited as a Mendelian dominant. It is a rare cause of presenile dementia, and is characterised by early development of social disinhibition due to frontal lobe degeneration. Focal neurological defects appear as the disease progresses. The characteristic neuropathological picture includes the presence of balloon-like Pick cells and atrophy of brain tissue with marked neuronal loss.

Neurological Disorders

When sufficiently diffuse, neurological disorders may cause dementia. When multiple sclerosis is accompanied by euphoria and emotional deterioration then some degree of dementia is also likely to be present. Whenever dementia occurs in middle age, in the absence of a history of brain damage, the possibility of tumour or GPI must always be considered, especially when focal or localised neurological deficit is present. Frontal tumours may present with disordered behaviour and social disinhibition: neurological signs may be minimal at first.

Differential Diagnosis of Dementia

Poor concentration due to any cause may lead to apparent impairment of memory and intellectual performance.

Depression may in this way present with complaints of memory disturbance and so simulate early dementia.

Schizophrenia may also be mistakenly diagnosed as dementia because of the deterioration in general behaviour due to intense social withdrawal and preoccupation with inner fantasy life. Kraepelin coined the term 'dementia praecox' for schizophrenia and highlighted the apparent intellectual impairment. In fact, provided the patient is prepared to co-operate adequately, psychological testing reveals that in this disease there is not necessarily any deterioration in performance of tests involving intellectual function.

Hysterical Amnesia is usually global or selective for painful material, and understandable as a reaction to stress in the life situation. The patient may also have shown previous histrionic personality traits.

Malingering, which involves a process of conscious deception by the patient who pretends to be disabled when he is not, occasionally takes the form of impairment of memory or other intellectual function. This is most often seen in persons trying to evade legal repercussions of their own misdoings: whatever the cause, the secondary gain is often obvious.

Investigation of Dementia

This is pursued vigorously in presenile cases when general health and longevity are more conducive to radical treatment. While many dementias are not susceptible to specific treatment, a thorough assessment is always necessary in order not to miss those due to treatable causes, for example GPI, myxoedema, or cerebral tumour. Clinical assessment may be followed, where indicated, by *radiological screening* (chest, skull); *metabolic investigations* (thyroid function, serology, blood sugar, insulin tolerance tests); *neurological investigation* (lumbar puncture, air encephalography, angiography or EEG – whilst the EEG may remain normal in advance dementia, in certain conditions such as subdural haematoma, it can be very useful in diagnosis); *psychological investigation* (tests of intelligence, memory and intellectual deterioration).

THE AMNESIC SYNDROME (KORSAKOW PSYCHOSIS)

In this condition there is a highly specific defect of recent memory without other impairment of intellectual function. It is not a dementia. The patient may behave normally, hiding his disability by confabulating false information, and he may be passed as normal unless memory function is specifically tested. Korsakow psychosis may follow beri beri, delirium tremens, severe cerebral anoxia (strangulation, cardiac arrest), ECT, epilepsy, or tumours in the region of the third ventricles. It is associated with degenerative changes in the mid and hind brain, most severe in the mammillary bodies and hippocampus.

B. PSYCHIATRIC REACTIONS TO SYSTEMIC DISEASE AND PHYSICAL EVENTS

Apart from mental phenomena due directly to organic brain disorders, the relationship between non-neurological physical illness and psychological disturbance is also very close. A variety of non-specific psychological reactions may develop in this way, and psychodynamic mechanisms usually play an important aetiological role besides the physico-chemical factors related to the systemic physical disease itself.

REACTION TO MAJOR ILLNESS

Many individuals bear severe illness with remarkable stoicism and from the psychological point of view may be said to have adjusted successfully to their disability. This occurs particularly when the illness develops slowly and takes a chronic course. Severe emotional reactions in terms of anxiety and depression occur more frequently when physical illness appears unheralded and leads to unexpected economic hardship. In the elderly, severe physical illness represents one of the factors predisposing towards suicide.

Convalescence from severe physical illness may be delayed because of secondary emotional factors: prolonged effort intolerance following an episode of cardiac infarction may be entirely psychological in origin and requires appropriate treatment in itself by exploration of the emotional factors involved, and commonsense reassurance that is not so inconsistent as to be rendered ineffective. Any disability that occurs during or after physical illness, and which seems excessive for the amount of physical disorder, should lead to a search for psychological causes.

Terminal illness produces many psychological problems, not the least of which concerns the patient's attitude to dying. In many cases, where the patient defends himself by denying the reality of the situation and does not raise the subject, it is wise to leave the topic alone. When the patient asks for the truth the doctor must decide in each case whether the personality concerned is resilient enough to face it and, if so, exactly how it should be presented.

ENDOCRINE DISORDERS

These are not associated with specific psychiatric syndromes although certain general patterns of psychological disturbance occur.

Thyrotoxicosis

This may closely simulate anxiety state, characterised by tremor, restlessness and agitation, with subjective tension and worry. An underlying thyroid disorder must be considered in any anxiety state when weight loss with good appetite, heat intolerance and high resting pulse are prominent clinical features. Thyrotoxicosis may also be accompanied by depression, and in acute crises there may be delirium: fortunately, this is rarely seen nowadays with adequate therapy.

Myxoedema

This may be complicated by depression, paranoid psychosis, impaired concentration and poor memory for recent events. The depressive symptoms often clear with adequate thyroid substitution, but occasionally this is in itself not sufficient and further measures such as antidepressant drugs or even ECT may be required. Paranoid symptoms if present usually consist of persecutory delusions. Intellectual impairment in myxoedema is at first reversible: excessive delay before institution of adequate therapy may lead to irreversible dementia.

Addison's Disease

This is associated with apathy and mild impairment of recent memory.

Cushing's Disease

This may be complicated by a variety of psychological disturbances: depression is found in 75 per cent of cases, accompanied by either agitation or retardation. Paranoid episodes may occur, or periodic excitement with grossly disturbed behaviour. Euphoria is rarely found; this is in contrast to steroid therapy (ACTH, cortisone, prednisone) which may be accompanied by elevation of mood (in 50 per cent of cases) or psychotic disturbance with delusions or hallucinations (in 5 per cent of cases) sometimes with disorientation.

Insulin

These effects have already been considered.

EPILEPSY

Related to Ictus

Preictal-epileptic Aura. These are characteristically short-lasting (seconds), and thus may be differentiated from migrainous phenomena such as teichopsia which may last up to an hour or so. Epileptic aura due to temporal lobe epilepsy may be experienced as recurrent episodes of anxiety and fear, often rising from the epigastrium.

Ictal. In temporal lobe epilepsy, the fit itself may involve complicated automatic motor behaviour which is not necessarily accompanied by convulsions.

Postictal. Temporal lobe epilepsy may lead to automatic behaviour and clouded consciousness over several hours (postepileptic automatism). Sometimes a series of epileptic fits is followed by an acute paranoid hallucinatory state.

Personality Changes

A long-standing epileptic sometimes presents the picture of irritability and slowness in mental activity. This is usually due to chronic oversedation, or a reaction to the disability imposed by the illness together with frustration at society's intolerance towards him.

Schizophrenic-like Psychosis in Temporal Lobe Epilepsy

A psychosis closely resembling schizophrenia develops in some cases of long-standing temporal lobe epilepsy: other types of epilepsy do not lead to this complication. The mental illness usually comes on some ten years after epilepsy began and often at a time when the epileptic fits have become less frequent.

PSYCHIATRIC COMPLICATIONS OF SURGERY AND CHILDBIRTH

Postoperative Psychosis

This is an acute mental reaction following a surgical operation. It should be seen as a reaction to the total situation, and psychological causes predominate. The true incidence and clinical picture are difficult to assess because minor upsets after surgery tend not to be referred for psychiatric opinion. Severe reactions sufficient to lead to admission to a psychiatric hospital have been estimated to complicate 1/1,600 surgical operations. The clinical picture in these cases may take a variety of forms, for example depression, mania, schizophrenia, or confusional state. The disturbance either follows immediately upon the operation or develops within a few days of it. Certain surgical procedures, for example hysterectomy or open heart surgery, tend to be associated with a higher incidence of subsequent mental upset than others, and it is relevant that the emotional significance of the operation is probably greater in these cases.

Puerperal Psychosis

This may be defined as a psychotic illness developing within six months after childbirth: most cases occur in the puerperium (four weeks immediately following the delivery). The causes are probably multifactorial. The sudden complex endocrine and other physical changes following upon childbirth, together with the emotional stress of the pregnancy, labour and the arrival of a dependent infant all contribute to precipitation of mental breakdown in a vulnerable individual.

Minor transient mood disturbance is common, almost universal, in the first few days after childbirth. Florid puerperal psychosis is much less common (0.7 per 100 live births, with a recurrence rate of 35 per 100 subsequent pregnancies).

The psychotic puerperal reaction can cause severe disturbance of behaviour, and may resemble confusional states, depression, mania, or schizophrenic illness. Occasionally, the child's safety is endangered. This applies in any case where a severely disturbed mother is left in charge of the infant, but it is a particular problem when severe depressive features are present. The mother may then entertain suicidal ideas possibly with homicidal impulses towards the child. These symptoms are an integral part of the depressed state, and they are usually accompanied by delusions of self-blame and futility about the future.

In the differential diagnosis of postoperative and puerperal psychoses, the three important alternatives to consider are organic mental states, drug withdrawal states or neurotic reactions.

It is important that postoperative and puerperal patients who develop psychiatric complications should be examined carefully for physical complications, especially when mental symptoms follow within a few days of the physical event. In a disturbed patient it can be difficult to differentiate a functional (non-organic) mental state from a confusion due to organic factors (e.g. blood loss, vitamin deficiency, metabolic disturbance, or

444

drug withdrawal in a habituated individual), and physical assessment should always be carried out.

One of the commonest causes of sudden and unexpected disturbance of mental state starting within a few days of hospital admission is alcohol withdrawal in an addicted individual. Restlessness, agitation, aggression, confusion, and delirium may be found. The true cause is often not recognised because the patient may not spontaneously admit to dependence on alcohol. Less commonly, withdrawal of sedative drugs (usually barbiturates) in an addicted individual may lead to a similar mental syndrome.

These may also be seen after operations or childbirth, and they are usually understandable in the light of the patient's previous personality. A rigid obsessional personality may develop accentuation of obsessional traits, with unreasonable fears, checking, or ritualistic behaviour. Obsessional fears, of harming the baby are not uncommon in the puerperium, and provided they have all the criteria of obsessional symptoms (*see* page 466) they are harmless, and can be distinguished from the true homicidal impulses of a severe depression reaction. Specialist advice should be sought if in doubt. The possibility that symptoms may have a hysterical basis should be considered when a patient has shown previous histrionic personality traits, especially if there has been a previous history of hysterical illness.

Treatment of postoperative and puerperal mental disorders should consist in the first instance of adequate therapy for any physical complications (infection, blood loss, metabolic or nutritional). The disturbance in mental state may require symptomatic treatment with tranquillisers (in grossly disturbed behaviour or schizophrenic reactions) or antidepressants. When depression is marked, ECT may be necessary, especially when the suicide risk is high. The patient may have to be transferred to a psychiatric ward because of behaviour disturbance. Where possible, a mother should continue to care for her baby, but when there is severe disturbance of mental state, and the baby is thought to be in danger, the mother should not be allowed full charge of the child until clinical assessment is reassuring on this point. Prevention of postoperative mental reactions might be possible by adequate preoperative psychological preparation of the patient, especially in vulnerable individuals with a history of previous episodes of mental illness or in operations such as hysterectomy or open heart surgery which carry an increased risk of psychiatric complications. When surgery is carried out in emergency situations such preparation is, of course, difficult to achieve. Puerperal psychosis is more common in those women who have entertained a considerable amount of somatic symptoms during pregnancy. The majority of postoperative

and puerperal reactions settle very quickly. Occasionally, a puerperal psychosis of the schizophrenic kind may lead to prolonged disability, but most resolve quickly and one short episode is not in itself an indication for termination of further pregnancies. However, a history of recurrent puerperal psychoses, or one severe schizophrenic-type puerperal breakdown might justify termination of a subsequent pregnancy on psychiatric grounds in view of the high probability that similar difficulties will recur.

C. THE PSYCHOSOMATIC ILLNESS

In this group of illnesses, although somatic disturbance may appear to be the most obvious clinical feature, it is likely that psychological factors are important both in the initiation and continuation of the disease. It is of course possible that any emotional upset which accompanies physical disease is merely secondary to the physical disability, and it can be difficult to prove retrospectively that mental disturbance antedated the somatic disorder. There is much evidence to suggest, however, that chronic emotional problems such as anxiety, unresolved conflict, suppressed hostility and anger may be contributory aetiological factors in the psychosomatic conditions. These include bronchial asthma, ulcerative colitis, rheumatoid arthritis, certain skin diseases, peptic ulcer, migraine, essential hypertension and possibly even coronary artery disease, to quote the best known examples. This view is supported by the fact that relapse in these conditions may be precipitated by acute emotional upset.

Inherent in the concept of psychosomatic disease is the principle that treatment must be aimed at both physical and psychological factors. The psychological approach can contribute very considerably and it pays particular attention to:

1. Emotional upset, particularly anxiety, depression, resentment and frustration due to difficulty in accepting the illness itself and its resulting disabilities.
2. Problems in relationship to other key individuals in the patient's life, perhaps themselves emotionally upset, or hostile and impatient when they in turn resent the illness. In such circumstances they may tend to attribute the patient's symptoms to deliberate manipulation.
3. Problems which antedate the illness, only to be accentuated by it: personality vulnerability and long-standing marital difficulties are perhaps the most common.

A careful history, with particular attention to the temporal sequence of symptom development should clarify these points. It should be remembered that the precise significance of a stressful event, its psychopathological impact, may vary considerably from one individual to another depending on the premorbid personality and particular life situation.

Though little success has been achieved in trying to associate specific personality characteristics with the various psychosomatic syndromes, some are worthy of mention. Migraine sufferers are often ambitious, tense and anxious, and chronic asthma may sometimes be related to suppressed anger and inability to verbalise feelings. In ulcerative colitis there may be traits of over-dependence and inability to express aggressive feelings directly. It is well recognised that relapse may be closely related to an upsetting life event. Interesting though these themes may be, there is much individual variation and there can be no substitute for a careful history in each case.

The patient with a psychosomatic problem may refuse to accept a psychological cause for his symptoms and he frequently continues to press for an organic explanation. Finding common ground which permits further psychological exploration is a challenging clinical task. Relaxation therapy which focusses on the somatic aspects of anxiety is often very useful in this respect and close collaboration with a clinical psychologist is the best approach.

PSYCHOLOGICAL DISORDERS OF FOOD INTAKE

These illustrate the close relationship that may exist between somatic and psychological aspects of disease. Bodily nutrition may become markedly disturbed as a result of a variety of psychiatric syndromes. *Depressive states* often lead to weight loss due to impairment of appetite, sometimes related to morbid guilt. Less often, depression is accompanied by weight increase due to overeating which relieves a feeling of unpleasant subjective tension. *Schizophrenic psychoses* often lead to gross malnutrition and weight loss through self-neglect. Occasionally, food is avoided because of paranoid delusions about being poisoned. *Alcoholism* may be complicated by obesity and avitaminosis due to high calorie intake in the form of alcohol without an adequate balanced diet. In the later stages there may be marked weight loss particularly when other physical complications have occurred. *Drug addiction* may cause severe weight loss due to neglect of diet or complicating physical illness. *Phobic anxiety* can lead to fears of choking which render the patient unable to swallow solids. Such fears may make it necessary to take only a milk diet over many years.

ANOREXIA NERVOSA

First described by Gull, 1874, and Lasegue, 1873, anorexia nervosa is a syndrome characterised by self-imposed starvation with particular avoidance of high calorie foods, and an intense preoccupation with a need to avoid fatness and to be thin. It may result in severe weight loss, alternating in some cases with episodes of overeating and obesity. When the illness occurs in the female, amenorrhoea is invariably found during its active stages and may actually precede weight loss.

Clinical Features

The illness usually begins in young adults aged 15 to 25 years. It occurs more commonly in the upper social classes and is ten times more frequent in females than in males. The onset may be sudden, when some life upset is usually significant, or gradual out of life-long behavioural difficulties. Intense preoccupation with a need to be thin or avoidance of fatness leads to reduction of food intake, particularly concerning foods high in calorie content, and to progressive weight loss which in extreme cases may become life-threatening. The limbs are cold and cyanosed, and bradycardia is common. Hunger is not necessarily lost. In many cases it may remain normal, or its intensity may cause the patient distress. Subterfuges such as hiding or throwing away food, self-induced vomiting or excessive exercising or purgation may be used as ways of avoiding calorie intake or countering its effects. Secondary sexual development (size of genitalia and breasts, presence of axillary and pubic hair) is normal. The patient may appear indifferent to her own emaciation, or she may show intense anxiety over her weight, usually concerning the possibility of being or becoming fat. There may be distortion of self-assessment of body image, in which the patient claims she is obese even when weight loss is severe. Depressive symptoms are also sometimes seen and obsessional features occur in about twenty per cent of all cases. No schizophrenic features are to be found in typical anorexia nervosa. The patient often shows an intense emotional involvement with the parents, who generally show much distress over her eating difficulties. She may try to control the food intake and other activities of relatives, pressing them to eat excessively and preparing food for them though she takes little herself.

Background

The severe cases seen in hospital practice are uncommon, but minor non-hospitalised forms of the syndrome occur much more frequently. A recent survey of female students in Bristol University revealed that two per cent had experienced an episode of anorexia nervosa at some time. There is some evidence that there has been a real increase in the incidence of this disorder in recent years. It is tempting to attribute some relationship between this and the current popularity of being slim, a fashion which is of course most common in upper class females.

Predisposing Factors. These consist of psychological difficulties which impair the individual's ability to cope with precipitating events. The causes of the predisposing vulnerability in persons destined to develop anorexia nervosa are obscure. The fact that mental illness is common in other members of the family (usually anxiety or depression) makes it likely that disordered family processes play a part in predisposing children to anorexia nervosa-type illness at puberty. It is always difficult to be sure whether family disturbance has antedated the illness, because secondary upset in relatives as a result of the patient's food refusal is usually in itself severe. The parents are often socially mobile upwards, with high aspirations both for themselves and for their children. In such a family a child may have an inordinate need to achieve instilled into it, and this may lead to anorexic psychopathology, especially when the child's ability is discrepant from the expectations of others. There is no convincing evidence to suggest any primary neurological or endocrine cause for anorexia nervosa.

Precipitating Factors. When vulnerability is severe, there may be no particular life upset to precipitate the illness, but other cases appear to become ill at a time of precipitating stress which probably acts in a non-specific way. It is commonly some aspect of adolescence, the stress of incidental physical disease or disharmony with family or peers.

Hysterical mechanisms have long been regarded as important in anorexia nervosa, probably because of the controlling influence the patient appears to exert on other persons or situations and the apparent unconcern she may show at her own condition. Thus the girl who fears sexual maturation may avoid what it entails by self-imposed weight loss which in itself lessens the chance of heterosexual contact by rendering her physically unattractive and reduces her own sexual interest. In others, the illness may lead to avoidance of emancipation from home, or in those who lack confidence in these respects, assumption of adult responsibilities. Under stress the vulnerable individual develops an abnormal investment in food avoidance and weight loss, equating it with self-control, a sense of achievement in the face of other real or imagined failures, and viewing it as an insurance, albeit a distorted one, against future difficulties.

The greater incidence of anorexia nervosa in females is not easy to explain. It may be that adolescence is more stressful in the female, reflecting not only biological but also personality differences between the sexes.

Differential Diagnosis

1. Depression in adolescence may lead to anorexia and weight loss, but fear of weight gain is absent.

2. Physical illness. Hypothalamic or pituitary disorders may cause amenorrhoea, but weight loss is not severe and there is usually poorly developed or loss of secondary sexual characteristics. Tuberculosis was at one time an important differential diagnosis: Gull pointed out that the emaciated tuberculous patient does not show the abundant physical energy and overactivity seen in anorexia nervosa. Persistent tachycardia, fever, marked anaemia or raised blood viscosity are not found in uncomplicated anorexia nervosa, and they indicate organic disease. Thyroid function tests are useful when thyrotoxicosis is suspected, because in anorexia nervosa there is no significant hyperfunction of the thyroid gland.

Complications

1. Peripheral oedema.
2. Electrolyte depletion (especially hypokalaemia when vomiting is persistent or purgative abuse present).
3. Moderate anaemia (Hb: 10 g/100 ml).
4. Follicular hyperkeratosis with lanugo-type hair on trunk.
5. Severe inanition which may be fatal.

Basis of Treatment

This is aimed at resolving both the emotional conflicts within the patient and the relevant environmental factors. The parents may need to be involved in therapy, especially when family pathology is thought to be significant. It is always difficult to break through the patient's psychological defences in order to achieve a radical change in attitudes. Discussion of causes is rendered ineffective if too much attention is paid to the rationalisation of the patient regarding the reasons for food refusal. Management varies from permissiveness, arising from recognition that eating difficulty is related to deeper emotional problems which themselves must be treated, to a firm control of dietary intake, which may in any case be necessary when weight loss is life-threatening. This authoritarian approach can in certain cases lead to a temporary rapid improvement in attitudes as weight increase occurs.

Admission to hospital is advisable if the body weight is falling persistently and rapidly. There is considerable danger of physical complications if the weight falls to the region of 60 per cent of what it would be in the average person of the same sex, age and height (Geigy Scientific Tables).

A patient who progressively loses weight in spite of hospitalisation is probably resorting to various subterfuges and should be confined to bed and allowed to get up only to the bedside commode until weight control is achieved. The use of tranquillisers such as chlorpromazine has been recommended as a way of increasing food intake presumably by reducing anxiety. Modified insulin has no valid place in therapy. There is usually no want of appetite in anorexia nervosa, merely anxiety as a reaction to it.

Prognosis

Cases of anorexia nervosa followed up several years after hospital treatment show a wide variety of outcome, ranging from recovery or considerable improvement with normal weight and menstruation (39 per cent), through intermediate degrees of disability (29 per cent), to poor outcome with continuing severe weight loss, menstrual and other difficulties (29 per cent). The mortality rate (5 to 10 per cent) is by no means negligible.

PSYCHOGENIC (FUNCTIONAL) VOMITING

This is a syndrome of persistent vomiting in the absence of organic disease. Sometimes the vomiting is mechanically self-induced, but often it appears to be involuntary. It occurs most often in young adult females, and is occasionally severe enough to cause weight loss, hyponatraemia and hypokalaemia. In a proportion of patients there may be a clear association with some kind of psychological upset, particularly in the nature of conflict. In others it may be a learnt mechanism of anxiety reduction. Occasionally, the vomiting may be part of the anorexia nervosa syndrome. Frequently there is no clear psychological cause, though concern over the vomiting itself is often marked. It is not always easy to exclude organic abdominal disease and if the patient complains of other gut dysfunction, abdominal discomfort or pain, then combined management between physician and psychiatrist may be necessary at least in order to follow all diagnostic possibilities. Not uncommonly, both psychological and organic factors are important, as in those patients with peptic ulcer who deliberately induce vomiting because it leads to relief of pain. Psychogenic vomiting can be a most intractable condition. When precipitating factors are clear and can be resolved, then recovery may be complete, although subsequent relapses may occur.

ABDOMINAL HYPOCHONDRIACAL SYNDROMES

Weight loss may occur when food intake is reduced as a result of hypochondriacal fears concerning the gastrointestinal tract. The precise content of such anxieties may vary within wide limits, although they most commonly involve worry that eating may reactivate or cause organic gut disease. Such fears are an important cause of delayed convalescence following abdominal surgery. Extreme food fads may occur and there may be eccentric and bizarre ideas concerning the effects of food intake on gut function. When the main preoccupation is with bowel evacuation, then chronic abuse of purgatives is a common complication.

A depressive illness sometimes presents with hypochondriacal fears, and it is important to search for symptoms indicative of severe depression in every patient. Careful assessment may sometimes reveal the hypochondriasis to be part of the anorexia nervosa syndrome.

Extended supportive psychotherapy is usually necessary with exploration of the life situation for possible precipitating events. Dietary guidance is indicated and it may be necessary to resort to a liquid diet initially if weight loss has been severe.

OBESITY

Obesity is more frequent in the lower social classes and its incidence increases with age, particularly in women. It is the commonest nutritional disorder in the United Kingdom, and its harmful effects on physical health are in themselves serious. Causes may be familial, possibly genetic in nature or related to faulty early family experience of food intake. Psychological disturbance is found in a small proportion of obese individuals, and it is not easy to determine whether it is causal or merely a secondary complication. Overeating may be a source of comfort in persons who are tense, anxious or depressed, and such distortion of the normal process of food intake by emotional factors is probably an important cause of chronic obesity.

Mild obesity of late onset may respond to group pressures and support, for example the kind offered by Weight Watchers, but those with emotional difficulties may need psychiatric help. The aim should be to provide individual support over an extended period, concentrating on the underlying psychological problems rather than direct confrontation over repeated failure to reduce food intake. Gradual weight reduction is probably better than sudden major loss, because it is more likely to be accompanied by a general readjustment in eating behaviour. Psychiatric assessment should always be carried out in those cases of resistent severe obesity in which more radical procedures such as jaw wiring or intestinal by-pass surgery are contemplated. The psychiatric complications of such operative intervention are themselves by no means negligible.

II. THE ADDICTIONS

Definition

Addiction to drugs or alcohol consists of an excessive dependence on them, resulting in repetitive intake of such a degree that it interferes with the patient's physical, interpersonal, and economic well-being.

Dependence of this kind has both psychological and physical components. In psychological terms the addictive agent is regarded by the patient as an indispensable prop in life and this attitude results in poor motivation towards abstinence. Chemical dependence is due to the direct effect of the addictive agent on the body: it results in unpleasant side effects when abstinence is attempted, and so furthers the continuation of the addiction. Most addictive agents lead to a state of chemical tolerance, whereby regular intake causes progressively less desired effect and so the addicted individual has to take increasing amounts to obtain adequate satisfaction.

CHRONIC ALCOHOLISM

Background

The distinction between socially acceptable drinking patterns and alcohol addiction is often difficult to make, because considerable cross cultural variation is found in the extent to which alcohol intake and intoxication is tolerated by society. The definition of alcohol addiction requires that the intake should be excessive, repetitive, and to an extent that it interferes with the person's physical, economic, and social (usually family) well-being. The presence of withdrawal symptoms often provides added confirmation of an addictive drinking pattern.

Estimates of incidence of chronic alcoholism range from 1/1,000 to 11/1,000 of the adult population. High-risk groups include business executives, publicans, barmen, and members of the armed forces. Alcoholism is a major problem in industry in terms of absenteeism and loss of efficiency. Surveys of patients in medical and surgical hospital wards have shown that about thirteen per cent have a 'drink problem' which is probably high in this group because it so often itself precipitates physical illness.

Predisposing Factors. The causes of alcoholism in terms of predisposing factors consist of personality difficulties which probably stem from genetic make up together with early family and childhood stresses. The parents of alcoholics show a greater than average incidence of chronic alcoholism. It is difficult to say whether this familial incidence reflects hereditary factors or is merely due to pathogenic effects of parental alcoholic behaviour on the children. The precise personality vulnerability which predisposes to alcoholism may take various forms. Anxieties of various kinds are often marked, particularly social anxieties and lack of confidence in meeting people. Any psychological difficulty that is eased by the relaxation induced by alcohol must be regarded as important in this respect.

Precipitating Factors. Precipitating factors usually take the form of *opportunity* and *example*. Occupations that involve regular contact with alcoholic beverages (e.g. handling them by publicans or their use in entertainment by executives) carry a high risk in this way. Example is important when a vulnerable individual finds himself in a group in which it is fashionable to

depend a great deal on alcohol intake to facilitate social activities (armed forces, clubs, business).

Symptoms

Acute Inebriation. Alcohol is essentially a depressant of the central nervous system. Severe overdose leads to loss of consciousness, even coma and death either due to direct chemical effects, or from complications such as inhalation of vomit, pneumonia, injury or exposure. Acute inebriation not involving loss of consciousness may range from relaxation with feelings of confidence, renewed energy and efficiency, to noisy, disinhibited, often aggressive, behaviour with gross inco-ordination.

Chronic Alcohol Addiction. This is usually punctuated by episodes of acute inebriation. The pattern may consist of regular sprees of drunkenness with intervening variable periods of complete abstinence (loss of control), or regular excessive daily intake over months or years, usually gradually increasing in amount (inability to abstain).

It is important to detect the disease in its early stages when it is easiest to reverse the harmful effects on the individual and others. Suspicions should be aroused when solitary drinking develops in a person who previously has drunk only in a social setting, particularly when he resents the fact being discussed, or he dismisses it in spite of obvious harmful repercussions on his job, family, or health. He may try to minimise the extent of his drinking by hiding bottles or other evidence of his drinking. The development of morning tremor, which necessitates alcohol intake before or instead of breakfast to 'steady his nerves', or amnesic spells in which he is unable to recollect events of the previous evening (although not very inebriate at the time), are useful as early diagnostic features. The patient's attitude in the early stages of the disease is usually one of rationalisation whereby he denies to himself the possibility that he might be an alcoholic. In the later stages, when the ravages of the disease are obvious to all, and regrettably sometimes irrevocable, he may accept more easily that he is ill. Occasionally, he resorts to the defence mechanism of projection, and blames all others except himself for his predicament. By this time he may have lost his job, and his wife has probably left him: the resulting social isolation reinforces his drinking. A vicious circle has then developed and treatment becomes doubly difficult. In some individuals, usually in those with severe predisposing personality vulnerability, the devastating social deterioration produced by the disease leads to the tramp-like existence of the 'skid row' alcoholic.

Investigations

Assessment of a patient suffering from chronic alcoholism must include interview with other informants (relative, friends) in order to obtain an objective view of the

449

severity of the problem. The account obtained from the patient himself is usually distorted by rationalisation, paranoid projection, and gross minimisation of the alcohol intake and its repercussions. In view of the large number of physical complications that may occur, it is necessary to supplement full physical examination with adequate investigations.

Complications

Acute Intoxication. This occurs episodically throughout the illness with increased risk of accidental self-injury or antisocial and violent behaviour. During subsequent remorse there may be suicidal impulses.

Withdrawal Syndrome. When alcohol is discontinued after prolonged daily intake that has led to a state of neurological tolerance, there may follow a series of symptoms due to resulting overactivity of the nervous system. Thiamine deficiency may be an added aetiological factor in some cases. Tremor begins in twelve hours, and there may follow epileptic fits and, in severe cases, full delirium tremens is seen, usually two or three days after alcohol withdrawal. The patient then shows severe restlessness, anxiety, visual hallucinations and illusions, disorientation and confusion. Minor confusional forms of this syndrome often occur in patients admitted to hospital for other reasons, e.g. medical or surgical emergencies, and the true cause is often unrecognised. Although usually self-limiting, delirium tremens requires careful treatment. Mortality rates in reported series have been in the order of fourteen per cent and death may be due to injury, hyperpyrexia, bronchopneumonia or status epilepticus.

Other Physical Complications. Peripheral neuropathy, cardiomyopathy, gastritis, peptic ulcer, hepatic cirrhosis, pancreatitis, pulmonary tuberculosis, cumulative effects of recurrent trauma.

Other Psychological Complications. Defect of recent memory (Korsakow psychosis), possibly more global types of dementia, paranoid attitudes, morbid jealousy, impotence. The risk of suicide is high. In one study, eight per cent of chronic alcoholics who had received in-patient psychiatric treatment committed suicide within a few years of discharge, their suicide rate being eight times the national average. Up to half of all cases of self-injury or self-overdose are carried out under the influence of recent alcohol intake, and up to one-third of such patients have a chronic drink problem. Persons suffering from recurrent depressive illness who use alcohol to excess are highly vulnerable with regard to suicide.

Basis of Treatment

Detoxification. It is usually necessary to admit a newly diagnosed case to hospital for full physical and psychological investigations. This is particularly important when acute withdrawal symptoms are anticipated (for example when daily intake of alcohol has extended over the immediately preceding three months or more: delirium tremens is unlikely to follow a shorter spell of daily drinking). In the acute stages, the aims are to remove alcohol completely and restore physical health and nutrition to normal. A florid withdrawal syndrome requires adequate sedation in the form of chlordiazepoxide (up to 50 mg four times if necessary). Promazine (up to 100 mg daily) may also be used in preference to chlorpromazine which tends to be more hepatotoxic. The extreme agitation may lead to injury unless it is fully controlled. Adequate fluid intake must be maintained, and if fits supervene it is necessary to use full anticonvulsant medication. These may be started immediately on admission in a preventive capacity if there has been a previous history of delirium tremens with fits. Insomnia is a frequent symptom in chronic alcoholism, and should never be treated with potentially addictive drugs such as barbiturates.

Antabuse is useful in certain patients who are reliable enough to appreciate the full implications of its use. It acts by blocking alcohol metabolism at the stage of acetaldehyde, which then causes severe vomiting when alcohol is taken. It should not be given unless there has been a test reaction in hospital, and its use is not appropriate if serious physical disease is present, particularly in the case of hepatic or cardiovascular disorders.

Treatment of the Addiction Itself. This is always difficult. It requires enthusiasm and persistence, and depends on individual and group psychotherapy. In the former, a one-to-one relationship is established between patient and therapist, in which it is necessary to point out the patient's rationalisation and plausible explanation for his behaviour. To succeed, it requires good motivation on the part of the patient.

Group support is perhaps the most effective form of therapy, whether in the form of Alcoholics Anonymous meetings or formal group psychotherapy with other alcoholic patients.

Hospitalisation, essential in the preliminary stages of detoxification, can have limitations in the treatment of the addiction itself. Unless special provisions are made it may even produce harmful effects by encouraging the patient to retreat from his problems, and to deny his illness, or by minimising self-help. A very useful setting for treatment of the addiction is in a hostel specifically devoted to this purpose, providing group support yet insisting that the patient adopts a self-helping attitude living and working in the community.

Prognosis

The eventual outcome depends on the patient's motivation and the amount of support available for him. Those who attend AA, request antabuse, still have their family support, and show good previous personality tend to have the best outlook. There may be several relapses before the patient becomes sufficiently well motivated. 'Skid row' alcoholics are usually so deteriorated that it may not be feasible to talk in terms of complete cure, although a hostel setting may achieve dramatic improvement by providing long term specialised support.

HEROIN AND MORPHINE ADDICTION

Addiction to opiate drugs is by far the most severe form of drug dependence. Heroin in particular tends to cause severe deterioration in personality and behaviour. Cocaine is often taken with heroin to counteract the inhibitory effects of the latter. So strong is the addiction that it exerts a marked control of the person's behaviour, and deception and theft will be committed if necessary in order to ensure a continuing supply of the drug. It follows, as in every type of addiction, that an objective appraisal of the drug intake may be obtained only by thorough checking, for example by interviews with others besides the patient, or assay of drug levels in body fluids.

Background

Until 1960, the problem of opiate addiction in the UK was small and circumscribed, occurring almost entirely in medical and nursing personnel (probably arising out of ease of access to drugs), or in persons who had received opiates in a therapeutic way for some chronic painful disease. The Brain Committee reported in 1961 that the problem was at that time contained, and it did not recommend the compulsory registration of addicts. The Committee was reconvened in 1965, when the situation had changed dramatically with a 500 per cent increase in known heroin addicts (68 to 342) and a 600 per cent rise in cocaine abuse (30 to 211). The rapid increase had occurred mainly in young persons who were neither members of the medical or nursing profession, nor had their addiction arisen out of the therapeutic use of opiates (Fig. 20.3). Overprescribing by a few medical practitioners was blamed by the Committee for the increase in drug addiction, and legislation followed concerning certain drugs in Part I of the 1965 Dangerous Drugs Act. Medical practitioners in the UK are now prohibited from administering, or authorising the administration of, heroin or cocaine to any person for the purpose of treating addiction, except under a licence issued by the Secretary of State. (This prohibition does not apply if an addict or any other person requires heroin or cocaine for the relief of pain due to organic disease or injury.) Medical practitioners are also now required to notify to The Chief Medical Officer of the Home Office, Whitehall, London SW1, particulars of persons with whom they have professional contact who

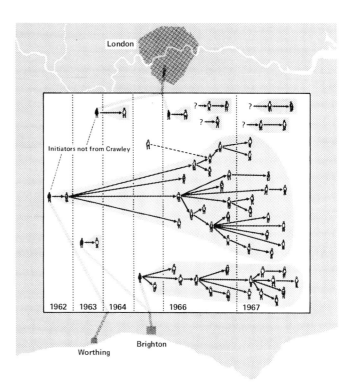

Fig. 20.3 Case to case spread of heroin abuse in Crawley New Town.
(*From* de Alarcon. *Bulletin on Narcotics,* **Vol XXI,** No. 3.)

are addicted to heroin or any of the compounds listed in the Schedule of the Misuse of Drugs (Notification of and Supply to Addicts) Regulations 1973. These are illustrated below.

Controlled drugs to which the Misuse of Drugs (notification of and supply to addicts) Regulations 1973 apply

1. The following substances and products:

Cocaine	Methadone
Dextromoramide	Morphine
Diamorphine	Opium
Dipipanone	Oxycodone
Hydrocodone	Pethidine
Hydromorphone	Phenazocine
Levorphanol	Piritramide

2. Any stereoisomeric form of a substance specified above, not being dextrorphan.

3. Any ester or ether of a substance specified above, not being a substance for the time being specified in Part II of Schedule 2 to the Misuse of Drugs Act 1971.

4. Any salt of any substance specified above.

5. Any preparation or other product containing a substance or product specified above.

As in chronic alcoholism, addiction to heroin arises out of a combination of predisposing and precipitating factors, in other words, personality difficulties combined with opportunities and example. Most, if not all, heroin addicts have severe personality difficulties which they try to solve by the addiction.

Symptoms

The early stages of opiate addiction may be characterised by secrecy of behaviour, reticence towards other members of the family and gross fluctuations in behaviour from placid contentedness to restless irritability. Blood staining on clothes (resulting from injections), coryza, red eyes, and rhinorrhoea may also occur. Physical examination should include a search for injection marks (particularly over veins), or multiple superficial venous thromboses.

In well-established opiate addiction, there is usually marked impairment of general efficiency, unemployment, and unstable social relationships. Only very few can find a stable solution to their problems in opiate drugs, because rapid tolerance effects usually necessitate progressive increase of dosage required to produce the desired symptoms.

Complications

Overdose. This is often accidental, and is most frequently seen when the patient has been discharged after a spell of abstinence in hospital. Loss of tolerance may result in dangerous coma if the previously accustomed dosage is used again immediately, and this is one of the reasons for the high mortality associated with opiate addiction (20 × expected for age).

Withdrawal Symptoms. Complete withdrawal in an addicted individual may be followed in 6 to 12 hours by anxiety, anorexia, perspiration, yawning, gooseflesh, tremors and, in severe cases, vomiting and diarrhoea, with raised blood pressure and tachycardia. It is out of consideration for these unpleasant effects that withdrawal, when attempted, should always be gradual. It is highly likely that the addict will overemphasise the severity of withdrawal symptoms and the doctor should not allow his medication to be controlled too easily in this way.

Sepsis. Local infection due to faulty injection technique may progress to septicaemia, which is occasionally a fatal complication in heroin addiction.

Virus B Hepatitis is also regularly seen due to faulty injection techniques.

Cocainism may result from excessive use of cocaine, and is characterised by paranoid delusions and paraesthesiae.

Suicide. Severe mood disorder and suicide may also occur, usually by deliberate massive overdose of the addictive agent or other drugs.

Basis of Treatment

Opiate addiction is one of the most difficult of all psychiatric conditions to treat. A patient presenting for the first time with this type of addiction should be offered hospital admission with a view to gradual withdrawal under the cover of tranquilliser drugs, if necessary with temporary transition to methadone before complete withdrawal. Many addicts refuse this regime and demand long term maintenance supplies of heroin or other opiates. It is doubtful whether this is justifiable in more than a very small proportion of addicts, if at all, and it should not be embarked upon without full hospital assessment. Most areas of the UK now have treatment centres to which opiate addicts should be referred. The 1968 Regulations in effect insist that heroin is not prescribed for the purpose of treating addiction except by specialists with relevant experience. All addicts require a great deal of continuing personal support and interest, particularly when they are attempting to give up the addiction.

Heroin addicts often present themselves in hospitals with urgent requests for supply of the drug, usually saying that they are temporary residents or have mislaid their prescriptions, messed up an injection, or lost their supply. Sometimes, of course, this story is true, but more often it is a fabrication. The first step is to check immediately by telephone with the centre currently supplying the patient's drugs, or with the Home Office Register. If the story then sounds true, and provided the appropriate agency agrees, it may be reasonable to offer methadone linctus (10 to 20 mg with repeat in twelve hours) provided the patient is not vomiting, with the advice that the patient should return to his treatment centre as soon as possible. It is never necessary to give morphine or heroin in such an emergency, and most cases can be adequately managed by giving only a tranquillising drug such as chlorpromazine. Only by adopting such stringent measures can overprescribing and resulting spread of addiction in the community be avoided. Unfortunately, stringent control of the availability of drugs through medical prescription is easily vitiated by burglaries of retail chemist shops that usually involve remarkably large amounts of drugs.

Prognosis

In opiate addiction the prognosis is often poor, particularly when heroin is the addictive agent and there is evidence of severe preceding personality problems. When the addiction is of long standing, treatment is particularly difficult because by this time the whole life pattern has become centred around the addiction and only very radical reorientation of attitudes and habits will effect a cure.

Follow-up studies suggest that about one-third of all opiate addicts may eventually stop drug misuse on their own initiative.

BARBITURATE ADDICTION

Although barbiturates are most effective sedatives, they should always be used with caution because of their addictive propensities. Their use is justified as hypnotics in acute illnesses for short periods when other sedatives fail, but they are not justified in long term management of insomnia or in the form of prolonged day-time therapy for anxiety. Tolerance may occur, and a typical withdrawal syndrome similar to that in alcoholism, including delirium tremens, may then follow sudden cessation of drug intake. Subcutaneous administration of barbiturates by addicts sometimes causes severe local tissue necrosis.

AMPHETAMINE, METHEDRINE ABUSE

These are stimulants that induce euphoria with a sense of abundant physical energy. True chemical dependence does not occur, but withdrawal may be accompanied by severe depression. Acute overdose may produce a paranoid hallucinatory state in which visual experiences predominate. Chronic amphetamine abuse may be complicated by a paranoid psychosis (with persecutory ideas and auditory hallucinations) resembling chronic schizophrenia, but in most cases the mental symptoms disappear when the drug is stopped. Treatment of amphetamine and methedrine abuse should consist, in the first instance, of admission to hospital. These drugs should never be prescribed to addicts.

MARIHUANA

Obtained from the Cannabis plant, marihuana is being used to an increasing extent in the UK, usually smoked as 'reefers'. It produces a sense of well-being and relaxation, but its use is not accompanied by physiological dependence. It has acquired a reputation that it facilitates escalation to 'hard' drugs such as heroin, but it is far from certain whether the drug itself rather than other social factors inherent in mixing with the 'drug set' is the important factor. The use of marihuana must be viewed with caution, however, because it can itself precipitate severe emotional upset (anxiety, panic, depression) or psychotic break with reality in vulnerable individuals. In the UK it is now illegal to possess any form of marihuana.

LSD

This is a hallucinogen which is also rapidly assuming increasing importance as a drug of abuse. The effects (often referred to as a 'trip') consist of euphoria, vivid visual hallucinations, and disorders of time experience. They are usually self-limiting, but in vulnerable individuals resolution of the experience may be slow, and occasionally a psychotic illness may be precipitated, either schizophrenic or manic depressive in type.

OTHER POTENTIALLY ADDICTIVE DRUGS

In order to lessen the likelihood of excessive dependence, long term courses of tranquillisers or sedatives should be used rarely, and never without good reason and specialist advice. New synthetic analgesics require careful scrutiny for addictive qualities: for example, dipipanone, when combined with diphenhydramine (as in Diconal) is rapidly becoming the most popular addictive agent in the UK.

III. MENTAL SUBNORMALITY (MENTAL HANDICAP)

Mental subnormality is a condition of arrested mental development. It is to be distinguished from dementia, in which deterioration from a previously higher level of intellectual function has occurred. The 1959 Mental Health Act dispensed with terms such as idiocy and imbecility, which have now acquired pejorative overtones, and defined two major clinical categories of mental subnormality:

1. **Subnormality.** This may be defined as a state of arrested or incomplete development of mind, which includes subnormality of intelligence, and is of a nature or degree which requires or is susceptible to medical treatment or other special care or training.

2. **Severe Subnormality.** This is present when a person is rendered incapable of living an independent life or of guarding himself against serious exploitation, or will be so incapable when of an age to do so. Defined in these terms, the emphasis is not so much on intellectual performance alone as general social ability, although subnormality tends to respond to an IQ range of 50 to 75, and severe subnormality below an IQ of 50. The emphasis on general personality function is important because the ability to fit into society does not necessarily correlate clearly with IQ level. An IQ of 50 with good personality may be compatible with free existence in society, whereas a person who has an IQ of 70 with marked behaviour problems might need institutional care.

Background

Most cases with severe mental subnormality declare themselves at an early age because of the obvious incapacity that ensues. It should be suspected when there is inability to acquire reading or writing, and it occurs with a prevalence of 3.6/1,000 of the general population. Severe mental subnormality is usually secondary to gross organic defect in the central nervous system and its causes may be as shown below:

Causes of severe mental subnormality

Genetic

Recessive: phenylketonuria, lipoidoses, Wilson's disease, carbohydrate metabolic defects.
Dominant: tuberose sclerosis.
Chromosomal: trisomy 21 (Mongolism), XXY, Klinefelter's syndrome.

Intrauterine

Infective: rubella, syphilis, toxoplasmosis.
Metabolic: cretinism, kernicterus
   (rhesus incompatibility).
Anoxic: antepartum haemorrhage.

At birth, infancy or childhood

Traumatic: brain injury.
Infective: meningitis, encephalitis.
Anoxic
Severe prematurity

Idiopathic

Probably the largest group. May be associated with gross anatomical defects of the CNS, e.g. hydrocephalus, microcephaly.

The incidence of mental subnormality as defined is more difficult to determine. Criteria such as employability are too dependent on the local economic situation to be satisfactory indicators of morbidity rate. Mental subnormality, particularly in less severe forms, is frequently a variation of the normal distribution of mental abilities in the population, and, in contrast to severe subnormality, tends not to be so regularly associated with organic disorders to the nervous system. All the listed causes of severe subnormality, if mild in degree, may also cause subnormality. Poor social conditions, characterised by lack of education stimulus, may be associated with an apparent mild degree of subnormality which is susceptible to improvement with adequate stimulus and opportunity.

Mental handicap associated with presumptive brain damage is evenly distributed amongst the different social classes (Fig. 20.4). On the other hand, when not accompanied by brain damage it is far more common in the lower social groups: it has been argued that there is

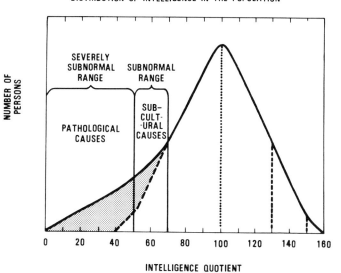

DISTRIBUTION OF INTELLIGENCE IN THE POPULATION

Fig. 20.4 Distribution of intelligence in the population. (*From* Forest *et al*. *New Perspectives in Mental Handicap*, Churchill Livingstone.)

a 'sub cultural' type of handicap which accounts for 75 per cent of persons with mild degrees of handicap (the educationally subnormal). If this is due to social factors itself, theoretically at least it is preventable.

Psychopathology

In severe mental subnormality there may be inability to distinguish between right and wrong, and antisocial behaviour may result. Secondary disability (emotional upset, aggressive behaviour) may arise as a reaction to the handicap, especially when the child has been handled wrongly, for example educationally misplaced and overstressed in school. The family of a handicapped child may also show emotional upset as a result of management difficulties.

Symptoms

In the most severe cases, life consists of a vegetable-like existence needing hospital care to prevent self-injury and to ensure an adequate level of personal care. The general personality structure is of great importance. Mongols, although usually in the severe mental subnormality range, are often very affectionate and tend to elicit a warm response from their families. This sympathetic atmosphere often permits their survival outside hospital during childhood. Less severe grades of mental subnormality may cause surprisingly little functional impairment, provided local employment facilities and social opportunities are good. On clinical assessment, the only findings may be a history of special education and poor educational achievement, manifest as inadequate command of general information and the basic academic skills.

Investigations

In infancy, these include recognition and vigorous treatment of rhesus incompatibility and infections, and metabolic screening for errors of metabolism. Adequate clinical examination will detect Mongolism at an early age and permit counselling of parents and appropriate management of the child. Regular assessment of school childrens' intellectual capacity permits early detection of mental subnormality and correct educational placement, thereby avoiding secondary reactions due to overstressing the handicapped child. Mental subnormality in adults and children is detectable by highly reliable psychological tests of intelligence.

It is important to distinguish childhood autism and psychosis from mental handicap. In the former, the child's physical appearance is normal and this may differentiate it from severe mental handicap related to brain damage, inherited chromosomal or metabolic deficit in which physical abnormalities are very common. Unsuspected deafness may also lead to a mistaken diagnosis of mental handicap, as may any other condition which interferes with the normal processes of skill acquisition, for example, blindness or developmental aphasia.

Complications

Severe Subnormality. Injury (lack of self-care or inadequate appreciation of common dangers).

Severe Subnormality and Subnormality. Antisocial behaviour and exploitation by others, prostitution, criminality, aggression when frustrated.

Basis of Treatment

Good obstetric and infant care can prevent many cases of subnormality which would otherwise arise due to trauma, prematurity, infection, anoxia, metabolic damage arising from errors of metabolism, or kernicterus complicating rhesus incompatibility. Hereditary causes are as yet difficult to anticipate by genetic counselling.

The importance of care in the community in preference to the institution has been emphasised in recent years. Even amongst the severely subnormal, 80 per cent of children and about half the adults are cared for at home.

All grades of subnormality do better, in terms of behaviour and level of functioning, with treatment which emphasises individual care and interpersonal contact combined with opportunity and stimulus as opposed to a custodial regime. Small family type units may lead to gratifying improvement in severe subnormality. For patients living in the community (subnormality grade) facilities such as day and training centres which are integrated with local firms and industry often

permit a stable and happy existence. No treatment is complete unless it involves the whole family, initially by getting it to accept the child's handicap and, later, in learning how to cope with a developing child whose potential and achievement will never be normal.

Management of mental handicap requires close co-operation between the family and social, education and medical agencies. In the majority the problem is primarily educational, and the educational psychologist needs to devise a programme for the individual child, taking into account perceptual and personality problems as well as cognitive deficits.

IV. THE FUNCTIONAL DISORDERS

The functional mental disorders are those acquired conditions for which there is no clear demonstrable physical cause either in terms of structural or physico-chemical disturbance. Although some illnesses at present included under this category may eventually turn out to be at least partly organic in orgin (certain types of schizophrenia, for example, could conceivably be related to biochemical defects in the nervous system) it is likely that psychological mechanisms play a much more important role both in the initiation and maintenance of all the functional disorders. Aetiology may prove to be multi-factorial in most cases, with predisposing and precipitating factors acting successively to produce the final picture of illness.

A. THE FUNCTIONAL PSYCHOSES

Psychosis is a pathological state of mind in which assessment of the self and one's situation is grossly impaired. We have already seen that in the organic psychoses, this is due to defect in cognitive function, especially that involving recent memory and intellect, with secondary phenomena such as visual hallucinations. In the functional psychoses there is no such cognitive impairment, and the patient's distorted assessment of reality usually occurs in a state of clear unclouded consciousness.

There are two main groups of functional psychoses:

1. **The Affective Psychoses** – in which a major disorder of mood appears to be the primary disturbance, with resulting secondary delusional ideas and sometimes hallucinatory experiences.

2. **The Schizophrenic Psychoses** – in which delusional thinking may be marked though not explicable by mood disturbance. There may also be a disorder of thinking and hallucinations, and these too do not appear to be related either to intellectual impairment or mood disorder.

THE AFFECTIVE PSYCHOSES (depressive, manic or manic depressive psychoses)

Definition

In these conditions the disorder of mood is the primary disturbance. It is usually the presenting and foremost clinical feature, and all other phenomena are understandable as secondary reactions to it. Although there is a strong tendency to recur, each spell of illness tends to be self-limiting, and complete reversion to the functional level of the previous personality is possible, even after many attacks have occurred. This contrasts with a schizophrenic illness in which recurrent episodes are usually followed by residual defects in personality.

Morbid change in affect may take the form either of depression or elevation of mood. Both types of disorder may occur successively in one individual (manic depressive or circular psychosis). Intellectual impairment does not occur as an integral part of the affective psychoses.

Background

The morbid risk of an individual developing an affective psychosis is 1 per cent. At any point in time the prevalence in the community is 0.4 per cent. The affective psychoses were long regarded as endogenous in origin, unrelated to life stress and due to inborn, constitutional defects of unspecified nature. Nowadays, this rigid dichotomy between endogenous and reactive illness is being discarded in favour of the view that each illness results from a combination of predisposing and precipitating factors, although varying in proportion from one individual to another.

Predisposing Factors. Familial predisposition towards affective psychosis undoubtedly can occur. The increased incidence of this type of illness in close relatives of a patient with affective psychosis (parents, children, siblings: 10 per cent) does not, of course, necessarily mean that the cause is genetic, because pathogenic influences arising from family disturbance and acting on a child in its early years could also lead to this kind of familial incidence. Personality types that are said to signify vulnerability towards affective psychotic breakdown include the cyclothymic individual whose mood swings regularly above and below the normal sufficiently to interfere with daily routine, or the highly rigid obsessional person who has to order his life excessively in order to retain his emotional equanimity. In many cases, however, the previous personality appears well integrated, with warmth and richness of affective response, and this contrasts with the flatness and emotional coldness in schizoid individuals who tend to develop schizophrenic breakdown.

Precipitating Factors. Although the affective psychoses occasionally appear to be unprovoked by upsetting life events, the absence of obvious stress factors in such cases may merely reflect the basic difficulty in deciding on what is stressful for the particular individual. Frequently, the difficulties may not become apparent until after recovery, when the patient and relatives can retrospectively give a more objective account of the situation. It is, therefore, necessary to search for precipitating factors in all cases. The depressed state may sometimes be understood as a protective reaction against stress. Experimental work has shown that recurrent frustration may lead to depressive type symptoms by a process of habituation. Personal crisis can sometimes precipitate a hypomanic illness, as if the mood swing may be precipitated in either direction in a non-specific way. Occasionally, physical illness, especially influenza, infectious hepatitis, or chest infection may appear to act as precipitant. A physical event such as childbirth may be followed by a puerperal affective psychosis. Psychological causes are the most common precipitants, often in the nature of object loss (job, friendship, financial support, status, bereavement) although a wide variety of emotional upsets may also act in this way.

Symptoms

The typical affective psychotic syndromes appear in adulthood, in 50 per cent of cases before 30 years of age, although in 25 per cent the onset is delayed until after 40 years. The male/female ratio is 1:2.

THE DEPRESSIVE PSYCHOSES

1. **Overt Depression of Mood.** This consists of unhappiness and loss of enjoyment in life, in severe cases amounting to profound misery. Tearfulness may be frequent, and is all the more significant when it is totally out of character for the individual. Diurnal variation in severity may sometimes be seen, with accentuation of depression in the early morning.

All other phenomena found in affective psychosis can be understood as secondary to the mood disturbance.

2. **Disorders of Thinking.** *Excessive self-blame and guilt* is a prominent feature, and consists of morbid preoccupation with minor misdeeds and indiscretions of the past. A middle-aged spinster who consulted her doctor because she had recently acquired the belief that she had contracted venereal disease through being kissed twenty years previously at a party, and felt very guilty about it, was in fact suffering from a depressive psychosis. Ideas of self-blame may be held with delusional intensity. The patient may not only feel that he deserves punishment, but he may actually request it or believe that he is about to receive it.

Suicidal ideas may complicate any severe depression, and the doctor should always satisfy himself on the risk of self-injury and suicide in every patient. No harm is done by tactful but direct discussion of this issue with the patient. A suitable introduction to the topic is the patient's attitude to the future and life in general. Undue pessimism and disinterest are congruent with real suicidal ideas. It has been estimated that one in six of all patients with affective psychosis eventually commit suicide. Occasionally, there is a risk of homicide, usually in the family, when the depressed patient feels he must commit suicide and cannot leave his relatives to face life without him. *Poor concentration* may be an early symptom, as may *mental slowness* manifest as delay in replying to questions. There is never incoherence or thought disorder of the schizophrenic kind. Hypochondriasis may be a prominent symptom in depressive illness. When it is the presenting clinical feature, the patient is sometimes subjected to a wide variety of physical investigations before the true depressive nature of the illness is recognised. In some cases the hypochondriasis is extreme and bizarre. For example, the patient may believe that his inside is rotting or dead. This type of picture is seen most often in older patients, and when accompanied by marked anxiety and agitation the syndrome is called *involutional melancholia*. This is merely a variant of depressive illness, the content of the symptoms reflecting the preoccupation with physical illness inherent in growing old. *Hallucinations*, usually auditory in type may accompany depressive psychosis, and most often consist of voices criticising or condemning the patient who accepts what is said uncritically. In rigid obsessional individuals a depressive illness may be accompanied by accentuation of obsessional compulsive symptoms.

3. **Motor Concomitants.** *Loss of weight and appetite* may be marked. Sleep disturbance is common, and in severe depression it is often resistant to hypnotics. Although the typical pattern of insomnia is said to consist of early morning waking, it is common to see a variety of sleep difficulties, including inability to get off to sleep and interruption during the night. Slowing of physical and mental activity is called psychomotor retardation. Occasionally, there may be *restlessness, agitation*, and a feeling of tension due to *superadded anxiety*; the patient is then unable to relax and appears to fidget or pace up and down incessantly. Constipation is also a fequent somatic accompaniment of depression: loss of libido may be an early symptom.

Special Forms of Depressive Illness

Grief Reaction. Normally the distress of bereavement follows a self-limiting course. There may be an initial numbness and a lack of full appreciation of what has happened. This is succeeded by episodic distress with depression, insomnia, anorexia and occasionally angry resentment against persons regarded as conceivably responsible. There may be a tendency to idealise the deceased, or even a feeling of the continued presence of the dead person, whose memory may remain an intense preoccupation for a month or more. Chance sounds may be misinterpreted in an illusory way. A widow may fleetingly assume that an opening door signals her dead husband's return, or she equates other sounds with his footsteps. In the normal grief reaction these symptoms do not lead to psychiatric consultation or social isolation and the degree of overt distress usually gradually declines, until after one to six weeks normal day-to-day activities can be resumed.

In morbid (atypical) grief reaction, the symptoms may lead to more severe disability by virtue of the fact that they are accentuated or unduly prolonged. Occasionally there may be a delay before a severe reaction ensues, perhaps not until the anniversary of the bereavement, or the reaction may be disguised in the form of psychosomatic symptoms.

Morbid reactions occur more often in women, and difficulty in accepting the loss, with feelings of guilt and marked hostility to individuals concerned with the death, are all more common than in normal grief. It is well recognised that grief is associated with an increased mortality risk, due to a greater incidence of suicide and death from a variety of organic diseases, particularly those of a cardiovascular nature during the first six months following bereavement. Excessive grief reactions are more common when the relationship with the deceased had been an unhappy one, or when the bereaved person is of vulnerable dependent personality.

Freud was one of the first to recognise that in order to learn acceptance of the loss of a loved person, the 'work of mourning' must be carried out. Grief is an active process whereby the loss is made real, and emotional bonds are altered accordingly. Various methods of ritualising the mourning period help this process of working through. During this time, outside intervention may not be sought and individual privacy should of course be respected. Help is however on the whole welcomed by the bereaved, especially if it is based on the recognition that simply sitting with, listening to and recognising the distress is itself often as helpful as any other kind of intervention. Some find self-help groups to be a welcome form of support. When grief is short-lasting no other help is required, but atypical reactions may need specialised psychotherapy, especially when there is marked depression and inability to relinquish the memory of the deceased or when an intractable sick role has developed.

Involutional Melancholia. This is merely a depressive illness coming on for the first time in the involutional stage of life, and often characterised by severe anxiety with hypochondriacal fears or delusions. It is not a separate disease entity, and management is identical with that of depressive illness in general.

Puerperal Depressive Psychosis. This follows closely on childbirth. The full syndrome of depression is present, and it is particularly important to assess the danger to the child because depressive infanticidal and suicidal ideas may be present.

Complications

1. Impaired judgement may lead to unwise decisions during the illness itself. For example, feelings of inefficiency may precipitate resignation from work. Patients with depressive illness should always be urged not to make major decisions affecting their life situation until the depressive symptoms have resolved.
2. Weight loss and malnutrition (neglect of diet and the self).
3. Chronicity was a common problem prior to the introduction of somatic treatment such as ECT.
4. Suicide and, fortunately rarely, homicide.

Differential Diagnosis

1. **Any Other Major Mental Illness** may present with depressive symptoms and so may lead to diagnostic confusion.

Dementia may lead to depression in the initial stages if the patient retains insight into his intellectual deficits.

Early schizophrenia may also be accompanied by severe depression, even suicide, possibly because at this stage insight is still present and, hence, there is alarm at the psychotic symptoms.

Chronic alcoholism is usually punctuated by depressive swings of mood, often in the stage of remorse after a drinking spree.

Personality disorder may lead to short-lasting depressive swings as reactions to life stress. They are not usually accompanied by self-blame typical of psychotic depression and generally improve rapidly when the difficulties are resolved.

2. **Physical Illnesses.** The hypochondriacal fears so commonly seen in depression usually have no organic basis, but it should be remembered that physical disease and depression can occur coincidentally in the same patient. Only full physical examination combined with appropriate investigations can clarify the situation. For example, thyrotoxicosis may easily be mistaken for an anxiety depressive state unless the true significance of the weight loss with good appetite, tremor, tachycardia, and eye signs is recognised.

3. **Drug Induced Depression.** Reserpine, when used widely as a treatment for hypertension, was found to precipitate severe depression in some cases. Amphetamine withdrawal after prolonged abuse, or sudden cessation of antidepressant medication, may also cause marked depressive symptoms. Long-acting depot phenothiazine preparations may also cause depression, especially when used inappropriately in illnesses other than schizophrenia.

Basis of Treatment

The general principles of treatment are the same whatever the severity of the depression, and both constitutional and reactive mechanisms are sought in each case. Many cases are treated in the community, but it is necessary to admit the patient to hospital when the symptoms are severe, especially when there is a risk of suicide, or the illness has failed to respond to outpatient treatment.

1. **Support and Psychotherapy.** During the severe stages of the illness, it is usually impossible and even dangerous to discuss causes and interpret behaviour, because while the psychotic depression persists the patient is unamenable to any change in attitude. Even at this time, however, regular sympathetic and reassuring interviews are appreciated by the patient who otherwise feels completely lost and hopeless. The value of more intensive interpretive psychotherapy in the affective psychoses is uncertain. It can be helpful inbetween attacks of illness in an attempt to prevent relapse, particularly on a conjoint basis with the spouse. In general, it is wrong to advise an expensive holiday such as a sea cruise for the really depressed patient. Indeed, until the depression has been fully treated a vacation might even make the patient worse.

2. **Social Work.** While the patient is receiving treatment it is important to work with relatives, particularly when their relationship with the patient is causing difficulties.

3. **Physical Treatment:**
(i) *Drugs: symptomatic.* Insomnia is often marked and distressing in the severe stages of depression. It may be justified to use a short course of barbiturate night sedation at this stage, but prolonged courses should be avoided. Anxiety may respond to minor tranquillisers but, occasionally, phenothiazines may be required if agitation is severe.

(ii) *Antidepressants.* Although a great deal has been claimed for the efficacy of so-called specific antidepressants it should be remembered that no group has received universal acclaim, and the results of controlled trials of these drugs are not always convincing. Depression is often self-limiting, and spontaneous improvement may sometimes be falsely attributed to the drug itself. The potential side effect of monoamine oxidase inhibitors may be so serious, and their beneficial effects are so uncertain, that this group is not recommended routinely in the treatment of depression. Tricyclic drugs (amitriptyline or imipramine 25 to 50 mg, three times daily) are well worth using, especially as their side effects are usually minor and not serious (*see* page 436).

(iii) *ECT* is indicated when there is a significant risk of suicide. In such circumstances ECT should not be delayed and it is not safe to rely for long on drugs. ECT may also be used when disabling depressive symptoms persist in spite of other kinds of treatment. This form of treatment is most effective in those cases where environmental factors are minimal or reversible, and the typical clinical picture of psychotic depression with sleep disturbance, self-blame and weight loss is seen. ECT is unlikely to prove curative when the environmental factors are severe and irreversible, for example in the case of intractable marital upset, although it may still have to be used in such cases if suicide risk is severe. Striking response to ECT is seen in typical involutional melancholia.

(iv) *Modified leucotomy.* This is said to be helpful in unremitting depression, accompanied by marked tension, in older patients of good previous personality. The use of leucotomy in this way must nowadays be very uncommon, and it should never be considered until all other forms of treatment have been thoroughly explored.

Prognosis

When affective psychosis begins in early adulthood, recurrent attacks throughout life are common, although in 25 per cent of cases no further breakdown occurs. Complete restoration to normal personality is possible even after many attacks of affective psychosis. Good prognostic factors include late onset, absence of organic or paranoid features, and good previous personality.

HYPOMANIA AND MANIA

Hypomania is characterised by marked persistent elevation of mood, manifest as elation out of proportion to the situation. The most extreme form of this disorder is called mania. The euphoria and good humour may last for weeks, months or even longer, and is accompanied by physical overactivity. The patient undertakes a large number of tasks both in his work and private life yet is unable to carry them out efficiently and completely. The happy good humour is punctuated by short-lasting spells of tearfulness and irritability. Considerable management difficulties may arise out of the patient's lack of insight and resulting refusal to be guided in decision-making, together with overactivity, ill-judged enthusiasm and ebullience. The serious impairment of judgement may result in rash overspending of large sums of money or in the establishment of inappropriate friendships, even engagement or marriage. The typical hypomanic speech (called flight of ideas) is rapid and discursive, tending to wander from the topic because of

distractibility by chance outside stimulus, rhyming, or punning. This contrasts with schizophrenic thought disorder which does not appear to be related to distractibility or chance associations. In some cases a paranoid attitude may develop, sometimes of delusional intensity.

Complications

1. **Undesirable Socio-economic Repercussions.** These may result from impaired judgement and must be prevented by adequate controlling measures.

2. **Depression.** This may follow immediately upon a hypomanic or manic illness in about 50 per cent of cases. It can be severe, and may require intensive antidepressant treatment. In view of this, close supervision should be provided in the convalescent stages.

Differential Diagnosis

Acute Schizophrenia, especially the catatonic type, may be accompanied by similar excitement and overactivity. The diagnosis may not be clarified until symptomatic therapy has reduced the level of disturbance.

Acute Organic Brain Syndromes. In these, any agitation and overactivity is accompanied by impairment of consciousness, memory disturbance and, possibly, disorientation; organic delirium is characterised by anxiety and fear rather than elation. Epileptic excitement is to be considered when there is a history of fits. Direct effect of stimulant drugs (e.g. amphetamines, methedrine) may also lead to euphoria and excitement. GPI occasionally presents as a hypomanic state, but evidence of memory loss and intellectual impairment is always found on close assessment.

Basis of Treatment

Most cases of hypomania require hospitalisation. Informal admission is usually adequate, but when the illness is severe and is causing serious socio-economic complications it may be necessary to place the patient on an observation or treatment order to ensure adequate control. Hypomania or mania can be among the most difficult of all psychiatric conditions to treat.

1. **Drug Treatment:**
Major tranquillisers (phenothiazines) may be required in high doses to control the disturbed behaviour (chlorpromazine up to 100 mg, fives times daily). Insomnia may be difficult to control even by barbiturate hypnotics.

Lithium carbonate may sometimes control a manic illness when phenothiazines have failed.

2. **ECT** may be effective in mania that has failed to respond to adequate drug therapy.

Prognosis

A first attack of mania is unlikely to be the last. Recurrent episodes do not lead to personality defect, although successive attacks tend to last longer. Rarely, a state of chronic mania develops. Lithium carbonate has been advocated as a prophylactic against recurrent attacks. Such treatment requires careful monitoring of dosage (blood levels should not exceed 2 mEq(mmol)/litre and it must be stopped if tremor, drowsiness or impaired renal function develops.

MANIC DEPRESSIVE PSYCHOSIS

This is characterised by a history of both depressive and hypomanic or manic illness in the same individual. No special clinical considerations apply to this condition other than those already described, except that a history of hypomania requires caution in the use of ECT in the depressive stage for fear of precipitating hypomania.

THE SCHIZOPHRENIC PSYCHOSES

In contrast to the manic depressive psychoses in which mood disorder is the primary disturbance, there are many psychotic illnesses that cannot be explained in this way. Kraepelin, in 1898, delineated a group that he called dementia praecox, characterised by delusions, hallucinations usually utterly non-understandable and alien, in a setting of clear consciousness, and tending towards chronic deterioration in some cases. In view of the fact that true intellectual deterioration, as usually found in dementia, does not occur in this group of illnesses, the name was later discarded and E. Bleuler introduced the concept of the schizophrenias, characterised by a fundamental disorder of mental association involving thought processes and their relationship to affect and drive.

Background

The prevalence of the schizophrenias in the general population is 0.8 per cent.

Aetiology

Genetic Factors. These may well be important. A high incidence of this illness is found in relatives of schizophrenic patients (in siblings 7 to 15 per cent, in parents 9 per cent, in children with one parent schizophrenic 7 to 16 per cent, or with both parents schizophrenic 40 to 60 per cent). The concordance rates among monozygotic twins is also said to be high. Such evidence is not conclusive in favour of genetic mechanisms because

shared pathogenic environment in childhood due to disturbed family interaction could also lead to a familial pattern of incidence. Recent studies answer this criticism to some extent. It has been demonstrated that children of schizophrenic parents, adopted into normal homes in infancy, still show an increased incidence of schizophrenia compared with controls. It has also been found that adopted children who develop schizophrenia have true parents who themselves are more often schizophrenic than controls.

Biochemical Theories. Many biochemical theories have been put forward to explain the aetiology of schizophrenia, but none has maintained wide acceptance for long. Recent theories have centred around a claim that 3:4 dimethoxyphenylethylamine (DMPE) has been detected in the urine of schizophrenic patients. Fig. 20.5

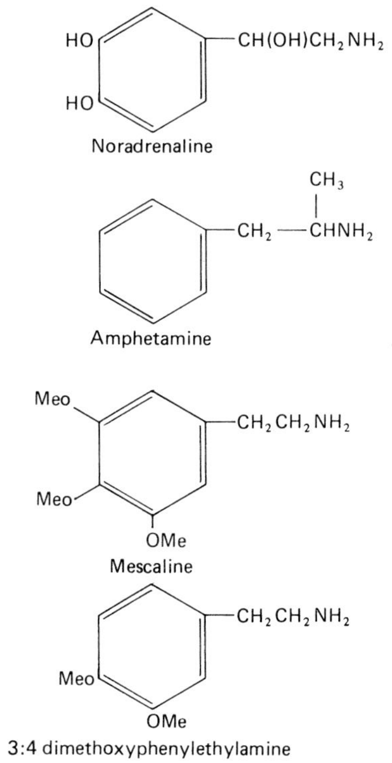

Fig. 20.5 Chemical structure of metabolites and hallucinogens relevant to biochemical theories of schizophrenia.

shows the close structural similarity of DMPE and the hallucinogen mescaline. A process of abnormal methylation might conceivably lead to DMPE formation from adrenaline as a result of metabolic defect in the nervous system. These experimental findings have not been reduplicated, and may have been due to coincidental uncontrolled factors such as dietary variation.

Environmental Factors. These have been suggested both in the form of predisposing disturbed family patterns acting in childhood, and as precipitating causes immediately preceding each psychotic relapse.

460

This approach implies that the psychosis may be an understandable reaction to an intolerable family situation (Laing). Work with the families of male schizophrenic patients suggests that certain interactions may be of particular importance. The schizophrenogenic mother (Lindz) is one who has fostered an exclusive and engulfing relationship with her son in a way which reflects her own inadequacies, particularly in her marriage, and which impairs her son's attempts to develop his own identity and autonomy. Bateson and his co-workers suggest that schizophrenic behaviour may arise because of 'double-bind' relationships in a family, which lead to chronic ambiguity and uncertainty because they involve a choice between two alternatives, both of which are liable to meet with disapproval or other unpleasant sequelae.

Certain personality deviations are regarded as common in those individuals who later develop schizophrenia, the most prominent being schizoid traits characterised by social isolation, lack of affective warmth and retreat into fantasy life. In about one-third of cases the premorbid personality appears, on clinical assessment, to be normal.

Psychopathology

Psychoanalysts explain the symptoms of schizophrenia as a regression to an early infantile stage of mental development. Psychological tests suggest loss of abstract thinking together with over inclusive and unusual associations without true intellectual deterioration or organic type impairment. Bleuler postulated a fundamental loosening of associations between various aspects of psychic life. The symptoms have also been explained as reactions by which the patient defends himself against intolerable life situations. Undoubtedly, some of the symptoms in chronic schizophrenia may be reactions to chronic institutionalisation rather than direct results of the illness itself.

Symptoms

About three-quarters of schizophrenic illnesses begin between the ages of 15 to 25 years. Onset may be insidious following months or years of increasing social isolation, loss of initiative and gradual deterioration in social, economic, and academic efficiency. In such cases, environmental precipitating factors tend to be insignificant or apparently absent. Acute onset, on the other hand, tends to follow upon some traumatic physical or psychological event, and may be preceded by good personality adjustment. Bleuler distinguished two main categories of schizophrenic symptoms:

1. **Fundamental Symptoms.** The fundamental disorders of association involve thinking, emotion, and drive.

Schizophrenic thought disorder is an impairment of cohesion between logical thought sequences. In the early stages, the patient's speech may merely appear vague and woolly: speech tends to slip imperceptibly yet illogically from one topic to another, although speed is normal; the change of topic is so subtle (often called the knight's move, as in chess) that the observer's first impression is that he himself is not concentrating on what the patient is saying. The speech sometimes exhibits *neologisms*, which are new words made up by the patient.

Thought blocking is said to occur when the patient's stream of thought suddenly and transitorily stops. He may complain of this spontaneously, but it is very difficult to assess the significance of this symptom and to elicit it reliably. In severe cases the speech may become completely incoherent. Schizophrenic thought disorder is distinguished from flight of ideas found in hypomania, in which the rate of speech is increased and changes of topic can be explained in terms of the patient's distractibility by his surroundings. It is important to remember that schizophrenic thought disorder occurs in the absence of impairment of consciousness or memory loss.

Disorder of abstract concept formation is very difficult to assess objectively. The patient may offer 'concrete' interpretation of proverbs. For example, when asked to explain the meaning of 'people in glass houses should not throw stones' he may say, 'They may break the windows'. The mentally subnormal or intellectually impaired also tend to respond in the same way, and this test can be difficult to interpret.

Autism, or intense withdrawal from social contact and preoccupation with fantasy life rather than the real life situation, may precede or accompany the psychosis, and may remain as a postpsychotic personality defect state.

Affective changes occur as flatness, lack of emotional warmth in relating to others, resulting in an appearance of cold, unfeeling detachment: it is difficult to establish *rapport* with the patient. There may be *incongruity of affect*, which appears as an apparent dissociation between mood and content of speech: he may giggle spontaneously even when discussing serious topics. This symptom probably reflects a preoccupation with fantasy life and hallucinatory experiences, rather than an actual dissociation between mood and thinking. Depression of mood may also occur, especially in the early stages of the disease when the patient has insight into his difficulties.

2. **Accessory Symptoms.** These take the form of delusional ideas, hallucinations and catatonic disorders of movement.

Delusions are often bizarre and not understandable in the light of mood disturbance. They may appear suddenly, apparently precipitated by commonplace perceptions. Thus, a dog walking down the road may suddenly signify to the patient that he himself is of special identity (e.g. a member of the Royal Family). Delusions of influence and passivity are common. The patient may feel controlled in some inexplicable way by abnormal outside influences, often bizarre in nature, such as a machine sending rays to control his thoughts, or even extracting them and inserting new ones into his mind. True paranoid delusions may occur, characterised by ideas of persecution resented by the patient who reacts with anger and sometimes aggressive behaviour.

Hallucinations are most often auditory in type, but any sensory modality may be affected. Most commonly, voices are heard, perhaps uttering banal comments, discussing him in the third person, commenting on what he is doing or commanding him to do things. They are not necessarily critical of him, as in depressive psychoses, but may even compliment or reassure him. Tactile hallucinations may be related to passivity ideas, and they are often related to the genitalia.

Catatonic symptoms are abnormalities of movement, posture and speech. They may present as stupor or excitement, with sudden impulsive outbursts of aggressive behaviour. Negativism, characterised by a tendency to oppose commands, or even to do the opposite to that which is requested is a frequent catatonic manifestation. Other types of catatonic symptoms include echolalia (repeating what is said by the examiner) echopraxia (copying the movement of others) mannerisms (odd, stilted way of carrying out movements) stereotypies (habitual useless movements) posturing and waxy flexibility (maintenance of fixed, unusual postures for long periods and a tendency to remain in positions placed by the examiner).

Schneider has emphasised that certain 'first-rank' symptoms are particularly frequent in schizophrenia, and these are:
1. Certain types of auditory hallucinations, i.e. audible thought, voices heard arguing and voices giving a running commentary on the patient's actions referring to him in the third person.
2. Somatic passivity phenomena – the experience of influences playing on the body.
3. Thought withdrawal and other interferences with thought.
4. Diffusion of thought (or thought broadcasting) where the patient experiences his thought as being also thought by others.
5. All feelings, impulses (drive) and volitional acts that are experienced by the patient as the work or influence of others.

Whilst these may be useful as diagnostic leads, they should not be taken to mean that schizophrenia can be diagnosed on the basis of single symptoms, because this pays insufficient regard to the very considerable amount of variation in normal experiences, particularly when cross-cultural factors are relevant. The diagnosis of schizophrenia can only be based on the total clinical picture, which includes not only the natural history of the illness, but also thought content, its cohesion, as well as the mood state and general behaviour.

THE CLINICAL SCHIZOPHRENIC SYNDROMES

Certain broad clinical types of schizophrenia can be delineated, according to the predominant type of symptoms present.

Hebephrenic Schizophrenia tends to occur in young people (aged 15 to 25 years): affective changes and thought disorder predominate, and hallucinations or delusions are minimal or even absent. The patient may be severely incapacitated by thought disorder, and his behaviour may consist of incongruous giggling, fatuous manner, even prankish behaviour. The prognosis is said to be poor in this type of schizophrenia.

Catatonic Schizophrenia is dominated by the typical motor disorders already described. Onset occurs at any time from teenage to 40 years. Other schizophrenic symptoms may also occur, either fundamental or accessory in type, but they are usually overshadowed by the motor disturbance.

In Paranoid Schizophrenia, florid delusions and hallucinations dominate the clinical picture. Onset occurs at any time from teenage to 60 years. Late onset schizophrenia is typically in this form, which may be compatible with normal social life over many years because personality deterioration tends to be slow. Late onset paranoid schizophrenia is most common in unmarried females, when the delusional ideas often have a sexual content. Some sort of sensory defect (partial deafness or poor vision) often acts as a precipitating factor in such cases.

Simple Schizophrenia occurs in young adults, and is characterised by insidious loss of drive, social withdrawal, and deterioration in performance in both academic and general behaviour. The patient may sink into vagrancy and chronic unemployment, appearing apathetic and emotionally flat. This is a highly unsatisfactory diagnostic entity, because positive evidence for schizophrenia in the form of clear-cut typical symptoms is rarely present. This clinical picture is probably due to many causes, and should not be automatically attributed to a schizophrenic process.

Childhood Schizophrenia. It is rare to see schizophrenia in childhood and never before 7 years of age at the earliest. The syndrome of early childhood autism probably bears no relationship to schizophrenia. Its onset occurs at birth or within the first three years of life, and a profound withdrawal of emotional contact with people is one of its main characteristics.

Complications of Schizophrenia

1. Chronic psychosis.
2. Residual personality defects, usually manifest as social withdrawal or lack of persistence and initiative.
3. Socio-economic impairment, family break up, deterioration in occupational status or unemployability.
4. Suicide, probably most common in the early stages of the illness.
5. Disturbed and possibly aggressive behaviour.
6. Adverse effects of treatment, e.g. side effects of medication, institutionalisation.

Differential Diagnosis

1. **Other Functional Psychoses.** In the **manic depressive psychoses** the mood disturbance is usually obvious, and all other clinical features are understandable as secondary to it. Many psychotic illnesses do not show the typical features of either manic depressive or schizophrenic psychoses and are preferably categorised in terms of their manifest phenomena, e.g. *paranoid psychoses* or *paranoid hallucinatory states* rather than assuming that they are atypical examples of manic depressive or schizophrenic psychoses. When depressive features are persistent and severe in a patient who also shows schizophrenic features, the illness is sometimes called schizo-affective.

2. **Personality Disorder.** This may take the form of life-long eccentricity of behaviour. This should not be regarded as schizophrenic merely because it is strange and peculiar. The search for identity which may accompany normal adolescence must also be distinguished from psychotic illness. Psychosis should not be diagnosed unless delusional ideas and/or hallucinations are present. *Morbid jealousy* is a paranoid syndrome of varied aetiology: some cases are due to schizophrenia, others are abnormal personalities in which traits of jealousy have become accentuated. Many arise in the setting of chronic alcoholism. The spouse becomes the centre of intense jealousy and suspicion of infidelity. The condition is important to recognise because it may lead to homicide.

3. **Psychotic States Complicating Physical Events and Illnesses.** Certain physical events and illnesses may be complicated by paranoid hallucinatory states in which the typical organic type of mental impairment (memory, orientation) may be minimal or absent.

Drugs. Excessive and habitual intake of amphetamines may lead to a paranoid state with auditory hallucinations in which persecutory ideas are prominent. Chronic alcoholism may occasionally be complicated by auditory hallucinations. Recovery from drug overdose may sometimes be complicated by transient paranoid reactions secondary to clouding of consciousness and confusion.

Epilepsy. A series of grand mal convulsions may sometimes precipitate an acute paranoid hallucinatory state. Temporal lobe epilepsy, in a small proportion of cases, may be complicated by a chronic psychosis which is hard to distinguish from schizophrenia. It is of interest that focal epilepsy originating in other cerebral areas is not complicated by psychosis in this way.

GPI is occasionally complicated by a paranoid psychosis in which grandiose ideas and delusions are prominent.

Myxoedema. Depressive symptoms are most common, but occasionally a paranoid psychosis is found.

Postoperative psychosis may take a paranoid form.

Basis of Treatment

The Psychotic State. Personal support should be provided in all cases, although it is, in general, difficult to establish close *rapport* with the patient. It is useless, even dangerous, to discuss the origin of the psychotic symptoms or to interpret their meaning in the acute psychotic stage of the illness.

Physical Treatments, usually in hospital, remain the mainstay of treatment. Occasionally, it may be necessary to utilise compulsory observation or treatment under the *Mental Health Act* if the patient is dangerous to himself or others or refuses essential treatment. In the acute illness the aim should be to remove the psychotic symptoms as quickly as possible, in order to reduce both the complications of the psychosis itself and the chance that it will become chronic. Phenothiazines are the drugs of choice: chlorpromazine (doses in excess of 500 mg daily, if necessary by injection, may be required in some cases) or trifluoperazine (up to 10 mg, four times daily) may rapidly control the acute stages of the psychosis. Haloperidol (3 to 5 mg, three times daily) is sometimes effective when phenothiazines have failed. Anti-Parkinsonian drugs (benzhexol 2 to 4 mg, three times daily, orphenadrine 50 to 100 mg, four times daily) should be used routinely with these drugs, especially when high doses are employed. When the psychosis persists in spite of three weeks adequate medication, ECT should be added. Improvement then often follows in the majority of cases of recent onset or acute relapse. It may be necessary to give ten applications for full beneficial effect, but usually five to seven treatments are sufficient. It is important not to over-treat with ECT in attempts to eliminate less responsive chronic symptoms.

Nursing and general management of acutely psychotic patients follows certain general principles. Restraint should not be used unless the patient presents an immediate and significant danger to himself or others, bearing in mind that excessive restriction in itself tends to produce aggressive behaviour. The ward should, where possible, accommodate both male and female patients in a non-custodial atmosphere.

Rehabilitation. This includes the prevention of relapse, once the acute psychosis has resolved, and the management of personality defect states and chronic psychosis. Prevention of relapse poses many problems because impaired insight leads to a reluctance to continue medication: this usually shows up as a failure to take tablets after discharge from hospital. To overcome this difficulty, certain long-acting intramuscular phenothiazine preparations (e.g. fluphenazine) have proved invaluable in those patients who lose their psychotic symptoms with adequate medication, yet relapse repeatedly because of failure to co-operate in taking it over prolonged periods. In most cases, it is necessary to continue drugs for one to two years after recovery from a psychotic breakdown.

The use of such long-acting preparations may lead to certain complications which it is important to recognise and treat quickly. Severe extrapyramidal symptoms such as muscular rigidity or tonic spasm may occur. When this involves bulbar and neck muscles, as frequently happens, there may follow speech or swallowing difficulty. Motor restlessness may be troublesome, and stupor and drowsiness have also been reported. It is not unknown for such symptoms to be mistakenly diagnosed as part of an acute neurological disorder such as encephalitis. Dysphagia may be thought due to an oesophageal neoplasm or other local obstructive lesion. An exacerbation of the underlying psychosis may also be erroneously diagnosed, especially when the psychotic illness had previously included catatonic symptoms; further phenothiazines may then be given in error, with serious results. In view of these difficulties a case can be made that all patients receiving phenothiazine or similar preparations should carry a card stating this fact, with dates of injection, and the address of the relevant clinic. Severe rigidity and muscle spasm complicating such treatment can be controlled quickly by procyclidine (up to 10 mg by intravenous injection).

The schizophrenic patient is especially vulnerable to institutionalisation. If kept in hospital for long, particularly in a large impersonal institution where it is necessary to conform to a monotonous routine and all needs for initiative are removed, he may develop severe secondary handicap whereby he is no longer able to cope with the demands of an independent existence outside

hospital. Some of the classical clinical features of chronic schizophrenia may be secondary to an institutional regime. In order to counteract these harmful effects, emphasis is now placed on treatment in the community, usually by means of day hospitals. In this way, the schizophrenic patient may live at home yet attend daily for treatment. Any hospital admissions, which of necessity involve a retreat from living in the community, should be as short as possible. A great deal remains to be done in assessing the stresses on both patient and his family which arise from community-based therapy. Sometimes the repercussions in both patient and family are severe. It must be recognised that a small minority of schizophrenic patients will require life-long hospitalisation, and these should not be denied the asylum they require. Many will require protected employment (sheltered workshops and industrial therapy units), particularly when the local economic situation does not offer good prospects of employment.

Prognosis

At the time of the first schizophrenic breakdown the prognosis has traditionally been accepted as follows:

15 to 25 per cent full permanent remission.
25 per cent infrequent relapses.
25 per cent multiple relapses with personality deterioration
25 per cent chronic institutionalisation.

With modern methods of treatment it should be possible to improve these figures considerably. Repeated relapses tend to leave increasing degrees of residual disability in their wake, and the analogy with the natural history of multiple sclerosis is a close one. Good prognosis in any individual is associated with acute onset with good previous personality, clear precipitating factors, a history of affective illness in the family, and atypical clinical features such as the presence of severe depressive symptoms.

OTHER FUNCTIONAL PSYCHOSES

It is not uncommon to find functional psychoses that do not conform strictly to the manic depressive and schizophrenic dichotomy. In such cases it is best, in the present state of knowledge, to be satisfied merely with a label that describes the symptoms involved. *Paranoid psychosis* is a syndrome in which there are delusions of self reference (persecutory, grandeur, litigation, jealousy, love, hate, honour), which cannot be immediately derived from the prevailing abnormal mood and are not associated with typical schizophrenic symptoms of other kinds. *Paranoid hallucinatory state* is also a useful descriptive label that does not hinder search for both functional and organic causative factors.

B. THE NEUROSES

The neuroses comprise a variety of mental syndromes in which contact with reality is retained at all times and psychotic symptoms such as delusional ideas and hallucinations do not occur. Insight is retained in the sense that the neurotic patient realises that he is ill, and this constitutes an important distinction from the psychotic state.

Neurotic illness is by far the most common form of mental illness. In one year, at least 1 in 10 of a family doctor's patients will consult him because of neurotic symptoms. These are most frequently in the form of anxiety and depressive states, but the obsessional and hysterical neuroses, though less common, also contribute significantly to the total picture of neurotic illness in the community. Unlike the psychoses, which may soon declare themselves because of the resultant disturbed behaviour, much neurotic disability never reaches the medical services and remains both undetected and untreated.

NEUROTIC DEPRESSIVE REACTION

This consists of an excessive reaction with depressive symptoms as a result of environmental difficulties. These may take the form of any life stress, either acute (e.g. quarrel, disappointment) or chronic (e.g. marital conflicts, work difficulties). The reaction is clearly understandable in the light of the person's life-long personality difficulties, for example in the form of anxiety, lack of confidence, rigidity of personality with obsessional traits, or intolerance of frustration. Such lack of resilience makes it difficult for the individual to cope with life in general, and sudden stress may precipitate a depressive reaction. Thus, a woman with long-standing anxiety about leaving home (agoraphobia) may become depressed if her husband has to work away from home. This type of depressive reaction usually has a clear understandable temporal relationship with stressful life events.

The clinical features include overt depression of mood, tearfulness, even suicidal impulses, but typically there are no psychotic depressive features such as morbid guilt, retardation, or delusional ideas. It can be difficult to distinguish a neurotic depressive reaction from a depressive psychosis. Such distinction ceases to be of crucial importance, provided in every case of depression it is remembered that both exogenous and endogenous factors usually play some part.

In the treatment of neurotic depressive reactions, psychotherapy is of paramount importance, and is aimed at helping the vulnerable personality to cope with the demands made upon him. This may involve either trying to change his reaction to them, or altering the exogenous stresses themselves. When the environmental precipitant takes the form of disordered interpersonal relationships it may be necessary to involve the other person(s) concerned (usually the spouse) in combined interviews. Somatic treatment (drugs and ECT) are used only when the reaction is severe; they are palliative rather than preventive or curative, because they do not treat the underlying causes.

ANXIETY NEUROSIS

Here the principal clinical feature is excessive anxiety, often amounting to panic. Sometimes the anxiety centres around certain specific situations towards which the person is then said to be phobic.

Background

Anxiety neurosis may develop out of long-standing personality difficulties, commonly in the form of undue anxiety and lack of confidence. Anxiety neurosis is said to be present when symptoms assume a magnitude sufficient to interfere with normal daily activities. Sometimes the neurosis appears suddenly, and some situational precipitant is then usually apparent. Anxiety may be learnt; for example, when a frightening situation leads to a long-standing phobia specific to it. Phobias may acquire an element of secondary gain, whereby a patient may ensure support from others; successful treatment must then take this factor into account.

Symptoms

Anxiety dominates the clinical picture, with subjective tension, foreboding, and restlessness. There may be intensive hypochondriacal fears of heart trouble, cancer, or other serious illness. The patient's persistence with somatic complaints often results in intensive physical investigations, and psychiatric referral may not then take place until all are negative. Phobic anxiety may be situational (open spaces – agoraphobia; closed spaces – claustrophobia), social contact (social phobia) or towards specific objects (e.g. insects and other animals), or apparently unrelated to the situation. Chronic neurotic anxiety is a common crippling disability. The housebound housewife is unable to leave the home because of intense anxiety on going out. Fears of choking are also common, and may prevent the patient from swallowing anything except liquids.

Complications

Chronic restriction of activities both occupational and social with dependence on others.

Differential Diagnosis

1. It must be remembered that anxiety is a common finding in all types of depressive illness. In such cases careful clinical assessment will detect the hallmarks of

depression, e.g. typical sleep disorder, self-blame, suicidal ideas with overt depression of mood.

2. Physical illness can only be ruled out by full physical assessment. The cardinal rule should be that patients are investigated strictly on clinical criteria and not merely to reassure the patient who in any case usually remains uncomforted by this approach. Thyrotoxicosis should be considered when weight loss, agitation, and tremor are marked.

Basis of Treatment

Symptomatic therapy with minor tranquillisers is justified when the patient is very distressed by anxiety. Unfortunately, these drugs are often then prescribed for prolonged periods of time, frequently with no real benefit to the patient. Such prescribed drugs are regularly involved in deliberate self-overdose, which in recent years has become a clinical problem of rapidly increasing magnitude. This suggests that such symptomatic therapy is often inadequate, and can be no substitute for more radical measures. An anxiety reaction must be understood as a product of personality and life situation, and psychotherapy is usually required to resolve the problem. Behaviour therapy may help, particularly in localised anxiety, e.g. insect phobias. It is less helpful in more generalised anxiety, e.g. in agoraphobia, which is often related to other difficulties, particularly in the family, and which may even have an element of secondary gain. Psychiatric services must be prepared to reach out into the community to help such patients, who often remain undeclared to helping agencies. Anxiety may be a concomitant of any mental disorder and some physical illnesses, in which case its treatment will be secondary to that of the primary condition.

OBSESSIONAL COMPULSIVE NEUROSIS

This type of neurosis is characterised by recurrent thoughts or impulses which are accompanied by a subjective feeling of compulsion. The anxiety level is high and the obsessional symptoms provide only short-lasting relief from it. On quiet reflection the patient regards his symptoms as pointless, even ridiculous, and accepts that they are part of his own mental processes. He never attributes them to outside influences, as might a schizophrenic patient with passivity ideas. The distinction between obsessional personality and obsessional neurosis is arbitrary. Neurotic illness is said to have developed when the symptoms impair to a significant degree the ability to carry out normal day to day activities.

Background

Personality difficulties in the form of obsessional traits often precede the development of the neurosis.

Although the rigid perfectionist individual appears to be extremely efficient, demanding high standards of himself and others, this may in fact signify vulnerability whereby uncertainty or change of routine can easily precipitate anxiety. Obsessional symptoms may sometimes be understood as defence mechanisms, having symbolic significance: a hand-washing obsessional neurosis may occur as a grief reaction following the death of a spouse with whom the patient had an ambivalent relationship. As in all neuroses, once the symptoms are established there may develop self-perpetuating mechanisms through secondary gain. For example, extra attention may be obtained from otherwise inattentive relatives and this may occur at either conscious or sub-conscious levels.

Symptoms

Onset may be gradual in the context of life-long obsessional traits, or sudden and unexpected in a good personality. The latter mode of onset is usually associated with severe environmental stress. The symptoms may take the form of motor activities (tics, or rituals of checking, washing, dressing) compulsive thoughts known as ruminations (counting numbers, recurrent phrases, musical tunes endlessly repeated in the mind) or fears of own impulses (such as harming others in some way).

In severe cases, the patient may be at all times preoccupied with his symptoms, and there is resultant marked limitation of normal activities. A dressing or washing ritual may effectively prevent the patient from getting ready in the morning. Hand washing may be so repetitive and thorough that severe excoriation of the skin ensues. Fears of doing harm to others form the content of many obsessional symptoms.

It is safe to assume that fears of carrying out some antisocial act are for all practical purposes unfounded if they are typically obsessional. Important in this regard is the young mother who consults a doctor because she fears she will harm her child. If she has depressive psychotic symptoms with self-blame and suicidal ideas she will regard her impulses as sensible and necessary. In contrast, an obsessional fear is regarded by the patient, on quiet reflection, as absurd, and she says 'I would never do such a thing; it's quite ridiculous but the thought repeatedly comes into my head.' In the absence of psychotic symptoms or aggressive personality disorder characterised by impulsive behaviour, an obsessional fear is for all practical purposes never acted upon by the patient. The evaluation of such depressive and obsessional symptoms or personality traits is not easy and should in general be referred for an expert opinion.

Differential Diagnosis

1. **Other Mental Illness.** Obsessional symptoms may complicate any major mental disorder. In depressive

psychosis there may be accentuation of obsessional personality traits, but the depressive symptoms are in this case clear and unequivocal. In the schizophrenias, there may be obsessional as well as psychotic symptoms.

2. **Organic States.** Some cases of obsessional neurosis may arise as late complications of encephalitis lethargica. Temporal lobe epilepsy may be associated with compulsive-type symptoms but the epileptic features are usually obvious.

Basis of Treatment

Many obsessional neuroses remit quickly, though a significant proportion follow a chronic, fluctuant course. Symptomatic therapy with tranquillising drugs, or antidepressants if the depressive element is marked, may control the disability in some cases. Psychotherapy, apart from simple supportive measures is difficult, even though the symbolic significance of the symptoms may seem crystal clear. Very exceptionally it may be necessary to consider leucotomy in some chronic incapacitating obsessional illnesses, where there is severe subjective tension. Whenever an illness seems unresponsive to treatment it is important to investigate the environment for elements of secondary gain that may arise out of the obsessional symptoms or for continuing stress which leads to perpetuation of the illness.

Prognosis

At the onset of the illness there is a 50 per cent chance of being completely well in five years. The danger of chronicity is greater:
1. The longer the illness continues.
2. When the previous personality had lacked resilience.
3. When environmental factors or intrinsic conflicts remain intractable.

HYSTERICAL NEUROTIC REACTION

Definition

The hysterical neurosis is a psychological stress reaction. The symptoms are of two kinds:

1. **Conversion Symptoms,** which are psychogenic disorders of bodily function. These may take the form of paralysis, ataxia, tremor, blindness, deafness, pseudoepileptic or syncopal attacks, in the absence of adequate explanation in terms of organic disease.

2. **Dissociative Symptoms,** which are psychogenic disorders of consciousness, again in the absence of an adequate explanation on the basis of organic disease. There may be episodes of amnesia, sometimes accompanied by wandering (fugue) or clouding of consciousness with apparent disorientation.

Background

The hysterical reaction should be assessed in terms of the individual's long-standing vulnerability to stress (as shown by his personality make up), and the effect of precipitating factors immediately preceding the breakdown. There is usually evidence of previous personality difficulties, although only a proportion show typical histrionic personality traits characterised by a tendency to react excessively and to 'act out' under stress. Such characteristics have been regarded by some as indicative of emotional immaturity in view of their similarity to behaviour common in childhood.

It is important to regard hysterical neurosis as a reaction to some pathogenic factor, whether it be psychologically upsetting environmental events or true or imagined physical illness. Charcot erroneously believed hysteria to be a disease in itself, but in fact his patients were merely reacting to the theatrical situation in which he placed them.

The hysterical reaction is typically an unconscious process, quite distinct from conscious and deliberate assumption of symptoms by the patient as seen in malingering. It can be difficult to distinguish the two. In both, there is some understandable gain inherent in the symptoms whereby the patient attempts to achieve control over the life situation through adopting the sick role.

Symptoms

Hysterical symptoms may appear with dramatic suddenness in stressful situations. Their disappearance may also be rapid, especially when the precipitating factors have been resolved.

Conversion Symptoms tend to be variable from time to time, and the objective clinical findings usually differ in certain crucial respects from true organic disorder. Hysterical sensory loss is often of glove and stocking distribution, and does not follow dermatome distribution; hysterical ataxia may fail to conform to typical neurological disorder; hysterical weakness may be accompanied by contraction of antagonist muscles. The hysterical pseudoneurological disorders usually conform more to the layman's notion of disease than true organic illness. Dissociation symptoms often take the form of global amnesia, in which there is gross memory loss extending over much or all of the patient's life, in some cases making it impossible to recall identity or address. Such amnesia is almost certainly at least partly psychogenic in origin, and hysterical mechanisms are often important. Only the most gross organic brain injury could cause memory impairment of this severity, but the possibility of underlying physical disorder with a superadded hysterical reaction should always be kept in mind. Hysterical amnesia may also be selective for certain events that are emotionally painful.

467

The 'belle indifference reaction' in hysterical patients refers to the bland, indifferent, even smiling attitude they sometimes maintain in the face of grossly disabling symptoms.

It is important to search for underlying causes in every hysterical reaction, both in terms of psychologically upsetting events or underlying organic disease. Amnesia or weakness may be hysterical accentuation of organic impairment due to, as yet, undeclared physical illness. It follows that thorough physical investigations must be carried out in all cases.

A diagnosis of hysterical reaction should never be made by a process of exclusion merely because organic disease cannot be demonstrated. Adequate psychological explanation must be found and the reaction should, ideally, be understandable in the light of the previous personality make up. Close questioning regarding the pattern of illness in the past is often useful. There may have been a recurrent series of similar reactions under stress throughout the years. Hysteria is no more complete as a final diagnosis than would be pyrexia or pain of unknown origin.

Differential Diagnosis

1. **Malingering.** The distinction between unconscious motivation and deliberate deception can be very difficult to make. Malingering is likely when the symptoms are grossly inconsistent, depending on situations and audience, particularly when the element of gain is gross and superficial.

2. **Physical Disease.** This may be closely mimicked by hysterical symptoms. Commonly, both may be present, the hysterical symptom accentuating the organic disability. It can be a fatal mistake to assume that once a diagnosis of hysterical reaction has been made, then underlying organic disease has been ruled out: subsequent regular physical review is necessary in all cases.

Basis of Treatment

This involves management of personal predisposing factors and environmental precipitants. Formal interpretive psychotherapy is the most important form of treatment, by which an attempt is made to give the patient insight into his abnormal way of reacting to difficulties and to devise more healthy ways of coping. In practice, it can be difficult to achieve these aims. The hysterical patient may disarm the therapist by a passive agreement with or rejection of all that he says, and there may be a complete unwillingness to make any effort to change the situation. Therapy is made all the more difficult by the manipulative propensities of the patient, whereby situations are used to maintain the illness and so avoid on-going therapy. Treatment must include examination of the life situation as a whole in an attempt

to recognise areas of difficulty such as work responsibilities or social relationships. When interpersonal factors are important, it may be necessary to involve other persons (usually a relative) in conjoint therapy.

Hypnosis has been used widely in the treatment of the hysterical reaction. The patient is often highly suggestible and in certain cases there may be dramatic resolution of symptoms. Hypnosis is open to the criticism that it merely treats symptoms and not their underlying causes. Because of this it is not uncommon to see rapid relapse following its use in hysterical illnesses with the appearance of further hysterical symptoms unless it is accompanied by adequate psychotherapy.

Prognosis

The hysterical reaction may vary from a transient completely reversible disturbance to a chronic incapacitating illness. Prognosis depends on the reversibility of precipitating factors and the amenability of the patient to constructive discussion of the problem. Adequate previous personality adjustment and short duration of illness are good prognostic features.

C. PERSONALITY DISORDERS

Definition

Personality is the life-long psychological make up of an individual. Although each person is unique in terms of detailed personality profile, it is possible to classify personalities into broad descriptive types, each having a characteristic constellation of psychological traits.

Normal personality adjustment varies between wide limits of behaviour. In assessing mental illness it is particularly important to determine the individual's previous (premorbid) personality in order:
1. To assess the degree and rate of change in behaviour from normal.
2. To determine whether the illness is a reaction understandable in terms of previous attitudes.
3. To set realistic aims in treatment.

Personality disorder is a gross accentuation of certain psychological traits leading to a life-long pattern of difficulty in coping with the stress of day-to-day life. Before a diagnosis of personality disorder is made, it is necessary to have evidence of a persistent disorder of psychological adjustment in an adult over a period of several years. No psychotic features are present although the recurrent crises may precipitate severe reactive depressive symptoms from time to time.

Symptoms

The main personality anomalies are as follows:

Affective. Persistent disturbance of mood: may be depressive, anxious, or euphoric and overconfident. In the cyclothymic form there is gross variability between depression and elation.

Schizoid. Excessive shyness and social withdrawal. May be eccentric in habits. Tends towards cold, unfeeling personal relationships.

Obsessional. Overconscientious, perfectionist, rigid, vacillating, prone to anxiety, predisposed towards obsessional compulsive neurosis or depressive breakdown.

Histrionic. Overdramatic. Attention loving. Difficulty in making deep enduring personal relationships. Social relationships superficial. Prone to hysterical dissociative or conversion symptoms under stress.

Asthenic. General lack of resilience in meeting life's demands. Low drive and persistence. Prone to depression and may resort to alcohol if under stress.

Antisocial (Psychopathic). The Bristol physician C. J. Prichard (1835) was the first to describe this concept and emphasised the 'loss of self-government and lack of decency and propriety in the business of life'.

The label 'psychopathic' is currently used far too loosely and widely. It should be reserved for those individuals having 'a persistent disorder or disability of mind (whether or not including subnormality of intelligence) which results in abnormally aggressive or seriously irresponsible conduct on the part of the patient, and requires or is susceptible to medical treatment' (*Mental Health Act, 1959*). In practice, such patients can be remarkably resistant to efforts aimed at changing their behaviour, whether by therapeutic or punitive measures.

Paranoid. Excessively sensitive, suspicious of others' motives, but not psychotic. Tends to feel hard done by and may spend much time in defending and promoting principles and rights.

Basis of Treatment

The diagnosis of personality disorder is in many ways unsatisfactory because its aetiological, and hence therapeutic, implications are so ill-defined. Recognition of a life-long pattern of psychological disturbance does, however, help to establish realistic therapeutic aims. It is very difficult to achieve any radical alteration in well-established personality traits; the older the patient the harder it becomes. If he is actively and voluntarily seeking change, it is worthwhile offering short term psychotherapy which is aimed as much at getting the patient to recognise, modify or avoid life situations that cause him difficulty as attempting to achieve any radical change in his psychological make up. Frequently, it is necessary to involve other key persons in his life,

particularly the spouse. The recurrent social crises found in certain personality disorders (particularly the asthenic and psychopathic types) constitute a considerable burden on the community. When an affected family is receiving help from several agencies, it is important that these should all be well integrated. Long term support, with intensive help in a crisis, is more realistic than intensive time-consuming psychotherapy aimed at achieving true personality change in these cases.

SEXUAL DEVIATION

This includes a group of well-defined anomalies of sexual inclination and behaviour which are not secondary to psychosis or any other mental or physical illness.

HOMOSEXUALITY

Homosexuality consists of a sexual attraction towards other members of the same sex. When physical relationship ensues, the condition is regarded as *overt*, but it may remain *latent* when it is confined to the patient's fantasy life without leading to actual sexual contact.

1. MALE HOMOSEXUALITY

Background

In an American survey, Kinsey found that 37 per cent of adult males had experienced orgasm during homosexual behaviour at some time, 10 per cent had been exclusively homosexual for at least three years and 4 per cent had been exclusively so throughout their lives.

It is likely that the cause of homosexuality consists of a subtle interaction between genetic predisposition which then sensitises the individual to early learning situations of two main types:

Push Factors, whereby the man is driven into homosexuality by difficulties he experiences in making heterosexual contacts, for example:
(a) Learnt inhibition in heterosexual situations.
(b) Incestuous feelings concerning the mother may lead to revulsion towards heterosexual contact. Mother may have dominated the family and patient then identifies with her.
(c) Fear of failure in heterosexual role, lack of confidence in own masculinity or fear of rejection by a female.

Pull Factors, directly attracting him towards homosexual activity for example:
(a) Security of relationship with older man, especially when relationship with own father is impaired. Here, emotional factors other than sexual feelings may be more important.

(b) To gain self-esteem. The partner may provide this when it has not been obtained elsewhere.
(c) Fears of other men. As a result he may adopt a sexual attitude towards them.
(d) Material gain, especially in an economically deprived individual.

Symptoms

The boundary between illness and health is nowhere more ambiguous than in homosexuality. The mere presence of such deviation should not necessarily be equated with illness. The Wolfenden Committee concluded that homosexuality between consenting adults in private should no longer be regarded as an offence, and this is currently the legal situation in the United Kingdom.

The most common forms of homosexual behaviour are mutual masturbation and anal intercourse. Occasionally, the relationship is predominantly one of companionship, especially when there is a gross disparity of ages between the individuals concerned. The male homosexual may be quite happy with his orientation, and may deliberately set out to live in a homosexual subculture and acquire female mannerisms. However, society in general is usually derisory towards him. The homosexual male often finds that his sexual relationships are unstable, because they lack the stabilising influences such as the acquisition of dependents inherent in a normal family situation. Depressive symptoms often develop in the homosexual in the setting of recurrent break-ups in sexual relationships.

Complications

1. Depressive reactions when stable relationships are not achieved, or guilt over deviant feelings.
2. Venereal disease when promiscuity is present.

Differential Diagnosis

1. Transient normal phase in adolescent.
2. Normal sexuality but indulging in deviant behaviour merely for monetary gain.
3. Combined with other sexual deviation.

Basis of Treatment

The first step is to establish why the patient has presented himself to the doctor. When he comes reluctantly, perhaps coerced by others such as a dissatisfied wife or the courts, and he himself has no real wish to change, then psychiatric treatment is usually ineffective. On the other hand, he may come on his own initiative, wanting to be changed. In this case treatment may be feasible, and it is necessary to examine all the possible aetiological factors. Transient adolescent homosexual behaviour is common, and in itself is not necessarily of pathological significance. In older persons, the prospect of successful change in sexual orientation is greatest when the personality is stable and some heterosexual drive is also present. Psychotherapy may then prove effective and involves discussion of the 'push' factors which drive him away from heterosexual contact, and the positive forces which 'pull' him towards the homosexual role. Specialised techniques based on behaviour therapy (desensitisation, aversion techniques) are now being developed in the treatment of sexual deviation. Up to 40 per cent of selected homosexual patients may benefit from this kind of approach, but its exact value, especially with respect to long term results, remains uncertain.

Prognosis

In those male patients who request a change in sexual orientation from homosexuality, treatment is most likely to be effective when:
(a) There have been previous heterosexual feelings and experience.
(b) Personality has been stable.
(c) The patient is less than 35 years of age.

2. FEMALE HOMOSEXUALITY

This has been subjected to less systematic study than male homosexuality. Lesbianism is often more related to companionship than sexual gratification and such relationships tend to be relatively stable compared with those between male homosexuals. Kinsey found that four per cent of American females admitted to some overt homosexual experience at some time in their lives, and most studies agree that lesbianism is much less common than male homosexuality. It is compatible with a happy stable life, but female homosexuals as a group tend to be vulnerable to episodes of depression and anxiety.

OTHER SEXUAL DEVIATIONS

Transvestism is the derivation of sexual pleasure from dressing and sometimes masquerading in clothes of the opposite sex. Such behaviour may lead to legal repercussions, usually because of theft of clothing. In **exhibitionism**, sexual pleasure is derived from exposing the genitalia to the opposite sex. **Paedophilia** involves the wish to engage in sexual activity with children of either sex. In **fetishism**, sexual excitation arises mainly from inanimate objects which may or may not be related to the body of the opposite sex.

Management of these conditions follows the same principles as described under homosexuality. Social repercussions and penalties may in some cases be very severe, especially in paedophilia and exhibitionism. When such aberrant behaviour begins in older males for the first time, the possibility of dementia or other organic brain disease must always be kept in mind. Intermittent deviant behaviour may be secondary to alcohol abuse, the treatment of which may be more relevant than that of an otherwise latent sexual deviation.

Impotence is a failure by the male to achieve or sustain an erection during sexual intercourse even though libido remains normal. In the *primary* type, satisfactory sexual function has never been established, and in the absence of obvious physical causes, the disorder is usually due to deep-seated anxieties related to sexual function or orientation. The prognosis here tends to be poor. The *secondary* type develops in the context of previously normal sexual function. This may be seen in depressive illness, although in this case, loss of libido is usually more relevant. Secondary impotence is often due to a vicious circle sequence of events, whereby impotence is maintained by secondary anxiety following some episode of trivial sexual difficulty, for example temporary poor performance due to excess alcohol intake. This type may respond to a directive that heterosexual contact may continue, but full sexual intercourse is prohibited. This aims to remove the anxiety-provoking aspect of the situation, and frequently normal sexual function takes over before the next clinic appointment. In all cases of sexual difficulties it must be remembered that the symptom may merely be the presenting feature of more general problems between the marital partners. Full physical examination is always necessary, especially in the primary type, in order to exclude lumbosacral anomalies such as spina bifida.

In **premature ejaculation** the male arrives at orgasm and ejaculation before he wishes to do so, often before his partner has reached orgasm or even before intercourse has been attempted. It may be useful to base treatment on the principle of reducing sensory stimulation, for example simply by the use of a condom or by varying the frequency and length of penile intravaginal movement. Repeated masturbation just short of ejaculation may also have the effect of delaying ejaculation in normal intercourse. The work of Masters and Johnson in recent years has explored in detail such mechanical approaches to the problems of sexual dysfunction.

V. SOME IMPORTANT CLINICAL PROBLEMS

SUICIDE AND OTHER ACTS OF SELF-INJURY

SUICIDE

Definition

An individual commits suicide when he deliberately kills himself while possessing full knowledge of the implications of what he is doing.

Background

The rate of suicide in England and Wales has been decreasing in recent years. In 1969 it was 8.9 per 100,000 for the total population aged 15 years or over. The proportion due to hypnotic overdose is, however, increasing. The medical practitioner must report to the Coroner all cases in which he suspects suicide. *The Suicide Act, 1961* made suicide no longer a crime against the law, and has encouraged an enlightened therapeutic approach to the problem. No rise in suicide rate has occurred as a result of this change in society's attitude.

Suicide must be understood as a function of personal predisposition and environmental factors.

Environmental Factors. The rate of suicide correlates highly with the degree of social isolation of the individual, both in terms of living conditions and the extent to which he shares the values of the community in which he lives. The fall in suicide rate in times of war may be due to the increase in cohesion and purpose which results in the community. Suicide rates are higher in the separated or single than in the widowed; married persons have still lower rates. This sequence may be partly explained on the basis of social isolation. High rates are found in urban living conditions, particularly where there is an over-representation of single-person households and rapid population turnover. It is not poverty itself, but rather loss of belongings or status that appears to be a predisposing factor. Certain sub-groups are at risk. Although the overall death rate in university students is low, some 37 per cent of them are due to suicide. Rates are higher in upper social classes: the medical profession tends to have a high incidence, and here the easy availability of drugs may be just as relevant as work stresses.

Personal Factors. The highest rates of suicide are to be found in the elderly; and the rate in men is greater than in women. Other individual precipitating factors are: the presence of mental illness of any kind (recent studies have shown that over 90 per cent of suicides may show some evidence of mental disturbance in the preceding few weeks; between 11 and 17 per cent of persons who suffer from manic depressive illness eventually commit suicide), alcoholism, intractable physical disease, recent bereavement, and previous pattern of self-injury.

Prevention

Suicide poses considerable challenges in terms of preventive medicine. While many cases occur without any warning whatsoever, a high proportion (78 per cent) makes some sort of contact with the medical profession in the months preceding the actual suicide. Recognition by the doctor of high-risk individuals is therefore crucial in the initiation of adequate early treatment. Psychiatric patients are particularly vulnerable in the months following their discharge from hospital and they require intensive follow-up during this time. More general measures include planning retirement and encouraging social contacts, where appropriate. The Samaritans, a voluntary agency that offers emergency help (initiated by telephone contact) by day and night to those tempted to kill themselves, probably prevent a significant number of suicides. In 1977 almost 230,000 new callers availed themselves of the Samaritan's help in the UK.

OTHER ACTS OF SELF-INJURY ('ATTEMPTED SUICIDE')

Definition

Under this category are included those intentional acts of self-injury (poisoning or mutilation) that do not result in death. Although some of these may be true failed attempts at suicide, it is often difficult to be sure of the individual's motive at the time, and it is preferable to use the general term 'non-fatal deliberate self-harm' to describe this behaviour.

Background

In contrast to the rate of successful suicide, which has been falling consistently in recent years, the number of acts of non-fatal deliberate self-harm appears to have increased very rapidly over the last decade, especially those due to overdose of prescribed psychotropic drugs (Fig. 20.6). The true incidence of 'attempted suicide' is difficult to assess, but it is probably at least six to eight times more common than suicide itself.

Persons who deliberately but not fatally injure themselves, whether by self-poisoning or mutilation, constitute a highly vulnerable group, and a significant number repeat the act (about 20 per cent within one year) or end up by committing suicide (1.6 per cent within one year). It is dangerous for the doctor to regard such patients as merely seeking attention, and he should recognise that this form of maladaptive behaviour is potentially lethal. In statistical terms, non-fatal deliberate self-harm patients differ from successful suicides in several ways. They tend to be young (22 to 44 years, Fig. 20.7), married, they are more often female than male, and more frequently suffer from personality disorders rather than other types of mental illness.

Basis of Assessment and Treatment of Persons who have 'Attempted' or Threatened Suicide

The first problem is to assess the danger of repeat self-harm in the immediate future. Following on this, the most appropriate treatment setting must be established. A full history is required both from the patient and other close friends or relatives. Three aspects in particular must be taken into consideration in assessing

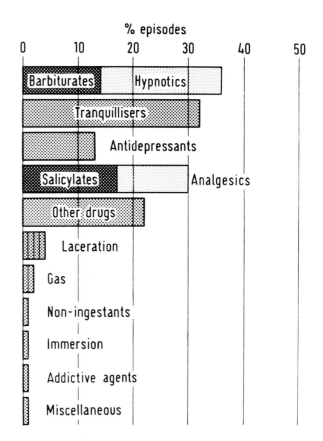

Fig. 20.6 Methods of deliberate self-harm in 368 interviewed patients.

any individual. Factors that indicate suicide risk include the following:

Predisposing Factors in the Patient Himself:
(a) Florid mental illness particularly depression (especially when there is agitation, self-blame, delusions of disease, and previous attempts at suicide).
(b) Alcoholism (8 per cent of chronic alcoholics commit suicide within five years of discharge from hospital).
(c) Elderly male.
(d) Intractable physical illness.
(e) Positive family history of suicide.
(f) Repeated serious self-injury in the past.

Predisposing Factors in the Environment:
(a) Social isolation and lack of support from others.
(b) Recent bereavement.
(c) Hostile reaction from others as a result of the self-injury (rejection by family and spouse, loss of accommodation, loss of job).

The Act of Self-harm:
(a) Serious rather than trivial act (size of overdose, extent of physical injury).
(b) Real attempts made to conceal (occurred at a time or situation which made discovery unlikely).

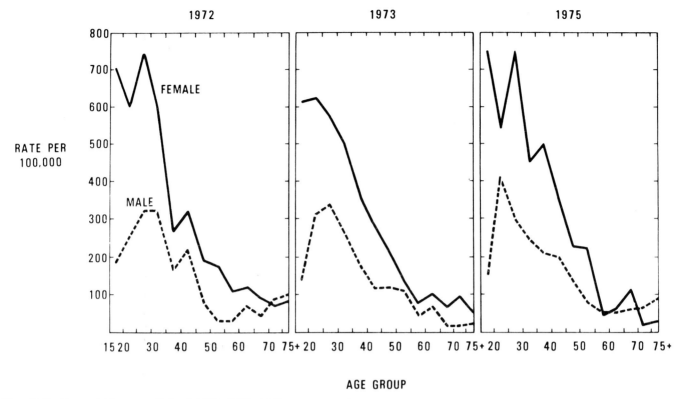

1972   1973   1975

Fig. 20.7   Parasuicide rates, Bristol 1972, 1973, 1975; patients referred to hospital casualty.

(c) Precautions taken to ensure success (e.g. blocking ventilation in attempted coal-gas poisoning).

(d) The patient's attitude suggests real suicidal intent (had fully intended to end life, regrets having failed, and wishes to repeat the act).

It is important that all cases admitted to hospital following acts of self-harm should receive adequate psychiatric assessment. A decision must then be made regarding the most appropriate treatment setting. In some cases it may be safe to arrange supervision by the family doctor or out-patient psychiatric support; other more serious cases may need immediate admission to a psychiatric ward.

MARITAL PROBLEMS

It has been estimated that about 50 per cent of marriages encounter early adjustment difficulties, although in most cases these resolve without outside help. About 10 per cent of married couples experience sufficient difficulty to contemplate or actually experience separation, and most of these problems arise in the first two or three years of marriage. Actual divorce is most frequent six to seven years after marriage.

Any satisfactory marriage demands a reciprocal understanding and close relationship between two individuals over an extended period of time. The rela-

tionship and life situation both undergo a gradual change, and the partners have to readjust their attitudes throughout the years. It is possibly for this reason that the most vulnerable marriages are those between very young people. Those who marry before 18 years of age have a re-marriage rate three times greater than those marrying later, especially when the young marriage takes place for inappropriate reasons (e.g. forced by pregnancy, or used as an escape from own family) or when the wife proves to be infertile. Adjustment difficulties in young marriages are probably related to the fact that personality development in the partners is still incomplete, with the result that unpredictable difficulties occur in forging an enduring relationship.

Legal Aspects

Marriage is a legal contract that can only be broken under very clearly defined conditions. The Catholic Church recognises divorce only in very exceptional circumstances. *The Divorce Reform Act, 1969* formulates grounds for divorce in terms of irretrievable breakdown of marriage. The traditional marital offences (desertion, adultery, cruelty, incurable unsoundness of mind) are now to be regarded only as possible components of a total breakdown in the relationship, and collusional manufacture of evidence of such misbehaviour by partners seeking divorce need no longer occur.

Clinical Features

In many cases of marital difficulties the fundamental causes are shared between both partners. Occasionally, the problem lies predominantly on one side, in the form of florid psychotic illness, alcohol addiction, personality disorder or neurotic syndromes which in themselves require treatment. Most frequently, the causes lie in the subtle interplay between two personalities each perhaps itself within the normal limits of adjustment. Each marital relationship is unique unto itself; because of the enormous variation to be found in marriages that appear viable and happy, no strict norms of behaviour can be laid down. Even a degree of aggressive behaviour is in certain social classes regarded as normal within a marriage. Sexual behaviour also varies a great deal. In assessing a marital problem it is necessary to take into account each partner's viewpoint before therapeutic aims are delineated.

Management

If one partner is suffering from gross psychological disorder then adequate treatment of this may itself alleviate many secondary marital problems. More commonly it is necessary to involve both man and wife in treatment. Regular therapy with one partner may serve a supportive function, but it rarely completely removes the difficulties between the two. It may even increase resentment in the other. It is sometimes useful in the initial stages of therapy for both partners to be seen individually by separate therapists, but the aim should be that combined interviews will begin as soon as possible. Ideally, the following criteria should be satisfied before conjoint therapy is initiated:
1. Both partners should have a genuine wish to improve their relationship by mutual discussion, and can accept that blame is not necessarily entirely on one side.
2. Neither partner is psychotic, or so aggressive and dominant as to overwhelm the other in discussion. Each must be able to represent his or her views, if necessary with the support of the therapist.

In conducting conjoint interviews, the therapist must not openly side with one or other partner. His role is to facilitate communication between them, and he should avoid giving authoritarian directive advice himself. The aim should be to get each partner to behave in a sympathetic and understanding way towards the other. The therapist must remember that his remarks will probably be relayed, often in distorted form, to others, and he should not permit himself to make any comment other than those directed at reconstruction of the marriage. Each conjoint interview should aim at resolving rather than fostering conflicts. Difficult issues must of course be discussed, but the interview has failed if it ends in an unresolved quarrel.

NON-ACCIDENTAL INJURY IN CHILDREN

The dramatic term 'battered baby syndrome' coined by Kempe in 1962 drew attention to the size and seriousness of this problem. It is not a specific clinical entity, merely a description of behaviour which may be due to a variety of possible causes. Child assault may stem from a wish to eliminate an encumbrance, or to relieve suffering (mercy killing), disordered thinking because of mental illness in a parent, displacement of anger, frustration and retaliation onto children, or it may be a response to some problem in the child itself.

Background

The incidence of non-accidental injury of course depends upon the degree of injury involved. Severe cases with major physical injury have been estimated to occur at an annual rate of 1 in 1,000 of children under four years of age in England and Wales. About two to four per cent of children in subnormality hospitals are brain damaged through assault by their parents, usually through violent shaking or battering. One-quarter of severely attacked young children are intellectually damaged as a result.

Clinical Features

Many factors may combine to prevent adequate recognition of non-accidental injury of a child.

The families come from all social classes and the parents may vary greatly in intelligence, attractiveness, mental stability, personality type and apparent efficiency in running the home. When non-accidental injury in a child is suspected certain points may provide useful leads.

In the Child. Evidence of successive injuries especially bruises of different ages in very young children or when the lesions are bizarre in nature. As a working rule all fractures in children up to two years of age must be viewed with suspicion. The child may be fearful towards certain adults, may show over-anxious concern for the parents' welfare and is often unhappy.

In the Parents. May be evasive and provide contradictory information, lack warmth towards the child and show inadequate confidence in handling it, or express overt criticism, for example concerning its refusal to be comforted or its excessive crying.

Prevention and Basis of Treatment

Much emphasis is rightly placed on the need for good and immediate communication between different branches of the caring services in dealing with non-accidental injury in children. Regional and Area Review

Source: Working Party of Royal College of Psychiatrists (1977) *Brit. J. Psychiat.* **131**: 366–380.

Committees have now been established for this purpose and all persons concerned should know how to communicate and share information when necessary. The use of case registers is also an important development. When there is suspicion of non-accidental injury to a child, a conference of all helping persons is called and further action agreed as a group decision. A key worker is nominated to integrate all subsequent activities. When the child is at immediate risk it may be necessary to act on an urgent basis. Admission of the child to a hospital ward for full assessment is usually the most acceptable procedure; occasionally when the parents object and the child is judged to be in danger, it may be necessary to remove it compulsorily to such a place of safety.

LEGAL ASPECTS OF PSYCHIATRY

1. Personal Liberty. Aspects of Compulsory Admission and Treatment

In certain circumstances, mental illness may make the patient such a danger to himself and/or others that it is then necessary to restrict his liberty by compelling him to receive appropriate care in hospital. The general approach of the *Mental Health Act, 1959* is to encourage assessment and treatment on a voluntary basis, but where no alternative is possible, certain sections of the Act make legal provision for the adoption of compulsory measures. The diagnostic categories covered by compulsory procedures are:
1. Mental illness.
2. Severe mental subnormality.
3. Mental subnormality.
4. Psychopathic disorder.

Only if the person is less than 21 years of age, unless referred through a court of law following an offence, do (3) and (4) above apply. It is made quite clear in the Act that no provision is made for compulsory measures based merely on grounds of promiscuity or other immoral conduct alone. All compulsory procedures whether for observation or treatment (except removal of mentally ill persons from public places by the police) necessitate two distinct steps:

(a) The medical recommendation.
(b) The application by a relative or mental welfare officer for admission to the relevant hospital. The order may apply in any hospital in the NHS.

A compulsory procedure is not merely the prerogative of the medical practitioner; his recommendation cannot be acted upon unless it receives the lay support in the form of application from a relative or authorised social worker. A great deal of responsibility is thus vested by the Act in the patient's nearest relative who must be the first choice signatory in any application. The authorised social worker may take on the relative's role in an emergency situation, but he must always consult the relative whenever it is practicable to do so.

The main compulsory procedures are outlined in Table 20.3.

The precise nature of the *medical recommendation* varies according to the compulsory procedure required:

Admission for Observation (Section 25). The medical recommendation here must state three things:
(a) The patient is suffering from mental disorder of a nature which warrants his detention in a hospital under observation (with or without other medical treatment) for at least a limited period.
(b) He ought to be so detained in the interest of his own health or safety or with a view to the protection of other persons.

Table 20.3 Compulsory procedures Mental Health Act 1959

Purpose	Section of Mental Health Act	Maximum duration	Persons making application	Medical recommendation
Hospital admission for observation	25	28 days	Nearest relative or authorised social worker	1. Registered medical practitioner 2. Recognised specialist in mental illness
Hospital admission for observation in emergency (when only one doctor is available and the degree of urgency does not permit delay to obtain a second medical opinion)	29	72 hours	Any relative or authorised social worker	Registered medical practitioner (if possible having previous knowledge of the patient)
Removal by police to place of safety Persons who appear to be mentally disordered in a place to which public have access. If in immediate need of care or control may be taken by police constable to a place of safety to await examination by doctor and authorised social worker	136	72 hours	Police officer	–
Emergency detention of informal patient already in hospital	30	3 days beginning with the day on which report furnished	–	The responsible medical officer (i.e. consultant psychiatrist in charge of the case). His deputy may act on direct instructions from the consultant if the latter is not able to see the patient immediately
Hospital admission for treatment	26	1 year May be renewed if appropriate Patient may appeal to a Mental Health Tribunal in the first six months	Nearest relative or authorised social worker. (The latter must, where practicable, first consult the nearest relative)	1. Registered medical practitioner with previous knowledge of patient (usually GP) 2. Recognised specialist in mental illness

(c) Informal admission is not appropriate.

If at the end of the 28-day period further treatment is needed, and the patient's consent cannot be obtained, the observation period cannot be extended, but a new application must be made under Section 26 of the Act, supported by a recommendation for treatment.

Admission for Treatment (Section 26). This may apply to a patient of any age, if suffering from mental illness or severe subnormality. If less than 21 years of age, it may also include subnormality or psychopathic disorder. When recommending treatment, the two medical practitioners must, in addition to the information required for observation, also:

(a) Give a clinical description of the patient's mental condition.

(b) State the form of mental disorder from which he is suffering and that it is of a nature or degree which

warrants detention in hospital for medical treatment.

(c) Indicate whether other methods of care or treatment are available, and if so, why they are not appropriate and why informal admission is not suitable.

2. Criminal Responsibility

For over 100 years the English criminal law regarding mitigation of responsibility on grounds of insanity has rested on the McNaughton Rules. By these, to establish a defence on the grounds of insanity it must be clearly proved that at the time of committing the act the party accused was labouring under such a defect of reason from disease of the mind, as not to know the nature and quality of the act he was doing, or if he did know it, he did not know that what he was doing was wrong. These rules have been much criticised, mainly on the ground that few certified insane individuals would fulfil these criteria. They force the court of law to consider the problem within the limiting framework of the rules themselves, and other relevant psychiatric aspects of the case may not be heard.

When a person has been tried for an offence in a court of law and is then judged to need compulsory treatment for mental illness he may be detained for this purpose under Section 60 of *The Mental Health Act*, either in a NHS psychiatric hospital or, if necessary, in a high security hospital. Mental illness may make a person unfit to plead if he:
1. Is unable to instruct his counsel.
2. Cannot appreciate the significance of pleading guilty or not guilty; cannot challenge the jurors or examine a witness.
3. Is unable to follow the evidence placed before the court and the court procedure.

The doctor in a court of law is not regarded as privileged: hence he may be forced on pain of imprisonment to divulge confidential information communicated to him by his patients. Many difficulties can arise when a doctor is asked to give psychiatric evidence in a court of law and he should, unless clearly called as an expert witness, merely state the facts of a case as known to him without offering theoretical interpretations of his own making.

3. Review of the 1959 Mental Health Act

There has recently been considerable discussion concerning possible ways of improving the 1959 Act. The main issues of contention centre around the restriction of individual liberty inherent in any compulsory admission procedure whether this be for observation or treatment. The National Association for Mental Health has been vociferous in this respect, and asks whether the Act places too great a responsibility and, worse still, too much power in the hands of the medical profession. The debate has been particularly concerned with the provision of clearer criteria for compulsory admission, as well as the problems which arise when treatment is imposed on someone who is either unwilling to agree or who does not understand the nature of the proposed procedure. Most are agreed that special provision should be made when such treatment is hazardous or irreversible. The recent DHSS review of *The Mental Health Act* discusses these problems in detail in the light of evidence submitted to an inter-departmental committee.

4. Testamentary Capacity

The ability to make a Will must be judged on the following criteria. The person concerned must:
1. Know he is making a Will and what this implies.
2. Know the nature and extent of his property.
3. Know the person who has claims on his bounty.
4. Possess judgment which is unimpaired regarding these persons.

The crucial issue is not whether the person is suffering from mental illness, but whether it impairs his ability to make a Will. Patients detained under the *Mental Health Act* in mental hospitals may make Wills if the mental illness leaves their judgment regarding property and its disposal unimpaired.

5. Management of Property

When a person is rendered unfit, because of mental disorder, to manage his property and affairs this may be undertaken by the Court of Protection (25 Store Street, London WC1) upon medical evidence furnished in the form of an affidavit. By appointing a receiver, the court thus provides a safeguard for the patient against exploitation. Such jurisdiction concerns property only, and the patient's liberty is in no other way affected.

TERMINATION OF PREGNANCY

The Abortion Act, 1967 specifies the circumstances under which pregnancy may be terminated on medical grounds. It states:
1. A person shall not be guilty of an offence under the law relating to abortions when a pregnancy is terminated by a registered medical practitioner if two such practitioners are of the opinion, formed in good faith:
(a) That the continuance of the pregnancy would involve risk to the life of the pregnant woman, or of injury to the physical and mental health of the pregnant woman or any existing children of her family, greater than if the pregnancy was terminated.
(b) That there is a substantial risk that if the child was born, it would suffer from such physical or mental abnormality as to be seriously handicapped.
2. In determining whether the continuance of a pregnancy would involve such risk of injury to health, account must be taken of the pregnant woman's actual or reasonably foreseeable environment.

A doctor who has moral or religious objections may refuse to advise a patient who seeks termination of pregnancy. However, such a practitioner can raise no objection if the patient consults another practitioner who may be prepared to consider the possibility of termination. The Act requires that two doctors' signatures should be sent to the Chief Medical Officer of Health when termination is recommended, and the operation should be carried out in an establishment that has been approved as being appropriate for that purpose.

Requests for termination of pregnancy pose problems for the psychiatrist who tries to adopt a consistent policy based on scientific principles. Under coercion such as threats of suicide or various social pressures, it is all too easy to attach psychiatric labels of convenience to patients. Interpretation of the Act then merely reflects the severity of the pressures placed on the psychiatrist rather than his own clinical opinion, which ideally should be the only basis for his decision. Firm scientific evidence on which the case must be judged on psychiatric grounds is scanty, and what is available poses a dilemma. The woman may change her mind and regret the termination once it has been carried out, and she who shows significant psychiatric disturbance at the time she requests termination is most likely to develop guilt and regret after it has been carried out. In one large series of patients refused abortions and followed up for seven to eleven years, it was found that 73 per cent subsequently stated that they were satisfied at the way things had turned out. A study of women who had received an abortion showed that although 75 per cent had no regret, a significant proportion (25 per cent) was self-reproachful, and those that had presented initially with psychiatric symptoms were heavily represented in this group. It should also be remembered that termination of pregnancy is a surgical procedure not without risk. Although the mortality rate is low (0.6 per 1,000) there is, even in the best centres, some kind of complication in a significant proportion of cases (e.g. pyrexia, haemorrhage, ruptured uterus). The risks are much greater after twelve weeks gestation.

Psychiatric Indications for Termination

In Mother:
1. *Recurrent puerperal psychosis* in the past, or a history of *one intractable puerperal illness*, especially if schizophrenic type. The risk of recurrence with further pregnancy is of such serious import that termination might be justified if requested by the pregnant woman.

2. *Acute emotional upset with suicidal risk.* In some cases, the pregnancy leads to emotional distress, with agitation, tearfulness and depression with talk of suicide. Although many patients (up to 20 per cent) talk of suicide whilst requesting termination, actual suicides in persons refused abortion is rare. Assessment of the risk in any individual requires expert psychiatric opinion and can be done effectively only by means of a short spell in hospital. The doctor should not allow himself to be pushed against his better judgement into complying with a request for termination when it seems that other kinds of help, particularly social support or treatment of depression are more appropriate. It is unwise to ignore talk of suicide when there are accompanying severe depressive symptoms, such as morbid guilt, or a history of recurrent serious self-injury at times of stress. Such patients should always be admitted to hospital for full assessment.

3. *Chronic mental illness.* A person suffering from florid, *chronic psychotic illness* may react adversely to the stress of pregnancy, especially if she is already experiencing difficulty in coping with family commitments, and her

claim for termination might be sympathetically considered. It must be remembered, however, that the risk of adverse mental reaction to the termination is high in this type of patient. *Mental subnormality* with a poor standard of care of the existing children may justify termination as a prophylaxis against family breakdown and child neglect. *Chronic neurotic illness* which causes severe impairment of function may on some occasions warrant termination. Depression and self-blame usually indicate that a subsequent adverse mental reaction is likely.

In considering a request for termination of pregnancy, psychiatric factors cannot be considered apart from social conditions, which themselves may hold the balance between health and breakdown. A request by a woman who is already under stress (e.g. isolated, overburdened with family commitments) will be considered more sympathetically than others, and the Act allows for this by stating that 'account may be taken of the pregnant woman's actual or reasonably foreseeable environment'.

The Child. Prior to the 1967 Act, the risk of fetal abnormality was regarded as relevant only in so far as the effect this would have on the mother's mental health. Fetal risk can now itself be regarded as an indication for termination. Situations in which fetal risk arises include rubella in the first 20 weeks of pregnancy, smallpox, vaccinia or exposure to cytotoxic drugs, X-rays (30 rad or more to the pelvis within the first trimester) and familial illness (phenylketonuria, galactosaemia, haemophilia, Christmas disease). Certain congenital abnormalities must also be considered. For example, the incidence of Mongolism increases with the age of the parents, and there is a 1 in 70 chance of a second Mongol child occurring in a family with one child already affected.

Sterilisation

Mental illness can rarely be regarded in itself as justification for sterilisation. This stems from the difficulty in predicting future psychiatric adjustment in any individual. Even chronic mental ill health may change dramatically as social circumstances alter. The danger of depressive reaction to sterilisation is, of course, particularly great in the mentally ill.

THE MENTAL HEALTH SERVICES IN ACTION

During the last four decades there has been a major change in emphasis with regard to the way mental health services are organised. The problems inherent in the institutional approach as represented by our mental hospitals have become readily apparent and determined attempts have been made to provide treatment, where possible, in the community.

The first advance was the acceptance that psychiatric out-patient clinics should be held in general hospitals,

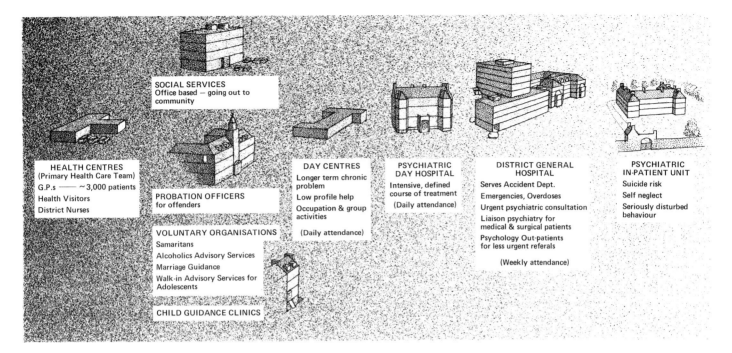

Fig. 20.8 The mental health services in action.

and more recently in-patient psychiatric units have been developed as an integral part of district general hospitals. Psychiatric day hospitals have been a further very important development, providing treatment for patients who may return home at night. Day centres which provide less active, but longer social support for persons who can live in the community but are chronically mentally disabled also play an important part. Sheltered workshops, industrial therapy and rehabilitation of a kind pioneered in Bristol afford some opportunity for mentally disabled individuals to compete for jobs in the community. The work of voluntary organisations and housing associations in providing group homes has also been most encouraging in recent years.

These developments have presented challenges to mental health care personnel who are gradually finding new roles that are less based on the institution and which are more community orientated. Psychiatric nurses are now playing a major part in visiting patients at home, hospital social workers (now employed by local authorities) and psychiatrists work increasingly in the community, for example holding clinics in health centres as opposed to the hospitals. The big challenge now is to define new working relationships between hospital based personnel, the primary health care teams and social service departments. Much uncertainty remains over the future role of our mental hospitals. Many feel that district general hospital psychiatric in-patient units will not be able to cater adequately for certain types of mental disturbance, especially when behaviour is severely disordered or the patient needs a long stay in hospital. If our mental hospitals lose their

role in treating acute psychiatric illness then we will be converting them into large, isolated and under-privileged institutions which we all want to avoid.

Psychogeriatric care presents us with a particularly difficult problem in the decades to come. Mental illness in old age may be unmasked by a social or medical crisis and rarely does the psychological disturbance stand alone. For this reason the health care of the elderly requires close co-operation between psychiatrists, physicians, social workers and nurses. Elderly patients with psychiatric illness make great demands on relatives and caring agencies. By 1991 the numbers of people of pensionable age will have increased by 15 per cent (a million more individuals) and those aged 75 years by 35 per cent. Demands for care of the elderly mentally ill are therefore likely to increase very considerably.

Against this background only a policy that gives priority to increasing domiciliary support will ease the strain on relatives and reduce the rate of increased demand upon residential care. In this field, therefore, the early ascertainment of disorder is of prime importance if crises are to be avoided. Future care of the individual should be planned to take account of all the factors involved. The approaches in management may be classified as social or medical in nature and in practice both strategies are combined together to help any individual.

It is important to remember that functional mental illness in the elderly, in the absence of significant organic mental impairment, can respond in a very gratifying way to conventional psychiatric treatment, and this should never be withheld or delayed merely because of a patient's advanced age. Even in the elderly, dementia is sometimes due to a treatable cause, for example myxoedema or subdural haematoma. The hallmark of good psychogeriatric care should be the assumption that nothing is completely untreatable. Early assessment is crucial together with efficient mobilisation of community resources, because residential services will for long remain grossly inadequate for the task in hand.

SUGGESTED FURTHER READING

Historical

Ackerknecht, E. H. (1959) *A Short History of Psychiatry*. New York: Hasner.
Barton, R. (1966) *Institutional Neurosis*. Bristol: Wright.
Hunter, R. A. and MacAlpine, I. (1963) *Three Hundred Years of Psychiatry*. London: Oxford University Press.

General

Department of Health and Social Services Interdepartmental Committee (1976) *A Review of the Mental Health Act 1959*. London: HMSO.
Hargrove, A. L. (1963) *The National Association for Mental Health Guide to the Mental Health Act 1959*. London: National Association for Mental Health.
Hooper, D. Roberts, J. (1973) *Disordered Lives: An Interpersonal Account*. National Marriage Guidance Council.
Russell Davis, D. (1972) *An Introduction to Psychopathology*, 3rd ed. London: Oxford University Press.

Russell Davis, D. (1971) Advances in Psychiatry. *The Practitioner* **207**: 474.

Specific Topics

Bancroft, J. H. J. (1970) Homosexuality in the male. *British Journal of Hospital Medicine* **3**: 168–181.
Bewley, T. H. (1970) An introduction to drug dependence. *British Journal of Hospital Medicine* **4**: 150–161.
Crisp, A. H. (1967) Anorexia nervosa. *Hospital Medicine* **2**: 713–718.
Crisp, A. H. (1978) Anorexia nervosa. *Medicine* **11**: 537–542.
Crown, S. (1976) Marital Breakdown: Epidemiology and Psychotherapy. In *Recent Advances in Clinical Psychiatry*, ed. K. Granville Grossman, 200–226. Churchill Livingstone.
Dominian, J. (1968) *Marital Breakdown*. Penguin.
Edwards, G. (1967) The meaning and treatment of alcohol dependence. *Hospital Medicine* **2**: 272–281.
Forrest, A., Ritson, B. and Zealley, A. eds. (1973) *New Perspectives in Mental Handicap*. Churchill Livingstone.
Home Office (1968) *Cannabis: Report by the Advisory Committee on Drug Dependence*. London: HMSO.
Joyce, C. R. B. (1970) Cannabis. *British Journal of Hospital Medicine* **4**: 162–166.
Kessell, Neil (1965) The Milroy Lectures: Self-poisoning. *British Medical Journal* **2**: 1265–1270, 1336–1348.
Kessel, N. and Walton, H. (1969) *Alcoholism*. Harmondsworth: Penguin Books.
Master, W. H., Johnson, V. E. (1970) *Human Sexual Inadequacy*. London: J. and A. Churchill.
McCulloch, J. W. and Philip, A. E. (1972) *Suicidal Behaviour*. Oxford: Pergamon Press.
Medical Defence Union (1968) Memorandum on the Abortion Act 1967. *British Medical Journal* **1**: 759–762.
Medical Protection Society (1969) *Proceedings of a Symposium on The Abortion Act 1967*. London: Pitman Medical.
Post, F. (1965) *The Clinical Psychiatry of Late Life*. Oxford: Pergamon Press.
Reed, J. L. (1971) Hysteria. *British Journal of Hospital Medicine* **5**: 237–249.
Roth, M. and Myers, D. H. (1969) The diagnosis of dementia. *British Journal of Hospital Medicine* **2**: 705–717.
Stengel, E. (1964) *Suicide and Attempted Suicide*. Harmondsworth: Penguin Books.
Wing, Lorna (1970) The syndrome of early childhood autism. *British Journal of Hospital Medicine* **4**: 381–392.
Wolfenden Committee (1957) *Report of the Committee on Homosexual Offences and Prostitution*. London: HMSO.

Treatment

Frank, J. D. (1963) *Persuasion and Healing*. New York: Schocken Books.
Goffman, E. (1968) *Asylums*. Harmondsworth: Penguin Books.
Schurr, P. H. (1973) Psychosurgery. *British Journal of Hospital Medicine* **10**, 53–60.
Shepherd, M., Lader, M. and Rodnight, R. (1968). *Clinical Psychopharmacology*. London: English Universities Press.
Silverstone, T. and Turner, P. (1974) *Drug Treatment in Psychiatry*. Routledge.

Neurology

21

R. LANGTON HEWER

Clinical neurology is concerned with the many diseases which affect the functioning of the central and peripheral nervous systems and the voluntary muscles. Common neurological disorders include epilepsy, stroke, migraine, multiple sclerosis, Parkinsonism, meningitis, head injury, cerebral palsy, and muscular dystrophy. Neurological disorders cannot, of course, be considered entirely in isolation and there is much overlap both with 'general medicine' and with psychiatry.

Some students used to think that neurology was a difficult subject – concerned mainly with the solving of medical jigsaw puzzles. Others thought that it was a subject concerned primarily with diagnosis and not with treatment. Happily the modern generation is more enlightened! Neurology is not difficult – assuming a basic knowledge of anatomy and physiology. It is a very logical subject and the diagnosis can usually be 'worked out' provided that a systematic approach is adopted. Many diseases can be successfully treated and although others are incurable in the ordinary sense of the word there is still a great deal that can be done to overcome disability.

During the last 30 years there have been great advances in the prevention and treatment of neurological disease. Poliomyelitis has virtually disappeared from Western countries due to the use of vaccine. Effective antibiotic treatment of pyogenic and tuberculous meningitis has greatly reduced both the mortality and morbidity arising from these conditions. Steroids have completely changed the outlook in disorders such as cranial arteritis and polymyositis. The neurosurgical management of much intracranial and intraspinal disease has improved greatly – partly due to advances in neurosurgical techniques and partly due to the introduction of new methods in diagnostic radiology. The last five years has seen the introduction of the CT (computorised tomography) scanner; this has totally revolutionised the diagnosis of intracranial disease.

Sometimes the diagnosis is made by the recognition of a clinical syndrome. Thus, migraine can be recognised by the association of stereotyped attacks of visual disturbance followed by headache and vomiting. Multiple sclerosis can be recognised by the occurrence in a young woman of transient episodes of neurological disturbance which may include blindness, double vision, tingling in one limb, and urinary urgency.

In most instances it is necessary to go through the orderly process of identifying the anatomical site of the lesion and then attempting to obtain information about the pathology. The example of a person with progressive weakness of the legs may be taken. It is first necessary to ascertain whether we are dealing with a lesion of the lower or the upper motor neurone.

In a lower motor neurone lesion there will usually be muscle wasting, weakness, hypotonia, and diminished tendon reflexes. The lesion may lie in a number of sites – the anterior horn cell, the cauda equina, the nerve plexuses, the peripheral nerves, or the muscle itself. A common example would be polyneuritis, in which there is frequently symmetrical weakness of the distal muscles of the legs (and usually of the arms) and in addition there may be distal sensory loss. The diagnosis is usually obvious clinically, but if necessary it can be sometimes confirmed by appropriate nerve conduction studies. Having made the primary diagnosis it is then necessary to ascertain the cause for the polyneuritis (for instance, diabetes, latent carcinoma, toxin, etc.).

In a lesion of the upper motor neurone there is no muscle wasting (except in the late stages – due to disuse). There is usually some degree of weakness, the muscle tone and tendon reflexes are increased (sometimes with clonus) and the plantar responses are extensor. Most cases of upper motor neurone weakness of both legs are due to a lesion of the spinal cord. Having decided that the disturbance lies within the spinal cord it is then necessary to ascertain at which level the cord is being affected. Spinal cord disease commonly involves ascending sensory, as well as descending motor, pathways. For this reason a disturbance in, for instance, the mid-thoracic region of the spinal cord may produce a 'sensory level' on the trunk – below which sensation is impaired or lost. Such a disturbance may be due to compression of the spinal cord from outside or to an intrinsic abnormality. In the former case a special radiological study (a myelogram) will usually demonstrate the compression. Once demonstrated it is necessary to ascertain its cause – for example a prolapsed intervertebral disc or a tumour. A normal myelogram virtually excludes a compressive lesion and, hence, the pathology is likely to be primarily within the spinal cord itself (for instance a plaque of multiple sclerosis).

It is not always possible to make an accurate pathological diagnosis; for instance, many types of headache defy precise classification. Similarly, in many cases of dementia it is not possible to be certain, in life, whether the condition is due to disease of the cerebral blood vessels or to one of the degenerative brain disorders. The clinician's most important task is to make certain that no treatable disease has been missed. He must be reasonably certain, for instance, that there is no underlying benign tumour or deficiency disease.

Having made a diagnosis in terms of anatomy and pathology, it is then necessary to undertake functional assessment. This is concerned with the ways in which the disturbance affects the patient's everyday performance. For instance, the patient with a common peroneal lesion may fall over repeatedly because his foot catches on the ground. He needs a foot drop support. The patient who has suffered an occlusion of one posterior cerebral artery will probably have an hemianopia. Unless he is warned about this he may get run over when he next tries to cross the road – having failed to see the oncoming traffic.

What of the future? The causes of such diseases as multiple sclerosis, motor neurone disease, brain tumour, and epilepsy so far elude us. It is greatly to be hoped that before long these disorders will yield up their secrets and a 'cure' be found. Prevention of disease is becoming increasingly important. Two examples of preventive neurology are: first, the hope that the incidence of hereditary disease can be reduced by genetic counselling and prenatal diagnosis; and second, that the effective detection and treatment of hypertension will result in a reduced incidence of cerebrovascular disease.

In some instances, neurological disease can be successfully treated but in others the damage to the nervous system is irreversible. Neurological disease is responsible for a very large proportion of the severe chronic physical disability affecting the community. Much time and energy goes into working out methods by which disability can be overcome and the patient helped to lead as normal a life as possible. The ways in which the damaged central nervous system recovers from injury are to a great extent unknown. The effect of physical forms of therapy (for instance physiotherapy) on recovery is likewise uncertain. This is a further fascinating field, ripe for exploration by the new generation of doctors.

INVESTIGATIONS IN NEUROLOGY

Special investigations are no substitute for careful and thoughtful clinical assessment. Some investigations are expensive and some involve an element of risk; they should not be undertaken without due thought. From the practical viewpoint investigations can be divided into two groups:

Group 1. This group can be undertaken on an outpatient basis and are uniformly safe. Many of them are simply an extension of the clinical examination.

Group 2. This group involves at least a short admission to hospital. All the investigations are associated with a small (usually *very* small) risk. They can be unpleasant.

Group 1 Investigations

Everyday screening investigations such as blood counts, plasma viscosity, WR and chest X-ray will frequently need to be done but will not be discussed further.

1. **Skull X-ray.** At least two views are usually taken – anteroposterior, and lateral. Additional views are taken in appropriate cases. A brow-down film (Towne's view) demonstrates the petrous temporal bones and the basal view demonstrates the skull base. Further special views may be required. For example, in a case of suspected acoustic neuroma it may be necessary to demonstrate the internal auditory meatus.

A skull X-ray may be required for a number of different reasons. The following are some examples:
(a) Fracture – in cases of head injury.
(b) Evidence of raised intracranial pressure – erosion of the posterior clinoid processes or sutural separation (in infants).
(c) Displacement of calcified midline structures. For instance, displacement of the pineal body may be produced by any supratentorial space-occupying mass.
(d) Erosion of the skull vault; for example by a tumour.
(e) Abnormal calcification; for example, in a tumour or aneurysm.

2. **X-ray of the Neck and Spinal Column.** Anteroposterior and lateral views are usually taken. Additional oblique views of the cervical spine will sometimes demonstrate abnormalities of the exit foramina – encroaching on the nerve roots. Abnormalities include:
(a) Degenerative changes in the vertebrae and disc spaces.
(b) Destruction of vertebral bodies by malignancy.
(c) Congenital abnormalities such as fusion of vertebrae.

3. **Computorised Transaxial Tomography (CT or EMI Scan).** The system includes a scanning unit, a computor, a magnetic disc unit, a viewing unit, a line printer and a teletype. The head of the patient is scanned as a series of cross-sectional slices approximately one centimetre thick by a tightly collimated narrow beam of X-rays. The readings are fed continuously to the computor which rapidly calculates the absorption values of

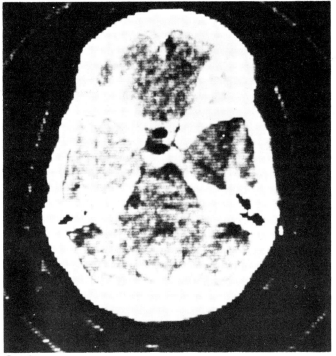

Cut 1

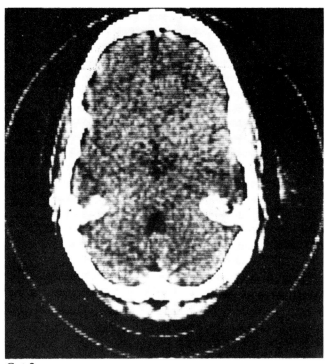

Cut 2

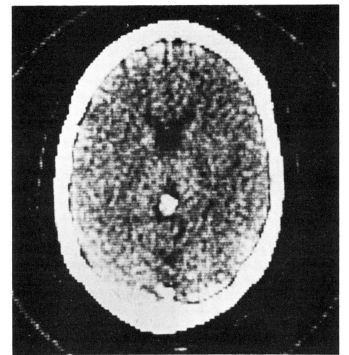

Cut 3

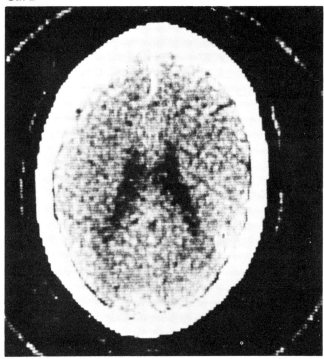

Cut 4

Fig. 21.1 Normal CT scans: Four horizontal cuts*

Cut 1: This is taken through the base of the skull and shows the sphenoid wing, the petrous temporal bone, and a central 4th ventricle.
Cut 2: This shows the top of the petrous temporal bones and the basal ganglia region.
Cut 3: This shows the anterior horns of the lateral ventricles and a calcified pineal gland. The thalami are on either side of the 3rd ventricle.

Cut 4: This shows the bodies and posterior horns of the lateral ventricles.

*These scans and those on pages 516, 517, 527, 529 and 539 were kindly supplied by Dr. J. L. G. Thomson, Consultant Radiologist, Frenchay Hospital, Bristol.

483

the material within each slice. The clinician is presented with a series of polaroid pictures. The value of the technique can be enhanced by giving an intravenous injection of a radioactive isotope (e.g. Conray) which is taken up by some tumours and occasionally by infarcts. CT scanning is particularly useful for detecting intracranial blood clots (e.g. after head injury), for demonstrating the ventricular system, and for identifying tumours.

Fig. 21.1 shows four normal CT scan pictures and these give an idea of what can be demonstrated. The CT scanner has totally revolutionised the investigation of intracranial disease. Those centres that are fortunate enough to have a CT scanner have found that they are performing fewer of the other investigative procedures, such as a gamma-encephalography, carotid arteriography and air-encephalography.

4. **Gamma-Encephalography.** This involves the intravenous injection of a radioactive isotope, usually technetium. Scanning of the brain is undertaken and the amount of radioactive emission from different areas of the brain is plotted. The technique is particularly useful in the diagnosis of multiple secondary tumour deposits and cerebral abscesses. A positive scan may also be produced by an ischaemic infarct. Some tumours, particularly meningiomas, may give a positive result but a negative scan does not exclude a tumour.

5. **Echoencephalography.** This involves passing an ultrasonic beam through the intact skull. The beam is deflected back as an echo, mainly from midline structures. A shift of the echo to one side occurs with supra-tentorial space-occupying lesions. The investigation is safe and in experienced hands can be used as a useful screening procedure.

6. **Electroencephalography (EEG).** Electroencephalography involves recording the electrical activity of the brain through the intact skull. This is done by using a series of small metal electrodes; either 8 or 16 electrodes are used in most centres. The normal EEG displays a number of different rhythms (alpha, beta, delta, and theta); the wave forms are categorised according to the dominant frequency. In the normal person the type of activity will depend partly on the area of the brain from which recordings are made and partly on the state of alertness of the patient. The EEG in young children displays a great deal of slow activity.

The principal clinical uses of the EEG are as follows:
(a) *The investigation of epilepsy.* This is discussed elsewhere (*see* 'The Epilepsies', page 517). It must be noted that a normal EEG does not exclude epilepsy.
(b) *The detection of focal abnormalities.* The finding of a marked 'focus' – particularly a slow wave focus – may be of particular value in the diagnosis of cerebral abscess, and sometimes of brain tumour. It must be emphasised however that the absence of a focal abnormality on the EEG does not exclude focal pathology – about 20 per cent of patients with cerebral tumours have a normal EEG.
(c) *Diagnosis of brain death.* Patients who have had a severe head injury, or have been subjected to a period of prolonged anoxia, may be kept alive indefinitely provided that artificial ventilation is maintained. A persistently 'flat' EEG – one showing no activity – over several hours practically always indicates that there is no hope of restoration of brain function. In such a situation there is no point in persisting with resuscitation.
(d) *Miscellaneous uses.* The EEG is useful in the diagnosis of encephalitis (diffuse slow waves) and for monitoring the state of brain activity in hepatic failure.

7. **Electromyography and Nerve Conduction Studies.** These are discussed in the sections on 'Diseases of the Peripheral Nerves' (*see* page 496), and 'Muscle Diseases' (*see* page 555).

8. **Psychological Testing.** Simple bedside tests of intellectual function should be part of the clinical examination of the patient. Assessment would take note of:
(a) Attention – the level of alertness.
(b) Cognitive skills. These include the ability to speak, understand speech, read, write, and perceive objects.
(c) Memory function. Both short and long term memory should be tested.
(d) Reasoning and problem solving.

A variety of detailed intellectual tests is available and these are usually applied by a trained psychologist. Such assessments are very valuable for the early detection of dementia and, sometimes, for picking out specific intellectual deficits that are not obvious on routine testing. For instance, sophisticated testing may reveal specific unrecognised deficits in the utilisation of language. Testing can be invaluable in cases of progressive dementia – enabling the clinician to assess improvement or deterioration.

9. **Plotting of the Visual Fields.** This is discussed elsewhere (*see* The Optic Nerve, page 486).

10. **Tests of Auditory and Vestibular Function** (*see* The VIIIth Nerve, page 493).

Group 2 Investigations

1. **Lumbar Puncture.** Lumbar puncture involves inserting a needle into the lumbar subarachnoid space below the termination of the spinal cord. The main indications for lumbar puncture are:
(a) To obtain cerebrospinal fluid for examination, for instance in cases of meningitis or subarachnoid haemorrhage.

The normal values for the chemical and cellular contents of CSF are given in the table of normal values (*see* Appendix I).

(b) To administer antibiotics.
(c) To inject air or positive contrast media (Myodil), as part of a radiological study.

Difficulty with obtaining cerebrospinal fluid is usually due to faulty positioning of the patient. Sometimes, however, severe spinal osteoarthritis or ankylosing spondylitis will prevent successful puncture. A lumbar puncture is, in general, a safe procedure. Some patients suffer severe headache, as a result of a fall in intracranial pressure due to leakage of cerebrospinal fluid from the subarachnoid space. Meningitis is a rare complication, but the puncture must always be undertaken under sterile conditions. *A lumbar puncture should never be undertaken if there is a suspicion of raised intracranial pressure.*

2. Carotid and Vertebral Angiography.
Carotid angiography is a routine neurological procedure and, in the hands of a competent person, is safe. It involves needle puncture of the cervical portion of the carotid artery and the subsequent injection of contrast medium. Vertebral angiography is technically a more difficult procedure.

Carotid angiography is the investigation of choice in many cases of focal cerebrovascular disease. The principal indications are as follows:
(a) Demonstration of an intracranial space-occupying mass, for example tumour, subdural haematoma, or abscess. The cardinal abnormality seen is displacement of vessels *away* from the swelling. Certain tumours, for example meningiomas, show a vascular 'blush'.
(b) Demonstration of a suspected intracranial aneurysm, for instance following a subarachnoid haemorrhage.
(c) Demonstration of arterial patency in patients with cerebrovascular disease, for instance, stenosis or occlusion of the internal carotid artery in the neck may be demonstrated.

There is a small but definite risk associated with angiography, especially in older patients, and the technique should not be used indiscriminately. The risks include inadvertent subintimal injection and dislodgement of a thrombus or artheromatous plaque.

3. Air Encephalography.
This involves introducing air into the subarachnoid space via a lumbar puncture needle. By suitable posturing of the patient it is usually possible to outline the ventricular system of the brain. The following are some examples of abnormalities found:
(a) Atrophy of the brain may be seen, for instance in cases of dementia. An increased amount of air may be seen over the surface of the brain, in the widened cerebral sulci. In addition the ventricles are usually dilated.
(b) Displacement or deformity of the ventricular system, for example by tumour or abscess.

(c) Dilatation of the ventricular system – in communicating hydrocephalus. In the case of obstructive hydrocephalus, the ventricular system will fail to fill.

The risks are those associated with lumbar puncture. Headache frequently occurs and may be severe. Patients with a cerebral tumour, especially if in the posterior fossa, may deteriorate rapidly after this procedure. Air encephalography is not now used very commonly in those centres possessing a CT scanner.

Air and Myodil can be introduced into the ventricular system directly, via a brain needle, through a burr hole in the skull. Radiographs (ventriculograms) are then obtained.

4. Myelography.
This procedure involves introducing positive contrast medium, usually 6 ml of Myodil, into the subarachnoid space via a lumbar puncture needle. By suitable posturing of the patient on a tilting table it is usually possible to outline the entire spinal canal from the foramen magnum downwards to the sacral area. The technique is used mainly to demonstrate compressive lesions of the spinal cord and cauda equina, for instance prolapsed intravertebral disc or tumour.

Myelography involves being tilted through a very wide angle and can be unpleasant, particularly when the patient is feeling ill. Some patients develop transient pain in the back of the legs and in the buttocks, following a myelogram.

THE CRANIAL NERVES

For ease of understanding we have divided the cranial nerves into arbitrary sections. The anatomy and pathology of each part will be discussed separately in order to facilitate understanding. The main cranial nerve syndromes are set out in Table 21.1.

1ST CRANIAL NERVE (OLFACTORY)

The olfactory nerve is entirely sensory. It lies in the olfactory groove in the floor of the anterior fossa. Central connections are made with the olfactory area of the cerebral cortex. There is a very close link between smell and taste, so that the loss of one of these functions is frequently accompanied by depression of the other.

Anosmia (loss of smell) may be due to any of the following causes:
1. Chronic rhinitis can cause unilateral or bilateral loss of smell.
2. Head injury. Anosmia may occur either with or without a fracture of the cribriform plate. The overall incidence of anosmia after significant head injury is about seven per cent, the occurrence increasing with the severity of the head injury.

Table 21.1 The main cranial nerve syndromes

Site of lesion	Nerves involved	Additional characteristics	Cause
Within the brain stem	IIIrd to XIIth, usually excluding VIIIth. A large number of different syndromes are described (*see* text)	Often long tract signs and multiple cranial nerve palsies	Vascular lesions Multiple sclerosis Poliomyelitis. Tumours Virus infection (e.g. *Herpes zoster*)
Cerebello-pontine angle	VIIth and VIIIth Sometimes Vth and VIth	Frequently signs of cerebellar and brain stem compression	Acoustic neuroma Meningioma
Apex of the petrous temporal bone	Vth and VIth	Pain	Infection in the middle ear may spread through the petrous temporal bone
Cavernous sinus	IIIrd, IVth and VIth plus the ophthalmic and maxillary division of the Vth	Proptosis	Cavernous sinus thrombosis. Aneurysm Tumours arising in the pituitary fossa and nasal sinuses
Orbital fissure	IInd, IIIrd, IVth, ophthalmic division of Vth and VIth	Proptosis	Sphenoidal wing meningioma. Aneurysm
Jugular foramen	IX, Xth and XIth (XIIth)		Tumours – especially carcinoma of the nasopharynx Fracture of skull

3. Compression of the olfactory nerve by tumour. A meningioma arising in the olfactory groove may produce unilateral anosmia. Anosmia may also be produced by frontal lobe tumours.

Olfactory hallucinations are a frequent feature of temporal lobe epilepsy (*see* page 518). Parosmia (distortion of smell sensation) sometimes occurs after head injury.

THE OPTIC NERVE AND OPTIC PATHWAYS

Anatomically, vision involves the retina, optic nerve, chiasm, optic tracts, the lateral geniculate body, the optic radiation and the occipital cortex.

Light from objects in the temporal half of the visual field falls on the nasal half of the retina. Similarly, light from the upper half of the visual field excites neurones in the lower half of the retina. Fibres in the optic pathway run in bundles and have a reasonably constant relationship to one another. In the optic chiasm, fibres carrying impulses from the temporal half of the visual field cross, but those carrying impulses from the nasal half of the field remain uncrossed.

Fibres in the optic nerve have two main destinations:
(a) The calcarine cortex – having synapsed in the lateral geniculate body.
(b) The upper mid-brain – this pathway is essential for pupillary light reflexes and reflex co-ordination of eye and head movements.
Testing of the optic nerve involves:

1. **Visual Acuity.** Do not forget to do this. The acuity should be tested with correction for refractive errors.

2. **Visual Fields.** These can be mapped out roughly with a small coloured pin. More accurate assessment requires the use of a perimeter and a special screen. Some of the commoner visual field defects are shown schematically in Fig. 21.2. The term hemianopia is frequently used. It means loss or diminution of vision in half the visual field. Two common examples, bitemporal and homonymous hemianopia, are shown in this figure. The term scotoma is used to describe an area of absent vision within the visual field.

3. **Examination of the Optic Fundi.** From the neurological point of view, two main abnormalities occur – papilloedema and optic atrophy (*see below*).

4. **Pupillary Reactions.** The reaction to light and to accommodation must be tested.

PAPILLOEDEMA

Definition

Swelling of the optic papilla (disc). Papilloedema is a physical sign which can be produced in several different ways.

Main Causes

1. Increased intracranial pressure. The optic nerve is surrounded by a subarachnoid space which is continuous with the intracranial subarachnoid space. Thus, any rise in intracranial pressure will be transmitted to the optic nerve with resultant venous and lymphatic

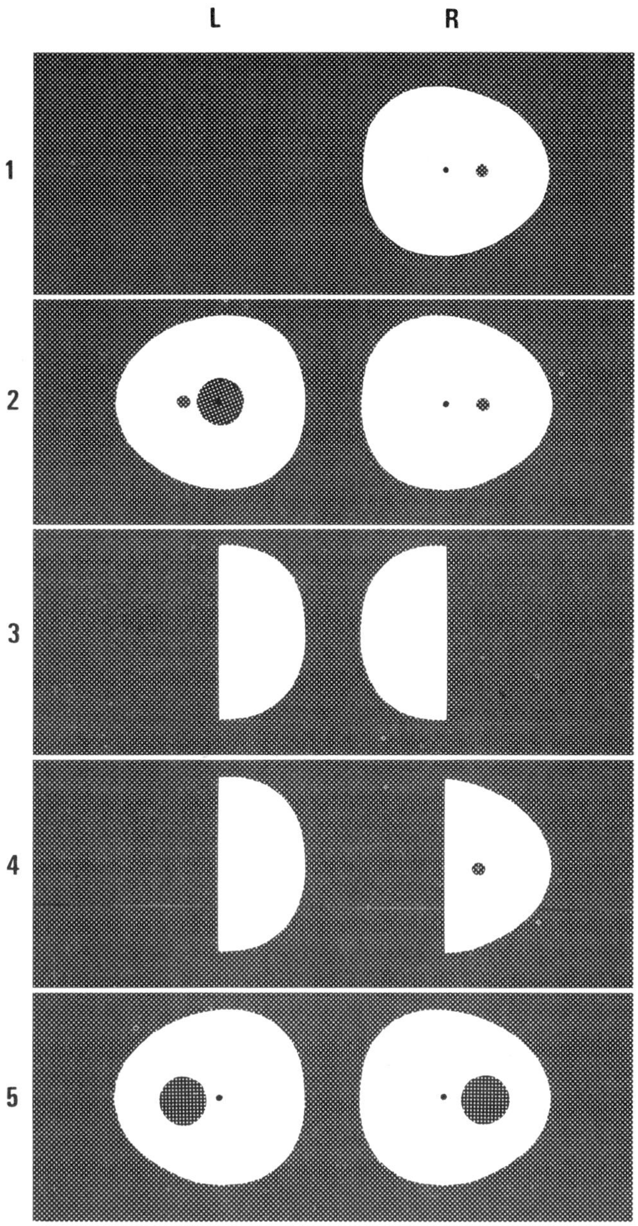

Fig. 21.2 Some common visual field defects (schematic).
1. Left side: total blindness. Normal visual field on the right.
2. Left side: central scotoma (due to a lesion of the optic nerve). Right side normal.
3. *Bitemporal hemianopia (due to chiasmal compression).
4. *Left homonymous hemianopia (due to a lesion of the right optic tract, radiation, or cortex).
5. Bilateral enlargement of blind spots (in papilloedema).

*It should be noted that the hemianopia may be incomplete and is not always symmetrical.

obstruction. Common causes of raised intracranial pressure include:
(a) Any intracranial space-occupying mass such as a haematoma, tumour, or abscess.
(b) Thrombosis of the cerebral venous sinuses.
(c) Hydrocephalus from any cause.

Other causes include meningitis, subarachnoid haemorrhage, and generalised brain swelling associated with head injury or encephalitis.
2. Inflammatory conditions of the optic nerve. Optic neuritis and retrobulbar neuritis are frequently due to acute demyelination in the optic nerve (see Multiple sclerosis, page 540). Sometimes the lesion does not involve the optic papilla, in which case there will usually be no papilloedema.
3. Obstruction of the central artery or vein of the retina.
4. Malignant hypertension.

Less common causes include anaemia of various sorts, bacterial endocarditis, hypoparathyroidism, and severe emphysema.

Symptoms and Signs

Symptoms
There may be none.
Blurring of vision is practically always noted with primary lesions of the optic nerve (such as optic neuritis).
Headache, vomiting, etc., if there is raised intracranial pressure.

Signs
The cardinal signs are as follows:
(a) The disc frequently becomes pinker than usual. This is an early sign.
(b) The disc margins become blurred.
(c) The optic cup becomes obliterated.

In gross papilloedema the edges of the disc may become invisible. In some cases there are profuse exudates and haemorrhages, particularly with malignant systemic hypertension and with vascular lesions of the retina and optic nerves. If the primary pathology lies in the optic nerve there will be poor vision and a central scotoma. When the papilloedema is due to raised intracranial pressure the visual acuity may be normal, or near normal, and there will be an enlarged blind spot but no central scotoma. At a later stage, however, secondary optic atrophy may occur.

Differential Diagnosis

Various conditions can simulate papilloedema. These include:
1. A normal optic disc. The optic disc varies enormously in appearance from patient to patient.
2. A high degree of hypermetropia. In this condition there is often a marked elevation of the optic discs. Haemorrhages and exudates do not occur and the blind spot is not enlarged.
3. Severe degree of myopia.
4. Opaque nerve fibres. Opaque nerve fibres are usually seen adjacent to the optic disc and may be mistaken for papilloedema.
5. Hyaline bodies (drusen) lying adjacent to the optic disc.

The diagnosis can be difficult. In doubtful cases an intravenous injection of fluorescein can be helpful. In true papilloedema the fluorescein leaks through the capillary walls and produces a diffuse fluorescence of the optic papilla. In other conditions capillary permeability is normal and no such changes occur.

Complications

Secondary optic atrophy with blindness may follow papilloedema due to raised intracranial pressure. When dealing with the patient who has papilloedema it is essential to plot the visual acuity at daily intervals in order to detect the first sign of deteriorating vision.

OPTIC ATROPHY

Definition

Atrophy of the optic nerve fibres with the production of a white, gliotic, optic disc. In gross cases partial or complete blindness occurs. In others (e.g. multiple sclerosis) the patient may have little, or no visual complaints.

Differential Diagnosis

1. **Normal Optic Disc.** Mild degrees of pallor of the disc, without corroborative evidence, should not be regarded as being diagnostic of optic atrophy.
2. **Chronic Glaucoma.** The disc frequently appears white due to atrophy of the optic nerve head and enlargement of the optic cup.

NEUROLOGICAL CAUSES OF VISUAL FAILURE

Neurological disturbance of vision may be produced by lesions anywhere along the course of the visual pathway. In each case it will be necessary to undertake a careful clinical assessment which will include measurement of the visual acuity, ophthalmoscopy and plotting of the visual fields. The pathway may be divided into three portions – the optic nerve, the chiasm, and the optic tract, radiation and calcarine cortex.

Lesions of the Optic Nerve

Most patients complain of difficulty with vision and in many instances there is a central scotoma. In the acute stage papilloedema and retinal haemorrhages may be seen on opthalmoscopy – particularly if the anterior part of the optic nerve is involved. The term optic neuritis is used to describe cases in which there is an acute disturbance of the optic nerve due to demyelination or to a toxin or an infection. The term retrobulbar neuritis indicates that the disturbance is proximally situated, so

that little or no abnormality can be seen on ophthalmoscopy. The two conditions are in reality identical. Optic neuritis and retrobulbar neuritis may be unilateral or bilateral and the condition is often accompanied by pain on moving the eye. The commonest cause is multiple sclerosis although in many instances no cause can be found.

We have divided the causes of optic nerve disturbance into acute and chronic. This is an arbitrary division and there is considerable overlap between the two groups.

Acute Lesions
1. Multiple sclerosis (*see* page 540).
2. Vascular lesions of the optic nerve.

When there is occlusion of the central artery of the retina the fundus looks pale, the retinal arteries are very thin and there may be papilloedema. Optic atrophy occurs late. Occlusion of the central vein of the retina results in a congested fundus with large flame-shaped haemorrhages radiating from the disc. There is usually marked papilloedema. Vascular lesions of the retinal arteries may be part of a generalised arteritis, as in cranial arteritis, polyarteritis, and secondary syphilis.

Ischaemia of the optic nerve (ischaemic optic neuritis) can occur without producing marked fundal changes.
3. Toxic and metabolic causes. (Many of these are more liable to cause gradually progressive blindness with optic atrophy). Sudden blindness may occur with methyl alcohol, quinine, and with tobacco amblyopia.
4. Miscellaneous causes. There are a wide variety of occasional causes, these include orbital cellulitis, encephalitis, and *Herpes zoster*. Glaucoma is an important cause.
5. Idiopathic. In some instances it is not possible to find a cause for optic neuritis – despite prolonged follow-up.

Chronic Lesions. Chronic lesions of the optic nerve are usually associated with optic atrophy. Diminished visual acuity and a central scotoma are usually present.
1. Compression from the outside. The optic nerve may be compressed from the outside by a tumour or aneurysm. It is vitally important to make the diagnosis. Failure to do so may result in avoidable blindness.
2. Glaucoma.
3. As a late result of any of the lesions mentioned in the above section on *acute* lesions.
4. Following papilloedema due to raised intracranial pressure. This type of optic atrophy is sometimes called secondary optic atrophy.
5. Syphilis – especially tabes.
6. Poisons – particularly methyl alcohol, quinine, arsenic, lead, and chloroquine. Tobacco amblyopia is probably produced by a deficiency of vitamin B_{12} – due to cyanide.
7. Various heredo-familial disorders.

(a) Leber's optic atrophy. This is an X-linked recessive disorder producing bilateral optic atrophy in young adult males.

(b) Retinitis pigmentosa. In this condition there is pathological pigmentation of the retina.

(c) Cerebral lipidoses.

(d) Hereditary ataxias. Most of the various forms of hereditary ataxia may occasionally be complicated by optic atrophy.

Lesions of the Optic Chiasm

Pressure on the chiasm from below is usually due to a pituitary tumour. Pressure from above may result from a midline tumour such as a meningioma or a craniopharyngioma. A large number of visual field defects can occur, but the most usual is a bitemporal hemianopia (see Fig. 21.2) due to interruption of the crossing fibres.

Lesions of the Optic Tract, Radiation and Cortex

Lesions in these sites may produce homonymous hemianopic abnormalities of the visual field. These may be complete or partial. Partial abnormalities are particularly liable to occur with lesions in the optic radiation where the fibres are widely dispersed. Vascular lesions and tumours of the temporal and parietal lobes are common causes. A homonymous hemianopia may be the only manifestation of occlusion of the posterior cerebral artery.

The patient with a complete homonymous hemianopia will be unable to see things on the affected side. He will probably bump into objects, such as tables and door-frames, on the hemianopic side. Unless warned, he will be liable to be knocked down when crossing the road, being unable to see the approaching traffic unless he makes a conscious effort to turn his head before crossing.

THE PUPIL

The constrictor muscles are innervated by parasympathetic fibres running in the third nerve while dilator fibres run in the sympathetic nerves. The pupil size depends on a large number of different factors and is a balance between the sympathetic and parasympathetic tone. Pupil size is readily altered by drugs.

1. ARGYLL-ROBERTSON PUPIL

The characteristics of this condition are:
1. Loss of light reflex.
2. Preservation of accommodation.
3. The pupils are small, irregular, and unequal with atrophy of the iris.

The condition occurs in neuro-syphilis, particularly in tabes dorsalis and GPI. The lesion is situated in the periaqueductal region of the mid-brain.

2. MYOTONIC PUPIL

Definition

A benign abnormality of one or both pupils in which there is pupillary dilation together with little or no reaction to light and a slow reaction to accommodation.

Background

This abnormality usually affects young women. When associated with depressed tendon reflexes it is called Adie's syndrome. Pathologically there is loss of cells in the ciliary ganglion.

3. HORNER'S SYNDROME

Definition

A syndrome due to interruption to the sympathetic nerve supply to one side of the head.

Background

The sympathetic fibres have a long course and may be interrupted at several different places:

Part 1: The Brain Stem. The fibres arise in the hypothalamus and run as a tract in the lateral medulla. Interruption in this position is usually associated with other features of the lateral medullary syndrome (see page 535). Vascular lesions, syringobulbia, and tumours are the commonest lesions in this area.

Part 2: The Cervical Cord. The fibres run through the cervical cord adjacent to the lateral column of grey matter and exit with the nerve roots from the upper thoracic cord. Interruption in these areas is usually associated with other evidence of spinal cord dysfunction. Common lesions include syringomyelia, trauma and gliomas.

Part 3: The Root of the Neck. The sympathetic fibres and stellate ganglion are situated on or near the neck of the first rib. Tumours at the apex of the lung may interrupt the sympathetic fibres at this point. A cervical sympathectomy is undertaken in this area.

Part 4: The Fibres that Run Through the Neck and Into the Skull. In this position they are wrapped around the carotid artery. Lesions include aneurysms and thrombosis of the carotid artery and malignant glands. A Horner's syndrome is occasionally seen after carotid angiography.

Lesions in the cavernous sinus and orbit are usually

associated with diplopia due to involvement of oculomotor nerves.

Symptoms

Usually there are no symptoms.

Signs

Small pupil (unopposed action of the parasympathetic).
Ptosis (never complete) – due to partial paralysis of the levator palpebrae superioris.
Enopthalmos – retraction of the eyeball into the orbit – due to paralysis of the orbital smooth muscle.
Lack of sweating on the same side of the face.

THE IIIrd CRANIAL NERVE (Fig. 21.3)

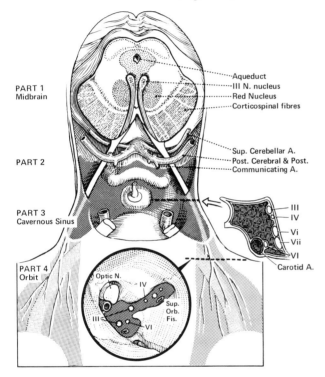

Fig. 21.3 The course of the IIIrd (oculomotor) cranial nerve (*see* text for description).

This nerve supplies the majority of the external ocular muscles (superior, medial, and inferior recti and inferior oblique), the levator palpebrae superioris and the sphincter pupillae.

The nerve may be considered in four parts:

Part 1: In the Mid-Brain. The nerve arises from a long nucleus lying near the aqueduct in the upper part of the mid-brain. It passes through the tegmentum and emerges on the medial side of the cerebral peduncle. Lesions in this position are sometimes partial, bilateral, and associated with long tract signs.

Part 2: In the Interpeduncular Cistern. It passes between the superior cerebellar and the posterior cerebral arteries and runs forward on the lateral side of the posterior communicating artery. Lesions in this site frequently produce no other neurological abnormalities.

Part 3: The Nerve Passes Through the Cavernous Sinus Lying in the Lateral Wall Above the IVth Nerve. Lesions in this site are usually associated with palsies of other cranial nerves especially the IVth, Vth and VIth.

Part 4: The Nerve Enters the Orbit Through the Superior Orbital Fissure. Lesions in the orbit are frequently associated with proptosis.

Symptoms

Inability to open the eye.
Diplopia (if the eyelid is elevated).

Signs

Complete or partial ptosis.
Dilated pupil, which may be fixed, showing no reaction to light or accommodation. The eyeball is noted to be pulled outwards and downwards (unopposed action of lateral rectus and superior oblique).

THE IVth CRANIAL NERVE

This nerve supplies the superior oblique muscle. Paralysis produces diplopia and inability to rotate the eyeball downwards and laterally.

The IVth nerve nucleus lies in the upper mid-brain (*see* Fig. 21.3). Its course, for practical purposes, is similar to that of the IIIrd nerve.

THE VIth CRANIAL NERVE

This nerve supplies the lateral rectus muscle.

Anatomy

Part 1. The cells of origin lie in the floor of the fourth ventricle in the lower pons, close to the facial nerve nucleus. The VIth nerve exits at the lower border of the pons. Lesions at this site may also produce a lower motor neurone VIIth nerve palsy, weakness of lateral gaze, and sometimes a contralateral hemiplegia.

Part 2. The nerve has a long course through the cisterna pontis and then crosses the apex of the petrous temporal bone.

Part 3. } As for the IIIrd nerve.
Part 4. }

Symptoms

Horizontal diplopia worse on looking to the side of the lesion.

Signs

Lateral movement of the eyeball is defective.

The causes of lesions of the oculomotor nerves (IIIrd, IVth and VIth) are shown in Table 21.2.

Table 21.2 Causes of lesions of the oculomotor nerves (IIIrd, IVth and VIth)

Site of lesion	Cause
1. Brain stem	Multiple sclerosis, poliomyelitis, syringobulbia, vascular disease, encephalitis, *Herpes zoster*, and tumours
2. Basal cisterns	1. Chronic meningitis (TB, carcinoma, sarcoid, syphilis) 2. Carcinoma of the nasopharynx 3. Aneurysm (an aneurysm of the posterior communicating artery is a common cause of a IIIrd nerve palsy) 4. Raised intracranial pressure (both the IIIrd and VIth nerves are particularly liable to be compressed or stretched – *see* Raised Intracranial Pressure, page 536)
3. Lesions at the tip of the petrous temporal bone	1. Infection may spread from the middle ear. Thrombosis of the petrosal venous sinus may occur. The VIth nerve is mainly affected 2. Carcinoma of the nasopharynx – this is a common cause of an isolated VIth nerve palsy
4. Cavernous sinus	1. Cavernous sinus thrombosis, usually complicating sepsis on the face or in the nasal air sinuses 2. Pituitary tumours extending laterally 3. Aneurysmal dilation of the intracavernous part of the carotid artery
5. Superior orbital fissure	A large number of tumours can occur in this region including meningiomas. In addition, there are a number of tumours of the orbit itself
6. Miscellaneous	1. Vascular lesions of the nerve trunk, especially in diabetics. 2. Guillain-Barré syndrome (acute polyneuritis) 3. Acute migraine
7. Other conditions which may cause diplopia	1. Myasthenia gravis (*see* page 556) 2. Thyrotoxicosis (*see* page 172) 3. Ocular myopathy

THE Vth CRANIAL NERVE – THE TRIGEMINAL

This is the motor nerve for the muscles of mastication and the sensory nerve for the skin of the face and the mucous membrane of the mouth and nasal cavities.

Anatomy

Motor Pathway. The motor nucleus lies in the upper part of the pons.

Sensory Pathway. The fibres of the sensory root arise in the trigeminal ganglion which lies at the apex of the petrous temporal bone. Peripheral branches travel in each of the three divisions of the Vth nerve. Central branches enter the brain stem where they divide into:
(a) Ascending branches – concerned with tactile sensation for the face.
(b) Descending branches – concerned with pain and temperature on the face. These form the spinal tract of the Vth nerve. This runs down through the pons and medulla and ends in the nucleus of the spinal tract of the Vth nerve.

Part 1. In the Brain Stem. Lesions in the brain stem sometimes produce dissociated sensory loss on the face, due to the different course taken by pain and temperature sensation, on the one hand, and tactile sensation, on the other. Other cranial nerve palsies, together with long tract signs, may be present. Causes include syringobulbia, pontine tumours, and vascular lesions.

Part 2: The Vth Cranial Nerve Exits From the Pons at the level of the middle cerebellar peduncle. The motor and sensory roots run together across the posterior fossa. Disturbance of function in this part of its course may be due to tumours (e.g. acoustic neuroma), chronic meningitis, and inflammation of the petrous temporal bone, usually secondary to middle ear infection.

Part 3. Trigeminal Ganglion. In this situation the motor root runs underneath the trigeminal ganglion. *Herpes zoster* is the commonest cause of a lesion at this site (*see* page 550).

Part 4. At the Trigeminal Ganglion the Nerve Divides into Three Main Divisions.

1. *Ophthalmic.* This is a sensory nerve. The nerve runs along the lateral wall of the cavernous sinus and then passes through the orbital fissure to supply the conjunctiva, cornea, some of the mucous membrane of the nasal cavity, and the skin of the crest of the nose, forehead, upper eyelids, and the area of scalp in front of the vortex.

2. *Maxillary nerve.* This is also a sensory nerve. This nerve passes along the lateral wall of the cavernous sinus and exits from the skull via the foramen rotundum. It crosses the pterygopalatine fossa, passes through the floor of the orbit in close relation to the maxillary sinus and emerges on the face at the infra-orbital foramen. Fibres are distributed to the skin of the nose, lower eyelid, cheek, and upper lip, and also to the mucous membrane of the palate, tonsil, nasal cavity, and cheek.

3. *Mandibular nerve.* This is a mixed nerve containing motor and sensory roots which pass through the foramen ovale and then fuse. The nerve subserves sensation to the teeth and gums of the mandible, and to the skin of the

temporal region, part of the auricle, and the lower part of the face including the lower lip. It is also the motor nerve to the muscles of mastication.

Common lesions affecting the peripheral branches of the Vth nerve include neoplastic diseases arising in the nasopharynx and nasal sinuses and fractures of the base of the skull.

Signs of a Vth Nerve Palsy

The earliest sign of Vth nerve damage is often an impaired or absent corneal reflex.

A total lesion of the Vth cranial nerve produces sensory loss on the face and on the mucosa of the mouth, loss of the corneal reflex, and paralysis of the masticatory muscles. Unilateral paralysis of the pterygoid muscles produces deviation of the jaw to the side of the lesion when the mouth is opened.

Trigeminal neuralgia is discussed on page 523.

VIIth CRANIAL NERVE (Fig. 21.4)

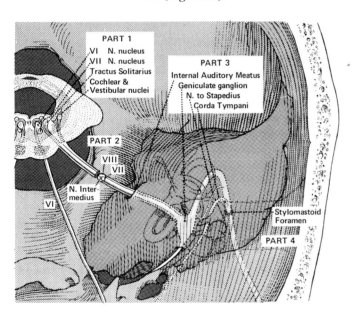

Fig. 21.4   The course of the VIIth cranial nerve.
Part 1: In the pons.
Part 2: In the cerebello-pontine angle.
Part 3: In the petrous temporal bone.
Part 4: In the face.
(For detailed description *see* text.)

The upper facial muscles have a bilateral supranuclear innervation. For this reason a lower motor neurone facial palsy can usually be easily distinguished from one due to an upper motor neurone lesion. In the former there is involvement of *all* the facial muscles on one side, whereas in the latter there is preservation of the muscles of the upper face (notably the frontalis).

The facial nerve may be conveniently divided into four sections –

Part 1: In the Pons. Fibres of the VIIth nerve encircle the VIth nerve nucleus. The nerve exits at the lower border of the pons. The facial palsy is frequently accompanied by a VIth nerve palsy. Sometimes there is a contralateral hemiplegia and paralysis of lateral gaze. Vascular lesions, tumours, and poliomyelitis are some of the commoner causes of involvement of the VIIth nerve at this site.

Part 2: In the Cerebello-pontine Angle. In this situation the nerve is in close relation to the Vth, VIth and VIIIth cranial nerves. Lesions at this site include acoustic neuroma and meningioma.

Part 3. In the Petrous Temporal Bone. The nerve enters the bone through the internal auditory meatus and has a long course through the facial canal. Its course includes a sharp bend (the genu), at which point is situated the geniculate ganglion. This is a sensory ganglion for taste fibres which join the facial nerve in the corda tympani and convey sensory impulses from the anterior two-thirds of the tongue. The facial nerve exits from the skull at the stylomastoid foramen. In the medial part of its course the motor and sensory components of the VIIth nerve run together with the VIIIth nerve and the auditory artery.

When the lesion is at, or proximal to, the geniculate ganglion there is frequently loss of taste on the anterior two-thirds of the tongue, and hyperacusis (due to disturbance of innervation of the stapedius muscle). With more distally placed lesions there is usually a pure VIIth nerve palsy without disturbance of taste and usually without hyperacusis.

Common lesions include skull fracture, infection (spread from the middle ear), *Herpes zoster* (Ramsay Hunt syndrome) involving the geniculate ganglion and tumours, for example glomus tumour.

Part 4: In the Face. Initially the nerve forms a plexus in the parotid gland and then supplies the muscles of facial expression. Common lesions include tumours of the parotid region and sarcoidosis.

The facial nerve may also be affected in polyneuritis, especially in Guillain-Barré syndrome and, occasionally, in diabetes. Bilateral facial palsies are particularly liable to occur in Guillain-Barré syndrome and in sarcoidosis.

BELL'S PALSY

Definition

Unilateral facial palsy that usually develops suddenly and is not associated with any other cranial nerve palsies.

Background

It seems likely that in most cases there is swelling of the facial nerve in the facial canal with resultant compression of the nerve.

Symptoms

Characteristically the patient wakes to find that his mouth has 'dropped'.
Dribbling from the corner of the mouth.
Food collecting between the teeth and lips.
Hyperacusis (sounds appear distorted and extra loud) – disturbance of taste may occur.

Signs

Complete or partial paralysis of all the facial muscles on one side.
Sometimes it may be possible to demonstrate disturbance of taste sensation on the anterior two-thirds of the tongue.
Always look for vesicles in the ear and in the mouth (geniculate herpes).

Investigations

Electrophysiological studies can be helpful with the early assessment of prognosis of Bell's Palsy. The tests are best done during the third week after onset. The facial nerve can be stimulated directly and the evoked response can be picked up with a concentric needle electrode in one of the facial muscles. The presence of an evoked potential during the third week indicates that there will be either partial or complete recovery. The absence of any evoked potential indicates that complete denervation is likely and the outlook is much more doubtful. Strength/duration curves may also be helpful in assessing prognosis.

Basis of Treatment

Acute Phase. ACTH or steroids are usually used in high dosage. They should be given as soon as possible, within the first 48 hours, for a period of about one week (e.g. prednisone 10 mg four times a day). The object of treatment is to reduce the oedema and swelling of the facial nerve.

Surgical decompression of the nerve in the facial canal and electrical stimulation of the paralysed muscles are not of proven therapeutic benefit. A small metal sling is sometimes helpful in maintaining a more normal facial appearance. A tarsorrhaphy is not usually required unless there is loss of corneal sensation (this would indicate that the case is not one of pure Bell's palsy).

Late. Cosmetic surgery can be very helpful in improving facial appearance.

Prognosis

About 65 per cent of cases recover completely. About 15 to 20 per cent are left with marked facial asymmetry from residual paresis, contracture, and associated movements. In addition, a small number of cases recover completely, apart from showing features of abnormal re-innervation (e.g. closure of the eyelids on attempting to smile).

HEMI-FACIAL SPASM

Definition

Regular, non-epileptic, clonic jerking movements of the facial muscles.

Background

The condition is usually idiopathic and usually occurs in middle-aged and elderly women. It is occasionally symptomatic and in this instance may be due to:
1. Any irritative lesion affecting the VIIth nerve, e.g. an acoustic neuroma.
2. Disseminated sclerosis.
3. Occasionally as a sequel to Bell's palsy.

Symptoms and Signs

The facial muscles on one, or both, sides display involuntary jerky movements in which the facial muscles go into spasm. The spasms may last for just a few seconds but may sometimes be much more prolonged than this. The eyelids are particularly liable to be affected and this may produce difficulty with vision.

Differential Diagnosis

1. **Focal Epilepsy.** In this case the history is usually short and the movements may involve the arm and leg on the same side. Epileptic movements usually start around the corner of the mouth.
2. **Habit Spasms** or tics.

Basis of Treatment

Mild Cases. Usually no treatment is indicated. A tranquilliser (e.g. diazepam) may be appropriate.

Severe Cases. Injection of alcohol or phenol around the VIIth nerve as it exits from the stylomastoid foramen may reduce spasms for a period of weeks or months. Surgical division of selected branches of the VIIth nerve is occasionally required.

THE VIIIth CRANIAL NERVE

The VIIIth cranial nerve has two components – cochlear and vestibular. The cardinal manifestations of disturbance of this nerve are deafness, tinnitus, and vertigo. The two portions of the nerve will be considered separately although many disease processes affect both components.

Cochlear Nerve

Auditory impulses are received by the organ of Corti and then travel in the VIIIth nerve to the cochlear nuclei in the pons. Their subsequent course involves the lateral lemniscus, the inferior quadrigeminal body, and the superior temporal gyrus.

The principal symptoms of cochlear nerve abnormality are deafness and tinnitus. Examination will be likely to show diminished hearing. Because the component parts of the middle ear are intact, air conduction will be as good as bone conduction. The ear drums appear normal. Audiometry involves testing the hearing using sounds of different frequencies and loudness. By this method a quantitative assessment of the degree of deafness can be obtained.

Vestibular Nerve

The vestibular nerve endings are in the labyrinth which consists of the three semicircular canals together with the saccule and utricle. The nerve travels with the cochlear fibres to the pons where they terminate in the four vestibular nuclei. These nuclei connect with the spinal cord via the vestibulospinal tract, the eye muscle nuclei via the medial longitudinal bundle, and the temporal lobe. Numerous other interconnections exist, notably with the neck muscles. Balance and equilibrium depend on a smooth flow of impulses traversing the vestibular system, which may be tested by running cold, and then warm, water into the ear and measuring the duration of the evoked nystagmus. In complete lesions of the vestibular system no nystagmus is produced (the condition of canal paresis). When the lesion is incomplete the duration of the evoked nystagmus is reduced.

The principal symptom of involvement of the vestibular nerve is vertigo (see below).

The VIIIth cranial nerve can be conveniently divided into four portions.

1. **End Organ.** The principal aetiological abnormalities involved are Meniere's disease, drugs (e.g. streptomycin), occupational causes (e.g. factory noise), spread of infection from the middle ear, and congenital (sometimes following rubella in pregnancy).

2. **Petrous Temporal Bone.** In this situation there is frequently an associated VIIth nerve palsy. Lesions include skull fracture and Paget's disease.

3. **In the Cerebello-pontine Angle.** There may be associated palsies of the Vth, VIth and VIIth cranial

nerves. There may also be unilateral cerebellar signs. Causes include acoustic neuroma and meningioma.

4. **In the Pons.** Deafness is very rarely produced by pontine lesions. Vertigo, however, is commonly produced by vascular lesions involving the brain stem.

VERTIGO

Vertigo is an hallucination of movement, of either the patient or his environment, and is usually due to a disorder of the vestibular system. Severe vertigo is accompanied by a gross disturbance of balance and frequently by vomiting. In the clinical setting it is essential to ascertain that the patient is complaining of true vertigo and not of the much commoner and totally non-specific 'giddiness'. (No two people mean the same thing when they use the term!)

Main Causes of Vertigo

Vertigo may be caused by any of the lesions affecting the VIIIth cranial nerve (see above).
1. Labyrinthine vertigo:
Meniere's disease (see below).
Streptomycin.
Benign positional vertigo. In this condition attacks of vertigo occur when the head is moved into a specific position, for example with stooping. It is due to an abnormality of the utricle and saccule. No specific treatment is indicated but the patient must learn to avoid the offending position.
2. Brain stem ischaemia:
Vertigo is one of the commonest symptoms of vertebrobasilar artery disease. Partial infarction of the brain stem may produce extremely severe vertigo.
3. Multiple sclerosis:
Attacks of severe vertigo are quite common.
4. Cerebellar disease:
Chronic cerebellar lesions are not usually associated with vertigo. However, acute bleeding into the cerebellum may cause very severe vertigo and vomiting followed rapidly by loss of consciousness.
5. Temporal lobe epilepsy:
Very occasionally, vertigo occurs as a manifestation of focal epilepsy, involving the temporal lobe.
6. Drugs:
Many drugs cause a transient vertigo. Alcohol is also an important cause.
7. Migraine:
Vertigo, frequently associated with nausea and vomiting, is a frequent component of migraine.
8. Acute vestibular neuronitis (epidemic vertigo):
This is a benign disorder of presumed viral origin. It is characterised by severe vomiting and vertigo. The site of the pathological process is not certain.

MENIERE'S DISEASE

Definition

A condition characterised by attacks of recurrent vertigo which is sometimes associated with tinnitus and vomiting. Progressive deafness occurs in the later stage.

Background

The condition is commonest between the ages of 40 and 50. Pathologically there is dilation of the endolymphatic system. The aetiology is unknown.

Symptoms

The attacks typically involve the sudden onset of vertigo with unsteadiness and vomiting. The patient frequently cannot stand. The attack may last for several hours during which time nystagmus may be observed. The attacks continue to occur at intervals of weeks, months, or years. In some cases complete deafness ultimately ensues and at this stage the attacks of vertigo usually stop.

Differential Diagnosis

Other causes of vertigo and deafness (see above).

Basis of Treatment

The medical treatment for this condition is not very satisfactory. Sedatives may be helpful in reducing the severity of attacks, but have little influence on their frequency. During an acute attack the patient will usually need to lie still in bed. Intramuscular chlorpromazine may be needed if there is profound vomiting. Prochlorperazine (Stemetil) 10 mg three times daily may be required.

Prophylactic management includes the regular taking of prochlorperazine (5 mg three times daily).

In severe cases of recurrent vertigo surgery may be required:
(a) Ultra-sound destruction of the labyrinth. This may be necessary in severe cases but deafness occurs in some instances.
(b) Surgical section of the vestibular nerve. The advantage of this procedure is that hearing is likely to be preserved.

THE IXth, Xth AND XIth CRANIAL NERVES

These nerves are considered together. The anatomy is complex and not of great importance in clinical neurology. All three nerves originate in the medulla and leave the skull via the jugular foramen.

The nerves supply the pharyngeal, laryngeal, and palatal muscles and also sensation in those areas. The vagi supply the abdominal viscera. The spinal portion of the XIth cranial nerve supplies the sternomastoid and trapezius muscles.

Common Lesions

In the Brain Stem. Motor neurone disease, acute polyneuritis, syringobulbia, poliomyelitis, vascular lesions, etc.

In the Jugular Foramen. Tumours, especially carcinoma of the nasopharynx.

In the Neck. Malignant glands, trauma, etc.

Symptoms

Difficulty with swallowing.
Choking with fluids ('going the wrong way').
Hoarseness of the voice.
Nasal regurgitation of fluids.

Signs

Weakness of the palate.
Depressed palatal sensation and absent gag reflex.
Paralysis of vocal cords.
Lack of explosive element to cough.
If the XIth nerve is affected there may also be paralysis of the trapezius and sternomastoid muscles.

RECURRENT LARYNGEAL NERVES

These are clinically very important branches of the vagi. The right branch arises at the root of the neck and in front of the subclavian artery. The left branch arises in the superior mediastinum and passes in front of the arch of the aorta. The nerves supply the intrinsic muscles of the larynx including the vocal cords.

Paralysis of the nerve produces dysphonia. The explosive element to the cough is lost.

Because the left recurrent laryngeal nerve is considerably lower than the right it may be involved by tumours of the mediastinum and aneurysms of the aorta.

In the neck, the nerve may be involved by injury (including surgery) and malignant glands.

THE XIIth CRANIAL NERVE

The hypoglossal nerve is the motor nerve to the tongue.

Anatomy

The nerve originates in the medulla in the floor of the fourth ventricle (see Fig. 21.16). It has a very short intracranial course and leaves the skull via the anterior condylar foramen. In this part of its course the nerve is in close proximity to the IXth, Xth and XIth nerves. It then passes deeply into the neck and towards the tongue.

Common Causes of XIIth Nerve Palsy

1. Brain stem. Syringobulbia and motor neurone disease.
2. Base of skull. Fracture, neoplasms.
3. In the neck. Trauma, malignant glands.

Symptoms and Signs of XIIth Nerve Palsy

Unilateral wasting and weakness of the tongue, with or without fasciculation.
The tongue is deviated towards the paralysed side.
If there is a bilateral supranuclear lesion the tongue will be seen to be lying in the floor of the mouth in a spastic fashion and almost incapable of protrusion. The jaw jerk will be exaggerated.

The features of upper and lower motor neurone lesions may coexist, in varying proportions, in motor neurone disease.

DISEASES OF THE PERIPHERAL NERVOUS SYSTEM

The peripheral nervous system is that part of the nervous system lying outside the pia-arachnid membranes. It includes the nerve roots, plexuses, and the peripheral nerves themselves. Diseases of the peripheral nervous system are characterised by muscle wasting and weakness, depressed tendon reflexes, and sensory loss.

It should be noted that disorders affecting the anterior horn cells (poliomyelitis and syringomyelia) also produce muscle wasting and weakness. Secondary changes occur in the roots and nerves. These primary abnormalities of the spinal cord itself are dealt with elsewhere (see 'Spinal Cord', page 506). In a few conditions (for example vitamin B$_{12}$ deficiency) there are abnormalities of the spinal cord *and* the peripheral nervous system.

When faced with a patient showing muscle wasting and weakness it is necessary to ascertain initially the distribution and anatomical extent of the signs. This assessment should indicate which part of the peripheral nervous system is involved. Affection of roots, plexuses and nerves give highly characteristic localised signs, and some knowledge of anatomy is necessary if an accurate anatomical diagnosis is to be made. In some instances there is symmetrical involvement of the distal parts of the limbs, notably in peripheral neuritis. Symmetrical, proximal wasting and weakness is most frequently due to primary disease of muscle.

During recent years much experimental work has been undertaken on the physiological and pathological changes occurring in disorders of the peripheral nervous system. The following principal pathological processes are recognised:

Wallerian Degeneration. Classically this occurs when a nerve trunk is severed. There is disintegration of the axon *and* myelin sheath distal to the site of severance. Electrically, there is no response when the nerve is stimulated. Recovery, if it occurs, is very slow and depends on regenerative growth of the proximal portion of the nerve.

Segmental Demyelination. This is a disturbance of Schwann cell function in which there is patchy segmental loss of myelin – between nodes of Ranvier. The axons remain intact. Electrically, there is marked slowing of conduction. Such a condition occurs in a large number of disorders including diphtheritic polyneuritis and acute polyneuritis. Remyelination often occurs quickly with rapid restoration of function.

Dying-back. In this situation the distal part of the nerve fibre degenerates; both the myelin sheath and the axon are affected. The process occurs particularly in some neuropathies of toxic and metabolic origin, and in some hereditary degenerative disorders, for example peroneal muscular atrophy.

Special Investigations

Electromyography. This may be helpful in distinguishing between denervation and primary disorders of muscle. The matter is discussed in more detail in the section on muscle disease.

Nerve Conduction Studies. Both motor and sensory nerve conduction can be measured. The particular *practical* uses of the technique are:
(a) Distinguishing between segmental demyelination and axonal disease. This is an important distinction because the prognosis is usually better in the former than in the latter.
(b) The investigation of compressive lesions of the peripheral nerve. For instance, compression of the ulnar nerve at the elbow may give localised slowing of conduction. Similarly, in the carpal tunnel syndrome abnormalities of sensory conduction and, sometimes, of motor conduction can be demonstrated.

Nerve Biopsy. This is not usually indicated. However, in occasional instances nerve biopsy is of diagnostic value; for instance, in leprous neuropathy and, sometimes, in neuropathy due to amyloid.

Muscle Biopsy. This is indicated only in selective instances, particularly when there is doubt as to whether muscle wasting and weakness is due to a primary disease of muscle fibres or to denervation.

Table 21.3 Cervical nerve roots

Root	Muscle	Action lost
C3, 4	Trapezius	Shrug the shoulder
C3, 4 and 5	Diaphragm	Inspiration
C4, 5	Rhomboids	Brace scapulae together
C5	Supraspinatus	Abduct arm against resistance
	Infraspinatus	External rotation of the arm
	Deltoid	Abduction of the arm
	Biceps	Flexion of the supinated forearm
C5, 6	Branchio-radialis	Flexion of the forearm in the mid-prone position
C5, 6 and 7	Serratus anterior	Fixation of scapula to chest wall
C6	Extensor carpi radialis	Extend the wrist (to the radial side)
C7	Extensor digitorum	Extend the fingers
C7 (C8)	Triseps	Extend the elbow
	Latissimus dorsi	Adduct the arm
		Muscle belly contracts palpably with coughing
C8	Long flexors of the fingers	Flexion of the fingers (grip)
T1	Small muscles of the hand	

LESIONS OF THE CERVICAL AREA

1. Lesions of the cervical nerve roots (Table 21.3).
2. Lesions of the brachial plexus.
3. Cervical spondylosis.
4. Shoulder girdle neuritis.
5. Thoracic inlet syndrome.
6. Effects of damage to single nerves in the cervical region and arm (Table 21.5).
7. Carpal tunnel syndrome.

LESIONS OF THE CERVICAL NERVE ROOTS

The common causes of cervical nerve root compression are cervical spondylosis, neoplastic disease of the vertebrae and surrounding area, and trauma. The patient complains of pain in the arm, shoulder, or up the back of the neck, usually in a 'root' distribution. Wasting and/or weakness of muscles occurs in a radicular distribution (see Table 21.3). There may also be signs of spinal cord compression.

LESIONS OF THE BRACHIAL PLEXUS

The brachial plexus is formed by the anterior primary rami of the C5, 6, 7, 8, and T1 nerve roots. The plexus consists of the three trunks (the upper, middle and lower) and three cords (the medial, posterior, and lateral). The plexus is liable to damage by trauma, tumour invasion, and compression by cervical rib or fibrous bands. The commonest parts of the plexus to be damaged are:

1. **The Medial Cord (C8, T1).** This cord is particularly likely to be damaged by hyperextension of the arm, with or without traction. When this injury occurs at birth it goes by the name of Klumke paralysis. Other causes of medial cord dysfunction include dislocation of the shoulder, compression by a cervical rib or fibrous band,

and tumour invasion (particularly tumours originating in the apex of the lung). The result is paralysis of the small muscles of the hand, and sometimes pain and sensory impairment in the medial part of the forearm and hand.

2. **Lateral Cord (C5, 6, 7 and 8).** This cord is likely to be damaged by trauma, especially a violent downward pull on the arm. The result is paralysis of the biceps muscle and flexors of the wrist and fingers, and sensory loss on the lateral aspect of the forearm and hand.

3. **Posterior Cord (C5, 6 and 7).** This is rarely damaged. The result is paralysis of deltoid, triceps, brachioradialis and extensor muscles of the wrist and fingers.

When traction injuries occur, the roots may be torn out of the spinal cord.

CERVICAL SPONDYLOSIS

Definition

Cervical spondylosis is the name given to degenerative changes that occur in the vertebrae and intervertebral discs in the neck. Sometimes there is secondary damage to the nerve roots (cervical radiculopathy) and/or to the spinal cord (cervical myelopathy).

Background

Degenerative changes occur predominantly in the lower half of the cervical spine. The most important pathological factors are:
1. Degeneration with resultant backward prolapse of intervertebral discs.
2. Local overgrowth of bone (osteophytes).
3. A congenitally narrow spinal canal. Even a minor degree of subsequent narrowing tends to produce damage to the spinal cord.

4. Pressure on the spinal roots and/or the spinal cord may result from the changes listed above. Secondary vascular changes frequently occur in the cord.
Note: Degenerative changes are always found in the cervical spines of older people. It is, therefore, unwise to assume a cause and effect relationship until other diseases have been excluded.

Symptoms and Signs

Pain and stiffness in the neck (*see* Table 21.4).

Table 21.4 Symptoms and signs of cervical spondylosis

	Symptoms	Signs
Root compression	Pain in the arm Weakness	Variable wasting, weakness, reflex change, and sensory loss in the arms (these frequently have a radicular distribution)
Spinal cord compression	Slow progressive difficulty with walking	Spastic paraparesis – weakness, spasticity, increased tendon reflexes, and extensor plantar responses

Investigations

1. X-ray neck. Look especially at the extent of osteophyte formation encroaching on the intervertebral foramina and the width of the spinal canal.
2. Myelogram. May slow compression of the spinal cord.
3. CSF. Usually normal unless there is a block in the spinal canal (very high protein).

Differential Diagnosis

1. Other causes of pain in the arm – carpal tunnel and thoracic inlet syndromes, etc.
2. Wasting in the arm – lesions of peripheral nerves, syringomyelia, etc.
3. Paraparesis or paraplegia – multiple sclerosis, spinal cord tumour, etc.

Basis of Treatment

Pain in the Arm. Medical measures include giving the patient a period of complete rest, supporting the arm in a sling, and use of a collar.

Myelopathy. An ordinary plastic or felt collar will sometimes prevent the progression of symptoms. Temporary complete immobilisation in a Minerva plaster may produce marked improvement.

Surgical Decompression:
1. *Posterior approach.* This involves undertaking a laminectomy and exposing the dura on the posterior aspect of the spinal cord. The results are usually disappointing.
2. *Anterior approach.* This involves removal of the affected intervertebral disc and its replacement by small fragments of bone (Cloward operation). Good results both for root and spinal cord symptoms have been reported.

Prognosis

Only a small proportion of patients with cervical spondylosis become severely disabled. In many instances the condition remains static over a period of years.

SHOULDER GIRDLE NEURITIS (NEURALGIC AMYOTROPHY)

Definition

An acute syndrome characterised by severe pain in the shoulder or arm which is followed by wasting and weakness of muscles around the shoulder.

Background

This condition frequently follows an acute non-specific virus infection.

The pathology is uncertain but probably involves acute inflammatory changes in the cervical nerve roots or, sometimes, more distally in the brachial plexus or its branches.

Symptoms

Acute onset of very severe pain in the shoulder and arm which may last for several days.
Later, muscle weakness.

Signs

Early – none.
Late – wasting and paralysis of one or more muscles around the shoulder girdle – particularly the deltoid and serratus anterior.

Investigations

X-rays of cervical spine and chest (to exclude other disease).

Differential Diagnosis

1. Any cause of severe pain in the neck and shoulder including *cervical spondylosis* and *acute inflammatory lesions.*
2. Serum neuropathy. This condition may follow on the injection of foreign serum (e.g. ATS). Wasting and

weakness of some muscles around the shoulder girdle may occur. Frequently there is associated fever and joint pains.

Basis of Treatment

None of proven value apart from analgesics in the acute phase. Steroid therapy is advocated by some.

Prognosis

The pain usually disappears completely within a few days. Muscle wasting or weakness may last for several months. Ultimate complete recovery is usual.

THORACIC INLET SYNDROME

Definition

A syndrome produced by pressure on the medial cord of the brachial plexus by a cervical rib or fibrous band.

Symptoms

Pain in the inner side of the arm especially after carrying a heavy basket, etc.
Weakness of the arm and hand.

Signs

Wasting of the small muscles of the hand.
Sensory loss on the inner side of the arm.

Investigations

X-ray the neck. A cervical rib may show up but fibrous bands do not.

Differential Diagnosis

Carpal Tunnel Syndrome. In this condition there is tingling in the lateral three fingers, and wasting, if present, has a median nerve distribution.

Cervical Spondylosis. This may closely mimic the thoracic inlet syndrome.

Basis of Treatment

The patient should be discouraged from carrying heavy loads. Surgical removal of a radiologically proven cervical rib and division of fibrous bands can cure pain, but wasting may remain.

EFFECTS OF DAMAGE TO SINGLE NERVES IN THE CERVICAL REGION AND ARM

These are shown in Table 21.5.

Table 21.5 Effects of damage to single nerves in the cervical region and arm

Nerve	Site of injury	Common causes	Result	Comment
Accessory (C3,4)	Base of skull	Fractures Tumours	Paralysis of the trapezius – inability to shrug the shoulders	Irritation of the nerve may cause spasm of the trapezius – 'wry neck'
	Neck	Inflamed or malignant glands		
Phrenic (C3,4,5)	Spinal cord	Poliomyelitis Vascular or neoplastic disease	Partial or complete diaphragmatic paralysis (can be confirmed by X-ray screening)	Irritation of the nerve may produce hiccough
	Neck	Trauma Inflamed or malignant glands		
	Chest	Neoplasms Operative		
Long thoracic nerve (C5,6,7)		Trauma Idiopathic	Winging of the scapula	
Circumflex (C5,6)		Dislocation of the shoulder 'Shoulder girdle neuritis'	Paralysis of the deltoid – inability to adduct the arm Sensory loss overlying the deltoid	

Table 21.5 continued

Nerve	Site of injury	Common causes	Result	Comment
Radial (C5,6,7,8 and T1)	Spiral groove	Fracture of the humerus Pressure on the nerve (Saturday night palsy!')	Inability to extend elbow, wrist and fingers Small patch of sensory loss on back of hand and at base of first and second digits	
	Below spiral groove	Trauma	As above, but triceps is spared	Uncommon
Ulnar (C8, T1)	Elbow	Repeated minor trauma – sometimes associated with an increased angle between the upper and lower arm Fracture dislocation of the elbow	Weakness of: Ulnar deviation of the wrist Flexion of the distal IPJs* of 4th and 5th digits Abduction and adduction of fingers Adduction of thumb Sensory loss: Front and back of half the 4th and the whole of the 5th digits plus medial part of hand Clawing of 4th and 5th digits	Surgical transposition of the nerve to the front of the elbow is sometimes indicated to prevent repeated trauma
	Wrist	Trauma (e.g. lacerations)	As above but: Forearm flexor muscles are all intact No sensory loss on back of hand	
	Palm of the hand	Trauma to the deep branch of the nerve	Weakness of: Abduction and adduction of the fingers Adduction of the thumb No sensory loss Hypothenar muscles intact	This lesion is sometimes produced by repeated use of a screwdriver
Median (C6,7,8, and T1)	Elbow	The nerve is rarely damaged at this site Trauma	Weakness of: Wrist pronation Radial flexion of wrist Finger flexion (grip) (flexion of the distal IPJs of the 4th and 5th digits is intact) Opposition, flexion and abduction of thumb. Sensory loss: Outer two-thirds of palm of hand plus palmar aspect of first 3 digits	The nerve is well protected in the upper arm and forearm
	Wrist	Lacerations Compression in the carpal tunnel	As above but forearm muscles are unaffected	This is the commonest site of compression of the median nerve (see 'Carpal tunnel syndrome')

*IPJ = interphalyngeal joint.

CARPAL TUNNEL SYNDROME

Definition

A syndrome due to pressure on the median nerve as it passes under the flexor retinaculum.

Background

The structures passing under the flexor retinaculum are tightly packed together. If the pressure in the compartment is raised evidence of median nerve dysfunction is likely to occur.

Two main types occur:

Idiopathic. This is particularly liable to occur in people who use their hands a great deal – housewives, plumbers, pianists, etc. Middle-aged women are most frequently affected.

Symptomatic. Tenosynovitis of the flexor tendons, injuries to the wrist, acromegaly, myxoedema, rheumatoid arthritis, and pregnancy.

Symptoms

Burning pain in the hand.
Tingling in the lateral three digits.
Aching – may involve the whole arm.
Later – numbness of the lateral three digits and weakness of the hand.

The sensory symptoms usually dominate the clinical picture and occur most frequently at night, often waking the patient.

Signs

May be none.
Slight sensory depression on the palmar aspect of the lateral three digits.
Wasting of the median supplied thenar muscles (especially lateral half of thenar eminence).
Percussion over the median nerve at the wrist may induce tingling in the affected fingers (Tinel's Sign).

Investigations

1. Nerve conduction studies may show evidence of slowing of motor or sensory impulses at the wrist.
2. X-ray of the wrist may show evidence of arthritis.

Differential Diagnosis

Other causes of tingling in the hand.

Cervical Spondylosis with root irritation. The symptoms are not usually localised to a median distribution and do not characteristically occur at night.

Thoracic Inlet Syndrome. Symptoms usually occur mainly in a T1 distribution.

Sensory Polyneuritis. All the fingers are equally affected.

Basis of Treatment

In mild cases it may be sufficient simply to advise temporary reduction in activities involving the hands; e.g. knitting, etc. A lightweight 'cock-up' splint when worn at night will frequently produce total disappearance of sensory symptoms (this can often be a useful diagnostic test).

Injection of hydrocortisone under the flexor retinaculum will sometimes produce relief of sensory symptoms but should be reserved for cases in which a splint produces insufficient relief.

Surgical decompression of the nerve is a safe and effective operation. It is indicated where the simpler medical measures have failed to relieve sensory symptoms or when there is muscle wasting.

LESIONS ARISING IN THE LUMBO-SACRAL REGION

1. Motor signs resulting from lesions in the lumbo-sacral region (Table 21.6).
2. Clinical syndromes produced by involvement of peripheral nerves in the leg (Table 21.7).
3. Cauda equina.

Table 21.6   Motor signs resulting from root lesions in the lumbo-sacral region

Root	Paralysis of
L2	Ilio-psoas – flexion of hip
L2,3	Adductors of hip
L3,4	Quadriceps femoris – extension of knee
L4 (5)	Tibialis anterior and posterior – dorsiflexion and inversion of foot
L5	Extensor digitorum longus and extensor hallucis longus – dorsiflexion of toes
L5, S1	Peronei – eversion of foot
L5, S1	Hamstring muscles – flexion of knee
L5 (S1)	Gluteus maximus – extension of hip
L4, 5, S1	Gluteus medius and minimus and tensor fascia lata – abduction of hip
S1, S2	Calf muscles – plantar flexion of foot
S1, S2	Small muscles of foot
S4, 5	Anal reflex

CAUDA EQUINA (Fig. 21.5)

The cauda equina is composed of a mass of vertically descending nerve roots from the lumbar and sacral portions of the spinal cord. The nerve roots are closely packed together and for this reason disease processes frequently involve more than one root. Lesions in the

Table 21.7 Clinical syndromes produced by involvement of peripheral nerves in the leg

Nerve	Site of injury	Causes	Result	Comment
Lateral cutaneous nerve of thigh (L2,3)	As the nerve leaves the pelvis	Compression as nerve passes under or through inguinal ligament	Syndrome of meralgia paraesthetica *Symptoms* Burning and tingling in the outer side of the thigh *Signs* Sometimes a small area of sensory depression	*Treatment.* Local injection of hydrocortisone or local anaesthetic Surgical decompression is usually successful
Obturator (2,3,4)	In the pelvis	Pelvic neoplasms Occasionally compressed in labour	Failure of adduction of the thigh	
Femoral (L2,3,4)	Rarely involved by trauma	Femoral neuropathy – diabetes, idiopathic	Syndrome of femoral neuropathy: Severe pain in the thigh Weakness and wasting of quadriceps Absent knee jerk Slight sensory depression on medial side of thigh and shin	*Treatment* Analgesics Control of diabetes if present *Prognosis* Ultimate complete recovery is usual – may take weeks or months
Sciatic (L4,5, S1,2)	Pelvis Buttock	Pelvic neoplasms Misplaced injection	Wasting and weakness: Hamstrings and all muscles below knee Absent ankle jerk Extensive sensory loss below knee except medial side of shin	Sciatica – may occur with lesions of the sciatic nerve but is more often due to irritation of L5 and S1 roots
Common peroneal (Lateral popliteal) (L4,5, S1)	As it passes subcutaneously around neck of fibula	Sitting with legs crossed Tight bandage or plaster Idiopathic	Wasting and paralysis: Dorsiflexors of foot and toes Evertors of foot (peronei) Sensory loss: Variable – on dorsum of foot and outer side of lower leg	A bad footdrop may necessitate the use of a below-knee iron or splint
Tibial (Medial popliteal) (L5, S1,2)	Rarely injured	Penetrating wounds Fracture of the ankle	Wasting and paralysis: Calf muscles (plantar flexors) Small muscles of the foot Anaesthesia on sole and outer margin of foot	

region of the lower thoracic and upper lumbar vertebrae may produce combined disturbances of the lower part of the spinal cord *and* the cauda equina.

Background

The common causes of cauda equina syndromes include:

1. Prolapsed intervertebral disc. A lateral protrusion of a prolapsed disc will frequently affect one root only (sometimes with the production of sciatic-type pain, down the back of the leg). Central protrusions may affect several nerve roots.

2. Fracture dislocation of vertebrae. This is particularly liable to occur in the upper lumbar and lower thoracic region and it is in this situation that the terminal portion

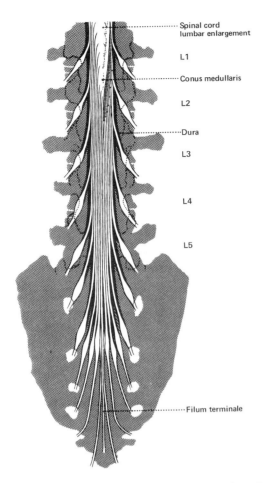

Fig. 21.5 The terminal portion of spinal cord and cauda equina.

Labels on figure: Spinal cord lumbar enlargement, L1, Conus medullaris, L2, Dura, L3, L4, L5, Filum terminale

of the spinal cord is sometimes injured.
3. Tumours.
4. Arteriovenous malformations.

Symptoms and Signs

The clinical picture will depend partly on the rapidity with which symptoms develop and partly on the anatomical structures involved. In severe cases there is flaccid paralysis of the legs with extensive sensory loss together with paralysis of sexual and sphincter function.

Symptoms

Pain in the leg (sometimes in a 'sciatic' distribution).
Difficulty with walking.
Retention of urine or incontinence.
Impotence.
Numbness – in the legs or in the sacral area.

Signs

Limitation of straight leg raising.
Muscle weakness.

Depression of tendon reflexes. ⎫ The distribution of
Sensory depression. ⎬ these will depend on which nerve roots
⎭ are affected.

Distended bladder.
Loss of anal reflex.

Investigations

When an acute cauda equina syndrome develops, and particularly when there is sphincter involvement, the situation must be investigated very urgently.
1. Plain X-rays of the lumbo-sacral area.
2. Myelogram.

Basis of Treatment

Surgical decompression is urgently indicated when there is sphincter involvement. Delay may produce permanent paralysis of bladder, bowel, and sexual function.

Compression of a single nerve root by a lateral protrusion of an intervertebral disc may respond to conservative measures such as bed rest, with or without traction. Surgical decompression is usually indicated if there is muscle wasting and when a central protrusion is present.

POLYNEURITIS

The term 'polyneuritis' is used to encompass a number of different conditions in which there is non-traumatic degeneration of the nerves of the limbs. The clinical picture is one of wasting and weakness of muscles, absent tendon reflexes and sensory loss. The following main clinical types are recognised:
1. Acute polyneuritis (Landry–Guillain–Barré syndrome).
2. Sub-acute or chronic distal neuropathy. This is the classical type of 'peripheral neuritis'. It is usually mixed, but may sometimes be purely motor or sensory.
3. Neuropathy of single nerve trunks.
(a) Compressive, traumatic, or occupational.
(b) Non-compressive. One or more peripheral nerves may be involved in the condition of 'mononeuritis multiplex'. Causes include diabetes, carcinoma, polyarteritis nodosa, amyloidosis and leprosy.

The following are some examples of the pathological processes that can be involved:
1. Acute swelling. This occurs in acute infective polyneuritis which is thought to have an allergic origin.
2. Occlusion of the vasa nervorum with focal infarction of nerve, e.g. polyarteritis nodosa.
3. Amyloid infiltration in the connective sheath of the nerves.
4. Segmental demyelination, e.g. diphtheritic polyneuropathy, diabetes.

5. Peripheral dying-back, e.g. hereditary neuropathies, poisoning with acrylamide.

The Main Causes of Polyneuritis

1. **Drugs.** Nitrofurantoin, isoniazid, Antabuse, vincristine.

2. **Other Toxic Agents:**
Lead affects the radial nerve particularly, with the production of wrist and finger drop. Usually, no sensory features. In children, encephalopathy may occur, with the production of convulsions and coma.

Other metals including arsenic, gold, mercury, zinc, bismuth, antimony and thallium. These metals usually produce a symmetrical distal sensory-motor neuropathy.

Triorthocresylphosphate. This was responsible for a very serious epidemic of polyneuritis in Morocco in the 1950s.

3. **Metabolic and Deficiency States:**
Alcohol. Alcoholic neuropathy is due to deficiency of B vitamins, including thiamine. The prognosis for recovery is good when alcohol is withdrawn and if thiamine is given.

Beriberi. The mechanism is similar to that occurring with alcoholic neuropathy.

Vitamin B$_{12}$ deficiency. Polyneuritis, usually combined with signs of spinal cord involvement occur (*see* section on 'Spinal cord', page 506).

Porphyria may be associated with a rapidly progressive severe symmetrical polyneuropathy. A less acute syndrome sometimes occurs.

Diabetes mellitus. At least 50 per cent of diabetics have signs of peripheral nerve involvement. The commonest manifestation is the finding of depressed or absent tendon reflexes and depressed vibration sense in the legs. Common syndromes are:
(a) Distal sensory neuropathy. This produces pains and tingling and numbness in the feet. Perforating ulcers and neuropathic joints may occur.
(b) Mononeuritis. One or more peripheral nerves may be picked out. In femoral neuritis there is severe pain in the thigh, together with wasting of the quadriceps and depression of the knee jerk. Recovery usually occurs after a few months.
(c) Autonomic neuropathy. This is common and manifests itself clinically by impotence, nocturnal diarrhoea, painless retention of urine, and postural hypotension.

(d) Ophthalmoplegia. Paralysis of one or more of the ocular motor nerves is common.
It is likely that control of diabetes is important in preventing progression of the neuropathy of diabetes. There is no other known way of influencing the course of the neuropathy.

4. **Uraemia.** Occasionally, in chronic uraemia, a subacute or chronic distal sensory motor paralysis of all four limbs occurs.

5. **Neoplasia.** The commonest neoplastic syndromes are a symmetrical sensory-motor neuropathy and mononeuritis multiplex.
Carcinoma. Non-metastatic involvement of peripheral nerves is quite common, especially with bronchial neoplasms. Polyneuritis may precede the finding of a neoplasm by weeks, months, or years. Removal of the primary neoplasm occasionally produces improvement in the neuropathy, but this is the exception rather than the rule.

Myeloma

6. **Connective Tissue Disorders:**
Polyarteritis nodosa. This is particularly liable to produce a mononeuritis due to involvement of the vasa nervorum.

Rheumatoid arthritis. Several forms of neuropathy have been described, including those due to entrapment of peripheral nerves as well as purely motor or sensory forms.

Disseminated lupus erythematosus. Neuropathy is uncommon.

7. **Infective Conditions:**
Acute infective polyneuritis (see below)

Diphtheria. This usually follows pharyngeal and laryngeal infections. Local action of toxins may produce paralysis of palatal and pharyngeal muscles – frequently within a few days of the primary infection. Blurred vision occurs a little later as a result of paralysis of accommodation. Four to six weeks after the throat infection a typical sensory-motor polyneuropathy may occur.

Infectious mononucleosis. The syndrome of acute infective polyneuritis may occur.

Leprosy. Lepra bacilli can usually be found in the nerves. Classically, leprosy affects multiple cutaneous nerves, producing areas of painless anaesthesia. Perforating ulcers and loss of digits may occur.

504

8. **Inherited Conditions.** A considerable number of uncommon inherited conditions affecting peripheral nerves are known. The commonest of these is peroneal muscular atrophy. This condition is usually inherited in a dominant fashion and produces very chronic wasting of distal muscles of all four limbs, frequently without sensory loss.

9. **Miscellaneous.** Serum neuritis (*see* page 498); neuralgic amyotrophy ('shoulder girdle' neuritis) (*see* page 498).

ACUTE POLYNEURITIS (LANDRY–GUILLAIN–BARRÉ SYNDROME)

Definition

A rapidly progressive, and usually fully reversible polyneuritis producing symmetrical paralysis of the limbs and sometimes of the bulbar and respiratory muscles.

Background

Approximately 50 per cent of cases have a history of a preceding non-specific virus infection during the previous two to three weeks. No single virus is implicated.

Acute polyneuritis has been known to be associated with almost every disease. Two diseases in particular, are associated with this syndrome – porphyria and infective mononucleosis. Occasionally, diabetes may be present.

Pathology

There is oedema and lymphocyte infiltration of the nerve roots and patchy demyelination of nerve fibres.

Symptoms and Signs

History of a recent upper respiratory tract infection.

Symptoms
Tingling in the extremities.
Weakness of arms and legs developing gradually.
Muscle pain and tenderness.
Dysphagia.

Signs
Weakness of arms and legs.
Absent tendon reflexes.
Minimal sensory loss.
Unilateral or bilateral facial weakness.
Any other cranial nerves may be involved.

In some cases (probably about five per cent) severe involvement of the bulbar muscles occurs with the production of dysphagia, choking with fluids, dysarthria, and a weak cough. Respiratory distress, cyanosis, and anoxia will occur if there is marked involvement of the respiratory muscles.

The disease has usually produced its maximum effect within four weeks, after which gradual recovery is usual.

Complications

Inhalation pneumonia, especially when there is bulbar paralysis.
Pulmonary embolus.
Severe hypotension, partly due to paralysis of vascular reflexes.
Cardiac arrhythmias and arrest.

Investigations

1. CSF. A raised protein is usual. There are rarely more than 30 cells per mm³.
2. Viral studies on blood and CSF.
3. Paul Bunnell test.
4. Test urine for porphyrins.
5. Glucose tolerance test.
6. Chest X-ray.

Differential Diagnosis

The diagnosis of acute polyneuritis is usually not difficult, particularly when there is involvement of the cranial musculature.
1. Poliomyelitis occurs in epidemics, is often asymmetrical, and there are no sensory features.
2. Acute paraplegia due to spinal cord disease. Usually the plantar responses are extensor and there is marked sensory loss.

Basis of Treatment

Acute polyneuritis is a self-limiting disorder. The majority of cases do not require any specific treatment. The object of treatment in severe cases, is to keep the patient alive until spontaneous recovery occurs. Steroids are often used but there is no positive proof that they are helpful and they can be dangerous.
Indication for tracheostomy:
1. Poor cough.
2. Marked dysphagia with evidence of inhalation of mouth contents.
3. Poor respiratory reserve. Assisted ventilation may be required and in these circumstances the patient should ideally be transferred to an Intensive Care Unit. Nasogastric feeding will be required in these cases. Because of the danger of pulmonary embolism, prophylactic anticoagulants may be indicated.

Prognosis

Acute polyneuritis is a self-limiting disease and most patients make a complete recovery. Approximately twenty per cent of those who require assisted ventilation will die during the acute phase. The vast majority of survivors recover completely. Even those who were once very severely paralysed, usually make a complete recovery. Occasional relapsing cases occur.

SUBACUTE OR CHRONIC DISTAL NEUROPATHY

Definition

A syndrome characterised by the gradual development of wasting and/or sensory disturbance in a symmetrical distribution in the distal part of the limbs.

Background

The syndrome is usually mixed – with motor *and* sensory features. Occasionally, pure motor (for example with lead) or pure sensory (with diabetes or nitrofurantoin) neuropathies occur. In most forms of neuropathy the legs are involved earlier and more severely than the arms.

A large number of different conditions may be associated with the syndrome. The commonest of these are:
1. Toxic causes including drugs and alcohol.
2. Diabetes.
3. Carcinoma, especially of the bronchus.
4. Vitamin B_{12} deficiency.
In at least 50 per cent of cases the cause is not found.

Symptoms and Signs

The syndrome usually develops insidiously.

Symptoms
Feet catching on the ground.
Weakness of the hands.
Numbness of the feet and hands.
Difficulty with 'fine' tasks, e.g. doing-up buttons.
Hypersensitivity and burning in the soles of the feet.

Signs
Weakness and wasting of muscles below the knees and of the hands.
Absent tendon reflexes.
'Glove and stocking' sensory loss.

Investigations

Remember to take a proper history relating to diet and possible exposure to drugs and toxins (especially ethyl alcohol!). A large number of investigations may need to be done if the causative diagnosis is not obvious.

1. Glucose tolerance test.
2. Chest X-ray.
3. Serum B_{12} level.
4. Test urine for porphyrins.
5. EMG. This confirms the presence of denervation (if there is doubt).
Nerve conduction studies – useful in distinguishing between primary demyelinating disorders and those involving axonal loss.
6. Examination of CSF. This is not usually necessary, but if done will frequently show a raised protein level.

Complications

Perforating ulcers on the feet. ⎫ Particularly liable
Gangrene. ⎬ to occur in
Neuropathic joints. ⎭ diabetes.

Differential Diagnosis

Other causes of wasting of the small muscles of the hands; for example compression of the first thoracic nerve root, syringomyelia and motor neurone disease.

Basis of Treatment

Treatment depends on the cause. If diabetes is found it should be properly controlled. In Vitamin B_{12} deficiency, regular injections are required.

In many instances treatment can only be symptomatic. If there is a marked foot drop, bilateral below-knee irons or splints will be required. A wrist and finger drop will require the use of a cock-up splint.

Prognosis

Most chronic neuropathies either progress slowly or appear to come to a virtual standstill. Some, such as those associated with alcoholism, drugs, and vitamin B_{12} deficiency, will improve when the correct treatment is given. Others, such as those associated with neoplasia, rarely improve.

DISEASES OF THE SPINAL CORD

The following conditions will be considered:
1. Syndrome of spinal cord compression (*see* page 507).
2. Injury to the spinal cord (*see* page 508).
3. Intrinsic tumours of the spinal cord (*see* page 508).
4. Vascular lesions of the spinal cord (*see* page 508).
5. Syndrome of myelitis (*see* page 508).
6. Syringomyelia (*see* page 509).
7. Subacute combined degeneration (*see* page 510).
8. Motor neurone disease (*see* page 511).
9. Multiple sclerosis (*see* page 540).
10. Friedreich's ataxia (*see* page 511).
Disease of the spinal cord is likely to produce damage to the anterior horn cells at the level of the lesion, and

evidence of tract damage below the level of the lesion. The following terms are in common use:
1. *Paraplegia.* Paralysis of the legs. By convention this term is reserved for paralysis due to upper motor neurone disturbance.
2. *Paraparesis.* Upper motor neurone weakness of the legs.
3. *Tetraplegia or quadraplegia.* Paralysis of all four limbs.
4. *Tetraparesis.* Weakness of all four limbs.

SPINAL CORD COMPRESSION

Compression of the spinal cord, whatever its cause, usually demands surgical relief. For this reason the condition is one of the greatest importance.

Causes

1. Prolapsed intervertebral disc – particularly in the neck.
2. Intradural tumour, particularly meningioma and neurofibroma.
3. Malignant invasion of the vertebrae, particularly secondary carcinoma (bronchus). Myeloma.
4. Infection, particularly with tuberculous infection of the vertebrae.
5. Epidural spinal abscess.
6. Spinal cord injury.
7. Skeletal deformities, for example kyphoscoliosis.

Symptoms and Signs

Spinal cord compression produces a transverse lesion of the cord with affection of all cord functions, motor, sensory and autonomic below that level. Involvement of roots *at* the level of compression produces pain and loss of function in a radicular distribution.

Spinal cord compression may occur acutely within minutes or over a period of several years.

Symptoms
Difficulty with walking.
Weakness of the legs (and sometimes of arms).
Numbness and tingling in the legs.
Radicular pain – sometimes in a girdle distribution.
Difficulty with passing urine.

Signs
Weakness of the legs.
Flaccidity in the acute stage.
Spasticity with markedly increased tendon reflexes in the chronic stage.
Extensor plantar responses.
Sensory loss below the level of the lesion.

In all cases it is essential to look for a 'level'. This may be:

1. *Motor.* For example wasting of the small muscles of the hand usually indicates involvement of the upper thoracic cord.

2. *Reflex.* Depressed or absent tendon reflexes are usual *at* the level of the lesion. Tendon reflexes *below* the level are increased.

3. *Sensory.* Depression of cutaneous sensation frequently occurs below a certain level. This level is most easily demonstrated when it involves the trunk.

Investigations

1. Chest X-ray, particularly if neoplastic disease of the vertebrae is suspected.
2. Plain X-ray of the spine centred on the appropriate level – vertebral collapse may be demonstrated.
3. Lumbar puncture. A spinal block may be present. The pressure of the CSF is low and does not rise with jugular compression. The CSF is yellow and contains a high amount of protein, but usually no cells.
4. Myelogram. Myelography is essential if compression of the spinal cord is suspected.

Differential Diagnosis

Acute Paraplegia:
1. Multiple sclerosis – a crisp sensory level is unusual.
2. Vascular lesions. Haematomyelia, in which bleeding occurs into the cord. Occlusion of the anterior spinal artery.
3. Myelitis of viral origin.

Subacute or Chronic Paraplegia or Paraparesis:
1. Multiple sclerosis. There is frequently optic atrophy, nystagmus and other evidence of diffuse involvement of the nervous system.
2. Intrinsic spinal cord tumour. The myelogram may show localised expansion of the spinal cord.
3. Subacute combined degeneration of the cord. Often a macrocytic anaemia and a low serum B_{12} level, etc.
4. Motor neurone disease. Fasciculation, generalised muscle wasting, and involvement of the bulbar muscles is frequent.

Basis of Treatment

Spinal cord compression practically always demands surgical relief. Even when compression has been present for many months a surprising degree of recovery may occur when the compression is relieved.

General Management in the Acute Phase:

Bladder function. In the acute stage, an indwelling catheter should be inserted using non-touch technique, to avoid infection. Early catheterisation is essential, and retention of urine with overflow must not be allowed to occur. Infections, if present, should be treated with sulphonamides or the appropriate antibiotic. In some instances, full recovery of bladder function will occur. In others, an 'automatic bladder' may be produced, the bladder emptying at regular intervals when the intravesical pressure reaches a critical level.

Bowel function. This does not usually present as large a problem as bladder function. Enemas, with or without manual evacuation, may be required.

Avoidance of bed sores. Frequent turning of the patient (at one to two-hour intervals) is essential, preferably using some form of bed that incorporates turning facilities.

Avoidance of contractures. The patient should be nursed in a well-supported bed so that the back is straight, the hips not allowed to become flexed, and the knees must not be allowed to become bent. If possible, the patient should spend some of his time sleeping on his face. This prevents excessive pressure on the buttocks and helps to avoid flexion contractures of the hips.

Later Management:

The patient should, ideally, be transferred to a paraplegic unit where intensive rehabilitation can be given. Active physiotherapy must be given. During the initial stage the legs may need to be splinted.

Postural hypotension may occur when the patient stands up, due to paralysis of vasomotor reflexes. Tight bandaging of the legs to encourage venous return is often helpful.

INJURIES OF THE SPINAL CORD

Most cases of spinal cord damage occur with fracture/dislocations in the cervical or in the lower thoracic regions. A relatively trivial injury may produce severe paralysis if there is pre-existing cervical spondylosis.

Basis of Treatment

Open operation is rarely called for because it is impossible to reverse damage already done. Treatment is directed towards preventing complications and creating the best conditions for natural recovery.

INTRINSIC TUMOURS OF THE SPINAL CORD

The most common tumours are ependymomas and gliomas of varying degrees of malignancy. The whole cord becomes swollen and the bony spinal canal is expanded. The clinical picture is usually that of a slowly progressive paraplegia.

Basis of Treatment

Surgical exploration is usually necessary for diagnostic purposes. If the tumour is found to be arising in the cord little can be done. Deep X-ray therapy is sometimes helpful. Occasionally, cystic tumours can be aspirated.

VASCULAR LESIONS OF THE SPINAL CORD

The spinal cord receives its blood supply via one anterior and two posterior spinal arteries. These vessels receive blood from the aorta and its main branches. The following principal syndromes occur:

Occlusion of the Anterior Spinal Artery. An acute paraplegia develops. The posterior column territory is usually spared, postural and vibratory sense remaining intact.

Haematomyelia. Spontaneous bleeding occurs into the substance of the spinal cord. The resultant clinical picture may resemble that of syringomyelia except that the onset is sudden.

Secondary Vascular Changes. This is probably the commonest cause of vascular disturbance to the spinal cord. In cervical spondylosis and in neoplastic disease of the vertebrae, the arteries supplying the spinal cord may be compressed.

MYELITIS

Definition

Acute inflammation of the spinal cord. When accompanied by inflammation of the brain the term encephalomyelitis is used.

Background

The main causes are:
1. Post-infective. The disorder may be due either to a virus infection of the cord or to demyelination (*see* 'Acute viral meningoencephalitis' and 'Acute disseminated encephalomyelitis', pages 547 to 550).
2. Poliomyelitis.
3. *Herpes zoster* (occasionally).
4. Multiple sclerosis.
5. Devic's disease. This is an uncommon variant of multiple sclerosis in which an acute demyelinating transverse cord lesion occurs together with retrobulbar neuritis.

508

Symptoms and Signs

There is usually an acute disturbance of the spinal cord function with the production of a paraplegia. In poliomyelitis, however, no 'long tract' signs appear.

Basis of Treatment

Apart from steroids in demyelinating cases no specific treatment is available.

SYRINGOMYELIA (Syrinx = pipe or tube)

Definition

A slowly progressive disorder in which cavitation occurs in the central part of the spinal cord and lower brain stem. The term syringobulbia refers to involvement of the brain stem.

Background and Pathology

The peak age of clinical onset is between 20 and 30.

Pathologically there is irregular cavitation involving the central grey matter of the cervical cord. In some instances the cavitation may extend into the lower brain stem. The cavitation is usually irregular and surrounded by considerable gliosis. Because of its central situation the crossing pain and temperature fibres are usually affected early. The process extends forwards and frequently destroys anterior horn cells (with the production of muscle wasting). Lateral extension occurs later with interruption of corticospinal fibres to the legs. Extension into the posterior columns usually occurs late. Abnormalities of the cervical vertebrae and lower part of the skull are frequent. It seems likely that some cases of syringomyelia are due to obstruction to the free flow of CSF in and out of the fourth ventricle. Thus, blockage at the exits of the fourth ventricle, for example by a congenital membrane or by adhesions, means that CSF is forced downwards into the middle of the spinal cord with each pulse beat. In other cases the cerebellar tonsils become prolapsed down into the cervical canal. Obstruction to free flow of CSF does not occur in all cases and it is likely that a proportion, at least, are due to maldevelopment or incomplete closure of the central canal of the spinal cord.

Symptoms and Signs (see Table 21.8)

The onset is usually insidious and the course fairly chronic.

Investigations

1. Plain X-rays of the skull and spine – normal in about 50 per cent. *May* show evidence of arrested hydrocephalus, platybasia, or abnormalities of vertebral fusion in the upper cervical region.

Table 21.8

Symptoms	Signs
Early:	
Painless burns on the hands.	*Dissociated anaesthesia in a suspended distribution over the shoulders and arms.
Wasting and weakness of one or both hands.	Wasting of the small muscles of the hands.
Spontaneous pain – this may sometimes be severe and felt in the back, chest, and arms.	Absent or depressed tendon jerks in one or both arms.
	Horner's syndrome.
	Sometimes a cervico-thoracic scoliosis.
Late:	
Severe pain may continue.	More extensive sensory loss in the arms and more severe wasting.
Increasing difficulty with using the arms.	Marked trophic changes in the hands (thick and discoloured skin together with unhealed ulcers)
Some difficulty with walking may be found but this is not usually severe.	
	†Charcot joints, especially shoulder and elbow.
	Legs – mild spastic paraparesis.
	There may be palsies of the lower cranial nerves, wasting of the tongue, palatal palsy, etc.

*Loss of pain and temperature sensation with preservation of other sensory modalities including light touch.
†Charcot joints: these joints show bony swelling together with an abnormal range of painless movement.

2. Myelogram. The spinal cord may appear widened. Prolapse of the cerebellar tonsils and/or evidence of CSF obstruction at the level of the fourth ventricle may be seen in some cases.

Differential Diagnosis

1. Tumour in the spinal cord. This may be very difficult to distinguish from syringomyelia. The course of a tumour is usually more rapid.
2. Haematomyelia (spontaneous bleeding into the centre of the spinal cord). This is usually of *sudden* onset.
3. Other causes of wasting of the small muscles of the hands, for example motor neurone disease (no sensory loss) and polyneuritis (sensory loss is not dissociated).
4. Cervical spondylosis. Dissociated sensory loss is rare but does occasionally occur.

Basis of Treatment

Surgical treatment may help cases in which there is obstruction to CSF flow at the level of the foramen magnum. In these cases removal of the posterior ring of the foramen magnum and opening up of the fourth ventricle is undertaken. Surgical aspiration of syringomyelic cavities has been disappointing.

Radiotherapy was given in the past but is not helpful in most cases. Its use is usually reserved for patients who have severe pain.

Medical treatment has little to offer apart from symptomatic relief of pain and the general measures applicable in cases of disability.

Prognosis

The condition is very slowly progressive and rarely kills the patient. The patient can usually still walk after many years although he may show marked weakness of the hands.

SUBACUTE COMBINED DEGENERATION

Definition

A disorder, due to deficiency of vitamin B_{12}, in which pathological changes occur in the spinal cord and in the peripheral nerves.

Background

This condition occurs in:
1. Addisonian pernicious anaemia (see page 379).
2. Following gastrectomy.
3. In other malabsorption syndromes (uncommon).

Pathology

The main sites of damage in this condition are:

1. **Spinal Cord.** The posterior columns and corticospinal tracts are maximally affected. A process of patchy spongy degeneration occurs.

2. **Peripheral Nerves.** Degeneration of the sensory ganglion cells and of peripheral motor and sensory nerve fibres occurs.

Symptoms and Signs (see Table 21.9)

The clinical picture is highly variable and depends mainly on the relative involvement of the spinal cord and peripheral nerves.

Other features include mental confusion and sometimes chronic dementia; visual deterioration and optic atrophy. There may also be the signs of Addisonian pernicious anaemia.
Note: The diagnosis should be suspected in all cases of:
1. Paraplegia and paraparesis.
2. All cases of polyneuropathy, particularly when this is mainly sensory.

Table 21.9 Symptoms and signs of subacute combined degeneration

Symptoms	Signs
Early:	
Tingling, pins and needles in the arms and legs.	Vibration sense lost in the legs. Tender calf muscles.
Later:	
Weakness of the limbs. Numbness, tingling, pins and needles in the limbs. Unsteadiness.	Tendon reflexes may be depressed or increased. Plantar responses often extensor. Vibration sense much depressed. Distal sensory loss for light touch in arms and legs. Ataxia – worse with eyes closed

It should be particularly suspected when (1) and (2) are combined.

Investigations

1. Full blood count. This may show macrocytosis and other features of megaloblastic anaemia.
2. Serum B_{12} level – below 140 pg per ml. ⎫ see
3. Schilling test – less than 5 per cent excretion. ⎬ page
4. Sternal marrow – megaloblastic picture. ⎭ 379
5. Analysis of gastric contents may show a histamine-fast achlorhydria.
Note: Subacute combined degeneration may occur when the blood count and sternal marrow are normal. If in doubt, give vitamin B_{12}.

Differential Diagnosis

1. Other causes of paraplegia, for example multiple sclerosis, spinal cord compression, etc.
2. Other causes of polyneuritis – diabetes, poisoning, etc.

Basis of Treatment

Injections of vitamin B_{12} (1,000 μg twice weekly initially) should be given without delay.

Treatment once started must be continued indefinitely (1,000 μg monthly).

Prognosis

If untreated, irreversible weakness of the limbs will occur. Great improvement is usual when vitamin B_{12} is given. The peripheral nerve component of the disorder tends to improve more than that due to spinal cord involvement.

MOTOR NEURONE DISEASE

Definition

A disorder of unknown cause in which there is degeneration of corticospinal tracts, corticobulbar tracts, anterior horn cells, and the neurones of the bulbar muscles.

Background

The disease mainly affects people between 40 and 60. It is rarely familial. The cause is quite unknown. There is a male preponderance of approximately 2.5:1.

Symptoms and Signs (Table 21.10)

In most cases there is evidence of involvement of more than one of the structures mentioned in the definition, but in occasional cases a reasonably pure syndrome emerges. There are very rarely any sensory symptoms and never any sensory signs.

Investigations

1. Electromyography. Frequently useful in obese patients to confirm the presence of fasciculation. A denervation pattern is likely to be seen. Normal nerve conduction – until terminal stages.
2. Muscle biopsy. This is not usually necessary but if done will show denervation.
3. Chest X-ray. The cachexia associated with neoplasms may resemble motor neurone disease.

Differential Diagnosis

1. Motor neuropathy. The muscle wasting is usually symmetrical and the tendon reflexes depressed.
2. Lesions of nerve roots and of peripheral nerves may be simulated, particularly when muscle wasting is asymmetrical.
3. Fasciculation due to other causes. Fasciculation can particularly occur when the patient is tense or cold.
4. Other causes of pseudo-bulbar palsy – vascular lesions of the brain stem and bilateral lesions in the internal capsule.

Basis of Treatment

No specific treatment exists. The dysarthria and dysphagia of pseudo-bulbar palsy can sometimes be helped by sucking ice before drinking or talking. Ultimately, a tracheostomy with or without a gastrostomy may be necessary.

When severe muscle weakness occurs the appropriate aids should be supplied including below-knee calipers and a wheelchair.

Prognosis

Motor neurone disease is a relentlessly progressive disorder. The average duration of the disease is about three years. The prognosis is worst in cases with severe bulbar involvement, inhalation pneumonia being an ever present danger.

FRIEDREICH'S ATAXIA

Definition

A familial disorder characterised by degeneration of cells in the posterior root ganglia with secondary

Table 21.10 Symptoms and signs of motor neurone disease

Syndrome	Symptoms	Signs
Bulbar palsy (degeneration of the cells of the cranial nerve nuclei)	Dysphagia Dysarthria Dysphonia	Wasting and *fasciculation of the tongue Weakness of the palate
Pseudo-bulbar palsy (involvement of cortico-bulbar fibres)	Dysphagia and dysarthria Emotional lability – laughing and crying inappropriately	Spastic tongue Increased jaw jerk
Progressive muscular atrophy (involvement of anterior horn cells)	Wasting and weakness of the limbs Twitching of muscles	Wasting of the limb muscles, frequently asymmetrical. This may be proximal or distal Brisk tendon reflexes Fasciculation
Amyotrophic lateral sclerosis (involvement of the cortico-spinal tract)	Stiffness of the limbs Difficulty in walking Frequent cramps	Spastic quadraparesis with very brisk tendon reflexes Extensor plantar responses (the features of a pseudo-bulbar palsy are frequently also present)

*Fasciculation – the spontaneous twitching of whole groups of muscle fibres.

changes in the peripheral nerves and in the posterior columns of the spinal cord.

Background

There are probably between 600 to 700 cases in the UK. The condition is inherited as an autosomal recessive.

Symptoms and Signs

The condition develops in a previously apparently healthy child. The age of onset is usually between 10 and 15.

Symptoms
Gradual onset of difficulty with walking.
Within a few years the child can no longer walk unaided.
Eventually a wheelchair is required.

Signs
Slurred speech.
Ataxia and weakness of the limbs.
Absent tendon reflexes.
Extensor plantar responses.
Defective postural sensation in the legs.

Complications

Heart failure is common.

Investigations

ECG. This is usually abnormal showing diffusely inverted T waves.

Basis of Treatment

Nil specific.

Prognosis

The mean age of death is about 35. The commonest cause of death is heart failure.

INHERITED AND DEVELOPMENTAL DISORDERS

VON RECKLINGHAUSEN'S DISEASE – NEUROFIBROMATOSIS

Definition

A dominantly inherited condition characterised by skin pigmentation and the presence of multiple neurofibromata.

Background

The neurofibromata arise from the neurilemmal sheath of nerves. They contain a great deal of fibrous tissue. Sarcomatous change is a rare complication.

Associated Conditions

Meningiomas and gliomas – multiple tumours occasionally occur. Both types of tumour occur more frequently in people with Von Recklinghausen's disease than in the general population.
Glioma of the optic nerve.
Stenosis of the aqueduct of Sylvius.
Phaeochromocytoma. Medullary thyroid carcinoma.
Scoliosis. This is usually associated with some structural abnormality of the vertebrae.

Symptoms and Signs

Von Recklinghausen's disease is frequently non-symptomatic. In some instances the disease is discovered at a routine medical examination. Other patients seek medical advice for cosmetic reasons. A third group present to the doctor because of compression of nervous tissue (for example brain stem compression due to an acoustic neuroma).

Skin pigmentation. The classical abnormality involves the presence of numerous pale brown macules – cafe-au-lait spots. These vary in diameter from less than 1 cm up to 14 or 15 cm. There may also be generalised spotty pigmentation in the axillae.

Skin tumours. These may be single or multiple. In some instances the patient's skin is very extensively involved. The tumours are situated subcutaneously and are soft, mobile, and sometimes lobulated.

Tumours at other sites. Acoustic neuroma. There are likely to be clinical features of a lesion in the cerebello-pontine angle, deafness, depression of facial sensation, and ataxia.

Tumours on spinal nerves. Symptoms of compression of the spinal cord (weakness of the legs, etc.) and of compression of nerve roots (segmental pain) will occur. Tumours in the thoracic region are sometimes found lying partly in the spinal canal and partly within the chest (dumb-bell tumours).

Basis of Treatment

No specific treatment is available. Tumours producing symptoms will need to be removed as necessary.

HYDROCEPHALUS

Definition

An increase in the volume of cerebrospinal fluid within the cranium.

Background

There are two basic types of hydrocephalus: non-communicating (obstructive), and communicating.

Non-communicating (Obstructive) Hydrocephalus.
This is due to a block within the ventricular system so that CSF cannot escape into the subarachnoid space. This produces dilatation of the ventricular system.

Causes:
(a) Stenosis of the aqueduct of Sylvius.
(b) Obstruction of the exit foraminae from the 4th ventricle by a congenital membrane or adhesions.

Communicating Hydrocephalus.
In this instance the ventricles and subarachnoid space are in communication. In many instances, however, some obstruction to CSF flow does occur, sometimes in the basal cisterns.

Causes:
(a) Obstruction to CSF flow in the subarachnoid space by adhesions, for example following meningitis or a subarachnoid haemorrhage.
(b) Thrombosis of the major intracranial venous sinuses.
(c) Idiopathic. It is possible that in some of these cases there may be excessive formation of CSF by the choroid plexuses.

Some cases of hydrocephalus are associated with congenital anomalies at the base of the skull or with spina bifida.

Symptoms and Signs

Children
Enlargement of the head.
Bulging fontanelles.
Convulsions.
Delayed milestones.
Spasticity of the limbs.
Pale optic discs.

In juveniles or adults
Gradual onset of intellectual deterioration.
Ataxia.
Convulsions.
Papilloedema, and other evidence of raised intracranial pressure.

Investigations

1. Plain skull X-ray will frequently show separation of the sutures. In adults a 'beaten silver' appearance of the vault is frequently seen, and erosion of the posterior clinoids.
2. Air or Myodil ventriculography is important in order to localise the level of the block and to exclude a tumour.

Basis of Treatment

Short-circuit operation to by-pass the block. A polythene tube may be inserted with one end in a lateral ventricle and the other in the cisterna magna (for example if there is aqueduct stenosis) or in a jugular vein in cases of communicating hydrocephalus.

Direct attack on the block – occasionally division of a membrane blocking the exit foramina from the 4th ventricle is possible.

Prognosis

Hydrocephalus in infancy has a high mortality. In some of the survivors the hydrocephalus arrests spontaneously. The majority of survivors have some degree of mental or physical handicap.

SPINA BIFIDA

Spina bifida is a condition in which there is incomplete closure of the vertebral canal, frequently in the lumbo-sacral region. In severe cases the cauda equina, terminal end of the spinal cord, and meninges protrude through the bony defect. In such instances there is a soft swelling over the lumbo-sacral area and there is frequently a skin defect. The chance of survival can be much increased by early closure of the skin defect. Most children with this defect are left with severe flaccid paralysis of the legs. Hydrocephalus frequently occurs also.

Lesser degrees of spina bifida occur. The least serious is a bony defect in the laminae of the sacral vertebrae unassociated with neurological deficits.

BASILAR IMPRESSION OF THE SKULL

This is a bony anomaly in which there is invagination of part of the foramen magnum into the skull. The result is some degree of compression of the lower cranial nerves, upper cervical nerves, and spinal cord. The condition is frequently associated with other bony anomalies. It may be congenital or acquired, sometimes secondary to bone softening diseases such as Paget's disease.

CEREBRAL PALSY

Definition

This term is used to describe a group of disorders in which brain damage is apparent at, or shortly after, birth. Affected children are sometimes called 'spastics', but it should be noted that not all those with cerebral palsy are spastic. Indeed, in some, the muscles are hypotonic. Ataxia or involuntary movements may be the main feature.

Background

There are many different causes for cerebral palsy. In many individual cases it is impossible to determine the aetiology. Causes include:
1. Intra-uterine anoxia.
2. Birth trauma.
3. Kernicterus – damage to the basal ganglia due to an abnormally high bilirubin level occurring shortly after birth.
4. Convulsions in early infancy.
5. Brain infarction due to arterial or venous occlusion.

Symptoms and Signs

The symptomatology will vary considerably and depends on the severity and anatomical extent of damage. The earliest manifestation is frequently a delay in achieving the normal milestones of physical and intellectual development. Later in childhood a number of recognisable variants occur –

Spastic Variety. This is one of the commonest types and involves spasticity of the limbs with the production of walking difficulty and a 'scissors' gait.

Athetosis. This involves facial grimacing and writhing movements of the limbs.

Ataxic Type. There is ataxia of the trunk and limbs.

Hemiplegic Type. A proportion of children have epileptic fits. Intellectual development varies – some showing an almost normal level while others are markedly backward.

Other defects include difficulty with speech, hearing, and reading. Sometimes these abnormalities occur without other clinical evidence of brain damage. It is of the greatest importance to identify such defects as it is only too easy to assume that affected children are mentally backward.

UNCONSCIOUSNESS

Normal consciousness is the condition of being fully awake and aware of oneself and one's environment. Fluctuations occur during the day from full alertness and deep concentration, on the one hand, to drowsiness and mind wandering (frequently after a large meal!) on the other.

Sleep is a state of physical and mental inactivity from which the patient can rapidly be aroused to full consciousness. A sleeping person has little awareness of himself or of his environment and in this sense may be said to be unconscious. On the other hand, he, or she, may respond to very small, unaccustomed stimuli such as the distant cry of a child or the opening of a door.

Various degrees of unconsciousness can be recognised. Coma is the most extreme state. The patient lies as if asleep but makes no response to external stimuli. In the deepest coma the patient will not even respond to the most vigorous painful stimulations. Corneal, pupillary, and tendon reflexes are absent. In lesser depths of unconsciousness these reflexes are preserved and the patient stirs or moans when shouted at or when the skin is pinched.

Stupor is a condition which may precede the development of coma itself. If stimulated vigorously, the patient will open his eyes and look around him. The response to spoken commands, however, is very slow. Stupor may be preceded by blunting of mental faculties so that the previously normal subject becomes unable to think clearly – a state of confusion. Frequently, for example with intoxicating conditions such as liver or kidney failure, this orderly sequence through confusion, stupor, light unconsciousness, and ultimately deep coma can be traced. In other instances, for example following head injury, the subject passes instantaneously from normal consciousness to deep coma.

The area most concerned with consciousness is the brain stem and thalamus. The cerebral cortex must be severely and extensively damaged before consciousness is lost. On the other hand, damage to the upper brain stem can produce profound loss of consciousness. The critical part of the brain stem, is the reticular formation. This is composed of widely scattered nerve cells whose processes form a net-like (reticular) mesh. The formation extends from the lower medulla upwards through the pons and mid-brain to the thalamus. The processes travel both upwards and downwards, linking together different parts of the reticular formation. The formation also has wide connections with the cerebellum, the cerebral cortex, the spinal cord, and other areas of the central nervous system.

We then come to the problem of sleep. It may well be asked why we should spend so much of our lives sleeping. The reason is unknown, but it is clear that the brain requires a minimum amount of regular rest. Those who attempt to reduce their optimal sleeping time do so at their peril. The brain will simply not work efficiently unless sufficient sleep is obtained. This fact is well known to interrogators. Experimental animals will die within a few days if completely deprived of sleep.

Present views of sleep mechanisms involve excitatory arousal systems in the reticular formation of the upper brain stem, on the one hand, being balanced against inhibitory impulses from other areas of the brain, on the other.

Diagnosis of the Unconscious Patient (Fig. 21.6)

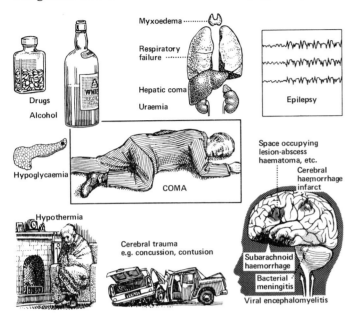

Fig. 21.6 Some important causes of coma.

When faced with an unconscious patient it is first essential to ensure that the patient does not get worse, or even die, while a diagnosis is being made. Some simple rules can be formulated:

1. Ensure that he is breathing properly and that the airway is clear. If not, intubation and assisted ventilation may be required.
2. Make sure that the blood pressure is satisfactory and that he is not bleeding.
3. If the case is one of trauma, make sure that he is not moved unnecessarily. Fractures of the neck are easily missed at this stage and unnecessary movement may produce irreversible damage to the spinal cord.
4. While the above measures are being undertaken make sure that the people who accompany the patient do not leave until they have been questioned. Early diagnosis may depend upon them.

Sometimes the cause for unconsciousness is obvious; for example when there is evidence of a head injury, when the patient has been observed to have an epileptic fit, or when there is clear evidence of a suicide attempt. None the less, the situation may not be as simple as it seems at first sight. Thus, the patient who appears to be in a state of alcoholic intoxication may also have had a head injury. The hypothermic old lady may also be suffering with barbiturate poisoning. If the diagnosis is obvious then treatment can be started immediately; for example, if the patient is known to have swallowed a large number of tablets in an attempt at suicide,

stomach lavage should usually be undertaken without delay (*see* page 204).

Often, however, the diagnosis is not immediately obvious. In these cases, once essential functions have been assured, the problem of diagnosis can be tackled. This must be done in a methodical manner, without undue haste, although obviously time must not be wasted.

The first essential is to question the ambulance men as to the circumstances in which the patient was found. For example, they may have found the patient in a gas-filled room. Sometimes, they will have found a suicide note. Secondly, the relatives must be questioned as to the patient's previous health. Thirdly, the patient's pockets must be searched for drugs and drug cards. Some epileptics and diabetics carry a card indicating the disease from which they suffer.

Examination of the patient must be thorough. It is frequently a good idea to observe quietly the patient for two to three minutes. The following points must be noted:

1. An assessment of the depth of unconsciousness. This must be made early so that a 'base line' assessment is available. It is important to note the patient's response to spoken commands and to other physical stimuli, including pain. These responses should be recorded in the case notes. An arbitrary grading might be:
(a) Stupor – drowsy but responds slowly to simple commands. Incapable of logical thought.
(b) Light coma – grunts only (no talking). Withdraws from pain.
(c) Deep coma – no verbal responses and no response to pain. Tendon reflexes may be depressed.

The Glasgow coma scale has been devised with the objective of standardising the grading of coma. The scale includes an assessment of eye opening, motor responses, and the results of verbal stimulation.

In assessing the depth of coma it is frequently helpful to elicit the oculocephalic and oculovestibular responses (*see* page 526).
2. Breathing. Note the rate and regularity.
3. Evidence of anoxia. Cyanosis may be present.
4. Temperature. Elevated or low.
5. Blood pressure. May be low in Addison's disease and in shock.
6. State of the skin. Sweating in hypoglycaemia, the skin is dry in dehydration and hypothyroidism.
7. State of nutrition. Rapid weight loss may occur in uncontrolled diabetes and in Addison's disease.
8. Odour of the breath; alcohol, ketosis, uraemia, liver failure, etc.
9. Signs of trauma. Note that bruising and lacerations on the scalp may be hidden by the hair.
10. Evidence of raised intracranial pressure; papilloedema, slow irregular breathing, etc.
11. Neck stiffness; e.g. meningitis, subarachnoid haemorrhage, and trauma to the neck.

12. State of the pupils. Unilateral dilatation may occur with one-sided space-occupying lesions. Bilateral, dilated and fixed pupils may occur with mid-brain lesions. Small fixed pupils occur in pontine haemorrhage.

13. Evidence of *focal* neurological disturbance; for example unilateral hypotonia of the limbs may be the only sign of a hemiplegia in an unconscious patient.

An idea of the cause of coma can usually be made after an evaluation of the history and the physical signs. However, some investigations are often required and these include:

(a) Aspiration of the stomach, if poisoning is suspected.

(b) Testing the urine for sugar.

(c) Estimation of blood levels of barbiturates, salicylates, urea, electrolytes and sugar.

(d) Liver function tests.

(e) X-ray chest and skull.

(f) Lumbar puncture. This should not be undertaken if there is evidence of raised intracranial pressure. A suspicion of meningitis or subarachnoid haemorrhage would be an indication for a lumbar puncture.

Common Causes of Unconsciousness

Poisons. Alcohol especially, barbiturates, aspirin and carbon monoxide.

Metabolic Disturbance:

Diabetic ketosis (*see* page 187). Deep sighing breathing, dry skin, breath smells of ketones.

Hypoglycaemia. This usually occurs in known diabetics. Sweating. Normal breathing. Low blood sugar.

Uraemia. Unconsciousness may occur during the terminal stages.

Hypoxia. Cyanosis *may* be present.

Hepatic coma. Look particularly for foetor and the other signs of parenchymal liver failure (jaundice, spider naevi, palmar erythema, etc.).

Addison's disease. Pigmentation, obvious weight loss, low blood pressure.

Epilepsy. The patient may be brought to hospital still convulsing or, more likely, in a state of post-convulsive unconsciousness.

Hypothermia. This usually occurs in the elderly and is sometimes accompanied by signs of hypothyroidism. There may also be evidence of alcohol or barbiturate intoxication.

Unconsciousness Following Head Injury

(a) **Concussion.** This is an abrupt transient loss of consciousness following head injury due, in part at least, to the enormous but short duration pressure rise that occurs in the cranium at the time of impact. Usually there are no focal neurological signs.

(b) **Cerebral Contusion.** Prolonged unconsciousness may be due to cerebral swelling with secondary brain stem compression or to primary damage to the upper brain stem region. Focal neurological signs may be present.

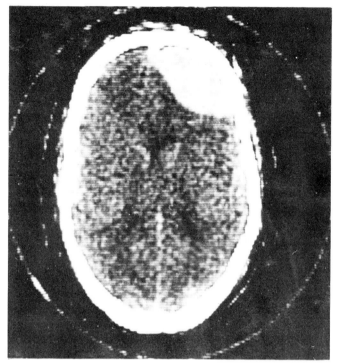

Fig. 21.7 Extradural haematoma.

(c) **Extradural Haematoma** (Fig. 21.7). There is usually a latent period of restored consciousness following recovery from concussion. The latent period is followed by a falling level of consciousness due to a collection of extradural blood formed from a ruptured middle meningeal artery. A fracture of the vault of the skull is usual. Immediate surgery is indicated.

Note: Always look for bruising and laceration of the scalp and bleeding from the ears (often indicative of a fracture of the skull base). A skull X-ray should always be done if head injury is suspected.

Acute Non-traumatic Intracranial Pathology

(a) **Cerebral Haemorrhage.** There is usually the sudden onset of loss of consciousness. There are often signs of a hemiplegia with extreme flaccidity of one arm and leg.

(b) **Subarachnoid Haemorrhage.** Classically, there is the acute onset of severe headache with neck stiffness and bloody CSF.

(c) **Cerebral Infarction.** This is often due to occlusion of a major cerebral blood vessel. A hemiplegia may be demonstrable.

(d) **Virus Encephalitis**

(e) **Bacterial Meningitis**

Both (d) and (e) can occasionally produce unconsciousness. Neck stiffness and appropriate CSF changes are present.

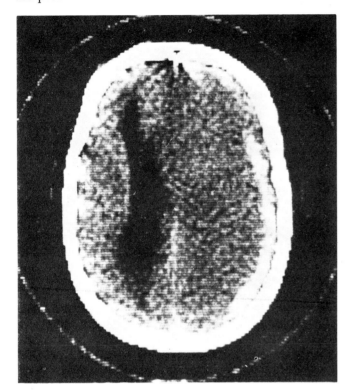

Fig. 21.8 Subdural haematoma with marked ventricular displacement.

Chronic Intracranial Space-occupying Mass

(a) **Cerebral Abscess**
(b) **Subdural Haematoma** (Fig. 21.8)
(c) **Cerebral Tumour**

In all these, the history usually extends over days or weeks. Papilloedema, periodic breathing, and other evidence of raised intracranial pressure may be present. Lumbar puncture can be very dangerous.

THE EPILEPSIES

Definition

Epilepsy is an intermittent disorder of cerebral function which is transient, starts and stops spontaneously, and is often accompanied by motor or sensory phenomena.

No definition of epilepsy is entirely satisfactory. The essence is that epilepsy is a paroxysmal abnormality of brain function, frequently accompanied by abnormal electrical activity on the electroencephalogram (EEG). The clinical manifestations are enormously variable and range from a generalised convulsion, on the one hand, to momentary staring into space, on the other.

Background

The human brain varies greatly in its tendency to produce convulsions. In some people a minor stress (such as prolonged sleep deprivation or lowering the blood sugar level) will produce epileptic activity. In others no such activity occurs, however severe the stress. This 'convulsive threshold' probably has a normal distribution throughout the population. Because of this variable threshold the population cannot easily be divided into epileptic and non-epileptic.

Aetiological Classification

Idiopathic

1. *Centrocephalic.* Major convulsions occur. The EEG shows symmetrical bilateral paroxysmal high voltage activity.

2. *Petit mal.* This starts in childhood. Attacks of transient blankness sometimes associated with myoclonic jerking and falling to the ground. The EEG shows a highly characteristic pattern – three per second spike and wave discharges.

3. *Uncertain.* In this group there is frequently, apart from the epilepsy, no clinical or EEG abnormality.

In Types (1) and (2) there is often a positive family history of epilepsy.

Symptomatic

1. *Focal brain damage.* Abscess. Tumour (primary or secondary). Infarct. Post-traumatic.

2. *Metabolic disorders:*
Anoxia, e.g. Stokes Adams attacks. These are transient episodes of cerebral ischaemia following asystole or severe cardiac slowing.
Hypoglycaemia.
Hypocalcaemia.
Drug withdrawal, e.g. barbiturates or alcohol.
Endogenous toxins – uraemia.
Exogenous poisoning, e.g. lead.

3. *Other:*
Encephalitis.
Meningitis – acute and chronic.
Febrile convulsions in children.
Porphyria.

Symptoms and Signs

From the clinical point of view attacks can be divided into the following categories:
1. Major seizures (Grand mal).
2. Petit mal.
3. Minor seizures, in which a large variety of epileptic manifestations occur.

Major Seizures (Grand Mal). The classical grand mal attack involves sudden loss of consciousness. During the early phase there is generalised rigidity of the body (tonic phase) and this is rapidly followed by a clonic phase in which there is generalised jerking. Attacks may be preceded by a momentary aura (warning phase). The attacks are frequently accompanied by profuse sweating, incontinence, and tongue biting. The attack itself is followed by a phase of flaccid unconsciousness which may last for anything from five minutes to several hours.

Petit Mal. This usually starts in childhood, but may continue into adult life. An attack of petit mal is generally momentary, the child suddenly breaking off from a conversation and staring into space for a few seconds before resuming as if nothing had happened. In some instances there is involuntary myoclonic jerking of the whole body, and other children fall to the ground without warning (akinetic attacks).

Minor Seizures. This group is not usually accompanied by full loss of consciousness. However, in some instances a minor seizure may be immediately followed by a grand mal epileptic fit.
1. A rhythmical jerking of one arm or leg which may spread to the other limb and to the face on the same side of the body. This type of attack occurs when the epileptic discharge involves the 'motor area' of the brain on the opposite side.
2. Tingling or other sensory disturbance may start on one side of the body and spread to involve the rest of that side.
3. Temporal lobe epilepsy. A large number of symptoms may be experienced including:
Hallucinations of taste and smell.
Abnormal and irritational emotional experiences – fear and hate.
Irrational and uncontrollable thoughts.
Déjà vu – a feeling of intense familiarity.
Feelings of unreality and depersonalisation.

The diagnosis of epilepsy depends on an accurate assessment of the clinical picture. It is essential to obtain an eye-witnessed account of any attacks if possible. Remember, unconscious people cannot tell you what was happening when they were unconscious!

The occurrence of focal fits (for example unilateral limb jerking) indicates a discharging focus in one particular area of the brain and usually merits full investigation.

Investigations

1. EEG. This is an extremely useful investigation in the assessment of epilepsy. It cannot be emphasised too strongly, however, that the clinical diagnosis of epilepsy depends on the clinical picture and not on the electroencephalogram. Normal EEGs may be found in people who have clearly had epileptic attacks and, conversely, an abnormal EEG may be found in non-epileptics. The following characteristic patterns are found.

(a) *Idiopathic centrocephalic epilepsy.* Bursts of high amplitude activity, sometimes lasting for several seconds are recorded over both sides of the brain. In some instances this activity can be produced by flashing a bright light at the patient at a frequency of 25 cycles/sec. This latter pattern is seen particularly in children who have fits when watching television.

(b) *Petit mal.* A highly characteristic pattern of 3 per second spike and wave discharges is seen symmetrically over both sides of the brain.

(c) *Focal discharges.* For instance, in brain abscess, a focus of abnormally slow waves may be seen overlying the abnormal area.

If the EEG shows either of the first two patterns mentioned above, then further investigations, directed toward the 'cause' are not likely to be helpful. On the other hand, the presence of a focal abnormality is a clear indication for further investigation.
2. Chest X-ray (secondary carcinoma may present with epilepsy).
3. Brain scan.
4. Full blood count, WR, serum calcium fasting blood sugar, and urine test for porphyrins, in appropriate cases.
5. Lumbar puncture – this is not indicated as a routine.

6. Carotid angiography $\left.\begin{array}{l} \\ \end{array}\right\}$ in appropriate cases, –
7. Air encephalography $\qquad$ particularly if a CT scan is not available

Differential Diagnosis

1. Other Causes of Unconsciousness:

Fainting attacks. These usually occur when the patient is standing or sitting. There is frequently a warning phase in which the patient feels sick and sweats. It must be remembered that occasionally fainting attacks are accompanied by minor epileptic phenomena such as transient jerking or stiffness.

Hysterical attacks. These are usually highly bizarre and frequently occur when other people are present.

Hypoglycaemia. Epileptic fits with or without periods of prolonged unconsciousness may occur. Sweating is usual, and there may be a clear relationship to meals.

Head injury.
Accidental gassing, poisoning, etc.

2. Other causes of focal disturbance of brain function without full loss of consciousness:

Transient ischaemic attacks (*see* section on 'Cerebrovascular disease').

Focal migraine. There is usually a past history of migraine and headache is usual.

A vast number of conditions can be confused with epilepsy. These include day-dreaming and falling asleep in appropriate places (for example when driving a car!)

Basis of Treatment

Patience and time are essential. The patient should be told that anyone can have an epileptic attack given the appropriate stimulus. It is most important that he should be made to understand that epileptics are not 'a race apart'.

The patient should be told, that with the help of drugs, epilepsy can usually be brought under excellent control. It is usually necessary to explore the background situation for there is no doubt that stress of various sorts can precipitate epilepsy and make control difficult. The more secure and stable the background the easier is proper control likely to be.

Driving. The question of driving will need to be positively discussed with the patient. In the United Kingdom an established epileptic must have been free from epileptic attacks whilst awake for three years before he can be granted a driving licence.

Employment. Certain occupations are unsuitable for epileptics. For example, those whose work involves driving or working at heights will probably have to change their employment. This is a very serious matter and urgent consideration must be given to the question of retraining and the finding of alternative employment.

Genetics. Idiopathic epilepsy does tend to run in families, although the exact mode of inheritance is not usually obvious. The patient will frequently wish to discuss the risk of epilepsy developing in his/her children.

The following advice should be given to patients:
1. An accurate record must be kept of the exact number of attacks that have occurred.

2. It is important to lead a reasonably well-ordered life with sufficient sleep and regular meals.
3. Drugs should never be stopped suddenly because of the danger of precipitating status epilepticus.

Medication. Certain simple rules can be enumerated for the physician:
1. The safest drug should be used first.
2. Drugs should be used to the limit of tolerance. They should not be changed until the full dose has been tried.
3. It is essential to know the side effects of the drugs being used and the patient should be warned about these (for example, phenobarbitone produces drowsiness).
4. The introduction and stopping of drugs should be undertaken *slowly*, usually over a period of days. Similarly, any change from one drug to another should be undertaken slowly. Failure to do this can produce intolerable side effects and/or increase in the frequency of the epileptic attacks.
5. Drugs should always be labelled. In addition, the patient should always have a card in his pocket listing the drugs he is taking.

Anticonvulsant drugs appear to have a threshold concentration below which they are ineffective. Considerable individual variation occurs in the rate of metabolism of drugs. It should be noted that measurement of circulating levels of individual anticonvulsants can be of great help in deciding dosage. Most anticonvulsants need only be given twice daily. This increases patient adherence (many people find it almost impossible to remember the midday dose). Folic acid and vitamin D deficiency may occur after prolonged use of some of the anticonvulsants, probably because of their hepatic microsomal enzyme inducing properties.

Grand mal attacks. The following drugs are used (in order of preference):
(a) Phenytoin. Many patients can be controlled on phenytoin alone. The commonest problem is failure of the patient to take his drugs, or inadequate dosage. The starting dose is 100 mg twice daily. Most patients are controlled on 300 mg daily, but occasionally it is necessary to use 400 mg daily. The effective plasma concentration is 40 to 80 μmol/l. If the dose is increased beyond this the patient is likely to become drowsy and to develop nystagmus, dysarthria, and ataxia. Other long term side effects include gum hypertrophy, acne, and hirsutism.
(b) Phenobarbitone. Starting dose is 30 mg twice daily increasing to 60 mg three times a day if necessary. The main side effect is drowsiness. The therapeutic plasma concentration is 40 to 120 μmol/l.
(c) Primidone (Mysoline). Some patients develop extreme drowsiness with only a small dose. For this reason a 125 mg test dose should be given initially. Thereafter the starting dose is 125 mg twice daily

increasing to 250 mg three times per day. The therapeutic plasma concentration is 40 to 90 μmol/l. It should be noted that this drug is partially broken down to phenobarbitone and should not be used in combination with that drug.

(d) Sodium valproate (Epilin): The starting dose is 200 mg twice daily. The maximum dose is 2.5 g daily. Most patients are controlled on doses of 1 to 1.6 g daily. The drug is relatively free from side effects. Drowsiness may occur.

(e) Carbamazepine (Tegretol): The initial starting dose is 100 mg twice daily. The maximum dose is 600 to 800 mg daily.

Petit mal attacks

(a) Ethosuximide. The initial dose is 250 mg daily. The dose is slowly increased up to a maximum of 1.5 g daily. The side effects include skin rashes, gastrointestinal disturbance and drowsiness.

(b) Sodium valproate (*see above*). Some workers now consider that this is the drug of choice for petit mal epilepsy.

(c) Troxidone. This drug is now rarely used. Dose 0.3 to 1.8 g daily. Side effects include marrow depression, nephrotic syndrome and exfoliative dermatitis.

Note: All doses given are for adults. Proportionately less is needed for children.

Prognosis

This is highly variable. In most cases excellent control can be achieved by the use of drugs, but in most instances treatment will need to be continued for a period of many years. Permanent brain damage is particularly liable to occur following status epilepticus.

STATUS EPILEPTICUS

Definition

A condition in which recurrent major epileptic attacks occur without recovery of full consciousness between attacks. The condition is dangerous and carries a high risk of death during the acute stage, from brain swelling and pneumonia. Permanent brain damage may result, particularly in children.

Basis of Treatment

It is essential to maintain an adequate airway and proper oxygenation. Hyperthermia, dehydration and electrolyte imbalance may all need to be treated. Remember also that it is important to elicit the underlying cause (for example status epilepticus may be caused by meningitis in infancy).

Drugs:

1. Diazepam. This is usually considered to be the initial drug of choice. Initially an intravenous injection of 10 mg should be given over five minutes (to adults). If the fits recur, then a constant infusion should be set up of 100 to 200 mg every twenty-four hours.

2. Paraldehyde. This is particularly useful for the emergency treatment of status epilepticus where the patient is seen in his own home. A dose of 5 to 10 ml is given initially and repeated every fifteen minutes if necessary. The drug should be given by deep intramuscular injection using widely separate injection sites (to avoid abscess formation). A glass syringe must be used.

Intravenous phenytoin or chlormethiazole can be used. If the above measures do not help then it may be necessary to curarise the patient and to provide assisted ventilation via an endotracheal tube.

HEADACHE AND OTHER PAIN SYNDROMES

The term headache is used to cover any condition in which there is pain or aching in the head. It may well be asked: Why does the head ache? The brain itself is not sensitive to pain. Much pain of intracranial origin is due to stretching of the arteries and veins. Because of their vascular origin these forms of intracranial headache are made worse by sudden movements and by straining.

Headache is one of the commonest symptoms in medicine. Acute headache, such as that due to subarachnoid haemorrhage or acute meningitis, rarely presents a diagnostic problem. Raised intracranial pressure (*see* page 536) and chronic meningitis may, however, present a considerable problem. The vast majority of chronic headaches have a benign cause, and a physician's first task is to separate the serious from the banal. Many people with headaches think that they have a cerebral tumour. The first step, therefore, is always to take the patient's complaints seriously and to give him a good hearing and a careful physical examination. Only when serious disease has, as far as possible, been excluded should the psychological aspects of the problem be explored.

Hypertension, sinusitis, and eye strain are among the three common diagnoses made when a patient presents with chronic headache. It is, however, likely that none of these conditions is an important cause of chronic headache.

MIGRAINE

Definition

A clinical syndrome, frequently familial, whose main features include episodic headache, vomiting, visual disturbance, and other transient abnormalities of neurological function.

Background

It is unfortunately true that no generally accepted definition of migraine exists. The pathological basis (*see below*) is not known for certain so that the definition must rely upon the clinical picture. The most important feature is that it is an *episodic* disturbance.

Incidence. 5 to 10 per cent of the population.

Inheritance. The exact mode of inheritance is not clear, but a positive family history is usual.

Mechanism. It seems likely that the pain of migraine arises from perivascular nerve endings in the meningeal and extracranial arteries. Two divergent vasomotor responses occur – constriction and dilatation. Neurological symptoms and signs (for example tingling in the limbs) may be due to transient focal ischaemia. Headache, on the other hand, is thought to be due to vascular dilatation. The cause of these abnormal vascular responses is uncertain, but may be related either to the altered body levels of circulating constrictor and dilator agents or to increased vascular reactivity to normal levels of vasoactive agents.

Among the *vasoactive agents* investigated is serotonin, but the importance of this substance in the genesis of migraine is still uncertain. However, on the basis of a hypothesis implicating it, a number of serotonin antagonists have been tried therapeutically (*see later*) with success in some patients.

Hormonal influence. The importance of such an influence is clear for the following reasons:
Attacks commonly start at puberty.
Attacks in women are often closely related to the periods.
The contraceptive pill sometimes increases the severity of migraine.

In some patients, migraine can be precipitated by the intake of high tyramine-containing foods such as chocolate and cheese.

Symptoms and Signs

Considerable variation in the pattern occurs from patient to patient. Overall, the picture is that of an episodic abnormality with complete normality between attacks. Common varieties include:
1. Transient disturbance of visual or neurological function, usually lasting for fifteen to twenty minutes, followed by headache and sometimes vomiting. This is the classical type.
2. Headache only.
3. Visual or neurological symptoms only, without headache.
4. Occasionally, the neurological features may start *after* the onset of headache.

Neurological Symptoms:
Visual symptoms: flashing lights (teicopsia); visual field defects; photophobia; blindness.
Tingling in the face.
Tingling or weakness in the limbs of one side of the body.
Headache. The severity of the headache varies considerably. It may be so bad that the patient cannot continue with his or her normal activities and must lie down in a darkened room. In other instances the patient is able to continue his activities, albeit with difficulty. Vomiting may occur at this stage. The headaches are frequently unilateral, but may be bilateral. The headaches may last for anything from between an hour and several days.

Variants of the Migraine Syndrome

1. **Hemiplegic Migraine.** Repeated attacks of unilateral paralysis may accompany migraine. This condition is frequently familial. Carotid angiography is usually necessary to exclude a vascular malformation.

2. **Ophthalmoplegic Migraine.** Paralysis of the eye muscles with diplopia occurs. The IIIrd nerve is most frequently affected. Occasionally, the syndrome is due to an aneurysm and, for this reason, angiography is usually indicated.

3. **Basilar Migraine.** The neurological symptoms occur mainly in the vertebro-basilar territory: vertigo, diplopia, facial tingling, etc.

4. **Migrainous Neuralgia** (*see* page 524).

5. **Status Migranosus.** Migrainous symptoms may occur continuously for days or weeks.

Investigations

In the vast majority of cases no investigations are indicated.

Differential Diagnosis

1. **Other Causes of Transient Disturbance or Neurological Function:**
(a) Sensory epilepsy.
(b) Transient ischaemic attacks.

2. **Other Causes of Headache:**
(a) Raised intracranial pressure. There are usually other features, including, papilloedema (*see* 'Raised intracranial pressure' page 536).
(b) Tension headache.
(c) Depression.

Arteriovenous malformations can produce a migraine-like headache. In this situation focal neurological symptoms and signs are usual and a bruit may be heard over the skull.

Basis of Treatment

General Management and Prophylaxis. Always remember that migraine is an unpredictable disorder frequently showing remissions which are not necessarily related to therapy.

Reassure the patient that no serious disease is present. Explain the nature of migraine as far as this is known. Ascertain whether there are any aggravating factors, such as:

(a) Depression and anxiety. Migraine may be precipitated by financial, family or other worries.

(b) The contraceptive pill. Migraine can be initiated and made worse in women on 'The Pill'. A change to a different brand, or sometimes stopping the agent entirely, may be necessary.

(c) Dietary factors. If attacks are precipitated by particular foods, such as chocolate and cheese, the diet should be modified accordingly.

(d) Premenstrual oedema. If there is fluid retention during the premenstrual phase a diuretic can be given.

Drugs Used to Reduce the Frequency and Severity of Attacks:

1. General sedatives and tranquillisers may be indicated if there is a lot of anxiety. Diazepam and prochlorperazine are appropriate.

2. Methysergide (Deseril) can be used, but is reserved for the intractable cases. The dose range is between 2 and 6 mg/day. Common side effects include nausea and weight increase. An occasional side effect is retroperitoneal fibrosis, and for this reason Deseril is not given for more than six months at a time.

3. Clonidine: dose 25 to 50 μg daily.

4. Sanomigran (pizotifen). Initial dose 0.5 mg daily; final dose 2 to 3 mg daily.

Treatment of the Acute Attack. A simple analgesic such as aspirin or paracetamol should be used first. Ergotamine preparations are useful in many patients, but it is essential to give a sufficiently large dose. Ergotamine should not be used in patients with vascular disease (for example, angina or intermittent claudication). Vomiting is an important side effect of ergotamine in some patients. The following are the main ways by which ergotamine may be given:

Orally. Ergotamine tartrate tablets, 1 mg; two to three tablets can be given at the beginning of an attack and the patient may take up to four at any one time. 'Cafergot' (caffeine 100 mg, plus ergotamine tartrate 1 mg); two to three can be taken at a time.

Rectally. 'Cafergot' suppositories. These are particularly useful in patients who vomit during the attack.

Inhalation. Via a medihaler.

Injection. A few patients learn to give themselves a subcutaneous, or intramuscular, injection of ergotamine tartrate, 0.25 to 0.5 mg.

CRANIAL ARTERITIS

Definition

A disorder in which there is inflammation of the extracranial arteries with the production of headache. A raised ESR, or plasma viscosity, is usual and the condition responds dramatically to steroid therapy.

Background

The condition affects older people; it is rarely seen under the age of 60.

Symptoms

Severe pains in the head.
Pain on chewing (if the facial arteries are involved).
Feeling ill.
Weight loss.
Anorexia.

Signs

Tenderness of extra-cranial arteries, particularly the superficial temporal, occipital, and facial arteries.

Complications

Blindness – due to involvement of the retinal arteries. Other evidence of occlusive vascular disease, including hemiplegia, myocardial infarction, etc.

Investigations

1. Blood count – frequently a normochromic anaemia.
2. ESR and plasma viscosity invariably raised (frequently above 100).
3. Biopsy of a scalp artery – evidence of active inflammation with giant cells.

Basis of Treatment

Because of the risk of blindness this condition is a medical emergency. Treatment must be started straight away even if the biopsy cannot be undertaken immediately. Prednisone 15 mg four times daily would be an appropriate starting dose.

Prognosis

The condition responds dramatically to steroids and within twenty-four hours the pain has usually disappeared completely. Treatment with steroids will usually need to be continued for one to two years. The dose of steroids should be reduced as quickly as possible (the exact dose should be determined by the level of the ESR which usually returns to normal within two weeks of starting treatment).

Cranial arteritis is a self-limiting disorder and at the end of one to two years it is usually possible to stop steroids completely without any recurrence of symptoms.

COUGH HEADACHE

This is a severe paroxysmal generalised headache precipitated by coughing. It is usually of benign cause.

TENSION HEADACHE

This, together with migraine, forms by far the largest proportion of chronic headaches. It is usually generalised, often continues for hours at a time, and is frequently accompanied by stabs of pain. Sometimes there are tender areas on the scalp, the pain being due mainly to chronic over-contraction of the scalp muscles. The diagnosis is usually reasonably easy. Reassurance, elimination of stress if possible, and treatment with a tranquilliser such as diazepam is usually helpful.

HEADACHE ASSOCIATED WITH DEPRESSION

The depressed patient often presents to the physician with headache. Characteristically, he wakes early in the morning with headache and will also frequently admit to morbid thoughts at this time.

FACIAL PAIN

Facial pain is another common symptom. The pain may arise in a number of different structures including the nasal sinuses, ears, and teeth.

Facial pain is a common symptom in patients who are anxious and depressed. Some specific forms of facial pain are mentioned below, but it must be noted that many cases do not fall neatly into any easily identifiable category.

TRIGEMINAL NEURALGIA (TIC DOULOUREUX)

Definition

A condition of unknown cause characterised by very severe stabbing pain in the face.

Background

In most instances the disorder affects older people and is of unknown cause. No constant pathological changes have been found.

Occasionally, the condition is 'symptomatic' especially in:
(a) Multiple sclerosis – with a plaque in the pons.
(b) Posterior fossa tumours.

Symptoms

There are sharp stabs of very severe pain that are often brought on by touching or even moving the face and also by standing in a cold wind. Sometimes the pain involves the inside of the mouth. There are frequently particular areas which, if touched, will produce the pain – 'trigger areas'.
The pain may affect one or more divisions of the Vth nerve but does not extend outside this area.
There may be a dull prolonged background ache but this is not usually severe.
The symptoms are often associated with severe depression.
Usually there are no signs.

Basis of Treatment

When treating trigeminal neuralgia two points should be borne in mind –
1. Trigeminal neuralgia is a phasic disorder and quite frequently significant periods of remission occur between attacks.
2. Depression is common and should be treated. The alleviation of loneliness and reassurance that there is no serious disease present can often be very helpful.

The simplest measures should be used first. Most cases respond to carbamazepine (Tegretol).
(a) Carbamazepine (Tegretol). This is usually given in an initial dose of 100 mg three times daily. The dose can rapidly be doubled. In most cases no other treatment is indicated. Allergic reactions including rashes and polyarthritis occasionally occur. Marrow depression may also occur.
(b) Blocking procedures and, if necessary surgical section of the peripheral parts of the affected nerve.
(c) Alcohol injection into the Gasserian ganglion, often very successful.
(d) Surgical section of the sensory root of the Vth nerve in the posterior fossa.
(e) Medullary tractotomy.

Some of the surgical procedures involve producing corneal anaesthesia. If this occurs, great care must be taken to protect the anaesthetic cornea against injury.

Addictive pain-killing drugs should be avoided as far as possible.

GLOSSOPHARYNGEAL NEURALGIA

This is an episodic severe stabbing pain which is felt mainly in the back of the throat, neck, and in the ear. It is often precipitated by swallowing. Apart from its distribution it has many of the characteristics of trigeminal neuralgia and responds to the same forms of treatment.

MIGRAINOUS NEURALGIA

Definition. A clinical syndrome of unknown cause characterised by severe paroxysmal pain in the eye and face.

Symptoms

Characteristically, the patient is awakened in the night with very severe pain in one eye. Associated features include reddening of the eye and blockage of the ipsilateral nostril. Attacks usually last for from three-quarters to two hours.

The attacks of pain occur in 'clusters', recurring nightly (or less commonly daily) for several weeks. The 'clusters' may occur at intervals of months or years and in the meanwhile the patient is free of symptoms.

Basis of Treatment

When the attacks occur at night prophylactic oral ergotamine, 1 or 2 mg should be given on going to bed. This will usually prevent attacks. Ergotamine should only be given for the duration of the 'cluster'. Methysergide may be used prophylactically.

COSTEN'S SYNDROME

This involves a severe shooting pain, felt in front of the ear with radiation to other parts of the face. It is usually precipitated by chewing. The exact mechanism is uncertain, but benefit can sometimes be obtained by altering the 'bite'.

POSTHERPETIC NEURALGIA

Definition

Segmental pain occurring at the site of previous *Herpes zoster* infection.

Symptoms and Signs

Clinically there are two main features:
1. Hyperaesthesia – increased sensitivity of the involved skin.
2. A deep dull continuous burning pain.

This condition is especially troublesome in the elderly; depression and loneliness are frequent important contributory factors.

Basis of Treatment

This can be an intractable condition and medical treatment is often disappointing. It is important to try to deal with background factors such as depression. Simple analgesics and injections of local anaesthetic may be helpful. Massage and vibration of the affected area may be used if the skin is markedly hypersensitive.

Prognosis

The condition usually shows some spontaneous improvement, but this may take several years.

CEREBROVASCULAR DISEASE

Cerebrovascular disease is the third commonest cause of death in the Western world. It is also the commonest cause of severe chronic disability in the community. The subject is therefore one of the most important in medicine.

The term 'stroke' usually denotes the rapid onset of some form of neurological deficit, most frequently a hemiplegia. It is the time course of the event that stamps it as being of vascular origin. The deficit may appear in a matter of seconds in some instances, although in others it develops over a period of hours or even days. When the development is very prolonged it may be difficult or impossible, on clinical grounds, to distinguish ischaemic brain disease from a tumour. About five per cent of people who present with a 'stroke' are ultimately found to have a tumour.

There is no completely satisfactory way of classifying strokes. Ideally the clinician will want to know:
1. The nature of the pathological process (haemorrhage or infarction).
2. The stage of development reached (whether the event is complete or whether it is still evolving).
3. The site of the lesion (for example cerebral hemisphere or brain stem).

The Nature of the Pathological Process

The principal pathological results of acute cerebrovascular disease are infarction of the brain and intracranial haemorrhage. Both processes frequently produce significant brain swelling with resultant brain stem compression. Infarction usually results from narrowing or occlusion of a major artery. Intracranial haemorrhage results from vascular rupture.

Atheroma is characteristically most severe in the basilar and vertebral arteries and in the arteries of the circle of Willis. In recent years there has been recognition of the frequency with which atheroma occurs in the extracranial arteries. Atheromatous change in an artery may produce three major abnormalities:

Stenosis. This must be gross before there is significant fall in cerebral blood flow.

Embolisation. Quite large thrombi may be produced at the site of atheromatous plaques. The thrombi may be dislodged and shot upwards into the cranium with resultant blockage of a major artery. Small platelet emboli are responsible for many transient disturbances of cerebral function.

Total Occlusion. This is usually due to thrombosis in an area of pre-existing atheroma.

It will quickly be realised that in any given case several different pathological processes may be found occurring together.

The Stage of Development Reached

It is obviously very important to know whether or not the stroke is still evolving. From this viewpoint we can recognise three types of stroke:

Transient Ischaemic Attacks (*see below*)

The Evolving Stroke. The neurological deficit may appear to fluctuate in severity or to be gradually progressing. This is a particularly important situation as there is the theoretical possibility of preventing development of a completed stroke.

The Completed Stroke. In this situation the neurological deficit appears to be static. A proportion of these patients are unconscious and in these cases both head injury and post-epileptic states come into the differential diagnosis.

The Site of the Lesion

The majority of strokes occur in the territory of the internal carotid artery and produce a hemiplegia. Brain stem strokes manifest themselves in a variety of ways – producing loss of consciousness in some patients, disturbed eye movements, dysphagia and weakness of all four limbs.

HYPERTENSION AND CEREBROVASCULAR DISEASE

In recent years it has been recognised that hypertension is extremely important in the genesis of cerebrovascular disease. This, and diabetes, are important causes of premature vascular degeneration. A stroke is the commonest cause of death in hypertensive subjects and all the principal forms of cerebrovascular disease, with the exception of embolic infarction, occur with increased frequency in hypertensive subjects. Intracerebral haemorrhage is the classical neurological manifestation of hypertension but ischaemic infarction also occurs with increased frequency, as does subarachnoid haemorrhage. Hypertensive encephalopathy is a very serious condition occurring in patients with malignant hypertension and is associated with severe headache, vomiting and convulsions.

Hypertension affects both large and small cerebral arteries. In both groups it encourages the formation of atheroma. The media of the small arteries is particularly affected. Hypertrophy of muscle fibres occurs early and at a later stage there is degeneration of the muscular and elastic elements, increase in connective tissue, and fibrinoid necrosis.

Two factors are of particular importance:

1. **Micro-aneurysms.** These are small aneurysms, up to 900 μ in diameter, which are found on the small lateral branches of the striate arteries in the region of the basal ganglia and internal capsule. It is rupture of these aneurysms that is responsible for most cases of primary intracerebral bleeding.

2. **Lacunes.** These are small cystic areas measuring up to 15 mm in diameter (usually less) and having a similar distribution to that of the micro-aneurysms mentioned above. Lacunes are thought to be produced by small areas of infarction. Clinically, they produce very localised lesions (for example, pure motor hemiplegia). Repeated lacune formation may produce a diffuse disturbance of cerebral function (for example dementia, pseudo-bulbar palsy, etc.).

In the normal person cerebral perfusion is maintained at a steady level and is not dependent on fluctuations in blood pressure. The relation between pressure and flow can be expressed thus:

$$\text{Cerebral blood flow} = \frac{\text{Blood pressure}}{\text{Cerebrovascular resistance}}$$

This system ensures that in healthy people cerebral perfusion is maintained over a wide range of mean arterial blood pressure. After an acute cerebrovascular accident this central control mechanism is disturbed and it is usually thought inadvisable to treat hypertension during the initial three weeks after an acute cerebrovascular catastrophe.

Two general points need to be made in relation to the treatment of the hypertensive subject. Firstly, adequate control of hypertension is important. Available evidence indicates that control of blood pressure produces a reduction in the likelihood of further strokes occurring both in symptomless patients and in patients who have already shown evidence of hypertensive vascular disease. Secondly, anticoagulants should be avoided in stroke patients who are hypertensive (because of the risk of bleeding from micro-aneurysms).

PREVENTION OF STROKES

As already mentioned hypertension should usually be treated. Transient ischaemic attacks are always a warning of impending stroke and should be dealt with appropriately (*see below*). There is some evidence that prophylactic aspirin or anticoagulants may be of use in selected groups of patients (*see below*). Lastly, the contraceptive pill is associated with an increased risk of cerebral thromboembolism. 'The Pill' should be avoided in all patients with a history of possible cerebrovascular disturbance and should symptoms occur, 'The Pill' should be stopped immediately.

Cerebrovascular disease will be dealt with under the following headings:
1. Intracranial haemorrhage:
(a) Primary intracerebral haemorrhage.
(b) Primary subarachnoid haemorrhage.
2. Cerebral infarction:
(a) Embolic.
(b) Non-embolic.
3. Recurrent cerebral ischaemia (transient ischaemic attacks).

SPONTANEOUS (NON-TRAUMATIC) INTRACRANIAL HAEMORRHAGE

There are two main types of non-traumatic intracranial haemorrhage – intracerebral haemorrhage and sub-arachnoid haemorrhage. It must be emphasised that there is considerable overlap between these two conditions. Thus, in a substantial proportion of cases with a primary subarachnoid haemorrhage there is destruction of brain tissue. Similarly, blood from a primary intracerebral haematoma may leak out into the sub-arachnoid space. Nevertheless, the two conditions are sufficiently distinct from pathological clinical, prognostic and therapeutic viewpoints that we shall consider them separately.

PRIMARY INTRACEREBRAL HAEMORRHAGE

Definition

Non-traumatic haemorrhage into the substance of the brain.

Background and Pathology

There is a strong association of primary intracerebral haemorrhage with systemic arterial hypertension. Small micro-aneurysms are found on the intracerebral arteries. These rupture, allowing blood at arterial pressure to be pumped into the substance of the brain. The principal sites of rupture are the internal and external capsules, the parietal white matter, and the centrum ovale. Occasionally, rupture occurs into the cerebellum or pons. About 90 per cent of fatal cases have blood in the CSF. Occasionally, a cerebral aneurysm will rupture into the brain, producing an intracerebral haematoma, without blood in the CSF.

Symptoms and Signs

The onset is usually abrupt. The clinical findings vary according to the size and site of the haemorrhage.

Symptoms
Weakness of arm and leg.
Headache.
Gradual loss of consciousness.

Signs
Unconsciousness.
Hemiplegia.
Neck Stiffness.
Hypertension.
Hypertensive changes in the fundi.
Left ventricular hypertrophy.

Brain Stem Haemorrhage
Deep coma.
Hyperthermia.
Inability to swallow.
Quadriparesis.
Eye signs. Any or all of the following may be produced:
(a) Very small pupils.
(b) No oculocephalic reflex (eyes do not move with head rotation).
(c) No oculovestibular reflex (no eye movements when the external auditory meatus is perfused with ice-cold water).
(d) Skew deviation of the eyes.
(e) Ocular bobbing (intermittent downward deflexion of the eyeballs).

Investigations
1. CT scan. A fresh blood clot usually shows up as a high density white area (see Fig. 21.9).
2. Lumbar puncture. The cerebrospinal fluid is blood-stained in 80 to 90 per cent of cases.
3. ECG. May show evidence of left ventricular hypertrophy.
4. Carotid angiography. Carotid angiography remains the most important investigation where a CT scan is not available. Persistent deep coma is not an indication for angiography after an abrupt cerebral episode with subarachnoid bleeding – surgical treatment at this stage being unrewarding. The angiogram would be expected to show the size and location of the clot. It should also show any underlying aneurysm or arteriovenous malformation.

Differential Diagnosis
The diagnosis presents no problem in a classical case.

Ischaemic Infarction. Factors favouring haemorrhage include severe headache and vomiting at the onset, rapid loss of consciousness, neck stiffness, and pre-existing hypertension.

Hypertensive Encephalopathy. This is very rare. It occurs occasionally in toxaemia of pregnancy, phaeo-chromocytoma, and in patients who are on monoamine

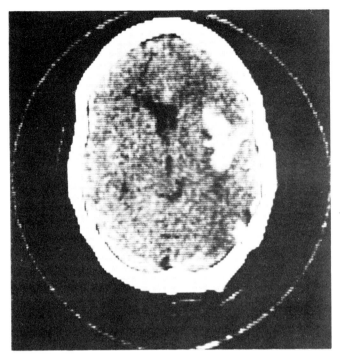

Fig. 21.9 Haemorrhage in the right Sylvian fissure produced by rupture of an aneurysm on the middle cerebral artery.

oxidase inhibitors who unwisely ingest tyramine containing foods (for example cheese) or incompatible drugs. The clinical picture usually develops over about twenty-four hours and if untreated progresses to coma and convulsions.

Head Injury. This may present a problem if the patient presents in an unconscious state and no history is available. Evidence of external injury and absence of dense focal neurological signs favour the diagnosis of head injury.

Other Causes of Unconsciousness (*see* page 514)

Basis of Treatment

The patient will frequently be in coma, and the routine medical and nursing measures appropriate in such cases must be instituted immediately. Hypotensive treatment is not indicated unless there is definitive evidence of malignant hypertension.

Surgery has nothing to offer the unselected case of cerebral haemorrhage, but occasional cases do benefit from removal of a localised accessible clot. Surgery may be indicated if the haemorrhage is localised to one temporal lobe, or occurs in the superficial part of one cerebral hemisphere, or in the cerebellum. Surgery is not indicated if the central part of the brain has been destroyed.

Prognosis

The overall mortality in cerebral haemorrhage is probably about 60 per cent. The vast majority of those who are deeply unconscious during the first twenty-four hours will die. However the mortality for small localised haematomas may be as little as twenty per cent.

SUBARACHNOID HAEMORRHAGE

Definition

Spontaneous bleeding into the subarachnoid space, usually with the production of severe headache and meningism.

Background and Pathology

Subarachnoid haemorrhage occurs most commonly in people between the ages of 40 and 60. The main causes of subarachnoid haemorrhage are:

1. **Rupture of a Saccular Aneurysm** (berry aneurysm). Seventy per cent of cases are due to rupture of saccular aneurysms. These aneurysms are probably due to a congenital defect in the media of the artery. The saccules are usually located at the bifurcation of a major artery, and rupture occurs at the dome of the aneurysm. Aneurysms are usually situated on one of the major arteries of the circle of Willis, usually on the anterior part. Aneurysms are multiple in approximately fifteen per cent of cases.

2. **Rupture of an Angioma.** These are developmental anomalies of cerebral blood vessels and are responsible for about ten per cent of cases of subarachnoid haemorrhage.

Other uncommon causes of subarachnoid haemorrhage include:

(a) Rupture of an aneurysm associated with subacute bacterial endocarditis or polyarteritis nodosa.
(b) Cerebral tumour.
(c) Bleeding diseases, for example haemophilia and thrombocytopenia.

Spinal subarachnoid haemorrhage is usually due either to a vascular malformation or to an intrathecal neoplasm.

A ruptured aneurysm may produce its effects in a number of ways:

1. The aneurysm may rupture into the subarachnoid space.
2. The aneurysm may rupture into the brain.
3. The aneurysm may rupture into the subarachnoid space *and* into the brain.

4. A haematoma may be formed. This is usually intracerebral, but is occasionally subdural. A clot in the ventricles will interfere with the free flow of cerebrospinal fluid and hydrocephalus may result.
5. Spasm of arteries. This is very important and may be extremely severe. Infarction of the brain may occur as a result of spasm.
6. A marked increase in intracranial pressure may occur with resultant brain stem compression.

Symptoms

The usual mode of onset is the very sudden development of severe headache, sometimes accompanied by feeling that something has snapped inside the head.
Unconsciousness – about 50 per cent.
Vomiting.
Epilepsy – about 10 per cent.
Severe lumbosacral pain (particularly in cases of spinal subarachnoid haemorrhage).

Signs

Neck stiffness. Kernig sign positive.
Papilloedema – about 15 per cent.
Sub-hyaloid haemorrhage (a large haemorrhage usually situated near the optic disc).
Focal signs in the limbs – about 20 per cent have a hemiplegia.
Skull bruit (this usually indicates an arteriovenous malformation).
Cranial nerve palsy (especially IIIrd and VIth).
Transient glycosuria.

Investigations

1. Lumbar puncture. If done within a few hours this will usually show a uniformly blood-stained CSF (take care not to confuse this with a 'bloody tap'). Blood disappears from the CSF in one to fourteen days. Xanthochromia (yellow colour) of the CSF is due to haemolysis and usually appears about 24 hours after the haemorrhage and lasts for two to three weeks. If the LP is undertaken two to three weeks after the haemorrhage a moderate number of lymphocytes may be found.
2. CT scan. A blood clot is frequently found localised to the area of bleeding. Thus a middle cerebral artery aneurysm may produce a clot in the region of the Sylvian fissure (see Fig. 21.9).
3. Carotid angiography. If a CT scan is not available then a carotid angiogram must be done if the source of the bleeding is to be identified. It is usually necessary to undertake bilateral carotid angiography in case there is more than one aneurysm. Carotid angiography fails to show an abnormality in about 20 per cent of cases. This may indicate either that the aneurysm has clotted or that it lies in the vertebro-basilar arterial territory.

Differential Diagnosis

1. Other causes of severe headache including migraine.
2. Other causes of a stiff neck including meningitis, cervical spondylosis, and neck injuries.
3. Other causes of coma. The patient with a subarachnoid haemorrhage may present to the doctor in coma. If there is glycosuria, diabetic coma may be simulated.
4. Other causes of sciatic-type pain.

Basis of Treatment

The patient should be nursed in bed. If headache is severe, appropriate analgesics must be given. Surgery may be undertaken in selected cases. The object of operation is to prevent a recurrence of the bleeding. Surgery is best undertaken one to three weeks after the haemorrhage and usually involves clipping the neck of the aneurysm. The best results are obtained with middle cerebral and posterior communicating artery aneurysms. Ligation of the internal carotid artery in the neck has been undertaken in some cases, but there is a substantial risk of producing a hemiplegia. Surgery is usually undertaken using controlled hypotension and hypothermia. There has been an increase in the success rate of aneurysm surgery following the use of the operating microscope.

In recent years there have been a number of studies with drugs designed to prevent clot lysis. It is thought that this is responsible for re-bleeding of aneurysms. The risk of re-bleeding is at its maximum around the end of the first week after the primary bleed. There is some evidence that EACA (epsilon aminocaproic acid) is effective in a dose of 4 g four-hourly. There is no definite evidence that hypotensive drugs are effective.

Prognosis

Approximately one-third of cases will die of the first haemorrhage, often within a few hours of the catastrophe. Between one-quarter and one-third will die during the next eight weeks and most of these die within three weeks of the first haemorrhage. Approximately one-third of the total survive eight weeks and only a small proportion of these have a further haemorrhage (approximately 20 per cent). A proportion of the survivors are disabled with epilepsy, residual neurological deficit including a hemiplegia, and anxiety symptoms. About one-half of the one-year survivors get back to full-time work. A poor prognosis is likely in the older age group, if there is severe persistent hypertension, and if there is prolonged unconsciousness.

CEREBRAL INFARCTION

Ischaemic cerebral infarction occurs when the blood supply to part of the brain is cut off or seriously diminished. Whether or not infarction actually occurs depends, in part at least, on the adequacy of the collateral circulation. The infarcted area frequently swells and brain stem compression may occur as a result of this. The principal vascular causes of infarction are embolic or thrombotic occlusion of a major artery and severe arterial hypotension.

EMBOLIC INFARCTION

Definition

Occlusion of a major cerebral artery by an embolus, with resultant infarction of part of the brain.

Background

About five per cent of strokes are clinically diagnosed as being due to embolisation, but at the autopsy the incidence may be as much as forty per cent. This disparity reflects the clinical difficulty in making a precise pathological diagnosis in life.

Emboli usually arise either from the origin of the internal carotid artery or from the heart.

The cardiac causes include:

1. **Arrhythmias.** Mitral stenosis with atrial fibrillation is associated with a high risk of arterial embolisation. Recent work on prolonged cardiac monitoring of active mobile patients has shown that episodes of dysrhythmia are more frequent than had previously been suspected. It seems probable that these give rise to emboli.

2. **Myocardial Infarction.** Complicated by arterial embolisation in up to 20 per cent of cases.

3. **A Miscellaneous Group.** Including, subacute bacterial endocarditis, atrial myxoma, cardiomyopathy, and following cardiac surgery.

The embolus is particularly liable to impact where a main artery divides. Common sites of impaction include the bifurcation of the common carotid artery, the carotid siphon, and the first major division of the middle cerebral artery. Occasionally, the vertebral artery is blocked. The embolus frequently fragments and at angiography the artery may appear to be patent because the embolus has dispersed. If the main artery remains occluded stagnation thrombosis will occur distal to the site of the occlusion. Later, organisation and occasionally recanalisation occurs. Infarcts are frequently multifocal and haemorrhagic.

Symptoms

The abrupt onset of a neurological deficit – usually with the preservation of consciousness.

Signs

(The neurological signs are determined by the location of the embolus).
Hemiplegia – usually.
Atrial fibrillation, mitral stenosis, or a bruit in the neck (usually representing stenosis of the internal carotid artery) provide some indication of the source of the embolus. Absent arterial pulses. Absent carotid and superficial temporal pulses indicate a blockage of the carotid artery proximally. Absence of leg pulses may indicate multiple arterial emboli.

Investigations

1. Carotid angiography. This is indicated particularly if the patient is seen early – with the possibility of surgical intervention.
2. CT scan (Fig. 21.10). This may be of use in determining whether or not a cerebral infarction has actually occurred.

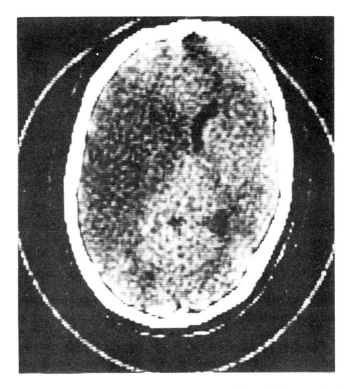

Fig. 21.10 Extensive infarction in the left middle cerebral artery territory with obliteration of the left lateral ventricle.

3. Lumbar puncture. The CSF is usually normal during the early stages. An increase in the white cell count may occur if there is infarction of brain tissue. A lumbar puncture is mandatory, in order to exclude bleeding, if anticoagulant therapy is contemplated.

Differential Diagnosis

The main differential diagnosis is non-embolic infarction. Factors favouring embolic infarction include the very rapid onset of symptoms, the rapid recovery from a severe deficit, evidence of a source for embolism, and evidence of systemic (non-cerebral) embolism.

Basis of Treatment

If there is reasonable certainty that the lesion is embolic then therapy with anticoagulants must be considered. There are two theories about this. One favours immediate anticoagulation in order to prevent further embolisation. The other view is that anticoagulants should be delayed for about three weeks in order to avoid the risk of precipitating haemorrhage into the infarct. The risk seems to be small, and for this reason immediate anticoagulation is advised provided that the CSF does not contain blood. Initially a heparin drip should be set up – followed by oral warfarin. Cerebrovasodilators have been used (for instance, inhalation of carbon dioxide), but have proved disappointing in practice.

It is technically possible to remove emboli from large and medium sized arteries. However, this procedure is dangerous if infarction has actually occurred as restoration of flow may well aggravate the damage. If the patient makes a reasonable recovery then surgery should be considered, particularly if there is evidence of stenosis of the internal carotid artery. Endarterectomy may then be undertaken with the objective of preventing a further stroke.

Prognosis

The immediate mortality is probably about ten per cent. There is, however, a considerable risk of further embolisation, but this risk can be reduced by the use of anticoagulants. Many patients make a good functional recovery, but others are left with severe permanent paralysis.

NON-EMBOLIC INFARCTION

Definition

Ischaemic infarction of the brain from causes other than embolisation.

Background

This group of cases was, in the older literature referred to as cerebral thrombosis. We intend to use the term non-embolic infarction. In using this term we recognise that the clinico-pathological correlation is not good and that some cases will be due to embolism.

A variety of pathological processes may occur in the same patient. These include severe narrowing of a major extra or intra-cranial artery and thrombosis. Thrombosis and stenosis may be associated with embolisation. Infarction may also be precipitated by hypotension associated with gastrointestinal haemorrhage or myocardial infarction. In many of these latter cases, severe cerebrovascular occlusive disease is also present – the hypotension being the 'last straw'.

There are also non-vascular 'causes of infarction', including severe hypoxia and metabolic disorders such as hypoglycaemic and metabolic acidosis. Certain areas of the brain are particularly vulnerable to hypoxia – particularly the 'watershed' areas (where two arterial territories abut).

The infarcted area of brain will frequently swell and thus act as a space-occupying mass. Such a sequence of events is frequently associated with drowsiness and unconsciousness.

Symptoms and Signs

These depend on the size and situation of the infarct. A large infarct may produce deep unconsciousness and a dense hemiplegia. A small infarct may produce only weakness of one limb.

Symptoms
Typically there is the gradual development of weakness of one arm and leg.
Alternatively, the patient may awake in the morning with a hemiplegia.
A headache is frequent.

Signs
Drowsiness and sometimes unconsciousness.
Dysphasia.
Hemiplegia.

Investigations

1. CT scan. During the first few hours no abnormality may be seen but after this the infarct usually shows up as a low u (black) area. Fig. 21.10 shows an infarct in the distribution of the middle cerebral artery.
2. Carotid angiography. Indicated for selected cases only.
3. Lumbar puncture. There is no indication for this unless anticoagulants are being considered (blood in the CSF strongly contraindicates anticoagulant therapy).

Other routine investigations which should be done in all cases include blood sugar, WR, plasma viscosity (occasional cases are due to diffuse arteritis), and chest X-ray.

Differential Diagnosis

Cerebral Haemorrhage. Most cases of cerebral haemorrhage have blood in the CSF.

530

Embolic Infarction. Factors favouring this include an abrupt onset and obvious source for embolism.

Cerebral Tumour (or other space-occupying lesions). In most cases there is a history of progressive neurological disturbance.

Subdural Haematoma. Usually there is evidence of progressing raised intracranial pressure frequently associated with drowsiness and mental confusion. A dense hemiplegia can occur, but is uncommon.

Basis of Treatment

Priority in the early stages must be given to life-saving measures. These include:
1. Maintenance of an airway.
2. Ensuring hydration and electrolyte balance.
3. Prevention of inhalation pneumonia (patients with dysphagia should not be given anything by mouth).
4. Regular turning of the patient to avoid bed sores.
5. The bladder should be catheterised if necessary.

Certain agents have been used in attempts to reduce the amount of brain swelling. Steroids, glycerol, and low molecular weight dextran have all been tried, without any positive benefit occurring. Anticoagulants have no place in the routine management of non-embolic cerebral infarctions. There is no place for surgery in the routine management of these patients. In occasional cases, however, endarterectomy may be undertaken if there is stenosis of the internal carotid artery in the neck with an uncompleted stroke.

Prognosis

About twenty per cent of patients die in the acute phase. Severe drowsiness or unconsciousness are poor prognostic signs. Indeed eighty per cent of people who are unconscious during the first twenty-four hours die. Recovery after brain stem infarction can be surprisingly good. The annual risk of having a further stroke is about ten per cent, but many people die as a result of a mycocardial infarction.

TRANSIENT ISCHAEMIC ATTACKS

Definition

A transient ischaemic attack is a focal disturbance of the cerebral circulation, frequently repetitive, resulting in a period of impaired function lasting for a short period (anything from a few minutes to twenty-four hours). Attacks can occur in the carotid and/or vertebral artery territories.

Background

The importance of transient ischaemic attacks is that they are often the forerunner of a permanent stroke. As many as 30 per cent of major strokes are preceded by a transient ischaemic attack during the preceding month. Approximately 33 per cent of patients with transient ischaemic attacks will develop a major stroke within the next five years.

It used to be thought that arterial spasm was responsible for these transient disturbances of cerebral function, but this is not now thought to be so. The commoner causes include:

1. **Embolism.** The best known example is that of platelet emboli which arise from a friable thrombus, frequently from an atheromatous plaque at the origin of the internal carotid artery in the neck. Minute fragments of thrombus composed of fibrin and platelets are dislodged and shot into the cranium. Transient ischaemic attacks are frequently highly stereotyped in their manifestations and it is thought that this is partly due to streaming of blood in the cerebral arteries, particles tending to travel in one particular layer of the blood.

2. **Compression of Extracranial Arteries.** The vertebral artery may become kinked by lateral protrusions of intervertebral discs and osteophytes.

3. **Arterial Stenosis.** Uncomplicated arterial stenosis is thought to be an uncommon cause of cerebral ischaemia. A stenosis has to be almost complete before there is a significant reduction in flow.

4. **Stealing and Re-distribution of Blood.** Reversal of blood flow in the vertebral artery can occur when there is a localised proximal occlusion, or severe narrowing, of a subclavian artery. Under these circumstances blood may pass to the arm via the vertebral artery, with resultant symptoms of brain stem ischaemia. Similarly, stealing can occur with an arteriovenous malformation within the cranium.

5. **Abnormalities of Blood Constituents.** Transient ischaemic attacks occasionally occur in polycythaemia, leukaemia, and dysproteinaemic states in which there are changes in blood viscosity.

6. **Systemic Hypotension.** Severe systemic hypotension usually results in unconsciousness due to generalised cerebral ischaemia. Occasionally, however, an abrupt change in cardiac output (due, for example, to a transient cardiac arrhythmia) can lead to focal disturbance of cerebral function. This is particularly likely to occur if there is an associated stenosis of one of the cerebral arteries.

Symptoms and Signs

The transient disturbances of cerebral function are usually of abrupt onset and last for a few minutes at a time. Some people have a single attack, others have several in a day. Most attacks are unprovoked and unpredictable. The symptoms vary according to the arterial territory maximally affected.

TRANSIENT CAROTID ISCHAEMIC ATTACKS

Symptoms

Dysphasia (if the left cerebral hemisphere is affected).
Weakness of the contralateral arm and/or leg.
Paraesthesia or numbness in the contralateral limbs.
Transient loss of vision in the eye contralateral to the hemiparesis (amaurosis fugax).

Signs

Usually there are no focal signs if the patient is examined between attacks.
If the patient is examined during an attack, the signs will match the symptoms – for example dysphasia, flaccid weakness of the limbs on one side of the body, etc.
Emboli in the retinal arteries may occasionally be seen with the opthalmoscope.
Bruit over the carotid artery.

TRANSIENT VERTEBRAL ISCHAEMIC ATTACKS

Symptoms

Vertigo (60 per cent).
Visual disturbance (50 per cent). The abrupt onset of dimness of vision and blurring – sometimes generalised and sometimes affecting only half of the visual field.
Ataxia on walking.
Diplopia.
Slurring dysarthria.
Headache – frequent.
Short periods of mental confusion.

Signs

There will usually be no signs between attacks.
If the patient is seen in an attack – the signs will match the symptoms.

Investigations

The first step is to exclude such disorders as polycythaemia, severe anaemia, valvular heart disease, severe hypertension, postural hypotension, and attacks due to vertebral artery narrowing – associated with neck movement.

1. Carotid arteriography. This should only be undertaken if carotid stenosis is thought likely and if the patient is thought fit for later surgery. Severe hypertension is usually a contraindication to arteriography. The needle must be inserted well below the bifurcation of the common carotid artery.
2. Arch aortography. This is an alternative to carotid arteriography. The main advantage is that the proximal parts of all four main arteries feeding the brain can be visualised.

Differential Diagnosis

1. **Focal Epilepsy.** There is often repetitive jerking of the affected limbs. The EEG is sometimes abnormal (usually normal in transient ischaemic attacks).

2. **Migraine.** This is a difficult differential diagnosis. Migraine can be regarded as being a particular type of transient ischaemic attack. Attacks usually occur in a person who has a history of previous migraine. Headache is usually, but not always, present.

3. **Hypoglycaemia.** Focal neurological disturbance can occasionally occur in diabetic patients who become hypoglycaemic.

4. **Other Causes of Vertigo.** Acute labyrinthitis and Meniere's disease can be simulated.
Note: It is always dangerous to diagnose transient ischaemic attacks in patients whose *only* symptom is that of vertigo.

Basis of Treatment

The main objective of treatment is to prevent the development of a completed stroke. An important secondary objective is to stop the transient ischaemic attacks themselves. Mortality appears to be little affected by either medical or surgical treatment.

1. **Surgery.** This usually involves disobliteration of the internal carotid artery in the neck with removal of friable thrombus (carotid endarterectomy).

2. **Anticoagulants.** There is reasonable evidence that anticoagulants reduce the incidence of completed stroke during the few years after the onset of transient ischaemic attacks.

3. **Aspirin.** The initial event in arterial thrombosis is adhesion of platelets to a region of damage in the blood vessel wall. *In vitro*, aspirin and other agents inhibit platelet aggregation. There is now considerable evidence that aspirin in a dosage of 300 mg four times daily is effective in reducing both the incidence of transient ischaemic attacks and the likelihood of a completed

stroke. It is not yet clear whether the use of anticoagulants or aspirin is more effective. Anticoagulants are contraindicated if the patient is hypertensive.

Prognosis

The overall annual risk of ischaemic infarction occurring in patients with transient ischaemic attacks is approximately seven per cent per year for the first five years. More than fifty per cent of the deaths occurring within the next few years are due to heart disease.

THE ANATOMY OF STROKES (Figs. 21.11, 21.12)

CAROTID ARTERY SYSTEM

Internal Carotid Artery (Fig. 21.11)

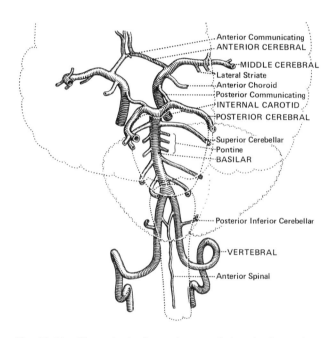

Fig. 21.11 The principal arteries supplying the brain (as seen from behind).

The internal carotid artery supplies most of the anterior portion of the brain via its main branches – the middle and anterior cerebral arteries.

The internal carotid artery is particularly liable to be obstructed in the neck, frequently just beyond the bifurcation of the common carotid artery. The common causes are:
1. Atheromatous narrowing.
2. Trauma to the neck.
3. Local inflammation, sometimes from infected tonsils in children.

The internal carotid artery may also be obstructed in the carotid syphon, usually due to atheroma.

Results of Narrowing or Occlusion of the Internal Carotid Artery:
1. There may be none if the collateral supply, from the other side, is good.
2. Transient ischaemic attacks (see page 532).
3. Dense hemiplegia (with dysphasia if the dominate hemisphere is affected).

Middle Cerebral Artery

The middle cerebral artery supplies much of the cerebral cortex (Fig. 21.12). It also supplies the posterior limb of the internal capsule and much of the basal ganglia via the striate arteries.

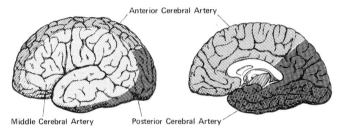

Fig. 21.12 Distribution of the three main cerebral arteries.

Results of Occlusion. A contralateral hemiplegia is likely to occur, sometimes with relative sparing of the leg. Dysphasia is likely if the dominant hemisphere is affected.

Anterior Cerebral Artery

The anterior cerebral artery supplies the medial part of the cerebral hemispheres (see Fig. 20.6). When the main trunk of the artery is occluded there is a contralateral hemiplegia, the leg frequently being more affected than the arm.

THE VERTEBRO-BASILAR SYSTEM

A large number of different syndromes arise from disease in the vertebro-basilar territory. Some anatomical knowledge is necessary in order to understand these and some simple diagrams of transverse sections taken through different levels of the brain stem are included (see Figs. 21.13, 21.14, 21.15, 21.16).

A lesion of one half of the mid-brain may produce a contralateral hemiplegia and an ipsilateral IIIrd nerve paralysis (Weber's syndrome). Paralysis of upward gaze may also occur.

A lesion affecting one side of the pons at this level will be likely to produce paralysis and loss of proprioceptive sensation of the arm and leg on the opposite side of the body. There may be ataxia of the limbs on the same side. In addition, there will probably be paralysis of lateral

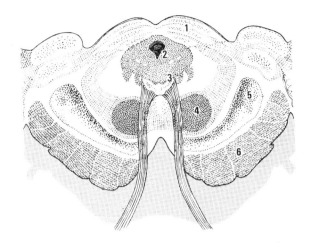

Fig. 21.13   Upper mid-brain.
1. Superior quadrigeminal body.
2. Aqueduct.
3. IIIrd nerve nucleus.
4. Red nucleus.
5. Substantia nigra.
6. Cortico-spinal fibres.

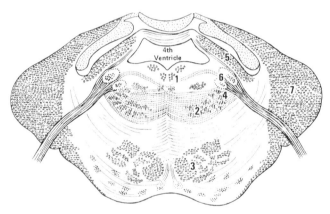

Fig. 21.14   Mid-pons.
1. Medial longitudinal bundle.
2. Medial leminiscus.
3. Cortico-spinal tract.
4. Lateral leminiscus.
5. Superior cerebellar peduncle.
6. Motor and sensory trigeminal nuclei.
7. Middle cerebellar peduncle.

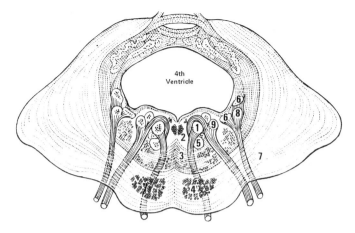

Fig. 21.15   Lower pons.
1. VIth nerve nucleus.
2. Medial longitudinal bundle.
3. Medial leminiscus.
4. Cortico-spinal tract.
5. VIIth nerve nucleus.
6. Vestibular nuclei.
7. Middle cerebellar peduncle.
8. Cochlear nuclei.
9. Tractus solitarius.

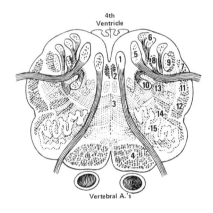

Fig. 21.16   Mid-medulla.
1. Hypoglossal nucleus.
2. Medial longitudinal bundle.
3. Medial leminiscus.
4. Pyramid.
5. Dorsal nucleus of the vagus.
6. Inferior vestibular nucleus.
7. Inferior cerebellar peduncle.
8. Tractus solitarius.
9. Descending nucleus and tract of trigeminal nerve.
10. Nucleus ambiguus.
11, 12. Dorsal and ventral spino-cerebellar tract.
13. Sympathetic fibres.
14. Spino-thalamic tract.
15. Inferior olive.

gaze (inability to turn the eyes laterally). In most instances, however, *both* sides of the pons are involved, with the production of extensive signs in the limbs and, sometimes, coma.

A lesion affecting one side of the lower pons will probably produce paralysis and loss of proprioceptive sensation of the opposite arm and leg together with ataxia of the limbs on the same side. There may also be an ipsilateral VIth and VIIth nerve palsy, nystagmus, and paralysis of lateral gaze.

The medulla contains many important structures. The resultant clinical picture tends therefore to be rather complicated. The following unilateral syndromes occur:

Medullary Syndromes

1. **Lateral Medullary Syndrome.** Many of the structures in the lateral part of the medulla are involved (5 to 14 on Fig. 21.16). Clinical features include some, or all, of the following:
Severe protracted vertigo and vomiting, nystagmus, dysphagia, hoarseness, and disturbance of taste.
Ipsilateral – depression of pain and temperature sensation on the face, palatal and vocal cord paralysis, Horner's syndrome, and ataxia of the limbs.
Contralateral – impairment of pain and temperature sensation over the arm and leg.

2. **Medial Medullary Syndrome** (involvement of structures 1 to 4 on Fig. 21.16).
Disordered eye movements.
Ipsilateral – paralysis and atrophy of the tongue.
Contralateral – hemiplegia with depression of light touch and postural sensation.
3. **Total Unilateral Medullary Syndrome.** There is a combination of lateral and medial syndromes.

Brain Stem Syndromes

Brain stem syndromes (Table 21.11) are frequently characterised by two features:

1. The presence of *bilateral* motor and sensory signs.
2. The presence of crossed syndromes with cranial nerve palsy on one side of the body and long tract signs on the other.

REHABILITATION OF THE STROKE PATIENT

The incidence of stroke in the Western World is approximately 2 per 1,000 per year. In England and Wales (population approximately 48.5 million) there are probably between 100,000 and 120,000 new 'strokes' each year. Approximately forty per cent will die within the first month. About 30,000 to 35,000 will be left with a significant neurological deficit which usually includes a hemiplegia. About seventy-five per cent of strokes occur in persons aged 65 or more.

What are the chances of recovery after a stroke? Between 60 and seventy per cent of those who survive the first four weeks will ultimately learn to walk again – with or without a stick or tripod. However, only ten to fifteen per cent regain normal arm function. About seventy per cent will regain independence in self-care. Adverse factors associated with an unfavourable functional prognosis include persistent mental confusion, defective comprehension, apathy, depression and lack of motivation. There is argument as to whether left or right cerebral hemisphere lesions carry a better prognosis. Left hemisphere lesions are frequently accompanied by a serious defect of speech. Right-sided cerebral lesions, on the other hand, are often associated with severe disturbance of a body image. Brain stem vascular lesions appear to carry a better outlook for functional recovery than cerebral lesions.

A number of general principles govern the management of disabled stroke patients:

1. **Assessment.** Every patient requires to be assessed. Assessment involves finding out as much about the patient as possible so that realistic objectives can be defined. Listed below are six major factors which need to be considered in each case.

2. **The Setting of Realistic Goals for Each Patient.** In this connection it is important to consider what the patient was like *before* the stroke. Remember that the patient is unlikely to be better after the stroke than he

Table 21.11 Brain stem arteries and their syndromes

Artery	Result of occlusion
Vertebral artery. The vertebral arteries supply most of the medulla and the inferior part of the cerebellum Frequently one artery is much larger than the other	May be 'silent' Lateral, medial or unilateral medullary syndromes may be produced (Fig. 21.16)
Posterior inferior cerebellar artery. Supplies the inferior part of the lateral medulla	May cause the lateral medullary syndrome (this syndrome is more usually caused by occlusion of the vertebral artery)
Basilar artery. This supplies the pons, upper part of the cerebellum and some of the mid-brain	Symptoms of arterial insufficiency include vertigo, ataxia, diplopia, and dysarthria. Occlusion produces a large number of different manifestations including paralysis or weakness of the limbs and bulbar musculature, diplopia, disordered eye movements nystagmus, and impaired vision Coma may occur
Posterior cerebral artery. This supplies the under surface of the temporal and occipital lobes together with the medial surface of the occipital lobe (including the visual area). It also supplies part of the thalamus, sub-thalamic area and part of the mid-brain	Contralateral homonomous hemianopia – complete or incomplete. Less common features include severe 'thalamic pain' and involuntary movements

was before it! For younger patients the goal may be return to work (about ten per cent of those who were working before the stroke will work afterwards). In older patients the objectives may be more limited – perhaps simply independence in self-care and the ability to go to 'the local'.

3. **The Planning and Implementation of a Properly Organised Treatment Programme.** This involves more than simply giving the patient a few minutes of physiotherapy and occupational therapy each day!

4. **Adequate Provision for Long Term Follow-up.** Many patients will be left with important residual disabilities and have to be helped to make a reasonable life for themselves.

5. **Integration and Maximum Co-operation Between the Various Personnel and Agencies.** This can be difficult to achieve. In hospital alone there may be as many as ten to fifteen different skill groups involved. The concept of the rehabilitation team which includes members of most of these groups has been evolved to deal with this problem.

6. **Adequate Recognition of the Psychological Impact of the Stroke on the Patient and His Family.** It is all too easy to forget what a devastating effect a stroke has on both the patient and his family. A variety of reactions experienced include shock, disbelief, anger, and depression.

7. **Avoidance of Complications.** Important complications include severe depression, painful stiff shoulder, contractures, peripheral nerve palsies and fractures of long bones (usually the femur). Many of these complications are avoidable.

The first person to be called when the patient has a stroke is usually the General Practitioner or his deputy. His first decision is whether or not to get the patient into hospital. Some patients are already in a moribund condition and are probably best left at home. Others have had a transient episode and are well on the way to recovery. In this group also hospital admission may not be considered urgent. For the remainder the desirability of hospital admission must be decided on the basis of diagnostic, therapeutic, nursing and social considerations. At the moment it appears that about forty per cent of stroke patients are admitted to hospital within the first week. The practical problems involved during this early stage include difficulty with transferring the patient from a chair to the commode, continence, dysphagia, and pressure sores. There is also the problem of how inexperienced people are to cope with their own, and the patient's, stress reactions. This problem is likely to be particularly difficult if the patient is dysphasic and/or confused.

During the three weeks following a stroke the medical situation is liable to change quite rapidly. Complications such as inhalation pneumonia and pulmonary embolism are common. After three weeks the situation is usually reasonably static and it is clear whether or not the patient is going to survive. The rehabilitation phase can be arbitrarily viewed as starting at this point.

At the end of the third week (sometimes earlier and sometimes later) assessment can usually be undertaken. Objectives need to be defined at this point. The first objective is usually independence in self-care activities. Most hemiplegic patients can be transferred from the bed to a chair and vice versa with the help of one person by about the sixth week after the stroke has occurred. It is at this point that hospital patients tend to be discharged home.

At the end of about four months it is usually considered that about eighty to ninety per cent of recovery has occurred and active therapy usually stops. For the disabled survivor this is the moment of truth. He now tends to feel rejected and let down by the medical and rehabilitation staff, particularly if he is still severely disabled. Depression is extremely common at this time. Recent studies of stroke survivors indicate a vast amount of residual frustration and unhappiness. The reasons include loss of the ability to lead a fulfilling life, loss of mobility, loss of self-respect, and loss of sexuality (in younger patients). It is this group of patients who require help with developing social and recreational activities.

RAISED INTRACRANIAL PRESSURE (Figs. 21.17, 21.18)

The skull is rigid, and any rise in intracranial pressure will tend to force the brain downwards through the tentorium and the foramen magnum. Herniation of the medial portion of the temporal lobe occurs through the opening in the tentorium, and the mid-brain becomes crushed against the opposite free edge of the tentorium. Similarly, the cerebellar tonsils are forced downwards

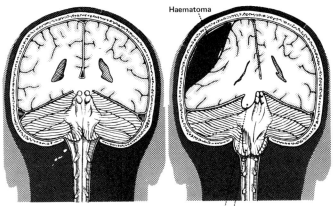

Fig. 21.17 Mid-brain and medullary compression resulting from an intracranial haematoma. Left: normal. Right: abnormal.

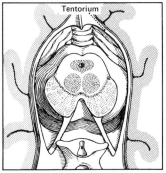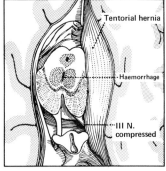

Fig. 21.18 Transverse section through mid-brain (from above), showing compression by a tentorial hernia. Left: normal. Right: abnormal.

between the free edge of the foramen magnum and the medulla. Medullary compression results. In both instances the vital brain stem centres concerned with consciousness, respiration, and circulation become damaged.

Some Important Causes of Raised Intracranial Tension

Acute (rapid onset of headache, vomiting and drowsiness):
1. Extradural haematoma – practically always a history of head injury and the skull X-ray usually shows a fracture of the vault.
2. Cerebral infarction with secondary resultant brain swelling.
3. Cerebral thrombophlebitis, for example due to thrombosis of the sagittal sinus.
4. Some forms of acute encephalitis, particularly due to *Herpes simplex*.

Sub-acute or Chronic:
1. Brain abscess.
2. Cerebral tumour.
3. Subdural haematoma.

4. Meningitis.
5. Hydrocephalus. Both communicating and non-communicating hydrocephalus may occur and may be due to a large number of different conditions, including obstruction to the exit foramina in the IVth ventricle (for example by tumour or meningitis) or to stenosis of the aqueduct.

Symptoms and Signs

Headache:
(a) The recent development of headache, or a change in the type of pattern of long-standing headache, should make one suspect raised intracranial tension.
(b) The headache is frequently, but not always, occipital in distribution. It is frequently present on waking in the morning and may actually wake the patient.
(c) The headache is sometimes accompanied by vomiting which may be effortless and not preceded by nausea.
Drowsiness. Always watch the state of consciousness when raised intracranial pressure is suspected. Coma may ultimately develop.
Slow pulse.
Slow and irregular breathing. If the raised intracranial tension is unrelieved then the patient may eventually stop breathing altogether.
Papilloedema. Raised intracranial pressure is one of the most important causes of this.
Note: However, gross rises in intracranial pressure *can occur* without papilloedema.
False localising signs. The distortion of brain stem structures due to raised intracranial pressure can produce certain signs which have no value whatsoever in localising the basic pathology. These include:
(a) Unilateral or bilateral VIth nerve palsy. This palsy is due to stretching of the VIth nerve.
(b) Unilateral IIIrd nerve palsy. This may be only partial; e.g. dilated or fixed pupil on one side (Fig. 21.18).
(c) Signs of unilateral or bilateral cortico-spinal tract involvement.

A large number of false localising signs can occur and, indeed, one should regard with suspicion any symptoms or sign that occurs at a stage at which there is a severe rise in intracranial pressure.

Investigations (*see* 'Intracranial tumours')

Differential Diagnosis

1. Other causes of papilloedema, including malignant hypertension and severe chronic emphysema.
2. Other causes of headache.

Basis of Treatment

Raised intracranial pressure always requires investigation. A lumbar puncture should almost never be undertaken and may have disastrous consequences. A differential pressure gradient can be produced between the increased intracranial pressure and the artificially lowered pressure in the spinal canal. The result is that the brain stem compression is increased, the brain being forced even further donwards, and the patient may die.

When the patient is drowsy and vomiting, neurological or neurosurgical advice should be obtained as a matter of the greatest possible urgency. Some lowering of intracranial pressure can be achieved for a short while by the use of:

(a) Intravenous frusemide – 120 mg.
(b) Intravenous mannitol – 500 ml of 20 per cent solution is usually given. It should be remembered that the patient may stop breathing, and for this reason some means of artificial ventilation must be readily available.

The neurosurgeon will usually make a burr hole in the skull and insert a cannula into one of the lateral ventricles, removing some CSF (which is usually under greatly increased pressure). When the intracranial pressure has been lowered diagnostic investigations, such as carotid arteriography, can be undertaken.

In some patients with chronic hydrocephalus, *permanent* ventricular drainage is necessary in order to keep the intracranial pressure within normal limits. A polythene tube is used, one end being inserted into one of the lateral ventricles, the other into the jugular vein or right atrium.

INTRACRANIAL TUMOURS

There is a very wide spectrum of intracranial tumour. This spectrum extends from the slowly growing benign compressive meningioma, on the one hand, to the highly malignant intrinsic invasive glioblastoma multiforme, on the other. Likewise, the prognosis varies from complete cure on the one hand to death within a few weeks on the other.

Background

The clinical picture produced by a brain tumour depends on a number of different factors–
1. The type of tumour, whether or not it is malignant, and the speed with which it grows. Tumours that grow slowly, such as meningiomas, can become very large indeed before producing symptoms. On the other hand, rapidly growing tumours tend to produce symptoms early. In some vascular tumours haemorrhage may occur.
2. Local infiltration, compression, and destruction of brain.
3. Oedema. Certain brain tumours, for instance secondary carcinoma deposits, generate a great deal of surrounding brain swelling.
4. Obstruction to CSF pathways. A tumour in the posterior fossa will tend to obstruct the aqueduct and the IVth ventricle, thus preventing the exit of CSF from the ventricular system. This will produce an internal hydrocephalus.
5. Site. A tumour involving the motor cortex may produce paralysis of the opposite arm and leg.
6. Raised intracranial pressure. A rise in intracranial pressure will be produced as a result of the space-occupying mass, and following obstruction to CSF pathways. Secondary brain stem compression will ultimately occur.

The commonest brain tumours, in order of decreasing frequency, are:

Gliomas. 60 per cent. These are intrinsic tumours which originate in the glia. The degree of malignancy varies enormously, some tumours being highly malignant and others growing very slowly.

Metastatic Tumours. 20 per cent. These arise particularly from carcinoma of the lung and breast.

Table 21.12 Intracranial tumours

Site	Clinical features
Frontal lobe	Dementia. Disinhibited behaviour. Contralateral grasp reflex
Fronto-parietal region	Contralateral hemiparesis. Dysphasia, if the dominant hemisphere is affected.
Occipital	Contralateral homonymous hemianopia.
In and around the pituitary fossa (e.g. pituitary adenomas and craniopharyngiomas)	All these tumours tend to compress the optic chiasm. A bitemporal hemianopia may be produced due to interruption of the decussating fibres of the optic nerve. Endocrine symptoms may occur and include features of panhypopituitarism and diabetes insipidus, Acromegaly may result from certain pituitary adenomas (*see* page 162)
Cerebello-pontine angle (e.g. acoustic neuroma – tumours arising from the sheath of the VIIIth nerve)	Disturbance of function in the Vth, VIth, VIIth and VIIIth cranial nerves Common features include deafness, facial palsy, and depression of the corneal reflex

Meningioma. 10 per cent. These tumours originate in the meninges and compress the brain. They are usually benign.

Acoustic Neuroma.

Pituitary Adenoma.

In children and young adults, tumours of the posterior fossa predominate. The commonest are medulloblastoma (highly malignant), cystic astrocytoma, and haemangioblastoma. The latter two tumours are usually benign. In adults, supratentorial tumours predominate, gliomas being the most frequent, and occurring most often in the fifth decade of life.

Symptoms and Signs

Tumours may present in a large number of different ways:
General, non-focal and non-specific symptoms:
Headache – this is enormously variable and sometimes absent.
Lack of concentration, irritability, emotional lability, depression and general slowing up.

It is in these patients with non-specific symptoms that particular care must be taken. It is important to obtain a history from someone who has known the patient for some while.
Convulsions. Approximately one-third of patients with supratentorial tumours have fits at some point. The fits may be of a focal nature.
Raised intracranial tension with the production of headache, vomiting, and papilloedema. Tumours that interfere with the free flow of CSF are particularly liable to present in this way.
Slowly progressive focal neurological signs. Many tumours present because of a localised disturbance of neurological function. The type of disturbance will depend upon the area of brain affected (Table 21.12).

Investigations

The nature and number of investigations will depend on the clinical assessment.
1. Chest X-ray. Exclude a bronchial carcinoma.
2. Skull X-ray. This may show displacement of a calcified pineal body, calcification in the tumour, and erosion of the posterior clinoid processes, indicating prolonged raised intracranial pressure.
3. EEG. The finding of a localised slow wave focus may indicate the presence of a tumour.
4. Linear brain scan. This is particularly useful in demonstrating secondary deposits, with multiple areas of increased uptake. Not all tumours show up on a brain scan.

5. CT brain scan. This is the investigation of choice. An example is shown in Fig. 21.19.
6. Carotid arteriography. This may show displacement of arteries. A 'blush' may occur in the region of the tumour, especially when this is very vascular.

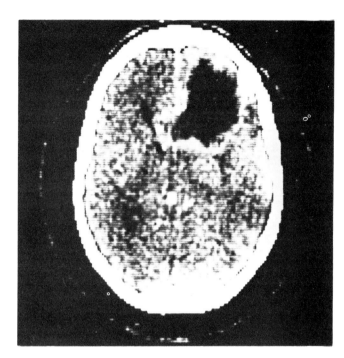

Fig. 21.19 Cystic glioma involving the right frontal region.

7. Air encephalogram. This may be required in some cases and should be done in a neurological centre.
8. Lumbar puncture. *This has no place* in the routine investigation of a patient suspected of having a cerebral tumour. The dangers of producing accelerated brain stem compression have already been mentioned.
9. Biopsy.

Differential Diagnosis

This includes other space-occupying lesions including cerebral abscess. Virtually every type of cerebral disease can mimic a brain tumour.

Basis of Treatment

Certain tumours, such as meningiomas, acoustic neuroma, and pituitary adenomas can be removed surgically. Intrinsic tumours can usually not be fully removed, but the diagnosis should be confirmed by biopsy unless a critical area of the brain is involved.

If there is evidence of raised intracranial tension a subtemporal decompression can produce a substantial and useful clinical improvement. Cystic tumours of the posterior fossa (particularly astrocytomas) can be frequently removed completely and the long term prognosis is usually good in these cases.

Radiotherapy. Certain tumours undoubtedly benefit from radiotherapy. This is a matter for expert assessment.

Steroids. In some cases, particularly where there is evidence of markedly raised intracranial tension, a dramatic improvement can be produced by the use of steroids. Dexamethasone (4 mg four times a day initially orally) will often produce a very substantial improvement in cerebral function so that a drowsy patient becomes alert and orientated. A maintenance dose of 0.5 mg twice daily is usually sufficient. The improvement may last for several weeks or even months.

Chemotherapy. A large number of antimitotic agents have been tried but on the whole the results are disappointing.

Prognosis

The prognosis in brain tumour depends on a large number of different factors. The person with a highly malignant invasive intrinsic tumour may well be dead within a matter of weeks. On the other hand, a meningioma involving the convexity of the brain can frequently be removed and a complete cure obtained.

DEMYELINATING DISEASES

This is a group of diseases characterised by demyelination in the central nervous system. By convention, demyelinating lesions of the peripheral nerves are not included. These latter are discussed in the section on 'Diseases of the peripheral nervous system'.

In the demyelinating diseases the myelin sheath is affected while the axon and nerve cell remain relatively intact. Three main groups of disease occur:
1. Multiple sclerosis.
2. Acute disseminated encephalomyelitis (*see* page 548).
3. Diffuse cerebral sclerosis (leucodystrophy). This is a group of diseases, usually presenting in childhood, in which there is progressive and massive demyelination affecting the cerebral hemispheres. A rapid deterioration of cerebral function occurs, with mental deterioration, weakness of the limbs, convulsions and blindness.

MULTIPLE SCLEROSIS

Definition

A disease of unknown cause characterised, pathologically, by areas of focal loss of myelin in the central nervous system and, clinically, by a course which is often relapsing and remitting and which extends over many years.

Background

Multiple sclerosis is slightly commoner in women than men. The first symptoms usually occur between the ages of 20 and 40 (mean age approximately 35).

There is a weak but definite genetic factor and first degree relatives are several times more liable to contract the disease than others in the population.

Multiple sclerosis shows an interesting geographical distribution. Its frequency diminishes as the Equator is approached. The disease is particularly common in Europe and North America and is uncommon in Africa and India.

The cause of multiple sclerosis is unknown, but a number of different theories have been propounded. It is currently thought that multiple sclerosis may be a disorder of virus origin, possibly a 'slow virus' infection acquired in childhood. Some patients show raised levels of measles antibodies in the blood and CSF, but the significance of this finding is not known. It is possible that multiple sclerosis represents a hypersensitivity response on the part of the central nervous system to an antigen, possibly of viral origin.

Pathology

Patchy loss of myelin is seen in the central nervous system and there appears to be a particular predilection for the optic nerves, the brain stem, the cervical spinal cord, and the periventricular white matter. Nerve cells are not primarily affected and, for this reason, muscle wasting is not seen (apart from that due to disuse), and the tendon reflexes are preserved and frequently increased. The myelin sheath of the peripheral nerves is not affected.

Table 21.13 Symptoms and signs of multiple sclerosis

Symptoms	Signs
Early:	
Diplopia	Nystagmus
Acute vertigo and vomiting	Pale optic discs
Tingling in the limbs	Ataxia of the limbs
Band-like sensations around the limbs	Increased tendon reflexes
	Absent abdominal reflexes
Sudden, or gradual, development of weakness of the legs	Extensor plantar responses
	Depressed vibratory sense in the legs
Urinary frequency or urgency	
Impotence	
Late:	
Disturbance of mood –	Tremor of the head
Euphoria or depression	(titubation)
Intellectual deterioration	Truncal ataxia
Poor vision (optic atrophy)	Ataxia of the limbs
Severe dysarthria	Paralysis of the legs with or without marked spasticity
	Total urinary incontinence

Symptoms and Signs (Table 21.13)

Classically the patient experiences acute symptoms which come on over a matter of hours or days and then clear up over a period of weeks. Recurrent attacks of neurological disturbance occur and frequently different parts of the nervous system are affected. In such patients it can truly be said that the lesions are 'disseminated in time and in anatomical location'. In other patients there is a slow progression of symptoms without obvious remission. In these cases diagnosis can be difficult. Thus, the development of a paraplegia without evidence of disturbance elsewhere in the central nervous system might also be due to a compressive lesion of the spinal cord or to some other intrinsic spinal cord disorder such as a vascular lesion or a tumour.

Optic neuritis. A considerable proportion of cases of multiple sclerosis have an episode of optic neuritis as the presenting feature. The patient notes partial or complete loss of vision which comes on over a period of hours or days. This may be accompanied by pain in the eye. Examination may show a central scotoma and, occasionally, there is some degree of swelling of the optic disc. Within two to three weeks the vision usually starts to recover and in over two-thirds it will recover completely or show substantial improvement.

Investigations

The diagnosis is made on clinical grounds, after other conditions have been excluded. However, various laboratory tests can be helpful although none can be regarded as being completely diagnostic.

1. CSF. During an acute episode there may be a lymphocytic pleocytosis, but rarely more than 100 cells/ml³. The total cell count is *usually* less than 20 cells/ml³. Between attacks the gammaglobulin fraction in the CSF may be raised. There may be a specific increase in the level of IgG.

2. Physiological tests. The most widely used procedure involves the recording of visually evoked cerebral potentials as a test of the integrity of the visual pathway. This technique involves stimulation of the retina with a checker-board pattern of black and white squares which is reversed at a frequency of about 2 cycles/second. The evoked response is recorded with scalp electrodes – using standard averaging techniques. The test is positive in about seventy per cent of cases of multiple sclerosis.

Other evoked potential studies can be of use (including auditory and somatosensory).

3. Myelogram. This may be required if the patient has a paraparesis – to exclude a compressive lesion of the spinal cord.

Differential Diagnosis

Practically all disorders affecting the central nervous system can be confused with multiple sclerosis.

Unilateral Blindness. Compressive, vascular, and toxic lesions of the optic nerve.

Paraplegia. Spinal cord compression, vascular lesions, etc.

Ataxia. Tumours and vascular lesions of the brain stem.

Three diseases, particularly, can be confused with multiple sclerosis – neuro-syphilis, subacute combined degeneration, and various collagen disorders (particularly polyarteritis nodosa).

Basis of Treatment

There is no specific treatment for multiple sclerosis. However, most clinicians agree that multiple sclerosis patients benefit from short courses of corticotrophin in the early active phase of the disease. The usual practice is to give 80 units of ACTH intramuscularly daily for two weeks. The dose is then gradually reduced over the next two weeks. There is no evidence that the long term use of ACTH is of any value in preventing relapses.

Various dietary regimes have been suggested. Many clinicians recommend that the diet should be supplemented by giving the essential fatty acid – linoleic acid. The usual practice is to give sunflower seed oil – two tablespoons daily. There is no evidence that a gluten-free diet is helpful.

The belief that there is an immunological basis to multiple sclerosis has led to trials of both immunosuppressive therapy and the administration of transfer factor. These forms of therapy are currently being evaluated.

Once the diagnosis has been made with reasonable certainty the patient should be told. At the same time some indication of prognosis should be given, together with assurance, in appropriate cases, that the prognosis is frequently not so bad as is commonly thought.

Symptomatic management of the established case is of extreme importance. Three of the main symptoms involve the following:

Bladder Function. Urgency can sometimes be diminished by the use of atropine-like drugs. Urinary infections should be treated with antibiotics. In cases of established incontinence, it will be necessary to provide some type of incontinence apparatus. Unfortunately, there is no entirely suitable apparatus available for women. In occasional cases it may be appropriate to establish an ileal bladder or to transplant the ureters into the colon.

Spasticity. No entirely suitable drug exists for the treatment of spasticity. However, Lioresal (a derivative of gamma-aminobutyric acid) does show considerable promise. The optimum dose range is 15 to 100 mg daily, most adults requiring 40 to 50 mg daily. Occasionally, the legs become hypotonic and this may result in a decrease in standing and walking ability. Diazepam (Valium) has been used for many years for the treatment of spasticity. Unfortunately, most patients are made intolerably drowsy by the dose that is required to control spasticity. Other measures include the use of intramuscular alcohol, intrathecal phenol, and surgical section of muscle, tendons or of nerve roots.

Intention Tremor. In some instances the amount of intention tremor can be in the arm and can be substantially reduced by applying lead weights to the limb – 500 to 600 g incorporated in a soft leather wrist band.

Physiotherapists and occupational therapists can be particularly helpful with retraining walking and in teaching the patient to transfer from his wheelchair on to the bed and vice versa. If the patient experiences difficulty with dressing it may be necessary to substitute zips of Velcro for buttons. Difficulty with feeding can sometimes be overcome by the provision of specially shaped plates and the use of non-slip mats.

Prognosis

The prognosis in multiple sclerosis is not as bad as is commonly thought. This is partly because morbidity and mortality statistics are frequently obtained by studying patients who have attended hospital. Patients with minor symptoms and little disability may never reach hospital. It therefore seems likely that hospital statistics provide us with an over-gloomy view of the prognosis, because of the including of a disproportionate number of patients who are severely affected.

It seems possible that some people have only one episode of demyelination. This certainly seems to be the case with retrobulbar neuritis. Some patients go on to develop widespread affection of the central nervous system, whereas others have no further episodes.

The average duration of disease in fatal cases is about twenty years. However, some patients are still ambulant twenty and more years after the onset of the disease.

INFECTIVE DISEASE OF THE CENTRAL NERVOUS SYSTEM

BACTERIAL INFECTION OF THE CENTRAL NERVOUS SYSTEM

ACUTE PYOGENIC MENINGITIS

Definition

Acute inflammation of the meninges as the result of bacterial invasion.

Background

Organisms can enter the subarachnoid space either via the bloodstream or from local disease. The commonest forms of meningitis are due to the following bacteria:

Meningococcus. Meningococcal meningitis occurs in epidemic form, particularly in overcrowded conditions. The condition is spread by droplet infection, the bacteria entering the body via the nose and pharynx. A septicaemia occurs initially and this may be followed by meningitis.

Pneumococcus. This may occur either as a complication of ear or sinus infection or associated with pneumonia.

Haemophilus influenza. This usually occurs in small children.

A large number of other organisms may also cause meningitis.

Meningitis may occur as a result of a skull fracture. For example, a fracture of the cribriform plate may produce recurrent meningitis. Spread of infection may also occur from an infected middle ear or from the nasal sinuses.

Bacterial meningitis may be associated with a thick exudate, which forms at the base of the brain and also over the convexities. This may be responsible for a communicating hydrocephalus – due to interruption of the free flow of CSF – and, also, for cranial nerve palsies.

Symptoms

Headache.
Fever.
Photophobia (dislike of the light).
Drowsiness.
Vomiting.

Signs

Early:
Rash (especially in meningococcal cases).
Fever.
Neck stiffness.
Positive Kernig's sign (resistance to straightening of the flexed knee).

Late:
May be drowsiness or stupor.
Confusion.
Fits (especially in children).

Complications

Early phase:
Cranial nerve palsies.
Epileptic fits.

Thrombosis of cerebral veins.

Cortical infarction, which may produce a hemiplegia.

Hydrocephalus, which may be communicating or non-communicating; for example when the exit foramina of the fourth ventricle become blocked.

Waterhouse–Freiderichsen syndrome – circulatory collapse, often with death, associated with haemorrhage into the adrenal glands (meningococcal cases).

Late phase:

Permanent brain damage which may follow any of the pathological processes mentioned above. A significant proportion of children with mental retardation have had meningitis.

Hydrocephalus.

Epilepsy.

Investigations

1. The diagnosis is made by undertaking urgent lumbar puncture. The CSF is usually under increased pressure and is found to be cloudy. Microscopy shows an excess of white cells (usually polymorphs), and, occasionally, organisms may be seen. The sugar level will usually be low. Identification of the organisms may need to await the results of bacterial culture.
2. Blood culture.
3. Chest X-ray.
4. Skull X-ray.

Differential Diagnosis

Viral Meningitis. The CSF is clear to the naked eye. There is a lymphocytic pleocytosis, normal sugar level, and negative bacterial culture.

Basis of Treatment

Antibiotic treatment must begin immediately the diagnosis has been made. If the CSF is turbid, 10,000 to 20,000 units of penicillin can be injected intrathecally if the patient is an adult, and proportionately less for children. *Special ampoules are usually available in the hospital pharmacy. The ordinary vials intended for intramuscular use should never be used.* Intrathecal antibiotic therapy need not be continued after the first injection provided that the organism is susceptible to an antibiotic known to penetrate the blood brain barrier.

The exact type of chemotherapy will depend upon the organisms involved and will be decided after consultation with the bacteriologist. If the organisms cannot be identified on the Gram film it will be 24 to 36 hours before a bacterial diagnosis can be made. In these instances systemic ampicillin or chloramphenicol can be used. After 36 hours the antibiotic therapy will depend on the type of organism.

Meningococcus. Benzylpenicillin 2 to 4 mega units four-hourly intravenously or intramuscularly together with sulphadimidine 4 g immediately and then 2 g six-hourly intravenously or intramuscularly (it can be given orally when vomiting has ceased). Treatment should be continued for at least ten days. Close contacts should be treated with sulphadimidine 1 g eight-hourly for three days.

Pneumococcus. Benzylpenicillin IV, 2 to 4 mega units four-hourly. Treatment must be continued for at least ten days.

H. influenzae. Chloramphenicol 75 mg/kg body weight is given IV or IM each twenty-four hours. Later the drug can be given orally.

Alternative treatment is ampicillin 200 to 400 mg/kg body weight per day.

It should be noted that some strains of *H. influenzae* are now resistant to ampicillin.

Staphylococcus aureus. Maximum treatment with benzylpenicillin, cloxacillin or other appropriate antibiotic.

Unknown infections. Give chloramphenicol or a combination of benzylpenicillin, ampicillin and cloxacillin.

Treatment must be continued for fourteen days in most cases although chloramphenicol should, if possible, be given for less than this time because of the danger of marrow depression. Serial lumbar punctures are required in all cases to ascertain the effects of the treatment.

Treatment of Complications

Cerebral oedema. This is usually responsible for the unconsciousness which occurs early in the illness. Give dexamethasone 10 mg immediately and thereafter 4 mg six-hourly.

Epileptic fits. Give phenytoin 100 mg three times daily. If frequent fits occur – intravenous diazepam is given.

Hydrocephalus. This may need to be treated with ventricular drainage.

Circulatory collapse. Intravenous steroids and fluids are given.

Prognosis

The overall mortality for all cases of pyogenic meningitis is around eight to ten per cent. The mortality is very high (around 80 per cent) in newborn infants. The prognosis is best in cases of meningococcal meningitis but is less good in pneumococcal and coliform infections.

Meningitis in children is particularly likely to be followed by permanent neurological damage as shown by epilepsy, deafness, and mental retardation. Serious morbidity is very much less common in adults.

Definition

Meningitis due to infection by the tubercle bacillus.

Background

This disorder is always secondary to tuberculosis elsewhere in the body and can complicate any form of the disease. It is most commonly seen as a complication of primary infection. Tuberculous meningitis can occur at any age. Coloured immigrants appear to be particularly at risk.

Infection usually reaches the central nervous system via the bloodstream although occasionally direct spread occurs from tuberculous osteomyelitis in a vertebra. It is probable that minute tuberculomata form in the central nervous system and that these eventually rupture into the subarachnoid space.

Pathology

Tuberculous meningitis is frequently associated with the formation of a very thick exudate at the base of the brain. Strangulation of cranial nerves may occur. CSF pathways may become blocked with resultant hydrocephalus and/or spinal block. Obliterative arteritis of both small and large arteries may produce infarction of brain tissue.

Table 21.14 Symptoms and signs of tuberculous meningitis

Symptoms	Signs
Early:	
Apathy	There may be none
Malaise	Low-grade fever
Anorexia	Usually no neck stiffness
Irritability	Papilloedema may be seen early
Amenorrhoea	Tubercles may be seen in the fundus of the eye (the pupils may require to be dilated)
Later:	
The patient feels and looks ill	Mental confusion
	Papilloedema
Headache	Neck stiffness
Fits	Cranial nerve palsies
	Hemiparesis
Late:	
Coma	Decerebrate rigidity
Blindness	Signs of extensive cranial nerve and cerebral damage

Symptoms and Signs (Table 21.14)

The onset is usually insidious – over a period of several weeks. The disease should be suspected when febrile symptoms do not clear and if there is a history of contact with tuberculosis.

Complications

Epilepsy.
Major neurological signs (for example).
Hydrocephalus.
Spinal block.

Investigations

1. CSF. Typically the CSF is clear to the naked eye, and microscopically shows a moderate pleocytosis (60 to 400 cells/mm^3), mainly lymphocytes.
The protein level usually parallels the number of cells (up to 400 mg per cent).
The sugar is low (except in diabetics).
A large volume (10 ml) CSF should be sent to the laboratory. Examination of the fibrinous clot or centrifuged deposit may show acid-fast bacilli. Fluorescent microscopy may be required. Culture and guinea pig inoculation are essential.
Note: Considerable variations in the CSF picture may occur – some cases showing very few cells (particularly in patients who are Mantoux negative, very ill, or taking steroids) and others showing large numbers (up to 1,000).
2. Chest X-ray. This may show evidence of tuberculosis (fifty to seventy per cent of cases).
3. Mantoux test. This is usually positive.
4. Bromide partition test. This is useful in difficult cases. The technique depends upon the knowledge that the blood/brain barrier is damaged in tuberculous meningitis. Normally, the relative concentration of bromide in CSF and blood, after a loading dose of bromide, is in the ratio 3:1. When the barrier is damaged equalisation tends to occur.

Differential Dignosis

Tuberculosis should be remembered as a cause of cranial nerve palsies, hemiplegia, paraplegia, and impairment of consciousness – particularly when the patient is febrile and when it is difficult to obtain a history.

Early
1. Almost any febrile illness.
2. Other forms of meningitis including viral, fungal, and neoplastic. In none of these are tubercle baccilli found.

Later. Many disorders can be simulated including cerebral tumour and cerebrovascular disease.

Basis of Treatment

Urgent and prolonged treatment with anti-tuberculous

drugs is essential. The starting of treatment should not be delayed until culture results are available.

Drug Treatment. It is usual to use three drugs simultaneously – because of the danger of drug resistance. The standard regime involves systemic streptomycin 1 g intramuscularly daily and isoniazid 300 mg daily. The third drug can be either rifampicin or ethionamide. PAS is not now usually used as it enters the CSF in low concentration and is difficult to take. The antibiotic treatment may need to be modified later if *in vitro* tests show that the organism is insensitive to the original antibiotic, or if there is a poor response to therapy, or if the CSF to drug concentrations are inadequate. Treatment with streptomycin is usually continued for six months. Oral therapy with two drugs is usually continued for a further eighteen months.

Most authorities recommend giving intrathecal streptomycin, 50 to 100 mg daily for the first two weeks and then thrice weekly for a further four weeks.

Oral corticosteroids can be helpful – especially when there is adrenal cortical failure or a severe drug reaction. It has been suggested that steroids should be used routinely to reduce the amount of exudative reaction. In general, however, the routine use of steroids is not recommended.

Throughout antibiotic therapy regular lumbar punctures should be undertaken to assess the response to treatment. During the early weeks after the introduction of therapy the patient often remains febrile and wild fluctuations in the CSF white cell count occur.

General Measures. This involves proper hydration via a nasogastric tube, and standard nursing care for severely ill patients.

Prognosis

Untreated, the mortality of tuberculous meningitis is one hundred per cent. The overall mortality today is now between fifteen and twenty per cent. The prognosis depends on:
(a) Quality of treatment.
(b) The stage reached when treatment is begun.
(c) Age. Prognosis is worst at the extremes of life. Recurrence of infection is uncommon, but can occur if the initial treatment is inadequate.

In a substantial proportion of patients there is some evidence of residual brain damage as shown by mental retardation and epilepsy. These complications are particularly likely to occur when the infection occurs in infancy.

INTRACRANIAL ABSCESS

Localised suppuration within the cranial cavity is most commonly found in the substance of the brain – 'brain abscess'. Abscesses occasionally, however, occur in other sites. An abscess in the extradural space is almost always associated with local osteomyelitis of the skull following sinusitis, middle ear infection, or an infected fracture of the skull vault. A subdural abscess is a rare complication of frontal sinusitis.

Definition

Localised suppuration within the substance of the brain.

Background

There are two main aetiological groups.
1. Spread from a local focus of infection. The two principal foci are:
(a) The nasal sinuses – usually with spread into the frontal lobe.
(b) Infection in the middle ear with spread either upwards into the temporal lobe or medially into the cerebellum.

Intracranial abscess may occasionally occur as a result of a penetrating injury.
2. Blood spread. This is particularly liable to occur with chronic lung infection such as abscess or bronchiectasis. Brain abscess is an important complication of cyanotic congenital heart disease.

Pathology

In the early stages an area of diffuse inflammation occurs. Later, this inflammation becomes localised, frequently with liquefaction. A capsule is formed containing fluid and semi-fluid pus. Abscesses are frequently multiple and loculated.

Symptoms and Signs

There may be evidence of sinusitis or of middle ear infection. The onset is frequently insidious and is often not accompanied by fever, especially if antibiotics have been used. Early symptoms include headache, 'feeling unwell', nausea, and anorexia. Later, there may be papilloedema and other evidence of raised intracranial pressure.

Focal features depend on the site of infection:

Frontal lobe:
Intellectual deterioration.
Disinhibited behaviour.
Dysphasia (if the dominant side is affected).
Contralateral hemiparesis.

Temporal lobe:
Dysphasia (if the dominant side is affected).
Quadrantic visual field defect.

Cerebellum:
Nystagmus.
Ataxia.

Investigations

1. EEG. This can be very helpful. A focus of localised slow waves is usually found over the affected area.
2. CT and linear brain scan.
3. Lumbar puncture. This must be avoided if there is any evidence of raised intracranial pressure. It is usually undertaken only if there are marked meningitic signs. Findings include a pleocytosis of 100 to 200 cells. Culture is usually sterile.
4. Blood culture. This is occasionally positive in metastatic cases.
5. Chest X-ray. Important in metastatic cases.
6. Skull X-ray. May show evidence of infection in the middle ear or nasal sinuses.
7. Aspiration of abscess. This is the only definitive way of making the diagnosis. Injection of radio-opaque material is usually undertaken to indicate the size of the abscess cavity.

Complications

Rupture into the ventricles.
Epilepsy.

Differential Diagnosis

1. **Any Other Space-Occupying Mass**, e.g. cerebral tumour, etc.
2. **Meningitis,** especially if headache and neck stiffness predominate.

Basis of Treatment

This is mainly surgical and involves aspiration of abscess cavities with instillation of antibiotics. Systemic antibiotics are also given.

Prognosis

Cerebral abscess is a dangerous condition with a high mortality and morbidity. The mortality rate is between 10 to 20 per cent. There is a high incidence of epilepsy (40 to 50 per cent) among survivors.

INTRACRANIAL THROMBOPHLEBITIS

Definition

Thrombosis of intracranial venous sinuses and veins.

Background

Any of the major intracranial sinuses can be affected. Septic and aseptic forms occur.

The septic form is usually associated with spread from a local focus of infection:
1. Cavernous sinus thrombosis usually occurs as a result of spread from a focus on the face or in the nose.
2. Thrombosis of the lateral sinus occurs as a result of spread of infection from the middle ear.
3. Thrombosis of the superior sagittal sinus occurs following infection in the nasal sinuses or elsewhere.

Aseptic thrombosis may occur in the post-partum phase, in women on the contraceptive pill, in polycythaemia, and, occasionally, in association with local infection, especially involving the middle ear.

Thrombosis of the superior sagittal sinus and lateral sinuses may lead to impaired reabsorption of CSF with resultant raised intracranial pressure and hydrocephalus.

Symptoms and Signs

In suppurative cases the patient is ill with evidence of pyaemia – rigors, high swinging fever, etc. The clinical features will depend on which sinus is primarily involved –

Cavernous sinus. Orbital oedema, proptosis, chemosis, palsies of the IIIrd, IVth and VIth cranial nerves together with the upper two sensory divisions of the Vth nerve. The signs may be bilateral in the later stages.

Lateral sinus. Headache. Papilloedema. Frequently no focal neurological signs.

Superior sagittal sinus. Headache and evidence of raised intracranial pressure. A single or double hemiplegia may be produced and, in some instances, the leg is more affected than the arm.

Investigations

The diagnosis is usually made by clinical assessment.
1. Carotid angiography. May show failure of filling of the relevant venous sinuses.
2. Blood culture, etc. may be required.

Differential Diagnosis

1. Other causes of raised intracranial tension including intracranial abscess.
2. Encephalitis.

Basis of Treatment

Thrombosis of the venous sinuses is frequently associated with evidence of bacterial infection. Antibiotic therapy is essential. Anticoagulants may be indicated in some cases.

Prognosis

Provided the infection can be eradicated the patient frequently makes a full recovery.

VIRUS DISEASE OF THE CENTRAL NERVOUS SYSTEM

Viruses may affect the central nervous system in a number of different ways:

1. A number of viruses attack particular nerve cells and for this reason are known as neurotropic viruses. Examples of this are poliomyelitis in which the anterior horn cells are picked out and *Herpes zoster* in which the cells of the dorsal root ganglion are involved.

2. Other viruses produce a more diffuse inflammation of the central nervous system or of its coverings.

3. In a third group of cases an acute demyelinating disorder can be initiated by the virus. It seems likely that this is an allergic response of the nervous system to an antigen, in some instances possibly the virus itself.

In many cases it can be difficult, on clinical grounds, to distinguish acute encephalitis due to virus invasion from an acute demyelinating reaction.

In recent years there has arisen the concept of 'slow virus infections'. Certain diseases, notably Kuru, seen in the natives of New Guinea, appear to be due to a transmittable virus particle which produces neurological disease with a very long incubation period – measured in months or years. It is possible that some other diseases, for example, multiple sclerosis, may eventually prove to have a similar aetiology.

The terms encephalitis, myelitis, and encephalomyelitis imply inflammation of the substance of the brain, spinal cord, and brain *and* spinal cord respectively.

ACUTE VIRAL MENINGITIS AND MENINGO-ENCEPHALITIS

Definition

Acute viral inflammation of the meninges and/or the substance of the brain.

Background

The distinction, both pathologically and clinically, between meningitis and encephalitis is blurred. Thus, in encephalitis there is always some meningeal reaction, and in meningitis there is frequently some inflammation of the underlying brain. From the clinical point of view, however, the meningitic form is almost always benign, whereas encephalitis may be followed by permanent brain damage.

Viruses involved in the meningitic form. Polio virus, Coxsackie, mumps, Echo, and the virus of lymphocytic choriomeningitis (whose major reservoir is in mice).

Viruses involved in the encephalitic form. Associated with systemic viral infection, particularly mumps, measles, rubella, varicella and influenza.

Herpes simplex – this produces a particularly severe form of encephalitis in which there is haemorrhagic necrosis and marked swelling of part of the brain (particularly the temporal lobe).

A large number of different viruses may produce encephalitis.

Symptoms and Signs

The severity of the illness varies considerably from patient to patient. Fever is present in most cases.

Meningitic form. Headache, neck stiffness, and photophobia. Usually no signs.

Meningo-encephalitis. Meningitis plus evidence of dysfunction of the brain – drowsiness, convulsions, hemiparesis, ataxia, etc.

Investigations

1. Lumbar puncture. CSF is crystal clear and shows a lymphocytic pleocytosis, slightly raised protein, normal sugar, and is sterile on bacterial culture.

2. EEG. Diffuse slow waves are seen on both sides in most cases of encephalitis.

3. Virological investigations as indicated.

4. CT brain scan in appropriate cases.

Differential Diagnosis

1. **Acute Disseminated Encephalomyelitis.** This may be impossible to distinguish on clinical grounds.

2. **Meningitic Form.** Bacterial meningitis. It is essential to exclude this first. CSF is cloudy, polymorphs++, low sugar, organisms seen on Gram film and grown.

Other causes of a clear CSF with a lymphocytic pleocytosis which is sterile on bacterial culture are:

(a) Cerebral abscess.

(b) Spirochaetal infection – syphilis, canicola fever, and Weil's disease.

(c) Infectious mononucleosis.

(d) Tuberculous meningitis.

(e) Carcinomatous meningitis.

(f) Sarcoidosis.

(g) Fungal infections; e.g. torulosis.

3. **Meningo-encephalitis.** Cerebral abscess, tumour, or other focal disturbance of brain function.

Basis of Treatment

In most instances no specific treatment is either indicated or available. Steroids have been used in some cases but are not of proven value.

Anti-viral agents – idoxuridine and cytarabine – are currently being evaluated for cases of *Herpes simplex* encephalitis.

Prognosis

A full recovery is to be anticipated in virtually all cases of viral meningitis and most of mild encephalomyelitis. A very poor prognosis (high mortality and morbidity) is found with *Herpes simplex* encephalitis.

ACUTE DISSEMINATED ENCEPHALOMYELITIS (ADE)

Definition

This is an acute disorder of the central nervous system characterised pathologically by perivenous demyelination and clinically by evidence of damage to the brain and/or the spinal cord.

Background

This syndrome may closely mimic acute virus encephalitis, but the pathology is quite different and the prognosis is, in general, worse.

The syndrome is characterised pathologically by perivascular cellular infiltration and by patchy demyelination in the white matter of the brain and/or of the spinal cord. It differs from acute virus encephalitis which mainly affects grey matter and is not accompanied by demyelination. The condition is thought to be an acute hypersensitivity reaction to some antigenic agent. A similar condition can be produced experimentally in animals by direct inoculation with a combination of brain tissue together with appropriate adjuvants.

Occurrence:
1. Following one of the acute childhood illnesses, especially rubella, varicella, and measles. The neurological features usually follow the primary illness by two to four days, but occasionally precede it.
2. Following vaccination against smallpox or rabies and, very occasionally, following other protective inoculations. It is likely that approximately 1 in 5,000 people vaccinated against smallpox will show some features of the disorder.
3. Idiopathic.

Symptoms and Signs

The clinical picture is very variable both in severity and in the distribution of lesions that may involve the brain, spinal cord, or both.

Encephalitic form. Symptoms and signs much the same as those listed under encephalitis (*see* page 547).

Myelitis. Paraplegia, etc. (*see* spinal cord, page 508).

Investigations

CSF. The findings are frequently the same as those in acute virus encephalitis.

Differential Diagnosis

As for meningo-encephalitis.

Prevention and Basis of Treatment

Smallpox vaccination should be carried out as early as possible in childhood; the incidence of ADE rises with increasing age. It appears likely that steroids and ACTH, when used in the acute phase, exert a beneficial effect.

Prognosis

This is variable. In mild cases there is virtually no mortality or morbidity. In severe cases, however, the mortality may be between 20 and 30 per cent, and survivors show a high incidence of permanent brain damage.

POLIOMYELITIS

Definition

An inflammatory disease of the central nervous system caused by one of three antigenically distinct poliomyelitis viruses. In the paralytic form the anterior horn cells are particularly affected, with the production of muscle paralysis and wasting.

Background

Three main types of polio virus are recognised – *Brunhilde, Lansing,* and *Leon.* Infection with a particular strain gives immunity against reinfection with that strain but not against other strains. Poliomyelitis used to have a world-wide distribution, but since the introduction of vaccination has almost disappeared from many areas, notably Europe and North America. Even in these areas occasional cases do occur but some of these are probably due to one of the *Coxsackie* viruses. Poliomyelitis is still widespread in tropical countries.

The disease is spread by faecal contamination of water and food. Flies are a frequent vector. The virus enters the body via the alimentary tract.

Poliomyelitis frequently occurs in epidemics and occurs with maximum frequency in July to September in temperate zones.

Pathology

A diffuse inflammation of the meninges and substance of the brain may be produced. The virus has a particular tendency to attack anterior horn cells and cells of the bulbar motor nuclei.

Symptoms and Signs

Poliomyelitis has an incubation period of six to twenty days. Four varieties of the disease are recognised and it must be noted that in the vast majority of cases muscle paralysis does not occur.

Sub-clinical. This is responsible for ninety-five per cent of cases. It involves the invasion of the body by the virus without the production of symptoms. The virus can usually be recovered from the stools.

Abortive form. This is a mild non-specific illness, frequently upper respiratory or gastrointestinal, without the production of neck stiffness or evidence of involvement of the nervous system.

Non-paralytic (meningitic) form. This is a meningitic illness with fever, headache and neck stiffness but no paralysis. Some cells are usually found in the CSF.

Paralytic form (see Table 21.15).

Complications

Severe bulbar paralysis, which may result in inhalation of vomit, pulmonary collapse, etc.
Respiratory paralysis, following paralysis of the intercostal and accessory respiratory muscles and the diaphragm.

Investigations

1. Stool examination will usually enable the virus to be isolated.
2. Blood. Rise in antibody titres.
3. CSF. *Early* – polymorphs (100 to 200), sugar normal, bacterial culture negative. *Later* – lymphocytes (up to 200). Protein raised. In the meningitic variety a very large number of cells may be found.

Differential Diagnosis

1. In the meningitic phase – any other form of meningitis.
2. In the paralytic phase:
(a) Acute polyneuritis (Guillain–Barré syndrome). This is usually symmetrical, sensory symptoms or signs are usual, and the CSF shows a marked elevation in protein but very few cells.
(b) Acute transverse myelitis. In this condition the plantar responses are usually extensor and there is loss of sphincter control.
(c) Acute rheumatic fever or acute osteomyelitis. These conditions may cause pain and tenderness.

Prophylaxis

In an epidemic, gammaglobulin should be given. Excessive exertion should be avoided as it is probable that this promotes paralysis in an infected person.

Routine prophylaxis involves the administration of attenuated live oral polyvalent vaccine of Sabin type. At least two doses are given, several weeks apart, and booster doses at occasional intervals. The virus multiplies in the intestinal tract and remains at this site. Oral immunisation is very safe and produces almost complete immunity against the disease.

Basis of Treatment

Once established there is no specific treatment for poliomyelitis. It is essential to watch out for respiratory and bulbar palsy. A tracheostomy may be required and indications for this are:
(a) Inability to swallow, with or without pooling of saliva in the pharynx.
(b) Very weak cough (with or without vocal cord paralysis).
(c) Respiratory insufficiency. In the latter instance assisted ventilation will be required.

Table 21.15 Paralytic type of poliomyelitis

	Symptoms	Signs
Pre-paralytic phase	Headache, feeling ill, muscle pains	Fever, neck stiffness, muscle tenderness
Paralytic phase	(Sometimes the disease shows a bi-phasic form so that the pre-paralytic phase appears to subside only to be followed suddenly by the features of the paralytic phase.)	
	Severe muscle pains Inability to move paralysed parts Bulbar palsy – dysphagia, and difficulty with talking	Fever Muscle tenderness++ Paralysis of muscles – frequently asymmetrical Bulbar paralysis (approximately 20%) – paralysis of facial, pharyngeal and palatal muscles Respiratory paralysis

Paralysis is usually complete within about twenty-four hours, but in occasional cases may continue for up to seventy-two hours

Prognosis

The mortality among paralytic cases is approximately five per cent if the patient is nursed in a good centre. Pneumonia, pulmonary collapse and embolism are the usual causes of death. The patient showing even very severe initial paralysis may make a reasonable functional recovery. Recovery may continue up to two years after the acute illness, but sixty per cent of recovery occurs during the first three months. In occasional instances severe permanent paralysis of the limbs and respiratory muscles remain.

HERPES ZOSTER (SHINGLES)

Definition

A disorder of virus origin characterised pathologically by unilateral acute inflammation of one or more posterior root ganglia and clinically by the appearance of painful vesicular eruption on the skin of the involved segment.

Background

The viruses of varicella and *Herpes zoster* are serologically identical.

The disease occurs at any age, but becomes more frequent with increasing age.

Secondary zoster occurs following trauma, tumours, and deep X-ray therapy. The vesicles frequently occur in the segment affected by the original disorder. Shingles also appears to be more common in persons who are unwell for any cause.

The majority of patients with *Herpes zoster* give a history of previous attack of varicella. It is probable that the virus lies dormant in the dorsal root ganglion for a long while until some factor activates it.

Pathology

The principal pathology is haemorrhagic necrosis in the dorsal root ganglion. The process may spread into the neighbouring part of the spinal cord.

Symptoms

Pain.
Paraesthesiae.
Hypersensitivity of the skin.

Signs

Vesicular eruption of the skin of the affected segment.

The commonest areas to be affected are the skin of the chest and upper abdomen (75 per cent) and the face.

Particular Forms of Herpes Zoster

1. **Ophthalmic Herpes.** This occurs when the ophthalmic division of the Vth nerve is affected. There is danger of corneal ulceration and scarring. If the infection is not controlled with antibiotics a panophthalmitis may develop, with permanent loss of vision.

2. **Geniculate Herpes.** This occurs when the geniculate ganglion of the VIIth nerve is involved. Vesicles occur in the external auditory canal and on the palate and tongue. Other features include severe pain in the ear and facial palsy (*see* page 492). The vesicles usually clear in three to four weeks, often less.

Complications

Local muscle wasting and paralysis, due to anterior horn cell involvement.
Post herpetic neuralgia (*see* page 524).

Differential Diagnosis

1. In the pre-eruptive phase, any cause of severe pain, for example appendicitis, fracture, etc.
2. *Herpes simplex*. This does not usually have a segmental distribution. Virological studies on the vesicular fluid may be undertaken if there is doubt.

Basis of Treatment

1. Idoxuridine (an anti-viral agent) may be applied locally if the patient is seen during the first few days.
2. Pain and discomfort should be treated with analgesics. Pethidine may be required if the pain is very severe (particularly in ophthalmic herpes).
3. Secondary bacterial infection may need to be treated with local and systemic antibiotics.

Cases of ophthalmic herpes should, if possible, be supervised by an ophthalmologist. Idoxuridine and steroids may be instilled into the conjunctival sac.

NEUROSYPHILIS

Involvement of the cardiovascular and nervous systems is responsible for the vast majority of deaths due to syphilis.

Different patterns of neurological syphilis appear, according to the length of time elapsing since the primary infection. In the early years involvement of the meninges and arteries predominates. Many years later, the parenchyma of the central nervous system is affected. Gummata occasionally occur in the CNS and may mimic other space-occupying lesions. Proper antibiotic treatment will stop the progression of inflammatory changes, but it is vital that this is given before

there is severe irreversible damage. The following types of neurosyphilis occur:
1. Asymptomatic neurosyphilis. In this there are no clinical symptoms or signs but lumbar puncture shows evidence of active inflammation in the meninges.
2. Meningitic form.
3. Meningovascular syphilis.
4. Tabes dorsalis. ⎤ Usually occur between
5. General paralysis of ⎬ ten and twenty years
   the insane (GPI). ⎦ after the primary
6. Gumma. infection.

Acute Meningitic Form. This usually occurs within two years of the primary infection and presents the features of an acute or subacute meningitis.

Meningovascular Syphilis. This tends to occur between two and five years after the primary infection. In this type of the disease chronic meningeal inflammation is combined with an arteritis which may affect the cerebral or the spinal arteries.

Meningeal form. In this type, all the features of chronic meningitis may occur with the production of headache, cranial nerve palsies and hydrocephalus. (The features are similar to those seen in tuberculous meningitis.)

Vascular occlusions. The clinical features produced will depend on the artery involved. They include hemiplegia, due to involvement of the middle cerebral artery, and paraplegia due to involvement of the anterior spinal artery.

CSF in Neurosyphilis

The CSF is abnormal in most cases of neurosyphilis. However, in some cases of tabes it may be normal.
1. Cells. A lymphocytic pleocytosis in most cases. Large numbers are found in the acute meningeal phase, less in GPI (up to 100) and a few in tabes.
2. Total protein content – usually somewhat elevated in most cases of untreated syphilis.
3. Lange curve – not very reliable. A paretic curve (first zone) is seen in GPI and sometimes meningovascular syphilis. A tabetic curve (mid zone) is seen in tabes.
4. CSF WR. This is positive in most forms of neurosyphilis. It is negative in about twenty per cent of cases of tabes.
5. Blood WR. This is usually positive in neurosyphilis but is occasionally negative. Thus, if neurosyphilis is suspected a lumbar puncture should be undertaken, even if the blood WR is negative.

Basis of Treatment

A three-week course of penicillin should be given in all cases of neurosyphilis. In some instances it may be necessary to give further courses of treatment. The response to treatment is measured by the number of cells and level of protein in the CSF. These should eventually return to, and remain, normal. The CSF WR, however, frequently remains positive despite treatment.

In GPI and tabes the spirochaetes are situated deeply inside the substance of the brain. For this reason some workers still recommend infecting the patient with benign tertian malaria to produce hyperthermia.

TABES DORSALIS

Definition

A form of neurosyphilis in which there is selective degeneration in the posterior roots of the spinal nerves with resultant secondary degeneration in the posterior columns of the spinal cord.

Symptoms

Lightning pains – severe, sharp, stabs of pain occurring in the limbs and elsewhere.
'Crises' of severe pain – rectal, vesical, or renal.
Painless retention of urine.
Impotence.
Falling over in the dark.

Signs

Argyll-Robertson pupils.
Bilateral ptosis.
Optic atrophy (ten per cent).
Absent tendon reflexes.
Depression of postural, vibratory and deep pain sensation in the legs.
Patches of hypalgesia on the face, front of the chest, and inside of the legs.
High steppage gait. Romberg's sign positive. Enlarged bladder.
Charcot joints.

Differential Diagnosis

Tabes can present in a large number of different ways and many different diseases can be simulated.

GENERAL PARALYSIS OF THE INSANE (GPI)

Definition

A condition characterised pathologically by progressive syphilitic inflammation of the substance of the brain and clinically by dementia and tremor.

Table 21.16 Symptoms and signs of GPI

Symptoms	Signs
Early:	
Lack of judgement	Evidence of intellectual
Personality deterioration	deterioration
Grandiose ideas	AR pupils, usually
(occasionally)	'Trombone' tremor of the
	tongue (the tongue moves
	in and out rapidly)
	Tremor of the limbs
	sometimes also present
Late:	
Gross dementia	Tendon reflexes frequently
	increased
	Extensor plantar responses

Differential Diagnosis

1. Other forms of dementia; e.g. arteriosclerotic.
2. Other conditions in which tremor occurs, for example Parkinsonism, disseminated sclerosis, etc.

TOXIC INFECTIONS OF THE CENTRAL NERVOUS SYSTEM

TETANUS

Definition

A disease caused by an exotoxin produced by the bacterium *Clostridium tetani* and characterised clinically by severe painful spasms of skeletal muscle.

Background

Clostridium tetani is a spore-forming anaerobic Gram-positive bacillus. The spores are found widely in soil and in the faeces of animals. They are very resistant to drying.

The tetanus bacillus usually enters the body by a wound of some sort and this is frequently trivial. Occasional cases follow the use of improperly sterilised catgut. Neonatal tetanus (associated with umbilical sepsis) is very common in some parts of the world (*see* page 584).

The tetanus bacillus multiplies locally but does not spread or invade nearby tissues. Toxin from the bacilli enters the bloodstream. This reaches the spinal cord and brain stem where it is thought to have a specific action on the Renshaw system, producing a reduction in central inhibitory activity. This results in a greatly intensified reflex response to afferent stimuli.

Table 21.17 Symptoms and signs of tetanus

Symptoms	Signs
Early:	
Difficulty with chewing	Recent wound
Discomfort in the jaws	Slight spasm of facial
Aching in the neck and	muscles
lumbar area	Slight muscle stiffness
Spasm of the jaw	
muscles (trismus)	
Later:	
Dysphagia	Marked facial spasms – risus
Difficulty with breathing	sardonicus

Painful muscle spasms: These are paroxysmal and involve the neck, trunk and limbs. They are often precipitated by noise and impeding injections. Sometimes continuous muscle spasm occurs between attacks

The incubation period is very variable; between 48 hours and several weeks. The period of development of symptoms also varies from a few hours to several days.

The duration of the disease varies considerably, from several days in mild cases up to ten weeks.

Complications

1. Asphyxia. This may occur due to a severe muscle spasm or to inhalation of vomit.
2. Respiratory arrest may occur as a complication of the above and also due to the action of the toxin on the respiratory centre in the brain stem.
3. Circulatory collapse. Hypotension and severe tachycardia are common in severe cases.
4. Deep vein thrombosis.
5. Pulmonary collapse, etc.

Investigations

The diagnosis of tetanus is made on the clinical picture. Bacteriological examination of the wound may reveal tetanus bacilli.

Differential Diagnosis

1. Other causes of trismus, for example dental abscess, etc.
2. Other causes of neck stiffness, particularly meningitis.
3. Dystonic reactions to the phenothiazine group of drugs which usually affect the facial muscles maximally.
4. Strychnine. Poisoning with strychnine gives a clinical picture very much like that of tetanus.

Prevention

Prevention is better than cure. Active immunisation with tetanus toxoid is both extremely effective and safe.

The initial course involves two injections at intervals of six weeks with a booster injection at one year. Booster injections of toxoid should be given whenever open wounds occur. Regular booster injections should be given at ten-yearly intervals.

Basis of Treatment

There is no specific treatment for tetanus. Once established the disease will pursue its course, although this may be modified with treatment.

General Measures. Nursing care is vital if the patient is severely ill, and he will probably require everything to be done for him.
1. Passive immunisation. Human anti-tetanus globulin should be given if this is available. If not, anti-tetanus serum 50,000 to 100,000 units should be given after the appropriate test dose. This can be expected to neutralise newly formed toxin but will not affect toxin that is already 'fixed' in the central nervous system.
2. Cleaning and debridement of the wound. Necrotic tissue must be removed and the wound should be excised.
3. Systemic penicillin should be given to kill the tetanus bacilli.
4. Assure the airway. Respiratory obstruction can easily occur in patients with tetanus and for this reason a prophylactic tracheostomy should be undertaken in all but the mildest cases.
5. Muscle spasms can be treated with large doses of intravenous diazepam (Valium) or with a specific muscle relaxant such as curare. In the latter instance, the ventilatory muscles will also be paralysed and it will be necessary to put the patient on a respirator.
6. Correction of sympathetic overactivity. In many instances there is evidence of marked sympathetic overactivity (tachycardia, excessive sweating, and marked variability in blood pressure). Adrenergic beta blocking agents have been found to be helpful in counteracting this state.

The above measures must be continued until clinical recovery occurs. When the patient has recovered he must be actively immunised with tetanus toxoid (an attack of clinical tetanus does not give immunity against subsequent attacks).

Prognosis

The mortality varies considerably and depends on the area of the world involved, the excellence of medical care, and the age of the patient. In individual cases a poor prognosis is associated with a short incubation period and a rapid onset of symptoms. A high mortality also occurs in the very young, the very old and the ill.

If the patient recovers, he does so completely, usually without any residua.

DIPHTHERIA (*see* page 24)

OTHER DEGENERATIVE DISORDERS OF THE NERVOUS SYSTEM

PARKINSONISM

Definition

An extrapyramidal disorder characterised by tremor, slowness of movement, and rigidity.

Background

The main clinical forms of Parkinsonism are as follows:

1. **Parkinson's Disease.** This is the commonest form of Parkinsonism. About one in every 100 people in Great Britain over the age of 60 suffer from this condition. The disease is caused by destruction of pigmented brain stem nuclei that contain neuromelanin, with loss of the neurotransmitters dopamine and noradrenaline. The basic cause of the cellular degeneration is not known.

2. **Postencephalitic Parkinsonism.** This develops as a late sequel to encephalitis. It occurred principally as a sequel to encephalitis lethargica but the last epidemic of this was 50 years ago. However, other forms of encephalitis are sometimes followed by Parkinsonism. This form of the disease is typically associated with oculogyric crises and dystonic disturbances of movement.

3. **Drug-induced Parkinsonism.** The drugs most likely to cause a Parkinsonian syndrome are phenothiazines and reserpine. Phenothiazine-induced Parkinsonism is particularly liable to be seen in psychiatric patients who are being given large doses of drugs. The condition usually disappears when the drugs are withdrawn.

4. **Miscellaneous Causes.** These include atherosclerotic Parkinsonism. The pathological basis for this disorder is uncertain, but it occurs in elderly hypertensive patients many of whom show evidence of other disorders including dementia. Occasional causes include head injury, chronic trauma (for example boxing), poisoning with carbon monoxide or manganese, and Wilson's disease.

Symptoms and Signs (*see* Table 21.18)

It should be noted that there is considerable variation in the clinical pattern from case to case which may partly depend on the aetiology, for example tremor frequently predominates in Parkinson's disease. In the early stages diagnosis may be difficult, particularly when tremor is absent. Lack of arm swinging is a particularly characteristic early feature.

In some instances the disease is markedly asymmetrical and, for example, tremor may be entirely confined to one arm.

Differential Diagnosis

1. Other forms of tremor, for example essential tremor.
2. Hypothyroidism and depression can be simulated when hypokinesia predominates.

In the late stages there is usually no problem about the diagnosis.

Basis of Treatment

L-dopa. The advent of L-dopa has completely changed the outlook for patients with Parkinson's disease. Previously, drug treatment was disappointing.

Dopamine is an important synaptic transmitter in the striatum. Studies have shown that the level of striatal dopamine is diminished in Parkinson's disease. Attempts were made to raise the level of dopamine in the brain artificially, by giving the substance orally. Unfortunately, dopamine does not cross the blood/brain barrier in large quantities. However, its precursor, L-dopa does. L-dopa is converted to dopamine by decarboxylation. Nowadays L-dopa, alone or combined with a decarboxylase inhibitor, is the most effective treatment for Parkinsonism.

Most patients with Parkinson's disease should be started on L-dopa provided that they are sufficiently disabled. Mild cases do not require treatment. L-dopa should always be introduced slowly so that any side effects can be identified before they become too severe and frightening. The optimal dose of L-dopa is usually between 2 and 4 g per day, but some patients need up to 8 g.

The principal side effects of L-dopa are:
1. Nausea, vomiting, anorexia and weight loss. Most patients experience nausea and to some extent this problem can be avoided by giving L-dopa with food.
2. Postural hypotension.
3. Involuntary movements. These include grimacing movements of the face and choreiform movements of the jaw, tongue and limbs. Most patients ultimately develop such movements which can severely limit the amount of L-dopa tolerated.
4. Confusional states. These are uncommon (occurring in about fifteen per cent of cases), but very important.

Nausea, vomiting and hypotension can be reduced by giving L-dopa combined with a decarboxylase inhibitor. Various preparations are available including 'Sinemet' and 'Madopar'. Once L-dopa therapy has been started it must be continued indefinitely. Withdrawal of therapy will be rapidly followed by deterioration.

Other forms of therapy comprise:

Anticholinergic Drugs. It has long been known that cholinergic activation aggravates Parkinsonism whereas anticholinergic drugs produce clinical benefit. This is the rationale for the use of such synthetic anticholinergic drugs as benzhexol and benztropine. Benzhexol (Artane) can be given in doses ranging between 2 and 20 mg per day in divided doses. The usual starting dose is 2 mg three times daily. Side effects include mental confusion and glaucoma.

Other Drugs. There are several ways in which the activity of dopamine systems of the brain can be increased with the object of reversing the symptoms of Parkinsonism. Dopamine receptor stimulant drugs (for

Table 21.18 Symptoms and signs of Parkinson's disease

Symptoms	Signs
Early:	
Tremor. This is the presenting symptom in approximately 70% of idiopathic cases	Tremor. This is characteristically present at rest at a frequency of 5 to 6 cycles per second. It is not usually made worse by intention
Deteriorating handwriting	Facial masking
Falling over for no apparent reason	Lack of arm swinging when walking
Late:	
Difficulty with talking	Immobile face
Dysphagia (occasionally)	Speech may be unintelligible, being slow and of low volume
Inability to write, feed, wash, and dress	Tremor++
Difficulty with turning over in bed	The limbs may show severe rigidity
Difficulty with walking and sometimes complete inability to walk	The gait may show the following features –
Mental confusion (sometimes this may be due to drugs)	1. difficulty with starting, stopping and turning
	2. may be shuffling
	3. tendency to fall, either forwards or backwards
	Deformities. A stoop frequently develops
	Contractures of the shoulders, elbows, hips and knees may occur

Other features. Usually there is no change in muscle power, deep tendon reflexes, or in sensation.
 Oculo-gyric crises may occur. These are sudden uncontrollable spasms of upward movement of the eyes.
 Excessive sweating and salivation.

example bromocriptine and apomorphine) or dopamine releasing drugs (for example amantadine and amphetamine) can be used. Dopamine turnover can also be increased by a number of hormones. None of the agents mentioned has found its way into routine clinical practice.

Surgical Treatment. Stereotactically produced lesions in the ventro-lateral nucleus of the thalamus have been found to be effective in alleviating tremor and rigidity. Hypokinesia is usually unaffected. Nowadays, surgery is usually reserved for patients who have made a poor response to L-dopa.

Prognosis

L-dopa results in improvement in about three-quarters of all patients with Parkinson's disease. Patients with arteriosclerotic Parkinsonism respond less well. L-dopa usually remains effective for five to six years. Parkinson's disease is slowly progressive in most subjects and there is no evidence that L-dopa significantly reduces the rate of progression. Prior to the advent of L-dopa, the average duration of life after onset of symptoms was about ten years.

HUNTINGTON'S CHOREA

This is a genetically determined disorder, inherited in an autosomal dominant fashion, and manifesting itself clinically by choreiform movements and intellectual deterioration. The disease usually presents in the third or fourth decades of life.

Pathologically there is a loss of cells in the basal ganglia, notably the caudate nuclei. The involuntary movements can frequently be controlled by tetrabenazine.

MUSCLE DISEASES

In recent years a large amount of research work has been undertaken on the ultrastructure, chemistry, and physiology of normal and diseased skeletal muscles. From the clinical point of view there has been considerable progress in the classification of muscle disease, but it must be admitted that there have been disappointingly few advances in treatment. A notable exception to this, however, is the treatment of polymyositis with steroids.

The term myopathy is used to cover all diseases which are thought to be due to primary abnormality of skeletal muscle fibres or of the interstitial tissue between the fibres. The group includes diseases that are degenerative, inflammatory, metabolic, and endocrine in origin. The term dystrophy is reserved for those forms of genetically determined degenerative myopathy in which the degenerative process is thought to develop primarily in the muscle fibres themselves.

Clinical diagnosis of suspected muscle disease is made easier by knowledge of the commoner syndromes. Thus, classical myasthenia gravis and Duchenne muscular dystrophy rarely present a serious diagnostic problem. In other instances, however, a 'staged' diagnosis must be made. In these cases it is necessary to decide whether one is dealing with a primary disturbance of muscle fibres, an abnormality of neuromuscular conduction, or an abnormality of innervation. In some instances it is impossible on clinical grounds to decide, and the diagnosis may depend on muscle biopsy, estimation of serum levels of muscle enzymes, and electromyography.

Muscle Biopsy

This is frequently a very useful investigation. In order to get the maximum information the muscle biopsy must be very carefully taken. The muscle must be chosen carefully. Avoid grossly wasted muscles (very few residual muscle fibres may be left). Choose a muscle with long parallel fibres (such as the deltoid or quadriceps). Avoid choosing a muscle that has been needled during electromyography.

The following characteristic histological pattern may be found:

Denervation. In recent denervation small angulated muscle fibres with normal striations are seen scattered randomly between normal fibres. In chronic partial denervation, groups of atrophic fibres may be seen together with areas of hypertrophied fibres, resulting from re-innervative sprouting of surviving motor nerves. Histochemical stains readily confirm this grouping into uniform metabolic types.

Myopathic Changes. Grouped atrophy does not occur. The muscle fibres are diffusely abnormal with loss of normal architecture, central nuclei and often necrosis with macrophage invasion. In some forms interstitial inflammation occurs especially surrounding vessels. Basophilic fibres with large vesicular nuclei, due to regeneration, are present only in myopathies. In late stages the muscle fibres are replaced by fat cells and collagen deposition.

Specific Changes. These may be seen occasionally, only, for example parasitic infestation in trichinosis, specific granulomatous nodules in sarcoidosis, and direct inflammation and necrosis of arterial walls in polyarteritis. Foci of inflammatory cell infiltration may be seen in a number of diseases but particularly in connective tissue disorders. In polyarteritis this is associated with muscle necrosis and regeneration.

Serum Levels of Muscle Enzymes

Primary muscle diseases such as Duchenne muscular dystrophy and polymyositis are associated with markedly elevated levels of serum muscle enzymes (10 to 15 × normal), but moderate elevation may also be found in chronic denervation disorders, for example, motor neurone disease. The creatine phosphokinase is the most useful enzyme to be measured, but elevation of aldolase and transaminases may also occur.

Electromyography

Electromyography (EMG) is the examination of the electrical activity in skeletal muscle with fine needle electrodes and its display on an oscilloscope. The main routine uses of this technique are:

1. **Distinguishing Between Primary Muscle Disease and Denervation.** In primary muscle disease there is no spontaneous electrical activity, the motor unit action potentials are reduced in amplitude and duration, but are generally normal in number. In denervation, on the other hand, the number of muscle potentials is markedly reduced and the remaining potentials may be enlarged and prolonged in duration. Spontaneous activity is a hallmark of denervation. Fibrillations are small spontaneous potentials of short duration. These represent spontaneous contraction of single muscle fibres. Fasciculations are large amplitude spontaneous discharges resembling normal units or more frequently of bizarre shape. They represent the spontaneous discharge of motor units either in whole or part. A visible movement in the muscle is usually seen, but in young children and obese women this may be hidden by subcutaneous fat. They are most commonly seen in motor neurone diseases but can occur in otherwise normal persons, in which case the units are of entirely normal configuration.

2. **Demonstration of Miscellaneous Abnormalities.** Myotonic discharges are high frequency oscillations which characteristically wane both in amplitude and frequency causing a dive-bomber sound in the loudspeaker. They are generally induced by needle movement and are commonly seen in myotonic dystrophy.

3. **Demonstration of Abnormalities of Neuromuscular Transmission** (*see* 'Myasthenia gravis').

Clinical Assessment

The assessment of a case of possible skeletal muscle disease must proceed along orderly lines. The following aspects should be considered:

1. **Family History.** A positive family history can be expected particularly in the sex-linked and dominantly inherited types of muscular dystrophy.

2. **Age of Onset.** Most muscle diseases have a tendency to manifest themselves at particular ages. Thus, Duchenne muscular dystrophy usually manifests itself between the ages of two and five years but very rarely in infancy. Similarly, the other types of muscular dystrophy usually manifest themselves in adolescence or early adult life. On the other hand, polymyositis has a much wider age-scatter although it most commonly occurs in the fourth and fifth decades of life.

3. **Speed of Onset.** Primary muscle diseases do not usually develop very quickly. Two disorders cause widespread rapidly increasing weakness of muscles – poliomyelitis and acute polyneuritis (Guillain-Barré syndrome). Polymyositis tends to come on over a few months, and muscular dystrophy has a more insidious onset, frequently extending over years.

4. **Muscle Fatiguability.** Rapidly increasing weakness on exertion with recovery after rest is characteristic of myasthenia gravis.

5. **Muscle Tenderness and Pain.** Tenderness is unusual in primary muscle disease. It does, however, occur in poliomyelitis and in some chronic neuropathies (for example the alcoholic). A spontaneous complaint of muscle pain is also unusual in primary muscle disease, with the single exception of McArdle's syndrome (*see* page 625).

6. **Palpable Abnormalities of Muscle.** Occasionally, abnormal muscle feels peculiar. Thus, the muscles in Duchenne muscular dystrophy sometimes feel doughy. Such differences are very difficult to quantify.

7. **Visible Abnormalities of Muscle.** Fasciculation does not occur in primary muscle disease with the possible exception of thyrotoxicosis. It is common in motor neurone disease. Myotonia may be seen as a very slow relaxation after voluntary contraction or when the muscle belly is hit gently with a percussion hammer. A dimple in the muscle may appear and slowly disappear.

8. **Muscle Wasting.** In most instances of muscle disease weakness is accompanied by wasting. The principal exceptions are myasthenia gravis and early Duchenne muscular dystrophy. In the early stages of the latter condition muscles may be enlarged but weak (pseudohypertrophy).

9. **Distribution of Muscle Weakness.** A careful systematic examination of each muscle group is essential. The principal groups are given in Table 21.19.

10. **Tendon Reflexes.** The tendon reflexes are lost late in the course of primary muscle disease. A slow contraction and relaxation is seen in hypothyroidism. In motor neurone disease the reflexes are generally brisk despite marked muscle wasting and weakness.

11. **Skeletal Deformities and Contracture.** These may occur in the course of muscle disease, and are sometimes severe.

MYASTHENIA GRAVIS

Definition

A disease characterised by abnormal fatiguability of voluntary muscle with improvement in power following rest or the administration of anticholinesterases.

Background

The disease affects women twice as often as men and starts most frequently between the ages of 15 and 35.

Table 21.19 Muscles affected by disease

Muscle group	Clinical features	Diseases in which muscles are commonly affected
External eye muscles	Diplopia	Myasthenia, Ocular dystrophy
Jaw muscles	Chewing difficult, jaw may hang open	Myasthenia
Facial muscles	Difficulty with whistling. Patient has flat forehead, weakness of eye closure, expressionless face and a horizontal smile (myopathic facies)	Commonly in myasthenia, dystrophia myotonica and facio-scapulo-humeral dystrophy. Occasionally in polymyositis, common in Guillain-Barré syndrome (GBS) but not in chronic polyneuritis
Palate Pharyngeal Laryngeal	Weak voice, weak cough, dysphagia	Myasthenia. GBS. Motor neurone disease, Polymyositis
Tongue	Dysarthria	Uncommon except in motor neurone disease
Neck fixator muscles	Difficulty with keeping the head up	Polymyositis, Duchenne dystrophy, Myotonic dystrophy
Respiratory muscles	Breathlessness on mild exertion, poor chest movement	Myasthenia and terminal stages of Duchenne dystrophy. Otherwise uncommon in primary muscle disease
Trunk muscles	Difficulty with getting up from a lying to a sitting position	Occurs in severe cases of GBS
Proximal arm muscles	Difficulty with doing hair and hanging out washing	Occurs in all the common primary muscle diseases and GBS
Proximal leg muscles	Difficulty with going upstairs, getting on a bus, and getting out of a low chair	
Quadriceps	Knees give way readily	Many muscle diseases
Distal arm muscles	Difficulty with fine movements, buttons, etc.	Rarely severely affected in the earlier stages of primary muscle disease except in dystrophia myotonica. Commonly affected in polyneuropathies and motor neurone disease
Distal leg muscles	Wearing out the tips of the shoes and tripping over curbs and carpets. Patient catches toes on the ground and may have a high steppage gait.	

The prevalence is 20 to 50 per million.

Between ten and twenty per cent of cases overall have a thymic tumour, but the incidence of tumour increases with age and as many as eighty per cent show abnormal thymic histology. It has been clear for a long while that there is abnormality of neuromuscular transmission in this disease. Until recently, however, the nature of the abnormality has been unclear. There have been extensive searches over the years for a neuromuscular blocking agent in the blood of patients with myasthenia gravis, but the results were always inconclusive. There is, however, now little doubt that the disorder is due to a reduced number of functioning acetylcholine receptors and that this results from immunological damage provoked by circulating antibodies to the acetycholine receptor.

Pathology

The commonest histological changes in voluntary muscle are collections of lymphocytes, atrophy of muscle fibres and abnormalities of the nerve terminals and motor end-plates.

Symptoms and Signs

The cardinal abnormality in myasthenia gravis is the presence of undue fatiguability with maximal contraction. Symptoms may develop toward the end of the day or after physical exertion and there is a marked variability in muscle strength from day to day and from hour to hour. The cranial musculature is usually involved early.

Symptoms

Diplopia.
Drooping eyelids.
Difficulty with chewing (particularly steak!).
Difficulty with swallowing (sometimes with choking due to aspiration into the trachea).
Nasal regurgitation of fluids.
Slurred speech.
Difficulty with combing hair and going upstairs.

Signs

Defective eye movements.

Ptosis.

Weakness of the jaw.

Weakness of the facial muscles with inability to whistle and an expressionless face.

Palatal palsy.

Weakness of the proximal limb muscles.

The tendon reflexes are preserved and there is no sensory loss. Muscle wasting is rarely seen early in the disease, but may occur later.

Investigations

The object of these is, first, to make the diagnosis of myasthenia, and secondly, to ascertain whether there is any associated disease such as thymic tumour or thyrotoxicosis.

Diagnosis of Myasthenia

1. Intravenous edrophonium chloride (Tensilon). A syringe is loaded with 1 ml (10 mg). Initially, 2 mg is injected intravenously to detect undue sensitivity. The remaining 8 mg is then injected two minutes later. Improvement in ptosis or squint should be noted within one minute, and may be dramatic, but it lasts only two or three minutes. Improvement in the power of the limb musculature is much more difficult to detect because of the short time available for testing muscle strength.

2. Intramuscular injection of neostigmine. Usually 1.25 mg of neostigmine is combined with 0.6 mg of atropine. Careful measurements of muscle strength are necessary both before and after injection. Serial tape recordings of speech can be helpful. Improvement starts in ten to fifteen minutes and may last for two to three hours. In cases in which the response is equivocal the test can be repeated with 2.5 mg of neostigmine. Occasionally, neostigmine can precipitate an attack of bronchial asthma.

3. Electromyography. Repetitive supramaximal nerve stimuli produce a rapid decrease in the size of the evoked muscle action potential.

4. X-ray of chest and superior mediastinum to detect a thymic mass.

5. Thyroid function studies to exclude thyrotoxicosis.

Differential Diagnosis

1. Psychogenic weakness. The weakness fluctuates from second to second. (*Note:* Myasthenia gravis is the only condition in which there is a dramatic response to neostigmine.)

2. Other causes of diplopia; for example multiple sclerosis.

3. Other causes of bilateral ptosis, for example ocular myopathy and dystrophia myotonica (page 560). Occasionally, the myasthenic ptosis may be unilateral or moderately asymmetrical, and in this instance the differential diagnosis includes a IIIrd nerve palsy and 'Horner's syndrome'.

4. Other causes of proximal limb girdle weakness; for example muscular dystrophy and polymyositis.

5. Familial periodic paralysis. This is a rare disorder in which there are attacks of severe muscle weakness associated with abnormalities in the serum potassium level.

6. Cataplexy. Muscle weakness or paralysis is precipitated by strong emotion; e.g. laughing. This is usually accompanied by narcolepsy – inappropriate episodes of sleep.

Basis of Treatment

Anticholinesterases are required in all but the mildest case of myasthenia.

The two most commonly used drugs are:

1. Neostigmine bromide. The standard tablet contains 15 mg. The dose varies between half a tablet (7.5 mg) three times a day to 3 (45 mg) tablets every two hours.

2. Pyridostigmine bromide. The standard 60 mg tablet is approximately equivalent to 15 mg of neostigmine. The effect lasts rather longer than that produced by neostigmine.

Principles in Using Anticholinesterases. Always match the time and size of each dose to the needs of the individual patient. The drugs should be given prior to times of particular need; for example before public speaking.

Most people do not require atropine. Indeed, the parasympathetic effects (especially colic) may act as a useful warning of overdosage.

Watch out for overdosage. A cholinergic crisis may result, increasing doses of anticholinesterases producing increasing weakness. This is extremely dangerous.

Remember that myasthenia is a highly variable disease and drug dosage needs to be kept under constant review, particularly early in the course of the disease. Remember, too, that infections, emotional upsets, and extremes of heat and cold can increase the degree of weakness. In some patients a profound degree of weakness is produced by antibiotics, notably – *the mycins*.

Steroids and ACTH. Corticosteroids are not required for the 'average' case controlled with neostigmine. However, the response to corticosteroids is often dramatic and a good response can be expected in about fifty per cent of patients. It should be noted, however, that a transient worsening of the myasthenia sometimes precedes the improvement. Patients should, therefore, not be treated with steroids or ACTH unless there are facilities for assisted ventilation. The usual initial dose is 30 to 60 mg of prednisolone daily, but some workers recommend giving the steroids on alternate days. A small maintenance dose is required in some cases.

Thymectomy. Thymectomy is now recognised as being very important in the management of patients with myasthenia gravis. The incidence of remission increases with the number of years after thymectomy – complete or substantial improvement can be expected in eighty per cent of cases who do not have a thymic tumour. However, it may take three to five years before the benefits of operation are apparent. In patients who do have a tumour, early operation is indicated.

The risks of thymectomy are now small, provided that the operation is undertaken in a centre with good facilities for intensive care and where there is considerable experience of the operation.

Management of Severe Myasthenia. These patients have dysphagia, weak cough, and a poor respiratory reserve. They are in great danger of dying from inhalation pneumonia and hypoventilation resulting in cardio-respiratory arrest. A tracheostomy with or without assisted ventilation may be required. ACTH or steroids, if given as a short intensive course, may produce a remission.

The increasing evidence of the immunological causation of myasthenia gravis has led to considerable interest in immunosuppressive therapy. Thoracic duct drainage has a beneficial effect. Plasma exchange improves muscle strength in patients with severe myasthenia and it seems that the beneficial effects can be maintained with subsequent immunosuppressive treatment (for example with azathioprine).

Prognosis

Myasthenia gravis varies greatly in severity both from case to case and from time to time in the same case. At one end of the spectrum are cases (approximately twenty per cent of the total) in whom the muscle weakness produces no more than ptosis and/or diplopia. At the other end are the cases of extreme widespread weakness of bulbar and limb muscles. Complete or marked remission occasionally occurs early in the course of the disease.

MUSCULAR DYSTROPHY (*see* Table 21.20)

Definition

A group of genetically determined disorders in which there is progressive degeneration of skeletal muscles.

DUCHENNE MUSCULAR DYSTROPHY
(PSEUDO-HYPERTROPHIC)

Background

Duchenne muscular dystrophy is usually inherited as an X-linked recessive, although thirty per cent of cases occur by spontaneous mutations. It is the most rapidly progressive of the commoner types of muscular dystrophy. The disease affects male children, and the onset is in early childhood, usually before the fourth year. However, female carriers can sometimes be shown to manifest a subclinical myopathy (*see below*).

Symptoms and Signs

The pelvic girdle is involved first. The earliest symptom is usually an inability to run. Later, the gait becomes obviously clumsy, and there is a tendency to fall. The child has difficulty in getting into an erect position and has to climb up his legs with his arms (Gower's sign). Weakness of the arms is usually noted by the age of 5 or 6. Pseudo-hypertrophy may be present (due partly to the large amount of intramuscular fat) and is usually seen in the calves. The disease progresses rapidly so that most children become severely disabled within a few years and chairbound by 10 years of age. Contractures ultimately develop (flexion deformities of the arms and legs, and scoliosis) making nursing difficult.

Investigations

1. Serum levels of muscle enzymes. The creatine phosphokinase (CPK) is usually grossly elevated (200× normal is not uncommon), particularly early in the course of the disease.
2. Muscle biopsy. The characteristic findings are:
(a) Enormous variation in the size of the muscle fibres, fibres that are both much smaller and much larger than normal being seen.
(b) Fibres undergoing necrosis, and others showing regeneration are common in early cases.
(c) A large increase in the amount of intramuscular fat.
3. Electromyogram (EMG). A myopathic pattern will be seen.

Prognosis

The cause of muscular dystrophy is unknown and no curative treatment is available. Most children are in a wheelchair within ten years of onset and survival beyond the age of 20 is unusual. Death is usually due to pneumonia or to heart failure (the myocardium is invariably involved by the myopathic process). There is a less common form of the disease, inherited as an autosomal recessive, in which the sexes are equally affected, and the progress of the disease is slower than in the classical form.

Basis of Treatment

Life can be made tolerable by thoughtful, sympathetic management.

In the early stages, prolonged bed rest (for example, after infections or surgery) invariably makes the disability worse. Activities that involve walking and the main-

Table 21.20   The common forms of muscular dystrophy

Type	Inheritance	Onset	Progress	Muscles particularly affected	Pseudo-hypertrophy	Serum level of muscle enzymes	Comments
Duchenne (pseudo-hypertrophic)	Sex linked Recessive Males affected (occasionally autosomal recessive)	Early childhood	Rapid Usually in a wheelchair by 10 and dead by 20 (pneumonia or heart failure)	Initially the pelvic girdle – later all the limb and trunk muscles Myocardium	Usual	Very high, especially early in the disease	Female carriers may also show a raised serum muscle enzyme level
Limb girdle	Autosomal recessive Sometimes sporadic	Very variable Usually 10 to 20	Variable Usually severe disability within 20 years Premature death	Muscles of pelvic and shoulder girdle	Occasionally	Slightly raised	
Facio-scapulo-humeral	Autosomal dominant	Variable Usually 10 to 20 but often later	Usually very slow. Patient not usually severely disabled Normal life expectancy	Starts in face and shoulder girdle Pelvic girdle affected later	Rare	Slightly raised or normal	This is the most benign of the commoner muscular dystrophies Very variable in severity
Dystrophia myotonica	Autosomal dominant	Variable 20 to 60 Rare congenital form	Most patients are unable to walk 20 years after onset Premature death (pneumonia or heart failure)	Facial Sternomastoids Distal limb muscles	Absent	Usually normal	Muscle weakness is only a *part* of the disorder Other features – Myotonia, one-third present with this Cataracts Testicular and ovarian atrophy

tenance of mobility should be encouraged.

Later, passive stretching of affected muscles and proper posturing of the patient is essential if contractures are to be avoided.

A light spinal support can prevent a severe scoliosis.

Over-eating must be avoided because obesity makes nursing very difficult and may embarrass breathing and cardiac function.

Respiratory infections are potentially lethal and require treating (poor respiratory reserve).

Genetic Advice. The most hopeful way of eliminating this disease is to detect the carriers of the abnormal gene and to advise strongly against pregnancies. A female having an affected brother has a 50 per cent chance of being a carrier. For a woman known to be a carrier there is a high risk that any pregnancy will result in an affected son or carrier daughter. Many, if not all, female carriers have a slight degree of myopathy which can usually be detected; about seventy per cent show an elevated serum CPK level. Some also show abnormalities on EMG and muscle biopsy.

LIMB GIRDLE AND FACIO-SCAPULO-HUMERAL MUSCULAR DYSTROPHY

Details of these two forms of muscular dystrophy are given in Table 21.20. The most benign of the muscular dystrophies is the facio-scapulo-humeral type, and people with this disorder have a virtually normal life expectancy.

DYSTROPHIA MYOTONICA

For full details *see* Table 21.20. This disorder is inherited as an autosomal dominant trait. It mainly affects the face, the sternomastoids, and the distal limb muscles. Myotonia can usually be observed and consists of delay in relaxation after a sustained muscular contraction. Thus, if the belly of the affected muscle is hit with a tendon hammer, extremely slow relaxation is noted to occur (percussion myotonia). Myotonia is not usually very troublesome, and treatment is not usually necessary. Phenytoin sodium is probably the drug of choice but procaine amide, quinine, and steroids are sometimes effective.

Dystrophia myotonica is associated with other, non-muscular abnormalities, the principal ones being frontal baldness, gonadal atrophy, and the occurrence of cataracts.

CONGENITAL MYOPATHY

A familiar problem to paediatricians is that of hypotonic weakness from birth. Some of the cases fall into the group known by the name of benign congenital hypotonia, the condition being non-progressive and sometimes showing complete recovery. Other cases show one of the rare forms of non-progressive myopathy such as central core disease. Occasional cases are due to Duchenne muscular dystrophy, although this is usually not evident in infancy. Muscle biopsy and estimation of the serum levels of muscle enzymes are of great importance in distinguishing these conditions.

POLYMYOSITIS

Definition

The term polymyositis is used to cover a group of disorders, of mainly unknown cause, characterised pathologically by non-suppurative inflammation and degenerative change in skeletal muscle and, clinically, by muscular weakness. About fifty per cent of cases have skin changes and for these the term dermatomyositis is sometimes used.

Background

A proportion of patients with polymyositis have evidence of a diffuse collagen disease such as rheumatoid arthritis, scleroderma or disseminated lupus erythematosus. This close connection with other connective tissue disorders has suggested that the disorder may have an autoimmune basis. Another group of cases is associated with carcinoma, particularly of the lung. The muscle disorder may antedate the discovery of the carcinoma by months or years. Again, it is suggested that the tumour may produce some substance which provokes an antigen/antibody reaction in the muscle. Other uncommon causes include sarcoidosis and various drugs (particularly chloroquine). Approximately fifty per cent of cases are unassociated with any other obvious pathological process or cause. Polymyositis can occur at any age but is commonest in the 4th and 5th decades.

Pathology

The histological findings in affected muscles may be summarised as follows:
1. Widespread destruction of muscle fibres.
2. Patchy collections of inflammatory cells. The number

of these is very variable and some cases show very little inflammatory infiltration while others show a great deal.
3. Regeneration with basophilic staining of the sarcoplasm.

Table 21.21 Symptoms and signs of polymyositis

Symptoms	Signs
Early:	
Difficulty with rising from a low chair, going upstairs, and combing the hair	Proximal muscle weakness Muscle tenderness is unusual
Late:	
Inability to walk or to use the arms Dysphagia Difficulty with breathing and coughing Breathlessness	Marked weakness of the limbs plus weakness of the bulbar, neck, and respiratory muscles Evidence of heart failure and cardiac arrhythmias

Symptoms and Signs (*see* Table 21.21)

Most patients show the insidious, painless, development of proximal limb weakness. Later, the bulbar muscles, and the heart, may be involved. A variety of skin changes occur. Particularly characteristic is the occurrence of a lilac-coloured change in the skin of the upper eyelids and forehead. Non-specific patches of dermatitis may occur. Raynaud's phenomenon occurs in some cases.

Investigations

The first problem is to make the diagnosis of polymyositis.
1. Serum levels of muscle enzymes, especially creatine kinase. These are usually elevated in the acute stage.
2. EMG. A myopathic pattern is found. In addition, fibrillation potentials and other evidence of neurogenic involvement can be demonstrated in some cases.
3. Muscle biopsy. This is very important. A good biopsy should be taken from a muscle that is moderately affected clinically.
Once the diagnosis of polymyositis has been made it is important, as a second stage, to look for a latent neoplasm and for evidence of more generalised disease.
4. Chest X-ray and barium meal examination.
5. Plasma viscosity or ESR. These are sometimes raised but are often normal.
6. Tests relevant in cases of possible connective tissue disease. – LE cells, antinuclear factor, and so on.

Differential Diagnosis

This is usually from other conditions that cause weakness of the proximal limb muscles.

1. **Muscular Dystrophy.** This usually starts in the first three decades of life, the development is much slower than polymyositis, and the family history is sometimes positive.

2. **Motor Neurone Disease.** This is rarely symmetrical and there is usually fasciculation in affected muscles. In addition, there may be brisk tendon reflexes and extensor plantar responses.

Basis of Treatment

As in other inflammatory conditions of unknown cause, steroids have been found to produce a beneficial effect. They are used initially in high dosage but need to be continued in lower dosage for a long period. Some workers have found that immunosuppressive drugs, for example azathioprine, are of benefit and exert a steroid sparing effect. It has been suggested that low doses of penicillin should be given prophylactically on a long term basis, but the value of this is unproven.

Once the diagnosis of polymyositis is made, prednisolone in a dosage of 40 to 60 mg/day should be started. The steroid dosage should be regulated by the clinical response and by the level of serum enzymes. This high dosage of steroids may need to be continued for two or three months and a lower dose may need to be continued for up to two years. A small proportion of cases of polymyositis associated with malignancy respond to steroids. Some of these may also respond to removal of the neoplasm, but both the response to steroids and removal of the primary tumour is unpredictable.

Prognosis

Most cases show some response to steroids, with evidence of marked improvement in muscle function. Only rarely does the disease progress to severe permanent disablement. Death, due to the disease, is uncommon, and when it does occur it is usually due to involvement of bulbar or respiratory muscles or to cardiac failure.

METABOLIC MUSCLE DISEASE

The limits of this group cannot be clearly defined. Many disorders produce some disturbance of function, albeit mild, of skeletal muscle. The most important ones, from a clinical point of view, are as follows:
1. Diseases of the thyroid gland – thyrotoxicosis and hypothyroidism.
2. Cushing's disease and corticosteroids therapy.
3. Changes in serum potassium levels.
4. Osteomalacia.
5. Myopathy induced by drugs or toxins.
6. McArdle's syndrome.

THYROTOXICOSIS

A mild degree of limb girdle weakness is extremely common in untreated thyrotoxicosis. In a few instances a *marked* degree of proximal muscle weakness occurs. Occasionally, the bulbar muscles are maximally affected. Considerable diagnostic difficulty may be encountered if the muscle weakness is the presenting feature and the other manifestations of thyrotoxicosis are not clinically obvious. Muscle biopsy is usually unimpressive. The weakness resolves completely when the thyrotoxicosis is treated.

Exophthalmic ophthalmoplegia involves weakness of the external ocular muscles with exophthalmos. The subject is dealt with elsewhere (*see* page 172).

Occasionally, myasthenia and periodic paralysis, associated with hypokalaemia may occur in thyrotoxicosis.

HYPOTHYROIDISM

Sluggish tendon reflexes with a reduction in the speed of contraction and relaxation are seen. There is rarely any complaint of muscle weakness, but very occasionally a proximal myopathy may occur.

CUSHING'S DISEASE, AND CORTICOSTEROIDS

A proximal limb girdle myopathy sometimes occurs in Cushing's disease and in people treated with corticosteroids (especially those containing a fluorine atom at the 9 alpha position) for prolonged periods. Few histological changes occur. Corticosteroid-induced myopathy usually recovers when therapy is stopped, but that occurring in Cushing's disease recovers less well.

CHANGES IN SERUM POTASSIUM LEVEL

The normal electrical polarisation of the muscle membrane is related to the high intracellular, and the low extracellular, concentration of potassium. The muscle action potential is accompanied by an outward movement of potassium ions from the muscle cells. Gross changes, upwards or downwards, in the level of serum potassium will affect this process and lead to clinical weakness. Skeletal, smooth, and cardiac muscle are all affected.

HYPOKALAEMIC FAMILIAL PERIODIC PARALYSIS

This is an uncommon disorder inherited in an autosomal dominant fashion. Attacks of severe weakness and paralysis of skeletal muscle occur and may last for several hours. The attacks may be precipitated by a heavy carbohydrate meal. The serum potassium is usually low during the attack. The attack frequency may be lessened by avoiding carbohydrates. Individual attacks may respond to oral potassium.

OSTEOMALACIA

Patients with osteomalacia may develop weakness of the limb girdles. The exact cause is unknown but vitamin D therapy may produce some improvement.

DRUGS AND TOXINS

Steroid therapy is frequently associated with muscle weakness and is discussed above. Chloroquine may produce a myopathy affecting mainly the pelvic girdle. Characteristic vacuolar changes occur in the muscle fibres. Myopathic weakness may sometimes occur in alcoholic subjects. Acute and chronic syndromes occur but are not common.

McARDLE'S SYNDROME

This is a rare recessively inherited disorder in which the patient experiences severe painful muscle cramps on exertion. Exercise fails to produce the normal elevation in blood lactate, due to an inability to break down muscle glycogen. This abnormality has been shown to be associated with a virtual absence of muscle phosphorylase.

SUGGESTED FURTHER READING

General

Adams, R. D. and Victor, M. (1977) *Principles of Neurology.* New York: McGraw-Hill Book Company.
Bickerstaff, E. R. (1973) *Neurological Examination in Clinical Practice.* 3rd ed. Oxford: Blackwell.
Harrison's Principles of Internal Medicine (1977), 8th ed, p. 69–157. McGraw-Hill Book Company. This section provides an excellent discussion of some of the main symptoms in neurology.
Holmes, G. (1971). *An Introduction to Clinical Neurology,* 3rd ed. Edinburgh: Churchill Livingstone.
Jennett, W. B. (1977) *An Introduction to Neurosurgery,* 3rd ed. London: Heinemann.
Matthews, W. B. (1975) *Practical Neurology,* 3rd ed. Oxford: Blackwell.
Walton, J. N. (1975) *Essentials of Neurology,* 4th ed. London: Pitman Medical.
Spillane, J. D. (1975) *An Atlas of Clinical Neurology,* 2nd ed. Oxford: Oxford University Press.

Cerebrovascular Disease

Adams, G. F. (1974) *Cerebrovascular Disease and the Aging Brain.* Edinburgh: Churchill Livingstone.
Gardner, H. (1977). *The Shattered Mind.* Routledge and Kegan Paul.
Marshall, J. (1976) *The Management of Cerebrovascular Disease,* 3rd ed. London: Churchill.
Russell, R. W. R. (ed.) (1976) *Cerebral Arterial Disease.* Edinburgh: Churchill Livingstone.

Coma and Head Injury

Plum, F. and Posner, J. B. (1972) *Diagnosis of Stupor and Coma,* 2nd ed. Oxford: Blackwell.
Potter, J. M. (1974) *The Practical Management of Head Injuries.* 3rd ed. London: Lloyd-Luke.

Cranial Nerves

Brodal, A. (1965) *The Cranial Nerves – Anatomy and Anatomico-Clinical Correlations,* 2nd ed. Oxford: Blackwell.
Hughes, B. (1954) *The Visual Fields.* Oxford: Blackwell.

Epilepsy

Laidlaw, J. and Richens, A. (1976) *A Text Book of Epilepsy.* Edinburgh: Churchill Livingstone.

Genetics

Pratt, R. T. C. (1967) *Genetics of Neurological Disorders.* Oxford: Oxford University Press.

Headache

Lance, J. W. (1978) *The Mechanism and Management of Headache,* 3rd ed. London: Butterworths.

Multiple Sclerosis

British Medical Bulletin, January 1977, **33**, No. 1. Multiple Sclerosis.
McAlpine, D., Lumsden, C. E. and Acheson, E. D. (1972) *Multiple Sclerosis – A Reappraisal,* 2nd ed. Edinburgh: Livingstone.

Muscle Disease

Lenman, J. A. R. and Ritchie, A. E. (1977) *Clinical Electromyography,* 2nd ed. London: Pitman Medical.
Walton, J. N. (1974) *Disorders of Voluntary Muscle,* 3rd ed. London: Churchill.

Peripheral Nervous System

Medical Research Council Memorandum (1976) *Aids to the Investigation of the Peripheral Nervous System.* London: HMSO.
Sunderland, Sir S. (1978) *Nerves and Nerve Injuries,* 2nd ed. Edinburgh: Livingstone.
Wilkinson, M. (1971) *Cervical Spondylosis,* 2nd ed. London: Heinemann.

Rehabilitation

Nichols, P. J. R. (1971) *Rehabilitation of the Severely Disabled: 2 – Management.* London: Butterworths.
Nichols, P. J. R. and Hamilton, E. A. (1976) *Rehabilitation Medicine.* London: Butterworths.

Spinal Cord

Guttmann, Sir L. (1976) *Spinal Cord Injuries,* 2nd ed. Oxford: Blackwell.
Hughes, J. T. (1978) *Pathology of the Spinal Cord,* 2nd ed. London: Lloyd-Luke.

Chronic Disease and Disability 22

R. LANGTON HEWER

Despite the best endeavours of modern medicine there are many patients who cannot be cured. Some have in front of them a future which may involve many years of chronic illness. Examples include rheumatoid arthritis and multiple sclerosis. In other instances, the acute event has long since past but the patient is left with permanent damage. Such a situation may exist after poliomyelitis or trauma. It is estimated that in Britain there are at least one and a half million physically handicapped people.

Before embarking upon a discussion of the problems of chronic disease it is necessary to define three terms that are in common usage – impairment, disability and handicap.

Impairment. The term impairment refers to physical defects and the loss of normal bodily mechanical functions.

Disablement. Disablement is a consequence of the impairment. Thus a patient with rheumatoid arthritis may have extensive disease, and deformity, of the joints producing a substantial impairment. The inability to write, feed, dress and walk represents the resultant reduction in functional capability and is referred to as disability.

Handicap. The term handicap is used to describe the social effects of impairment or disabilities. Thus a patient with rheumatoid arthritis may be handicapped by being unable to work or even to visit the shops.

The physically handicapped do not form a homogeneous group. For example, a patient with chronic painful rheumatoid arthritis will require very different help from one suffering from multiple sclerosis, chronic bronchitis or epilepsy. Nonetheless, disabled people do have certain common disadvantages. Restrictive mobility, loss of income and the prejudices of the able-bodied members of the population are all examples of phenomena which can deny disabled people a satisfactory place in the community.

Two developments in the field of physical handicap have been of particular importance. The first was the passing of the *Chronically Sick and Disabled Persons Act, 1970*. The second was the publication of a report entitled, *Handicapped and Impaired in Great Britain* (Harris *et al.*, 1971). This latter document gave the results of a comprehensive national survey of handicapped and impaired persons living in the community. It has provided the basic data so essential for setting up a rational system of help for this large and important group of people.

What Are the Chronic Diseases?

Thirty to forty years ago infectious diseases, such as poliomyelitis and tuberculosis were rampant, producing a large amount of disability. Cerebral palsy and spina bifida were bigger problems than they are today. Improved techniques for prevention and treatment of these various conditions have been developed and as a result there has been a marked reduction in the number of persons disabled because of these disorders. In addition there were large numbers of war wounded, many of whom have now died. The situation has now changed and 'degenerative disease' has become the major cause of chronic impairment. In Western Europe most physical limitations now occur amongst people aged 50 and over. In numerical terms those who become disabled before middle life form only a small, albeit very important, proportion of disabled people.

Some of the most challenging problems occur in children and adolescents. In the first few years of life serious physical disability and handicap is caused by spina bifida, hydrocephalus, cerebral palsy and muscular dystrophy. Other important childhood problems include chronic asthma, poliomyelitis, epilepsy and Still's disease. One of the main risks of becoming disabled during the latter years of childhood and in early adult life stems from accidents – either on the road or in the home. The problems encountered during childhood may persist through middle life. At this point a number of other disorders, such as multiple sclerosis and rheumatoid arthritis become evident. About 75 per cent of patients in units for the younger chronic sick are there as a result of neurological disease.

Most physical limitations, however, occur amongst people aged 50 and over. The main causes of impairment are arthritis, stroke and bronchitis. Coronary artery disease, lower limb ischaemia, Parkinson's disease and dementia are other important problems. Further significant causes of disability include blindness, deafness, congenital malformations, injuries (including amputations), chronic renal and hepatic failure, alcoholism, chronic ulcerative colitis and chronic anaemia (especially in tropical countries).

Although this chapter is concerned primarily with the long term effects of chronic physical disease, it is nevertheless important to record that psychiatric disorders also produce disability and handicap. Important examples are depression, schizophrenia and the obsessional states. Furthermore, there are a large number of mentally subnormal people. The majority of these patients live in the community but others require care and supervision in hospital or in some other form of residential establishment.

Main causes of severe and very severe handicap in adults of working age

Arthritis – including rheumatoid arthritis.
Stroke.
Parkinsonism.
Cardio-respiratory disorders – especially chronic bronchitis.
Trauma and amputations.
Disorders acquired in childhood – e.g. cerebral palsy.
Multiple sclerosis.

THE ELDERLY

The past few decades have seen a marked increase in the number of older people in Western countries. In the United Kingdom the proportion of persons over retirement age has risen from about 5 per cent at the beginning of the century to over 16 per cent now. This trend is expected to continue until at least the end of the century. The result is that the prevalence of degenerative disease has markedly increased. In addition, for reasons previously stated, the number of people with physical impairment and disability has risen markedly.

Old people are vulnerable to any change in the somewhat precarious equilibrium upon which their independence rests. An illness, such as pneumonia, may produce only a few days' incapacity in a young man. The same illness in an older person may result in collapse of the previous state of equilibrium with, for example, the development of incontinence, confusion and loss of mobility. Such a patient requires careful management in order to enable him to regain his former

independence. It is all too easy for him to become yet another 'chronic case'. Some of the particular medical problems affecting the elderly are shown in Table 22.1.

There are a variety of non-medical factors which affect the situation. These may be as important, if not more so than the medical ones. For instance, the spouse of an ill person may be frail and quite unable to undertake the extra duties involved in caring for an ill or disabled person. Housing is often unsuitable, particularly if there are stairs and no downstairs toilet. Frequently, the medical and social problems are inextricably intertwined. Thus the frail old lady who cannot afford proper food and warmth will be prone to develop deficiency diseases (for instance scurvy) and hypother-

Table 22.1 Particular medical problems affecting the elderly

Problem	Comment
Impaired homeostasis and defence mechanisms	Impaired resistance to infection, dehydration, and hypothermia are all liable to occur.
High incidence of degenerative disease	Examples include osteoarthritis, defective hearing and vision, brittle bones, and impaired circulation to the legs. Healing may be slow.
High incidence of cancer and vascular disease	The prevalence of vascular disease and cancer rises with age.
Likelihood of *multiple* disease	For example, the patient who has developed a stroke may also have diabetes, defective vision, *and* chronic heart failure.
Altered presentation of disease	Disease may present in a less florid and dramatic way in elderly people. For example, thyrotoxicosis may present only with atrial fibrillation. The patient with pneumonia may have no fever.
Intellectual failure	Mental slowness is common. The problem is frequently complicated by deafness. Acute confusional states occur readily and can be induced by drugs, infection, or a sudden change to unaccustomed surroundings.
Decreased tolerance to drugs	Old people do not tolerate drugs well. The doses which are appropriate in middle age may produce side effects in the elderly.
Immobility	Older people are frequently unsteady. Falls are common. The patient may become bedridden as the result of a minor illness.
Incontinence	Some degree of urinary incontinence is very common amongst the elderly. Causes include difficulty with getting to the toilet, prostatic enlargement, and urinary tract infections.

mia. Any attempt at rehabilitation must take into account *both* the medical and social problems. The care of the elderly requires much patience, sympathy and understanding. It also requires a knowledge of the special problems of the elderly and, above all, time.

THE CONCEPT OF REHABILITATION

Rehabilitation involves the management of those patients who have passed the acute stage of their illness but are left with residual problems. The term is used to describe the process of restoring a disabled person to a condition in which he is able to resume as normal a life as possible. Virtually every disorder which cannot be totally cured leads to some degree of disability, either temporary or permanent. The subject is therefore seen to be of concern to all clinicians, although with differing emphasis in different specialities.

The essence of rehabilitation, as in the rest of medicine, lies in accurate diagnosis and prognosis and in appropriate treatment and management. It involves co-operation with a number of professional groups including social workers and remedial therapists. It is also important to have some knowledge of the interrelated provisions of the Health Service, Local Authority, Department of Employment, Department of Education and voluntary organisations.

Many patients admitted to hospital do not require intensive rehabilitation. However, it is essential that the consultant, or his deputy, should indicate clearly to the patient, his relatives and the family doctor the expected prognosis of the disease, the likely outcome of treatment together with an indication of when he can be expected to return to work. Unless this happens, uncertainty prevails and the patient loses confidence in his medical advisers with resultant depression and prolonged invalidity.

It will be immediately realised that a large number of professional groups are involved in rehabilitation. These include the patient and his family, the general practitioner, the hospital consultant, the social worker, nursing staff and remedial therapists. Other people whose help may be required include the employment officer and psychologist. The doctor has a central role to play. In addition to being concerned with diagnosis and medical treatment, he will also be responsible for the medical care of the patient (prescribing drugs, etc.). It is also usually the doctor who is responsible for co-ordinating the activities of the various groups involved. The general practitioner occupies a key position and will be able to keep the patient and his family under close observation. He will also be in a good position to liaise with the various community services including particularly the Social Services, the health visitor and the District Nursing Service.

Assessment

The doctor's first job is always to make a precise diagnosis in terms of disease – for example, multiple sclerosis, rheumatoid arthritis, etc. He must ascertain whether the disease is still active, whether drug or surgical treatment is likely to be helpful, the prognosis (in terms of survival and progression of the disease) and the possible complications which may occur. It is also important to list those problems which affect the patient's functional status. Thus, for example, a patient with multiple sclerosis may have a number of distinct but interrelated problems which might include partial blindness, incontinence of urine, severe spasticity of the legs and pressure sores. Each of these problems must be identified and managed.

Table 22.2 Principal factors requiring assessment

Medical problems	For example – pain, continence, pressure sores, flexor spasms, contractures, amputation, breathlessness, angina, etc.
Mental state	Depression, motivation, confusion, realism, etc.
Mobility	Transferring, walking indoors, stairs, car-driver, bus-passenger, wheelchair, etc.
Communication	Vision, hearing, speech, writing.
Self-care activities	Feeding, toilet, washing, bathing, preparing meals etc.
Sexual activity	
Employment	
Housing	Stairs, access to toilet, width of door for wheelchair, etc.
Persons available to care for the patient	Wife, husband, child, etc. – note their state of health.
Recreational activities and hobbies	

The principal factors requiring assessment are given in Table 22.2. The assessment is undertaken by various members of the rehabilitation team. It is usual for an assessment meeting to be called – chaired by the consultant or his deputy. It should be possible to draw up a list of problems and to make an appraisal of the situation. It will be necessary to set realistic objectives and to make sensible recommendations about treatment and management. For some disabled patients it may not be practical to do more than aim for a reasonably pain-free existence in the confines of his own home. Others may need to be retrained for a new job.

Rehabilitation of the Elderly

Many years ago, when geriatric departments were first being established, it became recognised that the *chronicity* of the illness which affected many elderly people was the result of neglect. It was shown that much could be done for many of these seemingly hopeless cases. The result has been a considerable reduction in the number of old people in long-stay hospitals. This has been achieved by recognising the special problem of the elderly and by applying the principles of rehabilitation.

In recent years there have been two major innovations in the field of geriatrics. The first has been the increase in the number of day hospitals. These are day units whose main purpose is to reduce the length of in-patient stay for some patients and to obviate the need for admission of others. Another important function is the physical maintenance of old people who are likely to deteriorate following discharge from the therapeutic environment of the hospital. The second development is the establishment of the five-day geriatric rehabilitation ward. Rehabilitation of many elderly and disabled patients can be conducted on a five-day basis. This sharing of care by the hospital and family seems to have a beneficial effect on recovery and morale – adjustment to living at home being gradually achieved.

Regretfully, many old people and their relatives, and even some doctors, have an unduly pessimistic view of the outcome of treatment. The suggestion that there may be scope for improvement is often expressed as, 'What do you expect at my age, Doctor?' These prejudices need to be constantly counteracted. The benefits of energetic management of this age group have been convincingly demonstrated by several studies.

Summary of the Main Principles Involved in Rehabilitation

1. Clinicians should accept responsibility for the management of patients who have failed to respond to treatment and are left with permanent disability. Some disabilities, such as pressure sores and joint contractures are avoidable and every effort must be made to prevent them.
2. The rehabilitation of a patient requires team-work and the clinician should provide the leadership. He must not only understand how nurses and remedial therapists can help the patient, but should encourage them to evaluate their treatment objectively.
3. An accurate and detailed assessment of function should be considered as important as the diagnosis. Such an assessment can have a profound effect on a patient's capacity to be independent at home or to return to employment.
4. The patient and his close relatives have the right to be involved in decisions about treatment and resettlement.
5. The clinician should learn to recognise and assess psychological effects of injury and disease and to determine what motivates individual patients to achieve their maximum potential.

6. Medical care is not complete until the patient has been trained to live and to work with whatever capabilities remain.

SOCIAL AND PSYCHOLOGICAL EFFECTS OF CHRONIC ILLNESS

Some factors which influence the level of ultimate handicap

1. Nature of the illness.
2. Age of the patient.
3. Premorbid state of health.
4. Premorbid personality.
5. Practical effects of the disease.
6. Extent of support from spouse and family.
7. Financial state.
8. Quality and extent of help offered by medical, social work, nursing and paramedical staff.

It is a common observation that the degree of handicap is not always indicative of the severity of the underlying disease. Thus one individual can be back at work as though nothing had happened three months after a severe heart attack. Another may still be a cardiac invalid three years after a minor attack. It is clear that many factors influence the patient's ultimate degree of handicap. Prominent amongst these is his personality and his attitude to life in general. The term motivation is frequently used to describe the drive and enthusiasm shown by the patient in attempting to overcome his difficulties. Some of the factors that influence the ultimate level of handicap are discussed below.

Nature of the Illness

There are at least four features of the disease itself which can influence the patient's reaction to it. These include:

1. *Whether or not the illness is recognised as being potentially fatal*. Myocardial infarction and subarachnoid haemorrhage are two obvious examples of 'disease' which could cause sudden death. Feeling that one is at the edge of a precipice is bound to engender a certain amount of anxiety.
2. *Mode of onset*. Patients with gradually progressive disorders, such as rheumatoid arthritis, react differently to those in whom the onset is sudden. Thus, for example, many patients who have suddenly become paralysed as a result of a stroke seem to expect that the limbs will recover equally rapidly. Years after the stroke, patients may be found nursing the paralysed arm, 'I am waiting for it to come back, Doctor.'
3. *The prognosis*. Disorders which relapse and remit, such as multiple sclerosis and rheumatoid arthritis,

produce particular psychological problems. Despair and hope may occur at different times and are particularly difficult to manage. Even a severe degree of disability produced by a 'once and for all' cerebral insult (for example after trauma) is easier to accept than uncertainty.

4. *Whether the disease affects the brain directly*. Involvement of the brain (for example, by stroke or encephalitis) will probably have an important impact on the patient's ability to cope with his disability. The long term result may include defective judgement, intellectual function, memory and emotional control.

Premorbid State of Health

Older patients are particularly liable to suffer with a variety of physical problems. Thus, a stroke may occur in a person who is already obese, in heart failure and suffering with chronic osteoarthritis. Obviously these medical problems are likely to have an important effect upon the ultimate level of disability and handicap.

Premorbid Personality

Some people are more resilient to the effects of disease than others. When assessing the impact of personality, it is important to enquire about previous psychiatric disturbances – for instance episodes of aggression and depression. It is desirable to know how the patient has 'coped' with previous crises such as unemployment, family bereavement and financial difficulties. It is also important to enquire about any previous experience of disease. Thus, for example, the man who watched his father become progressively more disabled as a result of successive strokes may well have a particular dread of having a stroke himself. When he actually does so the effects may be catastrophic.

It is also important to find out about the patient's previous interests and hobbies. This is yet another factor which may have an important bearing on the outcome. Thus the busy business executive whose whole life has been devoted to his job and who has never had time for his family or for recreational activities, may become lost when he is disabled and unable to work. His whole *raison d'etre* has disappeared. Such people frequently find it difficult to adjust to a restrictive life-style. On the other hand, the patient with a wide range of hobbies and interests may find it easier to build a new life for himself.

Practical Effects of the Disease

A large range of problems can result from chronic disease including pain, immobility, incontinence, impotence, loss of employment and physical dependency. Much will depend on the patient's ability to tolerate and accept these difficulties. The severity of these problems and the patient's ability to come to terms with them are closely interrelated.

Extent of Support from Spouse and Family

Once again, much will depend upon the situation which existed *before* the illness developed. A shaky marriage may be totally disrupted by chronic illness. The spouse (whether husband or wife) may leave home with the result that nobody is available to care for the patient. On the other hand, a loving, capable spouse may be able to greatly help the patient to make the best of a difficult situation by providing physical and psychological support. However, at this point, it must be noted that the illness is likely to have profound indirect effects on the spouse, who may herself develop symptoms such as depression and anxiety.

As already noted, chronic illness frequently affects older people. Often the spouse will be frail and unable to cope with heavy nursing duties (which may include having to lift the patient). In other cases the patient may have been living alone before the illness occurred. In these instances the patient may require some form of long term residential care.

Financial State

Chronic illness in adults of working age is likely to have a serious impact upon the financial security of the family. Thus, the bread-winner becomes unable to work and may find that he is unable to meet financial commitments, such as mortgage and hire-purchase repayments. This is bound to produce considerable anxiety.

However, there may also be substantial *disincentives* to re-acquiring the maximum possible independence. For instance, an 'attendance allowance' is payable if the patient is at home and requires constant attention. Any improvement in the patient's condition may result in the loss of the allowance. Similarly, the total allowances payable to a man with a wife and several children may be substantially more than he earned while at work. A disincentive also exists when a compensation claim has been made for financial recompense, for example, for the effects of an industrial or road traffic accident.

Quality and Extent of Help Offered by Medical, Social Work, Nursing and Paramedical Staff

There seems little doubt that the efficient diagnosis and management of disease and the resulting disability can result in a much lower degree of handicap than would have otherwise existed. A good example is the highly organised management of paraplegic patients which has developed at Stoke Mandeville Hospital. The quality of life of paraplegic patients has been infinitely improved as the result of the approaches and techniques developed in that centre.

Patients and their families can be helped to overcome their fears and worries by informed and sympathetic handling by the hospital and community staff. Regretfully, it is all too easy to allow problems to go unrecognised, without specific provision being made for dealing with them. All the relevant staff, whether medical, social, nursing or remedial should be familiar with the patients' problems and it is important that someone should be *specifically* responsible for undertaking the supportive role to which we have alluded above. In hospital, this task often falls to the already overburdened ward sister. In other instances this is undertaken by the social worker or doctor.

STATUTORY AND NON-STATUTORY HELP FOR THE CHRONICALLY SICK AND DISABLED

There are a bewildering number of sources of help for the chronically sick and disabled. This section attempts to describe these and to indicate where help may be found. Some disabled persons are unaware of what is available and as a result there is an appreciable amount of unnecessary hardship.

Help may be provided by a number of different bodies and the most important are the various departments of the Local Authority, the Department of Health and Social Security (DHSS), the Area Health Authority, the Employment Services Agency and various voluntary organisations such as the Red Cross.

Registration of the physically handicapped is carried out by local authorities under Section 29 of the *National Assistance Act, 1948* and the *Chronically Sick and Disabled Persons Act, 1970*. The authorities are required to maintain a register of those who are receiving a service from the Social Services Department and those who request registration. Yearly returns are required by the Department of Health and Social Security of the numbers registered. The register helps the department to develop appropriate services and to help those most in need. A thorough assessment is made at the time of registration.

Financial Provisions

A considerable number of disabled people are living in or near poverty. A wide variety of allowances are available and to some extent these are dependent upon the severity of the handicap and the financial status of the patient. Three examples are the Attendance, Invalid Care and Mobility Allowances. The expert assistance of a social worker should be sought to ensure that the patient receives his full entitlement.

Local Authority Provision

Local Authorities are responsible for identifying the number of disabled and chronically sick people living in their area and providing them with information on the services available. Through the Social Work Service they supply advice, help and support for people living in their own homes, often in conjunction with voluntary organisations. Examples include the Home Help Service and Meals-on-Wheels. Aids (for example hoists and bath seats) and adaptations (for example ramps and sliding doors) may also be provided. The Local Authority also supplies residential accommodation and day centre care. Authorities are required to include some housing designed for the disabled in new housing schemes.

The Local Authority Service is undertaken by social workers who work in conjunction with occupational therapists and sometimes physiotherapists. It should be noted that the services provided are dependent upon adequate finances being made available within the Local Authority budget. There is considerable inequality between different authorities and furthermore authorities do not necessarily have the same priorities.

Residential Care

Local Authorities have a number of places available for elderly people in residential homes. In addition the Local Authority and the Area Health Authority have a number of residential units for persons under the age of 65. Most residential units are *custodial* and provide little opportunity for active rehabilitation.

Day Centre and Day Hospital Care

Day centres are run by the Local Authorities. Patients attend two to three times per week, sometimes less. The patient is able to take part in recreational activities, but no active rehabilitation is practised (there is usually no physiotherapy available). Day hospitals are usually run by the Local Geriatric Service. They provide the services of a rehabilitation unit including remedial therapy, nursing care and medical and social work support.

Education

Childhood disability may prevent or impair education with the result that many young disabled people are without specific qualifications and skills. It is now generally accepted that physically disabled children should be educated with normal children if possible. This means that the child must be able to move around the school with ease. Unfortunately, many ordinary schools are not suitable for severely disabled children, with the result that some children with normal intellectual faculties are sent to special schools where they are taught in the same class as children with low intelligence or who are slow to learn. It must be remembered that for a disabled child a first class education represents the only chance of succeeding and becoming integrated with society. If possible, children should be educated along with other children of comparable intellectual status.

A major problem arises when a disabled child leaves school. Some must attempt to find a job. Others may require further special training. There are a number of residential colleges for further education of the disabled (for example the National Star Centre, Cheltenham and the Queen Elizabeth Training College for the Disabled, Surrey). Once again, however, for reasons already stated, if possible the child should go to an ordinary college or institute.

The Open University provides excellent opportunities for disabled students.

Employment

Inevitably, the generally high level of unemployment has an adverse effect on the employment and re-employment of disabled people. Nevertheless, it is important for clinicians to recognise that many people are capable of work despite a severe degree of disability. Indeed, the sooner the patient starts to consider returning to work, and the sooner he begins active rehabilitation with an emphasis on work, then the sooner he will return.

The Manpower Services Commission has two executive arms, the Employment Services Agency and the Training Services Agency. The main task of the DROs (Disablement Resettlement Officers) is to find jobs for handicapped people. Disablement Resettlement Officers can also act as direct links between employers and disabled employees to prevent the loss of jobs and to help patients return to suitable work as quickly as possible. They will, if necessary, arrange for the patient to be assessed at an Employment Resettlement Centre and retrained at a Skill Centre. If necessary they can attempt to obtain placement in a Sheltered Workshop.

Voluntary Bodies

Voluntary bodies have a proud record of achievement and there are now at least 300 organisations in the United Kingdom which deal, in some way, with disabled people. A list of some of the main organisations appears at the end of this chapter.

In April, 1977 the British Council for the Rehabilitation of the Disabled and the Central Council for the Disabled merged and they are now known as the Royal Association for Disability and Rehabilitation (RADAR). This organisation acts as an educational, advisory, welfare and research body in matters concerned with disability. The British Red Cross Society undertakes some nursing duties and also provides a range of practical help for the disabled.

There are a number of organisations which deal with specific disabilities. Important examples include the Royal National Institute for the Blind, the Muscular

Table 22.3 Factors affecting mobility

Pain	*Feet* Important causes include 'corns', bunions, pressure sores on the heels, and unsuitable footwear. Regular care of the feet is particularly important in older patients and in diabetics. Surgical correction of foot deformities may be required (for instance hallux rigidus and pes cavus). *Knees and hips* Rheumatoid and osteoarthritis are common problems – sometimes made worse by obesity. Fractures of the femoral neck are easily missed, particularly in older patients. Simple measures such as weight reduction, and the use of weight-relieving aids (e.g. stick or walking frame) may be needed. *The lumbo-sacral region* Low back pain is common in patients with defective leg function due to the extra strain imposed by a defective pattern of walking. Many disabled patients have difficulty with finding a comfortable position in which to sit. Appropriate physiotherapy and advice about suitable chairs may be helpful.
Spasticity	This is discussed on page 573. Excessive use of spasticity reducing drugs may render the legs incapable of weight bearing.
Contractures and deformities	Contractures are the result of irreversible changes in the soft tissues around joints. They are particularly liable to occur with unrelieved spasticity and in rheumatoid arthritis. Contractures can frequently be prevented by good nursing and physiotherapy. Management of established contractures may necessitate surgery. Serial plaster-of-Paris applications may be required to straighten bent knees.
Weakness and instability of lower limb joints	Weakness may result from a wide variety of disorders including multiple sclerosis and motor neurone disease. Weakness of proximal muscles occurs in polymyositis, steroid-induced myopathy and muscular dystrophy. Weakness of distal muscles occurs particularly in polyneuritis and with lesions of the lateral popliteal nerve and of the fifth lumbar nerve root. Muscle weakness may result in instability of joints and in this case stabilising calipers may be required.
Miscellaneous disorders	A wide variety of problems may affect mobility and these include Parkinson's disease, ataxia, poor vision, and severe breathlessness.
Iatrogenic causes	Examples include drug-induced Parkinsonism (with phenothiazine drugs), over-sedation (for example with tranquillisers), postural hypotension (produced by hypotensive drugs or phenothiazines) and excessive bed rest.
Psychological causes	Fear, anxiety, depression and dementia are all common causes of reluctance to walk, particularly in older patients. The problem is made worse if the patient has already had a number of falls. Sympathetic management and physiotherapy may produce a marked improvement.
Environment	Many houses are unsuitable for disabled people. Obvious defects include uneven floors, worn carpeting, and poor lighting.

Dystrophy Group, the Multiple Sclerosis Society, the Ileostomy Association of Great Britain and Ireland, the Leukaemia Research Fund, the Coeliac Society, etc.

There are also a number of pressure groups including the Disabled Income Group (DIG) and the Disabled Drivers' Association.

Sport and Leisure Activities for the Disabled

A very large number of sports and recreational activities are available for disabled people. Many have specific clubs which promote the interests of members. Examples include angling, archery, chess, gardening, modelling, music and wine making. There is even a National Wheelchair Dance Association!

Information about the opportunities available for the disabled and the handicapped is given in an excellent book entitled 'Directory for the Disabled', compiled by A. Darnbrough and D. Kinrade and published in association with the Multiple Sclerosis Society of Great Britain and Northern Ireland.

IMMOBILITY

Lack of mobility is one of the most important problems facing disabled people. It may result in loss of employment and social isolation. It is essential at the outset to find out precisely why the patient cannot walk properly. Some of the potentially treatable factors are listed in Table 22.3.

Transferring

The term 'transferring' is used to describe movement of an immobile patient between his bed, chair and toilet. If the patient can stand and take one or two steps the problems are considerably reduced. The majority of

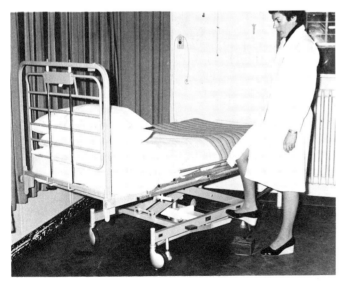

Fig. 22.1 Ellison King's Fund Bed (Hydraulic mechanism for adjusting height of bed from 15″ to 32″).

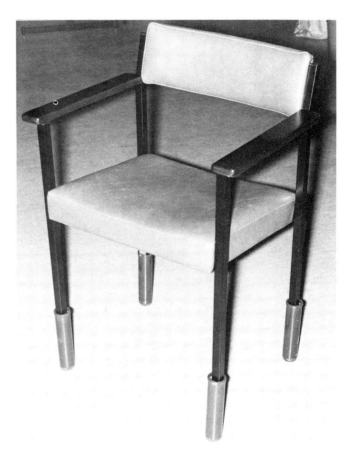

Fig. 22.2 Chair with 'sleeves' to raise the height of the seat.

patients can take some weight on their legs – thus making it possible for a 'standing transfer' to be used. Legs that will take no weight may require a hoist. When considering transferring several general points should be made:

1. The bed, chair, wheelchair and toilet should be at the optimal height. This height can only be determined by experimentation. It is not always possible to achieve this ideal. For instance, the standard hospital bed was designed for ease of nursing but is too high for getting on and off easily. For this reason, many hospitals use a variable height bed (e.g. the 'King's Fund' bed, Fig. 22.1). Similarly, many easy chairs and divan beds are too low. Putting a divan bed or a chair on blocks (Fig. 22.2) may elevate it sufficiently to enable an immobile patient to get to his feet with minimal help. Very soft mattresses and chair seats may also make it difficult to get from a sitting to a standing position. A raised toilet seat (Fig. 22.3) may make getting off the lavatory easier.

2. **Hand Supports.** There should always be something for the patient to hold onto – preferably with *both* hands. Examples of hand supports include monkey bars (over the bed), rope ladders (attached to the end of the bed) and grab-rails in the toilet (*see* Fig. 22.3) and on the stairs.

571

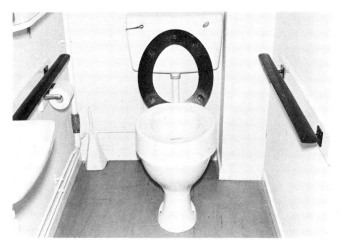

Fig. 22.3 Raised toilet seat (Derby).

3. **Help of Another Person.** In the majority of instances transferring can be achieved with the help of *one* other person. All medical and paramedical personnel should be able to undertake transferring of a disabled person with confidence.

4. **Sliding Board.** A sliding board can be used to bridge a gap between the seat of a wheelchair and a bed. The boards are usually made of polished wood. The patient sits on a cushion and slides from one surface to another.

Wheelchairs

Wheelchairs are necessary for patients who cannot walk a reasonable distance. The main causes of impairment necessitating the use of a wheelchair are osteoarthritis, rheumatoid arthritis, multiple sclerosis, cerebrovascular disease, lower limb amputations, cerebral palsy, paraplegia (including spinal injury and spina bifida), muscular dystrophy and cardiovascular/respiratory disease. The majority of wheelchair users are severely disabled and nearly two-thirds are totally dependent on a wheelchair for their mobility. Children and the elderly have special needs. For instance, the mother of a child may wish to take the child, and his wheelchair, on public transport.

A doctor's signature is usually required before a wheelchair can be supplied. Thus, whilst the detailed assessment of the type of wheelchair needed will usually be undertaken by the occupational therapist, it is important that the doctor should know what is required. It is salutary to recall that between one-quarter and one-third of wheelchairs supplied by the DHSS are returned or not used, because they are unsuitable for the patient.

Various medical conditions affect the choice of a chair. These include incontinence, spasticity, involuntary movements, the state of the upper limbs, and the presence or absence of spinal deformity. Thus, for example, a patient with severe scoliosis may require the provision of a specially shaped Sorbo cushion, into which the scoliosis can fit.

It is necessary to ask why the chair is needed. Usually the chair is required for use in the home and in the immediate environment. Sometimes there will be a need for it to be taken in the boot of a car, in which case a light-weight folding chair will be required. For indoor use the chair must be small enough to go through doors and it must not take up an excessive amount of space. If the patient is to sit in the chair for hours on end, particular attention must be paid to comfort. Finally, it is important to decide whether the chair is to be propelled by the patient himself and/or by an attendant. In patients with defective arm function it may be necessary to request the supply of an electric wheelchair.

Outside Mobility

Sometimes a powered chair for outdoor use is required. A number of such chairs are available for private use but the DHSS does not meet this particular need apart from providing the Mobility Allowance (*see* page 569). Such a vehicle must be robust and stable and it should be able to negotiate kerbs.

The DHSS no longer supplies cars for disabled persons. However, special provisions are currently being negotiated to allow disabled persons to purchase or hire specially adapted vehicles at concessionary rates. A major problem arises when a disabled person wishes to be tested to ascertain whether or not he is fit to drive. Unfortunately there are very few special centres where disabled persons can be assessed for driving.*

It is clear that management of immobility depends initially on an accurate assessment of why the patient cannot walk properly. Only when this has been done can appropriate recommendations be made. Help may be provided in a number of different ways – in the form of chiropody and the provision of suitable footwear on the one hand and the supply of a wheelchair and a hoist on the other. If possible the patient should be encouraged to walk, the essential qualities being speed and safety.

OTHER PHYSICAL PROBLEMS

A variety of physical problems may affect the disabled. Some of these are discussed in this chapter and are summarised below.

Pain

Pain is one of the main symptoms experienced by the disabled, occurring particularly in people with arthritis.

---

* Information can be obtained from the British School of Motoring Specialised Services Ltd., 102 Sydney Street, London SW3.

Pain in the weight-bearing joints has been discussed previously. Pain occurring in patients dying of terminal cancer is discussed in the section on 'Care of the dying', (see page 577). Pain in the shoulder is common in hemiplegic patients. It is usually due to faulty lifting techniques.

A wide variety of treatments is available for pain, including analgesics and anti-inflammatory drugs, joint replacements and correct positioning of the patient.

Spasticity and Spasms

Spasticity occurs in a large number of neurological disorders including multiple sclerosis and other spinal cord lesions. It also occurs in hemiplegia of vascular origin and cerebral palsy. The result is stiffness of the limbs – frequently with defective movement. Severe spasticity may make nursing extremely difficult. For instance, adductor spasticity may make perineal toilet impossible. Severe spasticity of the hand in hemiplegic patients may make washing of the hand difficult. Contractures may eventually occur. The following general principles of management apply:

Anxiety and Psychological Factors. Spasticity is made worse by anxiety. A tranquilliser may be helpful.

Avoidance of Physical Conditions which make Spasticity Worse. Bed clothes resting on the legs may increase spasticity – a cradle is often helpful. A full bladder, local infection and pressure sores are other important factors.

Drugs. A variety of drugs can be used. These include:
1. Diazepam (Valium) – in doses 10 to 30 mg daily. Unfortunately diazepam usually induces drowsiness before reducing spasticity.
2. Baclofen (Lioresal) – 10 to 50 mg daily.
3. Dantolene – 25 to 50 mg twice daily (up to 800 mg daily).

Phenol Injections. By careful positioning of the patient phenol can be brought into contact with the lumbar nerve roots. However, attempts to block the sacral roots may be complicated by bladder disturbance. Phenol and alcohol can be injected both around nerve trunks and into the motor points of spastic muscles.

Division of Nerves. Division of the obturator nerve can be useful in the management of severe adductor spasticity in the legs.

Division of Tendons. The Achilles tendon can be either divided or elongated in order to correct a fixed deformity of the ankle. Cutting of the adductor and flexor tendons around the hips may occasionally be necessary.

It is always necessary to start with the simplest procedures first. Only in occasional instances is it necessary to invoke surgery.

Urinary Incontinence

Incontinence may be due to very simple reasons such as loss of mobility or defective arm function. Thus the patient with urgency of micturition may be unable to get to the toilet in time because of impaired mobility. Defective arm function may make manipulation of clothes and urination difficult. Incontinence in older people is frequently due to faecal impaction.

Other common causes of incontinence include cerebral vascular disease, multiple sclerosis, disorders of the spinal cord and cauda equina and dementia. In addition, there are the problems of prostatic enlargement and pelvic prolapse.

Once a diagnosis has been made, a plan of management can be worked out. Some patients will need to be referred to a urologist. In most cases it is necessary to investigate the upper renal tract by doing an intravenous pyelogram. Urinary infection should always be excluded as this may both cause and complicate incontinence. Nocturnal incontinence can sometimes be prevented by restricting the evening intake of fluids. Marked urinary urgency can sometimes be helped by the use of Cetiprin, 200 mg three times daily.

Minor degrees of incontinence can frequently be managed with local padding and waterproof pants. Incontinence in men may necessitate the use of an incontinence apparatus, with a condom fitted to the penis and a collecting bag strapped to the inside of the thigh. In other instances it is necessary to use either a urethral or suprapubic catheter. Sometimes, however, the patient can manage by keeping a urinal with him at all times, even when sitting in a wheelchair.

573

Unfortunately, there is no effective incontinence apparatus available for women. Marked incontinence will usually need to be managed with a catheter. In a few instances it is found desirable to transplant the ureters into the bowel (sometimes by constructing a false bladder with a loop of ileum).

Incontinence is probably responsible for more misery amongst disabled patients than anything else. The problems must be managed energetically and sympathetically by the medical and nursing staff. Each patient needs thorough assessment and good advice. He also needs continued help from the district nurse and family doctor. The importance of extreme cleanliness must be emphasised.

The main principles of catheter management are given in Table 22.4.

Table 22.4 Catheter management: advice to patient and main carer

Hygiene	1. Wash skin around catheter. 2. Wash hands before and after changing collecting bag. 3. When not in use the bag should be soaked in soapy water.
Diet	Constipation may interfere with catheter drainage. Take bran with breakfast and use wholemeal bread.
Drainage of the catheter	1. Fluid intake: a reasonably high fluid intake is required to ensure catheter drainage. At least 4 pints per day are needed (equivalent to 12 cups of tea). 2. Avoid kinking the catheter. 3. Keep the bag below the end of the catheter.

Constipation

The vast majority of immobile patients suffer from some degree of constipation. Particular problems arise when there is difficulty with getting to the toilet quickly, where there is marked muscle weakness or paralysis (e.g. muscular dystrophy), or where there is marked spasticity (with involvement of the perineal muscles).

The general principles of management include a high roughage diet with added bran, a high fluid intake, avoidance of aperients if possible and ready access to the toilet. It should also be remembered that most analgesic tablets have a constipating action.

Faecal incontinence may be reversible or permanent. Reversible incontinence may occur when there is faecal impaction or when the toilet is inaccessible. Permanent incontinence is likely to occur when the anal sphincter is incompetent or when rectal sensation is defective.

The key to successful management of the bowels is adequate training. A proper bowel routine must be established. The management of the bowels is also closely related to the management of micturition. Constipation can precipitate urinary incontinence.

Menstruation

For the normal woman the monthly period is almost always a nuisance. Frequently it becomes a real burden and a physical drain, particularly when there is pain and/or a heavy flow. Severely disabled women sometimes have the greatest difficulty coping with these problems. Perineal toilet may be impossible. This causes not only physical distress but embarrassment at having to request the assistance of a relative or nurse at frequent intervals. It thus seems desirable to do everything possible to lessen the undesirable effects of menstruation.

General measures such as the treatment of anaemia, avoidance of constipation at the time of the period and appropriate management of pelvic pathology should not be forgotten. The blood loss and pain may be decreased by intermittent administration of the contraceptive pill. If necessary, menstruation can be stopped altogether either by a hysterectomy or by radiotherapy. The advice of a gynaecologist should be sought.

Sexual Problems

Disabled people have the same basic urges as everyone else, but until recently their sexual needs have been largely ignored. It is now recognised that many disabled people are able to lead a satisfactory sexual life. It is an important duty of the doctor to give guidance.

Difficulties may arise for a number of different reasons – physical and psychological. Arthritic disorders and abnormalities of the nervous system form the largest groups (see Table 22.5).

In addition to the physical problems itemised in Table 22.5 there are important psychological difficulties. Psychological factors play a vital role in the achievement of a sexual relationship in all humans – men and women. 'Normal' people frequently experience sexual problems of one sort or another during their lives (e.g. temporary impotence due to anxiety). The patient with physical disability has to cope not only with his mechanical problems but also with the impact that these have on his/her own self-confidence with a person of the opposite sex.

It is important for the doctor to remember the sexual needs of his patients. It is all too easy to assume that disabled people have no sexual requirements. Regretfully, this is an attitude that prevails widely. For instance, there are virtually no appropriate facilities in units for the younger chronic sick. It is also important for the doctor to remember that many disabled patients are physically capable of intercourse. Thus, for instance, those patients who have a clear-cut transection of the spinal cord in the spinal or thoracic region may retain the ability to produce an erection (although this is not necessarily well sustained and may appear at inappropriate times).

Table 22.5 Physical disorders and their impact on sexual function

Disorder	Result
Osteoarthritis	Pain and limitation of movement in the spine and limb joints.
Neurological disorders:	
(a) Traumatic paraplegia and tetraplegia	Paralysis and loss of sensation in the lower limbs. Many patients with cervical and high thoracic lesions are able to develop erections. Incontinence, flexor spasms, reflex hypertension and bradycardia may occur during intercourse.
(b) Lesions of the lower part of the spinal cord and cauda equina (e.g. spina bifida)	If interruption of the sacral reflex arc occurs there will be total impotence.
(c) Multiple sclerosis	Impotence is common (over 60 per cent in one series).
(d) Diabetes	An autonomic neuropathy is common – with resultant impotence (sometimes in *young* men).
Incontinence	Incontinence occurs for a wide variety of reasons. The fear that it will occur during intercourse can be important.
Angina and breathlessness	Occasionally these can be severe enough to limit intercourse.
Artificial stoma and catheter	An ileostomy, colostomy or catheter may inhibit intercourse for psychological reasons. A stoma should be covered with a towel.
Physical damage to the genitalia (extensive burns)	

The doctor must be well informed about the impact of disability on sexual function. He should be able to give guidance to his patients,* and this should include the ability to advise on such problems as techniques and positions of intercourse and also on the question of fertility and the production of children.

Obesity

Obesity is a common problem amongst disabled people, and results partly from lack of exercise. It interferes with mobility. Perivisceral and omental fat may make breathing difficult. Feelings of abdominal distension are common.

Unfortunately, weight loss is not always easy to achieve, partly because food plays such an important part in the lives of disabled people.

* Detailed advice can be obtained from the Committee on Sexual Problems of the Disabled, 49 Victoria Street, London SW1. This group produces a series of helpful advisory leaflets.

Pressure Sores

Pressure sores result from ischaemia of the skin and deeper tissues. The degree of damage depends on the intensity, duration and direction of the pressure. Sores usually occur in patients whose mobility is severely restricted so that they are confined to a bed or a chair.

Pressure sores are particularly liable to occur in patients with neurological disorders including spinal cord injury and multiple sclerosis. They also occur in patients who are unconscious for a prolonged period of time. Important contributory factors include incontinence, diabetes, generally poor physical condition (poor nutrition and anaemia) and extreme obesity or thinness. The elderly are particularly liable to pressure sores because of the fact that they may be in poor general health and that the skin is thin and does not heal well. In addition, elderly and disabled patients show considerable lack of spontaneous movement in sleep.

Sites. Pressure sores occur mainly over bony prominences. The most important areas affected are shown below:

Sites at which pressure sores commonly occur	
Sacrum Trochanters	Sores commonly occur in patients who are confined to bed.
Ischium (buttock)	Particularly in wheelchair-bound patients.
Heels	
Malleoli	
Inner surfaces of the knees	Particularly if there is marked adductor spasticity.

Prevention. The adage 'prevention is better than cure' might have been devised especially for this situation. It may, indeed, take months to heal a sore which developed over days. The most important principles are:

1. Regular inspection of the skin. It is important to look for redness, swelling and superficial excoriation. The patient himself can frequently be taught to carry out these inspections. The skin must always be kept clean and dry.

2. Frequent changes of posture are vital. Patients at risk should be turned every two hours by day and by night.

Turning can be made easier by using the Stoke Mandeville Egerton electrically controlled turning bed. Wheelchair-bound patients should be taught to lift themselves up for 20 seconds every five minutes (provided that they are fit enough to do so).

3. It is important to pay attention to the patient's general health. Anaemia and nutritional deficiencies should be corrected and obese patients should be encouraged to lose weight.

4. The patient should not be allowed to lie on wet or soiled bed clothes. If he does so the skin will rapidly break down.

There is then the next question of what preparations, if any, should be applied locally. Applications of talcum powder and spirit to the intact skin are thought by some to be of value. Probably, however, the friction of the nurse's hand is the main benefit, increasing the skin blood flow.

The quality of nursing and medical care on a ward can be judged by the incidence of pressure sores.

Treatment of the Established Sore. The most important rule here is – 'You can put what you like on a pressure sore, except the patient'. The general principles discussed above under the heading of prevention also apply when pressure sores have actually developed. Other general principles include:

1. Dead tissue should be excised.

2. Local infection should be treated. Systemic antibiotics may be required. Abscesses and sinuses should be opened and allowed to drain.

3. The wound should be packed with gauze soaked in saline. The whole area is then sealed with porous elastoplast to prevent reinfection, particularly by faecal material.

4. When granulation tissue has nearly filled the cavity, the area may sometimes be grafted. Some sores can be excised and sutured. Surgery is contraindicated in cases of local sepsis.

A variety of beds are available for nursing patients with pressure sores. Whatever type of bed is used, care must be taken to avoid creasing cotton sheets and waterproof protective sheeting. Ripple mattresses, water-beds and air-beds all have their advocates. One of the cheapest and most effective beds is a string hammock which fits on to the top of an ordinary hospital bed. Sorbo rubber packs may also be very effective.

A very large number of substances have been applied to pressure sores, from egg yolk to poultices of carrots and turnips! Every ward sister has her own particular foible. There is unfortunately very little evidence that any one preparation is better than another.

Complications. A number of complications of pressure sores can occur.

Local spread. Pus may track up fascial planes. For instance, pus may track into the groin where an abscess may occur.

Osteomyelitis. This is particularly likely to occur with trochanteric sores.

Septicaemia.

Secondary amyloidosis.

SELF-CARE

This section deals with the ability of the patient to look after himself. The problems of eating and drinking, washing, bathing, dressing and toilet will be briefly discussed. It is usually the responsibility of the nursing staff and the occupational therapists to help the patient overcome these problems.

Eating and Drinking

Social confidence often depends on the patient's ability to eat and drink in an acceptable way whilst in the company of other people. The patient wants to be able to eat with dexterity and without causing embarrassment. Many patients can be helped to eat more easily by the provision of one or two simple gadgets or adaptations. Examples include:

1. Weak or deformed hands (for instance) in rheumatoid arthritis. Large handled cutlery (Fig. 22.4) improve the patient's ability to grip. Wrist splints may provide stability.

2. Weak proximal muscles. Mobile arm supports (flexor hinged splints) provide support for the forearms, enabling the hand to be raised to the mouth.

3. Unsteadiness. Ataxic patients may spill food. This problem may be helped by using specially designed crockery and a non-slip mat (Fig. 22.4).

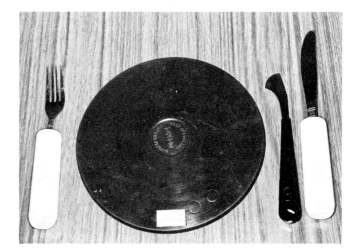

Fig. 22.4 Non-slip mat, Manoy knife and large handled cutlery.

4. Suitable furniture. A disabled person may find it very difficult to sit at a meal table in a chair. It may be necessary to raise the table slightly or even to purchase another.

Many patients find it easier to eat if their food is cut up. Drinking may be facilitated by the use of straws, polythene tubes or special non-spillable drinking mugs.

It should always be remembered that the disabled person usually wishes to look as normal as possible. Many people resent having to use gadgets.

Washing and Grooming

Disabled people, like everyone else, need to take a pride in their appearance. Unless they do so, social contacts may be difficult to maintain. For instance, disabled girls frequently need instruction and help in techniques of make-up. Mirrors and hand basins need to be of the correct height. Special holders with long handles for brushes may be required.

Bathing

Bathing can be extremely dangerous for severely disabled patients. For this group a suitably designed shower is better in every way.

If a bath is to be used, particular attention must be paid to its height. The height of the bath rim and of the wheelchair should be equal. A non-slip mat may need to be provided in the bottom of the bath. A bath seat may enable the patient to get out of the bath with reasonable ease (Fig. 22.5).

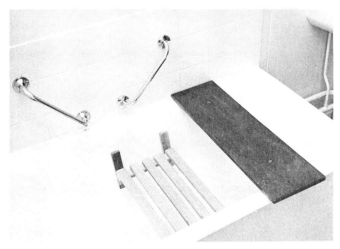

Fig. 22.5 Over-bath board, bath seat and safety grab bar.

Dressing

Clothing requirements must be assessed on an individual basis. Particular attention should be paid to comfort. Appearance is more important to some people than others (for instance young girls care greatly about what they wear). In general everything should look as normal as possible. However, clothing may need some modifications (for instance fastenings can be at the front). Velcro can be used instead of buttons and large buttons are better than small ones. Special one-handed shoelaces are available. Various types of dressing aid can also be helpful, such as a long-handled shoe horn.

Toilet

Toileting problems are made much worse if there are difficulties with micturition and defaecation. Three main problems need to be mentioned – access, transferring and the management of urination and defaecation.

Access. In some cases no downstairs toilet is available. A commode may be required on a short term basis, but most patients do not find this acceptable in the long term. A disabled person needs more room to manoeuvre than a normal person, particularly if he is in a wheelchair. Many toilets are narrow and some have steps. Some are in the garden. The following represents the ideal situation:
1. There should be no stairs or steps to the toilet (if necessary ramps should be provided).
2. There should be handrails around the toilet.
3. The room must be sufficiently wide to enable the patient to manoeuvre. A sliding door can sometimes be substituted for one that is hinged.
4. There should be a non-slip floor.
5. Lighting should be good.
6. The room should be heated, particularly if it is outside the house.
7. There should be a handbasin available for washing. This is particularly important as disabled people are liable to have accidents when using the toilet.

In some instances it is necessary to merge the toilet with the bathroom, thus making more efficient use of space.

Transferring On and Off the Toilet. Siting of the pedestal may be crucial. Access is easier if it is not placed too near the side or rear wall. The toilet seat may be raised by using a special toilet chair. The precise method of transferring will be different for each patient and the occupational therapist will be able to advise on this.

Use of the Toilet. The patient may require training from the remedial staff. Some adaptations to clothing may be required.

CARE OF THE DYING

It is necessary to discuss the management of those patients who have an incurable disease and are likely to die within the next few weeks or months. The most important incurable 'disease' is cancer. Others include very severe emphysema, intractable heart failure, the terminal stages of renal failure and motor neurone disease. In all these cases the inevitability of death is obvious. In other instances, for example, coronary artery and cerebrovascular disease, the prognosis is uncertain and although the patient may die soon, it is also possible that he may survive for several years. Patients suffering with these latter diseases cannot, therefore, strictly be said to be dying.

Thirty to forty per cent of patients die at home; the remainder die in hospital or in some other institution. Many patients are able to remain at home at least until the terminal stage of their illness. The majority of patients who die are over the age of 65. Unfortunately, there is considerable evidence to indicate that many patients suffer unrelieved physical discomfort and mental distress whether or not they are admitted to hospital. This is partly due to ignorance on the part of the medical and paramedical professions.

It is the doctor's job to ensure that the medical management is adequate and that the dying patient and his relatives do not experience unnecessary suffering. The patient must be helped to maintain his dignity and personality to the end. All this involves having an appreciation of the likely course of the disease, understanding the psychological and physical problems which may arise, and being willing to discuss the problems with the patient and his family. The doctor must also be willing to liaise closely with other professional groups, particularly the chaplain, nurses and social workers.

The primary objective is to minimise suffering. Therefore, the doctor must be able to exercise his judgement about such matters as treatment of infection with antibiotics or the administration of intravenous fluids. It is no part of good medicine to strive officiously to keep a patient alive.

During the past decade there have been considerable advances in the management of the dying. No longer does mystery surround the subject. A number of special hospitals have been established in the United Kingdom and as a result of their experience the principles of management have become firmly established.

Should the Patient Know?

Many people have a particular fear of cancer. The reasons include the nature of the disease itself, the belief that it is incurable (and therefore that death is certain), and the fear of pain. In addition, there are a number of general fears about death itself, including doubts about the unknown, the leaving of loved ones, and the humiliation and dependency of terminal illness. Each one of us has slightly different attitudes to death. For the young man in the prime of life who will leave a wife and several children the pill can indeed be hard to

swallow. For the elderly widower in poor health who has been living alone for years, death may come as a welcome relief from earthly cares. There is then the most important factor of religious belief and the added strength that this can give.

It is clear, therefore, that there can be no ready answer to our question – Should the patient know? Much will depend on the individual patient's attitude to life and death. There are some patients who are grateful to be told the full position and who then proceed to put their affairs in proper order whilst there is time. There are others who are shattered and they become depressed, withdrawn, sometimes suicidal. One thing is certain, deceit destroys the trust that exists between the patient and the doctor. There is no excuse for telling lies. The wisest approach is to discuss the situation gently with the patient and try to discover his attitude to illness and to death, and in particular whether he wants to know the diagnosis. There are some patients who ask outright, 'Have I got cancer?', 'Am I dying?' The answer will depend on the doctor's judgement as to whether or not the patient is ready to accept that he is dying. Sometimes the answer has to be given obliquely at the first interview and more clearly subsequently. A *gradual* dawning of truth is sometimes easier to bear than a blunt announcement. To handle the situation properly requires much tact, time, experience and sympathy. The relatives should always be brought into discussions and someone in the family (usually the spouse) must be told the correct diagnosis. Remember that if the spouse is told the full diagnosis and prognosis and if the patient is left in ignorance there will be a huge barrier erected between the two of them at a time when mutual help and support is essential. Remember too, that both in hospital and in the community there are a large number of staff involved (nurses, doctors, social workers, etc.). It is important that they too should know exactly what has been said to the patient and his family. It is particularly important that the general practitioner should be informed of the precise situation *before* the patient leaves hospital.

Drug Treatment of Pain in Terminal Cancer

Pain is an important symptom in about 50 per cent of cases of terminal cancer. In some instances localised pain can be treated with radiotherapy. The objective of drug treatment is to produce relief of distress whilst allowing the patient to remain mentally alert, at least until death is very near. The following general rules apply to drug treatment:
1. Give enough but not too much. The smallest possible effective dose should be given. If an excessive dose is given too early the patient may become unnecessarily confused and thus difficult to manage. Frequently, however, drugs are given in too small a dose, with

resultant avoidable distress. A fine balance exists between the two extremes. It is worth remembering that when dealing with dying patients there is usually no need for the physician to concern himself with the long term undesirable effects of drugs, such as addiction.

2. Drugs for pain relief should be given *regularly*. Pain can practically always be controlled provided the drugs are given in sufficient doses at regular intervals. In practice, for severe pain, this usually means four-hourly administration, although it is occasionally necessary to give drugs more frequently. It is not wise to wait until the pain has become established before giving drugs. It is also wise to avoid *suddenly* changing the dosage and frequency with which drugs are administered.

It is usually satisfactory to start with the weaker analgesics and to reserve the stronger drugs for the latter stages of the illness. Oral therapy is usually adequate initially. Intramuscular injections become necessary if there is intractable vomiting or if the patient cannot swallow. In the latter stages of the illness the effects of a powerful analgesic can be usefully augmented by alcohol and administration of a drug of the phenothiazine group (especially if there is vomiting). The main side effects of drugs are constipation, nausea and vomiting, heavy sedation and excitement. These symptoms are not usually severe and respond to appropriate management.

Mild Pain. Aspirin, codeine compound, dextropropoxyphen. Co.

Moderate Pain. Diconal (dipipanone hydrochloride 10 mg and cyclizine hydrochloride 30 mg). 1 to 2 tablets can be given four-hourly.
Phenazocine hydrobromide, 5 mg tablets. 1 to 3 tablets four-hourly.
Oxycodone pectinate suppositories (Proladone) 30 mg. 1 can be given every eight hours.

Severe Pain. The mainstays of treatment are diamorphine (heroin) and morphine itself. There is little difference between these two agents.

Oral therapy. Diamorphine and Cocaine Elixir, BPC (5 mg of each with 5 ml of chloroform water plus alcohol and syrup).
Morphia and Cocaine Elixir, BPC (5 mg of each with 5 ml of chloroform water plus alcohol and syrup).

If extra sedation is required, or if there is nausea or vomiting, it may be necessary to give added chlorpromazine (Largactil) 25 to 50 mg, or prochlorperazine (Stemetil) 5 to 10 mg. Additional alcohol may be added if necessary for its euphoriant effect.

Suppositories. Morphine Suppositories, BPC. Suppositories containing 10, 15, 20, 30 or 60 mg of morphine are available.

Intramuscular or subcutaneous therapy. Morphine Sulphate, BP. Ampoules of 1 ml containing 10, 15, 20 or 30 mg of morphine are available.
Diamorphine, BP. Vials of 5, 10 and 30 mg are available and must be freshly prepared by dissolving the powder in water for injection.

Management of Other Physical Symptoms

In general it is usually best to treat physical symptoms before mental distress. When this is done there is often a decrease in the amount of associated anxiety and apprehension. The use of large doses of sedatives, hypnotics and tranquillisers in such patients will usually do more harm than good, unless physical symptoms are treated first.

Anorexia. This is a very common symptom of malignant disease. An improvement in appetite can make a big difference to a patient's morale. Small helpings of appetising foods on small plates should be given. Small doses of steroids may improve appetite (e.g. prednisone 5 mg three times a day). Nausea is an important cause of anorexia and can usually be alleviated.

Dysphagia. Common causes include cancer of the oesophagus and motor neurone disease. For the former a Celestin tube may be required to maintain a clear passage for food. The dysphagia of pseudo-bulbar palsy due to motor neurone disease is associated with marked spasticity of the tongue and pharyngeal muscles. This can sometimes be reduced by sucking ice or iced drinks. Excessive accumulation of saliva in the mouth can be helped by atropine or hyoscine. A nasogastric tube may ultimately be required. Dysphagia is often made worse by anxiety and for this reason a sedative may well be required. Monilial infection of the mouth and oesophagus can cause dysphagia and is treated with amphotericin lozenges.

Intractable Vomiting and/or Nausea. This may be due to a variety of causes, including intestinal obstruction and biochemical disturbance (for instance uraemia or hypercalcaemia). Drugs are an important cause (including morphine).

A variety of anti-emetics are effective including prochlorperazine (Stemetil), chlorpromazine (Largactil) and metoclopramide (Maxolon), 10 to 20 mg.

Unpleasant Mouth and Halitosis. A foul mouth and halitosis can be very unpleasant for both the patient and relatives. Dehydration, drugs and mouth breathing can all cause dryness of the mouth. Monilial infections and sepsis are common.

Care of the mouth is therefore vital and includes frequent cleaning of the mouth and teeth, mouth washes, stimulation of saliva production by sucking pieces of fruit or lemon sweets. Infections must be treated. Cracked dry lips are treated with bland creams.

Hiccoughs. This is an irritating and exhausting symptom. It can be treated by chlorpromazine, orally or intramuscularly. Inhalation of 5 per cent carbon dioxide may be helpful.

Itching. This is a common symptom of unrelieved obstructive jaundice. Oral antihistamines may help as may cholestyramine. Methyl testosterone for men in a dose of 25 mg sublingually, daily, or norethandrolone (Nileven) 10 mg three times daily for women, may produce relief but will deepen jaundice. Itching may also be relieved by simple measures, including the local application of calamine lotion and the wearing of cotton rather than nylon clothes.

Breathlessness. This is a common symptom in patients dying of lung cancer and of respiratory failure due to emphysema. Because breathlessness is such a frightening symptom it may be necessary to give a sedative such as Valium. Bronchospasm, uncontrolled infection and large pleural effusions may require appropriate treatment. Excessive secretions may be dried up with intramuscular hyoscine, 0.4 to 0.6 mg, given with an opiate.

Cough. Intractable cough occurs with malignant disease of the larynx, trachea and upper air passages. It is very distressing to the patient and relatives and also to the other patients on the ward. Linctus Codeine, BPC, 5 to 10 ml, or morphine or diamorphine may be required.

A number of other problems arise, including insomnia, dehydration, constipation, incontinence and pressure sores. With good nursing care they should not present major problems. Mental confusion can cause difficulties and may require treatment with phenothiazine drugs, provided that a treatable cause such as infection or overdosage with drugs has been excluded.

Mental Distress

There is as much need to help our patients with their mental anguish as with their physical pain. Anxiety, anger, and depression are all common. Much can be done by calm, confident management by all concerned, particularly the nurses. The patient frequently has a need to talk to someone who is informed and who is able and willing to listen. The nursing staff on the ward are in a particularly good position to fulfil this supportive role. Kindness, calmness and efficiency are all equally important qualities. In certain instances, drugs can be of great value in relieving mental distress. For instance, diazepam (Valium) is particularly useful for agitation and anxiety. Antidepressants have a very limited use. Alcohol can be particularly beneficial. Many anxious patients are better if they have had something to drink. Diversional activities, such as knitting, playing cards and darts can be continued up to the end in some cases.

Those who have a strong religious conviction are fortunate. For them death is but the gate to something much better.

SUGGESTED FURTHER READING

Darnbrough, A. and Kinrade, D. (1977) *Directory for the Disabled*, Woodhead-Faulkner Ltd., in association with the Multiple Sclerosis Society of Great Britain and Northern Ireland.

Harris, A. I., Cox, E. and Smith, R. W. (1971) Handicapped and Impaired in Great Britain, Part 1. London: HMSO.

Nichols, P. J. R. (1971) *Rehabilitation of the Severely Disabled*, **vol. 2.** London: Butterworths.

Nichols, P. J. R. (1976) *Rehabilitation Medicine*. London: Butterworths.

Mattingly, S. (1977) *Rehabilitation Today*. Update Books.

Saunders, C. (1976) Care of the Dying, series of articles in *The Nursing Times*, July and August.

Aspects of Sexual Medicine (1976) BMA, Tavistock Square, London.

Coping with Disablement (1974) Consumers' Association, publishers of Which?

Help for Handicapped People (1975) Leaflet HB1. Issued jointly by the DHSS and the Welsh Office.

Housing Grants and Allowances for Disabled People (1975) A guide for disabled individuals to assist with home improvements and housing costs.

Physical Impairment: Social Handicap (1977) Office of Health Economics.

USEFUL ADDRESSES

The Family Fund,
PO Box 50,
York, YO3 6RB

The Spastics Society,
12 Park Crescent,
London, W1N 4EQ

Association of Spina Bifida and Hydrocephalus,
30 Devonshire Street,
London, W1N 2ED

Muscular Dystrophy Group,
26 Borough High Street,
London, SE1 9QG

National Society for Mentally Handicapped Children,
86 Newman Street,
London, W1P 8NS

British Red Cross Society,
9 Grosvenor Crescent,
London, SW1X 7EJ

Disabled Living Foundation,
346 Kensington High Street,
London, W14 8NS

Disablement Income Group,
Queens House,
180 Tottenham Court Road,
London, W1P 0BD

The Royal Association for Disability and Rehabilitation,
(merger April, 1977, Central Council for the Disabled
and the British Council for Rehabilitation of the Disabled),
25 Mortimer Street,
London, W1N 8AB

PHAB (Youth Clubs for Physically Handicapped and
Able Bodied),
30 Devonshire Street,
London, W1N 2AP

Councils for Voluntary Service,
26 Bedford Square,
London, WC1B 3HU

Voluntary Council for Handicapped Children,
c/o National Children's Bureau,
8 Wakeley Street,
London, EC13 7QE

Diseases in Tropical Countries 23

F. FAKUNLE

The pattern of disease in most tropical countries (Fig. 23.1) is made by two main strands. Neither of these strands is strongly represented in the highly developed nations of the temperate zones.

The first is one of diseases that used to be common in Europe and America, but which have been largely abolished by sound measures of public health, provision of clean water, plentiful food, good housing and preventive inoculations. In most tropical countries the problems of the infrastructure – roads, safe piped wat-

er, sewers, electricity, and trained health field-workers – have not yet been solved. Natural resources have not been developed to a point where preventive medicine can make its full impact. Consequently, we see in these countries all the diseases that once ravaged Europe.

The second strand is one of epizootic diseases and diseases carried by animal vectors from man to man. These diseases do not flourish in temperate climates, because animal vectors do not flourish in the cold. Again, the life of the predominant agriculturalist in tropical countries brings him into much closer contact with the animal vectors of disease.

Diseases common in the tropics can, therefore, be divided into:
1. Preventable infections occurring all over the world irrespective of climate.
2. Tropical infections, also preventable at a cost.
3. The diseases of malnutrition and toxicity.
4. Genetically determined diseases common in non-temperate climates.

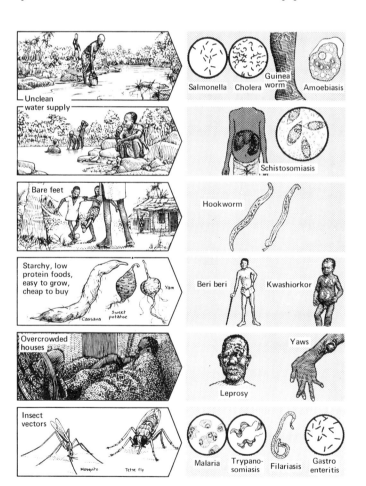

Fig. 23.1   Some special medical problems in the tropics.

PREVENTABLE INFECTIONS

SALMONELLA

Background

The great killers are typhoid and paratyphoid A and B, and since the spread of these diseases depends upon the contamination of food or water by organisms from human faeces, they are understandably common in communities where faeces are disposed of close to the water supply.

Symptoms and Signs

The normal picture of these diseases is described on page 25, but in tropical countries the presentation may be atypical. Fulminant typhoid may cause the rapid onset of delirium and coma, and by the time the patient reaches hospital a history may be unobtainable. Though blood culture, and later stool and urine cultures are necessary for diagnosis, time may not allow the clinician to procrastinate over the treatment. Clinical clues to the diagnosis are the slightly swollen, tense and tender abdomen, toxicity out of proportion to the rise of pulse rate, headache, confused thought process, and a palpable liver and spleen.

Basis of Treatment

After taking a specimen of blood for culture, treatment with chloramphenicol 500 mg at once, and then 250 mg four-hourly is started immediately. Ampicillin in similar doses can be used as a substitute, but is marginally less effective in fulminant disease. Both drugs can be given intramuscularly or intravenously. Corticosteroids may be usefully added to the antibiotic treatment in fulminant cases. Note that diarrhoea does not usually occur during the first week of the disease, and that it is a variable and unpredictable symptom. Perforation of the ileum, occurring usually in the second or third week (or earlier in the severe disease), can be treated by 'suck and drip' or by surgery if conditions allow. Because of its low toxicity and the emergence of chloramphenicol-resistant strains co-trimoxazole (Septrin) is also useful. Recent studies have shown that amoxycillin ('Amoxil' – a derivative of ampicillin) may also be a suitable alternative to chloramphenicol.

Note: If a patient has persistent tachycardia, pyrexia and is toxic after five days on an adequate dosage of chloramphenicol the organism is probably resistant and the antibiotic should be changed.

OTHER SALMONELLA INFECTIONS

Infections by *Salmonella typhimurium* and *Salmonella enteritidis* and other types are common causes of severe gastroenteritis in children or malnourished subjects, and since in hot climates fluid loss from the bowel is in addition to the usual sweat losses from the skin, dehydration with sodium or potassium depletion can kill quickly. In such situations, prompt intravenous medication and therapy with chloramphenicol is life-saving.

SHIGELLA

Background

In the past, bacillary dysentery was the most important cause of death in Europeans coming to live in tropical, subtropical, or desert countries. Flies carried the organisms from latrines to food. The disposal of faeces in such a way as to exclude flies from access, the screening out of 'carrier' food-handlers and the use of refrigerators and sealed food containers has dramatically curtailed both the incidence and the severity of dysenteric diseases in Europeans, but such diseases still contribute to the high mortality rates in native born children living perforce in less desirable conditions of hygiene.

Symptoms and Signs

Diagnosis is suspected clinically if there is a sudden onset of diarrhoea with blood appearing in the stools at an early stage.

Investigations

1. Microscopical examination of a wet specimen of stool reveals numerous polymorphs, red blood cells, and macrophages.
2. Rectal swabs of faeces grow shigella.

Basis of Treatment

This should not be delayed for the results of cultures from stool or rectal swab, and large doses (6 g daily) of a 'relatively' insoluble sulphonamide (sulphaguanidine) should be given. Treatment can, if necessary, be modified 24 hours later when results of stool culture and organism sensitivity are known. Alternative antibiotics are neomycin and oral streptomycin, but in the tropics tetracycline and chloramphenicol are more readily available.

TUBERCULOSIS

Background

It was long believed in Europe and North America that tuberculosis was a disease that had a predilection for people of certain races and that constitutional factors were the initial determinant of whether the disease took root, or was conquered by the body. The purely infectious nature of this disease was blurred over by the high host resistance in healthy adults and by the wishful thinking of medical observers.

The almost total eradication of the disease in Western countries has been achieved since 1948 by the treatment of carriers, so that the reserve of active bacteria has been drastically reduced, and by the protection of susceptible young adults with BCG inoculations. In such conditions, the likelihood of case-to-case spread is very small.

By contrast, the conditions in many tropical countries bear some resemblance to those pertaining in Ireland during the nineteenth century. There is a large pool of infective carriers, there is poverty and malnutrition diminishing host resistance, while domestic overcrowding favours case-to-case spread.

Symptoms and Signs

The pattern of the disease in tropical countries is somewhat different from that described in Western textbooks. For example, peritoneal tuberculosis of the 'wet' or 'dry' form, and of human origin, is common; miliary tuberculosis and tuberculous meningitis occur at any age, and tuberculous pericarditis is not rare. Pulmonary tuberculosis manifests itself in the same ways as in the West.

Investigations

Diagnosis is achieved by the same methods throughout the world, but a high index of suspicion is needed in tropical countries, for tuberculosis can be a great imitator. In many cases, especially peritoneal tuberculosis, the diagnosis must be based on the occurrence of fever, peritonism, or ascites with a high protein content, and a normal blood leucocyte count. Acid-fast bacilli are rarely found in the ascitic fluid and cultures take too long to grow, so that the therapeutic trial is often the only feasible method of diagnosis.

Basis of Treatment

Standard therapy with streptomycin 1 g daily in an adult, PAS 18 g daily and INH 200 mg daily, produces a dramatic fall of temperature, disappearance of ascites and gain of muscle weight within ten days. Alternative drug regimes are being introduced into tropical countries (see page 338).

The general problem of the treatment of tuberculosis in under-developed countries is linked with health economics and health education. As resources are scarce, schedules of treatment that would be unacceptable in the West have to be accepted in tropical countries. Health authorities have to design programmes aimed at adequate treatment of the greatest number at the least cost. Provision may have to be made for transport to and from treatment centres, or the establishment of injection clinics in remote rural areas. The duration of treatment with streptomycin may have to be brief, and one month only on the three drugs may be all that is possible, so that follow-up treatment with PAS, INH or a second line drug is very important. This is maintained with the help of local dispensaries and health workers for a succeeding year or more. Inevitably, with restricted schedules, there will be a higher risk of resistant strains of *Mycobacterium tuberculosis* developing, but so far, the positive health gains from making anti-tuberculous treatment widely available outweigh the disadvantages. Meanwhile, in the big drug houses the search goes on for cheaper and better oral drugs to combat tuberculosis, and in tropical countries the struggle is to train sufficient health personnel, so that BCG inoculation and case finding can cope with the pool of human carriers.

TETANUS (see also page 552)

Background

Rural populations have always been more susceptible to infection with the spores of soil bacteria, but whereas in the West mechanisation of agriculture has separated the worker from the soil, and preventive inoculation with tetanus toxoid has removed the worst risks of tetanus infection, the rural populations of the tropics have their bare feet and hands constantly exposed to soil, thorns, splinters and tools. It is not, therefore, surprising that tetanus is a major cause of serious illness in young people. In girls, puerperal and post-abortion tetanus is common. In neonates the unhygienic dressings applied to the umbilical cord at birth makes tetanus neonatorum an important cause of mortality in this age group.

Symptoms and Signs

The clinical diagnosis of tetanus presents little difficulty, and if the point of septic infection can be found the organism can readily be identified with Gram's stain. The all-important factor is prognosis, which is related to the time between infection and first onset of symptoms and to the time between first onset and first opisthotonus. If the former is greater than ten days and the latter greater than one day, the prognosis for ultimate recovery is good (80 per cent chance). If the figures are twenty days and three days, the attack will be mild and recovery certain, whereas if they are five days and six hours, the chances of recovery are very poor indeed. It stands to reason, therefore, that in under-developed countries where resources are scarce, the maximum effort should be concentrated on those patients in the middle range of prognosis.

Basis of Treatment

Sedation with diazepam 20 mg four-hourly, is the first requirement, provided the body weight exceeds 50 kg. The patient should, if possible, be nursed on his side with an absorbent pad underneath, and a nasogastric tube should be passed at the earliest possible moment. Complan 100 g and glucose 100 g, with 100 ml of normal saline, diluted to 1 litre, should be the basis of the nasogastric feeds. The patient should be disturbed as little as possible and the eyes should be shielded from injury by a non-irritant covering. Oral hygiene is impossible because of the clenched jaws, but if retained secretions and pulmonary ventilation become a problem, tracheostomy must be performed, the patient curarised, and artificial ventilation established by a hand-squeezed rubber bag if no other method is available. There is reluctance in tropical countries to perform tracheostomies, not only because of the subsequent difficulties of ventilation, but because tracheal stenosis by keloid scar may occur and if the patient recovers the repair of such defects is often beyond local resources. The peak of the disease is usually reached in fourteen days from the first onset of symptoms, and by three weeks the patient is out of danger. Overall mortality remains at 40 to 50 per cent. Details of passive immunisation required, the treatment of causative wounds, muscle spasm and sympathetic overactivity are given on page 552.

MEASLES AND PNEUMONIA

These diseases are a common cause of death in tropical climates for two reasons. First, babies infected by the virus are often malnourished or enfeebled by anaemia, so that the attack is a severe one. Second, bacterial superinfection is often severe and, due to the non-availability of medical advice and suitable drugs, antibiotic therapy is either not possible or given too late. All cases of measles in children under twelve should, if diagnosed, be treated prophylactically with penicillin V 250 mg four-hourly, and in the event of pneumonia developing despite this cover, ampicillin and cloxacillin should be given on the basis that a penicillinase producing staphylococcus or another penicillin-insensitive organism may be responsible.

MENINGITIS

Meningococcal meningitis has become a rare disease in the West, but it is still common in desert and tropical countries, where epidemics occur in approximately ten-year cycles, particularly when changes in climatic conditions or famine cause population movements or overcrowding.

As part of a generalised septicaemia or as a result of spread from infective sources in the ear, nose or throat, streptococcal, pneumococcal and staphylococcal meningitis may also occur, though less commonly in previously healthy young adults. Early diagnosis by lumbar puncture and prompt treatment with intramuscular penicillin and oral sulphonamides saves numerous lives. The strains of *Neisseria meningitidis* that cause epidemics in many parts of Africa are largely resistant to sulphonamides. Penicillin or chloramphenicol are the drugs of choice. The high mortality from pneumococcal meningitis remains enigmatic.

SPECIFICALLY TROPICAL INFECTIVE DISEASES

These are usually transmitted by insect vectors but occasionally by skin-to-skin contact (e.g. leprosy) of humans living at close quarters. They can be subdivided according to the nature of the infecting organism.

1. VIRAL INFECTIONS

SANDFLY FEVER

Background

This is transmitted by the sandfly (*Phlebotomus paptasii*) and is, therefore, common in desert and sub-desert areas (Palestine, Egypt, Libya).

Symptoms

Sudden onset of fever (up to 40.5°C subsiding in two to four days).

Frontal headache.
Ocular pain.
Neck stiffness.
Muscle pains.

Signs

Conjunctival injection.
Erythema of face and neck.

Investigations

There is no specific blood test for this disease, but a thin blood film stained as for malaria parasites shows a relatively low neutrophil population. If counted, the neutrophils rarely exceed 3,000/mm^3 and are usually much lower.

Basis of Treatment

Bed rest and simple analgesics only are required.

Prognosis

Towards the end of the second day the patient feels better, and the fever subsides to about 37.5°C. He needs less analgesics and demands food, but on the third and fourth days there is a recurrence of the original symptoms, usually in a less severe form. By the fifth day the patient is convalescent and it is rare for him not to be perfectly well within a week from the onset.

DENGUE FEVER

The disease, which is common in tropical countries such as India and Ceylon, is transmitted by a Culicine mosquito (mainly *Aedes aegypti*) and has a clinical course indistinguishable from sandfly fever. The main differential diagnosis in the early stages is vivax or falciparum malaria, but rickettsial diseases, typhoid, smallpox and influenza can begin in much the same way as Dengue. By the third day, the characteristic fever pattern of the disease is clear, and the diagnosis can be established. Undoubtedly, the modern and reprehensible temptation to diagnose 'clinical malaria' (*see below*) means that many cases of Dengue are wrongly treated with chloroquine and other drugs.

YELLOW FEVER

This is a virus infection also transmitted by *Aedes aegypti*. The disease is confined to certain areas (West and Central Africa, Central and South America) and thanks to stringent internationally agreed measures of active immunisation for travellers, not only has the spread of the disease been checked, but its seriousness has steadily declined in modern times. At the turn of the century the prevalence of and mortality from the disease in Central

America was such that the first attempt to build the Panama Canal was thwarted.

Symptoms

After three to six days incubation period:
Fever.
Backache.
Headache.
Prostration.
Nausea, vomiting.
Photophobia.

After four days:
Jaundice.
Haemorrhagic features.
Shock.
Coma and death (anuria).

Signs

Purpura.
Bleeding from mucous membranes.
Jaundice.
Renal failure.

Basis of Treatment

Supportive treatment and good nursing is all that is possible.
Note: Viral hepatitis (page 64), Lassa fever (page 21), and Marburg disease (page 21) are also important.

2. BACTERIAL DISEASES

LEPROSY

Background

This is a disease caused by *Mycobacterium leprae* and is spread by body contact. Poor housing, dirty floors and overcrowding favour its spread. There are two main clinical types, the 'lepromatous' in which the disease is more active and the bacteria can often be isolated from the lesions, and the 'tuberculoid' or 'closed' type which is essentially uncontagious. Impaired immune defences explain the florid disease in the former situation. The differences are indicated in Table 23.1.

Basis of Treatment

Dapsone (1–4 diaminosulphone) is effective in all forms of leprosy, though drug resistance has been observed in a few cases. It may be given orally or by injection, once or twice weekly. (This latter regime is a way of ensuring that treatment is really administered – always a problem in developing countries.) The recommended oral standard dose for adults is:

100 mg (one tablet) twice weekly for four weeks.
200 mg (two tablets) twice weekly for four weeks.
300 mg (three tablets) twice weekly for four weeks.
400 mg (four tablets) twice weekly for four weeks.

However, initial doses may be smaller, particularly as in borderline lesions the standard dosage may precipitate allergic 'lepra' reactions (erythema nodosum, fever iritis, etc.). These may be controlled with corticosteroids

Table 23.1 Leprosy

	Tuberculoid	Lepromatous
Basic lesion:	Vigorous reaction to small number of *M. leprae*.	Formation of granulation tissue and multiplication of *M. leprae* in peripheral nerves.
Histology:	Bacilli scanty. Giant cells, epithelial cells, lymphocyte infiltration.	Bacilli plentiful. Diffuse granulation tissue. Nerve damage.
Lepromin reaction: (Lepromin is an extract of lepromatous tissue)	+ or ++	—
Symptoms and signs	Single or multiple maculo anaesthetic areas. Affected areas dry, rough, scaly. Nerve involvement early and localised or absent. This causes contractions, casual burns and trophic ulcers, etc.	Diffuse infiltrative lesions affecting face, flexor aspects of arms – scapular regions, mucous membranes of upper respiratory tract, etc. Nerve involvement late.
Prognosis:	Healing ± scarring	Usually progressive
Infectivity:	Low	High

(whilst rifampicin is promising and does not have this problem of hypersensitivity). Surgical measures are possible for chronic neurological lesions such as drop foot, paralytic inversion of the foot, claw hand, etc., and plastic procedures are valuable where there is facial disfigurement.

3. PROTOZOAL DISEASES

MALARIA

Background

Differences in the distribution and clinical features of the four types of malaria are set out in Table 23.2.

Table 23.2 Malaria

Full name	Abbrev.	Parasite	Distribution
Malignant tertian	MT	*P. falciparum*	Equatorial
Benign tertian	BT	*P. vivax*	Equatorial Mediterranean
Quartan	Q	*P. malariae*	Equatorial
Ovale	O	*P. ovale*	N.E. Africa mainly

The life cycle of the malarial parasite is shown in Fig. 23.2, but to achieve some understanding of the manifold

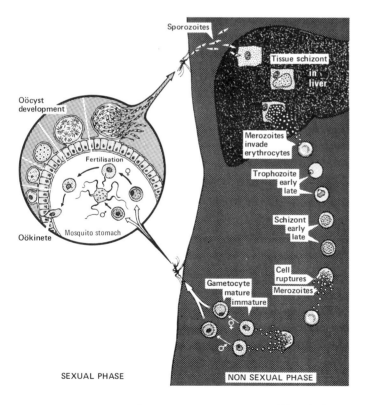

Fig. 23.2 The life cycle of the malarial parasite – BT malaria.

manifestations of these serious world-wide diseases, major textbooks on tropical medicine must be consulted. In general terms, it may be said that malignant tertian, quartan and ovale malaria are serious and potentially fatal diseases, whereas benign tertian malaria, though often a potent cause of ill-health and chronic anaemia, rarely causes death.

MT malaria, though carrying the highest mortality, is most easily eradicated as the parasite has no extra-erythrocytic cycle.

Partial immunity to malaria is widespread among those who have lived all their lives in one endemic region, and have not taken prophylactic antimalarials, but this biological 'advantage' is achieved only at the cost of a very high infantile mortality. The malaria mosquito bites at night or in deep shade.

Malariologists use terms such as hyperendemic, holoendemic, etc., referring to the parasite rate and incidence of splenic enlargement in adults and children in malarious areas, but a simpler division into 'stable' and 'unstable' malaria has practical importance (*see* Table 23.3).

Table 23.3 Differences between 'stable' and 'unstable' malaria

	Stable malaria	Unstable malaria
Regional occurrence:	Equatorial and West Africa	Ceylon, Upper Egypt
Incidence:	High	Low
Death rate:	Juvenile death rate increased	Death rate low
Herd immunity:	High	Low
Epidemics:	Not seen	Epidemics occur with high mortality
Control:	Difficult to eradicate	Easy to eradicate

Prevention

The principles only can be surveyed. Since the parasite spends part of its life in the mosquito and part in the human, vector control (killing of larvae or of adult mosquitoes in their daytime resting places) and the thorough treatment of humans infected with the parasite is the ideal solution, and there is good evidence that when money and organisation are applied malaria can be eradicated from an area. Ideal areas for such an eradication campaign are high density urban areas such as Singapore. The problem in the remote rural areas is insoluble for economic and cultural reasons only, and it seems unlikely that the resources of most under-developed regions will ever be enough to mount eradication campaigns, except in important cities and agricultural areas. However, pharmacological advances in recent years have made it possible to contemplate widespread prophylaxis by the use of injections of an antimalarial drug at long intervals of say, once a month. Whether countries with serious financial, transport and educational problems, who at the same time have an embarrassingly high birth rate will ever move into this prophylactic field remains to be seen. The fact is, however, that increasing numbers of African and Asian city dwellers are themselves moving over to personal prophylaxis. It is especially necessary for pregnant women, for homozygous sicklers, and for those with immunological deficiencies.

This personal prophylaxis is widely used by Europeans residing in malarial areas. The most convenient drug is pyrimethamine, a folic acid antagonist, 25 mg weekly for an adult. This destroys the pre-erythrocytic parasites in the liver so that the erythrocytic cycle is suppressed. It should be started a week before arrival and continued for four weeks after leaving the endemic area.

Pathology

A knowledge of the pathology of malaria is essential to the understanding of the protean features of the disease. The clinical features stem from the destruction of infected red cells with liberation of haemosiderin and malaria pigment and the blockage of capillaries by the parasites resulting in tissue anoxia. Immunologically induced cellular damage may complicate the process. In an acute case there is mild anaemia from the haemolysis with moderate enlargement of the spleen resulting from hyperplasia of the reticuloendothelial system. If haemolysis is severe the clinical picture is that of blackwater fever, with haemoglobinaemia and haemoglobinuria. Chronic, repeated infection leads to splenomegaly with hypersplenism and anaemia.

A more serious facet of the disease results from the obstruction of the micro-circulation by damaged erythrocytes and parasites, and the cellular reaction to these with vascular thrombosis and oedema is responsible for the clinical effects.

Symptoms

Acute onset of severe headache.
Nausea.
Vomiting, diarrhoea.
Chills.
Rigors, sweating.
Muscle pains.
Note: Repeated every second day for tertian or vivax malaria; repeated every third day for quartan malaria.

Signs

Rising temperature.
Tachycardia.
Herpes labialis.
Proteinuria.
Dehydration.
Splenomegaly.
Slight jaundice.

CEREBRAL MALARIA

In this deadly form of the disease, falciparum malaria involves particularly the cerebral micro-circulation. Capillary plugging results in thrombosis, petechial haemorrhage in the brain and oedema. Any neurological syndrome of acute onset with pyrexia, bizarre movements, acute confusional state, fits or coma, must always alert the examining doctor to the possibility of malaria as a cause. It is essential to enquire about overseas visits in the two to three weeks before the onset in all patients with this presentation, as early diagnosis is often live-saving in this otherwise rapidly fatal form of malarial infection.

BLACKWATER FEVER

This severe complication of malaria is almost entirely found in malignant (MT) malaria and is becoming rare since the introduction of modern antimalarials. The irregular use of suppressive doses of quinine may predispose to attacks. Blackwater fever is rare after a primary attack and rare in the population of areas of stable malaria. It may occur after return to a temperate climate. Acute haemolysis, haemoglobinaemia, haemoglobinuria, renal anoxia and oliguric renal failure may result.

Symptoms

Sudden onset of headache, rigors, loin pains, vomiting and dark urine.
Anuria develops after about eight days.
Relapses may occur.

Signs

Hyperpyrexia.
Enlarged painful spleen.
Icterus.
Convulsions, coma and possibly death.
Urine shows gross proteinuria, brown debris and granular casts.

Basis of Treatment

Uncomplicated Case of MT Malaria. Basic 'fever routine' with intravenous fluid therapy as necessary, chloroquine 600 mg (4×150 mg tablets) given in four separate doses over two hours, then 300 mg six hours later, and 600 mg daily for two days. In children, 25 mg/kg is given over four days.

If a chloroquine-resistant strain of malaria is suspected, then 500 mg of sulphadoxine (1 tablet) and 12.5 mg pyrimethamine ($\frac{1}{2}$ tablet) can be given in a single dose.

The treatment of BT, quartan and ovale malaria follows the same lines, but in BT malaria, suppressive therapy with proguanil 100 mg (1 tablet) daily is necessary afterwards, since the previously administered schizonticidal drugs will not eradicate the parasites in the liver. The alternative of giving primaquine 15 mg daily for fourteen days to eradicate the parasites is most suitable for Europeans developing the disease after return to a cold climate, but the drug carries with it the risk of exposing a pre-existing G-6PD deficiency, so is best avoided in endemic areas where G-6PD deficiency is common and reinfection likely (*see* page 386).

Cerebral Malaria. In this serious situation treatment must be prompt effective and given intravenously. Chloroquine 200 mg in 20 ml sterile water is injected slowly, or added to an intravenous drip, 200 mg chloroquine is then given intramuscularly. Alternatively, quinine 650 mg in 10 ml of distilled water should be given intravenously over ten minutes. Dexamethasone may be given intravenously (4 mg in 24 hours) to hasten recovery from the coma. 5 mg diazepam intravenously and 10 mg intramuscularly may be given if epileptic attacks occur.

Blackwater Fever. A single dose of sulfadoxine (500 mg) and pyrimethamine (12.5 mg) is used to eradicate the parasites and blood should be cross-matched for transfusion. An acute renal failure regime (*see* page 231) with or without dialysis is instituted. Steroids may be helpful.

AMOEBIASIS

Background

Entamoeba histolytica exists either in a vegetative amoeboid form or as a non-motile cystic form. The latter passed in the stools can contaminate food or water, so that new humans are infected. There is no animal reservoir and the disease requires a warm climate with primitive sanitation and water supply to flourish.

There are some curious anomalies in the distributions of this disease. In certain areas (Natal) it is very common, whereas in similar sub-tropical areas with a poorer infrastructure, the disease, though endemic, does not seem so virulent in its effects, and symptomless cyst passers are numerous. The prevention of the disease depends on a clean water supply, complete segregation of faecal waste, elimination of flies and carrier food-handlers. These conditions are almost impossible of fulfilment, except for privileged groups. The question of immunity to amoebic infection is ill-understood, but it is certainly true that white folk visiting tropical areas seem to be unduly susceptible to severe attacks of the disease.

AMOEBIC COLITIS (AMOEBIC DYSENTERY)

Pathology

The vegetative forms invade the mucosa, producing small ulcers with sharp, angular or undermined margins.

Symptoms

Usually insidious onset of diarrhoea with blood and mucus.
Abdominal pain.
Tenesmus.
Low-grade fever, headache.

Signs

Tender, palpable caecum or colon.

Complications

Toxic megacolon, perforation, and peritonitis have been observed in severe cases.

Investigations

The diagnosis can be made in either of two ways. The first and most satisfactory is to see the typical ulcers in the rectum with a sigmoidoscope and to take a swab of mucus from the ulcer, mix it with saline on a slide, cover the preparation with a slip, and look for the active amoeboid movements of the organism and the red blood cells within its cytoplasm. A fresh warm stool may be examined in the same way. Microscopy of cysts shows bar-shaped chromatoid bodies and iodine staining reveals one to four nuclei and a glycogen mass. The stool may be concentrated and cultural methods may assist isolation.

AMOEBIC HEPATITIS AND LIVER ABSCESS

Pathology

These are really stages of the same process which begins with the carriage of the organism by the portal vein to the liver. Histolytic action by the amoebae destroys liver cells, and pus accumulates. This mixture of pus and destroyed liver cells resembles anchovy sauce.

Symptoms

Fever.
Right upper abdominal pain.
Mild jaundice.
Prostration.
Nausea.
Night sweats.

Signs

Hepatomegaly.
Localised pain and swelling.
Rib pressure may produce pain.
Signs of right lower lobe lung collapse or effusion.

Investigations

1. X-rays of the chest often show a high right cupola, with or without a small pleural effusion.
2. A blood count shows a neutrophil leucocytosis.
3. Isotopic and ultrasonic liver scanning are of great value.

Differential Diagnosis

Leucocytosis and absent or slight jaundice distinguish it from viral hepatitis. The presenting features of hepatoma may resemble amoebic hepatitis, but the liver is harder and no pus is obtained on attempted aspiration. Isotope scanning is useful for localising an abscess in the liver, but not in distinguishing it from a tumour; ultrasonic scanning, however, is.

Basis of Treatment

The traditional treatment of amoebic dysentery used to be emetine hydrochloride 60 mg intramuscularly daily for three to five days accompanied by oxytetracycline 250 mg six-hourly, and then ten days of emetine bismuth iodine 200 mg daily by mouth. The latter is extremely difficult to tolerate because of nausea and vomiting. The introduction of metronidazole, a drug previously developed for the treatment of trichomonas infections, has enormously simplified the treatment of amoebiasis. In cases of colitis, 400 mg (2 tablets) can be given four-hourly for twenty-four hours and then six-hourly for five days. Symptoms rapidly abate, so that indigenous subjects accustomed to the disease may not complete the course of treatment. For them a single dose of 1 g (5 tablets) repeated in twelve hours may be adequate. The eradication of cysts in a largely symptomless patient may require longer periods of treatment and special precautions to ensure patient compliance. The toxicity of metronidazole in the therapeutic range of doses is low, but the urine turns orange-red while taking the drug. In amoebic hepatitis, the response to treatment with emetine hydrochloride, chloroquine, or metronidazole, 400 mg three times a day by mouth is equally dramatic. If pain and tenderness persist after twenty-four hours a long needle attached to a 50 ml syringe is inserted into the liver over the point of maximum tenderness and the anchovy sauce pus is aspirated. Occasionally, due to secondary infection, this material may be frankly purulent.

LEISHMANIASIS

Leishmania donovani the cause of kalaazar is transmitted from man or dogs to other men by sandflies. The organisms proliferate in the liver, spleen and marrow, causing hepatomegaly, splenomegaly, anaemia and leucopenia. There is often a skin eruption.

Diagnosis depends on finding a high level of gamma globulin in the serum, and *L.donovani* bodies in samples from marrow or spleen.

Treatment is difficult and usually with pentavalent antimony compounds.

Cutaneous leishmaniasis or oriental sore is caused by *L. tropica*, or in South America by other species. It can be suspected clinically by the appearance of the ulcerated nodule and diagnosed by the finding of *L. donovani* bodies in the serum from the margin of the ulcer.

AFRICAN SLEEPING SICKNESS

Two clinical varieties, *Trypanosoma gambiense* and *T. rhodiense*, occur, although they are morphologically identical

Distribution. West Africa, Sudan, Uganda (*T. gambiense*); Rhodesia, Mozambique (*T. rhodiense*).

Vector. Tsetse fly (various strains).

Symptoms and Signs

These include fever, malaise, headache with a skin rash (circinate erythematous rash), oedema of the eyelids, enlargement of cervical lymph nodes in posterior triangle (Winterbottom's sign), and later involvement of other lymph nodes. There are trypanosomes in the bloodstream for up to three weeks following the bite.

Later features include hepatosplenomegaly and a chronic meningo-encephalitis which causes apathy, intellectual deterioration, and somnolence (sleeping sickness). Diagnosis is made by gland puncture and demonstration of the trypanosome under light microscopy or by examining a CSF sediment by the same technique. High serum IgM and IgM in the CSF are highly suggestive of infection when no organisms are demonstrable.

Basis of Treatment

Treatment is more effective if begun before the nervous system is involved. Pentamidine isothionate is given intramuscularly on alternate days (10 doses). Central nervous system involvement is treated with arsenicals.

Prevention of the disease means destruction of the tsetse fly and the reservoir of infection in wild animals and cattle.

Note: T. rhodiense infection is severer and progression rapid. Serous effusions, myocardial involvement, high fever and local reactions at the site of the bite may occur.

CHAGAS DISEASE

Caused by *T. cruzi*, Chagas disease is endemic in Central and South America. The parasite is transmitted by the faeces of a house bug and its spread is favoured by primitive housing. There is a reservoir of parasite infestation in domestic animals. As the portal of entry is often through the conjunctiva, unilateral swelling of the eyelids is often the first sign of the disease, which soon reaches a generalised febrile state with lymphadenopathy, splenomegaly, etc. The central nervous system may be involved or the neurones in the myenteric plexus of the gut may be damaged, causing areas of dilatation or disordered peristalsis (*see* page 48). The disease is also an important cause of cardiomyopathy which may manifest with sudden death. Treatment is as yet not very satisfactory, but a number of different drugs have some effect in killing the parasite.

WORMS

TREMATODES – SCHISTOSOMIASIS (Fig. 23.3)

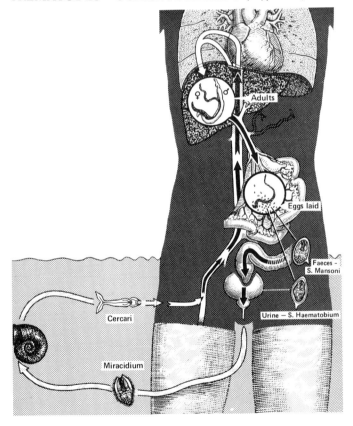

Fig. 23.3 Schistosomiasis – life cycle.

Background

After malaria, this is one of the most widespread and serious tropical diseases. Hundreds of millions of people are infected and in various degrees of ill-health. The life cycle of the parasite involves certain species of freshwater snails, and since life in tropical countries so often involves washing or growing crops in or near sluggish rivers, canals and ditches, it is easy for man both to pass the ova into the water and to expose himself to reinfection by the cercariae which have developed in the intermediate host, the snail. The parasite can thus maintain its life cycle.

Pathology

The adult female trematode lives in the portal, mesenteric or vesical veins accompanied by her ever-faithful male companion. Eggs are laid, and migrate to the wall of the bladder (*Schistosoma haematobium*) or rectum (*S. mansoni*). The terminally spined eggs of *S. haematobium* are voided mainly in the urine, while the laterally spined eggs of *S. mansoni* are voided in the faeces. Eggs of *S. japonicum* have no spines. The passage of these eggs through the wall of the bladder causes haematuria and, eventually, bladder fibrosis, granulomata, which may become malignant, and secondary damage to the kidneys. Rectal damage can cause bleeding and tenesmus, but the after effects are less serious. The passage of adults and eggs through the liver and portal vein may cause liver damage and predispose to cirrhosis. Egg output varies from 0 to 2,000 eggs/10 ml of urine or one gramme of faeces. A count greater than 500 is significant of active infection.

The eggs passed with the excreta hatch into a free swimming miracidium which enters a water snail. In the snail, the larva forms a sporocyst which forms daughter cysts, each of which grows into an active cercaria. This little beast with its forked tail is an active swimmer and can use enormous force to bore his head through the intact skin of humans wading in the water, or it can enter through the buccal mucosa. It then enters the lymph and bloodstream, and passes through the lungs to the liver.

Host-parasite Relationship. *S. mansoni* infection causes damage to the host by a complex immunological mechanism as illustrated (Fig. 23.4).

Symptoms

After an incubation period of one day:
Swimmers itch, i.e. itching, papular skin rash.
Then 20 to 60 days later:
Possibly fever, chills, hepatosplenomegaly (rare in *S. haematobium*).
Then: (a) Haematuria, dysuria (*S. haematobium*).
(b) Abdominal pain, diarrhoea (*S. mansoni*, *S. japonicum*).
Later: Haematemesis (from portal hypertension).

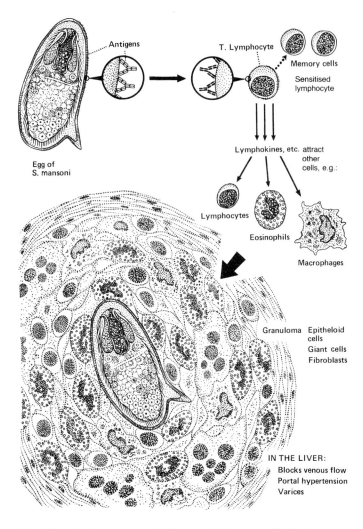

Egg of
S. mansoni

Antigens

T. Lymphocyte

Memory cells

Sensitised
lymphocyte

Lymphokines, etc. attract
other
cells, e.g.:

Lymphocytes

Eosinophils

Macrophages

Granuloma   Epitheloid
cells
Giant cells
Fibroblasts

IN THE LIVER:
Blocks venous flow
Portal hypertension
Varices

Fig. 23.4. Pathogenesis of disease in *S. mansoni* infection – a complex immunological reaction.

Signs

Skin rash on legs.
Late signs:
Bladder fibrosis, hydronephrosis, uraemia.
Hepatosplenomegaly.
Portal hypertension.
Late signs (S. haematobium):
Bladder calcification and granuloma formation, bladder cancer.

Complications

These are legion, but the most common are serious bladder scarring, secondary hydronephrosis and pyelitis, bladder cancer and anaemia. In *S. mansoni* infections, cirrhosis of the liver and chronic cholangitis are common. In all types of schistosomiasis the general malaise leads to loss of human efficiency.

Prevention

This is a serious challenge to any country, particularly those dependent on irrigation canals. Undoubtedly, the most effective method is to ensure by communal discipline that all urine and faeces are collected and allowed to ferment in closed chambers so that the heat produced kills the eggs of the parasites. Such discipline is hard to establish except under the guidance of a totalitarian regime, for example, China. Similarly, attempts to prevent children from wading and bathing in muddy rivers and from excreting on the banks are foredoomed to failure in most cultures. Snail control by chemical defoliation of canal and ditch banks is expensive and difficult. However, there is some hope that education and communal discipline can be effective in controlling the disposal of human excretion and that early treatment of infected children and adults may help to break the life cycle in such a way as to reduce the cercarial content of the water in which man must earn his living.

Basis of Treatment

The drug niridazole (Ambilhar) has largely replaced intravenous injections of sodium antimony tartrate which for years was the only effective means of eradicating the parasite. It is given orally as tablets in doses of 500 mg four times a day for seven days (25 mg/kg). Serious neuropsychiatric complications may occur in patients with established portal-systemic anastomosis and a low serum albumin. Reinfection is common in endemic areas.

OTHER TREMATODE INFECTIONS (*see* page 602)

Liver flukes parasitic upon sheep (*Fasciola hepatica*) may occasionally attack men who eat watercress or other aquatic plants. The symptoms are due to the passage of larvae through the liver. In South China *Chlonorchis sinensis* frequently infects man and is responsible for a great deal of chronic biliary tract disease. Both infections can be treated by chloroquine or emetine.

NEMATODE INFECTIONS

HOOKWORM (ANKYLOSTOMIASIS)

Background

This disease is widespread throughout the tropics and subtropical areas. The adult parasite attaches itself to the small intestinal mucosa, and each worm consumes about 0.1 ml of its host's blood daily. The ova passed in the stools germinate in the warm soil and the tiny thread-like larvae gain access to humans by penetrating the skin. They then travel via the bloodstream to lungs, up the bronchi and down into the intestine to form adults.

With such a life cycle it becomes clear why this disease affects mainly agriculturalists, whose faeces are passed directly onto the soil with which their bare feet are so often in contact. Since hundreds of millions of the world's population are in just such intimate contact with the soil, ankylostomiasis takes a vast toll of human health and energy.

Symptoms

Skin rash and itching.
Possibly transient 'asthma'.
Pallor, fatigue.
Ankle oedema.
Shortness of breath.
Upper abdominal pain.

Signs

Pallor.
Cardiomegaly.
Features of heart failure.

Prevention

The disease can be prevented by segregation of faeces and the wearing of shoes, but these measures are themselves dependent on wealth, energy and foresight in the population. The hookworm itself accounts in no small measure for these attributes being in short supply. The disease itself illustrates beautifully the interdependence of education, public health and agricultural improvement. The doctor may treat the infestation efficiently and restore the iron deficiency, but the patient who returns to the same village conditions will quickly be reinfected. Shoe-wearing town dwellers are rarely infected. Diagnosis depends on finding the ova in the stools.

Basis of Treatment

The eradication of the parasite can be achieved either by thiabendazole emulsion 7.5 ml twelve-hourly for four doses (900 mg/kg over two days) or by bephenium hydroxynaphthoate (Alcopar) 5 g in 40 ml water as a draught on three successive mornings. After eradication, iron deficiency anaemia must be treated thoroughly.

STRONGYLOIDIASIS

Though less common than ankylostomiasis, which it resembles in its life cycle, this parasite actually burrows into the intestinal mucosa and can eventually cause a severe malabsorptive state. The clinical picture is more varied. Urticaria, itching, perianal eruptions and abdominal pains may occur, in addition to anaemia and wasting. Diagnosis can be difficult. Blood eosinophilia is usually present, and motile larvae can sometimes be found in the faeces. Infestation is best treated by thiabendazole (*see above*).

ASCARIASIS

Infestation by the common round worm is universal in some tropical areas, but they cause few symptoms. The larval migration through the lungs, when it occurs in children, may cause cough, fever and malaise, and a heavy load of adult worms in the intestine can cause intestinal obstruction at the ileo-caecal valve or biliary tract involvement with jaundice. Diagnosis is by identification of the ova in the stools and a wide range of antihelminthics can eradicate the worm (*see page 599*).

FILARIASIS

Several thin nematodes of the family Filaridae may infect man, and the symptoms of the infestation vary from none to the most serious. The adult worms are more than an inch long and tend to live in lymphatics or to wander in the subcutaneous tissues, causing swelling, itching and even visual disturbances, when they cross the eye. The microfilariae, about $250\,\mu$ long, appear in the blood and can be readily seen under the low power of the microscope. *Vectors* (various types of mosquitoes and flies) transfer the microfilariae from man to man. The usual vectors, geographical distribution and common clinical manifestations of the different types of filariasis, are set out in Table 23.4.

Diagnosis depends on clinical features, eosinophilia and the finding of microfilariae in the blood or skin snip, or adults in the nodules.

Basis of Treatment

Treatment is with diethylcarbamazine (Hetrazan) 50 mg the first day, 100 mg the second, and so on, doubling the dose until an allergic reaction to the dead worms occurs or until the full dose of 500 mg daily is reached. Treatment is then usually continued for three weeks. The regime varies according to the type of worm, the site of main damage and whether there is likely to be an allergic response. If there is, antihistamines orally or cortisone eye drops may help to control it.

DRACONTIASIS

Caused by *Dracunculus medinensis* (guinea worm).

Distribution

India, Middle East, W. Africa, W. Indies. Infected cyclops (small crustaceans) are swallowed in drinking water and the adult worms migrate into various tissues before the gravid female (about a yard long) produces larvae which are discharged through a cutaneous ulcer, usually on the legs. The male worm dies.

Table 23.4 Dracontiasis

Parasite	Vector	Habitat	Manifestations
Wuchereria bancrofti	Culex fatigans (mosquito)	Coastal swamps, Africa, S.E. Asia, Pacific	Fever Lymphangitis Lymphadenopathy Elephantiasis Chyluria Hydrocoele

Diagnosis:
Microfilariae are found in the blood taken at night (2200 hours to 0200 hours). Thick blood films show sheathed microfilariae with discrete nuclei which do not reach the tail. Also found in hydrocoele, pleural, joint and ascitic fluid. Blood shows eosinophilia.

Parasite	Vector	Habitat	Manifestations
Brugia malayi	Mosquitoes (Mansonia and Anopheles)	Mangrove swamps, S.E. Asia, S. China	Similar to *W. bancrofti*
Loa loa	Chrysops (mango fly)	Slow-running streams, Central Africa	Conjunctivitis Lachrymation Urticaria Pruritis Calabar swellings (painless, non-pitting subcutaneous swellings)

Diagnosis:
Blood films during the day show microfilariae. Nucleus reaches tail. Tail bent on body. Adult worm may wriggle across conjunctiva. High eosinophilia 60 to 80 per cent.

Parasite	Vector	Habitat	Manifestations
Onchocerca volvulus	Simulium fly (coffee fly)	Fast-flowing streams, drier area of Central Africa, Tropical America.	Skin nodules (site related to biting habits of vector) *Blindness* – unusual before 30 and usually the result of iridocyclitis. *Skin lesions* – lichenoid lesions, thickened inelastic skin, 'Lizard skin'

Diagnosis:
Examination of skin snips. Microfilaria unsheathed head spatulate nucleus not extending to tail. Therapeutic trial with 50 mg Hetrazan (Mazotti test). An itching papular reaction to the skin 1 to 24 hours later strongly favours presence of microfilariae.

Symptoms and Signs

Generalised urticaria.
Coiled worm visible under skin producing marked burning and itching.
Secondary infection produces cellulitis, arthritis, etc.

Basis of Treatment

Niridazole is toxic to the worm which should also be extracted by knotting a silk thread round it and winding it gradually onto a small stick.

RICKETTSIAL

TICK-BORNE AND MITE-BORNE TYPHUS

These are endemic in many tropical and subtropical areas. The rapid onset of symptoms is similar to that of the classical louse-borne typhus, but there is usually an eschar (inflamed site of entry of the infection), with regional lymph node enlargement and ulceration. The rash often appears on the seventh day and is maculopapular. Treatment is with tetracycline.

SPIROCHAETAL

YAWS

This fast disappearing disease caused by *Treponema pertenue* is endemic only in communities where close body-to-body contact is frequent. The granulomatous skin lesions are highly infectious. It responds quickly to penicillin and can be eliminated in communities by cleanliness, education and improved housing.

RELAPSING FEVERS

Spirochaetes of the genus Borrelia can be transmitted by lice or ticks. About a week after infection there is high fever with severe body pains and conjunctivitis, often accompanied by jaundice and splenomegaly. The fever subsides in about a week, but may recur a week later again. The organisms can be identified in blood films. Tetracycline is curative.

LARVA MIGRANS

Defintion

Invasion of man by larvae of a variety of animal nematodes which are unable to develop further. They migrate either in the skin or viscera (*see* Table 23.5).

Table 23.5

Cutaneous Larva Migrans (larvae of cat and dog hookworms)	Visceral Larva Migrans
Ancylostoma caninum A. brazilliense, etc.	Toxocara canis Toxocara cati (*see* page 600)

These burrow in the skin producing an erythematous serpiginous track with intense puritis. The larvae die this can be accelerated by local application of CO_2 snow:

TROPICAL EOSINOPHILIA

This syndrome is caused by a filarial worm (*Brugia pahangi*) normally found in animals which, thus, cannot mature in man. The disorder occurs in many parts of the tropics. The microfilariae are sequestered in various organs particularly the lungs and each becomes surrounded by a granulomatous reaction.

The disease is commoner amongst young adult Indians (20 to 30 years). Males are affected more than females.

Symptoms

Weakness, loss of weight.
Chest pain and wheezing.
Cough with scanty sometimes blood-stained sputum.

Signs

Fever.
Rhonchi and rales over lung.
Splenomegaly.

Investigations

There is eosinophilia and miliary mottling of the lungs on X-ray, with hilar adenopathy.

Basis of Treatment

Diethylcarbamazine 12 mg/kg body weight is rapidly effective.
Note: Eosinophilia occurs commonly amongst tropical people, probably from multiple parasitic intestinal infestations.

TROPICAL PYOMYOSITIS

This is an acute bacterial infection of proximal muscles of the limbs or pelvic or pectoral girdle with abscesses in skeletal muscles. Males are affected more than females, and infection may follow trauma. *Staphylococcus aureus* is the commonest organism isolated. The disease occurs in hot humid areas of the tropics.

Symptoms

Fever.
Headache.
Aching muscles or joints.
Two to three days later:
Pain in a muscle or muscles.

Signs

Pyrexia.
Anaemia.
Tenderness.
Arthritis.
Jaundice, confusion, coma in those with associated septicaemia.

Investigations

There is leucocytosis. Culture of pus and blood may reveal the organism. X-rays should be taken to detect osteomyelitis.

Basis of Treatment

Incision and drainage and appropriate antibiotics.

Differential Diagnosis

The condition has to be differentiated from a guinea worm abscess. Polymyositis is unlikely to cause confusion as the latter presents with symmetrical weakness in proximal muscles. Fever and pain are rare and it is uncommon in most tropical countries.

TROPICAL SPLENOMEGALY SYNDROME

This term refers to gross splenomegaly with hyperplenism in immune adults in areas of the tropical world endemic for malaria. There is evidence that the syndrome results from an abnormal immunological reaction to infection with the malaria parasite. The occurrence in families in some instances suggests a genetic basis.

The major features of the syndrome are:
1. Occurs in areas of the world where malaria is endemic.
2. Patients are adults who have developed immunity to malaria.
3. There is gross splenomegaly with hypersplenism.
4. Liver may be enlarged with infiltration of the sinusoids with lymphocytes (hepatic sinusoidal lymphocytosis).
5. Serum IgM is grossly elevated.
6. There is regression of the symptoms and signs on malaria treatment and prophylaxis.
7. Full investigation does not reveal any disease known to cause gross splenomegaly.

Symptoms

Abdominal swelling.
Abdominal pain.
Weakness and loss of energy.
Swelling of legs – much less frequent.

Signs

Splenomegaly – usually gross (>10 cm), below costal margin.
Hepatomegaly – moderate.
Pallor.
Jaundice (infrequent).

Basis of Treatment

Chloroquine, 600 mg orally for three days. Proguanil 100 mg daily for life.

DISEASES OF MALNUTRITION AND TOXICITY COMMON IN TROPICAL COUNTRIES

Background

The causes of deficiency states in malnourished populations are complex. By no means all the malnourished are under-nourished, and what may be an adequate diet for a healthy person is inadequate for someone whose protein and haemoglobin stores are being leached away by hookworm disease or schistosomiasis. The combination of poverty, ignorance of food values and chronic infections causes a situation where a very slight decrease in food intake precipitates a deficiency.

In addition to the health problems of the individual, Society in tropical countries is faced with the difficulty of providing an even supply of food throughout the year, and of overcoming natural disasters like drought, flood and animal depredations. Food storage in tropical coun-

tries is difficult due to heat and humidity favouring a high prevalence of fungus spores and rapidly growing populations of weevils and cockroaches, etc. Food which may have been harvested in more than adequate supply may be so reduced in food value before it is eaten that the tribe or group has to spend several months on the edge of starvation. The shortage of roads, scarcity of cash and the absence of a sophisticated retail system make rural populations particularly vulnerable to temporary disturbances. The war in Nigeria in the late sixties occurred in a densely populated area normally self-sufficient in basic food stuffs, but the disruption of normal lines of distribution and the neglect of harvest and planting in areas affected by the war led very rapidly to those most vulnerable, women and growing children, developing protein–calorie malnutrition.

The factors producing malnutrition in individuals can therefore be summarised:

Inadequate Food Supply

Crop failure.
Storage wastage.
Storage disasters.
Toxic transformation in storage.
Group or individual poverty.
Social disruption and war.

Wrong Choice of Foods

Easily grown crops often of poor nutritive value (e.g. Cassava root which grows easily and can be harvested at any time).
Food taboos inhibiting protein intake in children.
Cheapness of carbohydrate compared with protein foods.

Increased Body Requirements for Food

Fevers increase metabolic rate.
Blood and protein wasting diseases deplete stores.
Manual labour in humid conditions demands high caloric intake.

KWASHIORKOR

The detailed clinical picture of protein–calorie malnutrition (Kwashiorkor) and of specific vitamin deficiences is dealt with on pages 102 to 104 but some examples are given here of the way in which mixed nutritional and toxic factors may give rise to some of the common clinical problems of the tropics. Clearly, the pattern of disease varies enormously from one area of the tropics to another, depending on the geographical distribution of parasites and vectors, the soil characteristics, the food habits and taboos of the people, and the burden of hereditary disease.

BERIBERI

Primarily due to a thiamine deficiency, this characteristically occurs in poor rice-eating populations. Polished rice purchased commercially contains inadequate thiamine, while a high carbohydrate diet demands high thiamine usage in the tissues. The symptoms are those of painful peripheral neuritis, mental confusion and cardiac failure due to cardiomyopathy.

PELLAGRA

This is particularly common in maize-eating populations, whose diet is otherwise deficient. Solar dermatitis, apathy, confusion, and a red sore tongue are the main features, and since the disease is often precipitated by gastroenteritis, diarrhoea and hypoalbuminaemic oedema often complicate the picture.

TROPICAL NEUROPATHY

This occurs characteristically in Cassava-eating populations and appears to be due to traces of cyanide in the root, which interfere with the metabolism of vitamin B_{12} in the central nervous systems so that the patients develop a peripheral neuritis, a sensory ataxia, and progressive optic and auditory nerve damage, similar in many respects to the outright B_{12} deficiency of pernicious anaemia.

CIRRHOSIS OF THE LIVER

The factors that lead to the high prevalence of subclinical liver cell dysfunction and of cryptogenic cirrhosis in tropical populations are still the subject of dispute. The answer probably lies in the two factors of liver cell vulnerability, perhaps due to a poor diet, and possibly by aflatoxins accumulating from mould contamination in bulk foods stored under suboptimal conditions, and to damage caused by the wide variety of pathogens – viral, protozoal and helminthic, that can at one time or another attack the livers of those living in the tropics. The importance of viral hepatitis is being demonstrated by surveys showing an increased incidence of HBsAg, and other markers of virus B infection.

Cirrhosis of the liver is, therefore, a common cause of disability, and the resulting ascites is the reason for many people seeking medical aid. Hepatoma, again perhaps related to chronic viral infection, is particularly common in the tropics.

GENETIC DISEASES COMMON IN NEGROID AND MEDITERRANEAN PEOPLES

HAEMOGLOBIN S AND C

Probably as a result of evolutionary developments caused by the effects of the malaria parasite on infant survival, haemoglobin S and haemoglobin C are widespread in the population of West and Central Africa. The homozygous form is normally lethal before the reproductive stage is reached, but the heterozygous condition may have some protective effect against death from falciparum malaria in infancy. The altered pattern of haemoglobins within the red cells causes malformation or sickling, and this causes cells not to flow smoothly along capillaries. The manifestations of the disease are due to a combination of haemolysis and microinfarctions (*see* page 387, for clinical details, diagnosis and treatment).

THALASSAEMIA

Thalassaemia (*see* page 388) occurring in the Mediterranean areas and S.E. Asia is due to inherited abnormalities either in the β or the a chain of the globin chain of haemoglobin. In the major form, chronic haemolytic anaemia (hypochromic with basophil stippling and target cells) leads to a perpetual loss of strength and energy. The spleen is often enlarged. The peripheral blood picture suggests iron deficiency but the serum iron is unaltered and iron therapy may be harmful.

GLUCOSE-6-PHOSPHATE DEHYDROGENASE DEFICIENCY

This is a common inherited abnormality in Mediterranean and African males. The deficiency makes them unduly susceptible to rapid haemolysis in response to toxic substances in food (e.g. favism) or to drugs (*see* page 386).

APPENDIX

Preventive inoculations and antimalarial prophylaxis for persons going and returning from the tropics.

On going to the tropics
Preventive inoculations
1. Anti-cholera vaccine by injection (useful for three months only and optional for most areas).
2. Anti-typhoid anti-tetanus (TABT), one injection four weeks before leaving, and two boosters. Tetanus immunisation the most important.
3. Smallpox vaccination (if not already in last three years).
4. Oral polio vaccine, one month before leaving and subsequent boosters (unless immunised).
5. Yellow fever vaccine, only required for certain areas (e.g. Central and South America).

On returning from the tropics
1. Continue anti-malarial prophylaxis for at least one month after return.
2. If diarrhoea and rectal bleeding occur, have fresh

stool samples examined for amoebae and for ova and cysts of parasites.

Antimalarial prophylaxis
Start pyrimethamine 50 mg weekly, two weeks prior to departure or proguanil 100 mg daily.

SUGGESTED FURTHER READING

General

Gillies, H. M. (1967) Medical care in developing countries. A review and commentary, *Lancet*, **i**; 718.

Amoebiasis

Adi, F. C. (1965) Clinical features of hepatic amoebiasis. *West African Medical Journal*, **14**: 181.
Adi, F. C. (1966) Complications and treatment of hepatic amoebiasis. *West African Medical Journal*, **15**: 43.

Hookworm

Gillies, H. M., Watson Williams, J. and Ball, P. A. J. (1964) Hookworm infection and anaemia, *Quarterly Journal of Medicine*, **33**: 1.

Leishmaniasis

Bryceson, A. and Leithead, C. P. (1966) Diffuse cutaneous leishmaniasis in Ethiopia. *Ethiopian Medical Journal*, **5**: 31.

Leprosy

Rees, R. J. W. and Waters, M. F. R. (1972) Recent trends in leprosy research. *British Medical Bulletin*, **28**: 1.

Malaria

W.H.O. (1967) Chemotherapy of Malaria. Tech. Report series, *World Health Organization*, No. 375.

Measles

Morley, D. C. (1969) Severe measles in the tropics. *British Medical Journal*, **1**: 279, 363.

Schistosomiasis

Davis, A. (1966) Field trials of Ambilhar in treatment of urinary bilharziasis in school children. *W.H.O. Bulletin*, **38**: 827.
Forsyth, D. M. and Bradley, D. J. (1966) Consequences of bilharziasis, *W.H.O. Bulletin*, **34**: 715.
Warren, K. S. (1972) The immunopathogenesis of schistosomiasis: A multidisciplinary approach. *Transactions Royal Society of Tropical Medicine and Hygiene*, **66**: 417.

Tropical Neuropathy

Osuntokun, B. O. (1968) An ataxic neuropathy in Nigeria – a clinical biochemical and electrophysiological study. *Brain*, **91**: 215.

Tropical Pyomyositis

Shaper, A. G., Kibukamusoke, J. W. and Hutt, M. S. R. (1972) Tropical myositis. *Medicine in a Tropical Environment*, p. 32, B.M.A., London.

Tropical Splenomegaly Syndrome

Marsden, P. D. and Crane, G. G. (1976) Tropical splenomegaly syndrome – a current appraisal. *Rev. Inst. Med. Trop. (Sao Paulo)*, **18**: 54.

Tuberculosis

East African/British Medical Research Council (1969) Pyrazinamide investigation. *Tubercle*. **50**: 81.
Roelsgaard, E., Iverson, E. and Blocher, C. (1964) Tuberculosis in Tropical Africa. An epidemiological study *W.H.O. Bulletin*, **30**: 459.

Typhoid Fever

Badoe, A. E. (1966) A review of 37 cases of perforated typhoid ulcer in Accra, 1964–1965. *Ghana Medical Journal*, **5**: 83.

Parasitic Diseases in Europe 24

P. BROWN

The incidence in Britain and Western Europe of diseases normally associated with tropical zones has increased steadily since the last World War for two major reasons:
1. Increased contact between tropical and temperate zones.
(a) Europeans working in the tropics for various periods.
(b) Tourists seeking more and more exotic holiday haunts.
(e) Immigration to various former colonial powers from their former colonies.

These facts explain the occurrence of exotic parasitic disease in various European countries (e.g. importation of filariasis into the Netherlands from Dutch Guyana).
2. Increased air travel. A sea voyage provided an excellent quarantine period, but travellers can now return home well within the incubation period of any infectious disease.

There are two groups of diseases which can be imported from the tropics.
1. Diseases which previously occurred world-wide, but because of improving socio-economic conditions have been largely eradicated from Western Europe, for example, smallpox, cholera, tuberculosis. These patients are at risk themselves, but also are a very real public health risk because of ease of transmission.
2. Specific tropical diseases may be a serious individual risk to the affected patient but they are not a risk to the community at large, as, without a vector, transmission in a temperate climate only occurs exceptionally (e.g. blood transfusion).

Perhaps the most important aspect of imported disease in developed countries is for the medical practitioner to be aware of such a possibility and ask the simple but vital question, 'Have you ever travelled abroad?'. This not only applies in the acutely ill patient with possible falciparum malaria, but also in more chronic conditions such as leprosy or schistosomiasis which may have been contracted many years previously.

The following imported diseases should be particularly borne in mind as they are potentially fatal and delay in diagnosis increases the risk to the patient and, in the case of smallpox, the risk to the community:
1. Falciparum malaria (*see* page 587).
2. Smallpox (*see* page 18).
3. Amoebic liver abscess (*see* page 589).
4. Visceral leishmaniasis (*see* page 590).
5. African trypanosomiasis (*see* page 590).

WORMS

Helminthic infections are of relatively minor importance in Britain. Only ascaris, enterobius, toxocara, trichuris, *Taenia saginata*, echinococcus and fasciola are native to this country. Imported worms are normally present only as a light infection causing, at the most, minor symptoms, and the chronic debilitating results of helminthiasis seen in the tropics do not occur.

NEMATODES (ROUNDWORMS)

Hookworm (*see also* page 592)

On a world-wide basis these are the most important of the intestinal nematodes, but are rarely a serious problem in this country. Two species, *Ancylostoma duodenale* and *Necator americanus* affect man, and although it was previously thought that the former worm occurred predominantly in Europe it is now uncommon. The main consequence of this infection is iron deficiency anaemia, but as the development of this depends on the intensity and duration of infection and on the iron content of the diet, it is rarely seen in Europe as infection is almost always light and dietary 'intake' is adequate.

Diagnosis is established by finding eggs in the stool and the number of eggs gives some idea of the intensity of infection. Treatment consists of the administration of antihelminthics and, if present, the correction of anaemia. Tetrachlorethylene, in a single dose of 0.1 ml/kg body weight to a maximum of 5 ml, thiabendazole or bephenium hydroxynaphthoate (Alcopar) 5 g, as a draught on three successive mornings, are most frequently used. Heavy infections or infection with *N. americanus*, which is less susceptible to bephenium may require a further course of treatment.

Ascaris Lumbricoides (*see also* page 593)

This infestation is uncommon in temperate countries, and is often only noticed when adult worms are passed in the stools. The presence of worms within the intestine can also be suspected by finding blood eosinophilia and the characteristic ova in the stools. Eradication can be achieved by a single dose of 4 g of piperazine with a saline purge the following day. Bephenium hydroxynaphthoate, as a single 5 g dose, or thiabendazole, 25 mg/kg body weight twice daily for two days, are possible alternatives especially if a mixed nematode infection is present.

Toxocariasis

This is an accidental human infection with the cat or dog ascaris (*Toxocara cati* or *Toxocara canis*, respectively). The popularity of domestic pets and the close, often oral contact between them and man leads to the accidental ingestion of ova which can hatch into larvae within the human intestine. The larvae burrow into the intestinal blood vessels and pass to the liver where the majority are filtered out. The remaining larvae die in the capillaries of the lungs, eye, muscle, and brain. The helminthic protein so released tends to set up an eosinophilic granulation reaction. The clinical importance of this is limited but there have been reports of ocular damage, of fever with eosinophilia, of hepatitis, and of eosinophilic granulomas in the liver as a result of this larval invasion. The adult worms do not develop in humans.

A heavy larval infestation is suggested by an otherwise unexplained eosinophilia in those with pets in the home, but the fact that a positive intradermal test, using toxocara antigen, is obtained in about five per cent of healthy adults suggests that this infestation is common and usually harmless.

The best form of management is to remove the source of infection by treating the affected animal with piperazine. Pets, especially puppies, should be wormed regularly if they are in contact with children.

Threadworm

These small worms (*Enterobius vermicularis*) are endemic in children of all races. The adult worm lives in the colon and rectum from where the gravid female which is about 1 cm long migrates, usually at night, to the anal margin to lay her eggs. This results in marked itching

---

Threadworm infection

Symptoms: Pruritus ani.
             Possibly enuresis.
             Insomnia and irritability.
Signs: Perianal excoriation.
             Worms occasionally seen in faeces.
             Demonstration of eggs from perianal region using adhesive cellophane.

---

and subsequent scratching by the child and this is very likely to lead to further auto-infection.

Treatment. Piperazine citrate in a daily dose of 300 mg for each year of life to a maximum of 1.8 g orally for seven days will kill off a generation of threadworms in a child, but this is pointless if the child immediately reinfects himself with eggs. To prevent reinfection, the child should have well-cut nails and have his fingers scrubbed in the morning. He or she should wear close-fitting pants at night, after a hydrocortisone cream has been applied to the anal area. If necessary, drug treatment and preventive measures should be applied simultaneously to all members of the family group.

Whipworm

Whipworm (*Trichuris trichuria*) is a very common parasite of man with a world-wide distribution. The adult worms are 30 to 50 mm in length and attach themselves by the head mainly in the caecum and ascending colon. Clinical symptoms are extremely uncommon, but massive infection in malnourished children may manifest itself as bloody diarrhoea or rectal prolapse.

Treatment. Thiabendazole 25 mg/kg twelve-hourly for three days may clear the infection.

Trichinosis

This worm (*Trichinella spiralis*) is essentially a parasite of the pig which acts as both the final and intermediate host and is the only important tissue nematode with a world-wide distribution. Man is infected by eating raw or partially cooked pork containing larvae. This results in a self-limiting infection of the intestine (adult worm) and of striated muscle (larvae). In the majority infestation is asymptomatic with clinical symptoms developing in less than five per cent, but, rarely, infection can be fatal especially if central nervous system symptoms predominate.

Treatment. Thiabendazole 25 mg/kg body weight for five to seven days produces symptomatic relief, but larvae can often still be found after treatment. Corticosteroids are useful for fever and myalgia, and essential if encephalitis develops.

Filariasis (*see also* page 593)

This term encompasses seven different nematodes belonging to the superfamily, filaroidea and are by far the most significant nematode infection with a worldwide incidence of over 200 million. As filariasis is only contracted in the tropics the incidence in Europe is low, but it must be remembered that certain types, for example onchocerciasis and loiasis, may present clinically many months after the patient leaves tropical Africa. In the chronic stage establishing the diagnosis may be difficult as the microfilariae may no longer be found in the blood. However, persisting eosinophilia, a positive skin test or a positive filarial complement fixation test may indicate the diagnosis.

CESTODES (Tapeworms)

Tapeworms normally share two hosts, the adult worm living in the intestine of one host and the larvae normally in the muscles of the other. The common important tapeworms can exist in man as adults (*Taenia saginata*), larvae (hydatid cyst) or both (*Taenia solium*).

Taenia Saginata

This is the commonest tapeworm affecting man, infection resulting from the consumption of beef containing a live larva (cysticercus). The cysticercus can survive a certain amount of cooking so that devotees of rare steaks are particularly at risk. In Britain about one per cent of beef carcasses are infected with cysticerci.

When a living cysticercus is ingested it attaches to the mucosa of the upper jejunum and a full grown, 5 m worm develops over the next three months. It is difficult to ascribe any symptoms to the presence of the worm although it has been postulated as a cause of weight loss, appetite disturbance and vague abdominal pain. The main problem is the distress and embarrassment caused to the patient by the passage of gravid segments of worm.

Taenia Solium

The pork tapeworm can be differentiated from *T. saginata* by the microscopical appearance of the uterus within the gravid segment, and by the head of the adult worm which has hooks as well as four suckers, whereas the head of *T. saginata* is armed only with suckers. The eggs of both species are morphologically identical. The adult worm is a strictly human parasite, but unlike *T. saginata* the larvae, while they normally occur in the pig, can develop in man (cysticercosis) which is why this parasite is so potentially dangerous. If the larvae spread in man they may lodge in striated muscle, connective tissue, subcutaneous tissue or in the central nervous system. Spread to peripheral tissue results in harmless but characteristic calcification, but although the larvae in the brain do not calcify they do swell as they degenerate and may result in epilepsy or psychiatric disturbances.

Treatment. Both species of taenia can be treated with niclosamide, two oral doses of 1 g, one hour apart, or with dichlorophen, two oral doses of 6 g, twenty-four hours apart. These drugs have the advantage that no lengthy bowel preparation is necessary and that they can be used on an out-patient basis. However, treatment results in disintegration of the head of the worm so that cure cannot be assumed until no further gravid segments are passed for twelve weeks. A more important potential risk when treating *T. solium* is that disintegration of the worm may result in larval spread. For this reason the older, more cumbersome treatment with mepacrine is still used. The patient is starved for forty-eight hours and on the night prior to treatment a duodenal tube is inserted through which 1 g of mepacrine in water is given, followed by 30 g magnesium sulphate. When the purgative acts a complete worm with an identifiable head is passed.

There is no treatment for cerebral cysts except in rare cases when isolated cysts may be removed surgically. Epilepsy, if present, is treated with the usual anticonvulsants (*see* page 519).

Echinococcus Granulosus (Hydatid Cyst, *see* Fig. 24.1)

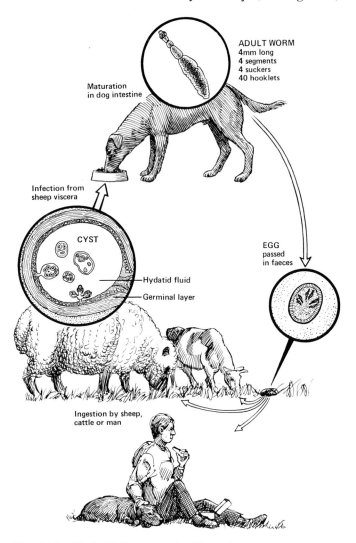

Fig. 24.1   Hydatid disease – the life cycle.

The adult worm lives in the small intestine of the dog which is the definitive host and is infected by eating larvae-containing remains of sheep or cattle which are the intermediate host. Sheep, cattle and, occasionally, man are infected by ingesting ova excreted by the dog. Hyatid disease is, therefore, commonest in farming areas such as Australia and Wales where up to 20 per cent of farm dogs carry the parasite. Infection manifests itself clinically in man by the local pressure effect of the developing cyst or by hypersensitivity reactions if a cyst ruptures spontaneously or at surgery. The commonest sites of cyst formation are the liver and lungs which account for about 90 per cent of cases. Hydatid cyst of the liver usually results in symptomless hepatomegaly, which must be differentiated from other causes of hepatic enlargement, while symptoms due to compression are commonest in the lungs.

Diagnosis should be suspected in patients with a hepatic or pulmonary lesion who have a persistent eosinophilia. A useful adjunct to the diagnosis is the Casoni skin test which involves the intradermal injection of antigen obtained from hydatid cyst fluid. A positive skin test, as indicated by a large weal and flare developing within 20 minutes is good evidence of hydatid disease, but a negative reaction does not exclude it. There is also a complement fixation test which is highly specific in the presence of live larvae.

Hydatid cyst should be excised surgically where possible because of the risk of rupture and subsequent anaphylaxis. Strict precautions must be taken at surgery to prevent spillage during cyst aspiration, and before removal the cyst should be refilled with formalin to kill any remaining larvae.

Diphyllobothrium Latum

The fish tapeworm encysts in fresh water fish and man is infected by eating uncooked fish flesh; the disease occurring only in Scandinavia, the Baltic and Canada. The main complication is megaloblastic anaemia due to the worms avidity for vitamin B_{12}. It can be treated with niclosamide or dichlorophen.

TREMATODES (Flukes)

Fasciola Hepatica

This is a hepatic hermaphroditic fluke which is less well adapted to man than the other hepatic fluke, *Chlonorchis sinensis* (widespread in the Far East), but which can infect man instead of its usual host, the sheep. It has a world-wide distribution and is particularly prevalent in low wet pastures where the miracidia, released from sheep faeces, invade lymnaea snails. Metacercaria, released from the snail, encyst on grass or watercress from where infection reaches sheep or man. In England, epidemics occur during wet summers, the most recent outbreak being in the Chepstow area in 1969. Jaundice, fever, urticaria and right upper quadrant pain are the usual initial symptoms and occasionally patients may present with biliary obstruction due to adult flukes in the common bile duct. Long term complications include cirrhosis and possibly malignant change in the bile ducts. The diagnosis depends on the demonstration of ova in faeces or duodenal aspirate. A useful diagnostic aid is a complement fixation test using an extract of adult fluke as antigen. Treatment is unsatisfactory, emetine and chloroquine having been used with equivocal results.

Schistosomiasis

Like filariasis, this is an infestation of minor importance in Europe, but on a world-wide basis is a disease of tremendous importance, with an overall incidence of more than 200,000,000. It is endemic in Africa, S.E. Asia and S. America and as the clinical manifestations may take years to present, the disease should be considered in the differential diagnosis of rectal bleeding, haematuria or cirrhosis if the patient has ever resided in an endemic area, especially if there is an associated eosinophilia. Diagnosis is by demonstration of the eggs in faeces or urine. However, in patients with chronic disease, especially cirrhosis, ova excretion may have ceased so that indirect immunological tests based on serological or skin reactions may be useful.

PROTOZOAN DISEASES

Of the four major protozoal infections, three (malaria, trypanosomiasis, leishmaniasis) have arthropod vectors so that, except in exceptional circumstances, the disease must be originally contracted in tropical areas where the insect thrives. The fourth infection, amoebiasis, is spread by the oro-faecal route and has a world-wide distribution although the incidence in any community depends mainly on socio-economic factors.

MALARIA

The incidence of imported malaria is increasing, with 5,590 reported cases in Europe in 1972. Of these 1,572 were falciparum malaria with 131 cases (including 7 of the 15 deaths) occurring in Britain (*see* page 587).

Falciparum malaria is the most important, as delay in diagnosis can be fatal. It must be considered in the differential diagnosis of any acutely ill patient who has passed through an endemic area in the preceding year. The incubation period is normally 8 to 15 days, but this may be markedly prolonged especially if the patient has had inadequate suppressive therapy or treatment. Fever, headache, malaise, nausea, vomiting and generalised arthralgia may be the only symptoms in an uncomplicated attack, but the patient can deteriorate rapidly, developing complications such as cerebral malaria or massive intravascular haemolysis with renal failure (blackwater fever). Relapses can occur for a limited time after a patient has left an endemic area (falciparum up to two years, vivax and ovale up to five years, quartan up to ten years).

Definitive diagnosis is by demonstration of the parasite in the blood and an indication of the likely severity can be obtained from the degree of parasitaemia. In the acutely ill patient, in whom the diagnosis is strongly suspected, treatment may have to be instituted without final proof.

Treatment (*see* page 588)

AMOEBIASIS (*see* page 589)

About 10 per cent of the world population harbour the causative organism, *Entamoeba histolytica*, the incidence varying from 1 to 5 per cent in Europe to 40 per cent in some tropical countries. In the vast majority of cases it is a symptomless commensal with no resultant tissue invasion, but intestinal amoebiasis and hepatic involvement occur.

Intestinal amoebiasis varies from a chronic mild intermittent diarrhoea to a fulminant dysentery which may progress to peritonitis and death. Numerous, ill-defined abdominal symptoms have been blamed on the presence of a few amoebic cysts in the faeces, but the evidence for pathogenicity in such cases is very slight. Diagnosis is based on the demonstration of the trophozoite in fresh faeces, in mucus or in sigmoidoscopic scrapings from mucosal ulcers. If the trophozoites contain ingested erythrocytes, then this is definitive evidence of tissue invasion. Specific serological tests are now available, but do not differentiate between past and present amoebic infections. Treatment with metronidazole, 800mg three times a day for five days, will cure about 95 per cent of patients. To confirm cure at least three follow-up specimens should be examined at intervals one month after treatment.

Amoebic liver abscess may present clinically years after initial infection which may even have been subclinical, and rarely it may occur in patients who have never left Europe. The patient presents with fever, weight loss and right hypochondrial pain, and there is usually tender hepatomegaly with localised lower right intercostal tenderness (most abscesses occur in the upper part of the right lobe). The lesion must be differentiated from a pyogenic abcess and primary or secondary neoplasia; definitive diagnosis depending on the demonstration of bacteriologically sterile pus (anchovy sauce) with, in about 75 per cent of cases, a small number of *E. histolytica*. Treatment is with metronidazole and, if the abscess is large, repeated aspiration.

GIARDIASIS (Fig. 24.2)

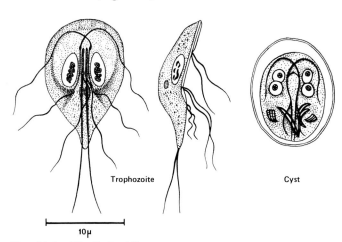

Trophozoite   Cyst

10μ

Fig. 24.2 *Giardia lamblia.*

Giardia lamblia is a flagellated protozoan which was first described by Leevenhoek as he examined his own stool with almost the first microscope. It has a world-wide distribution with an incidence of about five per cent in Europe, although the majority infected are asymptomatic. It presents as diarrhoea, especially in children, and is a cause of occasional outbreaks of travellers' diarrhoea. A recent well-documented epidemic occurred among a large group of American tourists in Leningrad who drank contaminated water. If the infection is severe enough it can cause steatorrhoea. Diagnosis is by demonstration of the trophozoite in a duodenal aspirate or in a diarrhoeal stool, or by demonstrating cysts in faeces. Treatment with metronidazole, 500 mg daily for five to seven days, is effective in 90 to 100 per cent of cases.

SUGGESTED FURTHER READING

Macgraith, B. (Ed.) (1976) *Clinical Tropical Diseases,* 6th Ed. Oxford: Blackwell Scientific Publications.

Principles of Antimicrobial Chemotherapy

25

W. A. GILLESPIE

AIMS AND LIMITATIONS OF CHEMOTHERAPY

The aim of chemotherapy is to help the body defences to destroy infecting micro-organisms. Success depends not only on a sufficient concentration of the drug reaching the lesion but also on the efficiency of the defences. There are several reasons why chemotherapy may fail, even when the pathogen is sensitive to the drug *in vitro*. The drug may be insufficiently absorbed when given by mouth, or the dosage may be insufficient to ensure penetration into the lesion. For example, tetracycline in a dosage of 1 g daily sometimes fails to reach an antibacterial concentration in the sputum in chronic bronchitis. Another cause of failure may be inactivation of the drug. Thus, sulphonamides are liable to inhibition by substances in blood and pus and are more effective in urine. Many drugs, including penicillins, form loose, reversible complexes with plasma proteins, but this does not prevent antibacterial action if dosage is sufficient.

Many drugs, including penicillins and tetracyclines, penetrate the blood/CSF barrier poorly, while others, e.g. sulphonamide and chloramphenicol penetrate well. Fortunately, in acute meningitis all these drugs pass the barrier more easily than in health; but even so, large doses of penicillin are required in treating bacterial meningitis. Chemotherapy of biliary tract infection requires a drug that is concentrated in the bile, e.g. ampicillin, tetracycline, erythromycin. The failure of tetracycline to cure typhoid fever while chloramphenicol does so (though no more active against typhoid bacilli *in vitro*) is perhaps explained by the readier penetration of chloramphenicol to the bacilli in the tissues.

Any interference with host defences hampers chemotherapy. Infections often cannot be cured, though they may be temporarily suppressed, when leucocytes or antibodies are seriously defective, as in acute leukaemia or hypogammaglobulinaemia; or if the entry of the defence agents into the lesion is prevented by a foreign body, or by fibrotic or necrotic tissue.

The free escape of secretions is important in defence against infection. Chemotherapy rarely cures an infection in the bronchus or urinary tract when function is abnormal because of obstruction or neurological disease. Chemotherapy will not remove an abscess, and is no substitute for surgical treatment.

DISADVANTAGES AND DANGERS OF CHEMOTHERAPY

No antibiotic is entirely free from the risk of causing undesirable, sometimes dangerous consequences:

1. Blind treatment of obscure pyrexia may delay the diagnosis. If the pyrexia is due to bacterial endocarditis, the patient's life will be jeopardised. This is perhaps the greatest danger of premature or uncritical use of antibiotics.
2. Toxicity, e.g. aminoglycosides and tetracycline in patients with renal insufficiency. Chloramphenicol may fatally damage bone marrow.
3. Allergic reactions, a special risk with penicillins. Though usually not serious they are occasionally fatal, even with oral administration.
4. Interference with the protection given by the normal bacterial flora. Thus, antibiotic treatment of salmonella gastroenteritis may damage the normal bacteria of the bowel more than the pathogen, and so delay recovery.
5. Resistant pathogens such as candida and antibiotic-resistant staphylococci may proliferate and replace the normal alimentary flora eliminated by antibiotics, especially broad spectrum ones like tetracycline. The consequence may be uncomfortable, e.g. stomatitis or, occasionally, a dangerous superinfection such as staphylococcal enterocolitis.

Table 25.1 Sensitivity of common organisms to antibacterial drugs *in vitro*
Note: **Successful therapy depends on several factors in addition to sensitivity (*see* text)**

	Penicillins G and V; Procaine penicillin	Ampicillin; Amoxycillin	Carbenicillin	Flucloxacillin; Cloxacillin; Methicillin	Cephalosporins	Aminoglycosides (Gentamicin; Tobramicin)	Tetracyclines	Chloramphenicol	Erythromycin	Clindamycin	Colistin	Fusidic acid	Vancomycin	Sulphonamides	Cotrimoxazole	Metronidazole	Nitrofurantoin (in urine only)	Nalidixic acid (in urine only)
A. Sensitivity patterns to favoured drugs fairly constant																		
Strep. pyogenes	1	1	–	–	1	5	3	1	1	1	5	4	1	3	1	5	–	–
Anaerobic streptococci	1	1	–	–	1	5	2	1	1	1	5	4	1	2	1	1	–	–
Pneumococci	1	1	–	–	1	5	3	1	1	1	5	4	1	2	1	5	–	–
Meningococci	1	1	–	–	–	1	1	1	1	1	5	–	5	2	1	5	–	–
Gonococci	2*	2*	–	–	4	–	1	1	1	4	5	–	5	3	2	5	–	–
Br. abortus	5	4	–	5	5	1	1	1	5	5	5	5	5	1	1	5	–	–
H. influenzae	4	2	–	5	4	1	2	1	4	4	1	5	5	2	1	5	–	–
Bacteroides fragilis	5	5	5	5	5	5	3	2	2	1	5	5	5	3	3	1	–	–
Clostridium spp.	1	1	–	–	1	5	1	1	1	1	5	5	1	–	–	1	–	–
B. Sensitivity often varies																		
Staphylococci (outside hospital)	3	3	–	1	1	1	2	1	2	1	5	1	1	2	1	5	1	5
Staphylococci ('hospital')	3	3	–	2	3	2	3	2	3	2	5	2	1	3	2	5	1	5
Viridans streptococci	2	2	–	–	1	4/5	3	1	2	2	5	–	1	2	1	5	–	–
Strept. faecalis	5	4	5	5	5	4	2	1	2	4	5	–	1	5	2	5	1	5
E. coli (outside hospital)	5	2	2	5	2	1	2	1	5	5	1	5	5	2	1	5	1	1
E. coli ('hospital')	5	3	3	5	3	2	3	2	5	5	1	5	5	3	2	5	3	3
Klebsiella spp.	5	5	3	5	3	2	4	4	5	5	1	5	5	3	2	5	3	2
Pseudomonas spp.	5	5	2	5	5	2	4	3	5	5	1	5	5	3	–	5	5	5
Proteus spp.	5	3	2	5	3	2	3	3	5	5	5	5	5	2	2	5	4	3
Salmonella spp.	5	2	–	5	2	1	2	2	5	5	1	5	5	3	1	5	–	–
Shigella spp.	5	2	–	5	2	1	3	3	5	5	1	5	5	3	1	5	–	–

Key: 1 = always or nearly always sensitive. MIC well below the blood concentration reached with recommended dosage.

2 = variable, usually sensitive.

3 = variable, often resistant.

4 = doubtful. MIC is usually near the blood concentration of the drug. It may be effective at urine concentrations.

5 = resistant.

– = irrelevant or uncertain.

* = some gonococci have become moderately resistant to penicillin. Others, that form penicillinase and are highly resistant, have recently appeared in several countries including the UK.

Antibacterial chemotherapy therefore should be avoided:
(a) For virus infections, unless complicated by secondary bacterial infection which though often feared, is rarely serious except in a few conditions, e.g. following upper respiratory viral infection in chronic bronchitic patients.
(b) For trivial bacterial infections.
(c) For localised infections that will recover with appropriate surgical treatment, e.g. superficial abscesses, uncomplicated appendicitis.
(d) Until an aetiological diagnosis has been made on clinical or laboratory evidence; or at least until the necessary specimens (blood cultures, etc.) have been obtained.

(e) For routine prophylaxis. (But there are important exceptions – *see below*).

CHOICE OF DRUG

The correct antibiotic cannot be chosen until a clinical diagnosis, at least presumptive, has been made. 'Blind' treatment should be avoided. The chosen drug should be one to which the pathogen is likely to be sensitive at a concentration that can be reached in the lesion. The properties of the more important drugs are summarised at the end of this chapter.

Bactericidal drugs, e.g. penicillins and aminoglycosides can destroy bacteria, unaided by the host's defence agents (though they will act more efficiently if the defences are normal). Bacteriostatic drugs such as sulphonamides, tetracyclines and erythromycin act mainly by preventing bacterial multiplication, and are therefore more dependent than bactericidal drugs on the integrity of the body's defences. In practice, the difference is unimportant when the lesion is in previously healthy tissue with a good blood supply and freely accessible to leucocytes, for example in streptococcal tonsillitis or uncomplicated urinary infection. However, a bactericidal agent must be used if the drug, unaided, has to destroy the organisms because leucocytes and antibodies are excluded from the lesion by dense avascular vegetations, fibrosis, necrotic tissue or foreign bodies. Thus, it is essential to treat bacterial endocarditis with bactericidal drugs.

Drugs with dangerous side effects should not be used except for serious infections for which they are the best available treatment, e.g. chloramphenicol in typhoid fever and in *Haemophilus influenzae* meningitis.

Ideally, the pathogen should be identified and its sensitivity determined before starting to treat an infection, but this policy is often impracticable. Acute infections such as bacterial meningitis are too serious to justify any delay and, once lumbar puncture has been performed, initial chemotherapy must be based on the probable aetiological diagnosis and modified if necessary according to the patient's progress and subsequent laboratory tests. Sometimes the causative organism cannot be isolated and sometimes a specimen such as sputum may contain more than one pathogen, with no certainty as to which is responsible for the patient's respiratory infection. Again, some infections are caused by mixtures of different organisms, including some that are delicate or slow-growing. Thus, a full bacteriological investigation of pus from acute peritonitis may take so long as to render the result clinically valueless (though microscopy of the pus may give a useful lead). In such circumstances antibiotic treatment must be initiated according to the inferred nature of the responsible organisms, rather than on the full bacteriology of a particular case. However, it is wise to check the sensitivity of the organisms whenever practicable. The usual antibiotic sensitivity patterns of important pathogenic bacteria are summarised in Table 25.1.

Note: The determination of sensitivity is only the first step in selecting a drug. Some that are active *in vitro* are not suitable for treating some infections because they cannot reach the lesion in effective concentrations, or for other reasons. Fortunately, the sensitivity to favoured drugs of pathogens such as pneumococci and haemolytic streptococci (*Streptococcus pyogenes*) seldom varies. Others such as staphylococci and coliforms are much more liable to vary in sensitivity and are often resistant to the best agents. Sensitivity testing is most rewarding with organisms such as these.

Cost should not be the deciding factor in prescribing

treatment but it should be borne in mind. The cost of different antibiotics varies greatly (Table 25.2). The

Table 25.2   Costs of some antibacterial drugs (July 1977)

Antibiotic	Daily dose (in grams, oral, unless otherwise stated)	Cost of one week's course £
Sulphadimidine	2.0	0.08
Tetracycline	1.0	0.17
Phenoxymethylpenicillin	1.0	0.30
Nitrofurantoin	0.2	1.00
Cotrimoxazole	4 tablets	1.89
Amoxycillin	0.75	2.06
Ampicillin	2.0	2.12
Metronidazole	1.2	2.66
Erythromycin	1.5	2.86
Clindamycin	0.6	3.67
Flucloxacillin	1.0	3.76
Nalidixic acid	4.0	4.70
Cephaloridine	2.0 im or iv	14.78
Fusidic acid	1.5	21.33
Cephazolin	2.0 im or iv	31.36
Gentamicin	0.32 im or iv	44.55
Amikacin	1.0 im or iv	141.96
Carbenicillin	30.0 iv	237.70

These are basic trade costs that may be different when the drugs are dispensed in general practice or hospital. The doses are examples, not necessarily suitable for all patients.

Department of Health and Social Security sends charts to doctors from time to time, illustrating the costs of equivalent preparations.

DOSAGE AND DURATION OF TREATMENT

The dosage should be high enough to ensure an adequate concentration in blood, tissue or urine, well above the minimum inhibiting concentration (MIC) for the organism. However, unnecessarily high levels may be dangerous. With some drugs, e.g. the aminoglycosides, the toxic concentration does not greatly exceed the effective therapeutic level. Special care must be exercised when these are given to patients with renal insufficiency, and dosage should be monitored by measuring blood concentrations.

The duration of treatment depends upon the natural history of the disease, the properties of the organism, and the accessibility of the lesion to the drug. The correct duration varies from about one week in acute infections caused by sensitive bacteria (e.g. uncomplicated cystitis due to *Escherichia coli*), to several weeks in subacute bacterial endocarditis and actinomycosis, nine to eighteen months in pulmonary tuberculosis, and much longer in leprosy.

Failure of an acute infection to respond to treatment in about four days suggests that the organism is resistant or that the drug is not reaching it.

607

ANTIBIOTIC COMBINATIONS

These should generally be avoided but sometimes are justified, as in the following circumstances:
1. Sometimes in treating mixed infections such as acute peritonitis.
2. To ensure adequate cover, in the initial treatment of dangerous infections, such as acute bacterial meningitis, before the causative organism has been identified.
3. To prevent the development of drug resistance, especially during prolonged treatment, e.g. in tuberculosis.
4. For *synergy*, in treating infections due to relatively resistant organisms, e.g. some cases of bacterial endocarditis. Pairs of independently-acting bactericidal drugs, such as penicillins and aminoglycosides, often kill bacteria much more rapidly than either drug alone, in the same concentration. The occurrence of synergy should be checked in the laboratory by tests on the organism isolated from the patient.

The possibility of *antagonism* between antibiotics should also be borne in mind. Bacteriostatic drugs such as tetracycline reduce the growth rate of bacteria and so may diminish the bactericidal activity of penicillins which are most active against rapidly multiplying organisms. Antagonism is easy to demonstrate experimentally, but its occurrence depends on the relative concentrations of antibiotics and it may be of less importance in clinical situations. However, potentially antagonistic pairs of drugs should not be prescribed without good reason (e.g. penicillins with tetracyclines or chloramphenicol).

PROPHYLACTIC CHEMOTHERAPY

A policy of routine antibiotic cover to protect all patients at risk may do more harm than good. No drug can prevent infection by all potential pathogens, with their varying sensitivity patterns, in patients whose resistance is diminished by surgical operations or other causes. Routine prophylactic chemotherapy may sometimes even increase the incidence of infection, especially when inappropriate drugs are given, and make it more difficult to treat. Thus, postoperative chest infection is usually caused by haemophilus or pneumococcus and requires antibiotics only if severe. Routine prophylactic chemotherapy (e.g. with ampicillin) will replace these sensitive organisms with more resistant ones such as *Staphylococcus aureus* or klebsiellae.

On the other hand, prophylactic chemotherapy is justified, and sometimes even mandatory, in order to protect selected patients against dangerous infection by particular pathogens of known antibiotic sensitivity. Only narrow spectrum drugs should be used. The dosage must be adequate and the timing appropriate to the duration of risk. The following are some examples of situations that justify prophylaxis:

1. Against relapse of rheumatic fever. Since *Streptococcus pyogenes* has remained sensitive to penicillin, a twice daily oral dose of phenoxymethylpenicillin greatly reduces the frequency of relapse, and may be continued for several years.
2. Malaria. An antimalarial drug (*see below*) is taken from the day before entering an endemic area until at least four weeks after leaving.
3. To prevent bacterial endocarditis during dental treatment in patients with congenital or previous rheumatic heart disease. Most oral streptococci are penicillin-sensitive, and penicillin cover for two days, starting about thirty minutes before the dental treatment, is effective. However, if the patient has recently been treated with penicillin, his mouth may contain many resistant streptococci. In these circumstances, or if the patient is allergic to penicillin, the best alternative is erythromycin.
4. Against clostridial gas gangrene in amputations and other bone-involving operations on the lower limb, in patients with arterial disease. *Clostridium welchii*, a sporing organism from the intestine, is often present on the thigh and no disinfectant can remove it completely. Since clostridia are moderately sensitive to benzylpenicillin, large doses should be given for about seven days, starting on the morning of operation. (The prophylaxis will not prevent wound infection by other, less dangerous organisms.)
5. To cover operations on a urinary tract that is already infected by an organism of known sensitivity. The appropriate drug, given from a day or two before operation, will usually prevent ascending infection and bacteraemia. On the other hand, antibiotic prophylaxis is usually better avoided in patients with sterile urine; and in all cases, strict asepsis should be observed, and a closed method employed if the bladder is drained by an indwelling catheter.
6. Recurrent upper urinary tract infection in children, associated with ureteric reflux, carries the risk of progressive renal damage. This may be reduced in selected cases, by the long term administration of cotrimoxazole in low dosage.
7. *Close* contacts of meningococcal disease should be given sulphadimidine for seven days. If the meningococcus is sulphonamide-resistant, minocycline (a tetracycline) should be given instead.

There are other circumstances in which prophylactic chemotherapy is probably justified but the timing and choice of drug are more debatable, e.g. open heart surgery, insertion of hip joint prostheses, and head injury with rhinorrhoea, to prevent meningitis.

ANTIBIOTICS IN RENAL FAILURE

After a loading dose (if necessary), maintenance treatment is adjusted according to whether the drug is mainly removed by renal or extra-renal routes and by the difference between therapeutic and toxic blood concentrations.

(a) Normal dosage: erythromycin, fusidic acid.

(b) Minor adjustment necessary: blood levels need not be checked: the penicillins, clindamycin, sulphonamides, cotrimoxazole.

(c) Major modification necessary, with repeated blood level estimations: aminoglycosides, colistin, vancomycin.

(d) Do not use: nitrofurantoin, tetracycline, chloramphenicol, cephaloridine.

LABORATORY CONTROL OF CHEMOTHERAPY

The role of the laboratory is to confirm the aetiological diagnosis and to test the sensitivity of causative organisms. The sensitivity of irrelevant organisms should not be tested (e.g. commensals in throat swabs and sputum specimens). To do so wastes laboratory time and may mislead the clinician.

Most sensitivity tests are performed by the disc method which allows many specimens to be tested quickly. Unfortunately, however, the simplicity of this test is matched by the difficulty of reliably interpreting its results. The diameter of the inhibition zones around the discs is determined by many factors in addition to the sensitivity of the organism. Unless these factors are understood by the laboratory worker and controlled by tests with standard organisms, gross errors will frequently occur, as several national surveys have shown. At best, the disc test demonstrates that an organism is either fully sensitive, doubtfully sensitive or resistant to the drug, and *it must be interpreted according to the site of the infection.* Thus, an organism may be resistant to the concentration of a drug that can be reached in the blood, while sensitive to the concentration normally obtained in the urine.

The disc test does not directly measure the minimum inhibiting concentration of the drug for the organism. When this is required, as it often is for the treatment of diseases such as bacterial endocarditis, it must be measured in a quantitative method by inoculating the pathogen into a series of culture tubes containing different concentrations of the drug. The minimum bactericidal level requires a still more elaborate method, especially when it is required to determine whether a mixture of drugs is synergistic. Finally, in controlling the therapy of bacterial endocarditis and other systemic infections due to organisms of marginal sensitivity, it is often helpful to measure the bactericidal titre of the patient's serum against his organism, during treatment. The results should be interpreted in consultation with the clinical bacteriologist.

Estimation of the concentration of antibiotic in the blood during treatment is rarely required except with aminoglycosides (*see below*).

SUMMARY OF ANTIMICROBIAL DRUGS

PENICILLINS

Penicillins act by inhibiting the synthesis of bacterial cell walls, rendering them susceptible to osmotic damage as they grow. Penicillins are bactericidal, especially against rapidly proliferating bacteria.

Penicillins are non-toxic, except with extremely high blood concentrations and in the central nervous system. Intrathecal injection is rarely needed and must *never* exceed 10,000 units (6 mg) of benzylpenicillin.

Allergy develops fairly often and, occasionally, is serious or even fatal. It may sometimes be detected by a skin test but this is not very reliable. A patient who is allergic to one penicillin will be allergic to the others and sometimes to cephalosporins also.

Penicillins are rapidly excreted, mainly by the kidney and less by the bile. The blood concentration may be increased by giving probenecid, a renal tubular blocking agent, provided renal function is normal.

Benzylpenicillin (Penicillin G) is given by injection. 1 mega unit (10^6 units) is equivalent to 600 mg. $\frac{1}{2}$–1 mega unit every six hours is a suitable dose for most purposes in adults. It is the most powerful penicillin against Gram-positive organisms, cocci and bacilli. However, many staphylococci destroy it by producing penicillinase (beta-lactamase). Of the Gram-negative cocci, meningococci are always sensitive but some gonococci have become resistant. *Treponema pallidum* is always sensitive.

Procaine penicillin is a slow-release compound of benzylpenicillin. It is more dangerous than ordinary penicillin in allergic patients.

Phenoxymethylpenicillin (Penicillin V) is acid-resistant and given by mouth on an empty stomach. The usual adult dose is 250 to 500 mg six-hourly. Larger doses may cause gastrointestinal upset and high blood levels are difficult to attain.

'Broad spectrum' penicillins are active against a wider range of bacteria than are penicillins G and V. They are destroyed by penicillinase and therefore are *not* active against penicillin-resistant staphylococci.

Ampicillin is acid-stable and usually given by mouth; the usual adult dosage is 250 mg to 1 g six-hourly. For serious infections it is given by intramuscular or slow intravenous injection. Ampicillin acts on organisms that are sensitive to penicillin G and is moderately active also against many strains of *H. influenzae* and *E. coli*. But pseudomonas and several other Gram-negative bacilli are resistant, and the proportion of resistant strains is increasing. *Amoxycillin* is similar and, being better absorbed is effective at about half the dose.

There is a high incidence of rashes following ampicillin; some are peculiar to it while others resemble the allergic rashes of other penicillins.

Carbenicillin is much less potent, weight for weight, than other penicillins. Its main use is in treating bacteraemia and other serious systemic infections by pseudomonas and some proteus strains.

Carbenicillin must be injected intravenously. Patients with normal renal function should receive 20 to 30 g daily in four to six divided doses by slow bolus injection, with oral probenecid to maintain high blood levels. Lower doses, without probenecid, are used in renal failure. Since carbenicillin is a disodium salt, care must be taken to avoid sodium excess.

Carfecillin is an ester of carbenicillin that is given orally. It is suitable only for treating urinary infection by carbenicillin-sensitive pseudomonas and proteus species.

Penicillinase-insensitive penicillins are less powerful than benzylpenicillin and their only indication is for treating serious infections that are known, or thought likely to be caused by penicillinase-producing staphylococci. It is difficult to achieve high blood levels of these penicillins, since large injections are painful. If preferred, one of them may be given together with benzylpenicillin when starting treatment, until the identity and sensitivity of the pathogen are known.

Methicillin, the first of this group to be introduced, has been largely replaced by *flucloxacillin* and *cloxacillin*, both of which may be given orally or by injection. Flucloxacillin is better for oral use; the usual dose is 250 mg six-hourly. Cloxacillin is suitable for injection, and given intravenously in serious infections; dosage 1 g every four to six hours.

The term 'methicillin-resistant' staphylococcus is used for strains that possess inherent resistance to *all* the penicillins; this does not depend on penicillinase which, however, they produce. So far, methicillin-resistant staphylococci have been found only among multi-resistant strains and are uncommon outside hospitals.

CEPHALOSPORINS

The cephalosporin molecule closely resembles that of penicillin and the drugs act similarly on bacteria. They are active against a rather wide range of organisms, roughly comparable with that of ampicillin; and they are relatively stable to penicillinase though less so than flucloxacillin or cloxacillin. Some patients who are allergic to penicillins are allergic also to cephalosporins.

The use of cephalosporins is limited by the availability of other drugs, e.g. penicillins, which have broadly similar ranges of activity and are cheaper. Cephalosporins therefore are generally only given in occasional, usually severe, infections when sensitivity tests show that they are suitable. Of the several cephalosporins available the most generally useful is **cephaloridine**, for intramuscular or intravenous injection (2 to 3 g daily in divided doses). It may damage the kidneys, particularly when there is already impaired renal function or when gentamicin or frusemide are given concurrently. **Cephazolin**, used similarly, is preferable when there is a possibility of impaired renal function.

AMINOGLYCOSIDES

These bactericidal drugs must be given by injection and are largely excreted by the kidney. When renal function is impaired, the blood concentration rapidly reaches a toxic level with damage to the inner ear or, occasionally, the kidney. Dosage is controlled by measuring blood concentrations. This precaution is essential when there is known renal damage and in the elderly, but is always very desirable since renal impairment may develop during the severe infections for which aminoglycosides are often used. Even more important, this precaution also avoids the risk of inadequately treating a dangerous infection. Concentrations should be estimated at times of 'peak' level (one hour after intramuscular dose, fifteen minutes after intravenous dose, taken from a different vein) and at 'trough' level (just before a dose).

Streptomycin is rarely indicated except in tuberculosis for which there are nowadays alternatives that often are more suitable (*see* Chapter 18).

Gentamicin is valuable, especially for serious infections (e.g. septicaemia) by aerobic Gram-negative bacilli and, sometimes, staphylococci, and also for some resistant urinary infections. The dose in patients with normal renal function is 2 mg/kg loading dose followed by 1.5 to 2 mg/kg eight-hourly, by intramuscular injection or intravenously (by injection over three minutes), for seven to ten days. When there is renal impairment the interval between doses must be increased, in consultation with the clinical bacteriologist. Satisfactory peak blood levels are 6 to 8 mg/litre falling to a trough level of 1 to 2 mg/litre. Trough levels above 2 mg/litre suggest that renal function is impaired. Levels above 12 mg/litre are potentially toxic.

Tobramycin resembles gentamicin but may be better in some pseudomonas infections.

Amikacin is active against some bacteria that are resistant to other aminoglycosides and should be restricted to treating serious infections by these. It is extremely expensive.

SULPHONAMIDES

These are bacteriostatic drugs that compete with p-aminobenzoic acid, an essential metabolite for folic acid synthesis by many bacteria. The many sulphonamide preparations show cross-resistance, but differ in their rates of absorption and excretion. Sulphonamides are inhibited by substances in pus and, to a lesser extent, in tissues and blood. They are more effective in urine and in CSF. Sulphonamides are still good first-line drugs and the cheapest, for treating uncomplicated acute urinary tract infections. Over 80 per cent of *E. coli* strains outside hospital are still sensitive. Adverse reactions, chiefly allergic, are uncommon.

Sulphadimidine (adult dosage 500 mg four times a day by mouth) gives satisfactory levels of drug in blood and urine.

'Long-acting' sulphonamides are strongly bound by protein and slowly released to give prolonged activity in urine with daily or even weekly administration. They may be used to treat urinary infections in patients who cannot be relied on to take tablets regularly. The risk of serious allergic complications such as the Stevens–Johnson syndrome is greater than with other sulphonamides.

COTRIMOXAZOLE

This is a mixture of sulphamethoxazole and trimethoprim, an inhibitor of the next step in folic acid synthesis by bacteria. The two ingredients are synergistic so that cotrimoxazole is more powerful than sulphonamide and sometimes is bactericidal. Bacteria do not easily acquire resistance.

Cotrimoxazole is active against many bacteria. It has a wider range of action than sulphonamides for treating urinary infections. However, sulphonamides alone are sufficient, and cheaper, for most cases of uncomplicated urinary infection outside hospital. Cotrimoxazole is also valuable in some respiratory infections by *H. influenzae* and in some systemic infections including enteric fever. Its toxic effects resemble those of sulphonamides and, in addition, it may cause folinic acid deficiency in patients with abnormalities of folic acid metabolism. Because the effect on the fetus is not yet fully known, it should be used with caution in pregnancy.

The normal adult dose of cotrimoxazole is two tablets twice daily. An intravenous preparation is available for serious infections.

TETRACYCLINES

The tetracyclines all act similarly on bacteria and differ only in their absorption and excretion. They are bacteriostatic against many organisms including some Gram-negative bacilli and Gram-positive cocci, mycoplasmas and rickettsiae. However, resistance develops rather easily. Many staphylococci, haemolytic streptococci and pneumococci are now resistant. *H. influenzae* is usually sensitive.

Tetracycline itself is given by mouth in divided doses amounting to 1 to 3 g daily for adults. If injected, the daily dose should not exceed 1 g. Because they are incompletely absorbed from the bowel and are concentrated in the bile, and because their wide range of activity includes not only *E. coli* but also the anaerobes that predominate in the colon, tetracyclines alter the bowel flora profoundly. This may account for the digestive upset that often accompanies treatment. Occasionally, multi-resistant staphylococci colonise the bowel after intestinal operations, causing staphylococcal enterocolitis.

Tetracyclines are incorporated in growing teeth and bone, and therefore are not given to children under seven years nor to pregnant women. High blood levels from parenteral dosage can damage the liver. The drugs can cause renal failure in patients with renal disease, and should be avoided if possible in the elderly.

CHLORAMPHENICOL

This bacteriostatic agent has a wide range of action, rather similar to that of tetracycline, but since it is used less often, fewer organisms are resistant to it. Its particular virtue is its easy penetration into tissues and cells, and into the cerebrospinal fluid (but not into bile). Because of its liability to damage the bone marrow, a rare but dangerous complication, chloramphenicol should be used only for those serious diseases for which it is still probably the best available antibiotic, e.g. typhoid fever, *H. influenzae* meningitis, and, occasionally, other life-endangering infections by organisms that are known, or thought likely to be resistant to other drugs (e.g. acute peritonitis). The oral adult dose is 500 mg to 1 g six to eight-hourly; the intramuscular dose is 500 mg six-hourly.

ERYTHROMYCIN

This drug is mainly bacteriostatic but has some cidal activity. It is best given as the stearate in oral doses of 250 to 500 mg four times a day. Its range of action is roughly similar to that of benzylpenicillin and it is a suitable alternative for patients with penicillin allergy. Erythromycin is also active against some mycoplasmas that cause respiratory infection. Bacteria may rapidly develop resistance.

CLINDAMYCIN

In its range of activity this drug resembles erythromycin and is useful in infections by staphylococci, streptococci and bacteroides. However, its use is restricted by the association between clindamycin and pseudomembranous enterocolitis. The oral dose is 150 to 300 mg four times a day; a parenteral preparation is also available.

FUSIDIC ACID ('Fucidin')

A powerful (and expensive) bactericidal drug with a limited range, it is sometimes indicated in serious staphylococcal infections and is often given together with a penicillin. Bacteria easily develop resistance. The usual adult dosage is 800 mg eight-hourly, by mouth or parenterally.

RIFAMPICIN

Though active against other organisms, this should be reserved for treating tuberculosis and leprosy (*see* Chapter 18).

VANCOMYCIN

A powerful bactericidal drug, vancomycin is occasionally life-saving when other antibiotics fail in septicaemia and endocarditis due to staphylococci or streptococci. Adults with normal renal function may be given 2 g daily in divided doses, intravenously. The main toxic effects are thrombophlebitis and, especially in patients with renal impairment, nerve deafness. Treatment should be controlled by blood assays.

COLISTIN

This is a polymyxin, active only against Gram-negative bacilli including pseudomonas but not proteus. Its effectiveness clinically is sometimes less than the *in vitro* sensitivity of the organisms would suggest. Dosage in adults is 50,000 to 100,000 units/kg daily, by divided intramuscular injections, or intravenously. It may be given as tablets by mouth in severe bacterial gastro-enteritis in infants.

METRONIDAZOLE

This was originally introduced as an antiprotozoal agent (*see below*) and was subsequently found to be active against anaerobic bacteria such as bacteroides. It is effective in Vincent's stomatitis. It may be given with other antimicrobial agents in treating serious abdominal infections by mixed intestinal organisms in which bacteroides often predominate. The usual oral dosage for adults is 400 mg three times daily for seven days. It may also be given in suppositories, or intravenously.

Alcohol should be avoided when taking metronidazole.

DRUGS ACTIVE IN URINE BUT NOT AT BLOOD CONCENTRATIONS

These are sometimes used for urinary infections instead of sulphonamides and antibiotics, when indicated by sensitivity tests.

Nitrofurantoin (adult dose 50 to 100 mg six-hourly) controls a wide range of organisms (but not pseudomonas). It may cause nausea. Prolonged treatment, especially in renal failure, may cause neuropathic and other toxic effects.

Nalidixic acid (adult dose 500 mg six-hourly) inhibits many Gram-negative bacilli but not pseudomonas. Bacteria may develop resistance. It has caused intracranial hypertension in babies and should therefore be avoided in small children and probably in pregnancy.

DRUGS USED FOR TREATING TUBERCULOSIS
See Chapter 18

ANTIFUNGAL DRUGS

Nystatin is applied locally for control of oral and vaginal infections by candida. It is not absorbed when swallowed, and is of no use for systemic infections.

Amphotericin B has a similar action. It may be given cautiously by slow intravenous injection, for serious systemic infections by candida and some other yeasts. Toxic side effects are common.

5-Fluorocytosine is active against many yeasts, but resistance may develop quickly.

Griseofulvin is given by mouth (adult dose 500 mg to 1 g daily) for some forms of ringworm, particularly that of the scalp and nails. It is useless for athlete's foot.

Clotrimazole can be applied locally for ringworm and candida infections. **Miconazole** is used similarly.
Note: Whitfield's ointment is generally as good as any modern agent for treating dermatophyte infections (except of nails and scalp).

SOME ANTI-PROTOZOAL DRUGS (*see also* Chapter 23)

Metronidazole (*see above*) is the best drug for treating amoebic dysentery and amoebic hepatitis. It is also effective in giardiasis and trichomoniasis, but not in infections caused by aerobic parasites such as malaria or trypanosomiasis.

Drugs for Malaria

Chloroquine largely replaced **quinine** for treating clinical attacks of malaria and is the drug of choice against sensitive parasites. However, the appearance of resistant strains of *Pl. falciparum* has restored quinine as a first line drug in life-endangering malignant tertian (MT) malaria in areas where chloroquine-resistant strains exist (e.g. South East Asia and South America). Combined treatment with **pyrimethamine** and **sulphadoxine** is a suitable alternative in clinically milder infections. In dangerously ill patients, treatment should be started with slow intravenous administration of quinine or chloroquine (*see* page 588).

In malaria due to species other than *Pl. falciparum*, chloroquine treatment is followed by **primaquine** to destroy parasites in the liver and prevent relapse.

For prophylaxis, proguanil (100 to 200 mg daily) or pyrimethamine (25 to 50 mg once a week) is taken from the day before arriving until at least four weeks after leaving a malarious area. Further advice about the best prophylactic drugs for particular areas can be obtained from the London School of Tropical Medicine and Hygiene, Keppel Street, London WC1 7HT (Tel: 01/636 8636).

SUGGESTED FURTHER READING

Up-to-date information about antibiotics and their use in treatment is to be found in articles published from time to time in the *Prescribers' Journal*, obtainable from Hannibal House, Elephant & Castle, London SE1 6TE.

Recent articles include:

Burslem, R. W. (1973) The treatment of trichomonal vaginitis, **13,** No. 1, 14.

Darrell, J. H. (1976) Current practice in systemic antifungal therapy, **16,** No. 1: 20.

Drew, Sir Robert (1972) Drug prophylaxis against malaria, **12,** No. 5: 109.

Forfar, J. O. (1973) Drugs to be avoided during the first three months of pregnancy, **13,** No. 6: 130.

Lorber, J. (1976) Treatment of neonatal meningitis, **16,** No. 4: 82.

Miller, J. (1973) Staining of the teeth by tetracyclines, **13,** No. 2: 39.

Reeves, W. G. (1972) Drug hypersensitivity, **12,** No. 4: 89.

Staffurth, J. S. (1972) The treatment of bacterial endocarditis, **12,** No. 4: 76.

Stirrat, G. M. and Beard, R. W. (1973) Drugs to be avoided or given with caution in the second and third trimesters of pregnancy, **13,** No. 6: 135.

Wise, R. (1975) The cephalosporins, **15,** No. 5: 119.

Recent articles in other journals include:

Garrod, L. P. (1975) Chemoprophylaxis. *British Medical Journal,* **4:** 561.

Johnston, H. H. (Nov. 1975) Antibiotics for urinary tract infection. *British Journal of Hospital Medicine,* p. 488.

Roe, F. J. C. (1977) Metronidazole: review of uses and toxicity. *Journal of Antimicrobial Chemotherapy,* **3:** 205.

Wise, R. (October 1975) The penicillins. *British Journal of Hospital Medicine,* p. 404.

Concise information about chemotherapeutic drugs and dosage is given in the *British National Formulary* (1976–78) published by the British Medical Association and the Pharmaceutical Society of Great Britain.

For a fuller account, with information about pharmacology and laboratory aspects, see *Antibiotics and Chemotherapy* (1973) Garrod, L. P., Lambert, H. P. and O'Grady, F. London & Edinburgh: Churchill Livingstone.

Molecular Disorders and Inborn Errors of Metabolism

26

R. F. HARVEY

A number of diseases are now known to result from a failure to synthesise specific proteins. If these are normal end-products, such as albumin or antihaemophilic globulin (AHG), a simple deficiency state results. If, as is usually the case, the protein is an enzyme, various types of abnormality may occur. There is often a metabolic block at the site of action of the enzyme. Normal precursor substances may then accumulate, being partially or completely metabolised by alternative pathways and excreted in the urine in increased amounts. If these substances are non-toxic there may be no clinical effects, but if toxic, various other sequelae (e.g. brain damage) may be seen. The metabolic block may alternatively result in absence of a normal end product, as occurs in albinism. In a few cases the defective protein is concerned not with a metabolic change, but with the active transport of a material across a cell membrane. The result may then be a failure to absorb the substance from the intestinal tract or excessive urinary losses due to a failure of renal tubular reabsorption.

INBORN ERRORS OF METABOLISM

In 1902, Archibald Garrod wrote a paper entitled 'The incidence of alkaptonuria: a study in chemical individuality', in which he drew attention to certain peculiar features of this condition: its onset could be dated to the first few days of life; it appeared to be due to a single chemical abnormality; and there was an unusual family distribution, many cases being siblings and often the offspring of marriages of first cousins. The parents were never affected. Some of these features were also seen in two other conditions, albinism and cystinuria. Mendel's laws of heredity had been 'rediscovered' in 1900, and William Bateson, one of the pioneers of the new science of genetics, pointed out that the familial distribution of these conditions could all be explained by a rare recessive gene which carried the trait. This was the basis on which Garrod, in 1908, was able to describe to the Royal College of Physicians the nature of what he called 'inborn errors of metabolism'. Since that time the number of known inborn errors of metabolism and

'molecular diseases' (a term coined by Pauling in 1949 for sickle cell anaemia) has increased rapidly. Well over 100 such conditions are described in this chapter (see Table 26.1) and many others in addition to these are

Table 26.1 Molecular disorders and inborn errors of metabolism

I	Defects of plasma protein synthesis: (a) blood clotting factors (b) immunoglobulins (c) plasma enzymes and inhibitors (d) transport proteins
II	Defects in the metabolism of amino acids
III	Defects in the metabolism of simple sugars
IV	Defects in the metabolism of lipids and steroids
V	Defects in the metabolism of purines and pyrimidines
VI	Intracellular storage disorders: (a) glycogenoses (b) mucopolysaccharidoses (c) lipidoses
VII	Defects in porphyrin and haemoprotein metabolism: (a) haemoglobinopathies (b) methaemoglobinaemia (c) acatalasia (d) the porphyrias (e) hyperbilirubinaemias
VIII	Defects in erythrocyte metabolism
IX	Disorders of cellular transport mechanisms: (a) kidney (b) intestine (c) thyroid
X	Inborn variations in the ability to metabolise drugs

known. For example, at least 130 different haemoglobin types have now been described, many being found in healthy individuals, but others in association with disease states of various types. They are included in this book because, although individually uncommon, their existence is important to the undergraduate as they illustrate the profound effects of minor changes in chemical structure on the expression of disease.

GENES AND PROTEIN SYNTHESIS

The manufacture of protein is controlled by information encoded in the genetic material deoxyribonucleic acid (DNA), found mainly in the nuclei of the cells, and transmitted by messenger ribonucleic acid (messenger RNA) to the ribosomes in the cytoplasm where protein synthesis actually takes place. The normal flow of genetic information is as follows:

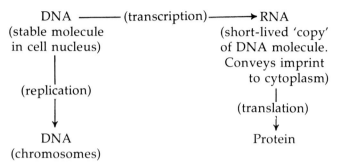

Genetic information is transmitted from parent to child in the chromosomes, which consist of a framework of long chains of DNA with protein attached. DNA is a simple polymer made up of a long backbone of alternating sugar and phosphate units with purine or pyrimidine bases attached to each of the sugar units. In DNA there are four such bases, adenine, guanine, cytosine and thymine, and the DNA in chromosomes is arranged in double helical strands joined by the bases. RNA is similar to DNA, but with ribose replacing deoxyribose and uracil replacing thymine.

That part of the DNA molecule concerned with synthesis of a protein is called the 'structural' gene locus. The sequence of amino acids in the protein corresponds to the sequence of bases in the DNA or RNA molecule at this site: one amino acid is represented by three bases in sequence. Thus, the base triplet uracil-guanine-cytosine in messenger RNA is the 'code' for synthesis of cysteine, and the triplet uracil-guanine-guanine corresponds to tryptophan.

A typical structural gene probably contains a length of DNA with a sequence of several hundred bases, i.e. three bases for every amino acid in the polypeptide or protein whose synthesis is determined by that gene locus. Gene mutations can be seen as events that result in a change in the sequence of bases. In the majority of cases the change probably consists simply in the substitution of one base for another at a single point in the sequence. In other cases there may be more drastic alterations with, for example, the deletion of a whole series of bases, or their complete rearrangement or reduplication.

RESULTS OF GENE MUTATION

A change (mutation) in the base sequence of DNA results in synthesis of an abnormal protein: in its simplest form this consists of a single amino acid substitution. Even such a slight change in the molecule may be enough to alter completely the properties of the protein. In sickle cell anaemia, for example, the gene corresponding to the β chain of haemoglobin has undergone mutation to produce an abnormal polypeptide with valine instead of glutamic acid at position 6. The haemoglobin so produced (HbS) has different physical properties from normal haemoglobin, and all the clinical features of sickle cell anaemia result from this (*see* page 387).

Many mutations lead to the formation of a structurally normal protein in considerably reduced (or less commonly increased) amounts. Such mutations affect not the 'structural' gene locus but 'regulator' genes on adjacent parts of the chromosome. These normally control the activity of the structural gene so as to produce the correct amount of protein. Other types of mutation result not in the production of an abnormal protein, nor in production of the normal protein in abnormal amounts, but in its complete absence. These may affect 'operator' genes which also modify the activity of the structural gene. The exact molecular relationships involved are still obscure. Once a mutation has occurred, the abnormality (if non-lethal) may be passed on from parent to child in a manner corresponding to the standard laws of genetics.

INCIDENCE OF MOLECULAR DISEASES AND INBORN ERRORS OF METABOLISM

The differences between human beings are largely due to individuality in our genetic make up. Many variations in protein constitution can be detected which are not accompanied by any clear abnormality of function. When common, these are regarded as normal variants – blood group and HLA antigens are familiar examples of proteins in which structural variations need not be associated with disease. Other traits may not produce symptoms unless some abnormal challenge (e.g. administration of succinylcholine to subjects with deficiency of pseudocholinesterase) is made. It is often difficult to decide whether such conditions should be considered as disease states or unusual but normal variants. Perhaps the best criterion is whether the condition is a potential cause of disability or death.

Most of these disorders are carried as autosomal or X-linked recessive traits, as potentially lethal dominant genes disappear rapidly because of an impaired survival fitness. Although the incidence of an individual inborn error may be quite low (e.g. phenylketonuria may be found in about 1 in 20,000 live births in the United Kingdom) the number of possible errors is quite large (over 1,500 genetically determined disorders were listed in 1971 by McKusick) so that in an obstetric unit with about 3,000 deliveries annually, a significant number of such disorders may be seen each year.

The overall incidence of monogenic disorders (those caused by a single dominant or recessive gene) is about 10 per 1,000 live births (about 7 per 1,000 dominant, 2.5 per 1,000 recessive and 0.5 per 1,000 X-linked). Common dominant genes are polycystic kidney disease and monogenic hypercholesterolaemia; common recessive genes are those for cystic fibrosis and sickle cell anaemia; and the commonest X-linked disease is Duchenne muscular dystrophy. In addition to these monogenic disorders there are many very common conditions with a strong genetic component, for example ischaemic heart disease, which currently kills about 1 in 4 of the population of the United Kingdom.

Abnormal recessive genes are seen with different frequencies in different races. There is a high incidence of various haemoglobinopathies (HbS, HbC and persistent HbF) in Africans, of acatalasia in Japanese, of lipid storage disorders (e.g. Tay-Sachs disease) in Jews, and of glucose-6-phosphate dehydrogenase deficiency and thalassaemia in Greeks and Italians. In the United Kingdom, the commonest autosomal recessive disorder is fibrocystic disease of the pancreas (1 in 2,500 births), with the adrenogenital syndrome probably second, followed by a number of conditions with a frequency of about 1 in 20,000 (e.g. phenylketonuria, albinism). The incidence of homozygotes with clinical disease is increased by inbreeding. A higher incidence of cousin marriages might be expected in relatively small isolated communities, and in these circumstances homozygotes for recessive traits may be quite common.

In South Africa the unique and very high prevalence of the dominant gene for varigate prophyria (about 1 in 400 or approximately 9,000 out of the total white population of three and a half million) has arisen because of the high fertility and low mortality of a small number of Dutch and French Hugenot settlers who arrived in South Africa 300 years ago. Today, the forty family names of the original forty burghers are shared by over one million of the white population. The families of present-day carriers of the gene can be traced back to the children of Gerrit and Ariaantje Jansz, a couple who married in 1688, he being one of the first free burghers and she one of a group of orphans sent from Rotterdam to be wives of the Cape settlers (Dean, 1963). It is only in the last 50 years, since the introduction of the barbiturates and sulphonamides, that the gene has been potentially fatal.

SCREENING FOR INBORN ERRORS OF METABOLISM

For a few inborn errors of metabolism effective treatment is available which, if started sufficiently early, may be life-saving or may prevent permanent brain damage. For many more of these disorders no completely effective treatment is known. Early identification of patients with treatable conditions is clearly of value and for this reason screening programmes have been organised in a number of countries. Two types of screening programme have been advocated (World Health Organisation, 1968):

1. Mass screening of all newborn infants for treatable disorders. This appears to be indicated:

(a) If the incidence of the condition is not excessively rare (e.g. 1 in 50,000 live births or more).

(b) If the untreated disease leads in most cases to a lasting physical or mental handicap.

(c) If effective treatment can be made available.

2. More extensive screening of specialised populations, for example:

(a) Inmates of hospitals for the mentally retarded.

(b) Children known or found to be retarded who come to the attention of the health or education authorities, or to hospital.

(c) Children in families with an affected member.

(d) Children of consanguinous marriages.

Considerable economic and administrative problems arise when mass screening programmes are undertaken. It has been estimated, for example, that the cost of detection and treatment of a single case of phenylketonuria may be similar to the long term cost of keeping an untreated phenylketonuric patient in a hospital for the mentally retarded. These high costs cannot be afforded by poorer countries, which in any case will not have the technical or administrative facilities to organise such a programme. In countries such as the United Kingdom, mass screening for less uncommon conditions such as phenylketonuria seems both desirable and economically feasible, and possibly more rewarding than the routine screening of asymptomatic adults for maturity onset diabetes, which is practised in most of our hospitals.

The cost-efficiency of a regional screening programme was studied in New England with five states participating. From January 1976 to June 1977, newborn blood specimens from 190,000 infants were screened. Forty-five individuals were found to have a congenital disorder of the type being looked for. Hypothyroidism (38 cases) was the commonest, with phenylketonuria (3 cases), homocystinuria (2 cases) and galactosaemia and maple syrup urine disease (1 each) much less common. The cost per infant screened was $0.80 for hypothyroidism screening and $1.20 for amino acid screening.

TREATMENT AND PREVENTION

In many of the inborn errors of metabolism no treatment has any effect on the course of the disease. In a small number the abnormality produces no clinical effects and is compatible with a normal life-span. The treatments available for the remainder are of various types (Table 26.2) depending on the underlying defect.

Many other forms of treatment are used and are described, where appropriate, in this chapter. It is possible that at some future date genetic deficiencies could be corrected by the direct transfer of genetic material (transduction). This can be achieved in bacteria, using selected viruses as transferring agents.

The incidence of abnormal recessive genes is likely to increase steadily if effective treatment of homozygotes results in their survival to adult life and production of offspring who are carriers of the trait. This could pose some problems in the future unless some way is found of replacing the balance of natural selection. Genetic counselling (Fuhrmann and Vogel, 1976) may help to reduce the incidence of homozygotes for certain lethal and sub-lethal genes. It is possible to detect carriers of some abnormal traits in affected families (e.g. phenylketonuria, galactosaemia, Hurler's syndrome) and such carriers can be advised of the potential risks to their children. In Italy, for example, a large network for thalassaemia detection provides facilities for the systematic diagnosis of heterozygotes and for premarital counselling. In practice, such programmes have had only limited success. Most parents who attend a genetic counselling centre do so only after the birth of an abnormal child. As about three-quarters of children with autosomal recessive disorders are born to parents who have had no abnormal children before, there may be no prior warning of such an event.

One more recent approach has provided a means for carriers of some abnormal recessive genes to have a family of normal children. Amniocentesis between the 12th and 16th week of pregnancy may show that the fetus suffers from the disease, and the parents may then be offered the possibility of an abortion. A number of conditions can already be directly diagnosed in this way, and others can be inferred by observation of linked genes such as the X chromosome in X-linked traits. The incidence of haemophilia could theoretically be decreased if affected men did not have daughters. Even assuming that only half the haemophiliacs and their wives wished to accept selective abortion as a compromise between childlessness and a risk of affected grandsons, the incidence of the condition could still be substantially reduced.

DEFECTS OF PLASMA PROTEIN

BLOOD CLOTTING FACTORS

Inborn deficiencies of the proteins concerned with blood coagulation (Table 26.3) result in bleeding disorders of varying degrees of severity. This group of disorders is particularly important for two reasons. Firstly, some (e.g. haemophilia A) are relatively common, and secondly, many may be treated by direct replacement of the deficient protein, a form of therapy possible in only a few of the molecular disorders. The clinical features and management of these disorders are described in Chapter 19.

IMMUNOGLOBULINS

Inborn deficiencies of immunoglobulin synthesis result in impaired resistance to infections. The severity of the disease and the outcome depend on the degree of deficiency and whether other elements (e.g. cellular immunity) are also affected. No official classification of this group of disorders exists as yet. The important varieties listed in Table 26.4 are as classified by Seligmann, Fudenberg and Good (1968).

PLASMA ENZYMES AND INHIBITORS

Plasma contains large numbers of different proteins for which no clear function is known. For others, enzymatic or anti-enzymic activities have been found and in certain disease states the plasma levels of these substances

Table 26.2 Forms of treatment available for inborn errors of metabolism

Type of defect	Possible treatment
1. Deficiency of plasma protein (e.g. haemophilia A)	Direct replacement (e.g. antihaemophilic globulin)
2. Metabolic block with accumulation of toxic precursors (e.g. phenylketonuria)	Reduce amount of precursors (e.g. diet low in phenylalanine)
3. Metabolic block with accumulation of non-toxic but insoluble substances (e.g. cystinuria, gout)	Encourage removal of substances (e.g. high fluid intake for cystinuria, uricosuric agents for gout)
4. Deficiency state due to failure of a transport system (e.g. iodine trapping defect in thyroid)	Replacement of deficiency (e.g. thyroxine)
5. Disease only manifest after exposure to certain agents (e.g. acute porphyria)	Avoid precipitating agents (e.g. barbiturates)
6. Any potentially serious defect	Enzyme replacement or genetic engineering may be possible in the future

may be abnormal. The exact relationship between the plasma enzyme deficiency and the disease is often unclear, but in at least one of the disorders shown in Table 26.5 (hereditary angioneurotic oedema) the disorder may be treated by replacement of the deficient protein.

TRANSPORT PROTEINS

Some of the plasma proteins do not behave as enzymes but act as carriers for various substances of low molecular weight. Absence of these proteins (Table 26.6) may not produce disease, but may lead to confusion in the

Table 26.3 Inborn errors of synthesis of blood clotting factors

Deficient protein	Factor number	Name(s) of deficiency state	Mode of inheritance*
Fibrinogen	Factor I	Afibrinogenaemia	Autosomal recessive
Prothrombin	Factor II	Congenital prothrombin deficiency	?
Labile factor	Factor V	Parahaemophilia	Dominant
Stable factor	Factor VII	Congenital Factor VII deficiency	Dominant, varying penetrance
Antihaemophilic globulin (AHG)	Factor VIII	Haemophilia A (classical haemophilia)	X-linked recessive
Plasma thromboplastin component (PTC); (Christmas factor)	Factor IX	Haemophilia B (Christmas disease)	X-linked recessive
Stuart-Prower factor	Factor X	Factor X deficiency	Autosomal recessive
Plasma thromboplastin antecedent (PTA)	Factor XI	Haemophilia C	Dominant
Hageman factor	Factor XII	Hageman trait	Autosomal recessive

*Some occur sporadically by new mutations, e.g. haemophilia A may be sporadic in up to 30 per cent of cases.

Table 26.4 Familial deficiencies of immunoglobulin synthesis

Disorder	Synonym	Laboratory findings	Clinical features	Inheritance
Infantile X-linked agammaglobulinaemia	Bruton's disease	All Ig classes extremely low Plasma cells absent Circulating lymphocytes normal	Recurrent pyogenic infections May survive for years if infections controlled	X-linked recessive
Autosomal recessive alymphocytic agammaglobulinaemia	Swiss type agammaglobulinaemia	All Ig classes extremely low Plasma cells absent Circulating lymphocytes very low or absent	Complete immunological incompetence Severe bacterial, viral and fungal infections from first weeks of life Seldom survive first year	Autosomal recessive
Primary lymphopenic immunological deficiency	Gitlin's syndrome	Ig deficiency, but classes affected vary, as does degree Plasma cells often low Lymphocytes always low	Similar to Swiss type – persisting bacterial, viral and fungal infections, with death in early infancy	X-linked or (less commonly) autosomal recessive
Selective IgA deficiency	–	Both circulating and secretory IgA absent, other classes normal Absence of IgA – producing plasma cells	Bacterial infections of respiratory tract; enteropathy with malabsorption of the coeliac type	Autosomal recessive(?)
Immunological deficiency with thrombocytopenia and eczema	Wiskott-Aldrich syndrome	IgM usually most affected Plasma cells normal Circulating lymphocytes low and decline progressively	Recurrent pyogenic infections (especially otitis media) with thrombocytopenic purpura and eczema Death in early childhood usual	X-linked recessive

618

interpretation of laboratory measurements (e.g. thyroxine-binding globulin).

Two of these 'disorders' have the interesting capacity to prolong life (by decreasing the risk of myocardial infarction), so might be regarded as advantageous.

DEFECTS IN THE METABOLISM OF AMINO ACIDS

A large number of disorders of amino acid metabolism are known, all presumably caused by the genetically determined absence of an enzyme, in most cases with consequent accumulation of the relevant substrate. In some (e.g. albinism) the substrate (e.g. tyrosine) is adequately metabolised by other pathways.

Diseases arising from inborn errors of amino acid metabolism are listed in Table 26.7. All are inherited as Mendelian recessive characters, as would be expected, for most involve some loss of survival fitness and many are lethal. Mutant genes tend not to survive if they produce a dominant character causing severe disability.

Several of these disorders (e.g. phenylketonuria, maple syrup urine disease, goitrous cretinism) are of particular interest because they are amenable to treatment, and early diagnosis may prevent permanent brain damage.

DEFECTS IN THE METABOLISM OF SIMPLE SUGARS

Galactosaemia is the most important of these disorders, with an incidence of about 1 in 50,000 live births. Accumulation of the toxic galactose-1-phosphate can be prevented by a galactose-free diet, so early detection of the condition may be life-saving. With the exception of hereditary leucine-sensitive hypoglycaemia (dominant) all these conditions are inherited as autosomal recessive characters (Table 26.8).

DEFECTS IN THE METABOLISM OF LIPIDS AND STEROIDS

THE HYPERLIPOPROTEINAEMIAS

No clear enzyme or protein deficiency has been demonstrated in any of this group of conditions except possibly Type I, which may be due to deficiency of lipoprotein lipase. All are characterised by variable increases in the plasma fat concentrations, and the classification, as given here in Table 26.9, is based on that of the World Health Organisation (1970). Not every case of hyperlipoproteinaemia can be fitted exactly into this classification on clinical grounds and there may be still some difficulty even after investigation of the serum lipids. This section is only concerned with genetically-induced

Table 26.5 Abnormalities of miscellaneous plasma enzymes and inhibitors

Enzyme	Normal function	Deficiency state	Clinical features	Inheritance
Alkaline phosphatase	Bone mineralisation	Hypophosphatasia	Abnormal bone mineralisation, often rather like rickets. Hypercalcaemia sometimes. Variable severity	Autosomal recessive
Pseudocholinesterase	Participates in destruction of some synthetic choline esters	Suxamethonium sensitivity	Succinylcholine (suxamethonium) is a popular muscle relaxant used in anaesthesia. Normal persons given the usual dose develop apnoea for 3 to 4 minutes. In homozygous pseudocholinesterase deficiency apnoea often lasts over half an hour, necessitating artificial ventilation	Autosomal recessive Heterozygotes are mildly affected
C1 esterase inhibitor	Inhibits activity of the complement component C1	Hereditary angiooedemá	Attacks of angioneurotic oedema and atypical abdominal pains. May be fatal if laryngeal oedema occurs. Fresh plasma has been used to interrupt a severe attack	Dominant
a_1-antitrypsin	Inhibits damaging effect of trypsin on lungs	Familial emphysema	Development of emphysema in adult life. a_1-antitrypsin deficiency is found in up to 50% of patients with 'pure' emphysema. Also liver disease	Autosomal recessive Heterozygotes are mildly affected
Caeruloplasmin	Oxidase activity Copper content 0.34% (8 atoms per molecule)	Hepatolenticular degeneration (Wilson's disease)	Low serum copper and increased copper absorption result in copper accumulation in tissues, with damage to liver (cirrhosis), kidneys (aminoaciduria, etc.) and basal ganglia (involuntary movements). Exact pathogenesis still uncertain	Autosomal recessive

hyperlipoproteinaemias, and it should be remembered that similar changes may be seen in patients with some acquired conditions (e.g. alcoholism, hypothyroidism, nephrotic syndrome).

DEFECTS IN CORTICOSTEROID METABOLISM

Congenital adrenal hyperplasia (adrenogenital syndrome) is an autosomal recessive disorder characterised by inborn defects in the biosynthesis of steroids. Several clinical and biochemical types have been defined. Defective synthesis of cortisol results in increased ACTH secretion and resulting adrenal hyperplasia. In most of the varieties there is increased androgen production bringing about premature virilisation in the male and masculinisation in the female (congenital adrenal hyperplasia is the commonest cause of female pseudo-hermaphroditism in the newborn). Salt loss occurs in

Table 26.6 Abnormalities of transport proteins

Protein	Function	Abnormality	Results	Inheritance
Albumin	Maintains colloid-osmotic pressure Transport protein for many substances of low molecular weight	Analbuminaemia	Slight oedema only. Treatment unnecessary	Autosomal recessive
		Bisalbuminaemia	Asymptomatic. Abnormal albumin (presumed due to substitution of a single amino acid) is normally functional, but differs in electrophoretic mobility, giving two peaks on electrophoresis. At least eight different albumin types are known	Dominant
α-lipoprotein	Lipid transport	Analphalipoproteinaemia Tangier disease	Hepatosplenomegaly, lymph-adenopathy, hypertrophy of tonsils with cholesterol deposition. Only about ten cases described. First patients lived on Tangier island, Chesapeake bay	Autosomal recessive
		Hyperalphalipo-proteinaemia	Decreased risk of myocardial infarction and increased life expectancy	
β-lipoprotein	Lipid transport	Abetalipoproteinaemia Acanthocytosis	Bizarrely-shaped erythrocytes (acanthocytes) with thorn-like projections. Steatorrhoea (failure of chylomicron formation). Ataxic neuropathy and retinopathy. Fewer than 40 cases described	Autosomal recessive
		Hypobetalipo-proteinaemia	Decreased risk of myocardial infarction with increased life expectancy	Dominant
Haptoglobin	Binds free haemo-globin, thus preventing undue urinary iron losses	Ahaptoglobinaemia	No ill effects. Iron deficiency a theoretical possibility	?
Thyroxine-binding globulin (TBG)	Transport of thyroxine	TBG deficiency	No clinical abnormality, but patient may erroneously be thought to have hypothyroidism as PBI and total serum thyroxine levels low	Dominant, men affected more than women
		Increased TBG	No clinical abnormality, but PBI and serum thyroxine levels raised, as in pregnancy, so patients may erroneously be thought to be thyrotoxic	Dominant, women affected more than men
Vitamin B_{12} binding protein	Transport of B_{12}	B_{12} binding protein deficiency	No clinical abnormality, but patients may erroneously be believed to have B_{12} deficiency as circulating levels are low	Dominant

Table 26.7 Inborn errors of amino acid metabolism

Condition	Defective enzyme	Biochemical and clinical consequences	Incidence*
Albinism	o-diphenoloxidase (tryosinase)	Lack of melanin in skin, hair and eyes, resulting in nystagmus, photophobia, skin carcinomas. Treatment symptomatic (avoid sun, wear dark glasses)	1:13,000
Phenylketonuria	Phenylalanine 4-hydroxylase	Phenylalanine accumulates in body fluids, phenylpyruvate and derivatives excreted in urine. Severe mental deficiency, epilepsy, eczema. Normal development possible if given low PA diet within first few months of life	1:20,000
Alkaptonuria	Homogentisic acid oxidase	Homogentisic acid accumulates in body fluids and is excreted in urine. Urine goes dark brown or black on standing, e.g. staining nappies. Cartilage and sclerae may darken (ochronosis) and osteoarthritis appears from 2nd or 3rd decade. Prognosis good without treatment	1:100,000
Homocystinuria	Cystathionine synthetase	Homocystine accumulates and is excreted in urine. Mental retardation, dislocation of lenses and tendency to arterial and venous thromboses. No proven treatment as yet	120 cases
Tyrosinosis	p-hydroxyphenylpyruvic acid oxidase	Tyrosine accumulates and is excreted. Rapid liver enlargement, cirrhosis and, usually, death in infancy due to hepatic failure. Chronic types known – these develop renal tubular lesion with acidosis and vitamin D-resistant rickets. Prognosis poor however treated	80 cases
Oxalosis (Hyperoxaluria)	Glyoxylic acid dehydrogenase(?)	Excessive conversion of glycine to oxalic acid. Calcium oxalate accumulates in tissues, especially kidney, giving nephrocalcinosis, renal stones and death from renal failure in childhood or adolescence. Treatment symptomatic only, e.g. high fluid intake	50 cases
Histidinaemia	Histidine deaminase	Slurred speech, mental retardation. No reports of wholly successful treatment	40 cases
Maple syrup urine disease	Branched chain ketoacid decarboxylase(?)	Accumulation of valine, leucine and isoleucine with urinary excretion of their derivatives (characteristic smell). Severe cerebral degeneration with early death. Milder form occurs which may be helped by diet low in the 3 amino acids	30 cases
Goitrous cretinism	(a) tyrosine iodinase (b) coupling enzyme (c) iodotyrosine deiodinase	All types develop goitre and cretinism of variable severity. Replacement therapy with /-thyroxine is completely effective	All types c. 75 cases

*Estimated incidence in UK live births; or total cases (approximate) reported in the world literature by 1978.

The following inborn errors of amino acid metabolism, almost all associated with mental retardation of varying degree, and often with early death, have each been described in ten or fewer patients, often in only one or two instances. The total number of reported cases of all these errors together is less than 120 (1978).

Alphaketoadipic aciduria
Argininaemia
Argininosuccinic aciduria
Aspartyl-glycosaeminuria

Carnosinaemia
Citrullinaemia
Cystathioninuria

Glutaricaciduria

Homocarnosinosis
Hydroxykynureninuria
Hydroxylysinuria

Hydroxyprolinaemia
Hyperammonaemia
Hyperbetaalaninaemia
Hyperglycericacidaemia
Hyperglycinaemina
(ketotic and non-ketotic types)
Hyperlysinaemia
Hypermethioninaemia
Hyperprolinaemia
Hypersarcosinaemia
Hypervalinaemia

Imidazole aminoaciduria
Isovaleric acidaemia

Lysine intolerance

Methylmalonic aciduria

Oasthouse urine disease
Ornithinaemia

Propionicacidaemia

Tryptophanuria

621

Table 26.8 Defects in the metabolism of simple sugars

Condition	Defective enzyme	Clinical features	Treatment
Galactosaemia	Galactose-1-phosphate uridyl transferase	Normal at birth. Symptoms after a few days or weeks of milk (lactose) ingestion. Galactose and Galactose-1-phosphate accumulate in body, with progressive hepatosplenomegaly, cataracts, mental deficiency, renal tubule defect. May die early but some survive for years	Galactose-free diet results in complete regression of liver, renal and eye lesions if started early (<3/12) Mental deficiency is irreversible
Galactose diabetes	Galactokinase	Hypergalactosaemia and galactosuria. Cataract formation main hazard. Brain and kidneys unaffected. Live to adult life	Galactose-free diet
Fructose intolerance	Fructose-1-phosphate aldolase	Accumulation of fructose and fructose-1-phosphate. Vomiting and hypoglycaemia after fructose ingestion. Progresses to hepatomegaly, cirrhosis, renal tubular lesion and metabolic acidosis	Avoid fructose and its precursors (e.g. sucrose). All changes potentially reversible except established cirrhosis
Fructosuria	Fructokinase	Urinary excretion of ingested fructose. Benign	None required
Pentosuria	*l*-xylulose reductase	Urinary excretion of *l*-xylulose and derivatives from oxidation pathways for glucuronic acid. Benign	None required
Hypoglycaemia (Leucine-induced)	Mechanism uncertain	The cause of about 50 per cent of cases of idiopathic hypoglycaemia of infancy. Protein (leucine) ingestion causes hypoglycaemia with resulting convulsions and cerebral damage	Adequate carbohydrate intake with every protein meal

Table 26.9 The hyperlipoproteinaemias

Classi-fication*	Synonyms	Appearance of fasting serum	Abnormally raised fats	Clinical features	Tendency to atheroma and coronary artery disease	Treatment
Type 1	Fat-induced hyper-lipidaemia. Familial hypertriglyceridaemia	Creamy	Triglycerides (++) Chylomicrons present even after overnight fast Cholesterol (++)	Uncommon Clinical manifestations usually present by 10 years of age Attacks of abdominal pain and pancreatitis Hepatosplenomegaly Eruptive xanthomas on face, buttocks and limbs Xanthelasma unusual	–	Very effective Low fat diet (10–25 g/day) produces fall in serum fats and regression of xanthomas Drugs unhelpful
Type 2a	Familial hyper-cholesterolaemia	Clear	Cholesterol (++) β-lipoproteins Phospholipids	50% of hyper-lipoproteinaemias this type. Xanthe-lasma palpebrarum, early (<35 years) arcus senilis, tendon xanthomas. Family history of coronary artery disease in 3rd–5th decade of life. Homozygotes get severe early manifestations, heterozygotes later	+++	Relatively ineffective except in heterozygotes treated before the age of 20. Low choles-terol diet with substitution of polyunsaturated for saturated fats. Clofibrate, cholestyramine may also help
Type 2b	–	Clear or milky	Cholesterol β-and pre-β lipoproteins	Similar to Type 4	++	As for Type 2a

Table 26.9 continued

Classi-fication*	Synonyms	Appearance of fasting serum	Abnormally raised fats	Clinical features	Tendency to atheroma and coronary artery disease	Treatment
Type 3	Broad Beta disease	Clear or milky	β-lipoproteins abnormally laden with triglyceride (broad band on paper elec-trophoresis). Cholesterol	Uncommon Xanthelasma palpebrarum, early arcus senilis, tuberose and eruptive xanthomas, yellow streaks on palms, accelerated atheroma and coronary artery disease. May have abnormal glucose tolerance	++ (especially peripheral vascular disease)	Moderately effective. If obese, diet to ideal weight, then diet as for Type 2. This. alone or combined with clofibrate, cholestyramine, often results in normal plasma lipid levels
Type 4	Endogenous hyperlipidaemia Carbohydrate-induced hypertriglyceridaemia	Clear or milky	Triglycerides (++) Pre-β lipoproteins (++) Cholesterol	Common. Usually overweight adults, often with abnormal glucose tolerance. Type 4 lipid patterns often found in patients with coronary artery disease	++	Effective. Diet to ideal weight: less than 35% of calories as carbohydrate, at least 50% of lipids as polyunsaturated fat. Response usually good. Clofibrate may help if not
Type 5	Mixed hyperlipidaemia	Creamy	Cholesterol Pre-β proteins Triglycerides Chylomicrons	Uncommon. Similar to Type 1 but usually presents in 2nd decade. Attacks of abdominal pain and pancreatitis, eruptive xanthomas. Xanthelasma unusual. May have abnormal glucose tolerance	−(?)	Effective Good response to weight reduction, low carbohydrate and fat diet. Clofibrate may help in some cases

*Based on World Health Organisation classification (Beaumont, J. L., Carlson, L. A., Cooper, G. R., Fejfar, Z., Fredrickson, D. S. and Strasser, T. (1970) *Bull. World Health Org.*, **43**, 891–903).

about one-third of all patients and may be life-threatening. With proper management the prognosis in most types is good, and fertility is possible. The known enzyme deficiencies are shown in Table 26.10.

DEFECTS IN THE METABOLISM OF PURINES AND PYRIMIDINES

Hyperuricaemia (gout) is one of the commonest of the inborn errors of metabolism. The association of gout with raised plasma uric acid levels was the first instance of a chemically-induced disorder and was described by the father of A. E. Garrod. Although some cases of adult gout may be due to deficiency of hypoxanthine-guanine phosphoribosyl transferase, as in the Lesch-Nyhan syndrome, the defect in most cases is still unknown. Uric acid synthesis is increased, presumably because one of the mechanisms regulating the synthesis of purines is faulty.

Xanthinuria and orotic aciduria are very rare. β-aminoisobutyric aciduria is much more common, especially in some racial groups, and is harmless. The genetic type is seen in healthy individuals, but β-aminoisobutyric acid (a normal breakdown product of thymine) is excreted in excess wherever there is increased tissue breakdown or DNA turnover (e.g. leukaemia). These conditions are described in Table 26.11.

INTRACELLULAR STORAGE DISORDERS

There are at least ten diseases due to abnormalities of glycogen metabolism (Table 26.12). There may be failure to form this substance, or a glycogen of abnormal structure may be laid down, or the glycogen deposited in the tissues may not be broken down normally. In most, a specific enzyme defect has been described.

In the majority of the mucopolysaccharidoses and

Table 26.10 Enzyme deficiencies in steroid metabolism

Simple virilising type (± salt losing)	21-hydroxylase deficiency
Virilising and hypertensive type	11-hydroxylase deficiency
Hypertensive type	17-hydroxylase deficiency
Severe salt-losing type	β hydroxysteroid dehydrogenase deficiency
Hereditary hypoaldosteronism	18-hydroxylase and 18-hydroxy dehydrogenase deficiencies

Table 26.11 Defects in the metabolism of purines and pyrimidines

Condition	Defect	Features
Purines		
Gout	Excessive synthesis of uric acid from precursors	Very common: hyperuricaemia in 1–2% of adults, clinical gout 0.3% (i.e. asymptomatic in 80% of cases). Acute attacks of crystal arthritis. Urate deposition in joints and elsewhere (tophi). Deposits in kidneys lead to renal failure. Autosomal dominant with variable expression, more in males
Lesch-Nyhan syndrome	Deficiency of hypoxanthine-guanine phosphoribosyl transferase	Gout, mental retardation, choreoatherosis and self-mutilating behaviour (e.g. biting lips, fingers) in children. Most die of renal failure due to urate deposition. Allopurinol may help. X-linked recessive
Xanthinuria	Deficiency of xanthine oxidase	Xanthine excreted in urine, calculi formed. Rare
Pyrimidines		
Orotic aciduria	Deficiency of orotidine 5 phosphate pyrophosphorylase	Severe megaloblastic anaemia. Orotic acid crystals in urine. Autosomal recessive. Very rare
β-amino isobutyric aciduria	Deficiency of enzyme responsible for β AIA degradation	Benign, no clinical effects. Autosomal recessive. Very common (up to 5–10% of some normal white populations)

Table 26.12 The glycogenoses

Type (Cori)	Synonym	Deficient enzyme	Results	Clinical features	Treatment
0	Aglycogenosis	Glycogen synthetase	Virtual absence of glycogen	Severe fasting hypoglycaemia with resulting fits and mental deficiency (no glucose stores)	Frequent carbohydrate feeds
1	Von Gierke's disease	Glucose-6-phosphatase	Excess normal glycogen accumulates in liver and kidneys	Retarded growth, hepatomegaly, hypoglycaemic attacks. High cholesterol, xanthomas, episodes of lactic acidosis. 50% die in the first year. 20% of glycogenoses are of this type	Frequent carbohydrate feeds. ?Portal venous by-pass operation
2	Pompe's disease	γ-1, 4-glucosidase (lysosomes)	Normal glycogen accumulates in all organs	Normal at birth. From 2 months to 6 months age progressive muscle weakness, cardiac failure and death in infancy. 20% of glycogenoses this type	All fatal. No treatment helps
3	Forbes' disease Limit dextrinosis	Debrancher enzyme	Abnormal glycogen with short branches accumulates in liver and muscle	Hepatomegaly and hypo-glycaemia. Similar to Type 1 but less severe. Many reach adult life. 30% of all glycogenoses this type	Frequent carbohydrate feeds. ?Portal venous by-pass operation

Table 26.12 continued

Type (Cori)	Synonym	Deficient enzyme	Results	Clinical features	Treatment
4	Andersen's disease Amylopectinosis	Brancher enzyme	Abnormal glycogen with long branches accumulates in liver, spleen, lymph nodes	Abnormal glycogen (very like amylopectin of plants) excites foreign body reaction. Severe cirrhosis and death from liver failure in early life	All fatal. No treatment helps
5	McArdle's syndrome	Muscle glycogen phosphorylase	Inability to mobilise muscle glycogen	Muscle pain and cramps on exercise, prevented by intra-venous sugars	Avoid strenuous exertion. Take oral glucose with exercise
6	Hers' disease	Hepatic glycogen phosphorylase	Normal glycogen accumulates in liver	Hepatomegaly, mild or moderate hypoglycaemia, slight growth retardation. Similar to Types 1, 3. Prognosis good	Carbohydrate feeds if hypoglycaemic
7	–	Muscle phosphofructokinase	Inability to metabolise muscle sugars	Very like Type 5	As Type 5
8	–	Muscle phosphohexose isomerase	Inability to metabolise muscle sugars	Very like Type 5	As Type 5
9	–	Hepatic phosphorylase kinase	Normal glycogen accumulates in liver	Very like Type 6	As Type 6

Table 26.13 The mucopolysaccharidoses

Type	Synonym	Mucopolysaccharide affected	Clinical features
I	Hurler's syndrome Gargoylism	Chondroitin sulphate B Heparitin sulphate	Dwarfism, characteristic coarse facies, bone changes, hepato-splenomegaly, clouding of cornea, mental retardation and death by age of 10 in almost all cases
II	Hunter's syndrome	Chondroitin sulphate B Heparitin sulphate	Milder than I, often survive to teens, some to 6th decade. Coarse facial features, bone changes and hepatosplenomegaly as in I. Deafness. X-linked recessive but often new single mutant as males never known to reproduce
III	Sanfilippo's syndrome	Heparitin sulphate	Severe mental retardation with relatively mild somatic changes. Somewhat coarse facies, stiff joints, mild hepato-splenomegaly. Often appear normal until 3 or 4 years old
IV	Morquio's syndrome	Keratosulphate	Characteristic skeletal involvement with knock-knees, short trunk and neck, pigeon chest, loose joints, broad jaw. Corneal clouding, aortic incompetence. Lumbar gibbus, spinal cord compression
V	Scheie's syndrome	Chondroitin sulphate B	Corneal clouding and stiff hands, coarse facies, as I, with broad mouth. Aortic valve disease. Compatible with normal intelligence and near-normal life span
VI	Maroteaux-Lamy syndrome	Chondroitin sulphate B	Severe skeletal and corneal changes, as in I, but intelligence normal. Usually die by the age of 20

lipidoses, the excessive intracellular storage is believed to result from metabolic defects in the scavenger organelles, the lysosomes. These are normally equipped with a range of enzymes capable of hydrolysing many structural materials. Failure to hydrolyse the stored substances has been attributed to the hereditary absence of specific enzymes. The deficient enzymes have been identified in Gaucher's disease, metachromatic leucodystrophy and some other storage disorders.

The mucopolysaccharidoses (Table 26.13) are charac-terised by deposition of mucopolysaccharides (the major components of ground substance) in various

Table 26.14 The lipidoses

Disorder	Pathology	Clinical features
Tay-Sachs disease (familial amaurotic idiocy)	Accumulation of ganglioside in cytoplasm of neurones in CNS and peripheral nerves	Progressive degeneration of cerebral function beginning in early infancy and resulting in dementia, paralysis, epilepsy and blindness (amaurosis). Retinal examination shows cherry-red spot in macular regions. Rarely survive beyond 5th year. Autosomal recessive. Two-thirds of cases occur in Jewish people (1 in 6,000 Jewish live births in USA)
Gaucher's disease	Accumulation of glucocerebroside (kerasin) in cells of reticulo-endothelial system, especially in spleen, liver, bone marrow	(a) *Infantile, acute type.* Rapid and progressive hepatosplenomegaly with brain involvement and early death (b) *Adult, chronic type.* Insidious onset in adult life with splenomegaly, later hepatomegaly, patchy brown pigmentation on exposed parts, pingueculae. May have normal life span. Typical cells seen in sternal marrow, liver, spleen and lymph nodes (50% of cases Jewish)
Niemann-Pick disease	Accumulation of phosphatide (sphingo-myelin) in many organs, especially liver, spleen and lymph nodes	Onset in first 6 months of life usually. Mental retardation, hepatosplenomegaly, cherry-red macular spot, brain involvement with death usual in first 5 years of life. Some variant types may survive longer. 50% are Jewish. Autosomal recessive. Typical foam cells (Niemann-Pick cells) present in marrow, lymph nodes, liver and spleen
Fabry's disease	Accumulation of galacto-sylgalactosylglycosyl ceramide in neurones in CNS and peripheral ganglia, and in media of small blood vessels	Punctate skin lesions, episodic fever, paraesthesiae and proteinuria. Early death from cerebrovascular disease (strokes) or renal failure
Metachromatic leucodystrophy	Accumulation of sulphatides, mainly in brain and kidney	Variable brain damage (2 clinical types). Dementia, spasticity and death either by 2 years or in late childhood/early adulthood, depending on type

tissues and excretion of mucopolysaccharides in the urine. All are transmitted as autosomal recessives except Hunter's syndrome (X-linked). There are probably several types not yet fully delineated. The lipidoses (Table 26.14) form an ill-defined group for which there is as yet no official classification. Some of these disorders (e.g. Gaucher's disease) consist of sub-types that are distinct genetically and in other ways. Tay-Sachs disease is the commonest recessive disorder in Jews.

DEFECTS IN PORPHYRIN AND HAEMOPROTEIN METABOLISM

The haemoproteins are compounds in which haem is conjugated to protein (e.g. haemoglobin, myoglobin and a number of enzymes, especially the cytochromes). Haem is made up of porphyrin subgroups. Complete failure of haem synthesis is incompatible with life but various other disorders of these compounds are known.

THE HAEMOGLOBINOPATHIES

Over 130 different types of haemoglobin have been described, many in association with diseases of various types, especially haemolytic anaemia. They are described in Chapter 19.

METHAEMOGLOBINAEMIA

Two types of hereditary methaemoglobinaemia are known (*see* Chapter 19). In one the condition is associated with an abnormal haemoglobin molecule (Haemoglobin M). In the other type there is deficiency of the enzyme methaemoglobin reductase which in normal persons maintains the methaemoglobin in the erythrocyte at a very low level. In hereditary methaemoglobinaemia the level is between 25 and 50 per cent of the total. Patients have diffuse cyanosis, sometimes with symptoms such as breathlessness, and may be thought to have congenital heart disease. Usually no treatment is required.

ACATALASIA

This condition, seen mainly in Japanese families, is characterised clinically by recurrent ulcers on the gums and gangrenous lesions of the alveolar ridge. The blood from affected subjects turns brown on standing and does not produce bubbles on contact with hydrogen peroxide. Catalase may protect the mouth against hydrogen peroxide-producing organisms in normal subjects. It is absent in affected patients.

THE PORPHYRIAS

The disorders of porphyrin metabolism (Dean, 1963) are described elsewhere (Chapter 19).

THE HYPERBILIRUBINAEMIAS

Various defects in the metabolism and excretion of bilirubin by the liver are known. They are described in Chapter 4 (page 62).

DEFECTS IN ERYTHROCYTE METABOLISM

A number of hereditary haemolytic anaemias are due to deficiencies in red cell enzymes. Those definitely identified include glucose-6-phosphate dehydrogenase, glutathione reductase, pyruvate kinase, triose isomerase, 2,3-diphosphoglyceric acid mutase, hexokinase and ATPase. In other types of glucose-6-phosphate dehydrogenase deficiency there is no haemolysis unless the patient comes into contact with certain drugs and other substances (see Chapter 19).

DISORDERS OF CELLULAR TRANSPORT MECHANISMS

KIDNEY

Many of the substances in the glomerular filtrate are reabsorbed actively in the proximal renal tubule. For amino acids there are specific transport sites. One type is concerned with the reabsorption of cystine, lysine, arginine and ornithine, and this is abnormal in cystinuria. Excessive urinary losses of these four amino acids therefore occur in the urine, with the formation of cystine stones. In Hartnup disease the defect affects the transport site for another larger group of amino acids, and in both cystinuria and Hartnup disease a similar abnormality occurs in the transport of these particular amino acids across the intestinal cell.

The presence of various other relatively specific transport systems within the kidney is inferred from the various abnormalities of reabsorption which occur; generalised aminoaciduria, glycosuria, phosphaturia and renal acidosis are examples.

INTESTINE

Some transport systems are similar to those found in the renal tubule. Others are specifically concerned with the absorption of dietary substances. Enzymes in the cell membrane of the enterocyte split various sugars (e.g. lactose) and are essential for their absorption (see Chapter 4).

THYROID

Iodine is concentrated in the thyroid gland by an active 'trapping' process which is disturbed in one type of goitrous cretinism.

The disorders of cellular transport mechanisms are summarised in Table 26.15.

INBORN VARIATIONS IN THE ABILITY TO METABOLISE DRUGS

The effect of drugs may be accentuated if their normal degradation pathways are interrupted (e.g. in any patient with severe liver or renal failure). Some patients have a genetic intolerance to certain drugs (e.g. suxamethonium in pseudocholinesterase deficiency, barbiturates in porphyria, primaquine in glucose-6-phosphate dehydrogenase deficiency). In other subjects a normal dose of the drug gives increased side effects due to very slow metabolism presumably because of an abnormality of the enzyme normally responsible for degradation and inactivation of the drug. Examples of drugs for which this has been demonstrated are given below.

Some drugs whose rate of metabolism by the liver is genetically determined

Bishydroxycoumarin
Diphenylhydantoin
Ibrufen
Imipramine
Isoniazid
Monosodium glutamate
Nortriptyline and desmethylimipramine
Phenylbutazone
Streptomycin
Sulphadimidine

Intolerance of the flavouring agent monosodium glutamate produces in susceptible people the 'Chinese restaurant syndrome'. Half an hour or so after starting a Chinese meal a burning sensation develops in the chest and jaw, with transient lacrimation and palpitation. The symptoms are transient and not dangerous, and there is no need for genetic counselling.

MARFAN'S SYNDROME (ARACHNODACTYLY)
Definition

This is a connective tissue disorder, exhibiting dominant inheritance, and characterised by excessive length of the long bones, skeletal deformities, dislocation of the lens of the eye, and abnormalities of the aorta.

Table 26.15 Some inborn defects of transport mechanisms

Disorder	Site of defect	Biochemical abnormality	Inheritance	Clinical effects	Treatment
Cystinuria	Proximal renal tubule and small intestine	Defective tubular reabsorption and jejunal absorption of dibasic amino acids (cystine, lysine arginine, ornithine)	Recessive	Formation of cystine calculi (about 1% of all urinary calculi, much greater proportion in children). Asymptomatic in many cases, these are usually heterozygotes	High fluid intake. Alkalinisation of urine
Hartnup disease	Proximal renal tubule and small intestine	Defective tubular reabsorption and jejunal absorption of most monoamino-monocarboxylic and acidic amino acids. Deficiency of nicotinamide (derived from tryptophan) results in pellagra	Recessive	Pellagrous rash of face and extremities, (photosensitive) and cerebellar ataxia with falling attacks	Nicotinamide
Glycinuria	Proximal renal tubule	Defective tubular reabsorption of glycine	Dominant	Probably benign	None
Glycine aminoaciduria,	Proximal renal tubule	Defective tubular reabsorption of glycine, proline, hydroxyproline	Recessive	Probably benign	None
Lignac-Fanconi or Debré-de Toni-Fanconi syndrome Cystinosis	Proximal renal tubule	Defective tubular reabsorption of most amino acids, urinary losses of glucose, phosphate (leading to rickets), bicarbonate, (leading to acidosis), and deposition of cystine in tissues	Recessive	(a) Acute childhood type. Presents in 1st year of life with vomiting, thirst, failure to thrive. Acidosis and vitamin D-resistant rickets. Usually dead in 1st decade. (b) Chronic type. Usually presents about 2 years of age with vitamin D-resistant rickets and photophobia (cystine deposits in eye). Cystine deposited in tissues, especially reticuloendothelial system. Progressive renal damage and death from uraemia (usually in 2nd decade)	Alkalis, vitamin D
Adult Fanconi syndrome	Proximal renal tubule	Renal glycosuria, aminoacidura proteinuria and excessive urinary losses of phosphate, bicarbonate, potassium and water in various combinations	Recessive	First symptoms in adult life (e.g. 30 years of age) with bone pain, etc., due to osteomalacia	Vitamin D, other supplements if appropriate (e.g. potassium)
Renal tubular acidosis	Distal renal tubule	Impaired H^+ exchange in tubule resulting in acidosis, hyperchloraemia increased calcium excretion	Various	Rickets or osteomalacia, sometimes asymptomatic	Alkalis, vitamin D

628

Table 26.15 continued

Disorder	Site of defect	Biochemical abnormality	Inheritance	Clinical effects	Treatment
Hypophosphataemia (hereditary vitamin D-resistant rickets)	Proximal renal tubule	Excessive urinary losses of phosphate, resulting in low plasma phosphate	X-linked dominant	Presents as rickets around 1 year of age	Very large doses of vitamin D or dihydro-tachysterol
Pseudohypo-parathyroidism	Proximal renal tubule	Tubules unresponsive to action of parathormone (para-thyroids are normal). Abnormally low phosphate excretion high serum phosphate, low calcium	Dominant, varying penetrance	Onset in 1st or 2nd decade. Tetany, fits, cramps, paraesthesiae, mental retardation. Calcification in basal ganglia and subcutaneous tissue. Short 4th and 5th metacarpals	Large doses of vitamin D. Calcium supplements
Nephrogenic diabetes insipidus	Distal renal tubule and collecting ducts	Tubules unresponsive to action of antidiuretic hormone. Copious flow of dilute urine, which continues even if patient becomes dehydrated	X-linked recessive	Dehydration, mental retardation	High oral intake of water Chlorothiazide has anti-diuretic effect in some cases
Renal glycosuria	Proximal renal tubule	Reduced tubular reabsorption of glucose	Dominant	None. May result in mistaken diagnosis of diabetes mellitus. Glucose tolerance test will distinguish the two	None required
Iodine trapping defect	Thyroid	Inability to take up iodide from plasma	Various	Goitrous cretinism	l-thyroxine
Congenital lactase deficiency	Small intestine	Inability to hydrolyse lactose. This type much less common than acquired lactase deficiency	?	Symptoms develop within a few days of birth, as soon as feeding established. Misery, abdominal colic and acid diarrhoea (lactic acid formed from unabsorbed lactose)	Lactose-free diet
Congenital sucrase-isomaltase deficiency	Small intestine	Inability to hydrolyse sucrose and isomaltose	Recessive	Most present in infancy, with diarrhoea at weaning, some later. Acid diarrhoea after sucrose and sometimes after starch	Sucrose free, starch-reduced diet

SUGGESTED FURTHER READING

Bondy, P. K. and Rosenberg, L. E. (eds.) (1974) *Diseases of Metabolism*. Philadelphia: W. B. Saunders.

Dean, G. (1963) *The Porphyrias*. London: Pitman Medical.

Fuhrmann, W. and Vogel, F. (1976) *Genetic Counselling*. New York: Springer-Verlag.

Garrod, A. E. (1902) The incidence of alkaptonuria: a study in chemical individuality. *Lancet* **ii**: 1616–1620.

Garrod, A. E. (1908) The Croonian Lectures on inborn errors of metabolism. *Lancet* **ii**: 1–7, 73–79, 142–148, 214–220.

Hers, H. G. and Van Hoof, F. (eds.) (1973) *Lysosomes and Storage Diseases*. New York: Academic Press.

Levy, R. I. and Fredrickson, D. S. (1968) Diagnosis and management of hyperlipoproteinaemia. *American Journal of Cardiology* **22**: 576–583.

McKusick, V. A. (1966) *Heritable Disorders of Connective Tissue*. St. Louis: Mosby.

McKusick, V. A. (1971) *Mendelian Inheritance in Man*, 3rd ed. Baltimore: Johns Hopkins.

Nyhan, W. L. (ed.) (1974) *Heritable Disorders of Amino Acid Metabolism*. New York: John Wiley and Sons.

Pauling, L., Itano, H. A., Singer, S. J. and Wells, L. C. (1949) Sickle cell anaemia, a molecular disease. *Science* **110**: 543–548.

Seligmann, M., Fudenberg, H. H. and Good, R. A. (1968) A proposed classification of primary immunologic deficiencies. *American Journal of Medicine* **45**: 817–825.

Stanbury, J. B., Wyngaarden, J. B. and Fredrickson, D. S. (eds.) (1972) *The Metabolic Basis of Inherited Disease*, 3rd edn. New York: McGraw-Hill.

World Health Organisation (1968) *Screening for Inborn Errors of Metabolism*. Technical Report Series No. 401. Geneva: WHO.

Diet

DIET AND DIABETES

The detailed management of diabetes mellitus is discussed elsewhere in this book (*see* page 186).

Diabetes is a condition of carbohydrate intolerance. All patients with diabetes require strict control of their *carbohydrate* intake.

Maturity Onset Diabetes

Patients with maturity onset type of diabetes are usually obese irrespective of their age of onset. Weight reduction alone is often the only measure required for control of the diabetes. Weight reduction is best achieved by control of carbohydrate intake.

Juvenile Diabetes

Patients with juvenile type of diabetes require insulin injections. The amount of daily insulin that is required will vary with the intake of carbohydrate. In order to be able to predict the amount of insulin that such a patient will require per day, the daily consumption of carbohydrate must be kept constant. By doing so, the daily insulin requirement is also kept constant and predictable, providing that energy expenditure in terms of muscular work per day is also kept relatively constant. Most insulin treatment regimes ensure that the effects of the injected insulin lasts throughout the working day. For this reason, carbohydrate intake should also be spread throughout the working day and not limited to one or two large meals.

THE DIABETIC DIET

Principles

A decision is first made on how much carbohydrate the diabetic patient should be allowed. This allowance must vary with the individual needs of the patient, taking into consideration the physical demands of his occupation and, in children, requirements for growth. As a guide, about 40 per cent of total calorie intake should be in the form of carbohydrate. For an average adult male with a non-manual occupation, this will approximate to 150 g of carbohydrate per day.

The total daily carbohydrate intake is best considered as being made up from a fixed number of smaller units. Each small unit contains an identical amount of carbohydrate. The small units are then interchangeable and known as a carbohydrate 'exchange'. Each exchange consists of 10 g of carbohydrate. A daily carbohydrate allowance of 150 g is, therefore, the same as an allowance of 15 carbohydrate 'exchanges'. The patient is provided with a comprehensive list of equivalent exchanges, each being equivalent to 10 g. The patient is then advised how to distribute his allowed number of exchanges throughout the day. An example of such a distribution is as follows:

Breakfast	4 exchanges
Mid-morning	1 exchange
Lunch	4 exchanges
Tea-time	1 exchange
Dinner	4 exchanges
Supper	1 exchange
Total	15 exchanges, equivalent to 150 g/day

From the list of exchanges, the patient may construct his own meals to suit his own taste. An illustrative list of carbohydrate exchanges is given in Table 27.1. From this list a patient may construct individual meals according to individual tastes.

Example: Breakfast

½ glass fruit juice	½ exchange
1 Weetabix with milk	1½ exchanges (Weetabix 1, milk ½)
1 egg on toast	1 exchange for the toast, eggs not restricted
1 slice buttered toast (small)	1 exchange
Coffee sweetened with saccharin	Not restricted
Total	4 carbohydrate exchanges

Table 27.1 Some equivalent carbohydrate exchanges

Each item = one carbohydrate exchange = 10 g carbohydrate

Bread	1 small slice
Potato	1 small
Crisps	1 small packet
Rice (cooked)	2 tablespoons
Baked beans	2 tablespoons
Spaghetti (tinned)	2 tablespoons
Porridge	1 small helping
Milk	1 large cup
Evaporated milk	½ small can
Malted milk (e.g. Horlicks)	2 teaspoons of powder alone
Soup – (except clear soups)	1 average helping
Fruit juice (unsweetened)	1 small glass
Beer	1 pint
Stout	½ pint
Biscuits (plain or semi-sweet only)	2
Crackers and crispbreads	2
Scone	1 small
Teacake	1 small
Plain cake	1 small piece

This system of carbohydrate exchanges is easy for patients to understand and allows considerable flexibility.

Some carbohydrates in the normal diet are presented for consumption in a highly concentrated form (*see also* the unrefined carbohydrate diet, page 635).

These foods are sugars and starches. Their exchange value is so high that they must be avoided (Table 27.2).

Table 27.2 Carbohydrate restricted (diabetic) diet

Foods to be avoided	Foods allowed freely
Sugar – glucose, fructose	Meats
Sweets – chocolates	Fish
Jams – marmalade, honey, treacle	Eggs
Sweetened condensed milks	Cheese
Canned fruits in syrup	Vegetables – except potato
Bottled coffees (Camp, Bev)	and beans
Cakes	Fruit – except apples
Puddings	and bananas
Sweet beverages – squash,	Nuts
lemonade, Lucozade, etc.	Unsweetened beverages
Sweet biscuits	Seasonings

Foods allowed in moderation only
Fats – butter, margarine, cream, cooking fat etc.

Non-carbohydrate Foods

The basis of a diabetic diet is carbohydrate restriction. Protein foods are freely allowed (Table 27.2). Fats are allowed in moderation but they have a high calorie density and may not be compatible with the need to lose weight in maturity onset diabetics.

Additional Considerations

Diabetic products are expensive and are not essential. However, they may offer additional variety which some patients may welcome.

Meals should be taken at regular times and not delayed. Alcoholic drinks such as sweet wines and sherry have a high carbohydrate content and are best avoided. One pint of beer, half a pint of stout and half a pint of cider are equivalent to one carbohydrate exchange.

Artifical sweeteners such as saccharin may be used, but other sweeteners such as sorbitol and Sucron are to be avoided. For patients on insulin who are unable to eat solid foods, the following may be substituted for one carbohydrate exchange:

Sugar or glucose	2 heaped teaspoons, 2 large or 4 small cubes
Honey, jam, syrup	2 level teaspoons
Lucozade	4 tablespoons

DIET AND OBESITY

The medical consequences of obesity are discussed elsewhere in this book. Obesity occurs when energy intake (food) is consistently in excess of energy expenditure. The major fuel for body metabolism is glucose. Over short periods of time, blood glucose is maintained by production of glucose from glycogen stores (glycogenolysis) or by synthesis from amino acids (gluconeogenesis). *These are reversible reactions.*

Glucose ⇌ Glycogen
Glucose ⇌ Amino acid pool

The body stores of glycogen are small and, except after an overnight fast, are saturated i.e. 'fully expanded'. This is a short term energy store. The body nitrogen (amino acid) pool is also optimally expanded. *Excess* production of glucose and amino acid from *excess* food intake, when these short term energy stores are saturated, results in the formation of a different form of energy store – fat (triglyceride), a long term energy store. *This reaction is not reversible.* Once triglyceride is synthesised, it may be consumed *only* by oxidation to CO_2 and water.

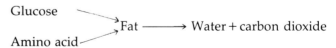

Glucose
Amino acid → Fat → Water + carbon dioxide

In order to achieve the oxidation of fat to carbon dioxide, the short term energy storage system must be insufficient to cope with energy demand; i.e. fat is oxidised only when short term energy stores are exahusted. In practice, this means that energy intake (food) must be *consistently* smaller than energy expenditure. Although the latter may be increased by exercise, experience shows that this is not a practical therapy for

631

the obese. The only alternative is to decrease intake either by voluntary effort or by more radical surgical approaches.

THE REDUCING DIET

Principles

The object of the diet is to reduce calorie intake to below the level of energy expenditure and to maintain it at this level. Because energy expenditure varies considerably, being high in an adult male performing heavy labouring work and proportionately less in a sedentary female, then the desirable calorie consumption will also vary considerably. As a guide, an average adult male in the United Kingdom may expend 2,000 kcal per day. Such a person may require a consistent calorie intake of 1,000 kcal/day to reduce weight.

Satiety

This is a pleasant sensation and the lack of satiety is unpleasant. To be consistently in a state of 'negative calorie balance' is, therefore, unpleasant and hence difficult for patients to maintain over prolonged periods. The factors which influence satiety are poorly understood. However, there is general agreement that the volume of food consumed, i.e. food bulk, influences *short term* satiety. In the average diet of the Western societies, many of the foods of high calorific value are of small bulk. It is, therefore, possible to decrease caloric intake considerably without seriously decreasing the total bulk of food consumed. This applies particularly to carbohydrate which forms 40 to 50 per cent of the total

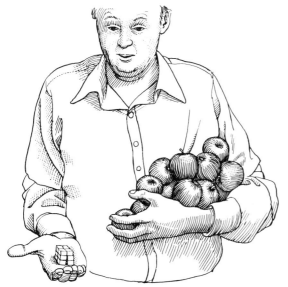

Fig. 27.1 The sugar cubes in the right hand (concentrated carbohydrate) are calorifically equivalent to the content of the left hand (naturally occurring carbohydrate).

calories of most Western diets. The processing of carbohydrate foods has evolved to such an extent that carbohydrate is consumed in a highly concentrated form – undiluted by the natural fibres which have been processed out (*see* Unrefined Carbohydrate Diet, page 635), e.g. sugar, cake, white bread, jams, syrup etc. (Fig. 27.1). Thus the elimination of foods of high calorie density is a simple method of achieving a large decrease in calorie intake without much change in food bulk.

However, some unprocessed foods have a high calorific value such as fats (as in creams, butter, some fatty meats) and potatoes. Unrefined carbohydrates (e.g. apples, Fig. 27.1), may produce short term satiety, because of bulk, with a low calorie load.

If the simple omission of foods of high calorie density fails to produce significant weight loss, many patients may benefit from more precise guidelines using charts of equivalent values, 'calorie exchanges', similar to the exchange system in diabetic diets. Table 27.3 gives some examples of calorie equivalents.

Table 27.3   Examples of equivalent calorie exchanges

1 slice of bread, thin
1 boiled potato
2 tablespoons cooked rice
3 tablespoons baked beans, spaghetti, sweet corn, parsnips
2 crackers or crispbreads
1 unsweetened yoghurt

Additional Considerations

The diet must recognise realistic targets for calorie consumption and weight loss. Unrealistic targets are depressing and depression causes failure. Daily weighings should be avoided. Small weight losses are discouraging – a weight loss of 2 lb (0.91 kg) per week sounds better than 1/3rd lb (0.15 kg) per day. Omitting meals should be avoided, as this causes hunger and increases the probability of failure. Sugar substitutes should be avoided; a preference for sweet tastes is an acquired characteristic which can easily be lost after quite a short time, but which is maintained if sugar substitutes are used. Diabetic food products should be avoided for the same reason. In addition they are expensive and often contain sorbitol – high calorie density. *Regular* rather than strenuous exercise should be encouraged to increase energy expenditure.

DIET AND KIDNEY DISEASE

As with hepatic disease, there is no indication for protein restriction in renal disease unless renal failure supervenes. In most instances of renal disease, a highly nutritious diet with adequate protein content is desirable except where indicated below:

1. ACUTE GLOMERULONEPHRITIS

In this condition, in which urinary output is severely decreased from the outset, uraemia is present, but to a variable degree. Some degree of protein restriction is usually indicated according to the severity of the accompanying uraemia (*see below*).

2. NEPHROTIC SYNDROME

In this condition, large quantities of albumin are lost in the urine. It is therefore imperative for all this protein to be replaced from dietary sources in order to prevent the catabolism of essential body proteins such as muscle. A high protein diet is, therefore, required. The total daily protein in the diet should be equivalent to the measured daily urinary protein loss plus 0.5 g/kg body weight. Such dietary treatment will not increase the serum albumin levels unless the protein leak is simultaneously corrected, but will prevent weight loss from the catabolism of tissue proteins. If the nephrotic syndrome becomes complicated by uraemia, then the principles of dietary treatment of renal failure apply (*see below*).

3. CHRONIC RENAL FAILURE

The normal kidney excretes the acid products which are produced when either endogenous (body) protein or exogenous (food) protein is catabolised. In the presence of renal failure, these products are retained in the body and acidosis and uraemia result. In mild renal failure, which is producing no symptoms, no dietary treatment may be indicated. In advanced renal failure, symptoms may be minimised by a low protein diet, i.e. a decrease in the intake of protein which is the major source of the toxic metabolites. However, sufficient protein must be eaten to allow the normal repair and replacement of essential and structural body proteins. Some protein *must* be eaten. The severity of dietary protein restriction required varies with the severity of the renal failure. Normal dietary protein intake is approximately 100 g. A commonly used low protein diet reduces intake to 40 g per day. Occasionally, very severe protein restriction to 20 g per day is indicated.

The body may use dietary protein either as a source of amino acids for the replacement and repair of essential tissue proteins – the desirable use, or merely as a source of calories – the undesirable use. To prevent protein from being burned merely to satisfy a need for calories, all low protein diets must contain at least enough calories from *non-protein* sources (such as carbohydrate) which will then be used as the fuel, thus sparing the smaller amounts of protein for the essential repair of muscle, essential enzyme systems etc. To exert this 'protein sparing' effect the diet must contain approximately 200 to 300 kcal in the form of carbohydrate or fat for each 1 g of nitrogen. Thus *increased* carbohydrate and fats are an integral part of a low protein diet.

The hypertension and fluid retention of advanced renal failure may in addition require a sodium restricted diet (*see* page 634).

LOW PROTEIN DIET (40 g PROTEIN DIET)

Principles

Meat, fish, eggs, cheese and milk are the major sources of dietary protein. They contain 'first class' protein, i.e. they are replete in the essential amino acids. However, other important sources of protein are foods containing flour (bread, cakes, etc.) cereals and potatoes. Protein from these sources does not contain all of the essential amino acids ('second class' protein). It is, therefore, important that most of the protein part of a protein restricted diet should be taken as 'first class' protein.

Commercially prepared low protein or protein-free products such as flour, bread, pastas etc. are available. To allow variation and individual choice, a system of protein exchanges is advised, similar to the carbohydrate exchange system described under the diabetic diet. Table 27.4 illustrates some equivalent protein exchanges. One 'first class' protein exchange contains 7 g protein, one 'second class' protein exchange contains 2.4 g protein. The patient is encouraged to take his protein allowance as 'first class' protein and to regard 'second class' protein as less desirable food. An average 40 g protein diet would contain three 'first class' protein exchanges and four 'second class' protein exchanges, but where severe restriction (20 g/day) is required, *only* 'first class' protein exchanges are used.

Table 27.4 Table of equivalent values for protein exchange

One 'first-class' protein exchange (7 g)	One 'second-class' protein exchange (2.4 g)
1 oz cooked lean meat	1 thin slice white bread
1 large sausage	3 biscuits
2 fish fingers	1 portion breakfast cereal
1 fish cake	3 small potatoes
1 egg	1 portion peas, beans
1 oz cheese	1 oz pastry (= 1 jam tart)
⅓rd pint whole milk	1 small bar plain chocolate

Additional Considerations

Because it is necessary to increase calorie consumption to 'protect' the dietary protein, non-protein foods of high caloric density are encouraged as follows:
1. Sugary foods – Jams, honey, syrup (but *not* peanut butter or lemon curds).
   Boiled sweets, barley sugars (but *not* milk-containing chocolate and fudge).

2. Flour-free starchy foods – Cornflour, tapioca, blanc-mange, sago.
3. Fats – Butter, margarine; double cream.
4. Fried foods should be frequently used.
5. Double cream thinned with water is an excellent milk substitute – high in calories (the fat content) and virtually no milk protein.

THE GIOVENETTI DIET

This is a diet very low in protein, and very high in calories. Protein content is approximately 7 g/day, equivalent to one egg. It is rarely used since the advent of dialysis.

DIET AND GASTROINTESTINAL DISEASE

1. LIVER DISEASE

Chronic Liver Disease

Some patients with acute or chronic liver disease suffer gastrointestinal discomforts such as flatulence or loose bowel actions after eating fatty foods which, due to bile salt deficiency, they may be unable to absorb effectively. In those cases who do suffer such symptoms, it is sensible to minimise these symptoms by reducing the fat intake – *a low fat diet*. This is particularly useful in conditions of chronic cholestasis, e.g. primary biliary cirrhosis, but these patients will then require parenteral supplements of the fat-soluble vitamins A, D and K.

Acute Liver Disease

Contrary to common misconception, patients suffering from acute liver disease, such as acute viral hepatitis or acute alcoholic hepatitis, do *not* require a low protein diet. In order to provide the nitrogen and calories to repair the damage to the liver in these conditions a high protein, high calorie diet is desirable. If vomiting is a problem, as in acute alcoholic hepatitis, the proteins and calories may be administered as tube feeds or, very rarely, as parenteral nutrition. Only if hepatic failure supervenes is there an indication for protein restriction.

Hepatic Failure

Hepatic failure may be manifest either as fluid retention (ascites, oedema) or as hepatic encephalopathy. Fluid retention occurs because of a failure to excrete sodium. Thus fluid retention is treated by decreasing sodium intake by using a *low salt diet* and, if necessary, by increasing salt excretion with an appropriate diuretic. The degree of salt restriction required varies with the severity of the hepatic failure, but in some cases the restriction may be extreme. There are three commonly used low salt diets:

1. No added salt diet – approximately 100 mmol/day sodium.
2. Low salt diet – approximately 40 mmol/day sodium.
3. Salt-free diet – approximately 20 mmol/day sodium. This can only be achieved by using bread, pastries etc. prepared from special salt-free flour.

Hepatic encephalopathy results from a failure of the liver to remove from the portal circulation the absorbed products of the metabolism of enteric protein by the bacteria in the colon. Much of the protein degraded in the colon by bacteria is endogenous (desquamated epithelium, etc.) but a *low protein diet* minimises the contribution of exogenous protein and forms one aspect of the treatment of hepatic encephalopathy. Normal daily protein intake is approximately 100 g. A diet of less than 20 g/day will result in negative nitrogen balance and muscle bulk will be consumed. A daily intake of 40 g/day of protein is a practical diet which is usually sufficient to control chronic hepatic encephalopathy without precipitating negative nitrogen balance. This should be taken as 'first class' proteins, (meat, fish, etc.) which are rich in essential amino acids rather than 'second class' proteins (cereal products, etc.). The low protein diets have already been discussed (*see* page 633).

THE SODIUM RESTRICTED DIET

These diets are used most frequently in hepatic and renal disease. The fluid retention of heart failure rarely requires strict control of sodium intake since the advent of the potent modern diuretics. However, when emptying a bath it seems sensible to turn off the taps in addition to removing the plug. Similarly, when trying to reduce the total body content of sodium, it seems sensible to reduce the intake by means of a sodium restricted diet in addition to promoting sodium excretion by means of diuretics.

The degree of sodium restriction required varies with clinical circumstances. Severe liver cell failure with ascites and oedema may require the strictest control of sodium and water intake.

Principles

No Added Salt Diet – 100 mmol/day sodium. All that is required for this diet is to avoid using salt at the table and to avoid eating very salty foods such as salty fish (e.g. kippers), salty meats (e.g. bacon), cheese, canned soups, and stock cubes. *Small* amounts of salt may be used in cooking.

Low Salt Diet – 40 mmol/day sodium. All salty foods must of course be avoided as in the 100 mmol/day diet. In addition, salt must not be added to foods in cooking, nor added at the table. Sodium is present in almost all foodstuffs to some extent. Because of this, the low salt diet must restrict some foods which, although not tasting 'salty', do in fact contain fairly large amounts of sodium. These restricted foods would include bread and any food containing baking powder (sodium bicarbonate). The average low salt diet would limit bread to three thin slices per day, milk to half a pint per day, eggs to one and unsalted meat or fish to two servings per day. Only salt-free butter is used.

Salt-Free Diet – 20 mmol/day sodium. It is not possible to achieve a diet entirely free from sodium because of the wide distribution of this element in nature. This diet contains approximately 20 mmol/day sodium and is the strictest that can be achieved. The diet lacks palatability. In addition to the restrictions imposed by the 40 mmol/day sodium diet described above, *only* salt-free bread is allowed. The diet excludes most prepared and processed foods but the allowance of unsalted meat, fish, eggs, milk, etc. is similar to the 40 mmol/day sodium diet.

Additional Considerations

Some milk substitutes are virtually salt-free. Salt substitutes and salt-free baking powder are available with which the stricter sodium restricted diets may be made more palatable. These salt substitutes usually are based on potassium salts instead of sodium and must, therefore, be used with caution in patients with renal disease. Many herbs may be usefully employed as flavouring for dishes lacking salt. *Beware of the many medicines which contain large amounts of sodium*, e.g. many antacid and antidiarrhoeal mixtures.

2. PEPTIC ULCER DISEASE

Gastric diets do not hasten the healing of peptic ulcers and are now obsolete. If a patient finds by his own experience that certain foods will cause symptoms (e.g. spirits, spices), then it is sensible to advise that patient to avoid those foods. Since food will often relieve symptoms and exerts some buffering effects on the gastric contents, it is usual to advise frequent, small meals in the management of peptic ulcer disease.

3. COLONIC DYSFUNCTION (SPASTIC COLON; FUNCTIONAL BOWEL DISEASE; IRRITABLE COLON)

The abdominal symptoms of this common condition are precipitated by the development of high intraluminal pressures in the region of the sigmoid colon. Increasing the bulk of the bowel contents increases the intraluminal diameter of the bowel which results in decreased intraluminal pressures. Faecal bulk may be increased by increasing the indigestible fibre in the diet. Fibre occurs naturally in all plant material (fruits, leaves, roots, etc.), but in varying amounts. Because of its high water-holding properties, wheat fibre (bran) is one of the most efficacious natural faecal bulking agents and forms the basis of the *high fibre diet* used in the symptomatic

treatment of this condition. The high fibre diet is a modification or extension of the *unrefined carbohydrate diet* which is also finding a role in the management of obesity and diabetes. The principles of this diet are to avoid highly refined foods, particularly 'concentrated carbohydrates', and to eat foods in their natural unrefined state, such as wholemeal bread, baked with unrefined flour.

THE HIGH FIBRE DIET

Principles

This diet is based on a diet of unrefined carbohydrate. Most of the carbohydrate consumed in developed countries is highly refined. This processing removes most of the naturally occurring fibre from the food and thus presents the food in a highly concentrated form (Fig. 27.1). Sugar and white flour are prime examples of this processing. The principle of the high fibre diet is to eat carbohydrate in its natural, unrefined state only. Thus sugar is excluded from the diet and *wholemeal* flour only is used in the bread, biscuits and cereal products included in the diet. If the patient does not eat much bread or food baked with wholemeal flour, then extra fibre may be added to the diet. Since all plant material contains fibre the additional fibre may be taken in this form (e.g. fruits, leaves, roots, nuts, etc.). However, wheat fibre (bran) which is normally processed out of flour is also cheap, relatively tasty, stable and easily available. It is by far the most popular method of artificially increasing dietary fibre content. It may be taken sprinkled on food such as breakfast cereals, used to thicken soups, sauces etc. or stirred into drinks.

4. COELIAC DISEASE

In coeliac disease, the epithelial lining of the small bowel is damaged by gluten. Gluten is the collective name given to the proteins of the wheat germ. The proteins which are toxic to patients with coeliac disease lie in the gliadin fraction of gluten and remain toxic even after peptic and tryptic digestion. The epithelium will recover if all gluten is withdrawn from the diet, thus the treatment for this disease is a gluten-free diet for life.

THE GLUTEN-FREE DIET

Principles

For a diet to be free of gluten, *all* foods that are produced from or that contain any wheat flour must be withdrawn. However, flour is such a basic food commodity that it is found ubiquitously in an extremely large number of foods either as a basic constituent (bread, cakes) or as an additive (thickening for soups, gravies, etc.), or as a form of garnishing (batter for fish, etc.). Moreover, being cheap and safe to normal people, it is found in foods where there may be no reason to suspect its presence – such as flavoured potato crisps, or as an innocuous diluent in some powdered coffees. For these reasons, the gluten-free diet is one of the most difficult of diets – even for an enthusiastic patient. Many manufactured, prepared and processed foods contain flour and, therefore, gluten.

However, the Coeliac Society of Great Britain maintains an up-to-date list of manufactured foods known to be gluten-free, but manufacturers may change their recipes without notice.

In order to maintain a patient on a strict gluten-free diet, frequent help, advice and discussion with physician, dietician and patient is recommended, particularly in the early stages of treatment.

In many instances, food that has to be omitted from the diet because of its gluten content may be substituted by a similar food that is baked or cooked with specially produced gluten-free flour. Gluten-free bread, gluten-free flour and a few other gluten-free products are available on prescription. Table 27.5 shows a few examples of gluten-free and gluten-containing foods.

Tables 27.5   Examples of gluten-free and gluten-containing foods

Gluten-free food (allowed)	Gluten-containing food (forbidden)
Cheese	Cheese spreads
Fish	Fish in bread crumbs or batter
Meat	Sausage, spam, some tinned meats, etc.
Plain potato crisps	Flavoured potato crisps
Fresh cream	Synthetic cream
Breakfast cereal made from maize (e.g. corn flakes)	Breakfast cereal made from wheat (e.g. Weetabix)
Tea, fruit squash, pure coffee	Ovaltine, Horlicks, chocolate drinks
Bread, pastry and cakes – baked with gluten-free flour	Bread, pastry, cakes, etc. – baked with normal flour
Rice, sweet corn	Spaghetti and all pastas

Additional Considerations

In addition to wheat protein (gluten), the proteins of barley are equally toxic to patients with coeliac disease. All diets that are gluten-free must, therefore, also exclude barley even though this is a cereal quite different botanically from wheat. However, barley is only infrequently used in Western diets, but may be found in certain drinks such as barley water and some coffee substitutes, and also in a few dishes such as pearl barley. Oats *may* be harmful to a few patients with coeliac disease, although opinion on this is divided. Oats are *not*, therefore, routinely excluded from the diet, but a trial of exclusion of oats may be appropriate in some patients who fail to respond well to a normal gluten-free diet. Oats may be a valuable source of fibre in a gluten-free diet which would otherwise be seriously fibre-deficient.

DIET AND HEART DISEASE

The commonest heart disease in the United Kingdom is ischaemic heart disease. The commonest cause of ischaemic heart disease is atheroma. Atheroma and ischaemic heart disease occur prematurely in the presence of obesity, some forms of hyperlipidaemia and hypertension. For these reasons, it is felt that weight reducing diets may have a role in the prevention of ischaemic heart disease. Some forms of hyperlipidaemia are exacerbated by diets high in carbohydrates (e.g. Frederickson Type IV), other forms by diets high in saturated fat (e.g. Frederickson Type II). For these reasons, diets that are carbohydrate restricted or that are low in saturated fats may have a role in the prevention of some cases of ischaemic heart disease. *However, it has not been proven that dietary treatment can prevent or reduce atheroma in man.*

The reducing and carbohydrate restricted diets have already been described.

LOW SATURATED FAT DIET

This diet is relatively easy and palatable.

Principles

Saturated fats are excluded or reduced in the diet and *exchanged* for unsaturated fats. Saturated fats are predominantly fats of animal origin. Unsaturated fats are predominantly fats of plant origin. The diet therefore requires the exclusion of butter, cream, fatty meat and eggs. Animal fats are commonly used for cooking (lard), for baking (butter), and milk is common in puddings, custard, blancmange, etc. These foods are, therefore, restricted, but it is easy to replace them with similar foods produced with fats from vegetable sources.

Milk	is replaced with skimmed milk.
Butter and margarine	is replaced with polyunsaturated margarine.
Cooking fat, dripping etc.	is replaced with corn oil, sunflower oil.
Cheese	is replaced with cottage cheese.

Meat is allowed freely, but lean cuts should be chosen and excess fat cut away.
Eggs are limited to two per week. Egg white is fat-free and unrestricted.
Fresh milk is limited to half a pint per day, but skimmed milk is unlimited.
Cottage cheese may be made from skimmed milk, as may custard, blancmange etc.
Many margarines contain unexpected amounts of saturated fats, so only those brands that have a high unsaturated fat content should be selected (e.g. Flora, Goodlife).

Pies, biscuits, cakes etc. may be baked using skimmed milk (e.g. Marvel) and polyunsaturated margarine (e.g. Flora).

OTHER DIETS

LOW RESIDUE DIET

This diet, once commonplace, is now rarely used. The only indication may be in the management of partial intestinal obstruction, such as may occasionally occur in a few cases of Crohn's disease, when a normal fibre-replete diet would risk converting a partial to a complete obstruction.

HIGH POTASSIUM DIET

Some foods such as citrus fruits, bananas, nuts, yoghurt and fruit drinks contain quite large amounts of potassium. They may be used as the basis for a high potassium diet. Such a diet may render unnecessary the potassium supplements normally prescribed for patients taking some diuretics. But the potassium intake is more predictable and patient compliance is felt to be better by administering potassium in tablet form. Potassium tablets are cheap.

HIGH PROTEIN, HIGH CALORIE DIET

This diet is useful in conditions of increased catabolism or of protein loss, e.g. nephrotic syndrome, inflammatory bowel disease. The requirements can be easily deduced from commonsense and need not be elaborated here. In addition to natural foods, commercially prepared protein concentrates are also available, e.g. Casilan, Complan.

LIQUID DIETS

Liquid diets are used predominantly for tube feedings.

ELEMENTAL DIET

This is a synthetic diet consisting of protein as amino acids and carbohydrate in the form of glucose with fat. The elemental diet is completely absorbed and requires no digestion. The diet can supply all the caloric, nitrogen and vitamin requirements of the body. The indications for the use of this expensive diet are relatively few, but it does have a definite role in medical practice. Because it is totally absorbed, it may be used in selected cases of 'intestinal failure'. It is a useful and safer alternative to intravenous feeding in some circumstances. The osmotic load from the elemental diet results in a tendency to diarrhoea. This is fairly easily overcome by controlling the rate of administration (over 24 hours) and appropriate dilution in the early stages of administration. The principles governing its use are very similar to those governing intravenous feeding.

SUGGESTED FURTHER READING

Cleave, T. L. and Campbell, G. D. (1969) *Diabetes, Coronary Thrombosis and the Saccharine Disease.* Bristol: J. Wright and Sons.
Bray, G. A. and Bethune, J. E. (1974) *Treatment and Management of Obesity.* London: Harper and Row.

APPENDIX I

NORMAL VALUES (SI UNITS) ABBREVIATED LIST

Specimen and test	Normal values	SI Units
S Albumin	35–47	g/l
P Ammonium (ion)	37–84	μmol/l
S Bicarbonate	21–28	mmol/l
S Bilirubin (total)	3–17	μmol/l
S Bilirubin (direct)	0–3	μmol/l
S Calcium	2.2–2.7	mmol/l
S Chloride	98–108	mmol/l
S Cholesterol	3.4–6.5	mmol/l
P Cortisol (9–10 am)	0.18–0.73	μmol/l
S Creatine	15–38	μmol/l
S Creatinine	53–106	μmol/l
P Fibrinogen	2–4	g/l
P Folate	16–36	nmol/l
S Free Fatty Acids	169–728	μmol/l
P Glucose	3.9–5.8	mmol/l
S Iron	11–27	μmol/l
B Lactate (arterial)	0.3–0.8	mmol/l
S Lipid (total)	4.0–7.0	g/l
S Magnesium	0.7–1.2	mmol/l
S Phosphate (as P)	1.0–1.5	mmol/l
S Phospholipids (as P)	2.3–3.6	mmol/l
B Pco$_2$	4.7–6.1	kPa
B Po$_2$	Average 13.3	kPa
P Potassium	3.5–5.3	mmol/l
S Protein (total)	60–82	g/l
B Pyruvate	58–196	μmol/l
P Sodium	135–148	mmol/l
S Triglycerides	0.34–2.26	mmol/l
S Urate	0.23–0.42	mmol/l
S Urea	2.5–6.4	mmol/l

S – serum   B – blood   P – plasma

CEREBROSPINAL FLUID COMPOSITION

	Normal values	SI Units
Pressure	70–160 mm water	
Volume (total)	120–140 ml	
Cells (lymphocytes)	0–5/mm^3	
Protein (total)	20–45 mg/100 ml	20–45 g/l
Globulin	0–6 mg/100 ml	0–6 g/l
Glucose	50–85 mg/100 ml	2.2–3.4 mmol/l
Chloride	120–130 mEq/litre	mmol/l

APPENDIX II

NORMAL VALUES – RENAL DATA

Renal blood flow	Approx. 1200 ml/min
*Glomerular filtration Rate (GFR)	105–132 ml/min per 1.73 m^2 body surface area
Range of urine diluting and concentrating ability	40–1400 mmol/ (SG 1002–1040)
Urine osmolality/Plasma osmolality ratio (Uosm/Posm)	3–4:1

Constituents of urine (per 24 hours except for urinary cell excretion rates):

Volume	600–2500 ml
pH	4.8–8.4
Protein	up to 150 mg
White cell excretion Red cell excretion	Approx. 200,000/hr
Urea	250–580 mmol (15–35 g)
Creatinine	9–17 mmol (1–2 g)
Sodium	10–200 mmol
Potassium	80–160 mmol
Calcium	2.5–7.5 mmol (100–300 mg)
Phosphate	16–48 mmol (0.5–1.5 g)
Uric acid	0.6–12.0 mmol (0.1–2.0 g)
Titrable acidity (H$^+$ ions)	20–40 mmol
Ammonium	20–70 mmol

*GFR decreases by 1 ml per year after age of 45.

NOMOGRAM FOR DETERMINATION OF BODY SURFACE AREA FROM HEIGHT AND WEIGHT

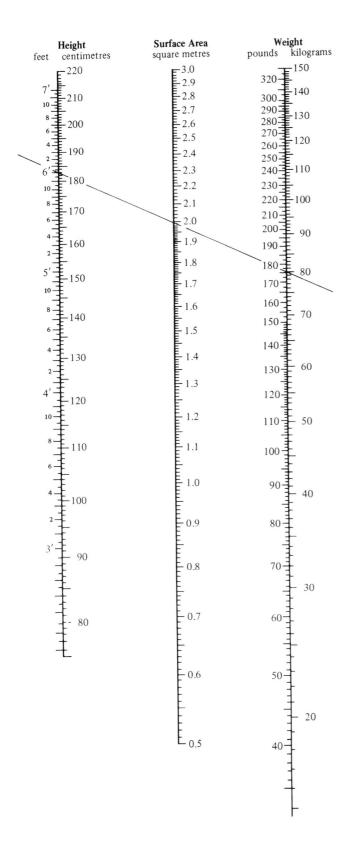

Height	Surface Area	Weight
feet centimetres	square metres	pounds kilograms

Example: Estimation of glomerular filtration rate from a creatinine clearance in a person six feet tall, and weighing 80 kg.

24 hr urine volume (V) = 2880 ml
Urine creatinine (U_{cr}) = 4000 μmol/l
Plasma creatinine (P_{cr}) = 80 μmol/l
Time (T) = 24 hr = 1440 min

i.e. From clearance formula: $Ccr = \dfrac{UcrV}{PcrT}$

$$Ccr = \frac{4000 \times 2880}{80 \times 1440} = \frac{50 \times 2}{1 \times 1} = 100 \text{ ml/min}$$

∴ uncorrected glomerular filtration rate = 100 ml/min

Correct for body size:
From nomogram surface area of subject = 2.0 m²

Normal reference man = 1.73 m²

∴ corrected glomerular filtration rate $= \dfrac{1.73}{2.0} \times 100$

$$= 86.5 \text{ ml/min}$$

Index

dystrophia myotonica 560–1
dysuria 228

Ebola (Marburg) fever 21–2
Echinococcus granulosus 602
echoencephalography 484
Echo virus 20
ECT 437, 459
ectopic ACTH syndrome 167
ectopic beats 270–1
eczema 128–32
    atopic 129–30
    discoid 130
    gravitational 130
    herpeticum 19
    infantile 129–30
    intertriginous 130
    nummular 135
    pompholyx 130
    seborrhoeic 130
    venous 130
Edward's syndrome 107
effort syndrome 268
EEG 484, 518
eighth nerve deafness, in congenital
    syphilis 156, 157
    in thyroid hormone deficiency 174
elation 429
elderly, medical problems of 565–6
    rehabilitation of 566–9
electrocardiogram (ECG) 270, 272, 274,
    275–6, 311–4
electroconvulsive therapy (ECT) 437
electroencephalography (EEG) 484, 518
electromyography 496, 556
embolism, of brain 529
    in chronic rheumatic heart disease 296
    in infective endocarditis 303–4
emphysema 341, 342, 344–5
encephalitis 15, 18, 19
    see also meningo-encephalitis
endocarditis 28, 29, 294, 303–4
endocrine disorders, psychiatric reactions
    to 443–4
endogenous hyperlipidaemia 623
endoscopy 97
Entamoeba histolytica 589
enterovirus infections 20
eosinophilia 391
eosinophilic pneumonia 350–1
epidemiology 5–8
    of chronic bronchitis 342
epiglottitis 328
epilepsy 517–20
    akinetic 518
    EEG in 518
    major (grand mal) 518
        treatment of 519
    minor 518
    petit mal
        treatment of 520
    psychiatric reactions to 444
    temporal lobe 518
    treatment 518–20
episodes of acute bronchial infection
    342–3
ergotamine tartrate 522, 524

erysipelas 23
erythema multiforme 144
erythema nodosum 154–5
erythrocyte metabolism, defects in 627
erythrodermia 132
erythromycin 611
erythropoietic protoporphyria 422
essential thrombocythaemia 395
ethambutol 338, 339
ethinyloestradiol 179
ethnic and cultural factors in disease 6
evolution, civilisation and diet 99
exhibitionism 470
exophthalmic ophthalmoplegia 562
expiratory flow rates 320–2
extradural haematoma 516, 537
extrasystoles 270–1
extrinsic allergic alveolitis 351–2

Fabry's disease 626
facial pain 523–4
facio-scapulo-humeral muscular
    dystrophy 560
factor assays 412
Factor II 419
    V 420, 421
    VII 419, 420
    VIII 416–8, 419, 421
    IX 419
    XII 420
faecal incontinence in disabled 574
fainting 268
falciparum malaria 603
familial amaurotic idiocy 626
familial hypercholesterolaemia 622
familial hypertriglyceridaemia 622
familial polyposis 86
Fanconi syndrome, adult 628
farmer's lung 351
Fasciola hepatica 592, 602
fat balance test 95
fatigue 268
fat-induced hyperlipidaemia 622
fats, absorption of 73
Felty's syndrome 35, 391
ferrous gluconate 376
ferrous sulphate 376
fetishism 470
α-feto protein 96, 115
fibre, deficiency of 101–2
    for irritable bowel syndrome 52
fibrin degradation products 412
fibrinolytic activity, tests of 412
fibrocystic disease of pancreas 73,
    of lungs 353
fibrosing alveolitis 34, 329
fibrosis of left ventricle 287
fibrositis 60
filariasis 593, 601
Flagyl 152
flapping tremor 69
flucloxacillin 610
flukes 592, 602–3
fluorescent treponemal antibody test
    (FTA) 157
5-fluorocytosine 612
focal glomerulosclerosis 238

folic acid (folate) 377–8
    deficiency of 381–2
follicle-stimulating hormone 160
food intake, psychological disorders of 446
food poisoning 25–6
Forbes' disease 624
forced diuresis, in poisoning 204–5
frequency of micturition 228
Friedreich's ataxia 511–12
frontal leucotomy 437–8
fructose intolerance 622
fructosuria 622
frusemide 279
Fucidin 612
fusidic acid 612
fungi, poisonous 212
fungus infections of skin 139–41

Gaisböck's syndrome 395
galactosaemia 619, 622
galactose diabetes 622
gall bladder, carcinoma of 88
    empyema of 91
gallstone ileus 91
gallstones 90–1
gamma BHC 143
gamma-encephalography 484
gangrene 288
gargoylism 625
gastric aspiration and lavage, in poisoning
    204
gastric biopsy 94
gastric function tests 94
gastric polyp 85
gastric ulcer *see* peptic ulcer, chronic
gastritis, acute 56
    atrophic (chronic) 57
        associated with cancer of stomach 85
gastrointestinal cancer 84–7
gastrointestinal symptoms in congestive
    heart failure 268
Gaucher's disease 626
generalised exfoliative dermatitis 132
generalised morphoea 122–4
general paralysis of the insane (GPI) 551
genes, dominant 111
    and protein synthesis 615
    recessive 112
    results of mutation of 615
genetic code 110
genetic counselling 114
genetic heterogeneity 111–2
genital herpes 19
gentamicin 610
geographical factors in disease 7
German measles 16, 23
giant follicular lymphoma 409
giardiasis 603–4
gigantism 182
Gilbert's disease 60
Giovenetti diet 634
Gitlin's syndrome 118
glandular fever 20, 24
Glanzmann's disease 416
Glasgow coma scale 515
globus hystericus 47
glomerular filtration rate 226

645

In Conjunction with this Book

SOUNDS IN MEDICINE

A one-hour compact casette, including the important respiratory and cardiac sounds, both normal and abnormal, including all the major cardiac murmurs

Prepared by the Department of Medicine, University of Bristol, and Mr A. Makepeace, Research and Development Consultant in Audio Visual Aids, University of Bristol

For further details apply to

The Secretary
Department of Medicine
University of Bristol
Bristol Royal Infirmary
Bristol BS2 8HW

NOTES

NOTES

NOTES

NOTES

NOTES

NOTES

NOTES

NOTES